Adolf Grünbaum

AMERICAN HANDBOOK OF PSYCHIATRY

Volume Six

AMERICAN HANDBOOK OF PSYCHIATRY

Silvano Arieti, EDITOR-IN-CHIEF

Volume One
The Foundations of Psychiatry
EDITED BY SILVANO ARIETI

Volume Two
Child and Adolescent Psychiatry, Sociocultural and Community Psychiatry
EDITED BY GERALD CAPLAN

Volume Three
Adult Clinical Psychiatry
EDITED BY SILVANO ARIETI AND EUGENE B. BRODY

Volume Four
Organic Disorders and Psychosomatic Medicine
EDITED BY MORTON F. REISER

Volume Five
Treatment
EDITED BY DANIEL X. FREEDMAN AND JARL E. DYRUD

Volume Six
New Psychiatric Frontiers
EDITED BY DAVID A. HAMBURG AND H. KEITH H. BRODIE

AMERICAN HANDBOOK OF PSYCHIATRY

SECOND EDITION

Silvano Arieti · Editor-in-Chief

VOLUME SIX

New Psychiatric Frontiers

DAVID A. HAMBURG AND H. KEITH H. BRODIE · *Editors*

BASIC BOOKS, INC., PUBLISHERS · NEW YORK

Library of Congress Cataloging in Publication Data
Main entry under title:

New psychiatric frontiers.

(American handbook of psychiatry, second edition;
v. 6)
Includes bibliographies.
1. Psychiatry. I. Hamburg, David A., 1925–
II. Brodie, Harlow Keith Hammond, 1939–   III. Se-
ries.
RC435.A562 vol. 6 [RC458] 616.8'9'008s [616.8'9]
ISBN 0-465-00152-1   75-26586

CONTRIBUTORS

George K. Aghajanian, M.D.
Professor of Psychiatry and Pharmacology, Yale University School of Medicine, New Haven.

Silvano Arieti, M.D.
Clinical Professor of Psychiatry, New York Medical College; Training Analyst and Supervisor, William Alanson White Institute of Psychiatry, Psychoanalysis, and Psychology, New York.

Jack D. Barchas, M.D.
Associate Professor of Psychiatry, Laboratory of Behavioral Neurochemistry, Department of Psychiatry, Stanford University School of Medicine, Stanford, California.

Patricia R. Barchas, Ph.D.
Assistant Professor, Department of Sociology, Stanford University, Stanford, California.

Samuel H. Barondes, M.D.
Professor of Psychiatry, School of Medicine, University of California at San Diego, La Jolla.

John Bowlby, M.D.
Honorary Consultant Psychiatrist, Tavistock Clinic and Tavistock Institute of Human Relations, London.

H. Keith H. Brodie, M.D.
Professor and Chairman, Department of Psychiatry, Duke University School of Medicine, Durham, North Carolina.

Bertram S. Brown, M.D.
Director, National Institute of Mental Health, Rockville, Maryland; Assistant Surgeon General, United States Public Health Service, Washington, D.C.

William E. Bunney, Jr., M.D.
Chief, Adult Psychiatry Branch, National Institute of Mental Health, Bethesda, Maryland.

Ewald W. Busse, M.D.
J. P. Gibbons Professor of Psychiatry, Duke University, Durham, North Carolina; Associate Provost and Director, Medical and Allied Health Education, Duke University Medical Center.

Enoch Callaway, III, M.D.
Professor in Residence, Department of Psychiatry, School of Medicine, University of California at San Francisco; Chief of Research, the Langley Porter Neuropsychiatric Institute, San Francisco.

Paul Chodoff, M.D.
Clinical Professor of Psychiatry, George Washington University, Washington, D.C.

Jack De Groot, M.D., Ph.D.
Professor of Anatomy, School of Medicine, University of California at San Francisco.

William C. Dement, M.D., Ph.D.
Professor of Psychiatry, Stanford University School of Medicine, Stanford, California.

Felton J. Earls, M.D.
Instructor and Macy Foundation Faculty Fellow, Harvard Medical School, Boston; Assistant, Children's Hospital Medical Center, Boston.

Merrill T. Eaton, M.D.
Professor and Chairman, Department of Psychiatry, University of Nebraska College of Medicine, Omaha; Director, Nebraska Psychiatric Institute, Omaha.

Leon Eisenberg, M.D.
Professor and Chairman, Executive Committee, Department of Psychiatry, Harvard Medical School, Boston; Senior Associate in Psychiatry, Children's Hospital Medical Center, Boston.

Jean Endicott, Ph.D.
Co-Director, Evaluation Section, Biometrics Research, New York State Department of Mental

Hygiene, New York; Research Associate, Department of Psychiatry, College of Physicians and Surgeons, Columbia University, New York.

Archie R. Foley, M.D.
Director, Division of Community and Social Psychiatry and Professor of Clinical Psychiatry, College of Physicians and Surgeons, Columbia University, New York.

Daniel X. Freedman, M.D.
Louis Block Professor of Biological Sciences and Chairman, Department of Psychiatry, University of Chicago Pritzker School of Medicine.

Charles M. Gaitz, M.D.
Head, Clinical and Sociological Research Division, Texas Research Institute of Mental Sciences, Houston; Clinical Associate Professor, Department of Psychiatry, Baylor College of Medicine, Houston.

David L. Garver, M.D.
Associate Director of Research, Illinois State Psychiatric Institute, Chicago; Research Associate, Department of Psychiatry, University of Chicago Pritzker School of Medicine.

Jane Goodall, Ph.D.
Director, Gombe Stream Research Centre, Tanzania; Visiting Professor of Psychiatry and Human Biology, Stanford University School of Medicine, Stanford, California.

Frederick K. Goodwin, M.D.
Chief, Section on Psychiatry, Laboratory of Clinical Science, National Institute of Mental Health, Bethesda, Maryland.

Chad Gordon, Ph.D.
Chairman, Department of Sociology, Rice University, Houston; Research Associate, Texas Research Institute of Mental Sciences, Houston.

Richard Green, M.D.
Professor, Departments of Psychiatry and Behavioral Science, and Psychology, State University of New York at Stony Brook.

Roy R. Grinker, Sr., M.D.
Director, Institute of Psychiatric and Psychosomatic Research and Training, Michael Reese Hospital and Medical Center, Chicago.

Ernest M. Gruenberg, M.D., D.P.H.
Research Director, Hudson River Psychiatric Center, Psychiatric Epidemiology Research Unit, Pough-

keepsie, New York; Professor of Psychiatry, College of Physicians and Surgeons, Columbia University, New York.

Beatrix A. Hamburg, M.D.
Assistant Professor of Psychiatry, Stanford University School of Medicine, Stanford, California.

David A. Hamburg, M.D.
Reed-Hodgson Professor of Human Biology and Professor of Psychiatry, Stanford University School of Medicine, Stanford, California.

Robert S. O. Harding, Ph.D.
Assistant Professor, Department of Anthropology, University of Pennsylvania, Philadelphia.

Harry F. Harlow, Ph.D.
Director, University of Wisconsin Primate Laboratory, Madison; Professor of Psychology, University of Wisconsin, Madison.

Sidney Hart, M.D.
Assistant Clinical Professor of Psychiatry, Albert Einstein College of Medicine, Bronx, New York.

Eric R. Kandel, M.D.
Professor of Physiology and Psychiatry, and Head, Division of Neurobiology and Behavior, College of Physicians and Surgeons, Columbia University, New York.

Seymour Kessler, Ph.D.
Adjunct Professor in Psychiatry, Stanford University School of Medicine, Stanford, California.

Lorrin M. Koran, M.D.
Assistant Professor of Psychiatry and Director, Undergraduate Training in Psychiatry, School of Medicine, State University of New York at Stony Brook.

Seymour Levine, Ph.D.
Professor of Psychology, Stanford University School of Medicine, Stanford, California.

Howard Levitin, M.D.
Associate Dean and Professor of Clinical Medicine, Yale University School of Medicine, New Haven.

Melvin Lewis, M.B., B.S. (London), M.R.C. Psychology, D.C.H.
Professor of Clinical Pediatrics and Psychiatry, Child Study Center, Yale University, New Haven; Attending Pediatrician and Psychiatrist, Yale-New Haven Hospital.

James W. Maas, M.D.
  Professor of Psychiatry, Yale University School of Medicine, New Haven.

William T. McKinney, Jr., M.D.
  Professor of Psychiatry, University of Wisconsin School of Medicine, Madison.

Arnold J. Mandell, M.D.
  Professor and Chairman, Department of Psychiatry, School of Medicine, University of California at San Diego, La Jolla.

Warren B. Miller, M.D.
  Director, Laboratory of Behavior and Population and Principal Research Scientist, American Institutes for Research, Palo Alto, California.

Merrill M. Mitler, Ph.D.
  Research Associate in Psychiatry and Lecturer in Psychology, Stanford University, Stanford, California.

Rudolf H. Moos, Ph.D.
  Professor, Department of Psychiatry, and Director, Social Ecology Laboratory, Stanford University School of Medicine, Stanford, California; Chief of Research, Psychiatry Service, Veterans' Administration Hospital, Palo Alto, California.

Arno G. Motulsky, M.D.
  Professor of Medicine and Genetics, and Director, Center for Inherited Diseases, University of Washington, Seattle.

Dennis L. Murphy, M.D.
  Chief, Section on Clinical Neuropharmacology, Laboratory of Clinical Science, National Institute of Mental Health, Bethesda, Maryland.

Frank Ochberg, M.D.
  Director, Division of Mental Health Service Programs, National Institute of Mental Health, Rockville, Maryland.

Gilbert S. Omenn, M.D., Ph.D.
  Associate Professor of Medicine, Division of Medical Genetics, University of Washington, Seattle.

Anthony F. Panzetta, M.D.
  Chairman, Department of Psychiatry, Temple University Health Sciences Center, Philadelphia.

Karl H. Pribram, M.D.
  Professor of Psychology and Psychiatry, Stanford University School of Medicine, Stanford, California.

Frederick C. Redlich, M.D.
  Professor of Psychiatry, Yale University School of Medicine, New Haven.

Julius B. Richmond, M.D.
  Professor of Child Psychiatry and Human Development, and Professor of Preventive and Social Medicine in the Faculty of Public Health and the Faculty of Medicine, Harvard Medical School, Boston; Director, Judge Baker Guidance Center, Boston.

Jurgen Ruesch, M.D.
  Professor of Psychiatry, School of Medicine, and Director, Section of Social Psychiatry, the Langley Porter Neuropsychiatric Institute, University of California at San Francisco.

Robert L. Sack, M.D.
  Assistant Professor of Psychiatry, Stanford University School of Medicine, Stanford, California.

Donald J. Scherl, M.D.
  Undersecretary of Human Services, Commonwealth of Massachusetts; Associate Professor of Psychiatry, Harvard Medical School, Boston.

Joseph J. Schildkraut, M.D.
  Professor of Psychiatry, Harvard Medical School, Boston; Director, Neuropsychopharmacology Laboratory, Massachusetts Mental Health Center, Boston.

Judith Scott, M.A.
  Research Associate, Gerontology Research Section, Texas Research Institute of Mental Sciences, Houston.

J. Fred E. Shick, M.D.
  Research Associate (Assistant Professor), Department of Psychiatry, University of Chicago Pritzker School of Medicine; Consultant, Illinois Drug Abuse Program, Chicago.

Albert J. Solnit, M.D.
  Director, Yale Child Study Center, Yale University, New Haven; Sterling Professor of Pediatrics and Psychiatry, Yale University School of Medicine, New Haven.

Robert L. Spitzer, M.D.
  Director, Evaluation Section, Biometrics Research, New York State Department of Mental Hygiene, New York State Psychiatric Institute, New York; Associate Professor of Clinical Psychiatry, College of Physicians and Surgeons, Columbia University, New York.

viii   CONTRIBUTORS

Albert J. Stunkard, M.D.
Professor of Psychiatry, Stanford University School of Medicine, Stanford, California.

Stephen J. Suomi, Ph.D.
Research Associate, University of Wisconsin Primate Laboratory, Madison; Lecturer, Department of Psychology, University of Wisconsin, Madison.

Sherwood L. Washburn, Ph.D.
Professor of Anthropology, University of California at Berkeley.

Herbert Weiner, M.D.
Chairman, Department of Psychiatry, Montefiore Hospital and Medical Center, Bronx, New York; Professor of Psychiatry and Neuroscience, Albert Einstein College of Medicine, Bronx, New York.

Frederic G. Worden, M.D.
Professor of Psychiatry and Director, Neurosciences Research Program, Massachusetts Institute of Technology, Cambridge.

Irvin D. Yalom, M.D.
Professor of Psychiatry, Stanford University School of Medicine, Stanford, California.

CONTENTS

Volume Six

PART ONE: *Basic Approaches to the Understanding of Human Behavior*

PART TWO: *The Development of Behavior*

PART THREE: *Frontiers in Psychopharmacology*

PART FOUR: *New Directions in Treatment and Care*

PART FIVE: *The Social Context of Psychiatry*

PART ONE

Basic Approaches to the Understanding of Human Behavior

CHAPTER 1

EVOLUTION AND HUMAN NATURE*

Sherwood L. Washburn
and Robert S. O. Harding

A s Mayr[28] has recently pointed out, acceptance of the concept of evolution through natural selection required the rejection of many previously held ideas. Not only were scientific beliefs about the age of the earth, the nature of geological processes and the causes of biological evolution changed, but since the theory of evolution applied directly to man himself, religion, ethics, and the very foundations of a moral society were challenged. It was not the idea of evolution that was so difficult for people to accept; the idea of steady progress toward perfection, perhaps aided by occasional intervention by a Creator, could be reconciled with traditional European beliefs. Since selection was central to the evolutionary process, however, it was no longer possible to believe in the inevitability of progress or the moral nature of the changing universe.

The development of modern genetics showed that the evolutionary process was based on chance mutation, selection, and the fate of genes in populations. The parts of Darwin's theories that were least acceptable to the average person were confirmed by an overwhelming body of experimental science. Now molecular biology has elucidated the nature of the gene and shed light on the way in which life may have originated. The fossil record has also provided some understanding of the nature of life and its history over the last 600 million years, and in the last 1 percent of that time there is now substantial fossil evidence of our own family, the Hominidae.

The new evidence suggests a solution to many of the traditional problems about the origin of man, some of which will be reviewed in this paper. We believe, however, that the

* Primate Behavior research is supported by National Science Foundation Grant No. GS-31943X. We wish to thank Mrs. Alice Davis for editorial assistance.

implications of the theory of evolution for the understanding of the biological nature of man are only beginning to become clear. At this point, we think it is more useful to speculate on the implications than to review the facts, although we will try to do both, keeping "fact" separate from speculation. In doing so, we will discover almost at once that such a separation may be more an illusion than a useful explanatory device. In a very fundamental sense, our society and our scholastic traditions are based on a pre-evolutionary view of man and his nature. At the social level, the fact that a custom exists does not prove that it is necessary, efficient, or desirable. At the individual level, the fact that a way of thinking may be logical, traditional and appealing does not mean that it is useful.

The essential point is that man evolved in response to conditions that no longer exist, that the human body and human nature are products of a succession of different ways of life, resulting in a peculiar, specialized kind of creature with great abilities and surprising limitations. In reviewing some of the major stages in our evolution, we will comment on the implications of these ways of life for modern man.

⟨ Apes and Men

The classic view of human evolution, as described by Huxley and supported by Darwin, was that mankind was particularly closely related to the African apes (the chimpanzee and the gorilla). In the intervening years most scientists abandoned this position and a wide variety of evolutionary theories were proposed. At present, the human lineage is considered to have originated anywhere from five to fifty million years ago, and the creature from which we evolved is visualized as anything from a tarsier to something very like the contemporary chimpanzee. Recent developments in molecular biology and immunochemistry have resolved these controversies, which could not be settled by traditional anatomical and paleontological methods.

Molecular Clues to Human Evolution

It has now become possible to compare the DNA of different animals and to directly assess the differences in their genetic material.[22,17] Using this method, man appears to be most closely related to the chimpanzee and gorilla, then to the Old World monkey, the New World monkey, and the prosimian, in that order.

A second method of estimating the similarity between two animals is to compare the number of differences in the sequence of the amino acids in a given protein. While there are no differences between man and chimpanzee in hemoglobin, for example, there are twelve differences between man and monkey. Similarly, there are no differences between man and chimpanzee in fibrinopeptides and an average of seven differences between man and monkey.

Immunological techniques have also been used to compare man with other primates; although this kind of experiment had been conducted for seventy years, neither anatomists nor paleontologists were convinced by its results. Immunological comparisons have recently been improved by the use of purified proteins and techniques that permit objective quantification. As Table 1–1 indicates, the re-

TABLE 1–1   **Differences between man and chimpanzee and man and monkey as measured by:**

	Man-Chimpanzee	Man-Monkey
DNA	2.5%	10.1%
Sequence of amino acids in:		
Hemoglobin	0	12
Fibrinopeptides	0	7
Immunology:		
Albumin	7	35
Carbonic anhydrase	4	50

sults are the same as those produced by DNA comparison or by amino acid sequencing: man and chimpanzee appear to be so closely related that the methods are at the limit of their usefulness. The order of relationship among the contemporary primates is: man, chimpanzee, gorilla, orangutan, gibbon, Old World monkey, New World monkey, and various prosimians, including the tarsier.[11]

This arrangement of the primates agrees with the classic nineteenth-century consensus and is the same as the pre-evolutionary ordering of these animals.[31] What must be emphasized is that the molecular data can be quantified and counted, and that the conclusions are the same regardless of which method is used or in which laboratory the tests are performed. In this sense, then, these results differ greatly from those obtained by traditional methods, which contain a large subjective element. What many scientists did not anticipate was how closely man appears to be related to the African apes, particularly the chimpanzee. The difference between man and chimpanzee is no greater than the difference between some species of macaques, or between species of *Cercopithecus* monkeys, which have never been regarded as particularly dissimilar. If one examines the tables summarizing the data,[11] the only animals as closely related as man and chimpanzee are such animals as the llama and vicuna, sheep and goat, and kinds of buffalo. Man and chimpanzee are more closely related than dog and fox.

It has been suggested that the small differences between man and the African apes may be due more to evolution slowing down than to any recent separation. But Barnicot[1] has noted that no reasonable explanation for such slowing down has been given. Fortunately, the immunological information provides a direct check on this hypothesis. Sarich and Wilson[39] compared various primates to carnivores. The distances separating them, measured in immunological units of albumin, are: man 169, gibbon 169, macaque 169, cebus monkey 169. Other experiments give similar results. Thus, there is no evidence of human evolution slowing down. Furthermore, the rate did become slower in a New World monkey (*Aotus*), and it is separated from carnivores by 150 units. If there is a slackening, this method detects it. In prosimians, small forms with short generation times, the distance from carnivores is: *Nycticebus* 143, *Lemur* 150, and *Tupaia* (a tree shrew) 163. Small, short-generation forms have changed less than monkeys, apes, or man. As in anatomy, the rate of evolution is independent of size or generation time.[42] Elephants have evolved more rapidly than rats.

Although the difference between man and other animals may be measured objectively by comparing DNA and amino acid sequences or by investigating various proteins with immunochemical techniques, converting these differences into years is more difficult. Attempts to relate molecular differences to dates when two evolutionary lineages may have separated have been discussed elsewhere,[52,46] and we will only estimate here that a "molecular clock" will be reasonably well calibrated in the next two or three years.

As far as the origin of man is concerned, the fossil record shows that lines leading to man and chimpanzee cannot have existed separately for less than 5 million years, while the biochemical data appear to rule out any date of over 10 million years. Unfortunately, there are not enough fossils to settle the matter. For example, in 1972 Kurtén[23] maintained that the separation of ape and human lineages must have occurred more than 35 million years ago. In 1970 another paleontologist insisted that the separation must have been in the Oligocene, some 25 million years ago, but by 1972 thought that the split might be as little as 10 million years ago. It is disagreements of this order that make it impossible to relate molecular change to the fossil record at this time.

Behavior and Anatomy

Until very recently little information has been available on the behavior of monkeys and apes under natural conditions. Most early descriptions of the behavior of nonhuman primates were based on travelers' tales and reflected the way people expected apes to behave. Over the last fifteen years a large amount of accurate data based on carefully planned field studies has become available. It fully supports the arrangement of the primates that the molecular information suggests.

The behavior of wild chimpanzees[47,48] reflects a close relationship to man. Chimpanzees are now known to use objects more extensively than any other mammal except man. They employ a variety of things for a variety of activities. They "fish" termites from their mounds with modified sticks and grasses, sponge rainwater from depressions in branches with crumpled leaves, clean their bodies with leaves, throw rocks and sticks, poke at things with sticks. Chimpanzees stalk, kill, and eat smaller animals, and adult males may cooperate in catching a prey animal. Chimpanzees will also share the meat with others, regardless of individual dominance status, unlike baboons, the only other nonhuman primate known to kill and eat an appreciable number of small animals. Finally, chimpanzees mature much more slowly than monkeys, and consequently the young are dependent upon and remain with their mothers for many years.

Chimpanzee and human anatomy is very similar in the arms and trunk,[49] which accounts for comparable motions at shoulder, elbow, and wrist as well as the similarity of many actions in moving and climbing. On the ground, both chimpanzees and gorillas walk quadrupedally, bending their fingers so that their knuckles touch the ground.[45] This is a specialized kind of locomotion derived from the way in which apes reach and climb about in trees. Both the field studies of behavior and man's close anatomical similarity to chimpanzees suggest that we developed from a ground-living, knuckle-walking apelike creature and that our ancestors moved about in this way before becoming fully bipedal. The problem of the origin of man has frequently been treated as the problem of how an arboreal ape came down to the ground, but the field studies clearly show that merely coming down to the ground does not result in bipedal walking.

In summary, recent molecular and immunochemical studies show that man is particularly closely related to the African apes. Field studies of behavior support this view. These show that many behaviors considered uniquely human are found among chimpanzees. This is in accord with our knowledge of ape and human anatomy. Using the few fossils available, we cannot determine the precise course taken by evolution. What evidence we have suggests that most of the higher primates at Miocene levels were apes (Pongidae). However, most of the apes became extinct in post-Miocene times. The monkeys became the common, successful arboreal primates, even producing several kinds of terrestrial monkeys that have proven to be far more successful than the knuckle-walking apes. Man is descended from one kind of ground-living ape, but men were not as numerous as monkeys until long after the advent of agriculture permitted human populations to expand. If the fossil record of the primates is examined,[41] we find no evidence of any general evolutionary trend toward man, nor, until very recently, any great human success.

⟨ The Human Way of Life

AUSTRALOPITHECUS

The first creatures in the fossil record that can definitely be identified as human (in the broadest sense) belonged to the genus *Australopithecus*. They lived in East and South Africa between one million and something over four million years ago.[16] The fossils suggest that at least two species of australopithecine existed: two jaw fragments found in Java, which may belong to the genus, indicate that they may have been much more widely distributed than can be proven from the fossil material now on hand. Although fragments of several hundred specimens have been found, the pieces are mostly teeth and jaws. Thus, reasonable disagreement exists over body size, proportions, and habits. The best guess is that these australopithecines were bipedal, hunted, and used stone tools. Since the deposits in which they were found show that they were living in dry savanna, the case for their human affinities is strong. A hand found at Olduvai Gorge, Tanzania has many attributes of a knuckle-walking hand, while a humerus from

East Rudolf, Kenya and an ulna from the Omo Valley, Ethiopia show that at least some australopithecines had very massive arms. Stone tools of considerable variety in size and form are found at many fossil sites.[18,25] In some sites, *Australopithecus* has been found with the bones of the animals he appears to have hunted; in others, both *Australopithecus* and numerous other animals seem to have been the victims of carnivores.[3]

One of the problems in attempting to reconstruct the australopithecines and their way of life has been the prevailing tendency to take each kind of new fossil man as it is discovered and make it appear as primitive as possible. Neanderthal man was first reconstructed in a very apelike manner, although many proportions of the European Neanderthals are ultrahuman, such as their large articular surfaces, short forearms and legs. Java man was depicted as halfway between man and ape, and Pekin man was regarded as too primitive to have made stone tools, although tools were found alongside his bones.

Australopithecus was a victim of the same bias. At first it was even denied that the ilium and the skull could belong to the same skeleton because the pelvis was so human and the skull had such a small cranial capacity. It is true, judging from the few well-preserved skulls found, that the brains of these bipeds were no larger than those of contemporary apes.[44] Holloway's[15] careful reassessment of their cranial capacities shows that australopithecine brains were even smaller than had originally been estimated. In any case, the fact that the brain was small made many scientists at first unwilling to think *Australopithecus* could be human, then unwilling to accept the notion that they could have made stone tools. In our opinion, the discovery of a nearly complete foot by Louis Leakey at Olduvai (see[5]) and of skulls, tools, and limb bones by Richard Leakey in the East Rudolf areas should have settled the matter.[19]

David Pilbeam[34] has provided a comprehensive review of these discoveries in which the human affinities of *Australopithecus* are evident.

Given the apelike size of the australopithe-cine brain, it is not surprising that the stone tools found with these creatures are both simple and easy to make. Furthermore, these tools do not increase in complexity over the two-million-year period in which they are found. Since both chimpanzees and contemporary hunter-gatherer peoples use wooden tools, not likely to be preserved in the fossil record over a long time, the lack of apparent progress in tool using may be misleading. Nevertheless, the small brains, roughly half the size of the brain of the beings that succeeded *Australopithecus*, and the simple, unchanging tools all suggest much less effective kinds of behavior than those of subsequent forms of man. If the separation of the human and ape lineages took place more than 6 million years ago, then by far the greater part of human evolution has been dominated by small-brained forms.

Early evolutionary theory held that the brain was the key element in human evolution, and that particularly intelligent apes saw the possibilities of life on the ground. The fossil record shows, however, that the large human brain first appears in the last phases of human evolution, a product of uniquely human evolutionary events. In short, for millions of years before large brains evolved man was a small-brained, tool-using biped who hunted.

The Genus Homo

The larger, more robust australopithecine species probably became extinct, while the smaller, gracile forms evolved into *Homo erectus*, the next stage in human evolution. These forms are known from skeletons found in Java and Pekin, and from more fragmentary remains found in Africa and Europe. Their brains were twice as large as an australopithecine brain, and their long, low skull with its large brow ridges was primitive but definitely human. *Homo erectus* teeth were also human, although often large, and their thigh bone is not exactly like that of modern man, but it is incontestably human in shape. These men hunted large animals and learned how to make fire. The distribution of *Homo erectus* stretched from eastern Asia across to western Europe and down to southern Africa, but in spite of the humanity of these creatures, the fossil record shows that cultural evolution proceeded very slowly.

A million years ago, more or less, complex stone tools appear over most of the Old World, in India, Africa, and Europe. In contrast to the tools found with *Australopithecus*, these tools (Acheulian and related forms) are very hard for a modern human to make. One can learn to make the earliest forms of tools in an afternoon, but an Acheulian bifacial flaked tool can only be made after months of practice. Some are so symmetrical and skillfully flaked that they are esthetically pleasing to modern eyes, and they may, in fact, be regarded as the first direct evidence of art. One of the evolutionary origins of artistic form might be the functional success of skillful manufacturing.[50] Nonetheless, these tools, which may be attributed to *Homo erectus*, continued with little change in form for hundreds of thousands of years.

Up until some forty thousand years ago these ancient forms of man persisted over much of the Old World. Then, in a relatively brief period of time, *Homo sapiens*, men anatomically like ourselves, appeared and history changed pace dramatically. Evidences of change are everywhere in the archeological record, in shelters, graves, and art. Boats exist, fishing goes on, and shellfish are eaten: water is no longer a barrier to man. Bow and arrow, spear throwers, and many other new tools and weapons are found. Man reaches Australia, conquers the Arctic, and peoples the New World. There is indirect evidence of language, complex social systems, and religion; in short, for human behavior as we know it today.

In summary, there appear to have been three major stages in the evolution of man: a very long early one, in which stone-tool-using bipeds evolve from the knuckle-walking apes; a million-year period, dominated by *Homo erectus*, in which human skills evolve; and, finally, a last stage, a moment in the whole process, in which *Homo sapiens* appears and the world as we know it begins to take form.

⟮ Interpretation

We have pointed out that increased intelligence did not cause the lines leading to man and ape to separate and that the large brain appears late in the fossil record, the result of adaptations to the final phases of human evolution. In this way, man resembles horses[6] and many other mammals.[37] The brain tends to follow in mammalian evolution, and this appears to be the case with man. Since the brain was evolving in a feedback relation with other aspects of human evolution, its structure now reflects this history. For example, the areas of the human brain concerned with manual skills[32,27] and language are very large compared to those of other primates. In both language and manual skills, control is limited to one side of the cortex. This lateralization is unique to man. Evolution has built structures in the brain that make it easy for man to learn both tool-using and speech. The structure of the brain does not precisely define the functions it makes possible, but it makes classes of learning extremely easy.

The relation of the brain to evolution may be stated in yet another way: since the complex structures of the brain have evolved, they must have important functions whether we know what they are or not. The great evolutionary increase in size of the frontal lobes and the corpus callosum should have made it obvious that these structures had important functions, even before these functions were known. Similarly, the thalamus and other basal ganglia are three times larger in man than in ape,[2] showing that evolutionary expansion is not limited to the newer parts of the brain. The cerebellum has also increased about the same amount, showing that the whole brain has evolved as a balanced, working system.

Learning of Skills

A comparison with some of the contemporary primates shows that humans have developed a unique ability to learn skills. It is well known that monkeys learn to be social,[13] and the importance of early learning has been shown in many experiments.[29] Chimpanzees mature about twice as slowly as monkeys and man about twice as slowly as chimpanzees.[40] This long period of maturation is necessary to accommodate the peculiarities of human learning. Skills can only be mastered through years of repetition, and the individual is motivated to repeat behaviors by social situations. For example, we may assume that throwing has been extremely important in human evolution. While chimpanzees may throw rocks or sticks, they do not make piles of rocks and practice throwing them, or play games that encourage throwing; nor do appreciative chimpanzee audiences gather to applaud a successful throw. On the other hand, if human adults use spears or bows, they practice these skills in games they play as children before they use them in dangerous situations. The mastery of skills is unique to man. Such behaviors are dependent upon hand-brain coordination, the structure of the brain, and social facilitation. In turn, social facilitation is important in man's unique ability to practice skills and man thus uses his biology far more effectively than any other mammal.

In other words, throughout human evolution there have been selective pressures for skillful performance. In the case of the hands, these pressures have operated to produce strong, effective holding; for example, the structure and proportions of the thumb itself, its muscles, and the areas of the cortex and cerebellum where manual skills are controlled. In the case of speech, as we shall see later, selection has improved the articulatory apparatus that makes the sound code possible, increased lateralization of control, and enlarged related parts of the brain. To be sure, individual skills must be seen as part of a complex socio-biological matrix which makes populations successful.

The Ability to Learn

The kinds of performance from which the selections have been made in the evolu-

tionary past have become easy to learn.[12,14] For example, humans may learn to speak with ease and will learn a language under almost any circumstances. However, the fact that something is easy to learn does not mean that it is learned quickly or that the final form is closely determined by the underlying biology. It takes a child years to learn to speak, and he may learn a wide variety of linguistic conventions in the process. Nevertheless, man is the only animal with a biology that makes this kind of learning possible.

Chimpanzees, our closest relatives, cannot be taught to speak.[21] Great efforts have been made to help them, including bringing young apes up with human children, but without success. The sounds nonhuman primates make under natural conditions are designed primarily to convey information about the emotional condition of the animal making the sound.[24] These sounds may be produced by stimulating the limbic system through electrodes implanted in the brain.[35,36] Neither sounds nor facial expressions are altered by removing large amounts of the cortex.[30] On the other hand, in man speech control becomes lateralized in the cortex during the first few years of life,[33,9] and lesions of the cortex may greatly affect speech.[10]

The communication system of nonhuman primates is multimodal, using sounds, gestures, and postures.[24] Gesture and tone are still important in man, especially for expressing emotion, but most communication is through the use of a sound code. That is, of combinations of a very few short sounds. This code allows an almost infinite number of combined sounds and thus an almost infinite number of meanings, although obviously the meaning assigned to any combination must be arbitrary. No nonhuman primate has anything resembling such a sound code, which helps to explain why these animals cannot be taught to speak.

Many attempts have been made to discover when the human kind of communication system with its sound code evolved. Unfortunately, no one has been able to demonstrate that the ability to make the necessary short noises and combine them can be functionally related in any way to a piece of bone that we might hope to find in the fossil record. The best guess is that languages as we know them today are some forty thousand years old.[43,7] But simpler modes of speech must have preceded the whole modern complex.

We have suggested that the necessity for practicing motor skills may have been a factor leading to selection for delayed maturation in man. It is equally likely that language influenced this development, since it takes years to learn a language, and participation in human social systems is not possible without it.

Language is not the only thing that man learns easily, however: because of our evolutionary past we have a biology that allows us to be social, to control rage and other emotions. The degree to which humans are able to control their emotions is remarkable, especially if man is compared with the nonhuman primates. Imagine an auditorium filled with several hundred chimpanzees, many of them in estrus! Control involves cost to the individual, however, for biology and social relationships do not operate on separate levels. Biological individuals learn from other individuals. The ability to learn is both a biological and a social concept, with a dimension in time as well. Learning may be both conscious and unconscious, but it always involves emotion as well as intellect (limbic system and cortex).

The ability to learn may be illustrated by the problem of aggression. If this term is limited to mean only inflicting damage or threatening to inflict damage on another human being,[4] then it is clear that man easily learns to be highly aggressive.[51,12] Johnson[20] has also given an excellent review of the nature of the biological and social causes of aggression. From the evolutionary point of view, aggressive behavior has been necessary in most human societies for a very long period of time. Livingstone[26] estimates that some 25 percent of adult males were killed in warfare among primitive societies. Killing people from other tribes was regarded as the way to social success and essential behavior for any real man. Until very recently, most fighting took place between individuals, victory often being followed by the torture of captives. The extent of human violence throughout history has been summarized by Freeman.[8]

Hunting and fishing are other examples of human behavior that man easily learns and enjoys. The most minimal success, or even hope of success, is all that is necessary to motivate a wide variety of human activities. Since hunting was important to man for millions of years, a biological base evolved that made learning to hunt easy and the act of killing enjoyable.

In times past, hunting was socially approved and techniques were practiced in play. Thus, a kind of behavior that was easy to learn was reinforced by the social reality. Since hunting and fishing are no longer essential forms of behavior for most people, selection pressures have altered and social reinforcement is lacking in most cases. Nonetheless, these forms of behavior continue to be easily learned because of our evolutionary past.

In general, men and most nonhuman primates will learn easily in response to a social reward. Experiments have shown that monkeys will respond even if their only reward is the sight of another monkey.[38] Juvenile humans who are apathetic in the classroom, where activities are maintained by discipline, may respond to sports, where the individual is rewarded by activity, support of others, emotional involvement, and in some cases, social position. Human ability to learn can only be maximized if the rewards are in accordance with man's nature and, in addition, involve social situations and emotions over substantial periods of time. Because we resemble nonhuman primates in these basic ways much can be learned from the behavior of our nearest relatives and little from the behavior of pigeons.

(The Primitive World

Man adapts through his social system, his technology, and his intelligence. Recently there have been enormous changes in technology and in the number of people in the world. But, as noted before, most of human evolution took place before the advent of agriculture, when men lived in small groups, on a face-to-face basis. As a result, human biology has evolved as an adaptive mechanism to conditions that have largely ceased to exist. Man evolved to feel strongly about a few people, short distances, and relatively brief intervals of time; and these are still the dimensions of life that are psychologically important to him. Children readily form deep attachments for a few individuals; they become familiar with small areas: the homesick child has no doubt of the importance of a small, psychologically meaningful world. Although man's perception of time changes with aging, no person can feel strongly about a period of more than a few years. Not only are millions of years of geologic time emotionally meaningless, but saving for one's old age must be enforced by law.

In discussing language, we pointed out that the meanings humans ascribe to combinations of the sound code are arbitrary. In the physical and biological sciences, the meanings of words are specified by the operations being performed; but in daily life and in the social sciences, words may have little or no meaning. The simple relation of word and referent in the primitive world is lost in our huge, complicated modern world, and our educational systems provide no guidance to understanding either languages or their relation to the brain. The reality of the present world is the many, the far, the complex, the impersonal. The human mind did not evolve to operate effectively under these conditions. To a person in a primitive society, the universe is small and the world is flat. Without access to a telescope, the human brain interprets stars as small, nearby objects, while the sun itself appears to travel across the sky. Simple, personal explanations are devised for complex natural phenomena; otherwise inexplicable events are thought to have been caused either by spirits or by other human beings. Other groups of humans are regarded as barbarians at best, as inhuman at worst.

Before scientific methods were developed, the human brain adapted to the small world of its experience through beliefs that were common to mankind. None of these folk beliefs corresponds to the nature of the world as it is revealed by scientific technology, and this is what is meant by the statement that the brain is an organ of adaptation, not an organ of truth. The apparently necessary beliefs of the primitive world about the nature of time, space, size, and cause, beliefs that were essential parts of human behavior, do not correspond in any way to the nature of the universe as seen by science. The human brain was simply unable to think its ways unaided to a more accurate way of looking at the world, and technology had to be invented to provide the necessary information for the brain to use in adapting.

Techniques developed in the physical and biological sciences have resulted in views that have expanded the limits of the primitive world. The belief in spontaneous generation has been superseded by an understanding of the function of DNA; bacteria have replaced spirits as the causes of some diseases; but in everyday life and in many of the social sciences, primitive ways of thinking still persist.

The study of evolution raises the issue of whether there can be a useful social science that pays no attention to the biology of the human participants in the social system. The doctrine that there are separate levels of understanding—physical, biological, and social—is a barrier to understanding the evolutionary process and, we think, a barrier to understanding human behavior. Future generations will probably regard such academic divisions as economics, political science, sociology, and anthropology as being as antiquated as the concept that the elements of the world are earth, air, fire, and water.

These categories, which seemed sensible in the nineteenth century, stem from the belief that man is a rational animal and that unaided human thought can arrive at some lasting truth. But the brain is a product of evolution. It evolved in response to the selection pressures of the primitive world, and it adjusted to the conditions of that world by adapting. The scientific-technical world is new. There is no more reason to think that the brain can judge the social scene correctly than to believe that astronomy could evolve without a telescope.

(Bibliography

1. BARNICOT, N. A. "Concluding remarks," in A. B. Chiarelli, ed., *Comparative Genetics in Monkeys, Apes and Man*, pp. 309–320. New York: Academic, 1971.

2. BLINKOV, S. M. and I. I. GLEZER. *The Human Brain in Figures and Tables*. New York: Basic Books, 1968.

3. BRAIN, C. K. "Who Killed the Swartkrans Ape-men?" *S. Afr. Mus. Assoc. Bull.*, 9 (1968), 127–139.

4. CARTHY, J. D. and F. J. EBLING, eds. *The Natural History of Aggression*. New York: Academic, 1964.

5. DAY, M. H, and J. R. NAPIER. "Hominid Fossils from Bed I, Olduvai Gorge, Tanganyika," *Nature*, 201 (1964), 967–970.

6. EDINGER, T. *Evolution of the Horse Brain*. Geological Society of America, Memoir 25. Baltimore: Waverly Press, 1948.

7. FOSTER, M. L. "American Indian and Old World Languages: A Model for Reconstruction." Paper presented at meeting of American Anthropological Association, New York, November, 1971. Unpublished.

8. FREEMAN, D. "Human Aggression in Anthropological Perspective," in J. D. Carthy and F. J. Ebling, eds., *The Natural History of Aggression*, pp. 109–119. New York: Academic, 1964.

9. GAZZANIGA, M. S. *The Bisected Brain*. New York: Appleton-Century-Crofts, 1970.

10. GESCHWIND, N. "The Organization of Language and the Brain," *Science*, 170 (1970), 940–944.

11. GOODMAN, M., J. BARNABAS, G. MATSUDA, et al. "Molecular Evolution in the Descent of Man," *Nature*, 233 (1971), 604–613.

12. HAMBURG, D. A. "Psychobiological Studies of Aggressive Behavior," *Nature*, 230 (1971), 19–23.

13. HARLOW, H. F. *Learning to Love*. San Francisco: Albion Publishing Co., 1971.

14. HINDE, R. A. and N. TINBERGEN. "The Comparative Study of Species-Specific Behavior," in A. Roe and G. G. Simpson, eds., *Behavior & Evolution*, pp. 251–268. New Haven: Yale University Press, 1958.

15. HOLLOWAY, R. L. "Australopithecine Endo-cast (Taung specimen, 1924): A New Volume Determination," *Science*, 168 (1970), 966–968.

16. HOWELL, F. C. "Recent Advances in Human Evolutionary Studies," in S. L. Washburn and P. Dolhinow, eds., *Perspectives on Human Evolution* 2, pp. 51–128. New York: Holt, Rinehart and Winston, 1972.

17. HOYER, B. H. "Polynucleotide Homologies of Primate DNAs." Paper presented at meeting of American Association of Physical Anthropologists, Lawrence, Kansas, April 1972. Unpublished.

18. ISAAC, G. Ll. "Chronology and the Tempo of Cultural Change During the Pleistocene," in W. W. Bishop and J. A. Miller, *Calibration of Hominoid Evolution*, pp. 381–430. New York: Scottish Academic Press, 1972.

19. ISAAC, G. Ll. and R. E. LEAKEY. "Hominid Fossils From the Area East of Lake Rudolf, Kenya: Photographs and a Commentary on Context," in S. L. Washburn and P. Dolhinow, eds., *Perspectives on Human Evolution* 2, pp. 129–140. New York: Holt, Rinehart and Winston, 1972.

20. JOHNSON, R. N. *Aggression in Man and Animals*. Philadelphia: W. B. Saunders Co, 1972.

21. KELLOGG, W. N. "Communication and Language in the Home-Raised Chimpanzee," *Science*, 162 (1968), 423–427.

22. KOHNE, D. E. "Evolution of Higher Organism DNA," *Q. Rev. Biophys.*, 3 (1970), 327–375.

23. KURTÉN, BJÖRN. *Not from the Apes*. New York: Pantheon Books, 1972.

24. LANCASTER, J. B. "Primate Communication Systems and the Emergence of Human Language," in P. C. Jay, ed., *Primates: Studies in Adaptation and Variability*, pp. 439–457. New York: Holt, Rinehart and Winston, 1968.

25. LEAKEY, M. D. *Olduvai Gorge: Excavations in Beds I and II, 1960–1963*. New York: Cambridge University Press, 1971.

26. LIVINGSTONE, F. B. "The Effects of Warfare on the Biology of the Human Species," in M. Fried, M. Harris and R. Murphy, eds., *War: The Anthropology of Armed Conflict and Aggression*, pp. 3–15. New York: Natural Hist., 1968.

27. LURIA, A. R. "The functional organization of the brain," *Sci. Am.*, 222 (1970), 66–78.

28. MAYR, E. "The Nature of the Darwinian

Revolution," *Science*, 176 (1972), 981–989.

29. MITCHELL, G. "Abnormal behavior in primates," in *Primate Behavior: Developments* in L. A. Rosenblum, ed., *Field and Laboratory Research*, Vol. 1, pp. 195–249. New York: Academic, 1970.

30. MYERS, R. E. "Neurology of Social Communication in Primates," in *Proceedings of the Second International Congress of Primatology*, Vol. 3, pp. 1–9. New York: Karger, 1969.

31. NAPIER, J. R. and P. H. NAPIER. *A Handbook of Living Primates*. New York: Academic, 1967.

32. PENFIELD, W. and T. RASMUSSEN. *The Cerebral Cortex of Man*. New York: Macmillan, 1952.

33. PENFIELD, W. and L. ROBERTS. *Speech and Brain Mechanisms*. Princeton: Princeton University Press, 1959.

34. PILBEAM, D. *The Ascent of Man*. New York: Macmillan, 1972.

35. PLOOG, D. "Social communication among animals," in F. O. Schmitt, ed., *The Neurosciences: Second Study Program*, pp. 349–361. New York: Rockefeller University Press, 1970.

36. ROBINSON, B. W. "Vocalization Evoked From the Forebrain in *Macaca mulatta*," *Physiol. Behav.*, 2 (1967), 345–354.

37. ROMER, A. S. *Notes and Comments on Vertebrate Paleontology*. Chicago: University of Chicago Press, 1968.

38. SACKETT, G. P. "Unlearned Responses, Differential Rearing Experiences, and the Development of Social Attachments by Rhesus Monkeys," in L. A. Rosenblum, ed., *Primate Behavior*, Vol. 1, pp. 111–140. New York: Academic, 1970.

39. SARICH, V. M. and A. C. WILSON. "Generation Time in Genomic Evolution in Primates," *Science*, 179 (1973) 1144–1147.

40. SCHULTZ, A. H. *The Life of Primates*. London: Weidenfeld and Nicolson, 1969.

41. SIMONS, E. L. *Primate Evolution*. New York: Macmillan, 1972.

42. SIMPSON, G. G. *The Major Features of Evolution*. New York: Columbia University Press, 1953.

43. SWADESH, M. "Linguistic Overview," in J. Jennings and E. Norbeck, eds., *Prehistoric Man in the New World*. Chicago: University of Chicago Press, 1964.

44. TOBIAS. P. V. *The Brain in Hominid Evolution*. New York: Columbia University Press, 1971.

45. TUTTLE, R. H. "Knuckle-walking and the Problem of Human Origins," *Science*, 166 (1969), 953–961.

46. UZZELL, T. and D. PILBEAM. "Phyletic Divergence Dates of Hominoid Primates: A Comparison of Fossil and Molecular Data," *Evolution*, 25 (1971), 615–635.

47. VAN LAWICK-GOODALL, J. "The behaviour of free-living chimpanzees in the Gombe Stream Reserve," *Animal Behaviour Monographs*, 1 (1968), 161–311.

48. ———. *In the Shadow of Man*. Boston: Houghton Mifflin, 1971.

49. WASHBURN, S. L. *The Study of Human Evolution*. Eugene: University of Oregon Press, 1968.

50. ———. Comment on "A possible evolutionary basis for aesthetic appreciation in men and apes," *Evolution*, 24 (1970), 824–825.

51. WASHBURN, S. L. and D. A. HAMBURG. "Aggressive Behavior in Old World Monkeys and Apes," in P. C. Jay, ed., *Primates: Studies in Adaptation and Variability*, pp. 458–478. New York: Holt, Rinehart and Winston, 1968.

52. WILSON, A. C. and V. M. SARICH. "Molecular Time Scale for Human Evolution," *Proceedings of National Academy of Sciences*, 63 (1969), 1088–1093.

CHAPTER 2

CHIMPANZEE BEHAVIOR AS A MODEL FOR THE BEHAVIOR OF EARLY MAN[*]

New Evidence on Possible Origins of Human Behavior

Jane Goodall and David A. Hamburg

THE SEARCH for information about man's evolutionary history has gradually yielded a wealth of fossil evidence that, together with accumulations of stone tools and detailed mapping of bones and other artifacts found on living sites, has given us an ever-growing understanding of man's physical and cultural evolution.[†] The fossil evidence, however, provides us with few clues as to the social behavior of our earliest known ancestors.

In recent years, an attempt has been made to reconstruct some aspects of prehistoric man's social life by drawing on our growing knowledge of the social behavior of the living primates.[72] Because baboons may live on the savanna in conditions similar to those which nurtured emerging man, these primates have often been selected as a model for the behavior of our remote ancestors. Certainly, baboons and men are both primates and thus share a variety of primate traits, and certainly we can learn much from studying the ways in which a nonhuman primate has adapted to savanna living.

The chimpanzee, however, is a much closer relative of man than the baboon.[70] This is suggested by many lines of research into the

* We are very grateful to the Grant Foundation and the Commonwealth Fund for making this work possible.
† See references 53, 74, 11, 29, 30, 76, 12, and 48.

biochemistry, physiology, anatomy, and behavior of the chimpanzee. In all these areas there are striking similarities between the chimpanzee and ourselves. Indeed, in some ways chimpanzees, along with the other African apes, the gorillas, are biologically closer to man than they are to the orangutan—certainly closer than to the baboon. Unless we postulate a remarkable case of parallel evolution in a whole variety of physical and behavioral traits, the African great apes must, at some time, have shared a common ancestor with man. Thus we are suggesting that an understanding of the biology and behavior of the living chimpanzee, while it certainly cannot give us an accurate model for the behavior of early man, may well be the best that is available to us.[6]

We suggest that these biological and behavioral characteristics which can be observed in the chimpanzee today and which show marked similarities to biological and behavioral characteristics of modern man are also likely to have been present both in the primate that served as the common ancestor and in the first true man.

An understanding of chimpanzee biology and behavior highlights those aspects which make man unique as a primate species. After we pinpoint these differences between ourselves and our closest living relative, we can then look for modes of behavior in the chimpanzee that might foreshadow human patterns. Next we can inquire about the environmental conditions in evolution that might, through natural selection, shape these precursors in a direction toward the ultimately human patterns. Clues to the evolutionary shaping of early man's behavior are relevant to the most fundamental considerations of human nature. A better understanding of the life of early man can lead to a recognition of crucial behavior patterns, which must have been highly adaptive in those times. A significant part of contemporary man's genetic and cultural heritage may lie in a readiness to learn such behavior patterns, some of which may not be appropriate to the problems we face today.

(Some Similarities in the Behavior of Man and Chimpanzees

Some of the more striking similarities between the chimpanzee and man are the following: (a) tool-using and tool-making; (b) hunting, cooperation, and food sharing; (c) the length of the period of childhood dependence on the mother; (d) the relationships between a mother and her offspring and between siblings; (e) some aspects of adolescence; and (f) some of the gestures and postures that form the nonverbal communication patterns of man and chimpanzee.

Behaviors described in this section very probably occurred, in a similar (sometimes very similar) form, in the common ancestor of the chimpanzee and man as well as in the earliest true men.

Before describing these behaviors it may be helpful to present a brief outline of the habitat, social structure, and daily behavior patterns of free-living chimpanzees. We are drawing on data collected during a longitudinal study of the behavior of chimpanzees in the Gombe Stream area in Tanzania, East Africa. This study was started by Jane van Lawick-Goodall in 1960. Since 1965 a growing staff has collected detailed information on many facets of chimpanzee behavior. Hugo van Lawick has developed an extensive record of chimpanzee behavior on 16-mm. film.

Chimpanzees live throughout the equatorial forest belt of west and central Africa, extending eastward to the northwestern forests of Uganda and for a few miles inland from the eastern shores of Lake Tanganyika. The Gombe National Park supports a population that is close to the easternmost limits of the species' range.

The Park comprises a narrow stretch of rugged mountainous country running for some ten miles along the eastern shores of Lake Tanganyika and inland only about three miles to the tops of the peaks of the rift escarpment. The rift is intersected by many steep-sided valleys that support permanent streams. In the valleys, riverine gallery forest is found. Between the valleys, the country is more open, supporting deciduous woodland; and many of the ridges and peaks are grass covered. The area supports a population of between 100 and 150 chimpanzees.

Chimpanzee populations may be loosely divided into communities of individuals who recognize each other. Within a community, which usually includes about forty individuals, chimpanzees move in small temporary associations, membership of which is frequently changing as individuals or groups of individuals split off to join other associations. These groupings may be all males, females and youngsters, or combinations of different age-sex classes. Some chimpanzees in a community meet only when circumstances, such as a local abundance of food or a female in estrus, throw them together; others meet more often; some show strong bonds of mutual attraction and frequently associate. A mother and her dependent offspring form the one association that may remain stable over a period of years; such a family unit frequently moves about for a while with other associations.

In the wild, chimpanzees probably always lived in male dominated societies though in captivity a female may have the highest social status in a group. Individuals of a community who frequently associate show a fairly well-defined dominance hierarchy; among chimpanzees who meet rarely the relative social status may be less clear. As yet there is little information on relationship between individuals of different communities.

Chimpanzees are omnivorous, feeding mainly on a variety of plant material, especially fruits; but they also consume insects, occasional birds' eggs or fledglings, and sometimes they actively hunt small mammals. They follow no set route, day after day, in their search for food. Within a fairly large home range (it may cover twenty square miles per year for a male) they are nomadic, sleeping wherever dusk finds them. They typically move on the ground when traveling and spend a considerable portion of each day on the ground. They also spend a good deal of time in the trees both during feeding and at night. They construct quite elaborate nests for sleep-

ing; each individual usually makes a new nest every night except for youngsters of up to five or six years (sometimes older) who share one with their mothers.

In the wild, a female chimpanzee does not give birth until she is about twelve years old, and she has only one infant every four or five years. Life expectancy in the wild is not yet known, but is probably approximately forty years. The longevity record for a captive chimpanzee, a female who was still fertile up to the time of death, is forty-seven years.

Tool-using and Tool-making

For many years the chimpanzee has been known to use objects as tools in captivity and, as far back as 1843, there was a report of a chimpanzee using a tool in the wild.[59] It is, however, only within the past decade that we have begun to learn something of the variety and frequency of chimpanzee tool-using and tool-making behavior in the natural habitat.

Tool-using in animals has been of much interest to students of human evolution because, for a long period, man was commonly referred to as "*the* tool-using animal." In fact, a variety of animals do use objects as tools, but it should be emphasized that tool-using ability on its own does not indicate any special kind of intelligence. The Galapagos woodpecker finch uses a cactus spine to probe insects from crevices in the bark.[8] This is fascinating behavior, but it does not make this bird more intelligent than the ordinary woodpecker, which uses its long beak and tongue for the same purpose. The Galapagos finch uses a behavioral adaptation while the woodpecker uses a morphological one. To further this argument we need only point out that there are some invertebrates that quite clearly use objects as tools. The ant lion who hurls grains of sand at prospective prey, causing it to fall into its pit in the ground, is a good example.

The point at which tool-using and tool-making in a nonhuman animal acquire significance, when viewed in relation to the evolution of tool-using behavior in man is, surely, when an animal can adapt its ability to manipulate objects for a wide variety of purposes and, in particular, when it can use an object spontaneously to solve a novel problem. Chimpanzees have shown themselves capable of using a wider variety of objects as tools for a wider variety of purposes than any other living creature except for man himself (Goodall, 1970[22]).

Research at Gombe has revealed that this one community of chimpanzees uses four different kinds of objects—grasses, sticks, leaves, and rocks—in a wide variety of different contexts during feeding, investigating, body care, and aggressive interactions. Moreover, if the object is not suitable for the specific purpose for which it is to be used, the chimpanzees will modify it accordingly. While they do not show any kind of sophisticated tool-making behavior, they certainly show the crude beginnings.

They use stems and grasses when feeding on termites. The tool is pushed down into the termite nest and then withdrawn, covered by termites clinging on with their mandibles. The chimpanzees pick these off with their lips. If they choose a leafy twig, they strip the leaves off prior to using the twig as a tool. Similarly, a wide blade of grass may be trimmed to size. The chimpanzees use larger sticks to push into ants' nests, and sometimes use a short stick to enlarge the opening to an underground bees' nest. In an earlier time when boxes with bananas in them were made available in a special area, the chimpanzees often used sticks to pry open the boxes. In these different situations, stick selection and modification are varied in accordance with the requirements of the situation.

Quite often during feeding a grass stem or twig may also be used as an investigation probe. For instance, a chimpanzee may push such a tool into a hole in a piece of dead wood and then withdraw it and intently sniff the end. After this he either leaves the wood or tears it apart; this usually reveals the larvae of some insect which is then eaten. Before working at a termite hole, a chimpanzee will commonly push the tool down and sniff the end, after which he either works the hole or moves to try a new one. Sticks are used in a similar

way to investigate objects that the chimpanzees are frightened to touch: one individual carefully touched a dead python with the end of a long stick and then sniffed the tip. Another, after his mother had repeatedly pushed his hand away, used a short stick to touch his newborn sibling.

These chimpanzees use leaves as a kind of sponge to sop up water that has collected in the hollow of a tree trunk and which they cannot reach with their lips. And this provides us with another example of crude tool-making. For the leaves are always briefly chewed before use to increase their absorbency. One individual used a similar sponge to clean out the last fragments of brain from inside the skull of a baboon. The chimpanzees also use leaves to wipe dirt from their bodies.

Individual tool-using performances (i.e., patterns that have been observed on one occasion only) were as follows: (1) an adult female used a short twig to pick at something stuck between her teeth; (2) an infant picked inside his nostril with a twig; (3) an adult male lined his hand with leaves before defecating into this "cup." He was then able to pick out small pieces of undigested flesh of a bushbuck he had fed on earlier without soiling his hand;[26] (4) an adult male used a stick to hit a banana from a human hand when he was too apprehensive to reach for it with his own hand; and (5) a juvenile killed a skink (a kind of lizard) and then laid leaves over it before stamping on it with his foot.

In addition to the use of objects as tools in feeding, self-care, and investigation, the chimpanzees at Gombe also use objects as weapons in aggressive contexts. Rocks and sometimes sticks may be hurled, often with considerable accuracy, during aggressive encounters with other animals. When baboons competed with chimpanzees for bananas at an artificial feeding area, the apes frequently threw rocks. Over a three-year period, more and more individuals began to throw objects as missiles, and they tended to select rocks that were larger and thus potentially more dangerous than the ones they had used initially. No baboon was observed to use any object as a missile during these encounters. Rocks and stones may also be thrown at conspecifics and humans. Sticks or palm fronds are sometimes brandished during aggressive displays and occasionally used as clubs to hit an opponent. One infant used a stick as a club to hit an insect on the ground.

In captivity chimpanzees often use objects quite spontaneously as tools. Wolfgang Köhler studied one group in which the individuals used sticks to pry open box lids and also to dig up roots to eat. They wiped themselves with leaves or straw, scratched themselves with stones, and pushed straws into columns of ants to feed on them. They also used sticks and stones as weapons. Sometimes they used bread to lure chickens close to their cage where they would suddenly prod the birds with sharp sticks, apparently in play.[40]

In another group poles were used as ladders to enable the chimpanzees to climb past electric wiring into trees and escape from the enclosure.[46] In the same group, several individuals used twigs or other material to remove loose deciduous teeth: one of them actually extracted a tooth of a companion with a short piece of stick.[45] Another captive individual was observed to push small slivers of sharp stick under his fingernail, apparently in order to try to relieve the pain caused by a very swollen finger tip. He used the slivers only after repeatedly sucking and biting at the affected area with his teeth.[9]

In laboratories many experiments have been designed to investigate the "tool-making" ability of chimpanzees. This work has shown that a chimpanzee can pile as many as five boxes, one on top of the other, to reach hanging food; that he can fit as many as three tubes together to make a tool long enough to reach food that has been placed outside his cage; and that he can uncoil a length of wire for the same purpose.[40] So far, no chimpanzee has been able to use one tool to make another. However, to our knowledge little experimental work has been attempted in this field. In one series of tests a chimpanzee was repeatedly shown how to use a hand ax to break off a splinter of wood for use as a tool. However, she was unable to do this and did not even try to manipulate the ax to achieve the desired

purpose. Instead she continued to try to break the wood with her hands and teeth—a method that had been successful in previous experiments with softer wood.[39] Before drawing conclusions from this experiment, it is important to realize that chimpanzee intelligence varies considerably from one individual to another. It is quite possible that further tests along similar lines, using different chimpanzees, might yield very different results. An orangutan did learn how to use a stone to chip a flake from a core: he then used the flake to cut nylon string to obtain a food reward.[80]

We think it would be particularly interesting for one chimpanzee to act as a model for another chimpanzee under experimental conditions in which: (a) the model made congenial movements (i.e., easy for a chimpanzee) in making (b) a relatively complex tool that then provided access to (c) a highly valued reward (d) under circumstances in which the reward could be obtained in no other way. Conditions of this sort would tend to elicit the full tool-making potentialities of chimpanzees, taking into account individual differences.

We know that observational learning and imitation play a highly significant role in the tool-using cultures of our own species. Can we say the same of the chimpanzee? The answer is almost certainly in the affirmative. For, while the ability to manipulate objects in a manner that enables them to be used as tools is undoubtedly genetically coded in the chimpanzee, there is increasing evidence that the different tool-using patterns of different chimpanzees are passed from one generation to another by observation, imitation, and practice.[24]

Infant chimpanzees, during their long period of dependency on their mothers, have much opportunity for watching tool use in their elders, particularly during termite fishing. In this context an infant of less than one year sometimes watches his mother intently for a few minutes, and he often picks up discarded tools and plays with them. During the following year's termiting season, he watches adult patterns more intently and during his play with grass and twigs he may "prepare" them for use as tools, stripping leaves off twigs, and so on. He may also make clumsy attempts to push tools into the nest—frequently where there is no hole. Initially, he tends to choose pieces of grass that are much too short: subsequently he uses longer tools, but ones that are too pliable. Gradually, during the next two years, his tool-using attempts mature. His movements become less awkward, and he begins to select material more suitable for use as a tool. This improvement is partly due to the maturation of the necessary motor patterns, but, almost certainly, it is also due to experience gained during practice. By the age of about five or six, the youngster is usually a skilled termite fisher.

It is not only in infancy that observational learning may play a role in the development of tool-using behavior. We mentioned earlier that at the special feeding area chimpanzees sometimes used sticks to try to pry open boxes containing bananas. This practice was first seen in three juveniles and for each of them it appeared to be an individual attempt to solve the problem. Subsequently, more and more individuals of the community began to use sticks, and it certainly appeared that they were gaining experience by watching the behavior of the others. However, until one adult female tried to open a box with a stick, on the *first* occasion that she dared leave the bushes surrounding the feeding area and venture into the open, proof was lacking. Since it is very unlikely that a chimpanzee with no prior experience of boxes would automatically use a stick to pry open a box, we may assume that she had learned the behavior by watching her companions from the bushes. The fact that she had been seen observing this behavior on previous occasions reinforces this assumption.

In captive colonies, it is an established fact that novel patterns may spread from one individual to another through observation and imitation. At the Yerkes Laboratory, for example, it was only necessary to teach one adult chimpanzee how to use a water faucet. All other members of the colony learned the pattern by observing him and each other.[81] In the colony mentioned earlier the pattern of poking at the teeth with twigs was an innovation of one adolescent female, and it was soon

transmitted to other individuals through observational learning.[45] Similarly, the use of poles as ladders was "invented" by one of these chimpanzees and subsequently imitated by the others.[46]

If tool-using behavior in the chimpanzee does represent a kind of primitive culture (where culture is defined as the passing on of information from one generation to the next by learning) then we would expect to find different tool-using patterns in different parts of the chimpanzee's range. As yet there are only two indications that this is so: (a) in two areas in west and central Africa, chimpanzees have been observed using rocks as hammers to open hard-shelled fruit or kernals[3,59] and (b) in Uganda, chimpanzees have been seen using leafy twigs as fly whisks.[63] At Gombe no chimpanzee has been seen to use a stone for any food-getting purpose although one infant, once, pounded at an insect on the ground with a stone. Nor have these chimpanzees been seen using twigs as fly whisks.

However, other tool-using patterns appear to be widespread throughout the range of the chimpanzee: termite-fishing behavior has been reported from another area in Tanzania,[65] in Rio Muni,[34] and in one individual of a group of wild-born, semicaptive chimpanzees in the Gambia.[10] The use of sticks or twigs during honey feeding has been seen in Western Tanzania[33] and the Cameroons[47] as well as at Gombe. The use of leaves for a drinking sponge has been observed also in one of the chimpanzees in the Gambia group.[10] The fact that some chimpanzee tool-using traditions are widespread should not be surprising since some identical stone-tool cultures of early man have been excavated in widely separated areas of the globe.

It seems sensible to suppose that early man used similar perishable tools (sticks, stems, and leaves) prior to his known use of stone implements. Indeed, the Bushmen of the Kalahari and one tribe of South American Indians use the leaf sponge to this day; and almost anyone will use a stick or some other long-shaped object to investigate a frightening object—to find out, for instance, whether a snake or a spider is alive or dead. And it is not only chimpanzees who hurl any object at hand in moments of rage.

Hunting, Cooperation and Food Sharing

Until the last decade, man was the only living primate known to hunt in organized groups, nor was it even suspected that hunting and meat eating might occur frequently in a nonhuman primate. Now, however, it is known that wild chimpanzees may hunt quite large mammals for food, sometimes in a quite organized manner. This has been observed at Gombe,[21,23,66] in other areas of Tanzania,[49,35,36] in Uganda,[64] and in a wild-born semicaptive group in the Gambia.[10]

The prey most frequently selected by the chimpanzees at Gombe is other primates—adult and young monkeys of three different species and infant and juvenile baboons. These chimpanzees also hunt young bushbucks and young bush pigs.*

Meat-eating behavior often occurs in clusters. Possibly an "accidental" kill (such as when a chimpanzee comes upon an unprotected infant prey) triggers off a "craving" for meat. Then a series of kills, together with a number of unsuccessful hunts, may follow in relatively quick succession. Such a meat-eating phase may stretch over a number of weeks and then either because the craving is assuaged, or, perhaps because the chimpanzees have a succession of failures, the cycle passes and the apes resume their usual plant and insect diet for the next few months. Up to twenty-two instances of meat eating have been recorded in one year for a community of about thirty-five to forty individuals; but in some years few predations occur. As yet, little is known of the factors governing the initiating causes, frequency, and duration of hunting periods.

Nearly all the hunting episodes observed during the past eleven years were initiated by males, but on one occasion two females were each observed to catch a baby bush pig.

* Some individuals regularly raid birds' nests for eggs and fledgling birds, but although small rodents and reptiles may be killed, no chimpanzee has been seen feeding from them.

Sometimes one chimpanzee chases after and seizes a small animal. The hunt is then an individual affair. At other times, however, a group of males may surround a potential victim, such as a young baboon temporarily isolated from its troop. This has been observed on five occasions. Although the eating of meat has been observed on many occasions, the actual hunt has been observed much less frequently. In each of the five instances of observed group hunting, a single chimpanzee (twice he was an adolescent male) climbed very slowly and silently up the tree toward the intended victim. The other males stationed themselves at the base of that tree and other trees that could be used as escape routes. Three times the victim managed to escape. On the two occasions when it did not, the waiting members of the hunting group then raced up to share in the meat.

Cooperation can also be observed when a group threatens a frightening object or when two or more chimpanzees challenge a chimpanzee who may be socially superior to most or all of them individually. In these instances, however, each individual of the group is playing a more or less similar role: each one is concerned with intimidating a potential predator or subduing an aggressive superior. The actual gestures used by the different individuals may vary, but the overall patterns are similar.

In the group-hunting incidents described above, it seems that the cooperative behavior is on a slightly different level since two quite distinct activities or roles are enacted: one chimpanzee is responsible for stalking and attempting to seize the prey, while the others are responsible for trying to prevent its escape. If each individual were solely concerned with *his own* chances of making the capture, one would expect a frenzied rush in which each chimpanzee tried to be the first one up the tree. But no such thing happens. Indeed, on one occasion, a group of adult males waited silently on the ground for over two minutes, staring intently up at a young male slowly chasing a juvenile baboon back and forth from the crown of one palm tree to another. Not one of the waiting males left his position on the ground in order to try to get closer to the prospective feast. Only when the victim finally took a wild leap to the ground and the direction of its flight became apparent, did the other chimpanzees run to converge on the baboon. We certainly cannot rule out the possibility that each of the males on the ground considered that his own chances of making the capture were just as good as those of the young male up in the tree. Whatever the motivations of such a group of individual hunters may be, the result is an effective demonstration of quite sophisticated cooperation. Detailed, sequential observation of complex cooperation has been made at Gombe in contexts of dominance interaction as well as hunting.[79]

Meat appears to be a much favored food: intense excitement is shown by all chimpanzees present at the time of a kill. They usually scream loudly and embrace or touch one another. The commotion is likely to attract other chimpanzees within earshot to the scene. In all cases when a kill was made and when other chimpanzees were present during or subsequent to the event, hunting resulted in food sharing. Prior to the observations at Gombe, no nonhuman primate had been reported to share food in the wild with the occasional exception of mothers with their infants.

After a kill at Gombe other individuals gather around the chimpanzee (or chimpanzees) in possession of the carcass or portions thereof and show a variety of begging gestures. They may reach out to touch the carcass, while looking at the male in possession as though seeking his permission to take some food. They may reach out to touch his mouth. Or they may hold their hand toward him, palm up, in the common begging gesture of man. The response of the feeding male varies with his personality, the amount of meat available, the amount he has already consumed, and his relationship with the begging individual. Sometimes a chimpanzee is permitted to feed from the carcass along with the male in possession; sometimes it is permitted to detach a piece of flesh; less often it is actually *given* a share of the meat that has been detached, the male in possession placing the

meat in the outstretched hand of the begging chimpanzee. During the eating of meat, the chimpanzee invariably puts a handful of leaves in with each mouthful of meat, and one of the most common forms of sharing occurs when an individual chewing such a wad is finally persuaded to spit it into the waiting hand of another.

There are, of course, many occasions when a chimpanzee in possession of a carcass responds unfavorably to begging, either by moving or turning away or by mildly threatening the begging individual. If fighting occurs during meat eating, it is usually when a male without a share of the carcass chases or attacks an individual subordinate to himself who is also without meat—an example of what is commonly referred to as redirected aggression.

Food sharing among adults does occur in some other contexts. We have repeatedly seen an old mother sharing bananas, another highly valued food, with her adolescent son. But it is during meat eating that food sharing is seen most frequently and most dramatically. Once, for instance, an adult and very high-ranking male actually tore in half the body of an infant baboon he had caught and handed one piece to a low-ranking adult male who had been begging and having tantrums for the previous ten minutes. An average-sized carcass, such as that of a young baboon, may well be shared by fifteen individuals, although the portions are by no means equal. The older males and the older and more persistent females or those in estrus are likely to get the largest pieces.

Period of Infant and Juvenile Dependency

Possibly one of the most striking findings to emerge from the longitudinal study at Gombe is the length of the period of infant and juvenile dependence on the mother. The infant is totally dependent on his mother for food, transport, and protection during the first six months or so. At about six months the infant takes its first tottering step. But steady locomotion does not occur until the third year and riding on its mother's back continues to be the main manner of getting from place to place until the fourth year.

The first minute amounts of solid foods are ingested at about six months of age, but milk continues to be the principal source of food for at least two years and possibly longer. Youngsters usually complete weaning during their fifth or sixth year; the youngest to be weaned, so far, was four and a half years. One male infant, early in his seventh year, is being finally weaned at the time of this writing. This weaning roughly coincides with the eruption of permanent dentition as with some human groups, e.g., Eskimos. (Schultz has argued that a higher percentage of well-worn deciduous teeth in early human children as compared with chimpanzee children indicates that early man had a longer childhood.[61] But perhaps extra wear from eating roots and other rough foods might account for the difference.) The weaning process may continue for over a year, the mother gradually rejecting her child more and more frequently but usually giving access to the nipple if it persists. Ultimately weaning appears to occur as a result of physiological changes in the mother, but these are not clear-cut since lactation may continue during pregnancy in some females.

Youngsters may continue to sleep with their mothers after being weaned. Usually they start sleeping in their own nests at night during the sixth or seventh year; if they are not already independent at night, they usually become so at the birth of a new sibling. One youngster continued to share his mother's nest at night until her death when he was eight and a half years old.

During its sixth or seventh year, a juvenile sometimes accidentally becomes separated from its mother. This usually results in obvious distress on the part of the child and sometimes the mother which may persist until the two meet again. During his seventh or eighth year, the male juvenile may begin to move about in a group away from his mother for a few hours or even days. But until he is at least nine years old, he does not spend long periods away from her except accidentally. The female offspring is likely to remain almost continuously with her mother for an even longer time.

As in man, the long period of dependency in the chimpanzee is adaptive in relation to social learning. When the youngster is traveling with and protected by its mother it has much opportunity for observation and learning. We have already presented evidence for the role played by observation, imitation, and practice in the acquisition of tool-using behaviors. Similarly the young chimpanzee frequently watches and subsequently imitates and practices a variety of other behaviors such as nest making, some kinds of feeding patterns as well as a variety of social patterns, notably maternal behavior for females and sexual behavior for males.

Indeed, we have a clear-cut example of the role played by observational learning in maternal behavior. A juvenile female, who spent long periods close to her mother and newborn sibling, carefully watching everything that went on, was one day offered a toy chimpanzee. She carried it pressed in the ventral position in the same way that her sibling was transported at that time. A month later, when her sibling had just commenced to ride on his mother's back, she was again given the toy. This time she immediately pushed it up onto her back when she walked off. This same female has now had her first infant and it is significant that several of her maternal practices show striking similarities to those of her mother.

Another aspect that should be considered here is that the long period of dependence prolongs the time when play is a frequent activity of the infant and juvenile chimpanzee. While play is a controversial category of behavior, both as to definition and function, there can be little doubt that the experience gained during locomotor and social play is valuable to the growing youngster. Compared to the playful activities of primates such as baboons, young chimpanzees exhibit an extremely rich variety of play patterns, both during social and solitary play. Once we observed how a novel mannerism, incorporated by one infant into her social play, spread to the other youngsters of her community in a few weeks. In this case, it was merely a nonfunctional facial expression (she sucked in her cheeks) and it was eventually dropped from the repertoire. But it remains a possibility that behaviors "invented" during play might sometimes lead to a new tradition or culture in the group.

It is apparent that just as observation, imitation and practice play a vital role in the development of human behavior,[2] so too these processes are important in the development of chimpanzee behavior, as well as in that of other nonhuman species such as Japanese macaques.[38]

Relationships within the Family

A chimpanzee "family" comprises a mother, her offspring, and any offspring of her daughters. This differs from the human family unit in that no father is included. In the wild, it has so far not been possible to know which chimpanzee has sired which infant. Even on those occasions when a female was presumed to have been with one male only at the time of conception, such a pair has never been followed long enough without interruption to obtain sure evidence of paternity. However, new data on this subject is becoming available.[44] In any event, the father plays no role in family life subsequent to the time of conception: the tasks of child raising lie solely with the mother, sometimes assisted by an older daughter.

An important finding of the long-term study at Gombe has been the realization of the strength and duration of the affectionate ties between a mother and her offspring and between siblings. Indeed, in most primate species, there is initially a close, affectionate relationship between a mother and her infant. But in those species where long-term studies have been carried out, these bonds have been found to be more persistent than was formerly supposed, particularly between mothers and their daughters. This applies to rhesus monkeys on Cayo Santiago,[58] Japanese monkeys,[38] and olive baboons.[20]

In the chimpanzee, however, the period of juvenile dependence on the mother is extremely long. It is characterized by a variety of affectionate behaviors and by a marked sparcity of pain-eliciting stimuli as compared with other mother-offspring relationships in primates such as baboons and macaques. Mother chimpanzees spend much time in grooming and playing with their youngsters and very seldom administer physical punishment. When they do, it is often followed by an embrace or some other reassuring gesture in response to the whimpering or screaming of the child.

The extent to which the young chimpanzee depends upon his mother is strikingly revealed when she dies. A three year old, who was probably still fairly dependent on maternal milk, survived her mother by some two and a half months. During this time she showed patterns similar to human depression—huddling, spending long periods in almost complete inactivity, almost total suppression of playful activity, and loss of appetite. She became increasingly lethargic. Finally she disappeared and was presumed dead. Two youngsters lost their mothers when they were between four and five years of age, and although both were "adopted" by elder sisters, they too showed signs of lethargy and abnormal behavior. One of them made a gradual recovery, and she behaved in a manner comparable to her peers a year after her mother's death. The other became increasingly abnormal and emaciated, and he finally died about one and a half years after losing his mother.

One juvenile male of about seven or eight years showed few signs of depression when he lost his mother and infant sibling. He was, however, fairly independent by this time and had quite frequently traveled on his own. An eight and a half year old who was still sharing his mother's nest at night and traveling with her constantly only survived her death by three weeks. He showed signs of severe depression by the second day and made only a few journeys away from the area where he last saw her body. He huddled, stopped playing, stopped eating, and was largely unresponsive to environmental stimulation. While in this condition, he developed gastroenteritis which probably contributed to his death twenty-five days after the death of his mother.

Even when young chimpanzees have attained some measure of independence and begun to move around for days or weeks with other individuals, they still spend much time in between such ventures associating with their mothers. A late adolescent male who was spending most of his time traveling apart from his mother began once more to move about with her frequently after cutting his foot badly. Another son of the same female, an adult male of some eighteen years, also traveled around constantly with her, away from other chimpanzees, after spraining his wrist in a status conflict. He only left her when he was fully recovered. This female was frequently accompanied by her three fully mature offspring until the time of her death, and the two other mothers known to have adult offspring were also often accompanied by them until death.

Mother chimpanzees not only actively protect their offspring during infancy, in common with mothers of all mammalian and avian species, but will usually try to protect their older offspring also. There is considerable variation in the extent to which individual mothers will attempt to assist their juvenile and adolescent daughters, but so far all mothers have at least hurried to the scene when their juvenile or adolescent sons were threatened or attacked by other chimpanzees. One mother rushed up when her young adult son was screaming and retreating from an older but rather low-ranking male. When she appeared, her son turned on his aggressor and together mother and son chased him away. This same female was observed to run half a mile, fast, when she heard her adult son (probably close to eighteen years) screaming during a serious attack. When she arrived, the action was over but her presence seemed to calm her son, who gradually stopped screaming. Similar behavior has been observed in rhesus monkeys.[57]

Adolescent sons have been observed to rush to their mother's defense in social encounters, and sometimes an entire family will present such a united front in the face of aggression that it is able to intimidate a male who would easily be able to dominate each of the members individually.

Of interest is the fact that we have never yet observed a physically mature male try to mate with his mother. Our sample size is too small for conclusions to be drawn about this, since it only involves two mothers, one with two adult sons and the other with one. However, during four days of estrus, the mother with two adult sons was mated by every mature male in her group *except* her two sons. Several adolescent males of lower rank than the two sons were observed mating with the female, so it cannot be argued that the sons were of too low a social status to mate with a popular female. There are indications that mother-son matings are infrequent in Japanese macaques[32] and rhesus macaques.[56,57] In these macaque species, the sons usually transfer out of their natal troops shortly after puberty, so there is less opportunity for sexual interactions with their mothers.

Mating does occur between a brother and his sister, but it is extremely rare. One female, when first she came into estrus, repeatedly ran off screaming on the few occasions when her two adult brothers tried to mate with her. Eventually she permitted them to copulate with her, but subsequently they have been observed to approach her sexually only a few times. Another brother-sister pair was seen mating only once during the two years when she had periods of estrus prior to conception. Another female who has been receptive to adult males for two years has not yet been seen having sexual relations with her elder brother.

The relationship between siblings is sometimes very strong and enduring. Juvenile and adolescent female chimpanzees may spend a great deal of time in watching, grooming, playing with, and carrying around their infant siblings, although this is not always the case. Some juvenile and even adolescent males may also pay much attention to their small siblings. On three occasions when mothers died their orphaned infants were adopted by older siblings, and this was the case even when the older sibling was a juvenile male.

Records at Gombe to date indicate that bonds between siblings of the same sex are likely to be stronger than those between brothers and sisters. Analysis of some of the recent data revealed that each individual of five adolescent and adult sibling pairs spent a greater percentage of observed time in association with a sibling than with any other chimpanzee of the same sex and similar age to that sibling. It also showed that brothers associated more with each other than with *any* other individual, at least during one year.⁷⁷

To date we have not been able to follow the development of a relationship between older sisters since the only known pair are both still traveling for most of the time with their mother.

At times a male may back up his brother during an aggressive social encounter. We have not yet seen mutual assistance between brothers and sisters. However, after a stressful incident an adolescent female hurried to sit close to her elder brother and this, in itself, seemed to have an immediate calming effect upon her. A juvenile female once ran to embrace her elder sister who was screaming and upset after being mated.⁵²

It is not only in chimpanzees that sibling bonds between males are known to extend beyond the infant and juvenile stage. A number of close associations between male siblings outside the natal group (that is, after they have transferred to another troop) have been reported among the rhesus on Cayo Santiago.⁵⁶ Indeed, at the time of his transfer, a young male is likely to join the group to which one or more of his brothers has already transferred.⁷

The above facts suggest that, whatever the precise structure of the family unit in our earliest ancestors, and whatever the role of the male may have been, it seems reasonable to assume that between mothers and their children and between siblings there were affectionate bonds of long duration, probably for the life span of the individuals concerned in many cases. If sufficient, reliable data can be gathered to show that incestuous relationships between mothers and sons in chimpanzee society do not occur, it will indicate that a similar inhibition was in operation among our stone age ancestors.

Adolescence

The period of adolescence in the chimpanzee commences at puberty (approximately seven to ten years of age) and ends when the individual reaches social maturity (about twelve or thirteen years of age in the female and fifteen or sixteen in the male). Adolescence is very often considered a culturally determined period unique to man. We shall attempt to show that, as in man, adolescence is an important stage in the life cycle of the chimpanzee, both biologically and psychologically.

It appears that this period is particularly difficult for the male chimpanzee. During puberty he has a growth spurt; he becomes more and more independent of his mother; and he is increasingly able to dominate females who, a short while previously, were able to subdue him with ease. On the other hand, he must behave with increasing caution in order to avoid arousing the aggression of adult males. One of the most interesting aspects of adolescence in the male chimpanzee is his ambivalent attitude to high-ranking mature males. On the one hand, he becomes increasingly fearful in their presence, often flinching at any sudden movement they make whether or not it was directed toward him. On the other hand, he increasingly seeks their company. When he first begins to travel with other groups, away from his mother, it is frequently with a group of adult males that he chooses to associate.

For the most part the early adolescent male occupies a peripheral position in a group of males, often watching them intently but seldom entering into their activities. For example, with regard to sex his behavior seems to be inhibited by the proximity of highly dominant males. Adolescent males certainly do mate, but seldom with a sexually popular female when there are mature males nearby.

All this suggests that the adolescent male, particularly during early adolescence, goes through a period of gradually changing relationships with many of the individuals of his community. It may well be that his relationship with his mother, which remains relatively constant, is the most stabilizing factor. Often, after associating for a while with males, and particularly when there have been frustrations involved (such as not being able to mate with a female in estrus) he returns to travel about with his mother for a while. Sometimes he may wander off completely on his own for some hours in the forest—e.g., after a thrashing by a dominant male.

During the last years of adolescence, the growing chimpanzee gradually begins to join in activities with the mature males; and he begins to challenge the status of the lower-ranking ones among them. Intense conflicts tend to occur at such times. Over a period of many months, or even several years, he gradually takes his place in the hierarchy of mature males of his community.

For the female chimpanzee, the period of adolescence is less demanding, and her relationship with other members of her community does not change markedly except during her periods of sexual receptivity. It is unnecessary for the female to leave her family group in order to learn her future role as a mother, and she typically associates with her mother for a more extended period than does the male. Most young adolescent females spend considerable time playing with, grooming, and carrying around an infant sibling or an infant of a nonrelated female.

For some females, the most stressful time of adolescence occurs when she has her first true estrus—that is, the first sexual swelling when she becomes attractive to adult males. Prior to this she has shown smaller swellings that attract the attention of infant males who are sexually precocious and start "mating" before they are one year old; toward the end of this phase she attracts juvenile males and the younger adolescents. Females show much variation in their initial responses to the sexual advances of mature males. Some are extremely fearful and, at least for the first few days, continually try to run from and avoid their suitors; others take such approaches as a matter of course.

In the female chimpanzee, there is a period of adolescent sterility. In wild chimpanzees, the duration of this period ranges from one to three years.

In most nonhuman primates, exchange of genes between groups seems to occur when males from neighboring ranges change groups. This has been observed in gorillas,[60] rhesus macaques,[57,7] baboons,[54,20] and it may occasionally occur in chimpanzees as well. However, we have also recorded a number of instances when young sexually mature female chimpanzees left their home communities during periods of sexual receptivity and mixed with and mated with males of neighboring communities.[24,44] In at least two cases, "stranger" females have been gradually integrated into the host community and finally abandoned their natal groups.

This may have significance for the understanding of the evolution of intergroup marriages in man. In many human cultures, it is the female who leaves her home and moves into new surroundings, often traveling miles to live with comparative strangers. Sometimes she must adopt a new culture also. In principle, such a major transition might have been facilitated by the evolution of love in the line leading to man, since love can overcome the concerns of strangeness. But most marriages in many cultures have traditionally been based not on love but on arrangements made either by the parents of the couple or by society. This discovery regarding chimpanzee adolescent female behavior, differing as it does from other nonhuman primates, raises questions about the evolution of human mating systems. More information is needed before we can adequately understand this behavior, but it does suggest that similar female restlessness may have been in operation in early man, may have contributed to the exchange of genes between groups, aided young women in coping with the stressful experience of being "given" to the son of a family in another group, or generally helped women through the difficulty of leaving what is familiar and going to what is largely unfamiliar.

Adolescence, in the chimpanzee as in the human, may be viewed as an extension of the learning period, a period when some of the skills and behaviors learned during childhood can be put to use in the adult context so that the developing individual will be fully prepared to handle the tasks of social maturity. It seems likely that the adolescent period of early man was more like that of the chimpanzee than the adolescent period of any human society after the advent of complex cultures.

Nonverbal Communication

Some of the most striking similarities in the behavior of chimpanzee and man are to be found in the gestures and posture of nonverbal communication. Thus chimpanzees may bow, kiss, hold hands, touch and pat each other, embrace, raise their arms in the air, bite, punch, kick, scratch each other, pull out each other's hair, and tickle. It is not only that some of these movements look remarkably similar to those of man, but also the behavioral contexts likely to elicit these patterns are similar in the two species.

When an adult chimpanzee is suddenly apprehensive or frightened, he may reach out to touch or even embrace another chimpanzee who happens to be nearby. Once two adult males were suddenly confronted with their mirror images: they responded with a variety of contact-seeking patterns, touching and patting each other, holding hands, embracing. In such a context, a high-ranking adult male may even embrace an infant or juvenile. Kortlandt and colleagues have filmed the responses of a wild chimpanzee group upon exposure to a stuffed leopard. One of the principal reactions was an intense outburst of mutual embracing, including adult males.[1] It is probable that the quick embrace a mother invariably bestows upon her infant if it utters a sound of fright may serve a mutually reassuring function, calming the fear of the infant and also the discomfort aroused in the mother by the distress signal of her child.

Humans, of course, show similar *contact-seeking behavior in stressful situations*, children and adults alike. Man carries his desire for contact in stress a step further and may caress or even embrace a pet when upset. In the human species, sudden anxiety often elic-

its self-contact patterns such as wringing the hands or clasping a hand to the breast or mouth. We have observed one wild chimpanzee who frequently clasps his genitals when suddenly fearful. Also, self-grooming is common in anxious chimpanzees.

Captive chimpanzees who have been raised without mothers, or who were separated from them at an early age, show self-contact patterns in moments of stress, mainly clasping themselves. Isolation-reared rhesus monkeys will actually bite themselves when suddenly alarmed.

The comfort adult chimpanzees and humans alike may derive from close physical contact with another individual must result from the years of infancy when, for so long, the embrace of the mother or contact with her body (or that of a mother substitute) serves to calm the anxieties of ape and human infants. As the child becomes increasingly independent of his mother he may, when suddenly frightened, seek contact with another individual—a temporary mother substitute—if his mother is not close by. Even an adolescent chimpanzee will seek contact with his mother, rather than another individual, if she is available. One adolescent male, after being threatened by a high-ranking male, hurried, whimpering, past several other chimpanzees to reach out toward his mother and hold the hand she extended.

When two or more chimpanzees become suddenly excited—if, for instance, they are confronted by a large pile of favored food—they often exhibit an outburst of contact-seeking behavior with their companions. Three or even four adults may pat each other, embrace, hold hands, press their mouths against one another and utter loud screams for several minutes before calming down sufficiently to start feeding.

This kind of behavior is similar to that shown by a human child, who, when told of a special treat, may fling his arms ecstatically around the bearer of the good news and squeal with delight. Similar adult responses in a variety of cultures are common experiences, though the intensity of expression is usually less exuberant.

Some chimpanzees consistently try to ingratiate themselves with more dominant animals. One female of our group seldom missed the opportunity of approaching an adult male who was passing anywhere near. Then, uttering submissive grunts, she would lay her hand on his head or back. Presumably, the sight of a high-ranking male makes such individuals uneasy: to calm themselves they approach and seek contact. There may be a similarity here to the uneasy human, who, during conversation, repeatedly reaches out to touch the person with whom he is talking.

A brief comment should be made here with regard to the human smile. It seems that we smile in two different contexts. We smile when we are pleased, happy or amused; and we smile also when we are uneasy and apprehensive. During a tense interview, a person may sit on the edge of his chair, clasp his hands, and smile. Indeed, he may smile at almost everything that is said, even when the content is unsatisfactory for him. This kind of tense, apprehensive smiling in man may be similar to the "grin" of the fearful or apprehensive chimpanzee in which the corners of the lips are drawn back and the lips slightly parted to expose the teeth.

After a chimpanzee has been severely threatened or attacked, particularly if the victim is a youngster, his need for physical contact is often dramatically illustrated. An adolescent may approach his aggressor after being attacked, still screaming, and obviously fearful. When he finally reaches the other, he will crouch, making gestures of appeasement or submission. In response, the aggressor will usually reach out and touch or pat the subordinate. He may continue patting gently until the youngster gradually stops screaming and whimpering. We have seen clear examples of conflict situations as adolescents approach an aggressor, so fearful that they keep turning away as though to flee, yet so much in need of a reassuring contact that they turn back and approach. In this manner they slowly come nearer and nearer the aggressor in a series of circles as the desire to flee is overcome by the desire for contact, and vice versa. Youngsters

have actually flown into violent tantrums, beating the ground and screaming, when the dominant chimpanzee did not respond with an appropriate contact behavior to their submissive gestures.

A very similar pattern is observed when a young human child who has been punished proceeds to follow the disciplinarian, crying, often clutching at legs or clothing, until he is picked up, petted, and forgiven. After a family dispute has been resolved, the people concerned often "make it up" with a kiss, embrace, or some other form of contact behavior. And the clasping of hands to denote mutual forgiveness and the renewal of friendly relations after a quarrel is common in many cultures.

However, this whole sequence of events— aggression, contact-seeking, and reassurance— is far from easy to understand in chimpanzees. Why should the dominant chimpanzee respond with a comforting gesture? When we think in human terms, this is the kind of action that we tend to regard as an expression of apology or sympathy or kindness. Does the dominant chimpanzee therefore show the beginnings of some kind of altruistic behavior? Does it show an enduring commitment of the individuals to each other?

There are certainly occasions when a human being reassures a friend with an encouraging pat on the back because the close proximity of a person in distress is disturbing. His unhappiness intrudes on his companion's sense of well-being and makes him uncomfortable. Thus the comfort given, while it results in calming his friend, may be made at least partially to relieve his own discomfort. It is equally possible that, for a chimpanzee, the sight and sound of a crouching, whimpering, or screaming subordinate may make him feel uneasy. He may have learned that he can calm the other with a touch. We have already mentioned that an agitated chimpanzee may seek reassurance by reaching out to touch a companion—such an action on the part of the uneasy superior would serve the double purpose of calming both.

It is also possible that both the submissive

posture of the subordinate and the reassuring touch of the dominant may have originated from social grooming. This is an activity which provides chimpanzees with long periods of relaxed physical contact and, as we shall indicate in a later section, grooming appears to calm apprehensive individuals. Thus, it is possible that the submission-reassurance sequence may be derived at least partially from the social grooming pattern. The crouching might be a ritualized invitation to groom; the touch of the superior a ritualized grooming response. There are, in fact, occasions when a few brief grooming movements do occur in response to submissive crouching.

When two chimpanzees meet after a separation, they may engage in gestures and postures that strikingly resemble forms of human greeting. Chimpanzees may bow, kiss, touch or pat one another, hold hands or embrace. A male may chuck a female or an infant under the chin. In chimpanzee society, reunion after separation often involves behaviors that serve to reestablish the relative social status of the individuals concerned. Originally greeting behavior in man probably served a similar function—and still does on some formal occasions. In general, however, greeting in man has become ritualized in a variety of cultures.

There are similarities, too, in some chimpanzee and human aggressive behaviors. A quick upward jerk of the arm serves as a threat in a chimpanzee, as does a level stare directed unwaveringly at a subordinate. A chimpanzee may adopt an upright posture when he is threatening and wave his arms above his head, and he may throw objects, overarm and underhand, toward whomever or whatever he is threatening. He may brandish a stick or make a downward clubbing movement. Attacking chimpanzees may bite, hit, and kick. Female chimpanzees sometimes scratch and pull out a handful of hair from their victim's head.

At this point, it should be noted that chimpanzees are not, on the whole, highly aggressive primates in the natural state as compared, for example, with baboons and macaques. Most aggressive incidents occur during status conflicts between males and these rather than taking the form of physical attack usually involve bluff—vigorous charging displays, often performed bipedally and with hair erect so that the actor looks as large as he can, waving sticks and branches, hurling objects. Two males competing with each other for status may "display" toward and around one another for up to thirty minutes, after which one of them either retreats or approaches and shows submission. Occasionally, such an episode terminates in a serious fight with grossly visible injury. Female fights occur also. Often they begin when squabbles occur during the play sessions of their offspring.

When the chimpanzees at Gombe were fed bananas on a regular basis, this resulted in the crowding together of relative strangers—individuals who would not ordinarily have met. These chimpanzees were competing for a favored food that was in relatively short supply. During these three years, aggressive incidents rose dramatically both in frequency and in intensity. When regular banana feeding was stopped, the chimpanzees, no longer crowded together in unusually large groups, quickly resumed their less violent way of life.[78] Lee has reported that Kalahari Bushmen who are usually nonaggressive become aggressive when several bands congregate around a water hole in time of drought.[13]

There are some similarities in the play patterns of humans and chimpanzees. Chimpanzees use their fingers in the same way as humans when tickling a playmate, and they respond to intense tickling with sounds not unlike those made by laughing children in a similar context. Chimpanzees turn somersaults and pirouette, and one youngster spent minutes at a time trying to stand on his head. Sometimes he succeeded if there were a nearby tree against which he could balance his feet.

Finally, what of the emotions? Most people who have become well acquainted with chimpanzees agree that these apes almost certainly have "moods" that are similar to those states which, in man, we call sadness, happiness, rage, grief, and jealousy. So far no one has tackled a scientific investigation of these states

in the chimpanzee; it will be an extremely difficult though very rewarding area of research.

❮ Some Major Differences in Chimpanzee and Human Behavior; and Possible Selection Pressures Leading in the Human Direction

In this section, we shall discuss several of the
more obvious differences between man and
chimpanzee that are highlighted by our understanding of chimpanzee behavior: (a) in
man hunting became a way of life rather than
an occasional luxury; (b) man developed a
characteristic bipedal gait; (c) the human female became constantly sexually receptive;
(d) humans began to show some forms of
contact behavior that differed in some ways
from those shown by the chimpanzee; (e)
man developed a language in which he could
communicate about events past and future
and about abstract concepts and theories. In
addition, man, at some point in his evolution,
lost most of his hair, an occurrence that might
have influenced a number of the changes
listed above.

Do we find traits in the chimpanzee today
that could be precursors of these uniquely
human characteristics? In some cases we do
and, with our understanding of chimpanzee
behavior in the natural habitat together with
information derived from the fossil record, we
are in a position to postulate some environmental and social pressures that might have
shaped such traits in the direction of their
present human form, i.e., conditions under
which natural selection might have favored
evolution from chimpanzeelike behavior in an
ancestral stock to humanlike behavior in a
later era.

During this discussion we shall refer, from
time to time, to a hypothetical group of chimpanzees, or chimpanzeelike creatures, living in
an area where gallery forests penetrate bush
or savanna country that is fairly rich in prey
animals. This will give a picture of a group of
beings that are undoubtedly similar in many
ways to our own ancestors, living in an envi-

ronment similar to that which is commonly
supposed to have nurtured early man. We
must remember that the patterns to be discussed undoubtedly evolved at different times,
different rates, and over many thousands of
years. In each case, therefore, we are considering an unknown span of time when crucial
changes were taking place. We are trying to
tease out factors that might have been responsible for changing a quadrupedal, tree-living,
mainly vegetarian ape into an upright, sa-
vanna-living hunter with a large repertoire of
tools and weapons, a more advanced culture,
and a language. Whether our hypothetical
group of apelike creatures are ancestral to the
first true men or early examples of *Homo* himself will probably vary with the aspect of behavior under discussion. Some features considered uniquely human today were probably
not yet apparent in the creatures that paleontologists would classify as *Homo*, while other
characteristics of man are, as we have seen,
present also in the chimpanzee and therefore
were undoubtedly present in the common
ancestor.

Hunting as a Way of Life

We have already described some of the
main hunting, cooperative and food-sharing
patterns occurring in the chimpanzee today.
Now we are concerned with the possible reasons underlying the change from a mainly
vegetarian to a mainly carnivorous diet in
early man. This change, if it forced our ancestors to spend more and more time on the savanna away from the comparative safety of
the forest, undoubtedly played a crucial role
in shaping human evolution. Behaviors most
likely to have been influenced directly were
the development of killing and cutting tools,
cooperation, food sharing, division of labor
and bipedal locomotion. In addition, a new
environment with its new challenges and dangers undoubtedly placed a high premium on
intelligence; individuals who were the most
quick-witted in times of sudden danger and
who were adept at problem solving were more
likely to survive.

Any clues we may derive from an understanding of the carnivorous behavior of the chimpanzee today that might help us toward understanding how and why early man or his ancestors adapted to a hunting way of life will be worthwhile. Firstly, then, we should ask what pressures operating on chimpanzees today might be expected to bring about an increase in hunting behavior. It is important to remember that chimpanzees appear to be extremely partial to meat. This is suggested by the intense excitement that always attends a successful hunt, the persistence of many individuals in trying to obtain a share of the kill, and the eagerness with which almost every scrap of carcass is consumed. Wild baboons also hunt and eat small mammals and birds with apparent satisfaction;[14,16,54,27] gibbons,[64] gorillas, and orangutans,[83] although so far they have not been observed eating flesh in nature, will readily accept it in captivity. We may, therefore, postulate an inherent tendency among higher primates to accept meat as food.

We should also consider the role of the individual in initiating any new tradition. Some chimpanzees like meat more than others or, at least, they seem to eat it more often. At Gombe, there was one old female who nearly always managed to be at the scene of a kill. She begged persistently and fearlessly from the adult males and nearly always managed to acquire quite large amounts of meat. In this case, at any rate, it seems that her offspring, probably as a result of early and repeated exposure to meat as food, have acquired her extreme interest in it. All of them, ranging from eight to over twenty years, also beg persistently at kills. Moreover, the two adult sons have both been actively involved in many hunts and have both made kills themselves, one of them even while he was still an adolescent and the other even after losing the use of one arm when he contracted poliomyelitis. Other individuals of the same age and sex as these four participate in meat eating and hunting less frequently.

These facts alone mean that it is not inconceivable that a trend toward increased hunting and meat eating might develop quite spontaneously in an area that was slightly richer in easily available prey animals than is Gombe. If, for instance, just a few individuals of our hypothetical group began to make frequent sorties into the neighboring savanna in search of young gazelle, the habit might, in time, spread through the community. If there was a particularly bad fruit crop one year, this might intensify such a hunting tradition.

There is another factor that might force chimpanzees to hunt more frequently. In the Kasakati Basin area, to the south of Gombe National Park, there is an annual migration of the group being studied. This apparently occurs as a result of the movements of a much larger group. The smaller group moves some twenty miles from the range it inhabits for about three quarters of each year, apparently to avoid the larger and more dominant group as it moves in.[50] In this particular area, the subordinate group simply moves on into another part of its range, which is ecologically very similar to the one it has been forced out of. But it is not difficult to imagine a situation in which such a group might be driven into an area that was ecologically different from its normal range—onto the fringes of the savanna where its very survival might depend on an increase in carnivorous behavior. The competing group might be a larger number of the same species, as is the case in the Kasakati Basin, or it might be of different species with larger or more aggressive individuals.

It is widely accepted today that the earliest men were already hunters. A great many bones and fragments of bones of animals presumed to have been the prey of *Homo habilis*, together with associated "pebble tools," have been found at living sites at Olduvai by Dr. L.S.B. Leakey and his colleagues. There is evidence suggesting that even the more primitive australopithecines were already hunters. There is, however, some controversy as to whether our ancestors became true hunters only after acquiring a taste for meat by scavenging or whether they were bona-fide hunters from the start. We firmly support the second hypothesis.

Although there is some evidence at Gombe that chimpanzees may seize a freshly killed victim from hunting baboons within a few moments of its capture, the apes normally catch their own prey. When we set out the body of a freshly killed bush pig, the chimpanzees appeared frightened and did not attempt to feed on it. At a time when the chimpanzees were in the habit of snatching domestic chicks for food, a juvenile female, after killing one, left it almost untouched. None of the other individuals who later passed the body touched it. The remains of a young bushbuck, probably caught earlier by baboons, was also ignored by the chimpanzees. Thus it seems that the prerequisites for chimpanzees feeding on flesh may be (a) the excitement attendant upon a kill (whether it be a chimpanzee or a baboon kill) or (b) the sight of another chimpanzee feeding on flesh.

It should be mentioned also that whereas baboons have been observed in many areas hunting and eating small mammals and birds, as mentioned above, we can find no reference of their scavenging from the carcasses of dead animals. Baboon troops have frequently been observed near the remains of kills on the Serengeti, but they were never seen to form a part of the attendant scavenger group,[69] and in Nairobi Park fresh carrion was ignored.[15]

Let us for a moment consider our hypothetical apes who are beginning to change to a more carnivorous diet, and imagine how they would fare as scavengers. Studies on the Serengeti Plains in Africa vividly reveal some of the problems and dangers attendant on a scavenging way of life.[69] Any appreciable amount of food available for scavenging consists of carcasses of animals that have died a natural death or the remains of the prey of other carnivores. One problem is to find such food. This may be done by sight, hearing, or smell. If the real killer is still finishing his meal, how can one get a share without being hurt? How can one get there before too many other competitors have arrived at the scene? It is not only vultures, jackals, and hyenas who feed on dead flesh—lions and leopards will do so readily.

In many ways the hyena is well adapted for a scavenging role. He has enormously strong teeth and jaws. Thus, he is able to chew extremely large bones and tough hide that he is subsequently able to utilize, thanks to a remarkable digestive system. He has acutely sensitive ears so that he can accurately locate far-off sounds made by other carnivores at a kill. He can run quite fast and he has great stamina. Yet even he does most of his own hunting. The jackal, too, though he is often successful in obtaining scraps from a kill even under the noses of larger carnivores, thanks to his lightning speed, nevertheless hunts insects and birds most of the time. In fact, the only creatures that are really successful at scavenging are the vultures and other winged carrion eaters. They can maintain vantage points high in the sky and keep watch over large areas of the country. When they see potential food with their exceptionally keen eyes, they can reach it much faster than a creature that must run on the ground. Indeed, it is by closely watching the movement of vultures in the sky that many earthbound predators are directed to available food sources.

Our hypothetical ape, in the process of moving onto the savanna and taking up a more carnivorous diet, might have been a reasonably fast runner, and he might have had great powers of endurance. But even though his hearing was probably keener than that of modern man, it is unlikely that his auditory capabilities could match hyenas or jackals. Nor would his sense of smell have been as acute as theirs. He would have been able to watch the sky for telltale movements of vultures and run to the scene of a kill along with other scavengers. If, on arrival, he had found only vultures there, or perhaps a couple of hyenas and jackals—or even a single lion—he might, if he was with a group of his kind, be able to drive them from their meal and appropriate it for his group. But in those early days when man (or his forebears) was just starting his hunting life, his weapons were probably nothing more than rocks and sticks, and it is unlikely that a small group of apelike creatures could have driven a large number of hyenas or a pride of lions from their kill. In those early days, there would have been little if any fear of man (found in most wild creatures today) to assist him in driving off competitors. Anyone who has watched the larger carnivores in action—seen a lion killing a hyena at a carcass, watched a group of hyenas chasing a lion from its prey, observed the deadly spring of a leopard—will be only too well aware of the dangers faced by scavengers.

We are not trying to say that, during his development into a hunter, man never scavenged. Man is, and undoubtedly always has been, an opportunist. Our Stone Age ancestors or their predecessors would have scavenged when the reward was worth it and the risks not too great. However, in view of the dangers attendant on scavenging, the difficulties involved, and the total absence of scavenging behavior in living primates today, it seems more reasonable to suppose that most of the meat early man consumed had been killed by his own group. Only when his weapons became more deadly and he had the means of intimidating the larger carnivores, would it have been practical to any great extent for him to try to supplement his meat diet by scavenging from the kills of others.

The environmental conditions favoring greater reliance upon the savanna need more specific attention.[31] Whatever these may have been, greater reliance upon the savanna would have meant more hunting and this in turn would have placed a premium upon cooperative behavior. As we have seen, cooperation is important in enhancing the effectiveness of chimpanzee hunting, and would probably have been much more important under open country conditions. So, whatever else an increasing reliance upon hunting may have meant for human evolution, we think it gave selective advantage to intelligently cooperative individuals.

Bipedal Locomotion

Man walks and runs in an upright position that is unique among living primates. Many speculations have been put forward as to: (1) the circumstances that might have given rise to the gait, and (2) the various ways it might have affected the subsequent development of man once it had been established.

How frequently does the bipedal stance occur in the chimpanzee today, and in what circumstances is it most likely to occur? For anatomical reasons the chimpanzee is a poor bipedal walker when compared to man: mostly he bends forward at the waist and shows a waddling gait. Usually he only moves for a few yards in this posture after which he resumes his quadrupedal, knuckle-walking gait. There are, however, exceptions to this: there are a few individuals in our community who walk upright with a posture that is almost that of a man, and one individual shows only the slightest sign of waddling. These chimpanzees tend to move farther in an upright posture than their companions. This suggests that there is ample biological variation in the locomotor system upon which natural selection could operate in a direction toward bipedalism, if environmental conditions favored such behavior.

Chimpanzees most often move bipedally when they are carrying food, performing aggressive displays, looking for a companion or some other object in long grass, or traveling over very wet ground. Two chimpanzees learned to travel almost constantly in an upright posture after each lost the use of one arm as a result of contracting a paralytic disease, probably poliomyelitis. One of these chimpanzees, in particular, has adapted to bipedal walking in a very dramatic manner. His posture is very upright, his strides are even, and he can travel in this way for many minutes. After he has taken a couple of tripedal steps using his one sound arm, he resumes the upright posture. In this way he can keep up with other chimpanzees even when they are traveling quite fast.

If our hypothetical group of chimpanzees living at the edge of the savanna only penetrated the grassland for very short distances, very infrequently, it is difficult to imagine that there would be any factors that would strongly select for more frequent adoption of an upright gait. If, however, their excursions from the forest became longer and more frequent, there would be much advantage for these individuals who were able to walk upright easily. (1) For one thing, they would be able to see over the grass and notice (a) the presence of dangerous carnivores, (b) the whereabouts of potential prey, and (c) the whereabouts of their companions, which would be especially important during cooperative hunting. Such behavior is striking among savanna baboons when they are in tall grass far from trees. (2) If these hypothetical chimpanzees made a kill, they would very likely want to carry the prey back to the forest. Chimpanzees are not equipped for eating meat quickly; moreover, they invariably eat quantities of leaves with flesh. They could carry the prey in a tripedal position, dragging it along the ground or slinging it over the neck or shoulder. But if they could not see over the grass, there would be the danger that some scavenger, such as a hyena, might sneak up and make off with their meat. (3) It is also possible that if the chimpanzees were not hunting but foraging the savanna for roots, berries, or even insects, they might still, particularly if they were close to the forest, return to feed in the safety and shade of the trees. A return journey of this sort would only be worthwhile if they could carry a large amount —that is, in both hands, and thus with a bipedal gait. At Gombe we have seen chimpanzees collecting handfuls of fallen fruit and then moving bipedally to sit and eat the meal in the shade of a tree. (4) Aggressive encounters with potential scavengers when the chimpanzees were still in the grassland would almost certainly result in aggressive bipedal displays. At Gombe encounters with baboons during competition for bananas at the open, artificial feeding area resulted in some of the most spectacular displays of this sort, when chimpanzees leapt upright in the air, waving their arms and hurling rocks or brandishing sticks. Baboons also eat meat, and we have seen a male baboon at Gombe try to take meat from a chimpanzee.

Thus, encounters with scavengers including baboons would have selected for increasingly vivid bipedal displays, since this form of bluff makes the chimpanzee appear bigger and more dangerous than he really is. Also, the upright posture is by far the best position for efficient throwing and stick wielding. If we envisage a situation in which the chimpanzee was confronted by another species of *ape*, a species that also specialized in bipedal bluff and throwing, then there would be a very powerful selective pressure for increasingly efficient bipedal display and weapon use. It is highly plausible that one of the main threats to early humans arose from other groups of early humans.[4,5]

In the chimpanzee still another factor would exert a strong selective pressure for the development of bipedal walking—namely, if infants were unable to cling to their mothers. Two factors that might have influenced this in human evolution are: (1) the loss of hair on the mother so that there was nothing for the infant to cling to, and (2) increased brain size necessitating earlier birth since the human pelvis will not permit the birth of a larger head. Thus, as human evolution progressed, infants were born in an increasingly immature condition, hence less able to cling effectively.

The development of some bipedalism might have been necessary to free the mother's hands sufficiently to hold the baby whose nervous system was too immature for firm clinging. Historically, there must have been a feedback relation among the major components of human evolution. The need to hold the immature, large-brained baby could have been a powerful stimulus to further improvement of bipedalism. We have evidence at Gombe that it is possible for a chimpanzee to adapt remarkably to an upright posture even during the life span of the individual. (We refer here to the two males who began to walk upright after each lost the use of one arm.) We suggest that it could also be possible for females to adapt in this way in order to carry their infants, particularly as this adaptation would take place slowly, over countless years with natural selection favoring those mothers who were effective in holding the infant.

It is frequently suggested that the development of tool use was one of the main factors that gave selective advantage to bipedalism. While we see the logic of this reasoning, we are inclined to think the point has been overemphasized in relation to the early phases of human evolution. As Tobias[67] has pointed out, the ability to sit in an upright position is all that is needed for the hands to be freed for tool use. The chimpanzees at Gombe do indeed carry out most of their tool-using performances in a sitting posture. Only when the tool-making cultures of early man were sufficiently advanced as to necessitate the carrying of premade tools from one place to another would bipedal locomotion become necessary for tool-using; and, as Leakey has pointed out, early stone tools were usually made on the spot rather than carried from place to place. However, as we have seen, more frequent use of weapons and the development of more sophisticated weapons would certainly give added selective advantage to upright locomotion.

Constant Sexual Receptivity in the Human Female

Another feature that is unique to the human primate is the constant state of sexual receptivity of the female. Other primates in natural habitats mate only during those periods when the female is in estrus or at least close to estrus. The human female is attractive and receptive to males throughout her reproductive life and beyond into the menopausal era. It is very difficult today to imagine a human society in which women were only sexually accessible once a month; and there has been a great deal of speculation as to the circumstances in which this unique development took place.

The most widely accepted suggestion is that a strong sexual bond was *necessary* to ensure that the male would return from his hunting sorties to share meat with waiting women and children and, in return, get his share of the berries and roots they had gathered during his absence. Once the sexual pattern of constant receptivity had been established, it enabled the formation of the typically human family structure.

It may be meaningful to review briefly the kinds of heterosexual relationships occurring in contemporary nonhuman higher primates, particularly in chimpanzees. The most usual monkey pattern is that in which each female in a troop is mated by a variety of males during at least part of her period of receptivity. In some species a high-ranking male is likely to monopolize her sexually during the peak of estrus—in other words, when she is most likely to conceive. In the hamadryas baboon, the local population is comprised of a number of "one-male groups".[41] In this species, each male acts as "overlord" to a number of females whom he zealously protects from sexual contact with other males of the troop. Nor does he seek sexual satisfaction other than with his own females. This system resembles the harem family group of many human cultures. There is only one example among nonhuman higher primates of a male and female forming a monogamous pair (which may be for life) and that is the gibbon, a small, tree-living Asiatic ape.

In chimpanzee society a variety of sexual behaviors are possible.[21,44] Sometimes a female may be mated by all the males available throughout her period of genital swelling. Sometimes she may go off with one male during the peak of estrus—the male may vary from one estrus period to the next. And sometimes a relationship develops in which a female will go off with the same male during successive periods of estrus. This is not to imply that the female will refuse the advances of other males nor that the male will not mate with any other females available to him. It does, however, suggest that there is some incipient tendency toward the formation of stable pair bonds in the species.

However, as female chimpanzees get older their periods of sexual activity become very widely separated. A young female is likely to show periodic swellings, when she is receptive to males, during most of her pregnancy; and she will resume sexual swellings again about two years after the birth of her infant, even though conception has not been known to occur until the previous infant was at least three and a half years old. But older females do not usually become sexually receptive either during pregnancy or until the infant is about four and a half years of age. These older females very frequently move about on their own, with only their dependent young, whereas younger females are much more often with groups of chimpanzees.

While it is not easy to see any particular

advantage for the chimpanzees at Gombe in the development of more stable associations between the sexes, this acquires a different significance for our hypothetical chimpanzee group that is moving frequently into the savanna from the forest. In this situation two factors that might select for longer and more frequent periods of sexual receptivity in the female suggest themselves. In the face of a potentially dangerous object or predator, it is the males who become especially aggressive, leaping about, calling, swaying branches, hurling rocks, brandishing sticks. For a society of chimpanzees cooperative protective bluff— and occasional serious fighting—would, presumably, become increasingly important to survival in the new and more dangerous environment of the grassland, where there are fewer trees and more carnivores. Females and youngsters wandering about far from the protection of adult males would be endangered; those with longer and more frequent periods of receptivity would travel more frequently with adult males and have a greater chance of survival.

We have already mentioned that a receptive female is very likely to obtain a share of meat when she begs from a male in possession of the carcass. If meat became a much more important item of chimpanzee diet—particularly in the face of any shortage of vegetable foods —it would become increasingly necessary for females to obtain adequate shares of each kill.

Previous discussions on the evolution of the unique human female sexual pattern have usually centered around that time in evolution when there already was a clear division of labor: when the men went out hunting and the women stayed behind gathering roots and berries.[42] But there is some overlap in the division of labor—e.g., in some hunting-and-gathering societies, women take part in the dismembering of the kill, especially if it is a large carcass such as that of an elephant.

If man's early ancestors showed incipient tendencies similar to those shown by the chimpanzees today toward stable pair-bonding, the further strengthening of those bonds between a man and woman would have been complicated by a change in life style from a mainly vegetarian to an increasingly carnivorous diet, from existence in the forest to existence on the grassland. When a male chimpanzee goes off with a female in estrus, they often stay away from all other chimpanzees for seven to ten days. But it might have been unsafe for an early human couple to go hunting alone in the savanna. Also, if meat was really important in the diet of these early ancestors, the pair could ill afford to remain away from the group for over a week each month since, on their own, they might achieve but little success in hunting. Life was difficult, there was probably a greater ratio of females to males as is common in most primate species, and in order to survive, early man could not afford to waste chances of reproduction by mating with one female only. It would have been important that all available females should be fertilized during the early struggle to survive in a new habitat. Thus, the effect of this great evolutionary transition on male-female attachments must have been complex. Our estimate is that it tended to strengthen them, but probably not to create a strictly monogamous society.

One other comment may be made in connection with the evolution of constant receptivity in the human female. There is evidence that social pressures can influence receptivity in some primates. Thus, in a hamadryas baboon society, where the female is forced to leave her mother and join a one-male group when she is only one year old, she develops a sexual swelling and becomes receptive to the advances of her male a whole year earlier than the females of other baboon species.

In the chimpanzee, there are numerous instances in which physiological and psychological stress can inhibit sexual swelling; and there is one case where psychological factors may have led to the development of a swelling. This occurred when an old female in our community was socially grooming with several adult males; suddenly a young female with a sexual swelling arrived. The males at once left the old female and hurried to groom the newcomer. For a few moments the old female simply stared at the young female, all her hair on end (a sign of aggression). Finally, she slowly approached the group and intently inspected the swelling of the other female. The following day, this old female had developed a small swelling, her first in a long time. The swelling was not large enough for any male to mate her, but several males were very interested, hurried up, inspected the swelling and groomed her vigorously as they had groomed the young female the previous day.

This incident is described here because any factors relating to the prolongation of receptivity in our closest relations may be significant to an understanding of the unusual constant receptivity of the human female. It is also worth emphasizing that the chimpanzee has probably progressed further than most other nonhuman primates in increasing the time when a *young* female is sexually receptive. She shows regular recurrent swellings for two to three years before she has her first infant; she continues to show cyclic swellings during six to seven months of her eight month pregnancy; and she may swell again when her infant is only fourteen months old, despite the fact that she will not conceive for another two and a half to three and a half years. It has been suggested that periods of estrus in baboons would be incompatible with caring for an infant owing to the complete disruption of other social patterns during that time. Among the chimpanzees, a mother continues to care adequately for her infant during repeated periods of sexual receptivity.

In captivity, when a chimpanzee male and female are housed together in a small cage with nothing to do, the male may copulate even when the female is anestrus and her sex skin is flat.[82] In similar laboratory conditions, rhesus monkeys also show an extension of the period in which copulations occur. Thus, it is possible that the evolution of a stronger bond between couples, with its enhancement of proximity, may in itself have provided conditions favoring extended receptivity in the women of early human societies.

Social Grooming

Social grooming, in which one individual looks through the hair of a companion and extracts, with lips or fingers, small flakes of dry skin, parasites, and so on, plays a very important role in the social life of most of the higher nonhuman primates. Chimpanzees may spend up to two hours in sessions of social grooming; these tend to be longest and most frequent between close associates such as adult males who travel around together, mothers and their older offspring, and some couples. Social grooming thus provides long sessions of relaxed, physical contact between friendly chimpanzees. Grooming also occurs in other contexts: it may serve to calm an excited or frightened chimpanzee and it is frequently seen during a greeting between two individuals or in response to a submissive present.

If our earliest human ancestors still had a fairly abundant supply of hair, it is almost certain that they, along with the other higher primates, would have groomed one another. But what would have happened when they gradually—or suddenly—lost their hair? For a while social grooming would undoubtedly have continued, first because of the important role it had played for so long, and second because there still are several hairy places left to groom on the unclothed body. Most of man's hairy patches, however, are not those parts of the body which are most frequently groomed by chimpanzees. Moreover, during a long grooming session between two chimpanzees each individual often searches through his companion's hair quite systematically, covering most of the body. With grooming restricted to the few parts of the human body that are fairly luxuriant in hair growth, a session could not be protracted except by covering the same areas time and again.

Perhaps for a while early man continued to make grooming movements on those places where it most pleased his companions to be groomed, even if they were areas such as the back, shoulders, and thighs, where there might have been very little hair. In time, however, such behavior might have become simply stroking movements. In place of the lips picking out small flakes of skin from the hair, kissing might have become more frequent. Individuals bored by stroking their hairless companions, might have merely laid their hands on the back or shoulders of their partners, and sat together in companionable, close physical contact. They might have held hands.

Social grooming, as such, has not disappeared entirely from the human repertoire. Waika Indians show intense mouthing of each other's skin during greetings, particularly of the face, and this behavior may well have derived from grooming with the lips.[17] Combing, brushing, or arranging a partner's hair, or searching for lice, may occupy some portion of each day in some cultures. There are many other examples of grooming activities, particularly between mothers and their young children and between young couples.

All these activities, however, play a relatively minor role in the social life of our own species. Yet in man, as in the chimpanzee, there is a need for friendly physical contact between closely associated individuals. What forms of contact behavior have we developed in place of social grooming?

In many cultures friends or close companions will hold hands, put their arms around each other's shoulders, or link arms. In many human societies such behavior is quite common between males despite the fact that, in Western culture, it is likely to be frowned upon. In heterosexual love relationships, touch, in the form of caressing, holding, and kissing, plays a very important role. Often, indeed, this kind of behavior may be as important to the feeling of well-being as sexual intercourse. And these are all forms of contact behavior which are almost entirely lacking in chimpanzees, though occasionally a mother may lay her hand on her child's back, or hold his hand for a while, and he may do the same. For the most part, in chimpanzee society, friendly contact is expressed in social grooming.

Human Language

Language, above all else, stands out as a unique evolutionary achievement of our own species, for it is chiefly through language that so many other human characteristics have been developed and refined—characteristics such as love, religion, self-respect as well as the most complex intellectual activities. While one may find simple precursors of such characteristics in the chimpanzee, without language it is impossible to conceive of their appearance in human form.

The chimpanzee has a large vocabulary of calls, each of which serves to convey specific information as to the context in which the call is given and the identity of the chimpanzee making the sound. Loud grunts are given when a chimpanzee finds a succulent food source; other chimpanzees can correctly interpret the calls, hurry along, and join in feeding. A youngster is attacked and screams; his mother hurries to the scene and defends him or provides support; but she will ignore the screams of another youngster of the same age and sex as her own offspring.

Recent research into the brain circuitry relating to speech suggests that the calls of the chimpanzee are not the direct precursors of human spoken language.[55,43] The neurobiology of speech is undergoing major clarification.[19,62] In considering the evolution of language, this is not the place to discuss the existing "vocabulary" of the chimpanzee. Instead we should look for circumstances that might have placed a very high premium on the need for a more precise exchange of information.[75]

Until recently it was believed that chimpanzees were unable to learn to talk partly because of deficiencies in the vocal apparatus but mainly because of their inability to conceptualize and think in abstractions. Current experimentation on teaching chimpanzees language by means of signaling or the use of plastic symbols indicates that the chimpanzee's capacity for concept formation has been underestimated. The young chimpanzee Washoe, trained in sign language by the Gardners, was able to recognize and identify her reflection in a mirror, thus indicating that the chimpanzee has at least a crude realization of "self."[18] Another chimpanzee, Sarah, trained in the use of plastic word symbols, showed that she could grasp the meaning of an abstraction.[51] She was taught that blue was a color and that red was a color. She was then able to work out for herself that green was also a color. Other research of this kind is steadily increasing our appreciation of the intellectual ability of the chimpanzee.

The development of hunting behavior in early man might have placed a high premium on the use of sounds that could be used to identify specific places and things.[71] They suggested that the first word may have been the name of a place where the group, having split into hunting parties, would meet in the evening. In addition to this possibility, other factors are worth considering. If man had evolved to the point where he could plan ahead to a meeting in the evening, he would probably have begun to use at least temporary shelters and would be likely to return there habitually. Washburn and Lancaster[73] have also suggested that as hunting increased it would have provided further selective advantage for the evolution of language. For it would have become more and more useful to communicate subtleties of the hunt for maximum cooperation. This could well be true, but many nonhuman animals have reached high levels of cooperation in hunting without the use of a spoken language. Moreover, while hunting, the Australian aborigines and the Kalahari Bushmen communicate by an elaborate series of signs—the kind of "language" that, as the experiments with Washoe suggest, might have evolved in the chimpanzee more readily than spoken language.

Bigelow[4] makes a similar point in relation to competition between early human groups. The need to defend themselves against enemies in order to survive must have put a premium on cooperation, and the efficacy of sustained cooperation might well have been enhanced by the advent of language. Here as elsewhere, multiple environmental pressures may coincide in a way that strengthens the selective advantage of a particular capacity. In the case of a truly remarkable capacity such as language, it seems likely that several advantages may well have coincided in a way that fostered its evolution. Therefore, we wish to suggest an additional set of circumstances that might have placed a high premium on the development of language.

Hayes raised an infant chimpanzee from birth for the specific purpose of trying to teach her to talk.[28] At the end of four years, Vicki's only accomplishments were softly uttered sounds that approximated papa, mama, and cup. The observers noted that it was exceedingly difficult for Vicki to make a sound—any sound—that was not directly induced by an accompanying emotion. To make a sound when she *saw* a plate of food was automatic; to make a sound when asked if she would like a plate of food was almost impossible for her. Yet the recent work with Sarah and Washoe demonstrates that the chimpanzee is quite capable of asking for things by gesture or of using plastic word symbols.

Let us now ask what circumstances might have arisen in evolution that would put a very high pressure on the uttering of sounds *not* associated with a sudden emotion? The chimpanzee infant, clinging to its mother and in close contact with her, utters very few sounds. But what if the infant were unable to cling to the mother? Unless the mother was already able to transport the baby in some kind of sling, she would have to put it down occasionally while she did other things. Such a situation might have arisen for the first time with the loss of extensive body hair. Or, if bipedal locomotion occurred earlier in evolution than the loss of hair, this would also produce an infant that was unable to cling to its mother, as Washburn has pointed out; for this led to a changed anatomy of the foot that would no longer permit hair gripping.

In a situation of this sort, there would be a very high premium on vocal communication between a mother and her infant. The contemporary chimpanzee mother and very young infant seldom utter sounds when communicating other than the occasional soft call of the baby as it searches for a nipple or feels its grip slipping—and the occasional distress scream which the infant may utter on falling or being startled. To both of these sounds, the mother may respond with a similar soft call.

If our hypothetical infant were lying on the ground while the mother was busy nearby and it uttered a cry of distress, the mother would very likely rush over to gather it up, probably uttering a sound herself. The sound would be an integral part of her emotion. But if the infant just gave a soft call, indicating that it was a little hungry or uncomfortable, there might well be a new element emerging in the pattern of mother-infant communication. The mother might want to make a reassuring sound even though she was not experiencing distress to indicate that she would come in a moment. As a result of the sound the baby might be quiet. Without that sound, it might call more and more loudly. In coping with the problems of a changing way of life, the mother might urgently need some way of communicating to her child that she was going away briefly but would be coming back soon: perhaps some way of telling him that if he made a noise he would attract prowling hyenas or lions.

Nowhere do we see more subtle, constantly changing and developing communication cues than between a mother and her growing infant; nowhere do we find a stronger affectionate bond. Many, if not all, of the communication signals used by adult chimpanzees are fundamentally learned in this mother-child relationship, though some are elaborated later in life. Thus, it seems logical to search for the evolutionary origin of language partly in this adaptively crucial relationship. Perhaps "Mummy" or "quiet" or "coming" would be just as likely candidates for the first spoken words of a new language as the naming of a place or a thing.

CONCLUDING COMMENTS

From our knowledge of the chimpanzees today, we cannot reconstruct the kind of society in which early man lived, nor can we determine the exact nature of his family structure. But we can assume that there were enduring affectionate bonds between a mother and her offspring, and between brothers and sisters. We can be confident that early man had a long childhood during which he explored his environment in play and learned the traditional behavior patterns of his group through watching and imitating and practicing the behavior of his elders.

We can be reasonably certain that early man went through a period of biological and social adolescence during which the male in-

creasingly took his place in hunting groups and learned the hunting techniques of the grown males, while the female spent much time in female society, probably with her mother, and helped to look after her own small brothers and sisters and sometimes the infants of other females of her group.

These early ancestors must have used simple tools of grass and stick and leaves before they developed any kind of sophisticated stone- or bone-tool cultures, and they must have been capable of fairly well-organized cooperative behavior when they hunted for small animals.

When they were frightened, they probably held hands and embraced each other. After quarreling or fighting they made up with a reassuring pat or clasp of hands. When they met again after separating, they kissed and embraced and held hands. They probably groomed each other for hours during their leisure time, or, as their hairy covering receded, made groominglike movements such as stroking each other.

In short, we have indicated a variety of reasons why the behavior of early humans must have resembled that of contemporary chimpanzees in important respects. A chimpanzeelike ancestor, common to *Homo sapiens* and to contemporary chimpanzees, must have had much genetically based behavioral variability in its populations. Some of this variability was inclined toward patterns of behavior characteristic of man—such as bipedalism and constant sexual receptivity. Drastic changes in environmental conditions, acting over long periods of time, must have given selective advantage in survival to some patterns in the "behavior pool" more than to others. We have tried to suggest some ways in which these steps toward man might plausibly have been facilitated—in light of rapidly emerging new facts in research on human evolution. Despite this recent progress, many serious information gaps remain. We hope this paper will serve as a stimulus to those interested in the quest for man's origins and the fundamental nature of the human species. This is an old quest, perhaps as old as man himself with all his insatiable curiosity. But today the opportunities for understanding are far greater than ever before, and the urgency of the task is greater as well.

(Bibliography

1. ALBRECHT, H. and S. C. DUNNETT. *Chimpanzees in Western Africa.* Munich: R. Piper and Co., 1971.

2. BANDURA, A. *Aggression, A Social Learning Analysis.* Englewood Cliffs, New Jersey: Prentice-Hall, 1973.

3. BEATTY, H. "A Note on the Behavior of the Chimpanzee," *J. Mammal,* 32 (1951), 118.

4. BIGELOW, R. *The Dawn Warriors.* Boston: Atlantic-Little, Brown, 1969.

5. ———. "The Evolution of Cooperation, Aggression and Self-Control," in *Nebraska Symposium on Motivation, 1972.* Lincoln: University of Nebraska Press, 1972.

6. BIRDSELL, J. B. *Human Evolution.* Chicago: Rand McNally, 1972.

7. BOELKINS, R. C. and A. P. WILSON. "Intergroup Social Dynamics of the Cayo Santiago Rhesus (Macaca mulatta) with Special Reference to Changes in Group Membership by Males," *Primates,* 13 (1972), 125.

8. BOWMAN, R. I. "Morphological Differentiation and Adaptation in the Galapagos Finches," *Univ. Calif. Berkeley, Publ. Zoo.,* 58 (1961), 1.

9. BREWER, S. In preparation.

10. ———. Personal communication.

11. CAMPBELL, B. G. "Conceptual Progress in Physical Anthropology: Fossil Man," *Annu. Rev. of Anthropol.,* 1 (1972), 27–54.

12. CLARK, J. D. *The Prehistory of Africa.* New York: Praeger Publishers, 1970.

13. COON, C. S. *The Hunting Peoples.* Boston: Atlantic-Little, Brown, 1971.

14. DART, R. A. "Carnivorous Propensity of Baboons," *Symposium Zoological Society London,* 10 (1963), 49–57.

15. DEVORE, I. and K. R. HALL. "Baboon Ecology," in I. DeVore, ed., *Primate Behavior: Field Studies of Monkeys and Apes.* Boston: Holt, Rinehart and Winston. 1965.

16. DEVORE, I. and S. L. WASHBURN. "Baboon Ecology and Human Evolution," in F. C. Howell and F. Bourliere, eds., *African Ecology and Human Evolution,* Viking Fund Publications in Anthropology, No. 36. New York: Wenner-Gren Foundation, 1963.

17. EIBL-EIBESFELDT, I. *Ethology: The Biology of Behavior.* New York: Holt, Rinehart and Winston, 1970.

18. GARDNER, B. T. and R. A. GARDNER. "Two-Way Communication with an Infant Chimpanzee," in A. Schrier and F. Stollnitz, eds., *Behavior of Non-human Primates.* New York and London: Academic Press, 1971.

19. GESCHWIND, N. "The Organization of Language and the Brain," in S. L. Washburn and P. Dolhinow, eds., *Perspectives on Human Evolution* 2. New York: Holt, Rinehart and Winston, Inc., 1972.

20. GOMBE STREAM RESEARCH CENTER RECORDS.

21. GOODALL, J. VAN LAWICK. "The Behavior of Free-Living Chimpanzees in the Gombe Stream Area," *Anim. Behav. Monog.* I, 3 (1968), 161–311.

22. ———. "Tool-Using in Primates and Other Vertebrates," in D. S. Lehrman, R. A. Hinde, and E. Shaw, eds., *Advances in the Study of Behavior,* Vol. 3. New York: Academic Press, 1970.

23. ———. *In the Shadow of Man.* Boston: Houghton Mifflin, 1971.

24. ———. "The Behavior of Chimpanzees in Their Natural Habitat," *Am. J. Psychiatry,* 130 (1973), 1–12.

25. ———. "Cultural Elements in a Chimpanzee Colony," in E. W. Menzel, ed., *Precultural Primate Behavior.* New York: Karger, 1974.

26. HALPERIN, S. "Aggressive Behavior of Free-Ranging Chimpanzees." St. Louis: Washington University, Ph.D. Thesis. Unpublished.

27. HARDING, R. S. O. "Predation by a Troop of Olive Baboons (*Papio anubis*)." Paper delivered at 4th International Primatological Congress, Portland, August 1972. Published in *Proceedings of the Congress, Am. J. of Phys. Anthropol.,* 38 (1973), 587–592.

28. HAYES, C. *The Ape in Our House.* New York: Harper and Row, 1951.

29. HOLLOWAY, R. L. and E. SZINYEI-MERSE, "Human Biology: A Catholic Review," in B. J. Siegel, ed., *Biennial Review of An-*

thropology, 1971. Stanford: Stanford University Press, 1972.

30. HOWELL, F. C. "Hominidae," in *McGraw-Hill Yearbook of Science and Technology.* New York: McGraw-Hill, 1971.

31. ———. "Recent Advances in Human Evolutionary Studies," in S. L. Washburn and P. Dolhinow, eds., *Perspectives on Human Evolution 2.* New York: Holt, Rinehart and Winston, 1972.

32. IMANISHI, K. "The Origin of the Human Family: A Primatological Approach," in S. A. Altmann and Yerkes Regional Primate Center, eds., *Japanese Monkeys.* Alberta: University of Alberta Press, 1965.

33. IZAWA, K. and J. ITANI. *Chimpanzees in Kasakati Basin, Tanzania,* Kyoto: Kyoto University Press, 1966.

34. JONES, C. and J. SABATER. "Sticks Used by Chimpanzees in Rio Muni, West Africa," *Nature,* 223 (1969), 100–101.

35. KANO, T. "Distribution of the Primates on the Eastern Shore of Lake Tanganyika," *Primates,* 12 (1971), 281–304.

36. KAWABE, M. "One Observed Case of Hunting Behavior Among Wild Chimpanzees Living in the Savanna Woodland of Western Tanzania," *Primates,* 7 (1966), 393–396.

37. KAWAI, M. "Newly Acquired Precultural Behavior of the Natural Troop of Japanese Monkeys on Koshima Islet," *Primates,* 6 (1965), 1–30.

38. ———. "On the System of Social Ranks in a Natural Troop of Japanese Monkeys: (1) Basic Rank and Dependent Rank," in S. A. Altmann and Yerkes Regional Primate Center, eds., *Japanese Monkeys.* Alberta: University of Alberta Press, 1965.

39. KHROUSTOV, H. F. "Formation and Highest Frontier of the Implemental Activity of Anthropoids," *7th Int. Congr. Anthropol.,* Moscow, 1964.

40. KÖHLER, W. *The Mentality of Apes.* New York: Harcourt, Brace, 1925.

41. KUMMER, H. *Social Organization of Hamadryas Baboons.* Chicago: University of Chicago Press, 1968.

42. LEE, R. B. and I. DeVORE. *Man the Hunter.* Chicago: Aldine, 1968.

43. MASLAND, R. L. "Some Neurological Processes Underlying Language," in S. L. Washburn and P. Dolhinow, eds., *Perspectives in Human Evolution 2.* New York: Holt, Rinehart and Winston, 1972.

44. McGINNIS, P. R. *Patterns of Sexual Behavior in a Community of Free-Living Chimpanzees.* Ph.D. dissertation. University of Cambridge, 1973.

45. McGREW, W. C. and C. E. G. TUTIN. "Chimpanzee Dentistry," *J. Am. Dent. Assoc.,* 85 (1972), 1198–1204.

46. MENZEL, E. W. "Spontaneous Invention of Ladders in a Group of Young Chimpanzees," *Folia Primatol.,* 17 (1972), 87–106.

47. MERFIELD, F. G. and H. MILLER. *Gorillas Were My Neighbors.* London: Longmans, 1956.

48. NAPIER, J. *The Roots of Mankind.* Washington: Smithsonian Institution Press, 1970.

49. NISHIDA, T. "The Social Group of Wild Chimpanzees in the Mahali Mountains," *Primates,* 9 (1968), 167–224.

50. NISHIDA, T. and K. KAWANAKA. "Inter-group Relationships Among Wild Chimpanzees of the Mahali Mountains," *Kyoto Univ. Afr. Stud.,* 7 (1972), 131–169.

51. PREMACK, D. "Language in Chimpanzees?" *Science,* 172 (1971), 808–822.

52. PUSEY, A. Personal communication.

53. RALEIGH, M. J. and S. L. WASHBURN. "Human Behavior and the Origin of Man," *Impact of Science on Society,* 33 (1973), 5–14.

54. RANSOM, T. W. "Ecology and Social Behavior of Baboons in the Gombe National Park." Ph.D. thesis. University of California, Berkeley, 1972. Unpublished.

55. ROBINSON, B. W. "Anatomical and Physiological Contrasts Between Human and Other Primate Vocalizations," in S. L. Washburn and P. Dolhinow, eds., *Perspectives in Human Evolution 2.* New York: Holt, Rinehart and Winston, 1972.

56. SADE, D. S. "Inhibition of Son-Mother Mating Among Free-Ranging Rhesus Monkeys," *Science Psychoanalysis,* 7 (1968), 18–38.

57. ———. "A Longitudinal Study of Social Behavior of Rhesus Monkeys," in R. Tuttle, ed., *The Functional and Evolutionary Biology of Primates.* Chicago: Aldine, Atherton, 1972.

58. ———. "Some Aspects of Parent-Offspring and Sibling Relations in a Group of Rhesus Monkeys, With a Discussion of Grooming," *Am. J. Phys. Anthropol.,* 23 (1965), 1–18.

59. SAVAGE, T. S. and J. WYMAN. *Boston J. Nat. Hist.,* 4 (1843–44), 383.

60. SCHALLER, G. *The Mountain Gorilla: Ecol-*

ogy and Behavior. Chicago: University of Chicago Press, 1963.

61. SCHULTZ, A. "Some Factors Influencing the Social Life of Primates in General and Early Man in Particular," in S. L. Washburn, ed., *Social Life of Early Man.* Chicago: Aldine, 1963.

62. SPERRY, R. W. "Mental Unity Following Surgical Disconnections of the Cerebral Hemisphere," in S. L. Washburn and P. Dolhinow, eds., *Perspectives in Human Evolution 2.* New York: Holt, Rinehart and Winston, 1972.

63. SUGIYAMA, Y. "Social Behavior of Chimpanzees in the Budongo Forest, Uganda," *Primates,* 10 (1969), 197–225.

64. SUZUKI, A. "Carnivority and Cannibalism Observed Among Forest-Living Chimpanzees," *J. Anthropol. Soc. Nippon.,* 79 (1971), 30–48.

65. ———. "On the Insect-Eating Habits Among Wild Chimpanzees Living in the Savanna Forest of Western Tanzania," *Primates,* 7 (1966), 481–487.

66. TELEKI, G. "The Omnivorous Chimpanzee," *Sci. Am.,* 228 (1973), 1.

67. TOBIAS, P. V. "*Australopithecus, Homo habilis,* Tool-Using and Tool-Making," *S. Afr. Archaeol. Bull.,* 20 (80), IV (1965), 167–192.

68. VAN LAWICK-GOODALL, J. *see* Goodall, J. van Lawick.

69. VAN LAWICK, H. and VAN LAWICK-GOODALL, J. *Innocent Killers.* Boston: Houghton Mifflin, 1970.

70. WASHBURN, S. L. "Human Evolution," in T. Dobzhansky, M. K. Hecht, and W. C. Steere, eds., *Evolutionary Biology,* vol. 6. New York: Appleton-Century-Crofts, 1972.

71. WASHBURN, S. L. and I. DEVORE. "Social Behavior of Baboons and Early Man," in S. L. Washburn, ed., *Social Life of Early Man.* Chicago: Aldine. 1963.

72. WASHBURN, S. L. and R. S. O. HARDING. "Evolution and Human Nature," in D. A. Hamburg and H. K. H. Brodie, eds., *American Handbook of Psychiatry,* Vol. 6, 2nd ed., New York: Basic Books, 1975.

73. WASHBURN, S. L. and C. S. LANCASTER. "The Evolution of Hunting," in S. L. Washburn, and P. C. Jay, eds., *Perspectives on Human Evolution 1.* New York: Holt, Rinehart and Winston, 1968.

74. WASHBURN, S. L. and E. R. McCOWN. "Evolution of Human Behavior," *Social Biology,* 19 (1972), 163–170.

75. WASHBURN. S. L. and S. C. STRUM. "Concluding Comments," in S. L. Washburn and P. Dolhinow, eds., *Perspectives in Human Evolution 2.* New York: Holt, Rinehart and Winston, 1972.

76. WEINER, J. S. *The Natural History of Man.* New York: Universe Books, 1971.

77. WRANGHAM, R. In preparation.

78. ———. In press.

79. ———. Personal communication.

80. WRIGHT, R. V. "Imitative Learning of a Flaked Stone Tendency—The Case of an Orang Utan," *Mankind,* 8 (1972), 296–306.

81. YERKES, R. M. *Chimpanzees. A Laboratory Colony.* New Haven: Yale University Press, 1943.

82. YERKES, R. M. and J. H. ELDER. "Oestrus, Receptivity and Mating in the Chimpanzee," *Comp. Psychol. Monogr.,* 13 (1936), 5–45.

83. YERKES, R. M. and A. W. YERKES. The *Great Apes.* New Haven: Yale University Press, 1929.

CHAPTER 3

PERSPECTIVES IN THE NEUROPHYSIOLOGICAL STUDY OF BEHAVIOR AND ITS ABNORMALITIES

Eric R. Kandel

T HE RECENT HISTORY of psychology has been characterized by alternate movements toward and away from biological explanations of behavior. The first rapprochement between psychology and biology dates with the work of Charles Darwin,[8,9,10] in the middle of the nineteenth century. Darwin's discovery of a behavioral continuum between animals suggested to him that the behavior of man might profitably be studied by examining its analogues in lower forms. This notion stimulated the comparative study of behavior and led to the development of animal models that could be used in relating the nervous system to behavior. This new perspective brought about the divorce of psychology from metaphysics and theology, and the acceptance

among psychologists of the idea, already established in neurology and psychiatry (see for example Meynert[55]), that even the most complex behavioral processes have their bases in the nervous system. This acceptance was exemplified in American psychology by the publication of William James' *Principles of Psychology* in 1890.[38] James' *Principles* generated a marvelous optimism about the capability of neurological science to relate brain mechanisms to behavior. But this optimism proved premature. During the first few decades of the twentieth century, studies of brain function failed to advance beyond a general localization of sensory and motor functions in various regions of the brain. The detailed mechanisms of behavior proved intractable to neural analysis. As a result, psychology and the neurological sciences drifted apart. Even psychologists with strong neurological interests often abandoned biological perspectives for a psychology that was free of commitment to ill-defined notions of brain mechanisms. This separation was, and continues to be, healthy for psychology. It has permitted the development of coherent systems of behavioral description that are not contingent on vague parallels with neural mechanisms. Freed from artificial neurological constraints, psychology has been able to develop a rigorous behavioral tradition and to establish bridges with social psychology and sociology. A very special interest and excitement, however, continues to reside in the analysis of the biological mechanisms of behavior. This area has recently undergone remarkable developments that have infused new hope for relating neural mechanisms to behavior.

Major progress in understanding the neurophysiological basis of behavior has resulted from the development of techniques for studying individual nerve cells and from the selection of appropriate experimental systems for studying a variety of behavior. Specifically, advances have been made in three related and progressively more complex areas. (1) The functioning of the nerve cell and the process of synaptic transmission—the mechanism by which one neuron communicates with another —are beginning to be understood. (2) The study of the interconnections among populations of nerve cells has begun to yield significant findings. Particularly good progress has been made in the sensory and motor systems where a beginning has been made in analyzing the cellular mechanisms of perception and motor coordination. (3) The application of cellular techniques to certain simple invertebrate animals, whose nervous systems are composed of relatively small numbers of cells, is making it possible to examine the total neural substratum of simple behavior. In these animals one can study not only the sensory information coming into the nervous system and the motor action coming out of it, but also the complete sequence of events that underlies a behavioral response.

These three developments provide a coherent framework of concepts and techniques that promises to clarify some basic relationships between brain functioning and behavior. While these concepts do not explain the complex behavior of man, they are beginning to prove useful in understanding certain elementary aspects of perception, motor coordination, and learning in animals.

In this chapter, I will try to summarize some of the main findings that have emerged from these three levels of investigation and to indicate the directions in which current research is going. I will particularly emphasize cellular studies both of sensory deprivation in newborn animals and of learning, two areas that are likely to provide useful and clinically interesting model systems of behavioral abnormalities. In being so selective, I hope to cover in detail some areas that are of potential interest to students of psychiatry. Unfortunately, this means that I must here exclude from consideration other currently active areas of neurobiology.

(The Cellular Biology of Neurons and Synapses

The properties of nerve cells that endow them with signaling capabilities stem from their ability to maintain a resting potential (membrane potential) that can be modulated by spike activity within the cell or by the synaptic activity of other cells. Until 1950, there were no satisfactory techniques for direct recording of the membrane potential maintained across the neuronal membrane or for the examination of the changes produced in it by synaptic activity and by spike generation. Technical advances made during World War II led to the development of the electronic instrumentation that could register and amplify small electrical signals recorded with minute high-resistance probes. This instrumentation led in turn to the development of the ultrafine glass microelectrode by Ralph Gerard and his colleagues.[53] These could be filled with a concentrated potassium chloride solution and used to record directly the activity from central nerve cells and muscle fibers.

In the decade that followed World War II, microelectrode techniques were applied extensively to the study of nerve cells and to synaptic transmission, and they led to the development of a general model of neuronal functioning that has provided the basis for much subsequent research (see[13,14,22]). According to this model, all neurons, regardless of shape, size, location, and function, can be considered to have four functional components: (1) an input (receptor) component; (2) an integrative (spike-initiating) component; (3) a conductile (long-range signaling) component, and (4) an output (transmitter–releasing) component. The input component consists of the external subsynaptic membrane that contains the receptors and the ionic channels for generating two types of graded synaptic potentials, depolarizing excitatory postsynaptic potentials (EPSPs) and a hyperpolarizing inhibitory postsynaptic potential (IPSPs). Excitatory synaptic potentials reduce (depolarize) the membrane potential and, if sufficiently large, will bring the membrane potential of the integrative component to the threshold for spike generation. Inhibitory synaptic potentials tend to increase (hyperpolarize) the membrane potential and to keep the integrative component from reaching the threshold for spike generation. Thus, the integrative action of a neuron resides in adding the sum total of excitation and inhibition and deciding whether or not to discharge an action potential. This decision is made at a specific site within the neuron, the integrative component usually being located at the initial segment of the neuron. The threshold of the integrative component is exceeded and an action potential is initiated if the net depolarization produced by the excitatory synapses exceeds the net inhibition produced by the inhibitory synapses by a certain critical minimum. Once initiated, the action potential propagates without decrement along the axon, the conductile or long-range signaling component of the neuron. At the terminal region of the axon, which abuts onto a specialized receptor site of the next cell, the action potential

in the output component of the neuron leads to the release of the chemical transmitter substance. The transmitter substance diffuses across the small space (synaptic cleft) that separates the presynaptic and postsynaptic elements of the synapse, and it interacts with the receptor molecules in the external membrane of the postsynaptic cell. Depending on the nature of the transmitter and that of the receptor, the interaction leads to current flow in the postsynaptic cell, which alters its resting potential by producing either an inhibitory or an excitatory postsynaptic potential.

A large number of recent studies of central nerve cells in both invertebrates and vertebrates have shown that this model is quite general. The conclusion is that, although neurons differ in detail, most of them are surprisingly similar in their general electrophysiological properties (see [13,14,22,71]).

These major insights derive largely from the work of Hodgkin, Huxley and Katz,[28,29] (for review see[27]) who developed the ionic hypothesis to explain how the electrical potential difference across the neuronal membrane (the resting potential) is generated, and how its sign is first quickly reduced and then reversed during the generation of the action potential. At rest, nerve cells maintain a potential difference across their surface membranes of about -60 mV, with the inside negative in relation to the outside. Working on the giant axon of the squid, Hodgkin, Huxley and Katz[28] demonstrated that this potential difference results from an unequal distribution of sodium, potassium, chloride, and organic anions across the semipermeable membrane of the nerve cell. This unequal distribution of ions leaves the inside of the nerve–cell membrane negatively charged in relation to the outside. The long-term distribution of ions is maintained by an active metabolic process, the "sodium-potassium pump," which keeps sodium concentration within the cell low and potassium concentration within the cell high by actively transporting sodium out of the cell and potassium into it. As a result of the constant activity of the sodium-potassium exchange mechanism, the potassium concentration inside nerve cells is about fifty times higher than that of the extracellular space and the sodium concentration is approximately ten times lower inside the cell than out. The resting–membrane potential results from the membrane's having a high leakiness (permeability) to potassium ions in its resting state and a relatively low permeability to sodium ions. Potassium is a positively charged ion. Because it is in high concentration inside the cell, it tends to be driven out under the influence of the concentration gradient, thereby making the cell membrane slightly more negative on the inside than the outside. The buildup of the negative charge on the inside of the cell tends to impede the further movement of the positively charged potassium ions. At a certain potential, the force due to the electrical charge on the membrane becomes equal to the oppositely directed force due to the concentration gradient and no further net movement of potassium ions occurs. This potential is called the potassium–equilibrium potential and is usually about −70 mV. The value of the resting potential is close to the potassium–equilibrium potential. Small deviations of the resting potential from the potassium–equilibrium potential are usually due to the slight leakiness of the membrane to sodium and other ions.

Most cells can generate a resting potential across their membranes. What differentiates excitable cells, such as nerve and muscle, from other cells is that the resting–membrane potential can be altered so as to serve as a signaling mechanism. When the membrane potential of a nerve cell is reduced by a certain critical amount, usually about 15 mV (from −60 mV to −45 mV) an all-or-none action potential is initiated. During the action potential there is a sudden reversal in the permeability characteristics of the nerve–cell membrane so that it suddenly becomes highly permeable to sodium. The resulting potential change is regenerative. Depolarization increases sodium permeability, which produces further depolarization, which increases sodium permeability even more. This explosive event abolishes and reverses the resting potential, ultimately driving the membrane potential to the sodium–equilibrium potential (about +60 mV). The sudden reversal of the membrane

potential is, however, transient and self-limiting. The progressive depolarization of the action potential leads to a shutting off (inactivation) of the enhanced sodium permeability. Concomitantly there is also a further increase in the already high permeability to potassium ions. These processes combine to bring the membrane potential back to the resting level.

The action potential, generated in the integrative component of the neuron, gives rise to the current flow necessary to depolarize and trigger an action potential in the next axon region, which in turn depolarizes the axon region ahead of it. In this way the action potential, once initiated, is assured faithful, undisturbed, all-or-none propagation without decrement along the whole length of the axon, the conductile element of the neuron. These several findings and their theoretical interpretation explain most of the major manifestations of electrical excitability of nerve and muscle. In all cases examined so far, the resting and action potentials have been found to be produced by a common mechanism, ions moving down their concentration gradient as a result of the selective permeability to one or more ion species.*

The pharmacologists Otto Loewi and Sir Henry Dales had previously shown that transmission at several peripheral synapses is chemical and involves the release of a transmitter substance such as acetylcholine or norepinephrine. In a major advance, Fatt and Katz[15,16] utilized the peripheral neuromuscular junctions of frog and crab as model systems and applied the ionic hypothesis to synaptic transmission. They found that the transmitter substance, released by the presynaptic terminals of a neuron, produces its action on the membrane potential of the postsynaptic cell by reacting with specific receptor molecules located on its external surface. This reaction leads to an increase in the permeability of the postsynaptic cell to certain ion species. By examining both excitatory and inhibi-

---

* In a few instances a small fraction of the total resting potential is maintained by an additional mechanism, the active, metabolically dependent extrusion of Na^+ from the cell by an electrogenic Na-K+ pump (see Thomas[76]).

tory junctions between nerve and muscle, Fatt and Katz found that the difference between synaptic inhibition and synaptic excitation depended upon which ionic permeabilities were increased. If the transmitter increased the permeability to sodium, the resulting action was invariably excitatory, even if other ionic permeabilities (e.g., potassium) were also increased. If the transmitter increased the permeability to potassium or chloride without altering sodium permeability, the resulting action was inhibitory. These differences in synaptic actions followed from the relationship of the threshold of the nerve cell (usually -45 mV) to the equilibrium potential of the ion whose permeability was increased. Any increase in the permeability to sodium would tend to depolarize the membrane beyond the threshold (-45 mV) in the direction of the sodium–equilibrium potential ($+60$ mV). By contrast, any increase in permeability to potassium or chloride would push the membrane potential away from the threshold voltage for spike generation toward the equilibrium potential for potassium (-70 mV) or chloride (-60 mV). Fatt and Katz thus showed that the difference between synaptic excitation and synaptic inhibition was in the relationship of the equilibrium potential of the specific ions involved to the threshold potential of the cell.

Subsequent work by Katz[45] and his colleagues del Castillo[11] and Miledi[46,47] and parallel morphological studies by de Robertis and Bennett[65] and by Palade and Paley[57,58] gave rise to the current morphological and functional view of how synaptic transmission at chemical synapses occurs (see[43,44]). Synaptic transmission takes place only at certain morphologically specialized points in the nervous system, where the presynaptic neuron and the postsynaptic cell come into appropriate apposition. Here, the generation of an action potential in the presynaptic terminal leads to the release of a chemical transmitter substance. This transmitter substance is stored in packets or vesicles, each of which is thought to contain several thousand transmitter molecules. As the action potential invades the terminals, it gives rise not only to the usual influx of sodium ions

but also to an influx of calcium ions from the extracellular space. The influx of calcium into the terminal region somehow increases the likelihood of transmitter packets combining with the cellular membrane. The fusion of the vesicle membrane with the inside surface of cell membrane is thought to be an essential step for an extrusion process known as exocytosis. Following membrane fusion the membranes open briefly to the extracellular space and the vesicles rapidly empty their contents into it. After the vesicle has extruded its contents, transmitter molecules diffuse across the synaptic cleft that separates the two cells, usually two hundred to three hundred Å wide. The transmitter then interacts with specific receptors in the postsynaptic cell to produce specific permeability changes that can be either inhibitory or excitatory.

In 1951, John C. Eccles took the bold step of applying the concepts that Hodgkin, Huxley, and Katz had developed in their study of resting and action potentials of the squid giant axon, and those that Fatt and Katz had developed from study of several neuromuscular junctions. He combined these separate conceptual schemes into a synthetic view of how central nerve cells function. This advance also required a well selected model system, and Eccles chose as his experimental object the large motor nerve cells (motor neurons) of the spinal cord. He found that the resting and action potentials of central nerve cells obeyed the predictions of the ionic hypothesis and that the function of central synapses could be explained by the Fatt and Katz model for peripheral synaptic transmission. In each case the electrical changes involved an increase in permeability to one or more ion species that then moved down their concentration gradients.

In 1953, Eccles summarized the ionic hypothesis and its applicability to central nerve cells in a book entitled *The Neurophysiological Basis of Mind*.[12] This remarkable book pointed the study of mammalian neural science in a new direction. Its major message was twofold. First, Eccles emphasized that to understand the brain requires that it be studied in terms of individual nerve cells. There are no short cuts to studying this complex computing system. Only by applying analytic techniques that can resolve neuronal processes on a unitary cellular level can one develop a useful, realistic, and synthetic understanding of how groups of cells and, ultimately, areas of the brain work. Second, Eccles emphasized, implicitly, something that is still not sufficiently appreciated, that studying the biophysical properties of nerve cells is necessary but insufficient for understanding how the brain works. To know how people perceive and think, feel and act, and how they relate to one another as human beings, it is essential to relate cellular function to behavior.

Within a few years of Eccles' pioneering work, cellular techniques were applied to a variety of brain structures, including the neocortex, hippocampus, thalamus, and the basal ganglia. This work moved surprisingly rapidly, in part because the model of neuron function derived from the study of spinal neurons proved to be general (see references [14] and [41]). As a result, it was possible to move slightly beyond studies of cellular properties and to describe a number of the key features of brain circuitry (see [14]). Relating cellular function to behavior has proven more difficult and has occupied much of the attention of researchers for the last two decades. One step in this behavioral direction was accomplished between 1955 and 1965, and was characterized by brilliant growth in our understanding of sensory physiology and its relation to perception. Another step has come in the period since 1965 and derives from the development of invertebrate preparations in which elementary behaviors and their modifications can be examined.

(The Neuronal Mechanisms of Sensation and Perception

Feature Abstraction and Binocular Interactions in the Visual System

In the decade 1955 to 1965, single cell techniques were applied with remarkable success to an examination of various stages in the vis-

ual and the somatosensory system. From this work it became clear that our brain "sees" the world around us not as a precise replication of reality but as an abstraction accomplished by neural transformations that occur at almost every stage in the hierarchy of relays in the sensory system, from the peripheral receptors onward. These insights stem primarily from the work on the somatosensory system by Vernon Mountcastle and his colleagues at Johns Hopkins, and from the work on the visual system by Stephen Kuffler, David Hubel, and Torsten Wiesel at Harvard. (For reviews see Hubel[30] and Mountcastle[56].) I will consider here only the visual system.

As early as 1942, Wade H. Marshall and Samuel Talbott[54] had used gross electrical recording techniques to show that the receptor sheet of the retina is represented in the visual cortex in an orderly, topographical manner and that by this means the brain achieves an anatomical representation of the external world. In 1953, Stephen Kuffler[49] applied single cell recording techniques to the visual system and carried this analysis one step further. Kuffler examined the output of the retina, the retinal ganglion cells (whose axons form the optic nerve) to see what kind of transformation of neural information occurs within the retina itself. The retina of mammals consists of receptors, the rods, and the cones. It ends on bipolar cells that in turn synapse on retinal ganglion cells. After forming the optic nerve, the medial (nasal) fibers from the retina cross in the optic chiasma to join the contralateral–optic tract and synapse in the contralateral geniculate. The fibers from the lateral (temporal) portion of the retina continue in the ipsilateral–optic tract and synapse in the ipsilateral lateral geniculate body. Neurons from the lateral geniculate body send axons to the striate visual cortex, area seventeen. Cells in this area project to the peristriate cortical regions, areas eighteen and nineteen. Cells from these two areas in turn project to the inferotemporal association cortex. The cells in the visual system are spontaneously active and fire occasional action potentials in the absence of visual stimulation. Kuffler found that the spontaneous activity of the retinal ganglion cells could be modulated by small spots of light projected onto the surface of the retina. He described the response characteristics of ganglion cells in terms of the *receptive field* properties of single cells. The receptive field of a cell (in the visual system) refers to the area of the retina that, upon stimulation with light, alters the firing pattern of a single cell. In anatomical terms, the receptive field of a retinal ganglion cell thus describes all the receptor and subsequent cells in the retina that converge upon and influence the firing pattern of a single ganglion cell. Kuffler discovered that the receptive fields of the retinal ganglion cells were round in shape and had distinct concentric excitatory and inhibitory zones. In the region of the macula, where most of these studies were done, the size of the receptive fields was small, ranging from 4 to 8° of arc in diameter. On the basis of the architecture of their receptive field properties, Kuffler divided all cells into two groups. One class of cells had a central excitatory zone and a surrounding inhibitory region ("on" center cells) whereas the other class of cells had an inhibitory ("off") central region and an excitatory surround region (off center cells). For example, cells with an on center receptive field responded very briskly to small spots of light aimed at the center of the receptive field but were inhibited if light impinged on the annular surround region. The most effective excitatory stimulus for a cell with an on center receptive field was therefore a circular spot covering the entire central region of the field. As the stimulus was enlarged to include some of the annular surround region, the effectiveness of the stimulus was reduced because of the mutual antagonism between the center and the surround region. The most effective inhibitory stimulus was a doughnut of light on the surround region. By contrast, cells with an off center receptive field were inhibited by light on the central region and excited by light on the surround region. Kuffler thus found that as early in the visual pathway as the retinal ganglion cells a significant amount of abstraction of sensory input had already occurred. The retinal ganglion cells did not

respond primarily to light intensity but to the contrast between light and dark.

This analysis was carried further by David Hubel and Torsten Wiesel,[32,34] who analyzed cells in the lateral geniculate and in the visual (striate) cortex (area seventeen). In the lateral geniculate cells, receptive field properties were very similar to the retinal ganglion cells. However, in the cortex Hubel and Wiesel found that the response properties of the cells were very much more complicated. Cortical cells could no longer be effectively stimulated by the circular–shaped stimuli that proved so effective in the retina and in the lateral geniculate. To be effective a stimulus had to have linear properties; the best stimuli were lines, bars, rectangles, or squares. On the basis of receptive field properties, Hubel and Wiesel grouped cortical cells into two classes: simple and complex. Cortical cells with simple receptive fields had discrete rectangular excitatory and inhibitory zones. A typical receptive field might have a central rectangular excitatory area with its long axis running from twelve to six o'clock, flanked on each side by similar shaped inhibitory areas. For this type of cortical cell, the most effective excitatory stimulus is a bar of light with a specific axis of orientation—in this case from twelve o'clock to six o'clock—projected on the central excitatory area of the receptive field. Since this rectangular zone is framed by two rectangular inhibitory areas the most effective stimulus for inhibition is one that stimulated one or both of the two flanking inhibitory zones. A horizontal or oblique bar of light would stimulate both excitatory and inhibitory areas and would therefore be relatively ineffective. Thus a stimulus that is highly effective if projected vertically onto a given area of retina so as to be on target for the excitatory zone would become ineffective if held horizontally or obliquely. Other cells had similar receptive field shapes but different axes of orientation (vertical or oblique). For a cell with an oblique field the most effective stimulus would be a bar of light running from ten o'clock to four o'clock or from two o'clock to eight o'clock.

The most interesting feature of the simple

cortical cells is that they are much more particular in their stimulus requirement than the retinal ganglion or the geniculate cells. For a stimulus to be effective for a retinal ganglion or a geniculate cell, it only has to have the proper shape, in general circular, and the proper retinal position so as to activate appropriate receptors in the retina. But in the cortex, in addition to shape (now generally rectangular) and retinal position, the effective stimulus has also to have a proper axis of orientation. Slight changes in the axis of orientation of the light-bar stimulus would make an effective stimulus ineffective. Thus the simple cortical cells not only have to represent all retinal positions and several shapes (lines, bars, rectangles) but also for each shape they have to represent all axes of orientation. These findings provide some insight as to why the visual cortex (or any cortex) needs so many cells for its normal functions. Cells are required to represent every retinal area in all axes of orientation so as to abstract the information presented to the cortex.

Another feature distinguishes striate cortical cells from geniculate cells. Geniculate cells only respond to stimulation of one or the other eye. In area seventeen of the cortex one begins to find cells responding to both eyes. These cells provide the neural basis for binocular fusion, essential for the stereoscopic vision of higher animals.

Hubel and Wiesel suggested that the simplest explanation for the response properties of a cortical cell with a simple receptive field was that they received innervation from a set of geniculate cells that had appropriate on center and off center properties and appropriate retinal positions.

Hubel and Wiesel also found a group of cells in the striate cortex with complex receptive field properties. For these cells the effective stimuli were also linear and had to have a correct axis of orientation, but the receptive fields of these cells did not have clearly delineated excitatory and inhibitory zones so that the exact position of the stimulus within the receptor field was not important. For example, a cell might have a fairly large rectangular receptive field (10° by 15° of arc) and respond to a vertical bar oriented at twelve o'clock to six o'clock and placed anywhere in its field. But this cell would not respond if the bar were tilted obliquely or horizontally. Hubel and Wiesel suggested that the simplest explanation for the generation of a complex receptive field was that these cells received excitatory projections from a set of simple cortical cells with similar receptive field positions and identical axes of orientation. In support of this idea is the finding that the visual cortex was organized into a series of narrow vertical columns, two cells to fifty cells wide, running from the surface of the cortex to the white matter. In a given column, cells had roughly similar receptive field positions and generally similar receptive field properties. Any one column contained both simple and complex cells and the properties of the simple cells in that column were such that they could account for the properties of the complex cells in the same column if one supposed that the simple cells of a column converged upon the complex ones. This finding not only provides some indirect support for the Hubel and Wiesel hierarchical scheme but also provides insight into the function of cortical columns. The columns seem to serve as elementary units of cortical organization designed both to bring cells together so that they can be appropriately interconnected and to generate from their interconnections the properties needed for cells with higher-order receptive fields.

Cells of area seventeen project to the peristriate cortex (areas eighteen and nineteen) and in these areas the visual message undergoes still further processing.[35] Cells in areas eighteen and nineteen have more sophisticated properties than those of area seventeen. Hubel and Wiesel refer to these properties as hypercomplex. Cells with hypercomplex properties have even more specific stimulus requirements and some respond only to a highly selective geometrical form such as a corner: two lines that meet at 90° to each other. As the angle between the two lines is changed from 90 to 180°, the stimulus becomes progressively less effective. As is area seventeen, areas eighteen and nineteen are organized into vertical columns that run from the surface of the cortex to the white matter. A given column contains cells with both complex and hypercomplex properties and, again, the properties of the complex cells are just what are needed to account for the hypercomplex ones, if one assumes that the hypercomplex cells receive their input from the complex cells in their own column. For example, in some columns the hypercomplex cells respond to a right angle whose base runs from three to nine o'clock. These columns contained complex cells that have two (but only two) types of axes of orientation. Some cells had an axis of orientation running from twelve to six o'clock whereas others had one running from three to nine o'clock.

From these studies Hubel and Wiesel have suggested a model for understanding how the cortex abstracts essential features from sensory stimuli. According to this scheme, the configuration of the effective stimulus that is necessary to excite (or inhibit) cells at various levels in the visual system varies. In the retina and in subsequent stages of the visual system, cells do not respond effectively to diffuse light but respond primarily to borders between light and darkness. Later in the system similar contrast detection is used in the analysis of lines. The hypercomplex cells respond primarily not to the linear properties of the stimulus but to changes in the direction of a line such as angles and corners. Thus hypercomplex cells may be serving as angle and corner (curvature) detectors indicating changes in the direction of a line. In higher cortical areas the linear aspects of a stimulus may be analyzed by measuring changes in its contour much as the light intensity for stimulus is analyzed at lower levels by measuring contrast between light and dark.

The studies of Hubel and Wiesel also suggest a function for the regional subdivisions of the visual system: the retina, the lateral geniculate, striate cortex (area seventeen), and the peristriate cortex (areas eighteen and nineteen). Each of these areas accomplishes one or more specific transformations of neural activity, and in each the transformations seem to occur within specific columnar systems that abstract some new features of the stimulus. In area seventeen the quality that is abstracted is receptive field orientation whereas in areas eighteen and nineteen it is angle and contour detection. Hubel and Wiesel propose that complex and hypercomplex receptive fields are the early building blocks of perception.

What occurs at a more advanced relay stop, the inferotemporal cortex? The inferotemporal cortex receives afferent input from the peristriate areas eighteen and nineteen as well as from the pulvinar region of the thalamus. Both of these structures are known to respond to visual stimuli. The available behavioral data (see Gross[19]) indicate that lesions of the inferotemporal cortex produce a severe impairment in the learning of visual discrimination, but do not affect visual acuity. At Princeton Charles Gross[19,20] has recently started to study the properties of neurons in the inferotemporal cortex of the monkey and found that they respond only to visual and not to other sensory stimulation. The receptive fields of units in the inferotemporal cortex were unusually large. Many were over $30°$ by $30°$ of arc in size. However, finding the effective stimulus for altering the spontaneous firing rate of these cells was very difficult, much more difficult than in the striate or peristriate cortex. Many cells showed a waning of response with repeated stimulation and it was often necessary to use stimuli separated by several seconds or more to get full recovery. Some of the cells encountered had the characteristics of the complex and hypercomplex units of the striate and peristriate cortex, but others had more unusual properties. By merely confining the stimulus to bars, edges, rectangles, and circles, Gross often was unable to describe the best stimulus for each unit. There were several cells that responded strongly to more complicated figures. Most striking were some units that responded weakly to dark rectangles but much better to a cutout of a monkey's hand: the more the stimulus resembled the hand, the more strongly the cell responded to it.

To summarize, the principle that emerges from the work of Kuffler, of Hubel and Wiesel, and of Gross is one of a series of hierarchical levels or stages in which cells, at each level, are converged upon by cells from the next lower levels. At each level cells abstract progressively more information, about the visual dimension of the world and its meaning to the animal, than at the preceding level. From this work we can begin to get an idea of the perceptual meaning of neural activity in the visual system. A retinal ganglion surveys the activity of bipolar cells that survey a group of receptors. A train of action potentials in a retinal ganglion cell signals that a spot of light is shining upon a particular part of the retina. The geniculate cell surveys a group of retinal ganglion cells and activity in the geniculate cell signals much the same. A simple cortical cell surveys a population of geniculate cells and the firing of a single cell signals that a bar of light is shining in the retina. These cells no longer signal just position but also a new abstraction, the orientation of the stimulus with respect to vertical or horizontal axis. The complex cell surveys simple cells and their activity means a stimulus with an axis of orientation without specific commitment to positions within the receptive field. The hypercomplex cells survey the complex ones and the activity of hypercomplex cells means a change in the axis of orientation, an angle or corner. Out of these kinds of transformations the brain can abstract more complex geometrical shapes and in the inferotemporal cortex (where cells receive input from both hypercomplex cells and thalamic cells) the brain seems to begin to endow these shapes with further meaning. The most striking aspect of this hierarchical processing is feature detection. Successive hierarchies or neural transformation help to analyze two-dimensional retinal space so as to represent simple aspects of light contrast and shape.

But an unresolved question that is now receiving increasing attention is, how far can this hierarchy go? Is there a special supercomplex cell or cell group on top of the hierarchical processing for each familiar face? Is there a group of cells that observes the hyper complex cells and makes one aware of the total pattern? And if so, is there a still higher group in the hierarchy that looks at combinations of complex patterns as these enter our awareness? There may indeed be other high-ordered cells combining the computational results of the inferotemporal—peristriate—striate cortices to produce even more elaborate abstractions. However, to discern the relatively simple features we have so far considered has already required an enormous amount of visual brain. It would appear curious to attribute progressively more important processing to a relatively smaller group of cells and ask them to do this incredibly complex abstraction. An alternative would be that at higher levels the mechanism of transformation changes, so that single units no longer serve to represent feature states (see Harmon [24]). To represent a familiar face or a landscape may require simultaneous combined states of a very large number of cells in the inferotemporal—peristriate—striate cortices. At this higher level of representation many cells are likely to be involved and their simultaneous signals may serve as the feature detector. The states of the parts taken separately may not represent the whole; rather it is the relation among them that is important. Harmon makes an analogy with the individual silver halide grains of a photograph: these do not represent the photograph of a face, but the ensemble of grains does. Thus a major question for future research in this area revolves around the "read out" of the abstracting process of the visual system. How do we ultimately perceive form? Is this information read out by a progressively smaller group of cells that sit progressively "higher" in a hierarchical system so that in the end one recognizes a face by the firing of a particular small set of feature detector cells that perceives as unique that particular face? Or does the hierarchical nature of the processing disappear and abstraction result from different combinations of neural populations firing in a certain temporal relation to each other? Recent work by Vernon Mountcastle and by W. A. Spencer indicates that in the somatosensory system the second process seems to be important for perception of tactile sensation. Mountcastle's work[56] has indicated the need to reconstruct the population activity of neurons to understand normal tactile sensation. Iwamura, Gardner and Spencer[36] show how perceptual distortion, created by certain tactile illusions, can best be explained by changes in the contours and spatial gradients of the population of neurons activated by the tactile stimuli. My own guess is that work in the visual system will also tend to move in this direction now.

In the next two sections, I will restrict myself primarily to the early stages of visual transformation where detailed knowledge is available, and illustrate how this understanding about the lower stages of visual function can provide insights into how abnormal environmental experiences can disturb the functioning of connections. But first let us briefly consider the formation of connections during embryonic development.

The Development of Connections in the Visual System

Much of our understanding of the development of connections in the visual system derives from the experiments of Roger Sperry[74,75] on the visual system of lower vertebrates: frogs, salamanders, and goldfish. These animals are useful objects for embryological investigation because, unlike higher vertebrates, cold-blooded vertebrates have remarkable regenerative capacities, not only in their larval states but also as adults. Thus, for example, Sperry found that he could cut an optic nerve in the frog, thereby separating the eye from the brain, place the eye back in the socket and still have regeneration of the optic nerve occur. These regenerated animals have complete restoration of visual function. Despite the formation of a scar, the newly regenerating fibers seem to find their way back to appropriate cells in the brain and to establish the connection necessary for normal vision. Sperry studied this regenerative process further and found that outgoing fibers from the retina had multiple opportunities to make contact with a variety of nerve cells at various points as well as with the glial cells and capillaries that they encountered along their path. Despite these many opportunities for synapse formation the outgoing fibers connected only

with the cells to which they were initially connected. Incorrect zones were consistently by-passed and left empty. Only when an outgoing nerve fiber reached the part of the brain where it had originally made connection did synapse formation occur. This specificity in the regeneration experiments suggested to Sperry that the presynaptic terminal of the optic nerve fibers, and the specific neurons they innervate, must have a complementary specificity so that the appropriate pre- and postsynaptic elements of the synapse are attracted to each other and maintained (for an alternative view see Gaze and Keating[18]). Sperry has done additional experiments that suggest that in lower vertebrates the development of appropriate synapses is due to a preprogrammed affinity between neurons that is fully present at birth. Synapse formation is not due to the pattern of impulses or to learning. For example, Sperry has cut the optic nerve in frogs, rotated the eye ball on its optic axis 180°, and found that regeneration still occurs. But now the animal's visual responses are inverted by 180°.[74] When such an animal reaches for an object placed in its upper temporal visual field, it will invariably reach toward its lower nasal field. These maladaptive responses persist indefinitely without correction. These findings seem to indicate that despite their current inappropriateness the optic nerve fibers of the rotated eye grew back and remained connected to the central cells initially appropriate for the eye when it was still right side up. Failure to re-educate the visual system suggests that the neural connections in the optic system of lower vertebrates seem to be laid down in a preordained manner, early in development, and these connections cannot be altered later even if they are nonadaptive. Jacobson[37] has recently shown that retinal cells are specified to hook up to definite central areas (in the tectum) before the axons of the retinal ganglion cells even begin to grow out toward the tectum.

Impressed with the importance of the detailed wiring necessary for the response specificity that they found in cortical cells, Hubel and Wiesel addressed themselves to the development of connections in the mammalian visual system.[33] They wanted to know whether hierarchical patterns of response to spots and bars of light that they found at different levels of the visual system in the adult animal were present at birth, prior to the animal's being exposed to pattern light. Hubel and Wiesel examined the major levels of the visual system in newborn kittens, and found that at each level the receptive field organization of the adult cat was present, at least to some degree. Although the results here are not completely clear, Hubel and Wiesel suggest that even in mammals the basic neuronal wiring necessary for complex perceptual behavior is built into the nervous system under genetic control. Newborn animals that have not been exposed to light show binocular interaction and some of their cells have specific axes of orientation.

These studies provided an interesting framework for examining two very different questions: (1) how is prewired neural architecture altered in early critical stages of development by abnormal sensory experiences and (2) how is this prewired nervous system affected in the adult by normal learning experiences? As yet these questions have only been examined in a few model systems. For the first question we are fortunate, however, in having experiments in the visual system of the cat on which there is already much useful information.

The Effects of Light Deprivation on the Functional Interconnections of Cells in the Visual System

Several clinical studies (see Senden[67]) suggest that people born with congenital cataracts that are not removed until maturity show permanent perceptual abnormalities. Such people may learn to recognize colors readily but show only the most rudimentary perception of visual pattern. Some require months to differentiate a square from a circle and have to count corners to distinguish a square from a triangle. Even after years of training they may never acquire the visual perception of people who have normal vision from infancy. Some of them may never learn to recognize people

whom they see daily, on the basis of visual clues alone.

These experiments have been carried an important step further by the imaginative research on chimpanzees by Austin Riesen.[64] Riesen found that at the age of four to seven months a normal chimpanzee has excellent visual perception and can readily learn to make selective responses to new visual stimuli. He will recognize those who care for him, welcoming their approach. He will fear and avoid strangers. A chimpanzee that has been reared in darkness from birth to age four to seven months behaves completely differently. These animals have a great deal of difficulty in learning to discriminate even simple objects. Weeks after being returned to a normal environment they cannot discriminate between strangers and friends and show no sign of curiosity and fear.

Riesen then brought up chimpanzees in an unbroken field of light, without the contours of a normal visual environment, by enclosing their heads in translucent plastic domes. These animals were just as blind as the animals reared in darkness. Thus it is not the absence of light but the absence of visual patterns that produces such devastating defects in visual perception. What emerges from Riesen's study is that the development of normal visual perception, the mere ability to distinguish between objects in the visual world, requires a prolonged early period of exposure to patterned visual stimulation.

The cellular neuronal mechanism of this important paradigm has now been probed in a number of studies (see Hubel[31]). In the first of these studies, Wiesel and Hubel examined the responses of newborn kittens who had one eyelid sutured closed so that the eye was not exposed to patterned vision.[79,80,81] If the lid was kept closed for three months following birth, a naive animal became permanently blind in that eye. In the normal brain most cells in the visual cortex respond to stimuli presented to either of the two eyes. In the cortex of a monocularly deprived animal, cells responded readily to appropriate stimuli presented to the normal eye, but no cell could be successfully stimulated from the eye that had been sutured closed. Closing the eyelid of an adult cat for a comparable period produced no effect.

The earlier experiments on newborn kittens suggested that the basic connections between the cells in the retina and the brain had been established at birth. Failure to find responses in the brain to stimulation of the eye deprived of patterned light suggests that something had happened in the visual system whereby previously interconnected neurons were now no longer in functional contact. This suggested to Hubel and Wiesel that, during this critical phase of development, immature synapses in the cortex need for their normal maintenance, stimulation via patterned light on the retina. Without exposure to patterned light the pre-existing connections can be disrupted.

This theoretical notion has now been supported in a number of elegant experiments that involved more subtle alterations of the visual environment. In one of these, Hubel and Wiesel[35] produced an artificial squint of the right eye by cutting an eye muscle, the right medial rectus, at the time of normal eye opening. These animals showed no behavioral defects three months later. When their visual cortices were examined, cells in the striate cortex still responded normally to stimulation of each eye. Binocular interaction was, however, absent. Normally 8o percent of cells in the cortex respond to stimulation of homologus spots in each of the two retinas. In animals with squint, only 20 percent of cells could be influenced from both eyes. A similar result was obtained when an opaque contact lens was placed on each eye on alternate days. These experiments suggest that the integrity of certain striate cortical pathways may depend not only on patterned light but also on the normal, presumably synchronous, presentation of patterned light to both eyes. The integrity of the striate cortical pathways necessary for binocular interaction seems to depend on the synchronous interrelation between the activity of the two eyes (see also [2] and [26]).

These studies provide a superb paradigm for relating cellular neurophysiology to psychology. Innumerable clinical studies have illustrated the devastating effect of early social deprivation on the social, intellectual, and emotional development of children. This work has now been extended into an animal model by the Harlows[23] who have documented the importance of maternal and peer interaction for the normal social and sexual development of infant monkeys. The Harlows have found that the first year of life is a critical period for simian social and sexual development. Isolation for more than six months during the first year has permanent and devastating effects. The studies of Hubel and Wiesel provide an extension of this approach to the cellular level. These studies begin to reveal the effect of the interaction between developmental processes and environmental stimulation on the formation of connections during the early stages of maturation. Developmental processes carry the potentiality for forming completely correct connections between the eye and the brain. But this potentiality can be disrupted by abnormal environmental stimulation. During this critical phase a normal pattern of environmental stimulation is essential for the maintenance and further maturation of preexisting connections. By developing more extensive animal models, using other modalities and progressively more complex social deprivation, one may begin to get some clues into the nature of the cellular and perhaps even the molecular mechanisms that underlie the destructive influence of early childhood deprivation.

Studies of sensory deprivation thus provide insight into the effect of normal and abnormal environmental stimuli on cellular functioning of the brain. They place Heinz Hartmann's concept of an average expectable environment[25] in a cellular biological perspective. But so far we have only considered studies involving profound changes in an animal's perceptive environment. We are, however, all constantly exposed to less traumatic stimuli that nonetheless affect behavior for long periods of time. How are these changes accomplished? Do they leave an obvious imprint on the brain that can be examined on the cellular level?

To answer questions of this kind neural scientists are beginning to examine the neuronal mechanisms of simple types of learning. These are the best experimental models for environmentally produced alterations in behavior. We have seen in the previous section that one can use simple instances of sensory deprivation to develop model systems for studying the effects of social isolation and its consequences for the developing organism. In the next section we will consider the analysis of simple behaviors and their modifications so as to gain insight into the kinds of changes that may occur in the brain, as a result of day-to-day behavioral experiences. These studies are useful in understanding how the normal acquisition of behavioral patterns occurs. They may also soon provide some insight about the acquisition of abnormal behavior patterns.

⟦ Cellular Neurophysiological Studies of Behavioral Modifications

Like the study of perception, the neurophysiological study of learning requires a detailed knowledge of the total neural circuit that mediates the behavioral response being examined. This requirement is difficult to meet in the intact brain of a higher animal because it contains an enormous number of cells—a billion—forming an even larger number of interconnections. In addition, the behavior of vertebrates is often highly complex. A way around these problems is to study simple behaviors that are controlled by numerically reduced neural populations, such as isolated portions of the vertebrate nervous system or invertebrate ganglia. Selecting an appropriately advantageous preparation for solving a particular problem is a common strategy in biology, but its application to psychology has not been fully explored. The most consistent progress comes from studies of two simple behavioral modifications, habituation and dishabituation, in two simple preparations: the spinal cord of the cat and the abdominal ganglion of the marine mollusc *Aplysia californica*.

Habituation, sometimes considered the most elementary form of learning, is a decrease in a behavioral response that occurs when an initially novel stimulus is presented repeatedly.[59]

When a sudden noise is heard for the first time, one's attention is immediately drawn to it and a number of concomitant changes may occur—e.g., one's heart rate and respiratory rate may increase. However, if the same noise is repeated, one's attention and one's bodily responses gradually diminish. As a result of habituation one can become accustomed to initially distracting sounds and work effectively even in a noisy environment. One also becomes habituated to the clothes one wears and to one's own bodily sensations. These enter our awareness rarely, in special circumstances. In this sense habituation is learning to ignore recurrent external or internal stimuli that have lost novelty or meaning. Habituation develops not only in reflex response systems but in instinctive response systems as well. For example, a fish will defend his territory against a nonspecific intruder. Upon repeated exposure to the intruder, however, the fish will gradually suppress his aggressive behavior, a maneuver permitting him to respond more effectively to other stimuli, such as sexual ones, that are more necessary for the survival of his species.[60] Deliberate habituation of emotional responses to anxiety–provoking stimuli is used clinically as part of behavior therapy.[82]

Besides being important in its own right, habituation is also frequently involved in more complex learning that consists not only in acquiring new responses but also in learning to reduce errors by eliminating incorrect responses to inappropriate stimuli. Once a response is habituated, two processes can lead to its restoration: (1) *spontaneous recovery* that occurs as a result of withholding the stimulus to which the animal has habituated, and (2) *dishabituation*, a restoration of the response that occurs as a result of changing the stimulus pattern, for example, by presenting another stronger stimulus to another pathway.

Habituation, recovery and dishabituation have been demonstrated for a wide variety of behavioral responses in all animals examined including man. Their general occurrence suggests that neuronal mechanisms underlying habituation may also prove to be quite general.

FLEXION WITHDRAWAL IN THE CAT

The first neural analysis of habituation was undertaken in the isolated spinal cord of the cat. The vertebrate spinal cord mediates the reflex responses underlying posture and locomotion. In the course of analyzing their neural mechanisms, Charles Sherrington[68,69] found that certain reflex responses, such as the flexion withdrawal of a limb to stimulation of the skin, decreased with repeated stimulation and recovered only after many seconds of rest. Sherrington had the great insight to appreciate that neural reactions within the spinal cord differ from those in the peripheral nerves because of the numerous synaptic connections within the cord. He therefore attributed the decreased reflex responsiveness of the withdrawal reflex to a functional decrease (which he called "fatigue") at the specific set of synapses through which the motor neuron was repeatedly activated. Thus, as early as 1906, Sherrington suggested that a change at central synapses could underlie response decrement.

Sherrington was able to show that the reflex decrement was central and not due to fatigue of the muscles or the sensory receptors, but he was not capable of testing his intriguing synaptic hypothesis because of the limitation of the neurophysiological techniques available to him. This problem was subsequently reinvestigated by Prosser and Hunter[63] and more recently by Spencer, Thompson, and Neilson.[72,73] They found that the habituated flexion withdrawal can be restored to full size (dishabituation) by applying a strong novel stimulus to another part of the skin. Indeed, Spencer et al. found that dishabituation is not simply a transient abolition of habituation but an independent facilitatory process superimposed upon habituation. Spencer and his colleagues studied the features of spinal-reflex habituation in some detail and found that these resembled the habituation of more complex behavioral responses. They also began the cellular analysis of habituation. By recording intracellularly from motor neurons, they showed that response decrement did not involve a change in the properties of the motor neurons but only in the synaptic impingement upon them. However, the central synaptic pathways of the flexion withdrawal reflex in the cat are complex, involving many as yet unspecified connections through interneurons.

GILL WITHDRAWAL IN APLYSIA

Further analysis of habituation required a still simpler system, one in which the behavioral response could be reduced to one or more monosynaptic systems. In search of such systems for behavioral studies, a number of investigators have been attracted to invertebrate preparations.[40,48] These animals' nervous systems contain relatively few cells, a property that simplifies neuronal analysis of behavior. The nervous system of opisthobranch molluscs is particularly advantageous because it contains cells that are unusually large (almost 1 mm in diameter) and therefore easy to study with intracellular microelectrodes. The most detailed behavioral work has been carried out on a marine mollusc, Aplysia. The central nervous system of Aplysia contains about twenty thousand cells. An individual ganglion such as the abdominal ganglion contains only about two thousand cells yet is capable of generating a number of biologically significant behaviors.

Working on Aplysia, Kupfermann and Kandel[51] studied a defensive withdrawal response that is in some ways analogous to the flexion withdrawal response in the cat. Aplysia has a gill, an external respiratory organ, analogous to the lung in man. The gill is partially covered by the mantle shelf, which contains this animal's residual shell. When either the mantle shelf or the anal siphon or spout (a fleshy continuation of the mantle shelf) is touched, the siphon contracts and the gill withdraws into the cavity underneath the mantle shelf. The defensive purpose of this reflex is clear. It protects the gill, a vital and delicate organ, from possible damage. Gill withdrawal is thus analogous to the defensive flexion withdrawal of a limb in the cat, or the withdrawal of a man's hand from a hot or potentially damaging object. As is the case for these other defensive responses, the gill withdrawal response habituates when repeatedly elicited by a weak or non–noxious stimulus.

Habituation in vertebrates is characterized by nine parametric features.[77] Seven of these features have been examined in the gill withdrawal response in *Aplysia* by Pinsker et al.[62] and found to be similar to habituation in mammals. These features include: (1) response decrement, typically a negative exponential function of the number of stimulus presentations; (2) recovery with rest; (3) dishabituation; (4) habituation of the dishabituatory stimulus with repeated presentations; (5) greater habituation with weak rather than with strong stimuli; (6) greater habituation with short rather than long stimulus intervals, and (7) greater habituation with repeated periods of habituation and recovery.

The existence of this satisfactory fit between short-term habituation in *Aplysia* and in mammals made it interesting to analyze the neural circuitry of this behavior. This analysis was a prerequisite for examining the functional modifications in the neural circuit that produce the behavioral modifications.

To analyze this reflex, Kupfermann and Kandel[51] developed a semi-intact preparation in which different neurons within the abdominal ganglion could be impaled with double-barrel microelectrodes for recording and direct stimulation and their function related to behavior. By firing different cells intracellularly and observing the movements of the external organs of the mantle cavity, Kupfermann, Carew and Kandel[49a,51] found ten motor cells that produced contractions of the gill, the siphon or the mantle shelf, the organs involved in the withdrawal response. Five of the ten motor cells produced movements limited to the gill. Four cells produced movement of the siphon and one cell produced movement of the gill, the siphon and the mantle shelf. Thus the motor component of this reflex consists of individual elements with both a restricted and overlapping distribution. This motor organization is highly redundant as are other motor systems described in vertebrates and in invertebrates. These ten cells are unique individuals. They are so characteristic in their location, in their electrophysiological properties, and in their motor function that they can be repeatedly recognized and examined from animal to animal. These cells and others like them have been termed "identified" cells; they are often referred to by specific numbers and letters. Uniquely identified cells have not been found to control other behaviors in *Aplysia* as well as in other animals including some lower vertebrates.[40]

Kupfermann and Kandel next analyzed the sensory component of the reflex. They mapped the tactile sensory receptive field of these motor cells and found that when the external organs of the mantle cavity were mechanically stimulated, causing the gill to withdraw, all five motor cells received large excitatory postsynaptic potentials producing a brisk repetitive spike discharge. The receptive field of these five motor cells involved the mantle shelf and siphon and was identical to that of the defensive withdrawal reflex. The excitatory input from this receptive field is in part monosynaptic and in part mediated by interneurons.[7] Although the population of sensory neurons that mediate this reflex (consisting of about twenty-five sensory neurons and three different interneurons) is larger than the motor populations, it would appear that the sensory neurons and interneurons may also be invariant. Byrne, Castellucci, and Kandel[3] have found that at least some sensory cells have invariant receptive fields and make invariant central connections to both interneurons and motor neurons.

These findings, and similar ones emerging from the study of reflex systems in the leech and the crayfish, support Sperry's idea of the specificity of neuronal interconnections. In vertebrates this specificity can only be examined on the level of groups of cells. In invertebrates, where the resolution is greater because of the reduced number of cells and the ability to identify unique cells, one can ask exactly *how* unique are the neurons and how precise are the interconnections between neurons that mediate a given behavior. From the few studies available, it would appear that for simple behaviors the neural wiring is surprisingly precise and invariant. This finding raises an interesting paradox. Given this constancy of cells and interconnections, how does behavior become modified? How is one to reconcile this apparent invariance of the wiring with known malleability of behavior? Are there unspecified cells—learning cells—that are set aside as "blanks" only to be called upon by the learning process and to be superimposed on the basic wiring of the behavior? Do behavioral modifications involve the outgrowth of new cells or new connections, or do they involve some functional change in the properties of the preexisting neurons and their interconnections?

To examine this question, Kupfermann et al.[50] studied the changes in the neural circuit that accompany habituation and dishabituation of the gill withdrawal reflex. They found that habituation, recovery, and dishabituation resulted from a functional change within the central nervous system. Thus, the excitatory postsynaptic potential, produced in the gill motor neurons by tactile stimulation of the skin, underwent characteristic changes that were causally related to habituation, to recovery, and to dishabituation. When a tactile stimulus was repeated so as to produce behavioral habituation, the excitatory postsynaptic potential in the gill motor neuron gradually decreased in size, and the amount and frequency of the evoked spike activity produced by the synaptic potential decreased correspondingly. With recovery of reflex responsiveness, produced either by rest or by a dishabituatory stimulus, there was an increase of the excitatory postsynaptic potential and a corresponding increase in spike activity.

In a more detailed examination of the mechanism underlying the change in the synaptic potential, Castellucci et al.[7] radically simplified the sensory component of the reflex pathway and examined individual sensory elements in isolation. They recorded simultaneously from one of the sensory neurons and from a gill motor neuron so as to reduce the gill reflex to its most elementary monosynaptic components and examined each element in turn as well as the interaction between them. Stimulation of one of the mechanoreceptor sensory neurons produced fairly large elementary excitatory synaptic potentials in the motor neuron. But repeated stimulation, at rates that produced habituation, led to a dramatic decrease in the amplitude of the excitatory postsynaptic potential; rest resulted in recovery. The synaptic potential produced by direct stimulation of the sensory neuron sometimes diminished so markedly that after a few stimuli it was barely visible. Similar changes have now been found in the connections between sensory neurons and several classes of interneurons.[6a] These data suggested that habituation is due to a change in excitatory synaptic efficacy of the central connections of the sensory neuron both to interneurons and motor neurons. This reduced synaptic effectiveness results from a decrease in the amount of transmitter released per unit impulse.[6a]

In the behavioral response of the intact animal, dishabituation occurs following the presentation of a strong stimulus to the animal's head or tail. On the cellular level, dishabituation is associated with a facilitation of the previously decreased effectiveness of the central excitatory synaptic connections of the sensory neurons. Thus, repetitive stimulation of tactile receptors of the siphon leads to habituation of the gill withdrawal reflex by producing a functional (plastic) decrease in the effectiveness of preexisting synapses made by branches of the sensory neurons (from the siphon) on the gill motor neurons and interneurons. Stimulation of the head leads to dishabituation of the gill withdrawal reflex by producing facilitation at the same set of synapses. Habituation is thus homosynaptic, involving a functional change in the synapses of the stimulated (habituated) pathway. On the other hand, dishabituation is heterosynaptic, involving a functional change in synapses of the habituated pathway (from the siphon) as a result of activity in a parallel pathway (the sensory pathways from the head or the tail). Castellucci et al.[7] have proposed a model that postulates that both habituation and dishabituation involve a common locus, a change in the synaptic terminals of the sensory neuron. These terminals are influenced by habituation and dishabituation so as to decrease or increase the amount of transmitter substance released per action potential.

An examination of the functional properties of the wiring diagram of a simple behavior undergoing habituation and dishabituation thus reveals that nonsynaptic properties of the neurons are not altered nor is there any fundamental change in their pattern of interconnections. No new connections appeared to be formed and no existing connections disappeared. What happened was that the functional effectiveness of certain connections was changed by the training procedure. The central synapses, made by various branches of the sensory neurons on the motor- and the interneurons, are endowed with remarkable plastic properties, so that transmission across these synapses was greatly depressed during habituation and recovered only after a rest of many minutes. But functional effectiveness could be returned immediately as a result of the presentation of a dishabituatory stimulus. These results are therefore consistent with the idea that genetic and developmental processes determine the properties of individual cells and the anatomical interconnections between cells. These processes leave unspecified, however, the degree of effectiveness of certain of these connections. Environmental factors, such as learning, produce their modifications in behavior by playing upon these "plastic" potentialities of neurons and their synapses (for review see [39]).

Cellular studies thus lead one to think of three ontogenetic stages of synaptic modification. The first stage, synapse formation, occurs primarily in the developing organism and is under genetic control. The second stage, maintenance of newly developed synapses, occurs during the critical early period of development and requires an appropriate pattern of environmental stimulation. The third stage, the regulation of the transient and long-term effectiveness of synapses, occurs throughout later life, and is determined by day-to-day behavioral experience. One of the implications of this view is that the potentialities for all behaviors of which man is capable are actually built into his brain under genetic control. What learning does is to alter the effectiveness of certain anatomically preexisting pathways, thereby leading to the expression of new patterns of behavior.

A cellular strategy can also be used to examine the biochemical mechanisms of behavioral modifications. Once the behavioral modification has been specified in cellular terms, it is possible to bring biochemical techniques to bear on the further analysis of the molecular mechanisms. This has been undertaken on the gill withdrawal response by Schwartz, Castellucci, and Kandel.[66] They have found that inhibition of protein synthesis for several hours does not interfere with either the acquisition or the retention of short-term habituation. This indicates that whatever the molecular mechanisms of short-term dishabituation and habituation may be, and we are still far from knowing them, they do not depend on the synthesis of new protein or on proteins that have remarkably fast turnover rates. This result is consistent with experiments on higher forms (see Chapter 4) that indicate new protein synthesis is not required for short-term learning.

THE MECHANISTIC RELATIONSHIPS BETWEEN DIFFERENT BEHAVIORAL MODIFICATIONS

Simple preparations are useful not only for examining the mechanisms of specific behavioral modification; they can also be used to examine the relationships between behavioral modifications. Previously these relationships could only be examined behaviorally, on a phenomenological level. I will consider here only two brief examples: (1) the relationship of habituation to dishabituation, and (2) the relationship of short-term to long-term behavioral modifications.

Pavlov,[59] who discovered habituation, and many subsequent psychologists have thought that dishabituation is merely a removal of habituation. As I have indicated above, the first new insight into this problem was provided by Spencer, Thompson, and Neilson.[73] They suggested that dishabituation of the flexion withdrawal response is an independent facilitatory process superimposed on habituation. Carew, Castellucci, and Kandel[4] have also examined these interrelationships, using the gill withdrawal reflex in *Aplysia*.[6] They used two independent pathways (siphon and mantle shelf) to elicit gill withdrawal and found that habituation of one pathway does not generalize to the other pathway. If one pathway (siphon skin) is repeatedly stimulated so that reflex responsiveness to stimulation of that pathway is habituated, the reflex responsiveness of the other pathway (mantle shelf) is unaffected. Carew et al. then habituated one pathway but not the other and examined the effects of a common dishabituatory stimulus on the two pathways. They found that whereas habituation was limited only to the stimulated pathway, dishabituation was much more widespread, involving not only the habituated pathway but the nonhabituated pathway as well. This evidence supports the work of Spencer, Thompson, and Neilson in showing that dishabituation is not merely the removal of habituation but is an independent superimposed excitatory process. Their findings and those of Carew, Castellucci, and Kandel indicate that dishabituation is a special case of sensitization, a form of behavioral arousal whereby a strong noxious stimulus can enhance a variety of reflex responses. Several investigators have now provided indirect evidence for the relation of dishabituation to sensitization in higher forms, including man. These findings suggest that the independence of habituation and dishabituation and the relationship of dishabituation to sensitization may be quite general (see Groves and Thompson).[21]

Another problem that may soon be amenable to investigation in cellular terms is the relationship of short-term to long-term memory. One would like to know whether these are two separate phenomena or whether one is merely an extension of the other. Carew, Pinsker, and Kandel[6] have begun to examine this question for habituation and for sensitization of the gill withdrawal reflex. Carew et al. found that if habituation training (ten trials a day) is repeated daily for four days, habituation of the reflex response builds up, so that it occurs more rapidly on each subsequent day. Thus on the fifth day, the mean duration of the reflex response was only twenty percent of its duration on day one. Habituation persists unchanged for a week and recovers only partially after three weeks. As is the case for complex behavioral modifications in vertebrates, massed habituation training (forty trials a day) was not as effective as spaced training (ten trials a day for four days). Thus habituation shows a sensitivity to the pattern of stimulation that resembles higher forms of learning. In a preliminary cellular analysis, Carew and Kandel[5] have found that the acquisition of long-term habituation is associated with prolonged changes in synaptic transmission that qualitatively resemble those found in short-term habituation. This suggests that long-term memory may not be a qualitatively different phenomenon but merely a quantitative extension of the short-term one. More extensive analyses are still required however to be certain of this point.

Recently, Pinsker, Carew and Kandel[61] found that sensitization of the gill withdrawal reflex can also be prolonged. If an animal is given four highly noxious stimuli daily for four days, the duration or reflex withdrawal to a weak or moderate stimulus is enhanced for several weeks. Long-term sensitization of reflex responsiveness is of particular interest because of its resemblance to chronic anxiety states. In a neutral environment *Aplysia* learns to ignore a mild tactile stimulus, particularly when it is repeated daily—that is, it habituates to such a "nonthreatening" stimulus and tends not to respond to it even when it is presented many days later. However, an animal that is presented with noxious stimuli for several days no longer lives in a neutral environment but in a potentially hostile one. As a result, even mild tactile stimuli can no longer be ignored but bring forth a maximal defensive response.

Since these long-term behavioral modifications involve a reflex response whose neural circuitry is relatively well understood it may be possible to provide cellular explanations for the relation of short-term to long-term habituation and dishabituation and thereby to shed some light on the relation of short- to long-term memory. In analyzing long-term sensitization one might also be able to develop a model system for the cellular studies of behavioral abnormalities. For example, it would be interesting to know whether other behavioral systems (heart rate, feeding, sexual behavior) are also affected by the sensitization procedure. What are the biochemical concomitants of sensitization? Can sensitization be reduced or abolished by drugs that can reduce anxiety in man? If so, what is the mechanism of action of these drugs?

❲ Perspectives

In a jocular moment Sidney Brenner described the dictum of modern biology as: "think small and talk big." I'm afraid I've indulged in both in this chapter. Although cellular studies of perception and of simple behavioral modification span more than a decade of research, they represent but a small beginning. We are still far from understanding the neuronal mechanisms of perception, of long-term memory, and of higher learning. But within the last years progress has quickened perceptibly. As a result cellular approaches may soon be usefully applied to more complex learning processes and even to behavioral abnormalities.

I have here considered only studies that combine cellular neurophysiological and behavioral approaches. However, much will be learned in the future from combining behavioral and genetic techniques. Molecular biologists have been highly successful in dissecting the network of cellular function in bacteria by using gene changes (mutations) in which one element is altered at a time. It thus seemed only natural to some molecular biologists that the network of the nervous system might also be successfully analyzed by the appropriate use of mutants. In an important series of studies, Seymour Benzer[1] has begun to dissect the neural network underlying behavior in the fly *Drosophila* using behavioral mutants. Benzer now has mutants with a variety of behavioral abnormalities, including visual disturbances, abnormalities in circadian rhythm and sexual behavior; muscular dystrophies, and sudden cessation of development. He has found that mutations can alter behavior in a variety of ways using a variety of mechanisms. These can affect the development and function of sensory systems, motor systems, and central

integrative systems. Mutations thus provide a powerful means for examining the component parts of a normal behavioral system. This approach promises to revolutionize behavioral genetics and in so doing will shed much light on the neural mechanism of behavior.

Looked at in the perspective of man's age-old search to understand himself and others, and of the relatively recent attempt of psychology and psychiatry to facilitate that search, one cannot help but view with optimism the accelerated progress in neural science. The long-sought merger between segments of psychology and neural science is becoming more of a reality. In this merger, neurobiology is likely to revitalize some segments of psychology much as molecular biology revitalized cellular genetics. In turn, contact with psychology is likely to provide a humanizing perspective for neurophysiology. This cannot but be helpful. For neurophysiology has, until recently, tended to be fascinated and satisfied with what the neurologist Francis Walshe once called, "the bloodless dance of action potentials."[78]

❲ Bibliography

1. BENZER, S. "From the Gene to Behavior," JAMA, 218 (1971), 1015–1022.
2. BLAKEMORE, C. and G. F. COOPER. "Development of the Brain Depends on the Visual Environment," *Nature*, 228 (1970), 477–478.
3. BYRNE, J., V. CASTELLUCCI and E. R. KANDEL. "Receptive Fields and Response Properties of Mechanoreceptor Neurons in the Siphon Skin of *Aplysia*." In preparation.
4. CAREW, T. J., V. F. CASTELLUCCI and E. R. KANDEL. "An Analysis of Dishabituation Sensitization of the Gill-Withdrawal Reflex in *Aplysia*," *Int. J. Neurosci.*, 2 (1971), 79–98.
5. CAREW, T. J. and E. R. KANDEL. "Rapid Acquisition of Long-Term Habituation: Behavioral and Cellular Neurophysiological Correlation." In preparation.
6. CAREW, T. J., H. M. PINSKER and E. R.

KANDEL. "Long-Term Habituation of a Defensive Withdrawal Reflex in *Aplysia*," *Science*, 175 (1972), 451–454.

6a. CASTELLUCCI, V. and E. R. KANDEL. "Aquantal Analysis of the Synaptic Depression Underlying Habituation of the Gill-Withdrawal Reflex in *Aplysia*," *Proc. Nat. Acad. Sci.*, 9 (1974), in press.

7. CASTELLUCCI, V., H. PINSKER, I. KUPFERMANN, et al. "Neuronal Mechanisms of Habituation and Dishabituation of the Gill-Withdrawal Reflex in *Aplysia*," *Science*, 167 (1970), 1745–1748.

8. DARWIN, C. *The Origin of Species*. New York: D. Appleton & Co., 1860.

9. ———. *The Descent of Man*. New York: D. Appleton & Co., 1871

10. ———. *The Expression of the Emotions in Man and Animals*. New York: D. Appleton & Co., 1872.

11. DEL CASTILLO, J. and B. KATZ. "Quantal Components of the End-Plate Potential," *J. Physiol.*, 124 (1954), 560–573.

12. ECCLES, J. C. *The Neurophysiological Basis of Mind*. Oxford: Clarendon Press, 1953.

13. ———. *The Physiology of Nerve Cells*. Baltimore: The Johns Hopkins Press, 1957.

14. ———. *The Physiology of Synapses*. New York: Academic, 1964.

15. FATT, P. and B. KATZ. "An Analysis of the End-Plate Potential Recorded with an Intracellular Electrode," *J. Physiol.*, 115 (1951), 320–370.

16. ———. "The Effect of Inhibitory Nerve Impulses on a Crustacean Muscle Fibre," *J. Physiol.*, 121 (1953), 374–389.

17. FRAZIER, W. T., E. R. KANDEL, I. KUPFERMANN, et al. "Morphological and Functional Properties of Identified Neurons in the Abdominal Ganglia of *Aplysia californica*," *J. Neurophysiol.*, 30 (1967), 1288–1351.

18. GAZE, R. M. and M. J. KEATING. "The Visual System and 'Neuronal Specificity'," *Nature*, 237 (1972), 375–378.

19. GROSS, C. G. "Visual Functions of Infero-Temporal Cortex," in R. Jung, ed., *Handbook of Sensory Physiology*, Vol. 7. Part 3. New York: Springer-Verlag, 1972.

20. GROSS, C. G., D. B. BENDER, and C. E. ROCHA-MIRANDA. "Visual Receptive Fields of Neurons in Inferotemporal Cortex of the Monkey," *Science*, 166 (1969), 1303–1306.

21. GROVES, P. M. and R. F. THOMPSON. "Habituation: A Dual Process Theory," *Psychol. Rev.*, 77 (1970), 419–450.

22. GRUNDFEST, H. "Electrical Inexcitability of Synapses and Some Consequences in the Central Nervous System," *Physiol. Rev.*, 37 (1957), 337–361.

23. HARLOW, H. F. and M. K. HARLOW. "Social Deprivation in Monkeys," *Sci. Am.*, 207 (1962), 136–146.

24. HARMON, L. D. "Neural Subsystems: An Interpretive Summary," in F. O. Schmitt, ed., *The Neurosciences*, pp. 468–493. New York: Rockefeller University Press, 1970.

25. HARTMANN, H. *Ego Psychology and the Problem of Adaptation*. D. Rapaport, transl. New York: Int. Universities, 1958.

26. HIRSCH, H. V. B. and D. N. SPINELLI. "Visual Experience Modifies Distribution of Horizontally and Vertically Oriented Receptive Fields in Cats," *Science*, 168 (1970), 869–871.

27. HODGKIN, A. L. *The Conduction of the Nervous Impulse*. Liverpool: Liverpool University Press, 1964.

28. HODGKIN, A. L., A. F. HUXLEY and B. KATZ. "Measurement of Current-Voltage Relations in the Membrane of the Giant Axon of *Loligo*," *J. Physiol.*, 116 (1952), 424–448.

29. HODGKIN, A. L. and B. KATZ. "The Effect of Sodium Ions on the Electrical Activity of the Giant Axon of the Squid," *J. Physiol.*, 108 (1949), 37–77.

30. HUBEL, D. H. "The Visual Cortex of the Brain," *Sci. Am.*, 209 (1963), 54–62.

31. ———. "Effects of Distortion of Sensory Input on the Visual System of Kittens," (Bowdich Lecture), *Physiologist*, 10 (1967), 17–45.

32. HUBEL, D. H. and T. N. WIESEL. "Receptive Fields, Binocular Interactions and Functional Architecture in the Cat's Visual System," *J. Physiol.*, 160 (1962), 106–154.

33. ———. "Receptive Fields of Cells in Striate Cortex of Very Young, Visually Inexperienced Kittens," *J. Neurophysiol.*, 26 (1963), 994–1002.

34. ———. "Receptive Fields and Functional Architecture in Two Non-Striate Visual Areas (18 and 19) of the Cat," *J. Neurophysiol.*, 28 (1965), 229–289.

35. ———. "Binocular Interactions in Striate Cortex of Kittens Reared with Artificial

Squint," *J. Neurophysiol.*, 28 (1965), 1041–1059.

36. IWAMURA, Y., E. P. GARDNER and W. A. SPENCER. "Geometry of the Ventrobasal Complex: Functional Significance in Skin Sensation," in W. Riss, ed., *Basic Thalamic Structure and Function.* Proceedings Downstate Medical Center Conference—Brooklyn. White Plains, N.Y.: Phiebig, 1972.

37. JACOBSON, M. "Development of Specific Neuronal Connections," *Science*, 163 (1969), 543–547.

38. JAMES, W. *The Principles of Psychology.* New York: Henry Holt & Co., 1890.

39. KANDEL, E. R. "Nerve Cells and Behavior," *Sci. Am.*, 223 (1970), 57–70.

40. KANDEL, E. R. and I. KUPFERMANN. "The Functional Organization of Invertebrate Ganglia," *Annu. Rev. Physiol.*, 32 (1970), 193–258.

41. KANDEL, E. R. and W. A. SPENCER. "Electrophysiological Properties of an Archicortical Neuron," in *Current Problems in Electrobiology, Ann. N.Y. Acad. Sci.*, 94 (1961), 570–603.

42. KANDEL, E. R. and L. TAUC. "Heterosynaptic Facilitation in Neurones of the Abdominal Ganglion of *Aplysia depilans*," *J. Physiol.*, 181 (1965), 1–27.

43. KATZ, B. *Nerve, Muscle, and Synapse.* New York: McGraw-Hill, 1966.

44. ———. *The Release of Neural Transmitter Substances.* Springfield, Ill.: C. C. Thomas, 1969.

45. KATZ, B. and R. MILEDI. "A Study of Synaptic Transmission in the Absence of Nerve Impulses," *J. Physiol.*, 192 (1967), 407–436.

46. ———. "The Timing of Calcium Action During Neuromuscular Transmission," *J. Physiol.*, 189 (1967), 535–544.

47. ———. "Tetrodotoxin-Resistant Electrical Activity in Presynaptic Terminals," *J. Physiol.*, 203 (1969), 459–487.

48. KENNEDY, D., A. I. SELVERSTON and M. P. REMLER. "Analysis of Restricted Neural Networks," *Science*, 164 (1969), 1488–1496.

49. KUFFLER, S. W. "Discharge Patterns and Functional Organization of Mammalian Retina," *J. Neurophysiol.*, 16 (1953), 37–68.

49a. KUPFERMANN, I., T. J. CAREW, and E. R. KANDEL. "Local, Reflex and Central Commands Controlling Gill and Siphon Movement in *Aplysia*," *J. Neurophysiol.*, 37 (1974), 996–1019.

50. KUPFERMANN, I., V. CASTELLUCCI, H. PINSKER et al. "Neuronal Correlates of Habituation and Dishabituation of the Gill-Withdrawal Reflex in *Aplysia*," *Science*, 167 (1970), 1743–1745.

51. KUPFERMANN, I. and E. R. KANDEL. "Neuronal Controls of a Behavioral Response Mediated by the Abdominal Ganglion of *Aplysia*," *Science*, 164 (1969), 847–850.

52. KUPFERMANN, I., H. PINSKER, V. CASTELLUCCI et al. "Central and Peripheral Control of Gill Movements in *Aplysia*," *Science*, 174 (1971), 1252–1256.

53. LING, G. and R. W. GERARD. "The Normal Membrane Potential of Frog Sartorius Fibers," *J. Cell. Physiol.*, 34 (1949), 383–396.

54. MARSHALL, W. H. and S. A. TALBOT. "Recent Evidence for Neural Mechanisms in Vision Leading to General Theory of Sensory Acuity," in H. Kluver, ed., *Visual Mechanisms. Biol. Symposium*, 7 (1942), 117–164.

55. MEYNERT, T. *Psychiatry.* New York and London: G. P. Putnam's Sons, 1885.

56. MOUNTCASTLE, V. B. *Medical Physiology*, 12th ed., St. Louis: C. V. Mosby, 1968.

57. PALADE, G. E. and S. L. PALAY. "Electron Microscope Observation of Interneuronal and Neuromuscular Synapses," *Anat. Rec.*, 118 (1954), 335–336.

58. PALAY, S. L. "Synapses in the Central Nervous System," *J. Biophys. Biochem. Cytol.*, 2, Suppl. 4, pt. 2 (1956), 193–201.

59. PAVLOV, I. P. *Conditioned Reflexes.* G. V. Anrep, transl. London: Oxford Press, 1927.

60. PEEKE, H. V. S., M. J. HERZ, and J. E. GALLAGHER. "Changes in Aggressive Interaction in Adjacently Territorial Convict Cichlids (*Cichlasoma Nigrofasciatum*): A Study of Habituation," *Behavior*, 40 (1971), 43–54.

61. PINSKER, H., T. J. CAREW and E. R. KANDEL. "Long-Term Sensitization of a Defensive Withdrawal Reflex in *Aplysia*," *Science*, 182 (1973), 1039–1042.

62. PINSKER, H., I. KUPFERMANN, V. CASTELLUCCI and E. R. KANDEL. "Habituation and Dishabituation of the Gill-Withdrawal

Reflex in *Aplysia*," *Science*, 167 (1970), 1740–1742.

63. PROSSER, C. L. and W. S. HUNTER. "The Extinction of Startle Responses and Spinal Reflexes in the White Rat," *Am. J. Physiol.*, 117 (1936), 609–618.

64. RIESEN, A. H. "Plasticity of Behavior: Psychological Aspects," in H. F. Harlow and C. N. Woolsey, eds., *Biological and Biochemical Bases of Behavior*, pp. 425–450. Madison: University of Wisconsin Press, 1958.

65. ROBERTIS, E. D. P. DE and H. S. BENNETT. "Submicroscopic Vescicular Components in the Synapse," *Fed. Proc.*, 13 (1954), 35.

66. SCHWARTZ, J. H., V. CASTELLUCCI and E. R. KANDEL. "Functioning of Identified Neurons and Synapses in Abdominal Ganglion of *Aplysia* in Absence of Protein Synthesis," *J. Neurophysiol.*, 34 (1971), 939–953.

67. SENDEN, M. VON. *Raum—Und Gestaltauffassung Bei Operierten Blindgeborenen Vor und Nach der Operation*. Leipzig: J. A. Barth, 1932.

68. SHERRINGTON, C. S. "Experiments in Examination of the Peripheral Distribution of Fibers of the Posterior Roots of Some Spinal Nerves," *Philos. Trans. R. Soc. Lond. Biol.*, 190 (1898), 45–186.

69. ———. *The Integrative Action of the Nervous System*. New York: Scribner's, 1906.

70. SOKOLOV, E. N. "Higher Nervous Functions: The Orienting Reflex," *Annu. Rev., Physiol.*, 25 (1963), 545–580.

71. SPENCER, W. A. and E. R. KANDEL. "Cellular and Integrative Properties of the Hippocampal Pyramidal Cell and the Comparative Electrophysiology of Cortical Neurons," *Int. J. of Neurol.*, 6 (1968), 266–296.

72. SPENCER, W. A., R. F. THOMPSON and D. R. NEILSON, JR. "Decrement of Ventral Root Electrotonus and Intracellularly Recorded PSPs Produced by Iterated Cutaneous Afferent Volleys," *J. of Neurophysiol.*, 29 (1966), 253–274.

73. ———. "Response Decrement of Flexion Reflex in the Acute Spinal Cat and Transient Restoration by Strong Stimuli," *J. of Neurophysiol.*, 29 (1966), 221–239.

74. SPERRY, R. W. "Mechanisms of Neuronal Maturation," in S. S. Stevens, ed., *Handbook of Experimental Psychology*, pp. 236–280. New York: Wiley, 1951.

75. ———. "Selective Communication in Nerve Nets: Impulse Specificity vs. Connection Specificity," *Neurosci. Res. Program Bull.*, 3 (5) (1965), 37–43.

76. THOMAS, R. C. "Electrogenic Sodium Pump in Nerve and Muscle Cells," *Physiol. Rev.*, 52 (1972), 563–594.

77. THOMPSON, R. F. and W. A. SPENCER. "Habituation: A Model Phenomenon for the Study of Neuronal Substrates of Behavior," *Psychol. Rev.*, 73 (1966), 16–43.

78. WALSHE, F. M. R. "The Brainstem Conceived as the 'Highest Level' of Function in the Nervous System," *Brain*, 80 (1957), 510–539.

79. WIESEL, T. and D. H. HUBEL. "Comparison of the Effects of Unilateral and Bilateral Eye Closure on Cortical Unit Responses in Kittens," *J. Neurophysiol.*, 28 (1965), 1029–1040.

80. ———. "Effects of Visual Deprivation on Morphology and Physiology of Cells in the Cat's Lateral Geniculate Body," *J. Neurophysiol.*, 26, (1963), 978–993.

81. ———. "Extent of Recovery From the Effects of Visual Deprivation in Kittens," *J. Neurophysiol.*, 28 (1965), 1060–1072.

82. WOLPE, J. "Reciprocal Inhibition as the Main Basis of Psychotherapeutic Effects," *Arch. Neurol. Psychiatry*, 72 (1954), 205–226.

CHAPTER 4

ESTABLISHING AND MODIFYING NEURONAL INTERACTIONS: SOME EXPERIMENTAL APPROACHES*

Samuel H. Barondes

ADVANCES IN BIOLOGY in the past decade have greatly clarified the mechanism of regulation of the metabolism of individual cells. This in turn has set the stage for analysis of cellular sociology—how certain cells come to associate with others and how neighbors regulate each other. Solution to these problems is particularly important for an understanding of the most societal of organs, the nervous system. The goal of this essay is to

* Supported by a grant from the A.P. Sloan Foundation and NIMH Grant 18282.

provide the reader with a sampling of several selected aspects of this work.

There are two areas of investigation which I will discuss briefly: (1) studies concerned with various aspects of the genetically determined "wiring diagram of the nervous system"; (2) studies concerned with establishment of new functial interneuronal relationships with learning. Since only a superficial discussion can be given here, it is hoped that the bibliography will be consulted. All that I will to do is to present work in several areas that is not usually called to the attention of psychiatrists. I will also emphasize the usefulness of various lower organisms for studies of this type. The least this will do is to remind us again of our humble origins.

⟮ Genetic Control of Nervous System Structure and Behavior

There is an obvious and striking constancy in the behavior of all members of a species and in the gross structure of their brains. Both reflect the genetically directed neuronal wiring diagram. Recent studies have been concerned with analysis of (1) the degree of precision of the connections between one nerve cell and another, and (2) the magnitude of the genetic change required to produce an observable change in behavior.

Work on these problems has been largely confined to organisms whose life history or nervous system structure makes them relatively easy to study. Although we will ultimately want to know the answers to these questions as they relate to man, favorable biological preparations are a prerequisite to any serious investigation. The following will provide some examples of what is being done.

Constancy in Structure of an Identified Neuron

Through extensive neurophysiological and behavioral studies it has been possible to identify the specific and often unique function of a number of identified neurons in the nervous systems of several marine organisms. Favorites for study are crustacea[18,23] and molluscs.[9] In both these groups of organisms there are a number of discrete ganglia, each of which contain relatively small numbers of nerve cells that can be identified in the living state. Identification is made both by the appearance of the neurons under the dissecting microscope and by characteristic electrophysiological properties that can be determined after introduction of a microelectrode into the nerve cell body. These ganglia are rich in interneurons and analogous to our central nervous system in that they perform complex integration. One, the stomatogastric ganglion of the lobster, contains only thirty neurons; yet it controls complex movements in the breaking up and transporting of food.[23] A number of interneurons in such systems have been shown to play a critical role in integrating inputs and directing outputs that control specific behavior.

Given the availability of such well–defined preparations, attempts have been made to determine the constancy of the microstructure and connectivity of specific neurons. Analysis of this type has been done by injection of Procion yellow, a fluorescent dye, into the soma of the same nerve cell in a number of specimens. The dye spreads through the axons and dendrites of the cell and permits direct visualization of the three dimensional structure of its branches.[23] These studies showed that a specific neuron has very similar microstructure from animal to animal, which reflects its synaptic connections with other neurons. Such anatomical constancy demonstrates the relationship between microstructure of a specific neuron and its participation in the regulation of a specific behavior.

Higher resolution studies of structural variability of an identified neuron have recently been initiated, using the small crustacean, *Daphnia*.[19] This organism was chosen since it can reproduce parthenogenetically. It is thus possible to study many animals that are genetically identical. Analysis was done by reconstructing the precise structure of the branches of an identified neuron after electron microscopy of serial sections. Although there were slight variations in the precise morphology of the terminal ramifications, a striking constancy in the branching of a single identified nerve cell was found. This is further evidence of the degree of genetic control of an identified neuron's precise structure.

Behavioral Genetics in Drosophila

The types of studies I have just mentioned seek to analyze organisms that are genetically identical, although they may ultimately be applied to analyzing the effects of genes on specific neurons. In contrast, genetic analysis has been concerned with the question: how small a genetic change can produce a grossly observable change in behavior? Whereas it is well known that different inbred strains of mammals may differ strikingly in their behavior,[13] it is not known whether or not these strains have extensive genetic differences. A more precise analysis of the genetics of behavior is presently being conducted in fruit flies. These organisms are a favorite of geneticists because they reproduce quickly and have many progeny. In addition, there is a vast technology that has been developed for analysis of genetic changes in this species. There are maps and markers that allow one to precisely determine where the genetic change is and how many genes might be affected.

In recent years an extensive series of behavioral mutants of *Drosophila* has been identified and investigated.[4] Some, with abnormalities in locomotion, have been named "sluggish" or "hyperkinetic." Some have an abnormal response to a perturbation. For example, the mutant called "easily shocked" responds to a mechanical jolt with something like a seizure. Still others exhibit abnormalities in courtship such as the male "savoir-faire" mutants.

One striking finding of these studies is that a mutation in a single gene can produce distinct behavioral changes. Although it is not yet known what modification of the nervous system is produced by these mutations, techniques are now being developed so that it may some day be possible to relate the effect of mutation in a single gene to morphological changes in the nervous system that mediate the altered behavior.[13]

⟨ Mechanisms for Development of Specific Intercellular Interactions

The studies thus far described have helped to identify the precision of connectivity of identified neurons and the susceptibility of gross behavioral systems to mutation at a single genetic locus. Another line of investigation has been concerned with the developmental mechanisms for establishing specific neuronal relationships. It has made use of embryological or biochemical techniques.

Experimental Embryology of the Retino–Tectal Connections in Amphibia

The retino–tectal connections of the amphibian are a particularly favorable system for studying how developmental forces determine specific interneuronal connections. The organism is a good choice since embryogenesis occurs outside the parent. This simplifies observation and manipulation. As for the system, it readily lends itself to investigation because of the relatively simple geometric arrangement of the retinal ganglion cells. These cells receive information about light from the photoreceptor cells and then transmit it directly to the contralateral optic tectum. There is a precise geometric correspondence between the location of a ganglion cell in the retina and the tectal region where it projects. The system is therefore ideal for experiments designed to determine how this correspondence is established during embryogenesis. Another favorable feature of this system is the ability of transected axons of the retinal ganglion cells to regenerate and reestablish functional synaptic connections with cells in the tectum, even in adulthood.

Sperry[24] was the first to take advantage of the system in an attempt to determine the mechanism for the establishment of retino–tectal connections. First he demonstrated that a transected optic nerve in the adult frog regenerated retino–tectal connections and that normal vision was reestablished. Regeneration also occurred when the eye was rotated 180 degrees after transection. In this case the retinal ganglion cells again established connections with exactly the same tectal cells they had sought out in embryonic development. Consequently, the animal now had inverted vision in the nasal-temporal and dorsal-ventral directions. If an object was presented to its dorsal visual field, it responded as if the object has been presented to its ventral visual field.

This experiment showed that the retinal ganglion cells connected with the tectal cells, for which they had a specific embryologically determined association. Despite the fact that this was now maladaptive to the organism, these connections persisted and the animal could not learn to respond normally to his visual environment. Clearly then the retinal cells and/or the tectal cells were immutably specified to make connections with each other.

To determine the mechanism of the specification of retinal and tectal cells, Gaze and Jacobson rotated the primordial eye at one of a number of times during embryogenesis.[11,16] If rotation was done early in embryogenesis, normal vision was found in the adult. This indicated that the retino–tectal system had not been specified at this stage of embryogenesis. If rotation was done late in embryogenesis, the results were the same as those in the adult. By varying the precise time of rotation, the critical developmental period when "specification" occurred was determined. It was also found that, after rotation at a specific stage in the adult, vision was normal in one dimension but inverted in the perpendicular dimension. This indicated that specification occurred first in one dimension and then in the other.

These findings have stimulated extensive work and speculation on the mechanisms of specification of cells during embryogenesis.[11,16] Two sequential processes may be operative. First it is proposed that there are foci within the embryo that release "inductive" substances to which retinal and tectal cells can respond. Cells are presumed to respond as a function of their relative proximity to this inductive source. Second it is proposed that the "inductive" substance specifies the type and number of surface molecules on the retinal and tectal cells that mediate their selective affinities for the surfaces of other cells. Both these notions and many others are considered in two recent books on this subject.[11,16] Speculations about the nature of putative cell surface molecules that mediate specific intercellular recognition have also been reviewed.[2] The use of other experimental preparations for evaluation of this problem is considered below.

Molecular Bases of Intercellular Recognition

Analysis of this problem has been begun in a variety of systems including the brain. Extensive experimentation indicates that the surfaces of vertebrate cells contain substances that favor association of cells from the same organ as opposed to cells from different organs.[20] For example, retinal cells will self–associate, but they separate from liver cells when the two cell populations are mixed together. More recently, cell extracts from different areas of the brain have been shown to promote association of cells from these areas as opposed to cells from other areas.[10] Thus far, however, purification and characterization of the molecules involved have proceeded more rapidly in simpler systems. For example, association of male and female yeast is apparently mediated by a cell surface glycoprotein.[7,8] The role of specific molecules in cellular associations of sponge and slime mold is beginning to be understood. The relative simplicity of the structure of these organisms greatly facilitates this work.

FACTOR MEDIATING ASSOCIATION OF SPONGE CELLS

Early in the century it was shown that when two species of sponge (whose cells happened to differ in color) were mixed together, the cells of each species self-associated but rejected association with cells of the other species. These results suggested that there were substances on the surfaces of the two species that mediated the selective association. Evidence for the existence of such substances was provided by the immersion of sponges in sea water from which magnesium and calcium had been removed. It was found that this led to the dissociation of the sponge cells and the appearance of a soluble factor in the medium.[14] When this factor was added to dissociated cells suspended in plain sea water, large aggregates were formed. The factor was species specific in that adding it to its own species promoted aggregation of that species but not that of other species. The soluble factor has since been purified,[15] although the mechanism whereby it mediates specific cellular aggregation is unclear. Since the factor mediates a species-specific intercellular aggregation, it may prove to be a model for similar substances in higher organisms.

STUDIES WITH SLIME MOLD

The cellular slime mold is a particularly favorable organism for studying cellular association, because it exists in both social and unsocial states.[6] In the presence of abundant food (bacteria) the slime mold cells show no interaction. However, when food is gone, the cells cohere and form a multicellular organism containing a stalk and a spore cap. When the spore caps are disseminated to a bacteria-containing medium, they de–differentiate and become single amoeboid cells again. Because of these properties it is possible to study the development of the factors responsible for cell cohesiveness by inducing this phenomenon through the removal of food. In addition, as with sponge, a number of species of cellular slime mold will, in the absence of food, segregate when mixed together.[6]

The presence of a factor on the surface of slime mold cells that mediates their self-association was demonstrated by making an antibody to slime mold cells. When this antibody was broken down into univalent fragments, it bound itself to the surface of the slime mold cells and blocked aggregation.[5] More recently a carbohydrate binding protein that could mediate this association has been isolated from slime mold cells.[22] The protein is made only when slime mold cells are deprived of food. It can be assayed by its ability to agglutinate sheep erythrocytes. This reaction occurs because the protein binds to specific sugars on the surface of the red blood cells and acts as a protein bridge between them. The nature of the binding is indicated by the fact that addition of N-acetylgalactosamine, a specific sugar that is a common constituent of cell surface glycoproteins, blocks the erythrocyte agglutination produced by this protein. The protein has been purified by affinity chromotography and its molecular characteristics have been studied. Although it has not been proven that this factor mediates cohesiveness of slime mold cells, the evidence is highly suggestive. Like the sponge factor, it may prove to be a useful model for similar substances in higher organisms.

❲ Memory: Modification of Functional Neuronal Connections

Although the nervous system is wired up under the influence of genetic forces, it retains the capacity for stable modification through the development of memory. The mechanisms whereby functional interneuronal relationships are modified for long-term memory storage are not presently known. As in the cases I have already discussed, it would be ideal if a simple preparation were available for the study of this process.

A relatively simple system that has been intensively investigated is the neuromuscular junction. It has been shown that repetitive stimulation of this junction at high frequency produces an increased sensitivity to subsequent stimulation. This phenomenon, called post–tetanic potentiation,[17] has been known for a number of years and is of considerable interest since the change in synaptic efficacy may last for up to several hours. Studies of changes of synaptic efficacy as a consequence of other forms of stimulation have been conducted in a variety of nervous systems, most notably the abdominal ganglion of the marine mollusc *Aplysia*,[17] which contains a small number of readily identified cells. It remains to be determined what the relationship is between relatively short-lived changes in such identified synapses and those which mediate long-term memory in mammals.

Because of the anatomical complexity of the mammalian brain, it is difficult to analyze modifications of the efficacy of specific synapses with learning. For this reason attempts have been made to design studies that will elucidate aspects of the mechanism of memory storage without a knowledge of the specific synapses involved. For example, it has been possible to test the hypothesis that memory is just another type of long–lasting cellular regulation;[1] and that it is therefore mediated by the synthesis of proteins that specifically facilitate the synapses involved in a specific behavioral event. Critical evaluations of this work have been published.[3,21]

This approach was made possible by the existence of specific antibiotics that inhibit protein synthesis in the nervous system as well as other cells. Administration of such drugs inhibits cerebral protein synthesis extensively for several hours with no long-term adverse effects for the animal. Since all cells in the nervous system are affected by these drugs, it is possible to examine the relationship of cerebral protein synthesis to memory in mammals without a knowledge of the specific neurons involved in the memory storage process.

In a typical experiment[3] mice are injected with cycloheximide, a potent inhibitor of protein synthesis, and trained half an hour later at which time their cerebral protein synthesizing capacity is reduced by 95 percent. The effects on learning and on memory at various times after learning can then be examined. When mice treated in this way are trained to escape shock by choosing the lighted limb of a T-maze, their learning curves are indistinguishable from mice injected with saline. Furthermore, in a typical experiment normal retention can be detected several hours after training. This result suggests that cerebral protein synthesis is not required for learning or for memory for hours after. If other groups of mice, trained in this manner, are tested for retention one day or seven days after training, they are found to have markedly impaired memory. Therefore, it appears that cerebral protein synthesis during training is required for a long–lasting memory. The critical cerebral protein synthesis presumably occurs during training or within minutes thereafter since injection of the drug thirty minutes after training has no effect on memory measured a day or seven days later.

The results of an extensive series of experiments of this type suggest that there are two processes in memory storage—a short-term process that lasts for hours and is independent of cerebral protein synthesis; and a long-term process that is dependent on cerebral protein synthesis. For the purposes of this discussion these experiments are also of interest because they indicate how tools developed for general biological studies may be applied to analysis of this special problem of mammalian brain function.

Conclusion

The goal of the essay is to provide a sampling of contemporary research on the establishment, consistency, and modifiability of functional neuronal wiring diagrams. Unlike studies of neurotransmitter metabolism or of psychoactive drugs, such work has not as yet provided any practical tools for psychiatry. It is concerned primarily with relatively primitive organisms and with general problems of differentiation and biological regulation. In a sense this work underscores our ignorance of the most fundamental processes involved in creating and molding the nervous system. It remains to be seen how analysis of these problems will influence our ability to predict or control behavior.

⟪ Bibliography

1. BARONDES, S. H. "The Relationship of Biological Regulatory Mechanisms to Learning and Memory," *Nature*, 205 (1965), 18–21.
2. ———. "Brain Glycomacromolecules and Interneuronal Recognition," in F. O. Schmitt, ed. in chief, *The Neurosciences: A Second Study Program*, pp. 747–760. New York: Rockefeller University Press, 1970.
3. ———. "Cerebral Protein Synthesis Inhibitors Block Long-Term Memory," *Int. Rev. of Neurobiol.*, 12 (1970), 177–205.
4. BENZER, S. "From the Gene to Behavior," *JAMA*, 218 (1971), 1015–1022.
5. BEUG, H., G. GERISCH, S. KEMPFF, et al. "Specific Inhibition of Cell Contact Formation in *Dictyostelium* by Univalent Antibodies," *Exp. Cell Res.*, 63 (1970), 147–158.

6. BONNER, J. T. *The Cellular Slime Molds,* 2nd ed., Princeton: Princeton University Press, 1967.

7. CRANDALL, M. A. and T. D. BROCK. "Molecular Aspects of Specific Cell Contact," *Science,* 161 (1968), 473–475.

8. ———. "Molecular Basis of Mating in the Yeast *Hansenula Wingei,*" *Bacteriol. Rev.,* 32 (1968), 139–163.

9. FRAZIER, W. T., E. R. KANDEL, I. KUPFERMANN, et al. "Morphological and Functional Properties of Identified Neurons in the Abdominal Ganglion of *Aplysia californica,*" *J. Neurophysiol.,* 30 (1967), 1288–1351.

10. GARBER, B. B. and A. A. MOSCONA. "Reconstruction of Brain Tissue from Cell Suspensions," *Dev. Biol.,* 27 (1972), 217–243.

11. GAZE, R. M. *The Formation of Nerve Connections,* New York: Academic Press, 1970.

12. HIRSCH, J. "Behavior Genetics and Individuality Understood: Behaviorism's Counterfactual Dogma Blinded Behavioral Sciences to the Significance of Meiosis," *Science,* 143 (1963), 1436–1442.

13. HOTTA, Y. and S. BENZER. "Mapping of Behavior in *Drosophila* Mosaics," *Nature,* 240 (1972), 527–535.

14. HUMPHREYS, T. "The Cell Surface and Specific Cell Aggregation," in B. D. Davis and L. Warren, eds., *The Specificity of Cell Surfaces,* pp. 195–210. Englewood Cliffs: Prentice-Hall, 1967.

15. ———. "Biochemical Analysis of Sponge Cell Aggregation," *Symp. Zool. Soc. Lond.,* 25 (1970), 325–334.

16. JACOBSON, M. A. *Developmental Neurobiology.* New York: Holt, Rinehart and Winston, 1970.

17. KANDEL, E. R. "Cellular Studies of Learning," in G. C. Quarton, T. Melnechuk, and F. O. Schmitt, eds., *The Neurosciences: A Study Program,* pp. 666–689. New York: Rockefeller University Press, 1967.

18. KENNEDY, D. "Nerve Cells and Behavior," *Am. Scientist,* 59 (1971), 36–42.

19. MACAGNO, E. R., V. LOPRESTI, and C. LEVINTHAL. "Structure and Development of Neuronal Connections in Isogenic Organisms: Variation and Similarities in the Optic System of *Daphnia Magna,*" *Proc. Natl. Acad. Sci. USA,* 70 (1973) 57–61.

20. MOSCONA, A. A. "Cell Aggregation: Properties of Specific Cell-ligands and Their Role in the Formation of Multicellular Systems," *Dev. Biol.,* 18 (1968), 250–277.

21. ROBERTS, R. B. and L. B. FLEXNER. "The Biochemical Basis of Long-Term Memory," *Q. Rev. Biophys.,* 2 (1969), 135–173.

22. ROSEN, S., J. KAFKA, D. SIMPSON, and S. H. BARONDES. "Developmentally Regulated, Carbohydrate Binding Protein in *Dictyostelium discoideum,*" *Proc. Natl. Acad. Sci. USA,* 70 (1973), 2554–2557.

23. SELVERSTON, A. I. and B. MULLONEY. "Synaptic and Structural Analysis of a Small Neural System," in F. O. Schmitt and F. Worden, eds., *The Neurosciences: A Third Study Program,* Cambridge: M.I.T. Press, 1973.

24. SPERRY, R. W. "Chemoaffinity in the Orderly Growth of Nerve Fiber Patterns and Connections.," *Proc. Natl. Acad. Sci. USA,* 50 (1963), 703–710.

CHAPTER 5

ELECTRICAL ACTIVITY OF THE CENTRAL NERVOUS SYSTEM*

Enoch Callaway, III

SHERRINGTON,[41] with his poet's eye, saw the brain as magically weaving a fabric of flashing and moving points of light. The passings of these fanciful shuttles in the enchanted loom of the cerebral cortex are in reality marked by shifting electrical potentials. In the brain itself the shifting potentials are exquisitely detailed and specific. Some are sharp, brief, and all-or-none; others are slow, persistent, and graded. At the surface of the head these potentials are attenuated and mixed. Much of the fine detail is blurred, but even so there is more than enough detail to go around since investigators are continuing to find new clues about what the brain is doing

* The author is indebted to Mrs. Keiko LeVasseur for her work on both the illustrations and the manuscript, to Dr. Charles Yeager for the EEGs in the figures, and to Mrs. Hilary Naylar for the AEP Figure.

by studying this cerebral electrical activity.

These shifting potentials on the surface of the head are referred to as the electroencephalographic activity and a recording of this activity is, of course, an electroencephalogram. The initials "EEG" serve to indicate both the activity and its record. The EEG was probably first described by R. Caton, in 1875, but the human EEG was the discovery of Hans Berger.[1] Berger was a psychiatrist and hoped the EEG would provide clues about the function of the mind. The logic is simple: if the EEG reflects operations of the brain, and if the brain determines functions of the mind, then the EEG should tell us something about the mind. That syllogism has sustained an amazing number of people in the faith that the EEG somehow contains clues as to mental processes. It sustained them during a long period when empirical support was scanty at best. Now, however, there is increasing evidence that the EEG does have psychological significance and there is even reason to hope that it may have practical applications in areas more psychological than neurological. But such was not always the case.

◖ The Physiology of the EEG, or Does It Come from the Brain?

People have seriously questioned whether the EEG really has anything to do with brain function. Thus, Kennedy[32] insisted that a lot of brain electrical activity could be the result of shock waves produced by the arterial pulse passing through the polarized jell of the brain. More recently Lippold[34] contended that oscillation of the eyeball produced a major part of the EEG. Without going into all the details, it seems now that these theories can by and large be rejected;[8] not that some of the EEG may not be due to things unrelated to neural activity. Muscles, eye movement, even mechanical events inside the skull may make their contribution to the EEG. Nonetheless, it seems fairly clear that most of the EEG originates in neural activity of the brain. The dendrites and cell bodies of neurons in the cortex are continually responding to incoming volleys by graded potential changes. These postsynaptic changes may be inhibitory or excitatory. The sum of these changes at the surface of the head probably account for much of the EEG. The orientations of the neuronal population, as well as the changes in dendritic polarization, influence what happens at the surface, and the possibilities in the cortex are large enough to account for almost anything that could occur. In special cases (the evoked responses, to be considered later) we know that certain arriving volleys depolarize apical dendrites that are oriented toward the surface of the head, and the result is a surface negative wave. In other cases, such as the far–field evoked potentials,[29] volleys coursing along deep tracks of white matter may produce a positive wave at the surface if the action potentials are not moving at right angles to the electrode. Usually these far–field waves are much smaller than the slow potentials. Thus we have a rough idea of how the EEG could be generated, if not a detailed picture of how it is actually produced. The actual EEG is much like what one might expect from the first of the two sources just described. In general, most of the EEG is made up of relatively high voltage—50 microvolts (abbreviated μv) slow waves—Hertz—up to 20 Hertz (abbreviated, Hz) or cycles per second—and these probably arise principally from the cortex.

◖ Form of the EEG

If you want to put an active electrode on someone's head to measure an electrical potential, you will of course have to decide where to put another electrode, for a potential is a difference between two points. Sometimes we try to find an inactive reference (monopolar recording) but this is always relative since there is no true electrically inactive site on the human body. Alternatively we can record between two active sites, but that has obvious problems, too, for it is very hard to tell whether a particular potential change is due to a drop in potential in one of the active electrodes or an increase in potential at the other.

Suppose, however, we choose the ear lobe as a relatively inactive site and put our so-called active electrode at the occiput. There we will usually be able to record a prominent sine-wavelike electrical activity at about 10 Hz in frequency and about 50 μv in amplitude. These are the alpha waves and they tend to appear when one is alert, relaxed, and ready to look but not yet visualizing anything. Close inspection of an EEG record will reveal other waves, including faster, lower voltage, so-called beta waves; slower theta waves; and occasionally even slower delta waves.

These Greek letter designations have now been formally defined by international agreement. Delta is below 4 Hz. Theta includes activity from 4 Hz up to but not including 8 Hz. Alpha goes from 8 Hz up to but not including 13 Hz, and beta goes from 13 Hz to above 30 Hz.

The form of the EEG can be described in terms of the visual impressions obtained by a trained encephalographer. One can also obtain an automatic frequency analysis which gives a power spectrum. This spectrum specifies the power at each frequency. The third common automatic approach is the period or line cross analysis which gives a measure of the abundance of waves with specific time periods between the instants that they cross the base line. "Period" is, of course, the reciprocal of "frequency," but conventional period analysis substitutes "abundance" for "power"—so although the two automatic analyses are related, they are not identical. Finally, if the power spectrum is obtained mathematically by Fourier analysis, one can also obtain coherence measures to specify relations between various areas of the brain.[4,15]

In general, children have high voltage and lower frequencies in the EEGs. Voltages fall and frequencies increase both with maturity and with arousal. The highly alert subject usually shows a low voltage beta record. When he is moderately alert but not specifically attending, higher voltage alpha waves appear. With falling alertness, alpha may disappear and slow theta waves may appear. When sleep commences, however, a complex sequence of EEG changes may be observed, and these will be considered in Chapter 8 on sleep.

The EEG from different sites on the head may also differ. As noted, alpha is most prominent at the occiput, and beta is more prominent frontally. The two hemispheres may also differ, and this also may be a function of the state of the subject.

For example, when the subject is engaged in a verbal task such as composing a letter, the EEG on the left, the "language" or "propositional"[2] hemisphere, is suppressed—much as alpha at the occipital "visual area" is suppressed by involvement in visual activity. By contrast, a nonverbal task such as mirror trac-

ing will suppress the EEG over the right or "appositional" hemisphere.[22]

⟨ The Neurologist's EEG—Epilepsy and Gross Intercranial Pathology

This basic EEG with its dominant occipital alpha was described by Berger.[1] The next developments, however, were of more interest to neurologists than psychiatrists. If there is a space-occupying lesion in the cranium, the EEG may reflect this. The EEG may be suppressed over the lesion itself and at the edges of the lesion irritation may cause sharp spikes and abnormal slow waves to appear. Thus the EEG can help in the localization of a brain tumor. Gross pathological alterations of consciousness are frequently reflected in the EEG just as are those gross normal alterations of consciousness referred to as sleep. Figure 5–1 shows a normal EEG and EEGs from patients in two common pathological states: the EEG of a patient in hepatic coma and that of a postalcoholic psychiatric patient receiving large doses of several tranquilizing drugs.

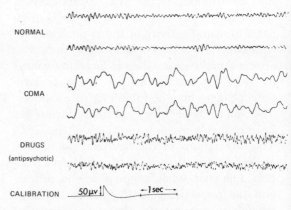

NORMAL

COMA

DRUGS
(antipsychotic)

CALIBRATION   50μv   ←1sec→

Figure 5–1.   Samples of EEGs showing a normal record, a record from a patient in hepatic coma, and a record from a patient with a history of alcoholism and psychosis who was receiving both phenothiazines and chlordiazepoxide.

Usually when patients have epileptic fits the EEG will also show signs of this. Petit mal attacks are characteristically accompanied by so–called spike and wave discharges, with typical alternating slow and fast waves. Grand mal seizures are marked by a buildup of activity that continues until the brain seems to be in the throes of an electrical storm. This is followed by deathlike stillness during the early parts of the postictal coma. Psychomotor fits may be accompanied by spiking discharges in the temporal area. These typical patterns are illustrated in Figure 5–2. Unfortunately, these pretty pictures are not as consistent as one would like. It may be very hard to catch an epileptic having a major fit and some people who have EEGs that look simply awful still manage to function surprisingly well. This imperfect correspondence between the EEG and

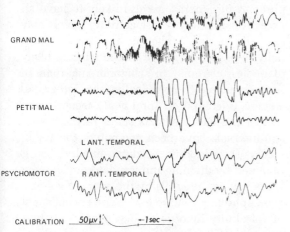

GRAND MAL

PETIT MAL

L ANT. TEMPORAL

PSYCHOMOTOR   R ANT. TEMPORAL

CALIBRATION   50μν   ←1sec→

Figure 5–2. Samples of EEG illustrating a brief major seizure (grand mal), spikes and waves accompanying an "absence" (petit mal), and a spiking discharge from the right temporal focus of a patient with psychomotor seizures.

clinical epilepsy is puzzling. The normal EEG in the clinical epileptic is not so bad; we can always rationalize that we've missed the fit or that the electrical signs of the fit are buried too deep in the brain to be picked up at the scalp. But the ability of some people to function when a large part of the brain is obviously having an electrical fit is unsettling for those of us who would like one-to-one correlations between behavior and the EEG.

If the above suggests the EEG may be a rubber crutch, this is not accidental. The surface EEG may give support to a clinical im-

pression and as such is justifiable. But the danger is that it may be used to justify poor clinical practice. For example, a geriatrics expert presented data on the EEG changes found in aging. Eighty percent of his cases who subsequently had demonstrable central nervous system (CNS) damage had an abnormal EEG. However, thirty percent who never developed evidence of CNS damage also had similarly abnormal EEGs. He concluded that the absence of EEG abnormalities should make one sensitive to the possibility of psychological problems. Should one also conclude that the presence of abnormal EEGs in a patient should allow one to ignore the possibility of psychological problems? I'm sure our geriatrics expert would be horrified at such a conclusion. No doubt he'd agree that optimum attention to psychological problems should be accorded to each person. Nonetheless, the EEG can be and, sad to say, often is an excuse for suboptimum clinical practice.

To summarize, we can say that the routine EEG arises mostly from graded potentials in the cortical feltwork. It reflects gross changes, such as sleep, space-occupying lesions, fits and death. An abnormal interictal EEG is common in seizure patients but not invariable, and abnormal EEGs can be encountered in people who never have had epilepsy. In short, outside of an overt major seizure, the correlation between epilepsy and EEG is statistical and not absolute. Most important, a normal EEG does not rule out gross cerebral pathology, nor does an abnormal EEG rule out psychologically mediated disability.

⟪ The EEG and Psychiatry

While the EEG was being applied to neurological problems (with more or less success), psychiatrists and psychologists worked, too, but with somewhat less to show for their efforts. Over the years, simple visual analysis of the EEG record has been supplanted by sophisticated and elegant computer-based systems, but psychologically relevant findings still remain controversial and meager on the whole.

Ellingson[16] and Vogel and Broverman[50,51] carried on an informative controversy about the relationship of the EEG to intelligence. Ellingson concluded that the EEG only correlated with intelligence by virtue of the fact that people with gross brain damage were more likely to have abnormal EEGs and to be less intelligent than people who had not suffered in this way. Vogel et al. marshaled considerable evidence to indicate that Ellingson was perhaps unduly pessimistic. But Ellingson's point is one to be taken seriously.

There has been some talk that slow EEGs (EEGs with lower frequency alpha) are associated with slower minds. Work on that continues,[46] but the best bet is that no such simple correlation will be found. Correlations between EEG variables and such psychological traits as rigidity, automatizing, etc., continue to be reported from time to time.[52] The EEG reflects the level of arousal, and since the level of a subject's arousal during specific situations will be related to such things as past experience, personality, and intelligence, it's not surprising to find that EEG–personality correlations occur.

The relations between the EEG and the level of arousal are also a factor in studies on the effects of psychotropic drugs. Using elegant computer techniques, Fink and Itil[20,21] have been able to show some more or less drug–specific EEG changes, but again, by and large, the EEG is more a function of the arousal of the subject than is the specific pharmacological agent employed. Social experience with alcohol should be sufficient for the reader to supply his own illustrations of how alcohol in equivalent doses can result in heightened interest and activity on one occasion (alcohol with friends at a cocktail party) and somnolence on another (alcohol alone in a strange hotel room). The EEG will in general reflect the state of the subject more than the dose of the drug.

EEG correlates in psychopathology also exist, and again the arousal factor may be important. There is some controversy about the correlation between the so-called six and fourteen EEG pattern and the psychopathic personality.[25] These six and fourteen patterns are made up of mixed slow and fast waves and occur rather commonly in adolescents and youths, particularly when the subject is drowsy. The specific relationship of this to psychopathology is questionable, but one might wonder if psychopathic teenagers get drowsy in a testing situation faster than non-psychopathic teenagers.

The schizophrenic syndrome has also been associated with specific EEG patterns. In chronic, process, organiclike schizophrenics who show poor responses to phenothiazine drugs, one is likely to encounter abundant hyperstable alpha activity.[27] In addition, schizophrenics in general are also likely to have an excessive amount of fast activity, which may give the record a choppy appearance.[11] Finally, integrated voltage of the EEG is likely to be less variable in schizophrenia than in normal people.[23] Specifically, the integrated voltage is computed for twenty-second samples of the EEG. After a series of these voltage intervals have been computed, the coefficient of variability is determined. This is obtained by dividing the standard deviation of these voltage integrals by the average voltage. Schizophrenics tend to have a lower coefficient of variability than do normal people. Average voltage itself does not distinguish schizophrenics from normal people so well, but the hyperstability does.

This again may be a function of arousal. The schizophrenic appears by many criteria to be in a chronic, poorly modulated state of hyperarousal. The normal person will show wide fluctuations in arousal during a testing session, and this may be reflected in a high coefficient of variability. The schizophrenic, on the other hand, is fixed in his anxious, defensive state and is notably lacking in adaptive plasticity, both by behavioral and by physiological criteria. This view, which attributes low coefficient of variability in schizophrenia to hyperarousal, finds support in the observation that amphetamine decreases and sedation increases the EEG coefficient of variability.

(Alpha Feedback

Behavioral modification by operant techniques is receiving more and more interest. Autonomic and other nonskeletal muscle (involuntary) responses were once supposed to be modifiable only by classical or Pavlovian conditioning. Some of the early attempts to test this dictum involved experiments intended to bring EEG alpha activity under operant control, since EEG alpha activity was considered a good example of involuntary behavior that was readily accessible to measurement. Although recently called into question,[24] the work of DiCara[12] and Neal Miller has apparently proved that involuntary behavior can be operantly conditioned. In the meanwhile, the pioneering work of Kamiya[31] indicated that the EEG alpha rhythm can also be brought under operant control. The method is fundamentally simple. The state of the EEG is made known to the subject. This can be done by providing a tone when the alpha waves are above a certain voltage. The subject is then asked to turn the tones on or off. Subjects learn to control the tones when they have no idea about the mediating physiological event.

The interpretation of these findings is something else. Eye position can affect alpha abundance, and just concentrating on tone bursts will also tend to increase alpha activity. Of equal interest, however, is the fact that subjects tend to enjoy turning on alpha, and they report subjective experiences similar to those described by subjects involved in religious meditation. Finally, certain religious men who have become expert at meditation (Zen Buddhist priests, yoga teachers, etc.) appear to have unusual abilities to control their alpha activity.

This work on alpha control has important implications both for research on states of consciousness and for studies of comparative religions. Because of its exotic nature, it has captured the popular fancy. Varieties of do-it-yourself alpha-control programs are available, and some promise to help the purchaser obtain Nirvana quickly and painlessly. Some of these popularizations are naive to say the least. Others are frankly fraudulent. The fundamental importance of this work, however, should not be obscured by the fringe of carnival fast-buck operators it has attracted.

(How to Average Evoked Potentials

The conventional EEG reflects global states. Death, fits, sleep, and general level of arousal can be determined with fair reliability. One suspects that correlations between more subtle psychological variables and the gross EEG also depend on indirect relations between the psychological variable, experimental conditions, and the resulting level of arousal in the subject.

The EEG, after all, looks at what the brain is doing moment by moment and since the waking brain is always busy at a variety of tasks, the potentials at the surface of the scalp are like a potpourri. Individual ingredients are hard to separate out and we notice principally the overall quality. How can we see potentials reflecting specific mental processes when they are buried in so much incidental activity? There are a variety of tricks, but most depend on getting the brain to repeat a specific act several times. If the incidental electrical babbling is random with respect to the specific activity in question, we can hope to distinguish between the repeating specific electrical events, and the other random or "noise" events.

The easiest trick is to average. As in all averaging procedures, the hope is that interfering variables will cancel out, leaving us with an accurate representation of the more or less consistent variable of interest. Specific brain responses can be seen in recordings from the cortex, and in some subjects, responses to single sensory stimuli are large enough to be apparent in the raw EEG in spite of all the background noise. Thus, evoked responses were known before averaging techniques were developed. The evoked response era, however, really began with averaging.

At first a variety of methods were tried. These included photographic techniques, magnetic tape methods, and so on. Condenser charging averagers are still used for special purposes, but today digital computers have pretty much won the day. The usual method demands that we know more or less precisely when an event is occurring in the brain. We present a series of events and after each event, we take a set of samples of brain electrical activity timed as precisely as possible with the event. These voltages are converted to numbers in a computer, and voltage-values for corresponding times–after–stimulation are averaged. The simplest illustration is a sensory–evoked response. If the stimulus is repeated over and over, we can hope that the subject will respond in more or less the same way to each repeated representation. Figure 5–3 illustrates how average brain wave samples

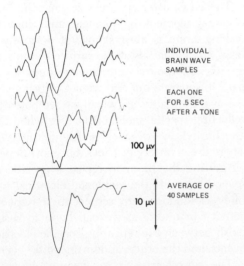

INDIVIDUAL BRAIN WAVE SAMPLES

EACH ONE FOR .5 SEC AFTER A TONE

100 μv

AVERAGE OF 40 SAMPLES

10 μv

Figure 5–3. The first five EEG samples of a set of forty samples are shown above the line, and the average of all forty are shown below the line. This subject had unusually large evoked responses in the first few samples.

taken during the half second following a click can be averaged to disclose the averaged evoked potential, or AEP. The AEP is almost the electrical by-product of the specific CNS event. We can only say "almost," however, because of the requirement of averaging. The whole averaging process is based on the idea that the same response is evoked repeatedly, so that it can be made to stand out against the background noise. In fact, the brain rarely

does anything exactly the same way twice, much less repeatedly, and the more important and complex the mental event is, the less likely it is to be repeated precisely.

❨ Sensory-Evoked Responses and Neonatal Audiometry

Since the closest approach to repetitive brain response is its response to a periodic, meaningless sensory stimulus, evoked responses to such stimuli were the first to engage the attention of investigators, and it is not surprising that the most generally accepted clinical application of the AEP uses sensory–evoked responses to test sensory function.

By and large, if you want to find out if someone has received a stimulus, the best way is to ask him. Evoked responses become clinically useful when the person cannot or will not talk, or when we need some extralinguistic point of reference. Neonates can't talk, and it's important to determine promptly if they have hearing loss so that steps can be taken to supply sensory stimulation. Otherwise, there may be a permanent loss of sensory function. As one might expect, the ability to obtain an auditory–evoked response from an infant is suggestive evidence that the child is able to hear.[10] It isn't proof since very large sounds can apparently produce an evoked response by their effect on the cochlear system, while, on the other hand, some children, and even adults, may fail to show demonstrable evoked responses and yet have intact hearing. In spite of these problems, evoked–response audiometry in neonates is in fairly wide clinical use today.*

Auditory–evoked responses have another practical application in the study of neonates. Gestational age can be measured in a number of ways. Best, of course, would be to know exactly when the child was conceived, but sometimes that isn't feasible. Weight at birth

* There now exists the ERA-Club (Evoked Response Audiometry) and the informative proceedings of their first international symposium have been published in English in Band 198, Heft 1, 1971 of *Archiv für Klinische und Experimentelle Ohren-Nasen- und Kehlkopfheilkunde.*

is also related to the gestational age, but some children are born unusually small or unusually large, even at term. Gestational age can be estimated from the raw EEG. This is best done by using EEG to determine stages of sleep and estimating gestational age on the basis of the nature of the sleep cycle. The auditory–evoked response can also be used to measure gestational age, since the latencies of the evoked response tend to be long at first and become progressively shorter, particularly over the first six months after birth.[18] Gestational age as estimated by the evoked response at birth predicts the time at which the child will walk.[28] Gestational age, however, has very little predictive validity when it comes to any of the later talents of a child.

Evoked responses have been obtained using all of the other sensory modalities. Visual-, olfactory-, gustatory-, tactile-, and vestibular–evoked responses have been studied and, in principle, the AEP could be used to test sensory function in any of these modalities. In practice, however, the practical applications have not been impressive, although the use of visual–evoked responses for perimetry and refraction in mentally retarded subjects may prove to be of practical importance. Finally, there is promise that function of various sensory pathways and of primary sensory–receiving areas may be tested by methodically changing the nature of the stimulus and the site of recording. Such a neurophysiologically sophisticated approach may offer a useful alternative to angiography and brain scan for localizing intercerebral lesions.

(Evoked-Potential Recovery Cycles

It is fortunate for us that Shagass,[40] one of the first psychiatrists on the evoked-potential scene, has published a book that combines a review of evoked-potential work relevant to psychiatry with a thorough presentation of his own work in the field.

Much of what Shagass and his followers have done involves recovery cycles. The basic notion is that one presents a conditioning stimulus and then, after a delay, a test stimulus. There tend to be periods of increased and decreased responsiveness in the interval following the conditioning stimulus, and these recovery cycles are probed by the test stimulus.

It is somehow intuitively appealing to consider that the impaired CNS of the psychotic patient might appear less efficient on neurophysiological measures. Thus, one would predict that psychosis would be associated with depressed recovery. The test stimulus should generally evoke a smaller response in the psychotic patient. That is to say, the post conditioning-stimulus depression should persist longer.

In general, " 'patienthood' appears to be associated with diminished amplitude recovery and earlier latency recovery. . . ."[40] However, the problem is complicated by the relationship of the test response to the general level of responsiveness (as shown by a response to a test-type stimulus with no preceding conditioning stimulus) and by the dependence of the whole recovery-cycle phenomenon upon relative intensities of test and conditioning stimuli.

More recent work has shown that schizophrenics and drug abusers with a history of psychotic drug reactions both showed a reduced range of responsiveness when the intensity of the conditioning stimulus was varied. In general, the more intense the conditioning stimulus, the smaller the response to the test stimulus.

The complexity of these recovery functions may make them seem less appealing than some other simpler appearing measures. However, studies of recovery functions have provided a variety of significant correlations with psychopathology. Also, recovery functions may seem more complex simply because we know more about them (and hence about their complexity). Thus, they lay serious claim to the interest of the psychiatric investigator.

(Cognitive-Evoked Potentials

The specific activity of sensory pathways is reflected in the early components and the

AEP. These early components are of great interest to the neurologist and neurosurgeon, but are relatively insensitive to psychological factors. In fact, it is a general practice to sedate children for AEP audiometry, and to record the AEPs while the child is asleep.

The AEP does, however, have components that reflect phenomena of greater subtlety than the mere patency of sensory pathways, and these components might well be referred to as cognitive–evoked potentials.

To oversimplify a little, one can consider that there are two cognitive components to the AEP: (1) the contingent negative variation or CNV: and (2) the third positive wave or P_3 (at about 300 msec.).

If one records from the vertex and uses recording equipment with a very long time constant (i.e., with a DC or very low–frequency response), one can detect a negative–going change between a warning signal and subsequent stimulus that demands some response (imperative stimulus). This negative variation is most striking when the subject knows the imperative stimulus is contingent on the warning stimulus. Thus, it is referred to as the contingent negative variation or CNV.[53]

Specifically, suppose we use a single click as a warning, and two seconds after each click we start a train of clicks that the subject must terminate by pressing a switch. The CNV will develop in the two seconds ready period. The magnitude of the variation may be as much as 15 to 20 μv and will depend on a variety of factors.[47]

For example, it is increased by: (1) certainty that the imperative stimulus will occur. Thus it builds up with experience. (2) Interest in the imperative stimulus; and (3) physical force required to respond to the imperative stimulus.

It is reduced by (1) distraction; (2) boredom; and (3) sleep deprivation.

The CNV is correlated with behavior. In the usual paradigm, the faster the response to the imperative stimulus, the larger the CNV.[26] But this is not always the case. For example, after sleep deprivation a subject can give normal reaction times, although his CNV is completely suppressed.[36]

Physiologically the CNV probably represents an excitation or "priming" that is relatively specific. Thus, if a subject develops a CNV in readiness for a signal of 100 Hz, an interposed probe stimulus of 1000 Hz will evoke a response that is larger during larger CNVs—as though the excited state represented by the CNV augments the "probe" AEP. Such an augmentation is not found in the probe stimulus of a flash, or even a 600 Hz time.[17]

The CNV holds some promise of practical clinical utility.[35] It is reduced or absent in persons with psychopathic character disorders; it is variable in schizophrenics; it may be absent in retarded individuals; and there may be a second negative "equivocation" wave after the imperative stimulus in schizophrenics and obsessives[48]—as though they tended to have afterthoughts following their responses.

At the moment, however, practical application is a mere possibility. The real value of the CNV lies in its use as a "convergent datum"[44] in psychological constructs. For example, does the CNV represent awareness of contingency, interest, or arousal? How do we operationally define and separate these concepts? In short, the CNV and P_3 bid fair to make honest men of heretofore loosely verbigerating psychologists.

This need for operational definitions of psychological constructs becomes even more obvious when P_3 is added to the general picture.[49] Generally, the more physically intense a stimulus is, the larger the AEP components that occur before 250 msec. and the shorter are the latencies of these components. The more psychologically intense the stimulus is, the larger are the AEP components occurring after 250 msec. and the longer their latencies. Perhaps this means that physically strong stimuli get into the CNS quicker and involve more neural circuits but that psychologically more intense stimuli require more processing time—although they also call into play more neural circuits. Whether or not that neurophysiological fantasy is true, it is a useful mnemonic.

This psychological augmentation in the AEP can be seen from about one hundred msec. on, but it is not seen in the negative wave which usually occurs around two hundred msec. That wave indeed may increase with light sleep! Cognition should take more time than simple sensory registration, and it is reassuring that psychological augmentation is most striking in the late positive component.

There is some confounding between the CNV and P_3.[14] Since the expectancy of a predictable but intrinsically interesting stimulus will produce both a CNV before the stimulus and a P_3 on stimulus delivery, the question arises whether the P_3 is the "resetting" of the CNV. The best answer is to say that one can vary P_3 independently of the CNV, for the P_3 reflects the information delivered by the stimulus and the CNV reflects the subject's expectancy. On the other hand, expectancy and its accompanying arousal can influence both the information delivered by the stimulus and —perhaps independently—amplitudes of some AEP components.

In studies of attention, words like contingency, arousal, interest, uncertainty, information, etc., have a tendency to float about without anchor. CNV and P_3 seem destined to provide some means of tying these concepts down.

❰ AEP and Intelligence

Having complained about the paucity of good correlations between the EEG and complex psychological processes, it would be worse than ungrateful to complain about the embarrassment of riches provided by the AEP. For example, while the EEG provided few convincing correlations with intelligence, this is not the case for AEPs. There are at least three (and perhaps four) different aspects of the AEP that correlate with the I.Q. The four AEP aspects are: (1) latency (short latency = high I.Q.); (2) plasticity (plastic or adaptive response = high I.Q.); (3) asymmetry (asymmetrical visual AEP = high I.Q.); and (4) variability (variable response under stable conditions = low I.Q.). We will consider the

first two in some detail to convey the flavor of the problems that still exist in this area.

The first work on the AEP and the I.Q. was done by Ertl,[19] who sought a measure of neural efficiency in measures of AEP latency. The logic is impelling. A fast brain should go with a fast mind. The speed with which AEP waves appear seems to reflect the speed of the brain in processing data at least in some cases, so the latency of AEP waves in general might reflect neural speed (or efficiency) and hence provide a measure of intelligence.

There is no doubt that correlations[38,40] (on the order of $r = -0.30$) can be found between visual AEP latency and I.Q. One needs to present from one hundred to eight hundred flashes that carry no special meaning to record the AEP from a central-parietal, bipolar–electrical pair, to measure latencies to the third or fourth wave—after defining "third wave" by counting peaks from stimulus onset.

But does AEP latency reflect neural efficiency? Perhaps. However, an alternate explanation can be found in AEP plasticity, which also correlates with the I.Q. Plasticity refers to the changes in the AEP that occur with changes in the demands of the occasion. Consider an experiment reported by Dinand and Defayolle.[13] While the subject faced a projection screen, flashes were presented at the periphery of his visual field. Most of the flashes were white and AEPs to the white flashes were recorded. Occasional flashes were red and the subject had to press a key when he saw a red flash. At one sitting the subject counted the white flashes and the AEP was large. At another sitting, complex logical problems were presented on the screen and, as would be expected, AEPs to the peripheral flashes were suppressed. The change in AEP amplitude (or AEP plasticity) correlated strongly with I.Q. ($r = 0.79!$).

Now it seems that "plasticity" explains, or at least plays a role, in the correlations between AEP latency and I.Q. Shucard[43] replicated Ertl's work, adding two conditions. First, subjects pressed a key to each flash, then they counted each flash, and finally, as in Ertl's procedure, they just watched. AEP amplitudes were highest and latencies longest, when the flashes required an immediate response. Latency-I.Q. correlations were smallest when subjects were alert and responding, and largest when the subject just watched the flashes. Finally, the drop in AEP amplitude from the first (attending) to the last (nonattending) condition also correlated significantly with I.Q. After the entire session, bright subjects rated themselves as more bored than did the dull subjects. If bright subjects become bored more quickly, then in a moderately boring situation, they would develop smaller AEPs with shorter latencies than would dull subjects. In other words, bright subjects, by being more "plastic," develop shorter latencies, and thus "plasticity" rather than "neural efficiency" may account for Ertl's finding.

The stories for the other AEP-I.Q. correlations are equally complex at this time but perhaps the above gives enough of the flavor of things to warn the reader against the uncritical ingestion of the brief survey that follows.

Rhodes et al.[39] found that differences in visual AEP amplitudes recorded over the left and right hemispheres are greater in bright subjects. Lairy et al.[33] also found alpha averages (averages triggered on alpha peaks rather than on stimuli) more asymmetrical in bright subjects. Conners,[9] on the other hand, found striking AEP asymmetry in severe dyslexia; so asymmetry cannot be taken uncritically as an indication of a good intellect.

Variability refers to the trial–to–trial changes in the individual evoked potential (EP), and it cannot be measured in a single AEP. Schizophrenic patients have more variable EPs than do nonschizophrenic patients.[6] Among schizophrenics, nonparanoids are more variable than paranoids. Over a period of time, a given patient will show increased EP variability when his thought–process disorder worsens, and decreased EP variability when he improves.[30]

In children, EP variability is high and measures of EP variability are inversely correlated with age from six years to sixteen years.

Since with more maturity and less schizophrenia, EPs tend to be more stable, it is not surprising that correlations between EP vari-ability and I.Q. can be found.[7] Here too, there are problems. Measurements of EP variability are complex and sometimes difficult to interpret. For example, EP variability and background EEG are inextricably confounded. Then, too, maturity and cognitive stability are not perfect correlates of intelligence. We all know very bright colleagues who are quite immature and who may even be a trifle schizophrenic.

⟮ Cognitive Style

Perhaps one of the hazards in the way of applying AEPs to psychiatric problems lies in our tendency to try to force the information we get from AEPs into psychological constructs like I.Q., which are not all that good in the first place.

We mentioned above how EP variability is high in schizophrenia. This tells us more about how a schizophrenic thinks than about any innate disease process. Everybody knows that schizophrenics tend to show more variability in almost every sphere of behavior than is normal. However, certain sorts of simple tasks will allow the schizophrenic to perform with as little variability as a nonschizophrenic. With such a task, the schizophrenic's EPs are also no more variable than normal.

Thus, the late components of the AEP may best be looked on as another way of examining cognitive process rather than as a way of looking at fundamental neuropsychological substrates.

There are many new studies using AEPs to examine relatively enduring patterns of cognitive functioning, which (to borrow a term popular among psychologists a decade ago) we may call cognitive style. There are fascinating AEP studies of attention deployment and field dependence, but some consideration of repression and augmenting-reducing will serve again to give the flavor of the field. The field is moving so fast that by the time this is published the fine details will be in need of revision anyway.

The concept of augmenting-reducing goes back to the work of Petrie,[37] but has been considerably elaborated by Buchsbaum and Silverman.[5] With increasing stimulus intensity, there is a tendency for all responses to increase, and this is true also for AEP amplitude. In many subjects, however, intense stimuli result in responses that may be smaller than those evoked with moderately strong stimuli. This seems to reflect the operation of a kind of automatic gain control whereby subjects who are particularly sensitive to low level stimuli can avoid being damaged by high level stimuli. Subjects with particularly active automatic vain controls will "reduce" their AEP amplitudes at high stimulus intensities and they are referred to as "reducers." Those with a more monotonic stimulus–intensity, AEP–amplitude function are called "augmenters." One's position on the augmenter-reducer continuum does seem to be a more or less enduring trait. It also seems to correlate with certain pathology. For example, lithium-responsive manics are augmenters while manic and lithium converts them into reducers.[3]

The concept of repression is much more familiar. Shevrin et al.[42] defined repression on the basis of Rorschach responses. For the evoked–response portion of the study, they used either meaningful or nonmeaningful stimuli and presented the stimuli tachistoscopically so briefly that the subject could not consciously recognize them. Repressed subjects tended to show smaller evoked responses to the meaningful stimuli and larger responses to the nonmeaningful stimuli than did the nonrepressed subjects. The repressed subjects also gave fewer responses in their free associations that could be related to the meaningful stimulus. By contrast, when the stimuli were presented supraliminally (i.e., when they were presented for thirty msec. so that the subjects could clearly recognize the content of the meaningful stimuli) repressed subjects then gave larger responses to the meaningful stimuli and smaller responses to the nonmeaningful stimuli. Although this work has no immediate clinical utility, it does provide valuable convergent data on the concept of repression.

(Conclusion

As this is written, there are no established clinical procedures using the EEG that are relevant to the diagnosis and treatment of psychological problems, but I suspect that this is a temporary state of affairs.

The EEG will continue to supply clues when one is tracking down epilepsy or considering a gross intercranial lesion. Soon evoked potentials and other computer-based techniques (i.e., cross spectra) may become routine tools to help select the proper medication for psychotic patients. We may use such techniques to distinguish between various forms of minimal brain dysfunction in children. In special situations, they may supplement more conventional intelligence tests.

Before all the details are agreed on, there will be a time when extravagant claims and unrealistic expectations will make optimum use of these new tools most difficult. To keep a proper perspective, it is useful to consider that the EEG and its computer-derived products (such as the AEP) are examples of brain-controlled behavior. Some such behavior is simple and stereotyped, like pupillary reflexes —or early components of sensory AEPs. Other such behavior may be complex and rich in psychological significance as, for example, language and cognitive-evoked responses. Although arcane electronic devices may be used to observe and record this electrical behavior, it is neither more nor less "biological" than any other sort of behavior. When a man says he is frightened, we look for other convergent data such as tremor, sweating palms, facial pallor, etc. to determine what inferences to make. We generally use several sorts of behavior to make inferences both about the structure of a person's brain and about its functions. EEGs and AEPs have more degrees of freedom than do the other types of behavior that don't depend upon skeletal muscles. So far there are only a handful of people who have voluntary control of their brain–electrical behavior. Thus, such behavior is resistant but not immune to mendacity.

In brief, newer techniques for observing and recording brain–electrical potentials give us access to a rich new set of behavior that can be used as other sorts of behavior are used, in the study of the human mind.

❪ Bibliography

1. BERGER, H. "Uber das Elektrekephalogramm des Menschen," *Arch. Psychiat. Nervenkr.*, 87 (1929), 527–570.
2. BOGEN, J. E. "The Other Side of the Brain I, II, III," *Bull. Los Angeles Neurol. Soc.*, 34 (1969), 73–105, 135–162, 191–220.
3. BORGE, G. F., M. BUCHSBAUM, F. GOODWIN et al. "Neuropsychological Correlates of Affective Disorders," *Arch. Gen. Psychiatry*, 24 (1971), 501–504.
4. BRAZIER, M. A. B. "Varieties of Computer Analysis of Electrophysiological Potentials," *Electroencephalogr. Clin. Neurophysiol.*, Supplement 26 (1967), 1–8.
5. BUCHSBAUM, M. and J. SILVERMAN. "Stimulus Intensity Control and the Cortical Evoked Response," *Psychosom. Med.*, 30 (1968), 12–22.
6. CALLAWAY, E., R. T. JONES, and E. DONCHIN. "Auditory Evoked Potential Variability in Schizophrenia," *Electroencephalogr. Clin. Neurophysiol.*, 29 (1970), 421–428.
7. CALLAWAY, E. and G. C. STONE. "Evoked Response Methods for the Study of Intelligence," *Agressologie*, 10 (1969), 535–539.
8. CHAPMAN, R. M., C. R. CAVONIUS, and J. T. ERNST. "Alpha and Kappa Electroencephalogram Activity in Eyeless Subjects," *Science*, 171 (1971), 1159–1161.
9. CONNERS, C. K. "Cortical Evoked Response in Children with Learning Disorders," *Psychophysiology*, 7 (1970), 418–428.
10. DAVIS, H. and S. ZERLIN. "Acoustic Relations of the Human Vertex Potential," *J. Acoust. Soc. Am.*, 39 (1966), 109–116.
11. DAVIS, P. A. "Comparative Study of the EEGS of Schizophrenic and Manic-Depressive Patients," *Am. J. Psychiatry*, 99 (1942), 210–217.
12. DiCARA, L. V. "Learning in the Autonomic Nervous System," *Sci. Am.*, 222 (1970), 30–39.
13. DINARD, J. P. and M. DEFAYOLLE. "Utilisation des potentiels évoques moyennes pour l'estimation de la charge mentale," Centre de Récherches du Service de Santé des Armées (Division de Psychologie), 1969. Unpublished paper.
14. DONCHIN, E. and D. B. D. SMITH. "The Contingent Negative Variation and the Late Positive Wave of the Averaged Evoked Potential," *Electroencephalogr. Clin. Neurophysiol.*, 29 (1970), 201–203.
15. DUMMERMUTH, G., P. J. HUBER, B. KLEINER et al. "Numerical Analysis of Electroencephalographic Data," *IEEE Trans. Audio Electroacoustics*, AU–18 (1970), 404–411.
16. ELLINGSON, R. J. "Relationship between EEG and Intelligence: A Commentary," *Psychol. Bull.*, 65 (1966), 91–98.
17. ELLIS, R. R. *Attention, Intention, and the Contingent Negative Variation Phenomenon*. Ph.D. thesis. University of Nebraska, 1970. Unpublished.
18. ENGEL, R., and B. V. BUTLER. "Individual Differences in Neonatal Photic Responses in the Light of Test Performances at 8 Months of Age," *Electroencephalogr. Clin. Neurophysiol.*, 26 (1969), 237.
19. ERTL, J. and E. W. P. SCHAFER. "Brain Response Correlates to Psychometric Intelligence," *Nature*, 223 (1969), 421–422.
20. FINK, M. "EEG Classification of Psychoactive Compounds in Man," *Psychopharmacology—A Review of Progress 1957–1967*. Washington: U.S. Govt. Print Off., 1968.
21. FINK, M. and R. ITIL. "EEG and Human Psychopharmacology," in *Psychopharmacology: A Review of Progress 1957–1967*. Washington: U.S. Govt. Print. Off., 1968.
22. GALIN, D., R. ORNSTEIN, K. KOCEL et al. "Hemispheric Localization of Cognitive Mode by EEG," *Psychophysiology*, 8 (1970), 248–249.
23. GOLDSTEIN, L., A. A. SUGERMAN, H. STOLBERG et al. "Electro–cerebral Activity in Schizophrenics and Non–psychotic Subjects: Quantitative EEG Amplitude Analysis," *Electroencephalogr. Clin. Neurophysiol.*, 19 (1965), 350–361.
24. HARRIS, A. H. and J. V. BRADY. "Animal Learning, Visceral and Autonomic Conditioning," *Annu. Rev. Psycho.*, 25 (1974), 107–133.
25. HENRY, C. E. "Positive Spike Discharges in the EEG and Behavior Abnormality," in

G. Glaser, ed., *EEG and Behavior*, pp. 315–344. New York: Basic Books, 1963.

26. HILLYARD, S. A. "Relationships Between the Contingent Negative Variation (CNV) and Reaction Time," *Physiology and Behavior*, 4 (1969), 351–357.

27. ITIL, T. M. *Elektroencephalographische Studien Bei Endogenen Psychosen und Deren Behandlung mit Psychotropen Medikamenten unter Besonderer Berucksichtigung des Pentothal–Elektroencephalogramms.* Istanbul: Ahmet Sait Matbaasi, 1964.

28. JENSEN, D. R. and R. ENGEL. "Statistical Procedures for Relative Dichotomous Responses to Maturation and EEG Measurements," *Electroencephalogr. Clin. Neurophysiol.*, 30 (1971), 437–443.

29. JEWETT, D. L., M. N. ROMANO, and J. S. WILLISTON. "Human Auditory Evoked Potentials: Possible Brain Stem Components Detected on the Scalp," *Science*, 167 (1970), 1517–1518.

30. JONES, R. T. and E. CALLAWAY. "Auditory Evoked Responses in Schizophrenia: A Reassessment," *Biol. Psychiatry*, 2 (1970), 291–298.

31. KAMIYA, J. "Conscious Control of Brain Waves," *Psychol. Today*, 1 (1968), 57–60.

32. KENNEDY, J. L. "A Possible Artifact in Electroencephalography," *Psychol. Rev.*, 66 (1959), 307–313.

33. LAIRY, G. C., A. REMOND, H. RIEGER et al. "The Alpha Average. III. Clinical Application in Children," *Electroencephalogr. Clin. Neurophysiol.*, 26 (1969), 453–467.

34. LIPPOLD, O. C. J. and G. E. K. NOVOTNY. "Is Alpha Rhythm an Artifact," *Lancet*, 1 (1970), 976–979.

35. MACCALLUM, W. C. and W. G. WALTER. "La Variation contingente négative en psychiatrie." Report presented at Colloque sur l'Etude de la variation contingente négative. Liège, 1967.

36. NAITOH, P., L. C. JOHNSON, and A. LUBIN. "Modification of Surface Negative Slow Potential (CNV) in the Human Brain after Total Sleep Loss," *Electroencephalogr. Clin. Neurophysiol.*, 30 (1971), 17–22.

37. PETRIE, A. *Individuality in Pain and Suffering.* Chicago: University of Chicago Press, 1967.

38. PLUM, A. *Visual Evoked Responses: Their Relationship to Intelligence.* Ph.D. thesis. University of Florida, 1969. Unpublished.

39. RHODES, L. E., R. E. DUSTMAN, and E. C. BECK. "Visually Evoked Potentials of Bright and Dull Children," *Electroencephalogr. Clin. Neurophysiol.*, 26 (1969), 237.

40. SHAGASS, C. *Evoked Brain Potentials in Psychiatry.* New York: Plenum Press 1972.

41. SHERRINGTON, C. S. *Man on His Nature*, 2nd ed. London: Cambridge University Press, 1952.

42. SHEVRIN, H., W. H. SMITH, and D. E. FRITZLER. "Repressiveness as a Factor in the Subliminal Activation of Brain and Verbal Responses," *J. Nerv. Ment. Dis.*, 140 (1969), 261–269.

43. SHUCARD, D. W. and J. L. HORN. "Evoked Cortical Potentials and Measurement of Human Abilities," *J. Comp. Physiol. Psychol.*, 78 (1972), 29–68.

44. SKINNER, P. and F. ANTINORO. "Auditory Evoked Responses in Normal Hearing Adults and Children Before and During Sedation," *J. Speech Hear. Res.*, 12 (1969), 394–401.

45. STOYVA, J. and J. KAMIYA. "Electrophysiological Studies of Dreaming as the Prototype of a New Strategy in the Study of Consciousness," *Psychol. Rev.*, 75 (1968), 192–205.

46. SURWILLO, W. W. "Relationship Between EEG Activation and Reaction Time," *Percept. Mot. Skills*, 29 (1969), 3–7.

47. TECCE, J. J. "Contingent Negative Variation and Individual Differences," *Arch. Gen. Psychiatry*, 24 (1971), 1–16.

48. TIMSIT, M., N. KONINCKY, J. DARGENT et al. "Variations contingentes et psychiatrie," *Electroencephalogr. Clin. Neurophysiol.*, 28 (1970), 41–47.

49. TUETING, P., S. SUTTON, and J. ZUBIN. "Quantitative Evoked Potential Correlates of the Probability of Events," *Psychophysiology*, 7 (1970), 385–394.

50. VOGEL, W. and D. M. BROVERMAN. "Relationship Between EEG and Test Intelligence: A Critical Review," *Psychol. Bull.*, 65 (1964), 132–144.

51. ———. "A Reply to 'Relationship Between EEG and Test Intelligence: A Commentary,'" *Psychol. Bull.*, 65 (1966), 99–109.

52. VOGEL, W., D. M. BROVERMAN, E. L. KLAI-
BER et al. "EEG Response to Photic Stimulation as a Function of Cognitive Style,"
Electroencephalogr. Clin. Neurophysiol.,
27 (1969), 186–190.

53. WALTER, W. G. "Slow Potential Changes
in the Human Brain Associated with Expectancy, Decision and Intention," *Electroencephalogr. Clin. Neurophysiol.*, Supplement 26 (1967), 123–130.

CHAPTER 6

THE LIMBIC SYSTEM: AN ANATOMICAL AND FUNCTIONAL ORIENTATION

Jack De Groot

(Introduction

MORE THAN three centuries ago, Thomas Willis[83] referred to a ring of cortical regions resembling a boundary zone or border (limbus) around the brainstem as "cerebri limbus." One illustration, ascribed to Sir Christopher Wren, the architect of St. Paul's Cathedral in London, corresponds in part to Figure 6–1(b). It is not clear whether Broca[14] was aware of this term in 1878 when he described the occurrence of a phylogenetically ancient portion of the cerebral cortex in several vertebrate species as "le grand lobe limbique"; in man, this designation included the subcallosal, cingulate, and parahippocampal gyri, as well as some portions of the hippocampal formation.

Extensive comparative anatomical studies*

* See references 31, 38, 41, 59, 65, and 74.

on the development and evolution of the forebrain followed Broca's investigation. Most of the descriptions were based on normal, that is nonexperimental material: the superficial relationships of the limbic lobe with the olfactory bulb, peduncle, and tracts on the basal aspect of the brain were readily apparent. No wonder that by the middle of this century the term "rhinencephalon" (olfactory brain or smell brain) was generally used to indicate the aggregate of these cortical regions with their fiber tracts, traditionally depicted as seen on the medial wall of the hemisphere (Figure 6–1 [a]). In a proposed reorientation[46] of this anatomical bias of the limbic system concept, the horizontal view from below is favored, hereby demonstrating anew that the limbic apparatus seen this way likewise forms a "limbus" encircling the brainstem (Figure 6–1 [b]).

It is of interest to note that early in mammalian phylogeny a more medially complete belt of cortex binds the hemispheres to the diencephalic portion of the brainstem. During ontogeny in man the structures surrounding the site of the laterally evaginated telenceph-alic vesicles, later becoming the cerebral hemispheres, become less readily recognizable as cortex. In the developing human brain these circumhilar structures are displaced down-

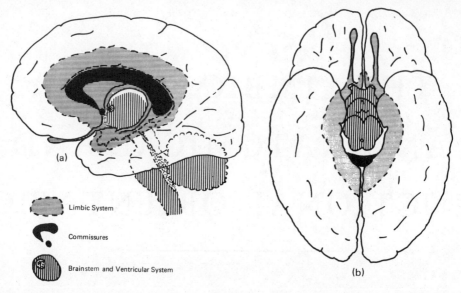

Figure 6–1. Diagrams of adult human brain surrounding the upper portions of the brainstem; (a) the right telencephalic hemisphere seen from its medial aspect to show the limbic system structures; (b) the whole forebrain seen from below.

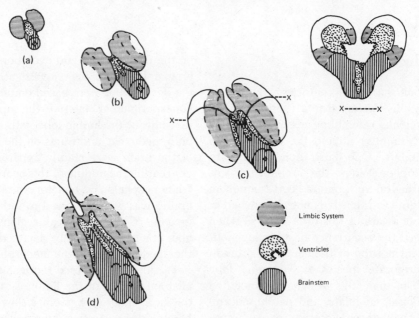

Figure 6–2. a–d: Schematic representation of the developing forebrain as seen obliquely from above, modified after Elliott.[25] The limbic cortex is seen restricted to the region where the hemispheres merge into the diencephalic portion of the brainstem. A coronal section x—x shows the relations to the ventricles in a plane behind the interventricular foramina (compare Figure 6–4).

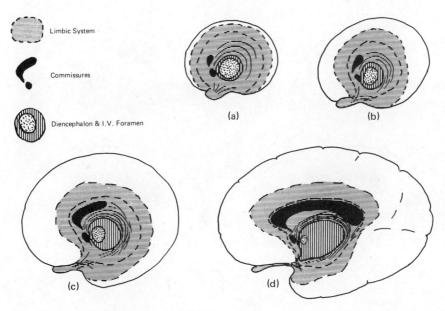

Figure 6–3. a–d: Schematic representation of the medial aspect of the developing telencephalon in man: the limbic system cortex surrounding the hilus of the hemisphere; the gradual displacement of the bulk of the inner cortical ring towards the temporal lobe; the semicircular fiber bundles in the limbic cortex; the development of the central olfactory structures; the overgrowth of the neocortex; the growth of the corpus callosum resulting in a partially "split" cortex.

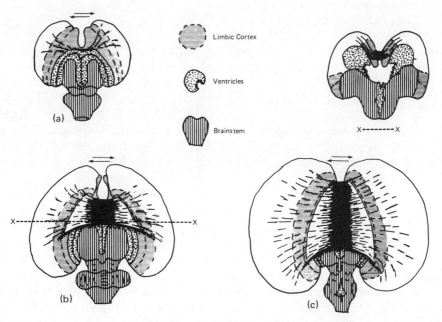

Figure 6–4. a–c: Diagram of the developing human forebrain as seen from above; the hemispheres have been pulled apart to show the formation of the neocortical commissure or corpus callosum (black) (modified after C. G. Smith[73]). The limbic system cortex is "split" into a supracallosal portion that is largely transitional cortex, and an infracallosal, older portion. A coronal section x—x shows the effect of this "split" in a plane behind the interventricular foramina, and with a corpus callosum (compare Figure 6–2).

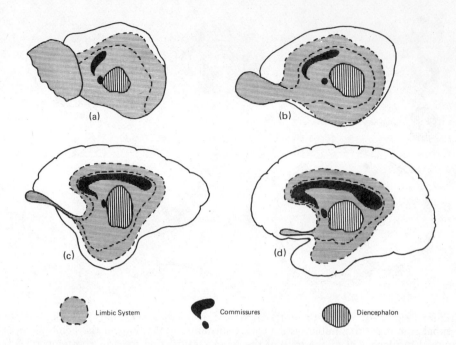

Figure 6–5. Diagrams to illustrate the medial aspect of the telencephalon in (a) hedgehog; (b) rabbit; (c) monkey; (d) man. Note the development of the corpus callosum, the decrease in size of olfactory structures, and concentric arrangement of old cortex around the hilus of the hemisphere (compare Figure 6–4).

ward and backward as they are stretched out and become overgrown with the massive neocortical regions on either side and their correspondingly conspicuous commissure, the corpus callosum (see Figures 6–2, 6–3, and 6–1 [a]).

The growing corpus callosum appears to split the "limbic" cortex into a supracallosal portion that is largely transitional cortex, and an infracallosal, older portion (Figures 6–3 and 6–4).

Vertebrate macrosmatic species with a keen sense of smell display a well–developed, primary olfactory brain apparatus. The degree of development of the sense of smell is not necessarily related to phyletic position, however, in contrast to the more constant pattern of evolution of the cortex as a whole. The more or less concentric arrangements in a medial view (compared by Broca[14] to a tennis racket with an olfactory "handle") are more obvious than in man: in lower forms, the limbic cortex represents a relatively bulky segment of the entire telencephalon, while with ascending phylog-

eny the neocortex expands unequally in every direction to all but obscure the ancient girdle of allocortex and other limbic system structures that lie as a junctional zone around the hilum of the hemisphere (Figure 6–5).

In the last few decades an increasing number of anatomical investigations* have shown that in higher forms the functions of much of the "olfactory brain" are not olfactory in nature, at least not directly or primarily. Aspects of autonomic nervous system physiology, certain features of neuroendocrinological regulation, expression of emotion, facets of learning and memory, patterns of behavior, "drives," as well as olfaction in the strict sense, all of these functions seem to have their neuroanatomical substrate in the "rhinencephalon." In view of such recent attempts to elucidate its physiology, several names have been proposed for this ancient portion of the mammalian brain, e.g., "visceral brain," "emotion brain," "vital brain," "limbic brain," or "limbic system."[48]

* See references 1, 3, 7, 16, 17, 18, 19, 20, 23, 54, 62, 64, 68, 79, and 81.

The last name is now widely accepted, although no unanimity exists concerning the exact definition and precise list of limbic–system components.[2,82]

In 1969, Brodal,[15] who in 1947 showed the error of including many nonolfactory structures under the designation "rhinencephalon," emphasized that "it is even less justifiable to speak of a 'limbic system.'" He stated[16] that "it becomes increasingly difficult to separate functionally different regions of the brain as research progresses, and that 'the limbic system' appears to be on its way to including all brain functions. As this process continues the value of the term as a useful concept is correspondingly reduced." It could be argued that in the strict sense the term rhinencephalon should now be limited to cerebral structures that are primarily involved in the reception, projection, and recognition of olfactory signals. However, since olfaction has been shown to influence affective and instinctual behavior as well as hypothalamic activity and since the limbic system indeed includes connections between true olfactory structures and other brain components, even the restricted use of the term rhinencephalon is, besides being confusing, not helpful. Perhaps for such reasons and in order to emphasize that in microsmatic man many limbic system structures do not subserve olfactory functions, the term rhinencephalon should be abandoned altogether, as was recommended in the reorganization of nomenclature pertaining to human anatomy (Paris, 1955).

The general term, limbic system, as used in this chapter is mainly based on its morphological merits; it includes phylogenetically ancient portions of the cerebral cortex and related subcortical derivatives, as well as intrinsic or

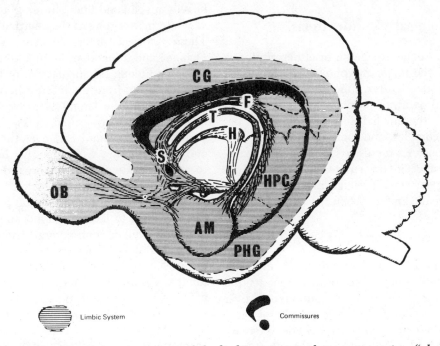

Figure 6–6. The major components of the limbic system in the cat as seen in a "phantom" diagram projected on a sagittal plane.

AM	= amygdaloid nuclear complex	OB	= olfactory bulb
CG	= cingulate gyrus	PHG	= parahippocampal gyrus
F	= fornix	S	= septum complex
H	= habenula	T	= stria terminalis
HPC	= hippocampus		

Medial forebrain bundle, olfactory tracts, stria medullaris, mammillary peduncle, habenulo-interpeduncular tract are sketched but not labeled.

intracortical fiber connections and extrinsic pathways linking these cortical components with the diencephalon and other areas in the brainstem (Figure 6–6). The aggregate of these structures constitutes the limbic system in the strict sense of the word. Efferent fiber tracts are to be included if the cells of origin are situated within gray components of the system. Afferent pathways can less readily be considered parts of the limbic system. However, through less than careful usage of the term or through emphasis on common functional manifestations, certain structures in the diencephalon (habenular complex, medial forebrain bundle) in the midbrain (ventral tegmental area) and in the frontal lobes are often included in the enumeration of limbic–system components. Transitional or junctional categories of cerebral cortex add to the difficulty of an explicit listing.

❨ Anatomical Considerations

In the subsequent pages, a brief description is given of the major morphological aspects of limbic system: cortex, subcortical gray derivatives, and pathways intrinsic to the system. In addition, the medial forebrain bundle, habenular complex, and some relationships with the neocortex are discussed in a few paragraphs, since in the strict sense these structures appear closely related in function to the telencephalic limbic system.

Hippocampal Formation

The hippocampal formation in man includes the hippocampus proper, the dentate gyrus with its attenuated continuation over the corpus callosum, called supracallosal gyrus or indusium griseum, intrinsic fiber systems, and a cortical transitional area, the subiculum: this area is located at the uncus, a surface landmark term referring to the most medial, somewhat hook-shaped portion of the temporal lobe. The hippocampal formation is derived from the anteromedial wall of the primitive cerebral hemisphere; its gray matter is allocortical or archicortical in nature. As the neocortical or isocortical portion of the hemisphere increases enormously in size during development, the major portion of hippocampal formation becomes displaced caudally, somewhat laterally, then ventrally, to lie as part of the temporal lobe along the juxtallocortical or mescocortical parahippocampal gyrus. In addition, the formation is rolled inward, with the result that the hippocampus proper forms a bulge in the floor of the inferior or temporal horn of the lateral ventricle.

The hippocampus, in certain planes of section, faintly resembles a sea horse or perhaps its tail; in earlier times, descriptive morphologists likened this structure to a dolphin, a silkworm, a triton, even an equestrian statue. A name often used in England is Ammon's horn or cornu Ammonis, referring to its curved shape as it follows the semicircular sweep of the lateral ventricle. The deepest layer of the hippocampal cortex is covered by heavily myelinated fibers forming a thin layer of white matter toward the ventricular lumen. These efferent fibers collect as fimbria (fringe) and it increases in bulk as more fibers are added along the medial rim of the hippocampus, rising from the inferior horn to about the atrium of the lateral ventricle. Here the fiber bundle, now called fornix (vault or dome) curves around and over the thalamus and joins its fellow from the other hemisphere to run alongside each other forward under the corpus callosum. A variable system of commissural fibers crosses the midsagittal plane as the fornices meet to link one hippocampal formation with similar, contralateral structures. The fornix bundles do not decussate; they curve rather sharply around the interventricular foramina (of Monro) to terminate in various regions of the diencephalon and in gray matter around the anterior commissure (cf. Figure 6–6). Many of the 1,200,000 fornix fibers reach the mammillary body nuclei; some have been traced to the rostral part of the periaqueductal gray matter, some to the septal nuclei, and others to the anterior thalamus directly.*

Most efferent fibers are contained in the

---

* See references 15, 21, 31, 54, and 79.

fimbria-fornix systems, although some afferent fibers reach the hippocampal by this route or by the somewhat longer trajectory from septum around the corpus callosum along the indusium griseum into the dentate gyrus.[23,81] Most afferent impulses reach the hippocampus by way of the fiber systems of the cingulum, a bundle coursing within the cingulate and parahippocampal gyri and reflecting the extent and shape of Broca's limbic lobe.[14,16,20,47] The cingulum receives inputs from adjacent cortical areas, as well as from the anterior thalamus,[7] which in turn is linked to the mammillary bodies by way of the mammillothalamic tracts. A special region of the parahippocampal gyrus, the entorhinal area, projects in rather specific ways to the various areas within the hippocampus. In recent years it has become evident that notwithstanding the relatively simple organization of the primitive hippocampal formation, differences exist between various areas—in terms of cytoarchitectonic composition—of efferent and afferent connections, of histochemistry, and probably also with respect to function.*

It must be clear from this brief description of the hippocampal formation and its associated fiber systems that it relates closely to many other regions of the brain, cortical as well as in the diencephalon. Moreover, it appears as if a circuitous trajectory of fiber connections is traversing a large part of the limbic system, without clear beginning or end. It is this circuit—hippocampus-fornix-mammillary body-anterior thalamus-cingulum-hippocampus—that Papez[56] described in 1937 as subserving a proposed mechanism of emotion. However, the subsequent detailed anatomical analyses as well as functional studies of the hippocampal formation have demonstrated that even the hippocampus proper cannot be considered a physiological unit.[2,9,34]

Olfactory Structures and Pathways

An elongated evagination of the primitive cortex on the basal surface of each hemisphere, known as the olfactory bulb, is connected to other limbic–system structures by way of flattened fiber bundles, which separate from the olfactory tract or peduncle.† In man, the medial bundle or stria reaches the region of the subcallosal gyrus, the septum, and perhaps the habenular complex, as well as the olfactory structures on the opposite side, by way of the anterior commissure (see Figures 6–1 and 6–6). The lateral bundle or olfactory stria appears to be the main projection pathway for the sense of smell. It courses along with a thin layer of gray via the limen insulae (the anterior threshold of the lateral fissure) to terminate in a limited area at the uncus, both in the rostral extent of the parahippocampal gyrus as well as in medial and cortical nuclei of the amygdala. Some fibers from the olfactory peduncle end in a triangular area of gray, cortical matter between the divergent lateral and medial olfactory striae, the olfactory trigone, approximately the anterior perforated space in the human brain. From this area, and from other structures where olfactory stria fibers terminate, a diffuse system of short neurons connects to the lateral region of the hypothalamus and hence further down the brainstem tegmentum.[1] This system of interconnected neurons, the medial forebrain bundle, receives additional afferents from other limbic-system areas and serves as a collection and distribution mechanism for reflexes triggered by olfactory sensations and other sensory signals.

Efferent projections from the primary olfactory cortex have not had a detailed analysis in all forms; connections with the amygdaloid nuclear complex and the entorhinal area of the parahippocampal gyrus have been described,[62,68] as forming other, more circuitous links with nuclei in the diencephalon. The contiguity of lateral olfactory stria terminations and efferent connections from the uncus to the hippocampus had led to the early concept that the latter structure represented the cortical projection area for the sense of smell. In the last few decades this concept, mainly extrapolated from comparative studies, has been shown to be erroneous on the basis of

---

* See references 2, 5, 20, 30, 43, and 53.

† See references 3, 31, 62, 68, and 84.

careful anatomical studies,[15] clinical case histories,[16] and experiments in animals.[3] It should be noted, however, that the primitive sense of smell is somewhat unique when compared to the other special senses: there are but two neurons involved in the pathway between olfactory receptor and primary projection cortex; there is no decussation, partial or complete; and there is no thalamic relay nucleus. On the other hand, subcortical reflex paths are abundantly present even in man and impinge on visceral regulatory centers in the brainstem, including the diencephalon. It is especially in this context that the terms rhinencephalon, visceral brain, and limbic system, sometimes used interchangeably, have unfortunately led to confusion, to controversial concepts, and occasionally even to contentious contradiction.

Amygdaloid Nuclear Complex (Amygdala)

In man, a surprisingly large subcortical gray mass, the amygdala, is found at the tip of the inferior horn of the lateral ventricle, just rostral to the hippocampus and under the uncus (see Figure 6–6). Mainly on the basis of comparative anatomical studies, this mass can be subdivided into (1) the corticomedial group of nuclei; (2) the basolateral group of nuclei (well–developed in man); (3) the anterior amygdaloid area; and (4) other aggregates of nerve cells. The various nuclei of the amygdaloid (almond-shaped) complex appear to have somewhat different fiber connections and correspondingly diverse functions, although the analysis is far from complete.*

Efferent projections from the amygdala include fiber systems of the stria terminalis, coursing alongside the caudate nucleus and paralleling the sweep of the lateral ventricle and the anterior commissure as well as diffuse amygdalofugal projections. These efferents terminate in the anterior hypothalamus, the septum complex, probably the habenular complex, possibly other nuclear groups, and they contribute to the medial forebrain bundle.

* See references 16, 17, 21, 32, 38, 60, and 78.

The amygdaloid nuclear complex receives afferents from the olfactory bulb by way of the lateral stria, terminating in the corticomedial group of nuclei, from adjacent regions of the parahippocampal gyrus (in some species named piriform cortex since the basal aspect of the temporal lobe resembles a pear) and possibly indirectly from various other cortical areas.[19,31,55] The amygdaloid complex, the olfactory gray structures, and an interconnecting band of cortex (diagonal gyrus, or band, of Broca[14]) are often described as paleocortical in nature, referring to a type of allocortex at the base of the forebrain.

Septum Complex

A mass of gray matter, mostly subcortical and derived from the medial wall of the primitive cerebral hemispheres, is found between and below the anterior horns of the lateral ventricles. It is well developed in most mammalian forms (cf. Figure 6–6). However, in primates and especially in man, it has been partially stretched out by the increase in bulk of the neocortical region and the corpus callosum. This thin portion is known as the septum lucidum. Other components include aggregates of gray matter around the anterior commissure, close to midplane and the transition to the mediobasal walls of the hemispheres and merging into subcallosal or paraterminal gyri.[1,65,74]

The septum complex is connected or adjacent to hypothalamus, preoptic area and medial forebrain bundle, amygdaloid nuclear complex and hippocampal formation, as well as to the habenular complex. No wonder that this component of the limbic system has invited investigation in recent years, not only by neuroanatomists and neuroendocrinologists but also by students of behavior and emotional reactions. An integrative function has been suggested by its very position, at the crossroads as it were, between limbic system, diencephalon, and neocortex. However, the complexity and limitations in size require strictly controlled experiments as well as a cautious interpretation of the results.

Limbic Lobe

As mentioned in the introduction to this chapter, the comparative neuroanatomical concept of a limbic lobe, viz., a convolution of cortical gray encircling the attachment of hemisphere to upper brainstem, can be traced back several centuries. The growth of the corpus callosum, concomitant with the development of the large lateral mass of neocortex and underlying white matter, seems to split through part of the border of primitive cortical gray (Figure 6–4). The result is a circular mass of allocortex and white fiber tracts (septum, fornix, and hippocampus) curving below the corpus callosum, and a histologically less primitive convolution above or outside it, with merged ends on either side; namely, in the subcallosal–gyrus area and in the hippocampus–parahippocampal–uncus region (Figures 6–1 and 6–3).

It is not immediately clear from the earlier descriptions whether or not the hippocampal formation in all cases was to be included in this lobe, also referred to as gyrus limbicus or gyrus fornicatus, since it showed a vaultlike extent; nor are its boundaries sharply defined. Two concepts are therefore encountered in the current literature concerning this.[14,16,31,74] There is (1) Broca's "grand lobe limbique,"[14] mostly juxtallocortical in nature, comprising subcallosal, cingulate, retrosplenial, and parahippocampal gyri or synonyms thereof; and (2) these structures as well as the allocortical structures described above as hippocampal formation.

In this chapter the first concept is preferred, although the transitional type of cortex found in much of this limbic lobe would indicate its more intermediary position between the innermost, truly limbic, more primitive or older, allocortical structures and more recent neocortex. The olfactory gray and gyrus diagonalis, linking septum complex and subcallosal area with amygdala and adjacent hippocampal formation, complete the innermost encirclement of the diencephalon (Figures 6–2, 6–3 and 6–5).

Mainly based on functional findings, some regions of the frontal lobe adjacent to the subcallosal area and connected by a well–developed association bundle (uncinate fasciculus) to the temporal lobe are sometimes mentioned as portions of the limbic system. However, these orbitofrontal gyri display cytoarchitectonic characteristics that suggest their neocortical nature.[31]

Pathways Linking Limbic-System Cortex with Diencephalon

It should be clear by now that extensive reciprocal connections exist between the limbic–system structures in the temporal lobe and the diencephalon, especially the hypothalamus. The conspicuous fimbria–fornix system, the less pronounced stria terminalis bundle from and to the amygdala through the anterior commissure, and more diffuse direct connections dipping under the limen insulae have been mentioned above. These links constitute well-developed, rather circuitous routes between the basofrontal and mediotemporal telencephalic components of the limbic system on the one hand, and the brainstem on the other hand, especially the basal diencephalon extending into preoptic area rostrally and ventral mesencephalic tegmentum caudally (see Figure 6–6).

It should be emphasized that these links are often both afferent and efferent with respect to the brainstem, albeit not to an equal degree. Also, the termination sites on the brainstem are not restricted to a few loci, but they are rather diverse and have been analyzed in several anatomical studies.[*] Equally interesting is the growing awareness that the major gray masses in the temporal lobe (hippocampus, amygdala, parahippocampal gyrus) are not homogenous in nature but appear to have different and often specific connections with other structures as well as typical histological and histochemical characteristics.[†]

Medial Forebrain Bundle

A multineuron, multisynaptic, often diffuse system of fibers can be found in the lateral

[*] See references 2, 9, 19, 55, 62, 64, and 79.
[†] See references 5, 20, 30, 43, and 53.

hypothalamus. This system extends from and connects with olfactory trigone gray, septum complex, uncus areas, and amygdaloid nuclei to the ventral gray of the tegmentum in the midbrain (see Figure 6–6). This medial forebrain bundle, as opposed to the lateral forebrain bundle or more modern internal capsule system, is essentially a limbic-system, projection pathway to the brainstem directions. Signals from several subcortical and cortical structures pertaining to the limbic system can thus be relayed to basal diencephalic and mesencephalic nuclei. Additional ascending fibers have been described, among these the mammillary peduncle, which is a discrete connection between ventral tegmentum and mammillary nuclei.[18] It has been postulated that the medial forebrain bundle constitutes the rostral portion of the reticular formation of the brainstem.[*] Its diffuse nature, consisting as it does of multiple short neurons and ascending and descending fibers, suggests that nonspecific stimuli as well as special sensory signals may influence the limbic–system function as a whole.[52] Conversely, discharges from the limbic system, triggered by olfactory cues or set off by primitive, basic cortical activity, may also reach the visceral and endocrine regulatory centers in the brainstem by way of the medial forebrain bundle.

Habenular Complex and Connections

The habenular complex, inconspicuous in man, consists of a long–stretched mass of nuclei and afferent fibers (stria medullaris) along either side of the roof attachment of the third ventricle (taenia thalami), the habenular commissure (coursing through the upper portion of the pineal stalk), and efferent fiber bundles.[21,31,49,51] The latter connect the epithalamic habenular complex with several ventral and possibly also dorsal tegmental regions in the midbrain. Among these the habenulo–interpeduncular tract (fasciculus retroflexus) can be readily identified in man. It is noteworthy that the habenular complex essentially parallels the medial forebrain bundle by span-

ning between preoptic, septal, and subcallosal limbic regions rostrally and ventral tegmental areas in the mesencephalon. The direction of conduction is mainly toward the midbrain, in contrast to the medial forebrain bundle. Another difference is that the latter, by traversing the hypothalamus, impinges on its many functions whereas the habenula does not nor does it appear to relate to thalamic activity. Neither the significance of the habenular commissure nor its relation to the pineal gland is clear.

Just as the medial forebrain bundle per se cannot be included in the limbic system, if one adheres to a strict morphological and anatomical definition derived from allocortex in the medial wall of the telencephalon, similarly the habenular complex cannot be considered a component of that system as it is treated in this chapter. Nevertheless, the intimate relationships, neuronally as well as functionally, of these two structures to limbic–system components make it possible to include them readily in the functional concepts of an extended limbic system. Insight into the functional importance of the habenular complex is far from complete; curiously, this is in contrast to its constant occurrence and conspicuous contours in many animal species. Recent investigations[22] have suggested that the habenula has a modulatory role in the regulation of pituitary hormone secretion and with respect to aspects of sexual behavior in rodents. So far, however, the habenular complex in man has not been related to any physiological activity.

Relationships with the Neocortex

In earlier discussions[4,42,48,54] of the concept of the limbic system, it is suggested that the neocortex functions almost independently from activity of the older limbic cortex. While that idea does not appear too difficult to accept, the reverse statement is. For, direct connections between the cortical portions of the limbic system and the rest of the telencephalic hemisphere have been reported[16,21,31,47] along large extents of the limbic lobe where juxtallocortex borders on neocortex. More specifically,

[*] See references 1, 48, 54, 59, and 65.

the parahippocampal gyrus is related to the fusiform and lingual gyri through short association bundles, the posterior and retrosplenial gyri to the precuneus, the anterior cingulate gyrus to the superior frontal convolution, and the subcallosal region to the ventromedial region of the frontal lobe. In addition, the thin gray band of primitive cortex extending along lateral olfactory tract, limen insulae, and uncus appears to relate to the posterior orbital gyri, the insula, and its opercula.

In short, the limbic system cortex is more or less connected with all secondary–sensory and many association areas but not with the primary projection areas for vision, audition, or general body sensation. These connections between the limbic system and neocortex are all mediated by short, mostly diffuse fiber systems that link the limbic lobe with the neocortex. Within the limbic lobe the distinct, long association bundles of the cingulum and the uncinate fasciculus impinge on many allocortical structures. Therefore, although the relations between neocortex and the oldest portions of the limbic system and hence the hypothalamus appear to be indirect ones by way of the limbic lobe or the thalamus, nevertheless, the neuronal substrate appears able to subserve and transduce neocortical influence on basic patterns of behavior and concomitant alterations in autonomic, endocrine, or motor activity.

⟨ Functional Considerations

For most of the structures discussed above the functional connotation of rhinencephalon was deemed too all–inclusive a few decades ago.[15] This was when experimental neuroanatomical investigations confirmed a nonolfactory function for much of the limbic system.[3, 42,48] Some have been tempted to substitute a term that either avoids the implication of a singular function by erring on the side of vagueness or that emphasizes anatomical characteristics.

No substitute has been entirely satisfactory. "Visceral brain," "vital brain," "emotional brain," all seemed to deemphasize olfaction without including enough in their associative functional terminology. As used here, limbic system appears to stress a neutral morphological concept, provided it does not conjure up some implicit, unified, systemic function. At a time when many seemingly diverse activities are shown to relate to one or more neuroanatomical substrates that comprise components of the limbic system, the dangers of spurious generalization may be replaced by the pitfalls of a too detailed analysis into unrelated facets of function, bodily or otherwise. Nevertheless, as information accumulates, attempts to synthesize our understanding of function should periodically accompany analysis.

Much of what is known today about the functions of limbic–system components is based on observation and experimentation in animal species, especially mammalian forms. Man may have analogous functions, but direct extrapolation is full of risks, even though phylogenetic development is well defined in this portion of the brain. For example, olfactory acuity may vary considerably, independent of the phyletic position. Animal investigations are cumbersome and they can be misleading when alterations in feelings or drives or aspects of memory are tested. On the other hand, controlled human experiments are rare and the clinical results often unreliable either because of a lack of circumscribed pathology or because of a protracted time element that allows for adaptation. In addition, since lower echelons often attempt to compensate for or stabilize dysfunction following experimental manipulation, the hierarchical organizations of basic, almost autonomous visceral functions and instinctual patterns of behavior, generally tend to resist clear-cut effects. Finally, confusion and redundancy in terminology versus incomplete insight in hodology and complexity of neuroanatomical substrate may result.

Nevertheless, even in microsmatic man, some progress in understanding the functional activities of the limbic system has been made in recent years. But there still is both a lack of clear comprehension and of comprehensive knowledge.

Olfaction

The sense of smell, one of the chemical senses, is a basic function for most lower vertebrate forms. It draws attention to potential danger from enemies or to possible prey; it can attract partners of the opposite sex[57] or differentiate between certain life–sustaining foodstuffs and nonedible material.[9,84] At the top of the phylogenetic scale, in *Homo sapiens*, the other senses are much more important in vegetative behavior.

Nevertheless, the ability of man to tell one smell from another is at least a useful adjunct in eating and drinking, pleasures that a bad nose cold can spoil. The continuation of the human race may not be so dependent on the sense of smell as many vertebrate species are, yet olfaction does not play a negligible role in our society as any perfume manufacturer or husband knows. Moreover, in primitive ethnic situations man's sense of smell may play an even bigger role with respect to social and reproductive behavior. Olfaction may not be a vital asset, but pleasant smells can make life more agreeable just as disagreeable smells can be very unpleasant and emotionally upsetting. While the human hippocampus and its connections are no longer considered olfactory substrates,[15] the regions at the rostromedial tip of the parahippocampal gyrus (uncus) and efferents to the brainstem have been shown to be important in this context. Irritation or stimulation of the temporal lobe may lead to so-called uncinate fits; olfactory cues may trigger patterns of behavior, emotions, even memories.

Aspects of Behavior

An extensive analysis of the role of limbic–system structures in human behavior is not within the competence of the author nor the organizational purview of this chapter. A few remarks should suffice.

First studied in animals,[17] later at least partially confirmed in man, the effects of bilateral lesions in the temporal lobe lead to characteristic changes in behavior as well as to altera-tions in the mechanism of memory (see below); the "Klüver and Bucy syndrome" consists of visual agnosia, absence of emotional responses, a tendency to examine objects by mouth, indiscriminate eating habits, increased reproductive behavior, etc.

Temporal lobe epilepsy is not uncommon,[34,35] but so far it has been difficult to match precise pathology with the symptoms. Olfactory or acoustic auras, some disturbance of consciousness, episodes of amnesia without loss of motor control, epileptiform seizures with a "march" of motor disturbances, all tend to make clinico-pathological analysis a formidable and arduous task.[17,60] Brodal states[16] that "in view of the ample interconnections and functional interrelations between the different structures contained in the temporal lobe, it is not astonishing that approximately identical disturbances may result from an abnormal activity starting in almost any of these structures. The initial symptoms may in some instances point to the site of origin (for example, olfactory sensations to the uncus)."

The simple, stratified nature of the allocortex has attracted fundamental neurocytophysiological investigations.[2,5,9,43] Electrophysiological studies[13,32,34,42] concerned with hippocampal potentials have shown that this structure has a very low seizure threshold, and that it is quite likely to show hypoxia– or hypoglycemia–induced changes in electrical activity. Hippocampal seizures, taking off from the intrinsic four–to–seven–second theta wave activity, may easily spread to other regions of the cortex. Thus, when hippocampal activity is desynchronized, the neocortex shows synchronization. Stimulation of the hippocampus in unanesthetized cats may result[33,63,69] in reduced reaction to external stimuli and increased attention, with bizarre motor manifestations, to "something" in the environment; this type of behavior has been compared to hallucinations, or "arrest," and sometimes may be interpreted as a prodrome for a temporal lobe seizure.

Other changes in behavior, notably altered drinking and feeding activities, have been described following destruction or irritation of limbic–system components, especially the lateral portions of the amygdala.* The oral behavior aspects of the Klüver-Bucy syndrome may be associated with this particular pathology. A review of the relation of limbic–system structures to hypothalamic regulation of food and water intake suggests that the role of extrahypothalamic structures in altered patterns of food intake is probably different from the regulatory function of relevant diencephalic structures.[4,52,84]

These past few years it has become evident† that a workable concept of a hierarchical organization of *autonomic nervous system functions* must include the "visceral brain," here referred to as the limbic system. This does not exclude a further cortical influence on autonomic function; indeed, there are easy examples of neocortically induced *emotional feelings*—shame, anger, fright, perhaps lust— "gut" reactions that may trigger visceral reflexes. Whether such manifestations of emotion are routed through the limbic system[56,72] or directly to the hypothalamic regulatory centers is not clear. However, experimental work of various nature suggests that stimulation of limbic structures may result in altered autonomic functions.[28,32,66,78] The increase in oral activity seen in the Klüver-Bucy syndrome—biting, licking, chewing, gagging— may be relevant in this context.

Aggressive behavior, with concomitant autonomic (sympathetic) reactions, and its counterpart *fear*, apprehension, or avoidance have found a neurological substrate in temporal lobe structures, especially the amygdala, as well as in other parts of the limbic system‡ Stimulation of the amygdaloid complex, which often occurs at the start of an epileptic seizure emanating from the temporal lobe, has produced feelings of anger or fear in conscious patients. It appears, therefore, that the amygdala is a nodal point, functionally related to emotional reactions and experiences.[16] However, the same can be said about other components of the limbic system such as the septum complex. Keepers and investigators attacked by laboratory animals with septum

lesions have suffered similar scars. Conversely, ferocious animals may exhibit a remarkable docility after temporal lobe ablation.[69] In this and other behavioral changes such as lack of discrimination, loss of memory, visual agnosia, absence of inhibition, the common threads may begin to weave themselves into an emerging pattern of a general limbic system function.

In an attempt to separate the various components of the Klüver-Bucy syndrome in male cats, Green and coworkers have suggested that the uninhibited and undiscriminating sexual activities displayed by their animals were due to lesions in parts of the amygdala and associated limbic cortex; a loss of the sense of "territory" was evident as well.[35] Similar profound changes in *reproductive behavior* have been reported in other species, including man, following the ablation of temporal lobe structures.§ The results of many of these studies, whether experimentally induced or clinical cases, are difficult to interpret, possibly because the pathology of the structures and the pathways involved are often surprisingly complex.[16,17,60]

Whereas in lower forms, olfaction or pheromones appear to play an essential role in the control of reproductive behavior as well as pituitary gonadotrophin secretion, little is known concerning such a mechanism in man. The exceptional and perhaps unexpected importance of smell has been reported[21,60,63] even in so-called microsmatic animals. In the comparative analysis of the interrelationships between pituitary function, behavior, and the olfactory component of the limbic system, it makes sense not only to pay attention to species differences in patterns of sexual behavior but also to consider factors such as emotional, experiential, visceral, hormonal, and perceptual correlates in any given setting within a species.

Endocrine System

In the past two decades, the role of nervous afferents to hypothalamic centers that control

---

* See references 4, 29, 35, 36, and 78.
† See references 2, 4, 42, 48, and 66.
‡ See references 35, 45, 71, 77, and 78.

§ See references 12, 21, 44, 61, 69, and 72.

mammalian pituitary function, which influence reproductive and other patterns of behavior as well as stress reactions, has received attention from an increasing number of investigators in various fields.* Important examples of these extrahypothalamic pathways impinging on the highly complex basal brainstem are the limbic–system efferents—especially the amygdalo–hypothalamic tracts—the olfactory afferents to the medial forebrain bundle, and the fornix system. In the broader sense, other portions of the limbic system such as the habenula, the cingulate gyrus, and possibly Nauta's limbic midbrain area[54] appear to contribute little to human pituitary function, although in experimental animals some suggestive evidence has been reported.[21]

In suitably primed animals, stimulation of the amygdala, its efferent fibers or pertinent hypothalamic nuclei may result in ovulation; the opposite phenomenon, i.e., the impairment of a nervous mechanism that normally enhances luteinizing hormone output by the pituitary gland, has been described, with lesions occurring in these regions.[11,21,24,26] The secretion of other hormones may likewise be influenced by limbic–system activation.[39,76]

The effects of lesions in the hippocampal formation, or of stimulation there, impinge on a diversity of manifestations: endocrine, visceral-autonomic, behavioral, related to aspects of memory, etc. Of interest for neuroendocrinologists is the course of some efferent fornix fibers toward posterior portions of the hypothalamus, a small bundle of fibers, described by Cajal[65] in normal rodent material in 1901, ending in the tuber cinereum close to the pituitary infundibulum. Changes in diurnal variation of adrenocortical activity, of recent interest because of the so-called jet–lag phenomenon, have been reported in some species after fornix transection or hippocampal pathology, but these changes are not generally confirmed.[16,22,27,34]

The notion of feedback arcs in neuroendocrinology now appears to be complemented by the concept of bias-setting mechanisms. Such unquestionably complex mechanisms,

* See references 2, 4, 9, 21, 22, 32, 52, 54, and 63.

investigated profitably only if one regulatory factor can be isolated to the stable exclusion of all others, must contain morphological substrates and circuits with certain properties: they must be phylogenetically old; they must be linked (in a functional sense) to "higher" cerebral centers mediating e.g., stresses or emotions; and they require prolonged stimulation in order to produce their effects. The suggestion has been made[21,34] that the effects of stimulation, ablation, or manipulation of limbic–system components point to the possibility that the morphological substrate and the circuits for the bias-setting mechanisms as well as the switch for the hypothalamo-pituitary "homeostat" might be among the phylogenetically old parts of the brain. This could explain both the lack of a conspicuous role, under "normal" conditions, and the pronounced effects, in certain situations, of lesion or stimulation of the limbic system.

Memory

In recent years, the role of the hippocampus in certain aspects of remembering has attracted considerable attention.[6,58,70,80] Surgical ablation of temporal lobe structures, including large portions of the hippocampus, may result not only in an inability to retain current experiences or to learn but, in addition, a significant forgetting of things past.[58] Ischemia of medial–temporal areas has been associated with episodes of transient global amnesia. It is quite likely that the hippocampus is involved although the actual vascular etiology has not been clearly proven. The well-known vulnerability of this structure to anoxia may underlie this phenomenon. Persistent memory defects have been described,[80] with infarction in the hippocampal formation and fornix as well as in the mammillary bodies. As seen in cases of Wernicke-Korsakoff encephalopathy, the amnestic confabulatory syndrome is usually associated with lesions in the mammillary bodies and medial–anterior thalamic areas. A severe loss of memory of things in the recent past is often present while events from the distant past can be easily recalled. There need be no concomitant deterioration in personality or general intelligence.*

The current view, therefore, is that the integrity of the hippocampus is essential to memorizing recent events. Brodal[16] cautions that this statement may be too explicit. Isolated damage to the hippocampus is rare and, in cases of Korsakoff's syndrome, there are often other changes in addition to those seen in the mammillary bodies. Bilateral transection of the fornix in man may be without demonstrable defects in recent memory, a term itself not easy to define. Besides, there is no evidence that the function of recent memory belongs to the hippocampus alone. Memory as well as learning disturbances have been described following bilateral ablation of the anterior cingulate gyrus or other limbic-system structures.[10,33,75]

Associated in some way with memory mechanisms and the limbic system is probably the instinctive behavior shown in animal species as well as the concepts of drives or motivational appetitive behavior such as hunger, thirst, sexual appetites, anger, fear, and so on. This is less clear in contemporary man, although it could lead to intriguing speculation. That is, a more or less fixed pattern of behavior, triggered by a certain cue, sometimes olfactory in nature, often involving extensive participation of autonomic nervous and musculoskeletal systems.

(Conclusion

The relatively recent introduction of modern neuroanatomical techniques has resulted in a clarification of the reciprocal neural pathways linking phylogenetically ancient parts of the telencephalon with diencephalic nuclei as well as certain other brainstem areas, thus necessitating a reappraisal of the neural control of pituitary function, of visceral activity, of appetitive or motivational mechanisms, of patterns of behavior and of expressions of emotion. The anatomical substrates for the function of olfaction have been (re)defined; the in-

* For recent reviews see references 8, 16, 27, 37, 40, 50, and 60.

fluence of olfactory reflexes awaits further elucidation.

From the foregoing pages two things should begin to emerge: on the one hand, a continuing clarification of the morphology, hodology, phylogeny, and ontogeny of the limbic system; on the other hand, an almost overwhelming wealth of semirelated functional facets of this system. Activities pertaining to neuroendocrinology of reproduction, stress and associated behavior; autonomic nervous function and olfactory reflexes; certain patterns of visceral behavior, all these can be aggregated as basic contributions to two somewhat conflicting major vital processes: preservation of the individual versus continuation of the species.[48] Certain memory and learning mechanisms, or electroneurophysiological manifestations characteristic of temporal lobe structures (e.g., forms of psychomotor epilepsy) do not readily fit into a unified concept of limbic-system function.

It is fashionable to contemplate how much has been studied and learned since Papez's[56] speculation on the "mechanism of emotion" in 1937 released a wave of investigations, interest and insight about the form and function of the olfactory brain in man. It is fascinating to speculate whether or not the next decade or two will demonstrate that a simplified, general approach to the significance of these temporal lobe structures and their outflow *is* feasible. It seems likely that some retrenchment and further analysis, anatomical as well as functional, will have to occur before a refined concept of the human limbic system is either accepted or put to rest alongside the rhinencephalon.

False facts are highly injurious to the progress of science, for they often long endure; but false views, if supported by some evidence, do little harm, as everyone takes a salutary pleasure in proving their falseness.

Charles Darwin
The Descent of Man

(Bibliography

1. ADEY, W. R., C. W. DUNLOP, and S. SUNDERLAND. "A Survey of Rhinencephalic

Interconnections with the Brain Stem," *J. Comp. Neurol.,* 110 (1958), 173–204.

2. ADEY, W. R. and T. TOKIZANE, eds., *Structure and Function of the Limbic System.* Progress in Brain Research, Vol. 27. New York: Elsevier, 1967.

3. ALLISON, A. C. "The Morphology of the Olfactory System in the Vertebrates," *Biol. Rev.,* 28 (1953), 195–244.

4. ANAND, B. K. "Functional Importance of the Limbic System of the Brain," *Indian J. Med. Res.,* 51 (1963), 175–222.

5. ANDERSEN, P., T. W. BLACKSTAD, and T. LÖMO. "Location and Identification of Excitatory Synapses on Hippocampal Pyramidal Cells," *Exp. Brain Res.,* 1 (1966), 236–248.

6. ANDY, O. J., D. F. PEELER, J. MITCHELL et al. "The Hippocampal Contribution to 'Learning and Memory': Information Retrieval and Comparison," *Cond. Reflex,* 3 (1968), 217–233.

7. ANGEVINE, J. B., Jr., S. LOCKE, and P. I. YAKOVLEV. "Limbic Nuclei of Thalamus and Connections of Limbic Cortex," *Arch. Neurol.,* 10 (1964), 165–180.

8. BARBIZET, J. "Defect of Memorizing of Hippocampal-Mammillary Origin: a Review," *J. Neurol.,* 26 (1963), 127–135.

9. BARGMANN, W. and J. P. SCHADÉ, eds. *The Rhinencephalon and Related Structures.* Progress in Brain Research, Vol. 3. New York: Elsevier, 1963.

10. BARKER, D. J. and G. J. THOMAS. "Ablation of Cingulate Cortex in Rats Impairs Alternation Learning and Retention," *J. Comp. Physiol. Psychol.,* 60 (1965), 353–359.

11. BAR-SELA, M. E. and V. CRITCHLOW. "Delayed Puberty Following Electrical Stimulation of Amygdala in Female Rats," *Am. J. Physiol.,* 211 (1966), 1103–1107.

12. BERMANT, G., S. E. GLICKMAN, and J. M. DAVIDSON. "Effects of Limbic Lesions on Copulatory Behavior of Male Rats," *J. Comp. Physiol. Psychol.,* 65 (1968), 118–125.

13. BRAZIER, M. A. "Studies of the EEG Activity of Limbic Structures in Man," *Electroencephalogr. Clin. Neurophysiol.,* 25 (1968), 309–318.

14. BROCA, P. "Anatomie comparée des circonvolutions cérébrales: le grand lobe limbique et la scissure limbique dans la série des mammifères," *Rév. Anthropol.,* Série 2, 1 (1878), 385–498.

15. BRODAL, A. "The Hippocampus and the Sense of Smell," *Brain,* 70 (1947), 179–222.

16. ———. *Neurological Anatomy in Relation to Clinical Medicine.* New York: Oxford University Press, 1969.

17. BUCY, O. C. and H. KLÜVER. "An Anatomical Investigation of the Temporal Lobe in the Monkey (*Macaca mulatta*)," *J. Comp. Neurol.,* 103 (1955), 151–253.

18. COWAN, W. M., R. W. GUILLERY, and T. P. S. POWELL. "The Origin of the Mammillary Peduncle and Other Hypothalamic Connexions from the Midbrain," *J. Anat.,* 98 (1964), 345–363.

19. COWAN, W. M., G. RAISMAN, and T. P. S. POWELL. "The Connexions of the Amygdala," *J. Neurol.,* 28 (1965), 137–151.

20. CRAGG, B. G. "Afferent Connexions of the Allocortex," *J. Anat.,* 99 (1965), 339–357.

21. DE GROOT, J. "The Influence of Limbic Structures on Pituitary Functions Related to Reproduction," in F. A. Beach, ed., *Sex and Behavior,* pp. 496–511. New York: John Wiley & Sons, 1965.

22. ———. "Limbic and Other Neural Pathways that Regulate Endocrine Function," in L. Martini and W. F. Ganong, eds., *Neuroendocrinology,* Vol. 1, pp. 81–106. New York: Academic Press, 1966.

23. DE VITO, J. L. and L. E. WHITE. "Projections from the Fornix to the Hippocampal Formation in the Squirrel Monkey," *J. Comp. Neurol.,* 127 (1966), 389–398.

24. ELEFTHERIOU, B. E. "Effect of Amygdaloid Lesions on Plasma and Pituitary Levels of Luteinizing Hormone," *J. Reprod. Fertil.,* 14 (1967), 33–37.

25. ELLIOTT, H. C. *Textbook of Neuroanatomy.* Philadelphia: J. B. Lippincott, 1963.

26. ELWERS, M. and V. CRITCHLOW. "Precocious Ovarian Stimulation Following Interruption of Stria Terminalis," *Am. J. Physiol.,* 201 (1961), 281–284.

27. ENDRÖCZI, E. *Limbic System: Learning and Pituitary-Adrenal Function.* Budapest: Hungarian Academy of Sciences, 1973.

28. FENNEGAN, F. M. and M. J. PUIGGARI. "Hypothalamic and Amygdaloid Influence on Gastric Motility in Dogs," *J. Neurosurg.,* 24 (1966), 497–504.

29. FISHER, A. E. "The Role of Limbic Struc-

tures in the Central Regulation of Feeding and Drinking Behavior," *Ann. N.Y. Acad. Sci.*, 157 (1969), 894–901.

30. FRIEDE, R. L. "The Histochemical Architecture of the Ammon's Horn as Related to its Selective Vulnerability," *Acta Neuropathol.*, 6 (1966), 1–13.

31. GASTAUT, H. and H. J. LAMMERS. *Anatomie du rhinencéphale*. Paris: Masson et Cie., 1961.

32. GLOOR, P. "Amygdala," in *Handbook of Physiology*, Sec. I., Neurophysiology, Vol. 2. Washington: American Physiological Society, 1960.

33. GODDARD, G. V. "Amygdaloid Stimulation and Learning in the Rat," *J. Comp. Physiol. Psychol.*, 58 (1964), 23–30.

34. GREEN, J. D. "The Hippocampus," *Physiol. Rev.*, 44 (1964), 561–608.

35. GREEN, J. D., C. D. CLEMENTE, and J. DE GROOT. "Rhinencephalic Lesions and Behavior in Cats," *J. Comp. Neurol.*, 108 (1957), 505–545.

36. GROSSMAN, S. P. "Hypothalamic and Limbic Influences on Food Intake," *Fed. Proc.*, 27 (1968), 1349–1360.

37. HALSTEAD, W. C., W. B. RUCKER, and J. P. MCMAHON. "Memory," *Annu. Rev. Med.*, 18 (1967), 1–14.

38. HASSLER, R. and H. STEPHAN. *Evolution of the Forebrain*. Stuttgart: Georg Thieme Verlag, 1966.

39. HAYWARD, J. N. and W. K. SMITH. "Influence of Limbic System on Neurohypophysis," *Arch. Neurol.*, 9 (1963), 171–177.

40. JOHN, E. R. "Higher Nervous Functions: Brain Functions and Learning," *Annu. Rev. Physiol.*, 23 (1961), 451–484.

41. JOHNSTON, J. B. "Further Contributions to the Study of the Evolution of the Forebrain," *J. Comp. Neurol.*, 35 (1923), 337–481.

42. KAADA, B. R. "Somato-motor, Autonomic and Electrocorticographic Responses to Electrical Stimulation of 'Rhinencephalic' and Other Structures in Primates, Cat and Dog." *Acta Physiol. Scand. Suppl.*, 24 (1951), 1–285.

43. KANDEL, E. R., W. A. SPENCER and F. J. BRINLEY, JR. "Electrophysiology of Hippocampal Neurons: I. Sequential Invasion and Synaptic Organization," *J. Neurophysiol.*, 24 (1961), 225–242.

44. KLING, A. "Behavioral and Somatic Development Following Lesions of the Amygdala in the Cat," *J. Psychiatr. Res.*, 3 (1965), 263–273.

45. LISS, P. "Avoidance and Freezing Behavior Following Damage to the Hippocampus or Fornix," *J. Comp. Physiol. Psychol.*, 66 (1968), 193–197.

46. LIVINGSTON, K. E. and A. ESCOBAR. "Anatomical Bias of the Limbic System Concept," *Arch. Neurol.*, 24 (1971), 17–21.

47. LOCKE, S. and P. I. YAKOVLEV. "Transcallosal Connections of the Cingulum of Man," *Arch. Neurol.*, 13 (1965), 471–476.

48. MACLEAN, P. D. "Psychosomatic Disease and the 'Visceral Brain,'" *Psychosom. Med.*, 11 (1949), 338–353.

49. MARBURG, O. "The Structure and Fiber Connections of the Human Habenula," *J. Comp. Neurol.*, 80 (1944), 211–233.

50. MEISSNER, W. W. "Hippocampus and Learning," *Int. J. Neuropsychol.*, 3 (1967), 298–310.

51. MITCHELL, R. "Connections of the Habenula and of the Interpeduncular Nucleus in the Cat," *J. Comp. Neurol.*, 121 (1963), 441–458.

52. MORGANE, P. J. "The Function of the Limbic and Rhinic Forebrain-Limbic Midbrain Systems and Reticular Formation in the Regulation of Food and Water Intake," *Ann. N.Y. Acad. Sci.*, 157 (1969), 806–848.

53. NAFSTAD, H. J. "An Electron Microscope Study on the Termination of the Perforant Path Fibers in the Hippocampus and the Fascia Dentata," *Z. Zellforsch. Mikrosk. Anat.*, 76 (1967), 352–542.

54. NAUTA, W. J. H. "Hippocampal Projections and Related Neural Pathways to the Midbrain in the Cat," *Brain*, 81 (1958), 319–340.

55. ————. "Neural Associations of the Amygdaloid Complex in the Monkey," *Brain*, 85 (1962), 505–520.

56. PAPEZ, J. W. "A Proposed Mechanism of Emotion," *Arch. Neurol. Psychiatry*, 38 (1937), 725–743.

57. PARKES, A. S. and H. M. BRUCE. "Olfactory Stimuli in Mammalian Reproduction," *Science*, 134 (1961), 1049–1054.

58. PENFIELD, W. and B. MILNER. "Memory Deficit Produced by Bilateral Lesions in the Hippocampal Zone," *Arch. Neurol. Psychiatry*, 79 (1958), 475–497.

59. PETRAS, J. M. and C. R. NOBACK, eds., "Comparative and Evolutionary Aspects of the Vertebrate Central Nervous System," *Ann. N.Y. Acad. Sci.*, 167 (1969), 1–513.

60. PILLERI, G. "The Klüver-Bucy Syndrome in Man. A Clinico-anatomical Contribution to the Function of the Medial Temporal Lobe Structures," *Psychiatr. Neurol.* (Basel), 152 (1966), 65–103.

61. POECK, K. and G. PILLERI. "Release of Hypersexual Behaviour Due to Lesion in the Limbic System," *Acta Neurol. Scand.*, 41 (1965), 233–244.

62. POWELL, T. P. S., W. M. COWAN and G. RAISMAN. "The Central Olfactory Connexions," *J. Anat.*, 99 (1965), 791–813.

63. PRIBRAM, K. and L. KRUGER. Functions of the "Olfactory Brain", in: Conference on Basic Odor Research Correlation, *Ann. N.Y. Acad. Sci.*, 58 (1954), 109–138.

64. RAISMAN, G., W. M. COWAN and T. P. S. POWELL. "The Extrinsic Afferent, Commissural, and Association Fibers of the Hippocampus," *Brain*, 88 (1965), 963–996.

65. RAMON Y CAJAL, S. *Studies on the Cerebral Cortex*. L. M. Kraft, transl. Chicago: The Year Book Publishers, 1955.

66. REIS, D. J. and M. C. OLIPHANT. "Bradycardia and Tachycardia Following Electrical Stimulation of the Amygdaloid Region in Monkey," *J. Neurophysiol.*, 27 (1964), 893–912.

67. ROBERTS, D. R. "Functional Organization of the Limbic System," *Int. J. Neuropsychiatr.*, 2 (1966), 279–292.

68. SCALIA, F. "A Review of Recent Experimental Studies on the Distribution of the Olfactory Tracts in Mammals," *Brain Behav. Evol.*, 1 (1968), 101–123.

69. SCHREINER, L. and A. KLING. "Rhinencephalon and Behavior," *Am. J. Physiol.*, 184 (1956), 486–490.

70. SHAPIRO, N. M., A. GOL and P. KELLAWAY. "Acquisition, Retention, and Discrimination Reversal After Hippocampal Ablation in Monkeys," *Exp. Neurol.*, 13 (1965), 128–144.

71. SIEGEL, A. and J. P. FLYNN. "Differential Effects of Electrical Stimulation and Lesions of the Hippocampus and Adjacent Regions upon Attack Behavior in Cats,"

Brain Res., 7 (1968), 252–267.

72. SINGER, M. "Emotional and Psychiatric Aspects of the Limbic Lobe," *Dis. Nerv. Syst.*, 27 (1966), 309–317.

73. SMITH, C. G. *Basic Neuroanatomy*. Toronto: University of Toronto Press, 1971.

74. SMITH, G. E. "Morphology of the True 'Limbic Lobe', Corpus Callosum, Septum Pellucidum and Fornix," *J. Anat.*, (London), 30 (1895), 185–205.

75. TEITELBAUM, H. "A Comparison of Effects of Orbitofrontal and Hippocampal Lesions upon Discrimination Learning and Reversal in the Cat," *Exp. Neurol.*, 9 (1964), 452–462.

76. TINDAL, J. S., G. S. KNAGGS, and A. TURVEY. "Central Nervous Control of Prolactin Secretion in the Rabbit: Effect of Local Oestrogen Implants in the Amygdaloid Complex," *J. Endocrinol.*, 37 (1967), 279–287.

77. URSIN, H. "The Effect of Amygdaloid Lesions on Flight and Defense Behavior in Cats," *Exp. Neurol.*, 11 (1965), 61–79.

78. URSIN, H. and B. R. KAADA. "Functional Localization Within the Amygdaloid Complex in the Cat," *EEG. J. Clin. Neurophysiol.*, 12 (1960), 1–20.

79. VALENSTEIN, E. S. and W. J. H. NAUTA. "A Comparison of the Distribution of the Fornix System in the Rat, Guinea Pig, Cat, and Monkey," *J. Comp. Neurol.*, 113 (1959), 337–363.

80. VICTOR, M., J. B. ANGEVINE, JR., E. L. MANCALL et al. "Memory Loss with Lesions of Hippocampal Formation. Report of a Case with some Remarks on the Anatomical Basis of Memory," *Arch. Neurol.*, 5 (1961), 244–263.

81. VOTAW, C. L. and E. W. LAUER. "An Afferent Hippocampal Fiber System in the Fornix of the Monkey," *J. Comp. Neurol.*, 121 (1963), 195–206.

82. WHITE, L. E., JR. "A Morphologic Concept of the Limbic Lobe," *Int. Rev. Neurobiol.*, 8 (1965), 1–34.

83. WILLIS, T. *Cerebri Anatome*. London: Martzer and Alleftry, 1664.

84. WOLSTENHOLME, G. E. W. and J. KNIGHT. *Taste and Smell in Vertebrates*. Ciba Foundation Symposium. London: J. & A. Churchill, 1970.

CHAPTER 7

THE ISOCORTEX

Karl H. Pribram

The important role of neocortical mechanisms in cognitive behavior has been a focus of scientific interest for the past century and a half. In the early 1800s, arguments raged between physiologists (e.g., Flourens[21]) and phrenologists, many of whom were good anatomists (e.g., Gall and Spurzheim[22] as to whether the cerebral mantle functions as a unit or whether a mosaic of cerebral suborgans determines complex psychological events. During the intervening period data have been subsumed under one or the other of these two views—almost always with the effect of strengthening one at the expense of the other. In the recent past, the accumulation of data has so markedly accelerated that a reevaluation of the problem promises to prove fruitful. Specifically, the data obtained by the use of electronic amplifying devices to study neural events has raised questions concerning the validity of concepts generated by neuroanatomical techniques; the adaptation to subhuman primates of measures of choice behavior has stimulated discussion of the validity of concepts derived from clinical neurological material.

❨ Problems of Neural Organization

First, let us take a look at some *neural* data and see how they fit current conceptualizations of cerebral organization. Explicitly or implicitly, most of us tend to think of the brain as being composed of receiving areas (sensory cortex) that function in some fairly simple fashion to transmit receptor events to adjacent areas of "association" cortex. Here, these neural events are "elaborated" and associated with other neural events before being transmitted to the motor areas of the brain; these motor areas are said to serve as the principal effector mechanism for all cerebral activity. This model was proposed some seventy-five years ago by Flechsig[20] on the basis of the then available anatomical information. As we shall see, the neural data available today make it necessary to modify this model considerably.

But, before we can come to grips with a new conception of brain organization, it is necessary to clarify some definitions. Over the years many of the terms used in neurology have been imbued with multiple designations.

Neocortex is such a term. Comparative anatomists use this word to describe the dorsolateral portions of the cerebral mantle since these portions show a *differentially* maximum development in microsmatic mammals (such as primates) as compared with macrosmatic mammals (such as cats). In other branches of the neurological sciences (see Grossman[25]) the term neocortex has come to cover *all* the cortical formations that reach maximum development in primates. The definition as used in these sciences subsumes portions of the cortex on the medial and basal surface of the cerebral hemisphere, which, though well developed in macrosmatic mammals, do show *some* additional development in primates. Since this mediobasal limbic cortex has been related[58,60] to behavior rather different from that which concerns us in this paper, it seems worthwhile to find an unambiguous term that delimits the dorsolateral cortex. As reviewed in an early publication,[58] the cerebral cortex may be classified according to whether or not it passes through a six-layered embryonic stage. The medial and basal limbic structures do not pass through such a stage and are called allo or juxtallocortex; the dorsolateral portions of the cerebral cortex do pass through such a stage and are called isocortex.

It has been fashionable to subdivide isocortex according to cytoarchitectonic differences; difficulties in classification have been pointed out[4,32,60] that question the immediate usefulness of distinctions based solely on the histological picture of the cortex. I should prefer, therefore, to subdivide isocortex on the basis of thalamocortical relationships since these relationships are determined by the most reliable neurohistological technique available to us: namely, retrograde degeneration of neurons in the thalamus following cortical resection. But, if we are to use this criterion of subdivision of cortex because it is a reliable one, we are forced into looking at the organization of the thalamus as the key to the organization of the cortex. Rose and Woolsey[65] have divided thalamic nuclei into two classes: (1) those receiving large tracts of extrathalamic afferents and (2) those receiving the major portions of their direct afferents from

within the thalamus. The former they called extrinsic (primary projection) and the latter, intrinsic (association) nuclei. Thalamocortical connections, demonstrated by retrograde degeneration studies[9,12,57,75] make possible the differentiation of isocortical sectors on the basis of their connections with extrinsic (primary projection) or with intrinsic (association) thalamic nuclei.

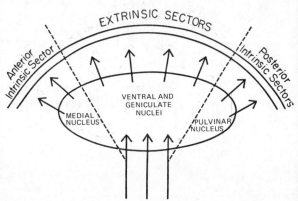

Figure 7–1. Diagrammatic scheme illustrating the division of isocortex into extrinsic (primary projection) and intrinsic (association) sectors on the basis of thalamic afferent connections. The ventral and geniculate thalamic nuclei which receive major direct afferents from extracerebral structures project to the extrinsic sectors; the medial and pulvinar thalamic nuclei do not receive such afferents and project to the intrinsic sectors.

It can be seen from Figure 7–1 that the portions of the cortex labeled as "extrinsic sectors" correspond essentially to those usually referred to as "primary projection areas," while those labeled "intrinsic sectors" correspond essentially to those usually referred to as "association areas." However, the terms association cortex and primary projection areas have their drawbacks: (1) Association cortex implies that in these portions of the cortex convergent tracts bring together excitations from the "receiving areas" of the brain. As we shall see, this implication is unsupported by fact. (2) Electrophysiological experiments, which will be discussed below, have demonstrated a topographical complexity of organization that necessitated labels such as Areas I and II. Should the term primary projection areas be used to denote the Areas I only or should it cover such areas as II as well? Additional confusion arises since the intrinsic (association) sectors *do* receive a thalamic projection, so that the term "secondary projection areas" has been suggested for these sectors.[67] These considerations have led me to substitute the currently less loaded terms, "extrinsic" and "intrinsic."

Can the subdivision of cerebral isocortex into extrinsic (primary projection) and intrinsic (association) sectors be validated when techniques other than retrograde thalamic degeneration are used? Figure 7–3 shows the extent of the cortical connections when myelinated fibers are traced by the Marchi (osmic-acid) staining technique from peripheral structures, such as optic tract and dorsal spinal roots, through the thalamus to the cortex. As can be seen by comparing Figures 7–2 and 7–3, there are, thus, at least two anatomical techniques that permit approximately the same subdivision of isocortex: one derived from cell body stains; the second, from nerve fiber stains. Further support for the classification comes from electrophysiological data. When receptors are mechanically or electrically stimulated or when peripheral nerves are electrically stimulated, an abrupt change in electrical potential can be recorded from portions of the brain that are connected to these peripheral structures. Under appropriate conditions of anesthesia, maps may be constructed on the basis of size of the potential

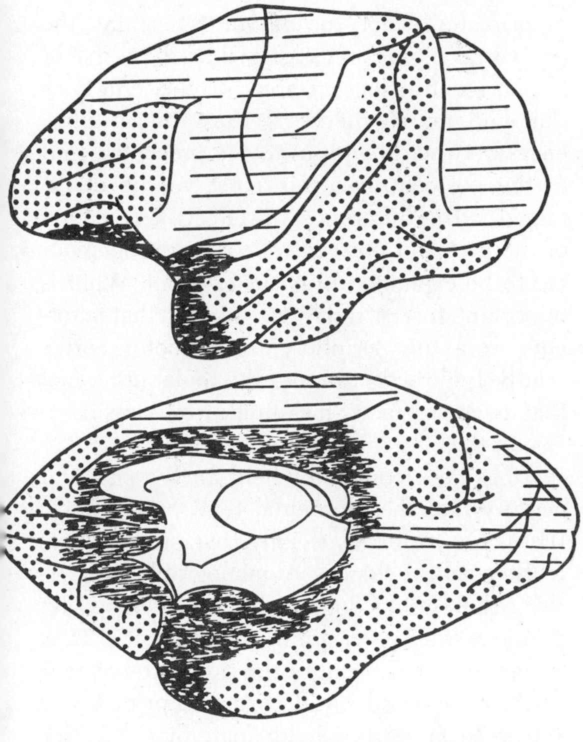

Figure 7–2. Diagrams of the lateral (above) and mediobasal (below) surfaces of the monkey's cerebral hemisphere showing the divisions discussed in the text. Shaded indicates allo-juxtallocortex; lined indicates extrinsic (primary projection) isocortex; dotted indicates intrinsic (association) isocortex. Boundaries are not sharply delimited; this is, in part, due to minor discrepancies which result when different techniques are used and, in part, to difficulties in classification due to borderline instances and inadequate data (e.g., how should the projections of *n. ventralis anterior* and of *lateralis posterior* be classified?)

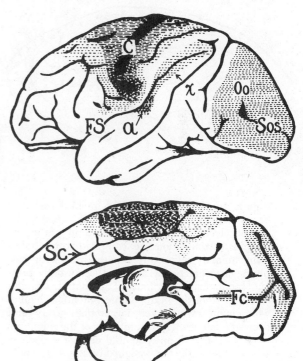

Figure 7–3. Extrinsic (primary projection) sectors as mapped by staining degenerating axons following thalamic lesions.

changes evoked and the latency that intervenes between the time of stimulation and the
recording of the potential change (Figure
7–4). As can be seen from the comparison of
the maps made by the histological and electrophysiological techniques, there is considerable, though by no means complete, correspondence between various delineations of
the extrinsic (primary projection) from the intrinsic (association) sectors of the isocortex.

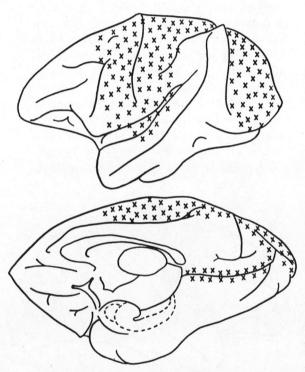

Figure 7–4. Diagrams of the monkey cerebral
hemisphere as in Figures 2 and 3. This map of the
abrupt electrical changes induced in cortex by
peripheral stimulation was compiled from studies
using animals sufficiently anesthetized with barbiturates to practically abolish the normally present spontaneous rhythms of potential changes
recorded from the brain. Those potential changes
were counted which were larger than 50 μv. and
showed a latency within 3 millisec of the minimum
latency of any abrupt potential change evoked in
the particular afferent system investigated. These
criteria were chosen as the most likely to indicate
major direct afferents from periphery to cortex.
The correspondences and minor discrepancies between this figure and Figure 3 indicate the approximate range of such similarities when different
techniques and brain diagrams are used.

(Input–Output Relationships

Enough of definitions. I am sure you are convinced by now that the cerebral isocortex may
usefully be divided according to whether its
major input derives, via the thalamus, directly
from the periphery or whether that input is
largely intracerebral. But have you noticed
that, according to all of the techniques mentioned, input from extracerebral structures
reaches the portions of the cortex usually referred to as motor as well as those known as
sensory areas? Electrophysiological experiments demonstrate that somatic afferents are
distributed to both sides of the central fissure
of primates. Since the *afferents* reaching the
precentral motor areas as well as those reaching postcentral sensory areas originate in both
skin and muscle nerves,[37] the critical differences between the input to the precentral and
to the postcentral cortex must yet be determined if the differences in effect of resection
of the pre- and postcentral cortex on behavior
are to be explained in terms of input. What is
important for us today is the fact that afferents from the periphery reach motor cortex
relatively directly through the thalamus, a fact
that becomes more meaningful on consideration of the efferents leaving the isocortex.

It has been commonly held for the past half
century that the pyramidal tract originates in
the motor cortex, especially that portion close
to the central fissure. A monograph by Lassek[33] thoroughly documents the evidence for
a more extensive origin of the pyramidal tract
from the entire extent of the precentral as well
as from the postcentral cortex of primates: a
return to an earlier held anatomical position
that had become submerged during the first
half of this century. Another conception held
during this latter period, the distinction between pyramidal and extrapyramidal, has repeatedly been questioned in the light of these
and other data. Woolsey[80] has shown that the
differences in movement brought about by
electrical stimulation of the various parts of
the precentral cortex may be ascribed to differences in somatotopic relationships rather
than to differences in the complexity of or-

ganization of the movement. Thus, Woolsey finds that stimulations in the more forward portions of the precentral region, which had formerly been called premotor, activate the axial musculature, while those close to the central fissure activate appendicular musculature. Since axial muscles are larger, the movements they produce appear grosser than those produced by such discrete appendicular muscular units as those found in the hand—one need not invoke different orders of coordination or complexity to distinguish between the posterior and anterior portions of the motor cortex. Thus, the distinction between motor and premotor cortex fades and, as a result, makes unnecessary the classical distinction between the locus of origin of the pyramidal and extrapyramidal systems, which has already been called into question by anatomical data.

On the other hand, evidence from ablation and stimulation experiments in both man and monkey indicates the continued necessity for differentiating precentral motor from postcentral sensory mechanisms.[27] Certainly the distinction cannot be thought of simply in terms of afferents reaching the postcentral and efferents leaving the precentral cortex. Thus, with these data in mind, a thorough reinvestigation is needed of the organization of the input–output relationships of the extrinsic (primary projection) system related to somatic structures.

The marked overlap of input–output is not limited to the somatic extrinsic (primary projection) system. With respect to vision, eye movements can be elicited from stimulation of practically all the striate cortex;[76] these eye movements can be elicited after ablation of the other cortical areas from which eye movements are obtained. With respect to audition, ear movements have been elicited;[3,73] respiratory effects follow stimulation of the olfactory receiving areas.[26,58] Thus, an overlap of afferents and efferents is evident not only in the neural mechanisms related to somatic function but also in those related to the special senses. The overgeneralization to the brain of the law of (Bell and) Magendie,[36] which defines sensory in terms of afferents in the dorsal-spinal and motor in terms of efferents in the

ventral-spinal roots, must, therefore, give way to a more precise investigation of the differences in internal organization of the afferent-efferent relationship between periphery and cortex in order to explain differences such as those between sensory and motor mechanisms. As yet only a few experiments toward this end have been undertaken.[1,14,64]

The afferent-efferent overlap in the *extrinsic* (primary projection) system suggests the possibility that the intrinsic (association) systems need not be considered as association centers upon which pathways from the extrinsic sensory sectors converge to bring together neural events anticipatory to spewing them out via the motor pathways. Unfortunately, there are few reliable anatomical data concerning the connections of the intrinsic sectors so that our analysis of the organization of these systems relies largely on neuropsychological data. Let us turn, therefore, to experiments that manipulate cerebral isocortex either by stimulation or resection, and observe the effects of such manipulations on behavior.

(Classification of the Amnestic Syndromes

I want to take this opportunity to dispel the myth that experimentally produced local brain lesions (especially ablations) do not affect memory functions, that is, learning and remembering. This conception, like so many in neuromythology, derives its strength from the fact that it is a half-truth. In this instance, the idea rests largely on Lashley's[28] contribution, *Brain Mechanisms and Intelligence*, and derives support from his later publication,[31] "In Search of the Engram." Lashley presented evidence and made interpretations. I shall show here that his data have been superseded —thus the fanciful aspect of the current myth —but that his interpretations were extremely shrewd—thus the myth's persistence. To make the counterargument I will describe data from experiments made over the past twenty-five years. In my laboratories alone some twelve hundred behaviorally tested rhesus monkeys have been subjected to selective brain operations during this period. These studies provide evidence that makes me think that the impairments in memory functions produced by local experimental lesions are best subsumed as deficiencies in input processing, and I will describe the evidence that demonstrates that memory traces become distributed widely within a sensory projection system. I will then argue that the mechanism of remembering critically involves input coding, both during storage and retrieval.

As noted earlier, the experimental analysis of subhuman primate, psychosurgical preparations has, contrary to popular opinion, uncovered a host of memory disturbances. The initial technique by which these brain-behavior relationships were established is called the method of the "intersect of sums,"[44] an extension of what Teuber named the method of "double dissociation" of signs of brain trauma. The intersect-of-sums method depends on classifying the behavioral deficit produced by cortical ablations into *yes* and *no* instances on the basis of some arbitrarily chosen criterion; then plotting on a brain map the total extent of tissue associated with each of the categories —*ablated:deficit; not ablated:no deficit*—and finally finding the intersect of those two areas (essentially subtracting the *noes* from the *yeses-plus-noes*). This procedure is repeated for each type of behavior under quantitative consideration. The resulting map of localization of disturbances is then validated by making lesions restricted to the site determined by the intersect method and showing that the maximal behavioral deficit is obtained by the restricted lesion (see Table 7–1 and Figure 7–5).

Once the neurobehavioral correlation has been established by the intersect-of-sums technique, two additional experimental steps are undertaken. First, holding the lesion constant, a series of variations is made of the task on which performance was found defective. These experimental manipulations determine the limits over which the brain-behavior disturbance correlations hold and thus allow reasonable constructions of models of the psychological processes impaired by the various surgical procedures.

Second, neuroanatomical and electrophysiological techniques are engaged to work out the relationships between the brain areas under examination and the rest of the nervous system. These experimental procedures allow the construction of reasonable models of the functions of the areas and of the mechanisms of impairment.

Two major classes of memory disturbance have been delineated by these operations: *specific* and *contextual* amnesias.

TABLE 7–1. **Simultaneous Visual Choice Reaction** *

Operates without deficit		Operates with deficit		Nonoperate controls	
Pre	Post		Pre	Post		Pre	Post
OP 1	200	0	PTO 1	120	272	C 1	790	80
OP 2	220	0	PTO 2	325	F	C 2	230	20
OP 3	380	0	PTO 3	180	F	C 3	750	20
LT 1	390	190	PTO 4	120	450	C 4	440	0
LT 2	300	150	T 1	940	F		
H 1	210	220	T 2	330	F		
HA	350	240	VTH 1	320	F		
FT 1	580	50	VTH 2	370	F		
FT 3	50	0	VTH 3	280	F		
FT 4	205	0	VTH 4	440	F		
FT 5	300	200	VT 1	240	F		
FT 6	250	100	VT 2	200	F		
DL 1	160	140	VT 3	200	890		
DL 2	540	150	VT 4	410	F		
DL 3	300	240	VT 5	210	F		
DL 4	120	100					
MV 1	110	0					
MV 2	150	10					
MV 3	290	130					
MV 4	230	10					
MV 5	280	120					
CIN 1	120	80					
CIN 2	400	60					
CIN 3	115	74					
CIN 4	240	140					

* Pre- and postoperative scores on a simultaneous visual choice reaction of the animals whose brains are diagrammed in Fig. 5, indicating the number of trials taken to reach a criterion of 90% correct on 100 consecutive trials. Deficit is defined as a larger number of trials taken in the "retention" test than in original learning. (The misplacement of the score H 1 does not change the overall results as given in the text.)

❨ The Specific Amnesias

Between the sensory projection areas of the primate cerebral mantle lies a vast expanse of parieto-temporo-preoccipital cortex. Clinical observation has assigned disturbance of many gnostic and language functions to lesions of this expanse. Experimental psychosurgical analysis in subhuman primates, of course, is limited to nonverbal behavior; within this limitation, however, a set of sensory-specific agnosias (discrimination disabilities and losses in

thinking, and experiments that led to our present view of the function of the inferior temporal cortex in vision.

VISUAL CHOICE REACTION

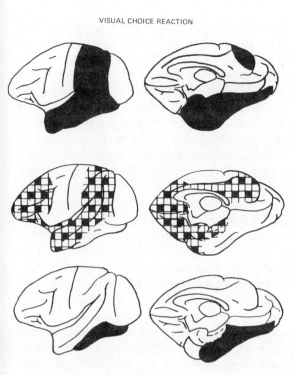

Figure 7–5. The upper diagram represents the sum of the areas of resection of all of the animals grouped as showing deficit. The middle diagram represents the sum of the areas of resection of all of the animals grouped as showing no deficit. The lower diagram represents the intersect of the area shown in black in the upper diagram and that *not* checkerboarded in the middle diagram. This intersect represents the area invariably implicated in visual choice behavior in these experiments.

the capacity to identify cues) have been produced. Distinct regions of primate cortex have been shown to be involved in each of the modality–specific mnemonic functions: anterior temporal in gustation,[3] inferior temporal in vision,[39] midtemporal in audition,[77,17] and occipitoparietal in somesthesis.[43] In each instance, discriminations learned prior to surgical interference are lost to the subject postoperatively and great difficulty (using a "savings" criterion) in reacquisition is experienced, if task solution is possible at all.

The behavioral analysis of these "specific" amnesias is still underway, but an outline of the psychological process involved can be discussed. Perhaps the easiest way to communicate this outline is to detail the observations,

❨ Search and Sampling

All sorts of differences in the physical dimensions of the stimulus—for example, size (Figure 7–6)—are distinguished less after the lesion,[38] but there is more to the disability than this as illustrated in the following story.

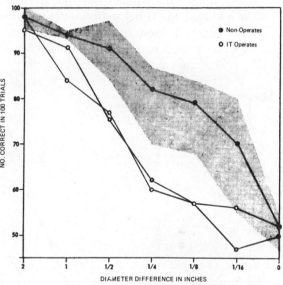

Figure 7–6. Scores for two operates and four controls on the first run of size discrimination. Shaded area indicates the range of performance of the four nonoperate controls. IT operates monkeys with resections of inferior temporal cortex.

One day while testing monkeys with such lesions at the Yerkes Laboratories in Orange Park, Florida, I sat down to rest from the chore of carrying a monkey the considerable distance between home cage and laboratory. The monkeys, including this one, were failing miserably at the visual discrimination task being administered. It was a hot muggy, typical Florida summer afternoon and the air was swarming with gnats. My monkey reached out and caught a gnat. Without thinking I also reached for a gnat—and missed. The monkey reached out again, caught a gnat, and put it in his mouth. I reached out—missed! Finally, the paradox of the situation forced itself on me. I took the beast back to the testing room: He was as deficient in making visual choice as ever. But when no choice was involved, the monkey's visually guided behavior appeared to be intact. This gave rise to the following experiment (Figure 7–7), which Ettlinger[18] carried out. On the basis of this particular observation, we made the hypothesis that choice was the crucial variable responsible for the deficient discrimination following inferotemporal lesions. As long as a monkey does not have to make a choice, his visual performance should remain intact. To test this hypothesis, monkeys were trained in a Gantzfeld made of a

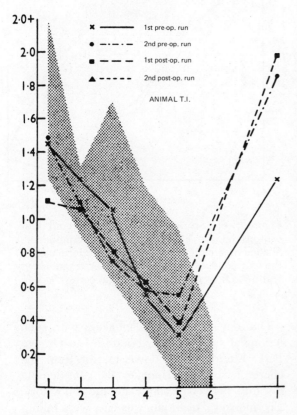

Figure 7–7. Single manipulandum performance curves of a single animal in a varying brightness situation. Shaded area indicates variability among groups of four animals.

translucent light fixture large enough so the animal could be physically inserted into it. The animal could press a lever throughout the procedure but was rewarded only during the period when illumination was markedly increased for several seconds at a time. Soon response frequency became maximal during this "bright" period. Under such conditions no differences in performance were obtained between inferotemporally lesioned and control animals. The result tended to support the view that if an inferotemporally lesioned monkey did not have to make a choice he would show no deficit in behavior, since in another experiment[39] the monkeys failed to respond differentially to differences in brightness.

In another instance[60] we trained the monkeys on a very simple object discrimination test: an ashtray versus tobacco tin (Figure 7–8). These animals had been trained for two or three years before they were operated on and were therefore sophisticated problemsolvers; this, plus ease of task, accounts for the minimal deficit in the simultaneous choice task. (There are two types of successive discrimination: In one the animal has either to go or not to go, and in the other he has to go left or right.) When given the same cues successively, the monkeys showed a deficit when compared with their controls, despite this demonstrated ability to differentiate the cues in the simultaneous situation.

This result further supported the idea that the problem for the operated monkeys was not so much in "seeing" but in usefully manipulating what they saw. Not only the stimulus conditions per se but the whole range of response determinants appear involved in specifying the deficit. To test this idea in a quantitative fashion we next asked whether the deficit would vary as a function of the *number* of alternatives in the situation.[41] The hope was that an informational measure of the deficit could be obtained. Actually something very different appeared when the number of errors was plotted against the number of alternatives (see Figure 7–9).

If one plots repetitive errors made before the subject finds a peanut—that is, the number of times a monkey searches the same cue

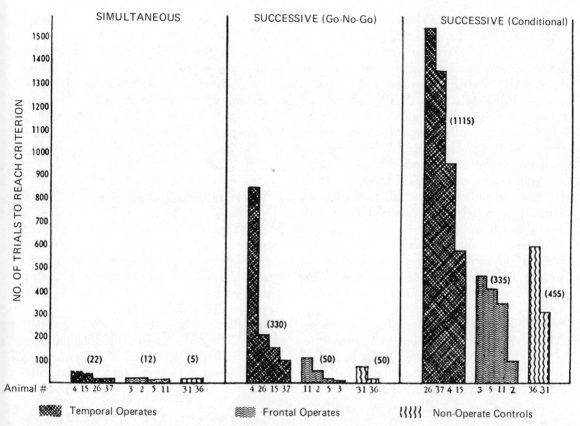

Figure 7–8. Comparison of learning scores on three types of object discrimination by three groups of monkeys. Note that though the cues remain the same, changing the response which was demanded increased the deficit of the inferotemporal groups.

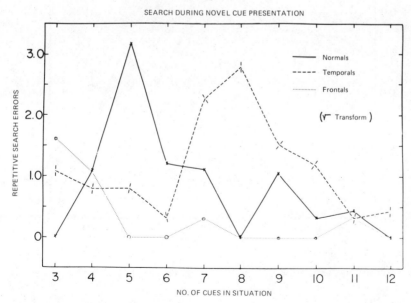

Figure 7–9. Graph of the average number of repetitive errors made in the multiple object experiment during those search trials in each situation when the additional, that is, the novel, cue is first added.

—versus the number of alternatives in the situation, one finds there is a hump in the curve, a stage where control subjects make many repetitive errors. The monkeys do learn the appropriate strategy, however, and go on to complete the task with facility. What intrigued me was that during this stage the monkeys with inferotemporal lesions were doing better than the controls! This seemed a paradox. As the test continued, however, after the controls no longer made so many errors, the lesioned subjects began to accumulate an error hump even greater than that shown earlier by the controls.

When a stimulus sampling model was applied to the analysis of the data, a difference in sampling was found (Figure 7–10). The monkeys with inferotemporal lesions showed a lowered sampling ratio; they sampled fewer cues during the first half of the experiment. Their defect can be characterized as a restriction in the visual field; however, the limitation is not in the visual-spatial field but in the information-processing field. That is, in the

number of alternatives they can sample or handle at any one time.

In short, the modality-specific defect that results from a posterior "association" system lesion appears to produce an information-processing defect best described as a restriction on the number of alternatives searched and sampled.

⦅ The Contextual Amnesias

The second major division of the cerebral mantle to which mnestic functions have been assigned by clinical observation lies on the medial and basal surface of the brain and extends forward to include the poles of the frontal and temporal lobes. This frontolimbic portion of the hemisphere is cytoarchitecturally diverse. The expectation that different parts might be shown to subserve different functions therefore is even greater than that entertained for the apparently uniform posterior

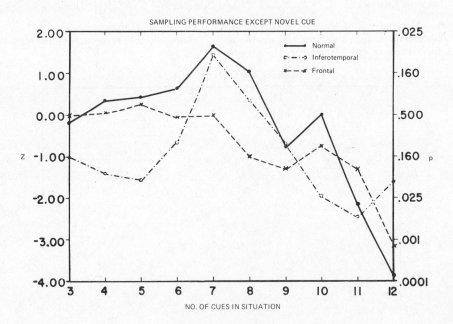

Figure 7–10. Graph of the average proportion of objects (cues) that are sampled (except novel cue) by each of the groups in each of the situations. To sample, a monkey had to move an object until the content or lack of content of the food well was clearly visible to the experimenter. As was predicted, during the first half of the experiment the curve representing the sampling ratio of the posteriorly lesioned group differs significantly from the others at the 0.024 level (according to the nonparametric Mann–Whitney U Test).

cortex. In the case of the posterior cortex, the diversity of lesion effects nonetheless allowed classification: differential discriminations were always involved, and the defects turned out to be sensory-mode specific. In the same manner, lesions of the frontolimbic region, irrespective of location (dorsolateral frontal, cingulate-medial frontal, orbitofrontal-caudate, temporal polar-amygdala, and hippocampal) have been shown to produce disruption of "delayed alternation" behavior. The alternation task demands that the subject alternate his responses between two cues (for example, between two places or between two objects) on successive trials. On any trial the correct response is dependent on the outcome of the previous response. This suggests that the critical variable that characterizes the task is its temporal organization. In turn, this leads to the supposition that the disruption of alternation behavior produced by frontolimbic lesions results from an impairment of the process by which the brain achieves its temporal organization. This supposition is in part confirmed by further analysis, but severe restrictions on what is meant by temporal organization arise. For instance, skills are not affected by frontolimbic lesions, nor are discriminations of melodies. Retrieval of long-held memories also is little affected. Rather, shorter term mnestic processes are singularly involved. In animal experiments these are demonstrated especially clearly when tasks demand matching from memory a cue (as in the delayed response problem) or outcome (as in the alternation task) that in the past has shown some complexity in the regularity of its recurrence. Rather than identify an item, the organism must fit the present event into a context of prior occurrences, only some of which relate directly to the situation at hand.

As noted, different parts of the frontolimbic complex would, on the basis of their different structures, be expected to function somewhat differently within the category of short-term mnestic processes. Indeed, different forms of contextual amnesia are produced by different lesions. But these relationships between the structures of the limbic forebrain and behavior are beyond the scope of this paper. Let us

therefore examine more closely the effects of frontal isocortical resection on problem solving.

❲ The Parsing Problem

Classically, disturbance of immediate memory has been ascribed to lesions of the frontal pole. Anterior and medial frontal resections were the first to be shown to produce impairment on delayed response and delayed alternation problems. In other tests, frontal lesions also take their toll: Impairment of the orienting galvanic skin response (GSR) is found, and of conditioned avoidance behavior, as well as of classical conditioning. Furthermore, error sensitivity was tested in an operant conditioning situation (Figure 7–11). After several years of training on mixed and multiple

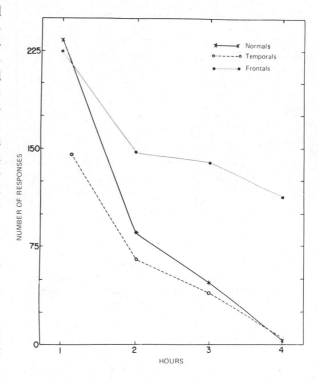

Figure 7–11. Graph of performance of three groups of monkeys under conditions of extinction in a mixed schedule operant conditioning situation. Note the slower extinction of the frontally lesioned monkeys.

schedules, four hours of extinction were run, that is, the reinforcement (peanuts) was no longer delivered, although everything else in the situation remained the same. Note that the frontally lesioned animals failed to extinguish in the four-hour period, whereas the control monkeys did.[49]

This failure in extinction accounts in part for poor performance in the alternation already described (Figure 7–12): the frontally lesioned animals make many more repetitive errors. Even though they do not find a peanut, they go right back and keep looking.[44]

This result was confirmed and amplified in a study by Wilson.[79] He analyzed the occasions for error: did errors follow alternation or nonreinforcement? To determine which, he de-

vised a situation in which both lids over the food well opened simultaneously, but the monkey could obtain the peanut only if he had opened the baited well. Thus the monkey was given "complete" information on every trial and the usual correction technique could be circumvented. With this apparatus the procedure was followed with four variations: correction-contingent, correction-noncontingent, noncorrection-contingent, and noncorrection-noncontingent. The contingency referred to is whether the position of the peanut depended on the prior correct or incorrect response of the monkey or whether its position was alternated independently of the monkey's behavior. Wilson then analyzed the relationship between an error and the trial preceding that error. Notice (Table 7–2) that for the normal monkey the condition of reinforcement and nonreinforcement of the previous trial makes a difference, whereas for the frontally lesioned monkey this is not the case. Alternation affects both normal and frontal subjects about equally. In this situation, frontal subjects are simply uninfluenced by rewarding or nonrewarding consequences of their behavior.

Now let me return to the multiple choice experiment discussed earlier.[46] (p. 114). Here also this inefficacy of outcomes to influence behavior is demonstrated; it is illustrated

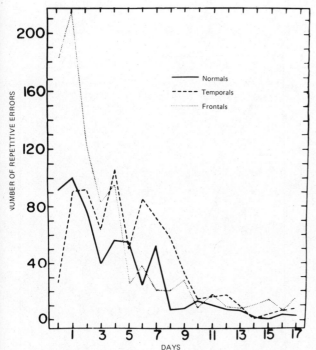

Figure 7–12. Graph showing the differences in the number of repetitive errors made by groups of monkeys in a go, no-go type of delayed reaction experiment. Especially during the initial trials, frontally operated animals repeatedly return to the food well after exposure to the "nonrewarded" predelay cue. Note, however, that this variation of the delay problem is mastered easily by the frontally operated group.

TABLE 7–2. **Percentage of Alternation as a Function of Response and Outcome of Preceding Trial** [*]

S	Preceding trial [†]			
	A-R	A-NR	NA-R	NA-NR
Normal				
394	53	56	40	45
396	54	53	36	49
398	49	69	27	48
384	61	83	33	72
Total	55	68	34	52
Frontal				
381	49	51	41	43
437	42	46	27	26
361	49	48	38	35
433	43	39	31	32
Total	46	46	33	33

[*] Comparison of the performance of frontally ablated and normal monkeys on alternations made subsequent to reinforced (R) and nonreinforced (NR) and an alternated (A) and nonalternated (NA) response.

[†] A, alternated; NA, did not alternate; R, was rewarded; and NR, was not rewarded.

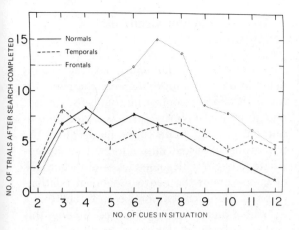

Figure 7–13. Graph of the average number of trials to criterion taken in the multiple object experiment by each group in each of the situations after search was completed, that is, after the first correct response. Note the difference between the curves for the controls and for the frontally operated group, a difference that is significant at the .05 level by an analysis of variance (F = 8.19 for 2 and 6 df) according to McNemar's procedure performed on normalized (by square root transformation) raw scores.

(Figure 7–13) by an increased number of trials to criterion after the monkeys have first found the peanut. The procedure calls for the strategy of return to the same object for five consecutive times, that is, to criterion. The frontally lesioned animals are markedly deficient in doing this. Again, we see that the conditions of reinforcement are relatively ineffective in shaping behavior once the frontal eugranular cortex has been removed, so that the monkeys' behavior is relatively random when compared to that of normal subjects.[55] Behavior of the frontally lesioned monkeys thus appears to be minimally controlled by its (repeatedly experienced and therefore expected) consequences.

Frontal lesions work their havoc on yet another contextual dimension. This is best demonstrated by manipulating the alternation task in a special way: Instead of interposing equal intervals between trials (Right-5″-Left-5″-Right-5″-Left-5″-Right-5″-Left-5″ . . .) as in the classic task, couplets of RL were formed by extending the intertrial interval to 15 seconds before each R trial (R-5″-L-15″-R-5″-L-

15″-R-5″–L-15″ . . .). Immediately the performance of the frontally lesioned monkeys improved and was indistinguishable from that of their controls.[62] I interpret this result to mean that for the subject with a bilateral frontal ablation, the alternation task becomes something like what this page would seem were there no spaces between words. The spaces, and the holes in doughnuts, provide some of the structure, the parcellation, parsing of events (doughnuts, alternations, and words) by which they became codable and decipherable.

⟨ An Alternative to the Transcortical Reflex

Models of cerebral organization in cognitive processes have, heretofore, been based to a large extent on clinical neurological data and have been formulated with the reflex as prototype. Such models state that input is organized in the extrinsic sensory, elaborated in the intrinsic associative, and from there relayed to the extrinsic motor sectors. I have already pointed out that the afferent-efferent overlap in the extrinsic (primary projection) system makes such notions of cerebral organization suspect. A series of neuropsychological studies by Lashely,[30] Sperry,[67,69] Chow,[10] Evarts,[19] and Wade[74] in which the extrinsic (primary projection) sectors were surgically cross-hatched, circumsected, or isolated by large resections of their surround, with little apparent effects on behavior, has cast further doubt on the usefulness of such a transcortical model. Additional difficulties are posed by the negative electrophysiological and anatomical findings whenever direct connections are sought between the extrinsic (primary projection) and intrinsic (association) sectors.[6,59] These data focus anew our attention on the problem faced repeatedly by those interested in cerebral functions in cognitive behavior. Experimentalists who followed Flourens in dealing with the hierarchical aspects of cerebral organization—e.g., Munk,[41] Monakow,[40] Goldstein,[24] Loeb,[34] and Lashley[28]—have invariably come to emphasize the importance of the *extrinsic* (primary projection) sectors not only in "sensorimotor" behavior but also in the more complex "cognitive" processes. Each investigator has had a slightly different approach to the functions of the *intrinsic* (association) sectors, but the viewpoints share the proposition that the intrinsic sectors do not function independently of the extrinsic. The common difficulty has been the conceptualization of this interdependence between intrinsic (association) and extrinsic (primary projection) systems in terms other than the transcortical reflex model—a model that became less cogent with each new experiment.

Is there an alternative that meets the objections leveled against the transcortical reflex yet accounts for currently available data? I believe there is. The hierarchical relationship between intrinsic (association) and extrinsic (primary projection) systems can be attributed to a convergence of the *output* of the two systems at a subcortical locus rather than to a specific input from the extrinsic cortex to the intrinsic. Some evidence supporting this notion is already available. Data obtained by Whitlock and Nauta,[78] using silver staining techniques, show that *both* the intrinsic and extrinsic sectors implicated in vision by neuropsychological experiments are *efferently* connected with the superior colliculus. On the other hand, lesions of the intrinsic thalamic nuclei fail to interfere with discriminative behavior.[11,42] Thus, the specific effects in behavior of the intrinsic (association) systems are explained on the basis of output to a subcortically located neural mechanism that functions specifically (e.g., superior colliculus in vision). This output, in turn, affects input to the extrinsic (primary projection) systems either directly or through the efferent control of the receptor (e.g., in vision, mechanisms of eye movement, accommodation). According to this conception, the associative functions of the central nervous system are to be sought at convergence points throughout the central nervous system, especially in the brain stem and spinal axis, and not solely in the intrinsic (association) cerebral sectors.

(How the Brain Controls Its Input

Recently much of our effort has been channeled into an attempt to increase the evidence for such efferent control mechanisms. To this end, a series of experiments was undertaken to find out how the brain cortex might affect the processing of visual information. It is appropriate to begin with some facts—or rather lack of facts—about the neuroanatomical relationships of the inferotemporal cortex. There is a dearth of neurological evidence linking this cortex to the known visual system, the geniculostriate system. There are no definitive anatomical inputs specific to the inferotemporal cortex from the visual cortex or the geniculate nucleus. Of course, connections can be traced via fibers that synapse twice in the preoccipital region, but connections also exist between the visual cortex and the parietal lobe, the excision of which results in no change in visual behavior (as shown above). In addition, massive circumsection of the striate cortex does not impair visual discrimination.[11,56] Further evidence that these "corticocortical" connections are not the important ones can be seen from the following experiment. I performed (Table 7–3) a crosshatch of the inferotemporal cortex, much as Sperry[68] had done earlier for the striate cortex, and found no deficit either in visual learning or in performance. On

TABLE 7–3.   **Comparison of the Effects of Undercutting and Crosshatching Inferotemporal Cortex of Monkeys on Their Performance in Several Discriminations**

	Animal	3 vs 8	R vs G	3 vs 8
Crosshatch	158	380	82	0
	159	180	100	0
	161	580	50	0
	166	130	0	0
Undercut	163	[1014]	100	300
	164	[1030]	200	[500]
	167	704	50	0
	168	[1030]	150	[500]
Normal	160	280	100	0
	162	180	100	0
	165	280	100	0
	170	350	100	0

the other hand, undercutting the inferotemporal cortex made a vast difference: it precluded both learning and performance in visual tasks. This suggests that the relationships essential to visual behavior must be cortico-subcortical.

This proposal can be tested, viz that the essential relations of the posterior association cortex are centrifugal, or efferent.[45] There is physiological evidence to suggest and support such a notion. In addition to an output to the superior colliculus (mentioned above), a large system of connections leads from the inferotemporal cortex to the ventral part of the putamen, a basal ganglion usually considered motor in function.[63] How would an efferent mechanism of this sort work? To find out we performed the following experiment.

Instead of making ablations or implanting an epileptogenic lesion, we now chronically and continuously stimulate the brain. Dr. D.N. Spinelli in my laboratory designed the stimulator (Figure 7–14) and the recording equipment.[70] The stimulator is sufficiently

small so that it can be implanted under the scalp. It puts out a square-wave bidirectional pulse, 1 msec. in duration and about 3 v in amplitude. The frequency of stimulation is approximately 8 to 10 pulses/second. The batteries that drive the stimulator are rechargeable.

Records were made in the awake monkey (Figure 7–15). Paired flashes are presented and recordings are made from electrodes implanted in the occipital cortex. The response to fifty such paired flashes are accumulated on a computer for average transients. The flash-flash interval is varied from twenty-five to two

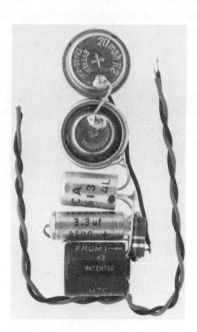

Figure 7–14. Stimulator and batteries for chronic brain stimulation. Batteries are rechargeable nickel-cadmium and are available in different sizes from the manufacturer.

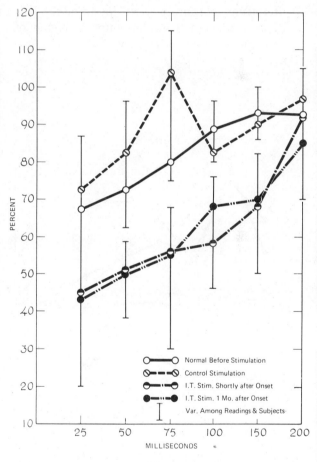

Figure 7–15. A plot of the recovery functions obtained in five monkeys before and during chronic cortical stimulation: relative amplitude of the second response as a function of inter-flash interval.

hundred msec. All are records from striate (visual) cortex. The top traces were recorded prior to the onset of stimulation and the lower ones after stimulation of the inferotemporal region had begun. Note that with cortical stimulation the recovery function is depressed, that is, recovery is delayed.

Figure 7–16 shows the average of such effects in five subjects. Chronic stimulation of the inferotemporal cortex produces a marked increase in the processing time taken by cells in the visual system.

A parallel experiment in the auditory system was done in collaboration with Dr. James Dewson. In this study, made with cats, removals of the auditory homologue of the inferotemporal cortex were performed. This homologue is the insular-temporal region of the cat. Dewson[15] had shown that its removal

impairs complex auditory discrimination (speech sounds), leaving simple auditory discriminations (pitch and loudness) intact. Removal, in addition, alters paired-click recovery cycles recorded as far peripherally as the cochlear nucleus. Bilateral ablation shortens the recovery cycle markedly. Of course, control ablations of the primary auditory projection cortex and elsewhere have no such effect. Thus, we have evidence that chronic stimulation of the intrinsic (association) cortex selectively prolongs, while ablation selectively shortens, the recovery time of cells in the related primary sensory projection system.

These results have been extended in both the auditory and visual modes. Electrode studies have shown alterations of visual receptive fields recorded from units at the optic nerve, geniculate and cortical levels of the visual projection system produced by electrical stimulation of the inferotemporal cortex. The anatomy of the corticofugal pathways of these controls over sensory input also is under study. In the auditory system the fibers lead to the inferior colliculus and from there (in part via the superior olive) to the cochlear nucleus.[16] Definitive results as yet have not been achieved in our studies of the visual pathways, but preliminary indications lead to the putamen, as already noted, and to the pretectal-collicular region as the site of interaction between the corticofugal control mechanism and the visual input system.

The contextual amnesias only recently have become subject to neurophysiological analysis. Again, as in the case of the specific amnesias, corticofugal efferent control mechanisms have been demonstrated. Results obtained in my laboratory show that in many instances these controls are the reciprocals of those involved in the sensory–mode specific processes.[71] Others (*Brain Res.*[7]) have shown that the most likely pathways of operation of the frontolimbic mechanisms involve the brain-stem reticular formation. Here, however, as in the case of the specific amnesias, control can be exerted as far peripherally as the primary sensory neuron.[71,72]

In general terms, the model derived from these experiments states that the operation of

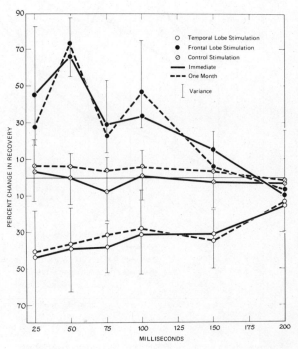

Figure 7–16. This figure plots the percent change in recovery for all subjects in the various experiments. It is thus a summary statement of the findings.

efferents from sensory-specific posterior intrinsic (association) systems tends to reduce and from the frontolimbic systems to enhance redundancy in the input channels, that is, the extrinsic (primary projection) systems. This presumably is accomplished by inhibition and disinhibition of the ongoing interneuronal regulatory processes within the afferent channels, both those by which neurons regulate the activities of their neighbors and those which decrease a neuron's own activity.

(The Distribution of Information in the Brain

As noted, this is not the first time in the history of experimental brain research that data have led investigators of complex mnestic disorders to focus on the primary projection systems. Munk,[41] von Monakov,[40] and Lashley[29] pursued this course from an early emphasis on the "association" to a later recognition of the importance of the organization of the input systems. Of special interest in this pursuit are the experiments of Lashley that demonstrated that pattern vision remains intact after extensive resection—up to 85 percent—of the optic cortex. These results make it imperative to assume that input information becomes widely distributed within the visual system. Two types of mechanism have been proposed to account for such distribution.[52,54] Here I want to present evidence that it indeed does occur.

We trained monkeys to discriminate between a circle and a set of vertical stripes by pressing the right or left half of a plastic panel upon which the cues were briefly projected (for 0.01 msec.). Transient electrical responses were meanwhile recorded from small wire electrodes. The electrical responses were then related by computer analysis to the stimulus, response, and reinforcement contingency of the experiment.[61] Thus we could distinguish from the record whether the monkey had looked at a circle or at the stripes, whether he had obtained a reward or made an error, and whether he was about to press the right or the left leaf of the panel. Interestingly

enough, not all of these brain patterns were recorded from all of the electrode locations. From some input-related patterns were obtained best; from others the reinforcement-related patterns were derived; and still others gave us the patterns that were response–related. This was despite the fact that all placements were within the primary visual system, which is characterized anatomically by being homotopic with the retina. It appears therefore not only that optic events are distributed widely over the system but that response and reinforcement-related events reliably reach the input systems. Such results surely further shake one's confidence in the ordinary view that input events must be transmitted to the "association" areas for associative learning to be effected.

(The Mechanism of Remembering

The experimental findings detailed here allow one to specify a possible mechanism to account for the lesion–produced amnesias. On the basis of the neurobehavioral and neuroanatomical data, I had suggested earlier[48] that the posterior association cortex by way of efferent tracts leading to the brain stem (most likely to the colliculi or surrounding reticular formation)[45] partitions the events that occur in the sensory–specific system and classifies these events. During the course of our joint work, Dr. Spinelli would repeatedly ask: "What do you mean by 'partitioning'? What is partitioning in neurological terms?" Until we had accomplished our electrophysiological experiments, I really had no idea just how to answer. But once we saw the results of these experiments, the neurophysiological explanation became evident: partitioning must work something like a multiplexing circuit. In neurophysiological terms, when the recovery time of neurons in the sensory–projection system is increased by posterior intrinsic (association) cortex stimulation, fewer cells are available at any given moment to receive the concurrent input. Each of a successive series of inputs thus will find a different set of cells in the system available to excitation. There is a good deal of evidence that, in the visual system at least, plenty of reserve capacity—redundancy—exists so that information transmission is not, under ordinary circumstances, hampered by such "narrowing" of the channel.[2] Ordinarily, a particular input excites a great number of fibers in the channel, ensuring replication of transmitted information. Just as lateral inhibition in the retina has the effect of reducing redundancy,[5] so the operation of the sensory–specific posterior intrinsic (association) cortex increases the density of information within the input channel.

Conversely, the functions of the frontolimbic mechanism enhance redundancy, making more cells available at any given moment to concurrent input. This diminishes the density of information processed at any moment and enhances temporal resolution.

The model has several important implications. First, the nonrecovered cells, the ones that are still occupied by excitation initiated by prior inputs, will act as a context or short–term memory buffer against which the current input is matched. A match–mismatch operation of this sort is demanded by models of the process of recognition and selective attention spelled out on other occasions.* These "occupied" cells thus form the matrix of "uncertainty" that shapes the pattern of potential information, that is, the "expectancy" that determines the selection of input signals that might or might not occur. The normal functions of the posterior cortex are assumed to increase the complexity of this context while those of the frontolimbic systems would simplify and thus allow readier registration and parsing.

Second, in a system of fixed size, reduction of redundancy increases the degree of correlation possible with the set of external inputs to the system, while enhancement of redundancy has the opposite effect. The number of alternatives or the complexity of the item to which an organism can attend is thereby controlled.[23] This internal alteration in the functional structure of the classic sensory–projection system thus allows attention to vary as a

function of the spatial and temporal resolution that excitations can achieve, with the result that events of greater or lesser complexity can be attended to. The sharper the spatial resolution, the greater the uncertainty and, thus, the more likely that any set of inputs will be sampled for information. Conversely, the greater the temporal resolution, the more likely that attention is focused and that events become grouped, memorable, and certain. In the extreme, the sharpening of the appetite for information becomes what the clinical neurologist calls stimulus–binding. Its opposite is agnosia, the inability to identify events because they fail to fit the oversimplified context of the moment.

Third, this corticofugal model of the functions of the intrinsic (association) systems relieves us of the problem of infinite regress—an association area "homunculus" that synthesizes and abstracts from inputs, only to pass on these abstractions to a still higher homunculus, perhaps the one that makes decisions, etc. Former ways of looking at the input–output relationships of the brain invariably have come up against this problem (implicit or explicit) of little men inside little men.

According to the model presented here, there is no need for this type of infinite regress. The important functions of perception, decision, etc., are going on within the extrinsic (primary–sensory and motor–projection) systems. Other brain regions such as the posterior sensory-specific intrinsic ("associated") systems and the frontolimbic systems exert their effects by altering the functional organization of the primary systems. Thus these *associated* intrinsic systems are not association systems; they simply alter the configuration of input–output relationships processed by the projection systems. In computer language, the associated intrinsic systems function by supplying *subroutines* in a hierarchy of programs, subroutines contained within and not superimposed from above on the more fundamental processes. In this fashion the infinite higher order abstractive regress is avoided. One could argue that in its place a downward regress of sub- and subsub-subroutines is substituted. I would answer that this type of regress,

* See references 13, 66, 8, 35, 47, 50, and 51.

through progressive differentiation, is the more understandable and manipulable of the two.

A final advantage of the model is that the signal itself is not altered: the invariant properties of a signal are unaffected unless channel capacity is overreached. It is only the organization of the channel itself—the matrix within which the signal is transmitted—that is altered. Thus the same signal carries more or less information, depending on the width of the channel. I am here tempted to extrapolate and say that the signal carries different meanings, depending on the particular structure or organization of the redundancy of the channel.

Concretely, the intrinsic (association) cortex is conceived to program, or to structure, an input channel. This is tantamount to saying that the input must be coded by the operation of this cortex. In its more fundamental aspects, computer programming is in large part a coding operation: The change from direct machine operation through assembler to one of the more manipulable computer languages involves a progression from the setting of binary switches to conceptualizing combinations of such switch settings in "octal" code and then assembling the numerical octals into alphabetized words and phrases and finally parceling and parsing of phrases into sentences, routines, and subroutines. In essence, these progressive coding operations minimize interference among like events by identifying and registering unique structures among the configurations of occurrence and recurrence of the events.

The evidence presented here makes it not unlikely that one function of the posterior and frontolimbic formations of the forebrain is to code events occurring within the input systems. As already noted, the distribution of information (dismembering) implies an encoding process that can reduplicate events without recourse to widespread random neural connections. Regrouping the distributed events (remembering) also implies some sort of coding operation—one similar to that used in decoding binary switch settings into an octal format.

An impaired coding process therefore would be expected to produce grave memory disturbances. The question is thus raised whether lesion–produced amnesias, specific and contextual, primarily reflect malfunctions of the mechanism of coding and not the destruction of localized engrams. (See Pribram.[53])

⟮ Conclusion

Conceptions concerning neocortical mechanisms in cognitive behavior have been re–evaluated in terms of recently accumulated data. Since the designation neocortex has become ambiguous, isocortex is substituted; relations to cognitive processes are inferred from discriminative and problem–solving behavior.

Isocortex has been classified according to the input it receives from the thalamus. When a sector of isocortex receives fibers from a thalamic "relay" nucleus that, in turn, receives its major afferents from outside the thalamus, the sector is called extrinsic. When a sector of isocortex receives fibers from a thalamic nucleus that receives no such extrathalamic afferents, that cortex is classified as intrinsic.

Neurally distinct portions of the *extrinsic* (primary projection) isocortex are known to serve distinct classes of behavior. The distinctions are in part related to differences in input from different peripheral receptor mechanisms (e.g., sense organs). Other distinctions such as between motor and sensory cortex *cannot* be attributed to such gross anatomical differences (e.g., that only afferents reach sensory and efferents leave motor cortex). Rather, differences in detail of the organization of the overlapping input to and output from *each* of the extrinsic (primary projection) sectors must be investigated.

Intrinsic (association) isocortex can also be divided according to demonstrated relationships to one or another class of behavior. Discriminative behavior (response to invariants) in specific modalities is affected when particular subdivisions of the posterior intrinsic cortex are removed. When the anterior intrinsic (frontolimbic) cortex is ablated, those discriminations are affected which are based primarily on recurring variable events which are not contemporaneous with the choice, irrespective of modality.

In several instances, intrinsic (association) and extrinsic (primary projection) systems are related to the *same* class of behavior. In these instances, the organism is limited in the possible complexity of cognitive behavior when the intrinsic cortex is resected—a limitation that is, however, not as severe as that resulting from extensive damage to the extrinsic system nor as that resulting from gross interference with receptor mechanisms. The hierarchical relationship described by these data has, heretofore, been attributed to specific afferents originating in subdivisions of extrinsic, and connecting to subdivisions of intrinsic, isocortex. Experiments have been quoted that make it unlikely that such *specific afferents* exist. Instead, the specificity of function of subdivisions of the intrinsic (association) isocortex is, in this analysis, attributed to *convergence* on a common subcortical mechanism of *efferents* from hierarchically related intrinsic (association) and extrinsic (primary projection) systems. The output from the intrinsic systems has been shown to influence, via regulation of the peripheral sensory mechanism, the input to the extrinsic systems.

Thus, experimentally produced local brain damage does demonstrably impair memory function. However, the impairment apparently is not so much a removal of localized engrams as an interference with the mechanisms that code neural events so as to allow facile storage and retrieval. The evidence shows that anatomically the memory trace is distributed within a neural system by means of an encoding process, while as a function of decoding the engram is reassembled, that is, re-membered. What and whether something is remembered is in large part dependent on how it is—and that it is—adequately coded.

(Bibliography

1. AMASSIAN, V. E. "Interaction in the Somatovisceral Projection System," *Res. Publ. Ass. Nerv. Ment. Dis.*, 30 (1952), 371–402.

2. ATTNEAVE, F. "Some Informational Aspects of Visual Perception," *Psychol. Rev.*, 61 (1954), 183–193.

3. BAGSHAW, M. H. and K. H. PRIBRAM. "Cortical Organization in Gustation (Macaca mulatta)," *J. Neurophysiol.*, 16 (1953), 499–508.

4. BAILEY, P. and G. VON BONIN. *The Isocortex of Man*. Urbana: University of Illinois Press, 1951.

5. BARLOW, H. B. "Possible Principles Underlying the Transformations of Sensory Messages," in W. Rosenblith, ed., *Sensory Communication*, pp. 217–234. Cambridge: MIT Press, 1961.

6. BONIN, G. V., H. W. GAROL and W. S. McCULLOCH. "The Functional Organization of the Occipital Lobe," *Biol. Symp.*, (1942), 7.

7. BRAIN RESEARCH. "Forebrain Inhibitory Mechanisms," special issue (1967).

8. BRUNNER, J. S. "On perceptual readiness," *Psychol. Rev.*, 64 (1957), 123–152.

9. CHOW, K. L. "A Retrograde Cell Degeneration Study of the Cortical Projection Field of the Pulvinar in the Monkey. *J. Comp. Neurol.*, 93 (1950), 313–340.

10. ——. "Further Studies on Selective Ablation of Associative Cortex in Relation to Visually Mediated Behavior," *J. Comp. Physiol. Psychol.*, 45 (1952), 109–118.

11. ——. "Lack of Behavioral Effects Following Destruction of Some Thalamic Association Nuclei in Monkey," *Arch. Neurol. Psychiat.*, 71 (1954), 762–771.

12. CHOW, K. L. and K. H. PRIBRAM. "Cortical Projection of the Thalamic Ventrolateral Nuclear Group in Monkey," *J. Comp. Neurol.*, 104 (1956), 57–75.

13. CRAIK, K. H. W. *The Nature of Explanation*. New York: Cambridge University Press, 1943.

14. DELL, P. "Corrélations entre le système végétatif et le système de la vie de relation: Mesencèphale diencéphale et cortex cérébral," *J. Physiol. Path. Gen.*, 44 (1952), 471–557.

15. DEWSON, J. H., III. "Speech Sound Discrimination by Cats," *Science*, 3619 (1964), 555–556.

16. DEWSON, J. H., III, K. W. NOBLE and K. H. PRIBRAM. Corticofugal Influence at Coch-

lear Nucleus of the Cat: Some Effects of Ablation of Insular–temporal Cortex," *Brain Res.*, 2 (1966), 151–159.

17. DEWSON, J. H., III, K. H. PRIBRAM and J. LYNCH. "Effects of Ablations of Temporal Cortex upon Speech Sound Discrimination in the Monkey," *Exp. Neurol.*, 24 (1969), 579–591.

18. ETTLINGER, G. Visual Discrimination Following Successive Unilateral Temporal Excisions in Monkeys, *J. Physiol.* 140 (1957), 38–39.

19. EVARTS, E. V. "Effect of Ablation of Prestriate Cortex on Auditory–visual Association in Monkey," *J. Neurophysiol.*, 15 (1952), 191–200.

20. FLECHSIG, P. *Die Localisation der Geistigen Vorgänge Insbesondere der Sinnesempfindungen der Menschen.* Leipzig, 1896.

21. FLOURENS, P. *Récherches Expérimentales sur les Propriétés et les Fonctions du Système Nerveux dans les Animaux Vertébrés,* Paris: Crevot, 1824.

22. GALL, F. J. and G. SPURZHEIM. "Research on the Nervous System in General and on That of the Brain in Particular," in K. H. Pribram, ed., *Brain and Behavior I*, pp. 20–26. Middlesex: Penguin Books, 1969.

23. GARNER, W. R. *Uncertainty and Structure as Psychological Concepts.* New York: Wiley, 1962.

24. GOLDSTEIN, K. Die Topick der Grosshirnrinde in ihrer klinischen Bedeutung. *Dtsch. Z. Nervenheilk.*, 77 (1923), 7–124.

25. GROSSMAN, S. P. *A Textbook of Physiological Psychology.* New York: Wiley, 1967.

26. KAADA, B. R., K. H. PRIBRAM and J. A. EPSTEIN. "Respiratory and Vascular Responses in Monkeys from Temporal Pole, Insula, Orbital Surface and Cingulate Gyrus: A Preliminary Report," *J. Neurophysiol.*, 12 (1949), 347–356.

27. KRUGER, L. "Observations on the Organization of the Sensory Motor Cerebral Cortex." Unpublished Ph.D. dissertation, Yale University School of Medicine, 1954.

28. LASHLEY, K. S. *Brain Mechanisms and Intelligence.* Chicago: University of Chicago Press, 1929.

29. ———. "The Problem of Cerebral Organization in Vision," in *Visual Mechanisms.* Biological Symposia, Vol. 7, pp. 301–322. Lancaster: Jacques Cattell Press, 1942.

30. ———. "The Mechanism of Vision: XVIII: Effects of Destroying the Visual 'Associative Areas' of the monkey," *Genet. Psychol. Monogr.*, 37 (1948), 107–166.

31. ———. "In Search of the Engram," in *Physiological Mechanisms in Animal Behavior,* pp. 454–482. Society for Experimental Biology. New York: Academic Press, 1950.

32. LASHLEY, K. S. and G. CLARK. "The Cytoarchitecture of the Cerebral Cortex of Ateles: A Critical Examination of Architectonic Studies," *J. Comp. Neurol.*, 85 (1946), 223–305.

33. LASSEK, A. M. *The Pyramidal Tract. Its Status in Medicine.* Springfield: Charles C Thomas, 1954.

34. LOEB, J. *Comparative Physiology of the Brain and Comparative Psychology.* London: Murray, 1901.

35. MACKAY, D. M. "The epistemological problem for automata," in *Automata Studies,* pp. 235–252. Princeton: Princeton University Press, 1956.

36. MAGENDIE, F. Expériences sur les fonctions des racines des nerfs rachidiens. *J. Physiol. Exp.*, 2 (1822), 276–279.

37. MALIS, L. I., K. H. PRIBRAM and L. KRUGER. "Action Potentials in 'Motor' Cortex Evoked by Peripheral Nerve Stimulation." *J. Neurophysiol.*, 16 (1953), 161–167.

38. MISHKIN, M. and M. HALL. "Discriminations Along a Size Continuum Following Ablation of the Inferior Temporal Convexity in Monkeys," *J. Comp. Physiol. Psychol.*, 48 (1955), 97–101.

39. MISHKIN, M. and K. H. PRIBRAM. Visual Discrimination Performance Following Partial Ablations of the Temporal Lobe: I. Ventral vs Lateral. *J. Comp. Physiol. Psychol.*, 47 (1954), 14–20.

40. MONAKOW, C. VON. *Die Lokalisation im Grosshirn und der Abbau der Funktion durch Korticale Herde.* Wiesbaden: Bergmann, 1914.

41. MUNK, H. *Uber die Funktionen der Grosshirnrinde: Gesammelte Mitteilungen aus den Jahren.* Berlin: Hirschwald, 1881.

42. PETERS, R. H. and H. E. ROSVOLD. "The Effect of Thalamic Lesions upon Spatial Delayed Alternation Performance in the Rhesus Monkey." M.D. thesis. Yale, 1955. Unpublished.

43. PRIBRAM, H. and J. BARRY. "Further Behavioral Analysis of the Parieto–temporo–

preoccipital Cortex," *J. Neurophysiol.*, 19 (1956), 99–106.

44. PRIBRAM, K. H. "Toward a Science of Neuropsychology: (Method and Data)," in R. A. Patton, ed., *Current Trends in Psychology and the Behavioral Sciences*, pp. 115–142. Pittsburgh: University of Pittsburgh Press, 1954.

45. ——. "Neocortical Function in Behavior," in H. F. Harlow, ed., *Neocortical Function in Behavior*, pp. 151–172. Madison: University of Wisconsin Press, 1958.

46. ——. "On the Neurology of Thinking," *Behav. Sci.*, 4 (1959), 265–287.

47. ——. A Review of Theory in Physiological Psychology," *Annu. Rev. Psychol.*, (1960), 1–40.

48. ——. The Intrinsic Systems of the Forebrain," in J. Field and H. W. Magoun, eds., *Handbook of Physiology*, Vol. 2, *Neurophysiology*, pp. 1323–1344. Washington: American Physiological Society, 1960.

49. ——. "A Further Experimental Analysis of the Behavioral Deficit That Follows Injury to the Primate Frontal Cortex," *Exp. Neurol.*, 3 (1961), 432–466.

50. ——. "The New Neurology: Memory, Novelty, Thought and Choice," in G. H. Glaser, ed., *EEG and Behavior*, pp. 149–173. New York: Basic Books, 1963.

51. ——. "Reinforcement Revisited: A Structural View," in M. Jones, ed., Nebraska Symposium on Motivation, pp. 113–159. Lincoln: University of Nebraska Press, 1963.

52. ——. "Four R's of Remembering," in K. H. Pribram, ed., *The Biology of Learning*. New York: Harcourt, Brace, and World, 1969.

53. ——. *Languages of the Brain*. Englewood Cliffs: Prentice–Hall, 1971.

54. ——. "How Is It That Sensing So Much We Can Do So Little?" in F. O. Schmitt and T. Melnechuk, eds., *The Neurosciences*, Vol. 3, pp. 249–261. Cambridge: MIT Press, 1974.

55. PRIBRAM, K. H., A. AHUMADA, J. HARTOG and L. ROOS. "A Progress Report on the Neurological Processes Disturbed by Frontal Lesions in Primates," in J. M. Warren and K. Akert, eds., *The Frontal Granular Cortex and Behavior*. New York: McGraw–Hill, 1964.

56. PRIBRAM, K. H., S. BLEHERT and D. N.

SPINELLI. "The Effects on Visual Discrimination of Crosshatching and Undercutting the Infero–temporal Cortex of Monkeys," *J. Comp. Physiol. Psychol.*, 62 (1966), 358–364.

57. PRIBRAM, K. H., K. L. CHOW and J. SEMMES. "Limit and Organization of the Cortical Projection from the Medial Thalamic Nucleus in Monkey," *J. Comp. Neurol.*, 98 (1953), 433–448.

58. PRIBRAM, K. H. and L. KRUGER. "Functions of the 'Olfactory Brain'," *Ann. N.Y. Acad. Sci.*, 58 (1954), 109–138.

59. PRIBRAM, K. H. and P. D. MACLEAN. "Neuronographic Analysis of Medial and Basal Cerebral Cortex: II. Monkey," *J. Neurophysiol.*, 16 (1953), 324–340.

60. PRIBRAM, K. H. and M. MISHKIN. "Simultaneous and Successive Visual Discrimination by Monkeys with Inferotemporal Lesions," *J. Comp. Physiol. Psychol.*, 48 (1955), 198–202.

61. PRIBRAM, K. H., D. N. SPINELLI and M. C. KAMBACK. "Electrocortical Correlates of Stimulus Response and Reinforcement," *Science*, 157 (1967), 94–96.

62. PRIBRAM, K. H. and W. E. TUBBS. "Short-term Memory, Parsing and the Primate Frontal Cortex," *Science*, 156 (1967), 1765–1767.

63. REITZ, S. L. and K. H. PRIBRAM. "Some Subcortical Connections of the Inferotemporal Gyrus of Monkey," *Exp. Neurol.*, 25 (1969), 632–645.

64. ROSE, J. E. and V. B. MOUNTCASTLE. "Activity of Single Neurons in the Tactile Thalamic Region of the Cat in Response to a Transient Peripheral Stimulus," *Johns Hopkins Med. J.*, 94 (1954), 238–282.

65. ROSE, J. E. and C. N. WOOLSEY. "Organization of the Mammalian Thalamus and its Relationships to the Cerebral Cortex," *Electroencephalogr. Clin. Neurophysiol.*, 1 (1949), 391–404.

66. SOKOLOV, E. N. "Neuronal Models and the Orienting Reflex," in M. A. B. Brazier, ed., *The Central Nervous System and Behavior*, pp. 187–276. New York: Josiah Macy, Jr. Foundation, 1960.

67. SPERRY, R. W. "Cerebral Regulation of Motor Coordination in Monkeys Following Multiple Transection of Sensorimotor Cortex, *J. Neurophysiol.*, 10 (1947), 275–294.

68. ——. "Preservation of High–order Func-

tion in Solated Somatic Cortex in Callosum–sectioned Cats," *J. Neurophysiol.*, 22 (1959), 78–87.

69. SPERRY, R. W., N. MINER and R. E. MEYERS. "Visual Pattern Perception Following Subpial Slicing and Tantalum Wire Implantations in the Visual Cortex," *J. Comp. Physiol. Psychol.*, 48 (1955), 50–58.

70. SPINELLI, D. N. and K. H. PRIBRAM. "Changes in Visual Recovery Functions Produced by Temporal Lobe Stimulation in Monkeys," *Electroencephalogr. Clin. Neurophysiol.*, 22 (1966), 143–149.

71. ———. "Changes in Visual Recovery Function and Unit Activity Produced by Frontal Cortex Stimulation," *Electroencephalogr. Clin. Neurophysiol.*, 22 (1967), 143–149.

72. SPINELLI, D. N., K. H. PRIBRAM and M. WEINGARTEN. "Centrifugal Optic Nerve-Responses Evoked by Auditory and Somatic Stimulation," *Exp. Neurol.*, 12 (1965), 303–319.

73. SUGAR, O., J. G. CHUSID and J. D. FRENCH. "A Second Motor Cortex in the Monkey (Macaca mulatta)," *J. Neuropath.*, 7 (1948), 182–189.

74. WADE, M. "Behavioral Effects of Prefrontal Lobectomy, Lobotomy and Circumsection in the Monkey (Macaca mulatta)," *J. Comp. Neurol.*, 96 (1952), 179–207.

75. WALKER, A. E. *The Primate Thalamus.* Chicago: University of Chicago Press, 1938.

76. WALKER, A. E. and T. A. WEAVER, JR. "Ocular Movements from the Occipital-Lobe in the Monkey," *J. Neurophysiol.*, 3 (1940), 353–357.

77. WEISKRANTZ, L. and M. MISHKIN. "Effects of Temporal and Frontal Cortical Lesions on Auditory Discrimination in Monkeys," *Brain*, 81 (1958), 406–414.

78. WHITLOCK, D. G. and W. J. H. NAUTA. "Subcortical Projections from the Temporal Neocortex in Macaca Mulatta," *J. Comp. Neurol.*, 106 (1956), 185–212.

79. WILSON, W. A., JR. "Alternation in Normal and Frontal Monkeys as a Function of Response and Outcome of the Previous Trial," *J. Comp. Physiol. Psychol.*, 55 (1962), 701–704.

80. WOOLSEY, C. N., P. H. SETTLAGE, D. R. MEYER et al. "Patterns of Localization in Precentral and 'Supplementary' Motor Areas and Their Relation to the Concept of a Premotor Area," *Res. Publ. Assoc. Nerv. Ment. Dis.*, 30 (1952), 238–264.

CHAPTER 8

AN OVERVIEW OF SLEEP RESEARCH: PAST, PRESENT AND FUTURE*

William C. Dement and Merrill M. Mitler

(Introduction

THIS CHAPTER may be regarded as a revision of the chapter on the "Psychophysiology of Sleep and Dreams" that appeared in Volume III of the first edition of the *American Handbook of Psychiatry*.[64] A gulf of nearly a decade separates the two. In the original chapter, the 258 citations listed in the bibliography represented a reasonably

* We wish to thank Mary Carskadon and Dr. Vincent P. Zarcone for their help with the manuscript. Thanks are due our collaborators Drs. Jack Barchas, Colin Pittendrigh, and Phillip Sokolove. Preparation of this chapter was supported by NINDS grant NS 10727, Career Development Award MH 5804 to W. C. Dement and a postdoctoral fellowship to M. M. Mitler from NIH Training Grant MH 8304. The UCLA Brain Information Service facilitated the bibliographic search.

complete coverage of work in the so–called modern era of sleep research inaugurated by the discovery of REM sleep. However, in the intervening years, perhaps ten thousand publications dealing with some aspect of sleep have appeared. In the face of this avalanche, our goals must be much more circumspect and modest than reviewing the field of sleep research. Furthermore, Volume VI will appropriately have two chapters devoted to aspects of sleep. The other chapter will be devoted mainly to clinical descriptions and issues. Considering all this, we have elected to give a somewhat personalized overview of the sleep –research field with special emphasis on issues that seem particularly relevant to psychiatry. We have also tried to fulfill an interpretive function, one of putting some things into perspective. In this regard, we feel that understanding of material presented under the rubric, "process view," is mandatory. We feel it is only through this conceptualization of the realities of sleep mechanisms, that the findings of sleep research can be meaningfully applied to such diverse problems as hallucinations, thought disorders, cataplectic seizures, insomnia, sleep apnea, and so on.

Another issue is tangentially raised by Frederick Bremer, the great Belgian neurophysiologist, in his introductory remarks to the proceedings of the First International Congress of the Association for the Psychophysiological Study of Sleep (APSS).[29] He says that the congress

. . . marks the date when 'sleep research' became a discipline unto itself. In the long way of man's endeavor to understand his body and his soul, the search for the neurophysiological mechanisms underlying the sleep phenomenon began very late, as if we had been paralyzed by an obscure feeling of awe in the face of these obligatory pauses in our busy life and by the magic appearances of the dream phantasmagoria.

Bremer may have repressed his prior acquaintance with the work of Sigmund Freud, but the point we wish to underscore is the notion of sleep research as a discipline unto itself. In the United States at least, sleep research has clearly been the foster child of psychiatry. Much of the work on sleep mechanisms has been conducted in the guise of clarifying the role of these mechanisms in mental aberrations. However, as will be seen in this chapter, there are a number of concerns that have to do only with sleep both on a basic and a clinical level. A case in point is the sleep apnea–insomnia syndrome recently described by Guilleminault et al.[116,117] This is clearly an organic sleep disorder. Yet, we may presume that many of these patients will find their way to the psychiatrist's consulting room. Who or what discipline is really responsible for such a patient? We have just about reached the point in time where the foster child is grown up and should either be formally adopted to share in the support and heritage of its foster parents, or should be cast out into the world, entirely on its own, to make its own way, to establish its own heritage, etc.

Before going to more specific topics, we would like to recommend a number of general references. Books and symposia dealing with sleep continue to be published at the rate of several per year. *The Sleeping Brain*, edited by Chase,[41] brings the field up–to–date in a number of specialized areas. Webb has edited a book[292] that ties together the work of a decade by having investigators comment upon earlier experiments in the light of present–day knowledge. Also of recent vintage are two volumes with entirely different purposes by Freemon[105] and Dement.[67,*] In addition, the National Institute of Neurological Diseases and Stroke has established information networks that include the Brain Information Service at UCLA. In addition to the monthly "Sleep Bulletin" and "Sleep Reviews," the service has begun publishing a yearly volume entitled *Sleep Research*, which will include the proceedings of the annual APSS meetings, and complete yearly cumulation of "Sleep Bulletin" and "Sleep Reviews." Other more general references will be cited from time to time throughout the chapter.

❨ Historical Perspectives

Sleep and wakefulness are essentially behavioral states and, as such, involve the whole organism. Further, they represent functional changes vastly extended in the temporal dimension. Scientific observation is ordinarily either cross–sectional or longitudinal, but the very essence of research on sleep is that it is simultaneously longitudinal *and* cross-sectional.

Perhaps the major factor that limited the ultimate validity of the earliest "laboratory" work on sleep was the natural assumption that

---

* Since this chapter has begun its editorial processing, the first of an excellent review series has appeared which deserves special mention here: E. D. Weitzman (Ed.), *Advances in Sleep Research* Vol. 1, New York: Spectrum Publications, 424 pages.

sleep was a single totally uniform state. With the often ignored exception of the occasional fleeting disturbance of a dream, sleep was viewed as the "off" condition of the organism and, accordingly, it was felt that a *single* observation of some variable would suffice to describe the behavior of this variable for the entirety of the nocturnal sleep period. A great many interpretations were made on this basis. For example, Pietrusky[240] published a "definitive" study of eye position during sleep in human subjects. He made single observations on three hundred individuals. From these data he concluded that the characteristic stationary resting position of the eyes during sleep was in divergence. In addition, this conclusion may have been predisposed in the sense that Pietrusky saw divergence during sleep as an inevitable consequence of predominant ocular convergence during wakefulness. By nightfall, he reasoned, the more fatigued internal recti could not maintain the midposition against a slight tonic pull of the less fatigued lateral recti. We now know that the eyeballs *do not* maintain a single characteristic resting position during sleep. Actually, much of Pietrusky's data could have been duplicated by making observations on one individual at three hundred different points in a single night. Any position in which we might find the eyeball is simply one of the relatively brief pauses separating the countless episodes of slow and rapid motility.[60]

Thus, any description of sleep must also take the temporal dimension into account. In this sense, sleep is something like a river— basically the same, yet different at every point depending upon the shape of its bank, the size of projecting boulders, the presence or absence of tributaries, the traffic upon it, the rate of flow, and so forth.

Obviously, a moment–to–moment description of the entire mammalian organism over the entire sleep period is an enormous task. It is possible that some aspects of the description will be quite trivial. However, we must guard against premature assumptions that this or that function is not important, or worth the effort of thorough study. As we shall see later in this chapter, certain physiological variables

that are quite easy to record during sleep, but have not been closely scrutinized in recent years because of a lack of interest, are today the subject of a second look and, in some cases, have pointed the way to whole new investigative realms. A case in point is respiration during sleep. Long taken completely for granted, the revelations of the discoveries involving the sleep apnea syndromes* have made us ask how we manage to continue breathing when we fall asleep and have made us realize how vulnerable this vital function really is during the complex functional adjustments that characterize the incredible transition from wakefulness to sleep.

In addition, there is a natural tendency for scientific investigators in any field to favor experimental approaches—direct attacks upon mechanism and function—at the expense of patient, comprehensive, unbiased passive observation. Again, sleep research is an outstanding example of a general principle: when pure description is not the goal, certain dramatic transients are easily overlooked among the myriad variables that constitute the behavior of the whole organism in time. There were innumerable experimental studies on the mechanisms of sleep before anything like the true nature of mammalian sleep was fully comprehended—that is, before the existence of rapid eye movement (REM) sleep was known. It is a great mystery how REM sleep was so long overlooked, given the techniques available in many studies, and particularly the fact that it can be seen with the naked eye! One explanation, as we have implied above, may lie in the fact that descriptive work generally holds second–class citizenship vis–à–vis experimental work, and the latter is, by definition, narrow (focused) and biased (hypothesis testing).

The EEG and the ARAS

The somnolent state has occupied the attention of laboratory scientists for more than a hundred years. During this time, the one thing that, more than any other, stimulated research

---

* See references 116, 117, 109, 110, 84, and 281.

was the development of electroencephalography (EEG). This tool permitted continuous observation of the electrical activity of the brain during sleep without disturbing the sleeper.

Berger[16] quickly noticed after his discovery of the presence of brain waves in humans that they always underwent qualitative changes when passing from wakefulness to sleep or vice versa. As is well known, Loomis's group at Harvard and Blake's group at the University of Chicago produced an exciting series of papers* that presented relatively detailed descriptions of the various EEG patterns during sleep in humans. These workers did not oversimplify their observations. Although they used sampling procedures, they nevertheless recognized dramatic differences in sleep EEG patterns as functions of time of night and time from sleep onset.

In the thirties and forties it was generally held that EEG waves represented a kind of integrated display at the scalp level of unit activity. Therefore, it was felt that the important parameter in sleep and arousal was EEG synchrony, assuming that frequency and amplitude are generally inversely related. Thus, it was logical that neurons would be discharging slowly and synchronously in deep sleep.

The work of Magoun's group strengthened this notion.[196,197,225] EEG desynchronization (cortical activation) was equated with arousal. Degree of cortical activation was assumed to depend upon the activity level in a hypothetical ascending extralemniscal system in the brain stem, the so–called ascending reticular activating system (ARAS). For these workers, the whole continuum of sleep and arousal was presumed to be controlled by a unitary mechanism residing in the brain–stem core.

Further, the ARAS was known to receive fibers from all sensory pathways. Thus, its activity could reflect the amount of stimulation impinging upon the organism. By interposing the ARAS between external stimulation and the cerebral cortex, one could hypothesize a certain amount of organismic independence from immediate sensory stimulation since the

ARAS could amplify, modulate, and reverberate input. This formulation seemed to explain so much and seemed so amenable to experimental manipulation in laboratory animals that it was reified before all the descriptive facts were available.

The ARAS concept also allowed for variation in the "depth" of sleep. Thus, the bigger and slower the EEG waves, the deeper the sleep. This was also consistent with the notion that cortical units were discharging slowly and synchronously, in contrast to their presumed patterns in response to the evocations of wakefulness. Figure 8–1 depicts this concept of the continuum of sleep and wakefulness.

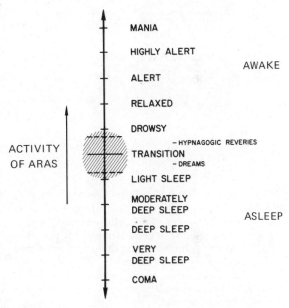

Figure 8–1.   The vertical continuum of human existence.

Several studies were also done that presented evidence supporting a relationship between EEG patterns and arousal threshold.† Here again, the relationship was reified before all the evidence was gathered. For example, in their otherwise superb *Atlas of Electroencephalography,* the Gibbs[113] eschewed numbers or letters to name the EEG stages of sleep, preferring instead a nomenclature based on the depth of sleep.

* See references 119, 54, 22, 23, and 24.

† See references 22, 55, 119, 225, 48, and 270.

Figure 8–2 presents classic examples of the typical EEG patterns seen during human sleep and will serve to make the point that the current classifications of sleep rhythms are not very different from the major descriptive categories set forth by the Loomis group. These workers originally used letter designations: the letter "A" designated waking alpha rhythm; "B" through "E" corresponded roughly to our EEG sleep Stages 1 through 4.

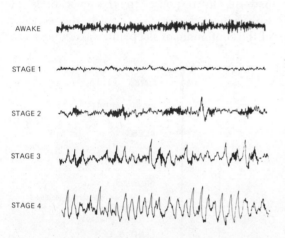

AWAKE

STAGE 1

STAGE 2

STAGE 3

STAGE 4

Figure 8–2. Examples of the recorded tracings of EEG stages of sleep for the same subject over a period of a single night. The recording paper was moving under the pens at one-third the standard speed, which means that the waves are somewhat pushed together. However, this also means that only one third as much paper is needed during the night, a considerable saving in eight hours of continuous recording.

The top line shows the ten-per-second alpha waves characteristic of the Awake EEG. Their mean amplitude, for comparison with the sleep patterns, is about fifty μv. The second line (Stage 1) shows a mixture of low voltage, irregular, relatively fast waves. The sample of Stage 2 in the third tracing shows the characteristic waxing-waning bursts of regular waves (sleep spindles) lasting one to two seconds. The frequency of the spindle waves is about twelve to fourteen per second, which causes them to be somewhat blurred at this paper speed. Nonetheless, they stand out sharply from the low voltage, irregular background rhythms. A moderate amount of high–voltage, slow activity is seen in the Stage 3 tracing. Stage 4, shown in the bottom line, is characterized by continuous high–voltage, slow activity. The frequency is about one per second.

REM Periods and the Temporal Course of Events during Sleep

We have pointed out that EEG patterns during sleep have long been known to vary throughout the sleep period. Nevertheless, a thorough study of the temporal course of events during sleep did not develop until Aserinsky and Kleitman[6] made their original observations on the occurrence of rapid, binocularly synchronous eye movements during sleep in human adults. This discovery, together with the additional observation that dream recall was very likely when such eye movements were present, fundamentally changed the focus of attention; now the temporal course of events throughout the night became critical. Intense interest in the temporal position and physiological concomitants of the rapid eye movement dream periods led to continuous monitoring over many hours instead of intermittent sampling. The ink writing electroencephalograph or polygraph was the perfect instrument for such work because it enabled continuous monitoring not only of brain–wave patterns but of eye movements as well, *without* disturbing the sleeper. Furthermore, the permanent paper record could be scrutinized carefully at a later date. One of the first reliable EEG instruments was available in Nathaniel Kleitman's laboratory at the University of Chicago, and with it we were able to inaugurate a period of intense observation of a relatively small number of physiological variables. This observation was aimed at a detailed, minute by minute description of the eight-hour nocturnal sleep period in man.[74,75,188] Because of the importance we naturally attributed to brain processes in sleep, EEG patterns were emphasized.

It is really unclear why the so–called Dement–Kleitman classification of sleep stages utilizing numbers became so popular. We always felt that it was really trivial whether numbers or letters were used. The reason may have been that the Dement–Kleitman classification was the first relatively precise description of brain–wave patterns during sleep. There were fairly specific descriptions of frequency, amplitude, and wave forms, which permitted scoring patterns fairly reliably into one of the four stages. In addition, these stage definitions helped in dealing with the huge mass of data that always accumulated from all–night sleep recordings before the advent of computer scoring.

It was soon apparent that all sleep epochs would fit comfortably into these four levels. More importantly, it was also obvious that the four stages seemed to alternate in a kind of cyclic fashion. With rapid eye movement periods as guideposts, repetitive sequences were clearly seen. Further understanding of the relationship between rapid eye movement periods and dreaming led to the first longitudinal generalization about the nature of sleep, the so–called basic rest activity cycle (BRAC).

The characteristic all–night EEG changes were viewed as cyclic alternations in depth of sleep. Moreover, central nervous system activity at the peak of the cycle (signaled by the appearance of low voltage, relatively fast EEG patterns) seemed consistent with the concomitant psychological experience of dreaming. In turn, such psychological activity was presumed to be responsible for other manifestations occurring at the peak of the cycle such as rapid eye movements and certain other physiological events. Thus, in 1958 it seemed that the only aspect of the rapid eye movement (REM) period that might give it importance for the human organism was its apparent association with dream activity. Although interesting quantitative data were compiled on lengths and locations of REM and Stage 4 periods, there was, as yet, no concept of two kinds of sleep.

⟨ Two States of Sleep

REM Sleep versus NREM Sleep

Several observations led to a drastic modification in the monolithic cyclic concept of sleep. First was the finding that rapid eye movement periods also occurred in the laboratory cat,[57] which stimulated much subsequent experimental work. In the next year, Jouvet and Michel[153] made one of the most remarkably simple and far-reaching observations in the history of sleep research. Jouvet and Michel found that the electromyographic (EMG) was quite active during slow wave periods, but when EEG activation with rapid eye movements appeared, EMG activity was totally suppressed! Berger[17] confirmed this finding in man. Thus, there was for the first time a strong suspicion that sleep was not a unitary state. These data are especially significant since every precedent favored closer scrutiny of the brain and diminished scrutiny of peripheral events; yet Jouvet and Michel had the temerity to observe the electrical activity of the muscles. Up to that point, most researchers assumed that EMG activity would more or less parallel depth of sleep and level of EEG activation.

Finally, Jouvet and his colleagues[154] discovered a very unique electrical activity in the pons of the cat during REM sleep. They initially referred to this activity as "spindles," but later recognized it as bursts or clusters of individual monophasic sharp waves, or spikes. Brooks and Bizzi[31] found the same activity in the lateral geniculate nucleus, and Mouret, Jeannerod, and Jouvet[227] completed the implication of the visual system in REM sleep by describing these waves in the visual cortex. Even in human scalp recordings, it is possible to identify unique features in the EEG of REM sleep. Schwartz[267] was the first to see bursts of peculiar waves that had escaped the notice of everyone else. These waves were related to rapid eye movements and have come to be known as saw-tooth waves. Thus, it became clear that some very unique phenomena were part of the spontaneous electrical activity of the brain during REM sleep, in addition to nonspecific arousal[57] or hyperarousal.[268]

Sleep researchers now realized that sleep was two processes. This was truly a revolutionary shift in viewpoint. It ran counter to the personal experience of sleep and was a complete departure from all previous thinking about sleep. Oswald[232] was probably the first to actually state this radical new notion in print, but we think that Jouvet probably deserves the most credit because of the impact of his epochal paper,[149] which appeared later in the year. Jouvet summarized a tremendous amount of anatomical, physiological, and behavioral work, and clearly established the brain–stem origins of REM sleep.

Thus, the regularly recurring REM period was recognized as one kind of sleep, and all the rest, albeit encompassing several very different EEG patterns, was recognized as another kind of sleep to which the term, non-rapid eye movement (NREM) was applied. Though outwardly very similar in terms of recumbency, quiescence, increased response threshold, etc., these two kinds of sleep are totally dissimilar when observed more closely. Indeed, as we all know, and as has been demonstrated repeatedly, nearly every physiological variable observed longitudinally during sleep shows markedly contrasting behavior as a function of REM periods versus NREM periods.

The Concepts of State and Stage

Some confusion still exists regarding the idea that REM sleep is a state and all other sleep (four stages) also comprises a state. The term *state* usually refers to a condition in which something exists that is qualitatively different from other possible conditions in which it may exist. A specific condition or state is usually recognized by the necessary presence of one or more attributes that are essentially absent at other times. For example, when water exists in the frozen state, it possesses attributes of solidity and rigidity that are present at no other time. In complex living organisms, the taxonomic problem of defining states becomes, to some extent, a matter of judgment and consensus. As a rule, a single variable will not suffice to define a state; a cluster of attributes whose simultaneous and repeated occurrence is highly unique must be present. It is commonly accepted that there are two, and only two states of sleep. As noted above, they are called REM and NREM sleep and they appear to be present in nearly all mammals.

The word *stage* usually refers to a relatively

precise, but arbitrary subdivision in the course of a continuously progressing quantitative change. Thus, water in the liquid state between 0° and 10° centigrade could be called Stage 1, from 10° to 20° could be called Stage 2, and so on. It is obvious that almost any number of stages could be defined arbitrarily within a state. In the case of the sleeping human, only four stages defined by the EEG have been commonly accepted as subdivisions of NREM sleep. There are *no* commonly accepted subdivisions of REM sleep.

To be useful, stage designations should have functional or organizational significance. The putative functional significance of the NREM EEG stages is that they represent levels in a NREM continuum of depth of sleep. These stages also show quantitative changes in several clinical conditions.

Are there stages in REM sleep? It may be presumed that no stage subdivision of REM sleep has been widely accepted because a clear-cut functional significance does not exist, or has not yet been conclusively shown to exist. Certain divisions of REM sleep have been used from time to time to facilitate an experimental approach. Most frequently, such a division is used for the study of the correlation between a REM sleep–associated variable and some aspect of dreaming. For example, epochs of REM sleep have been differentially classified according to the absolute frequency of individual eye movement potentials, heart rate changes, respiratory changes, so forth.

The realization that two entirely independent states of being alternated during the period of bodily quiescence (sleep) gave rise to two kinds of questions. One set of questions dealt with the biochemical underpinnings of the two states. These issues were extensively addressed by the Lyon group. Their early work led to the proposals of Jouvet that NREM sleep might be dependent upon serotonergic neurons, while REM sleep might involve catecholaminergic systems.[150,151] The second group of questions concerned the age–old problem of the function of sleep. If one could distinguish two kinds of sleep, what then were their respective functions? It was necessary to repudiate the total sleep deprivation studies because they had confounded the effects of the loss of both REM and NREM sleep. It was felt that functional clarity would come only as a result of selective sleep deprivation.

The first such study involved the selective deprivation of REM sleep. The early experiments[58,61] were rather successful in eliciting the postdeprivation REM rebound, which seemed to suggest some sort of need for REM sleep. In addition, there was a feeling that the rebound served a quantitative makeup function. While clarification of the specific role of REM sleep in the biological economy of the mammalian organism has remained controversial,[66] the mere fact that one could conceive of a possible need for a certain amount of REM sleep led to an augmented concern with quantification of sleep states and stages. Parenthetically, there was also a notion that Stage 4 might have some unique functional significance and it was also subjected to quantitative manipulation.

Accordingly, great consternation developed when Monroe first presented the results of his study of inter-rater reliability in the scoring of sleep stages.[220] To wit, he found that the numbers (minutes of Stage 4, REM, etc.) everyone had been presenting as experimental data did not have a generally reliable meaning. Monroe had distributed copies of exactly the same all–night sleep recording to a number of laboratories, and the results showed significantly different values for the sleep states and stages among the laboratories.

Primarily as a result of this debacle, the UCLA Brain Information Service sponsored a specific project to develop a standard manual for the scoring of human sleep stages. Under the chairmanship of Allan Rechtschaffen and Anthony Kales, a committee was formed to set forth absolutely precise definitions of the sleep states and stages so that anyone, at least in theory, should get identical results scoring human adult sleep records. This manual was completed and published in 1968.

The "Standard Manual"[251] not only details definitions of the sleep stages, but illustrates standard techniques and procedures for human sleep recording as well. Instructions are included for recording the three chief modalities used in sleep research, EEG, EOG, and EMG. Ample figures are presented in the manual for illustrating all the criteria and special rules for scoring sleep stages. To give a general idea of the thoroughness of the manual, we abstract from one of the sleep stage definitions:

Stage 1:   This stage is defined by a relatively low voltage, mixed frequency EEG with a prominence of activity in the 2 to 7 cps range. The faster frequencies are mostly of lower voltage than the 2 to 7 cps activity. Stage 1 occurs most often in the transition from wakefulness to the other sleep stages or following body movements during sleep. During nocturnal sleep, Stage 1 tends to be relatively short, ranging from about 1 to 7 minutes. The highest voltage, 2 to 7 cps activity (about 50 to 75 μv), tends to occur in irregularly spaced bursts mostly during the latter portions of the stage. Also during the latter portions of the stage vertex sharp waves may appear . . . (whose) amplitude is occasionally as high as 200 μv . . . Stage 1 requires an absolute absence of clearly defined K–complexes and sleep spindles . . . Stage 1 . . . is characterized by the presence of slow eye movements . . . Rapid eye movements are absent. Tonic EMG levels are usually below those of relaxed wakefulness . . . When the amount of the record characterized by alpha activity combined with low voltage activity drops to less than 5% of the epoch and is replaced by relatively low voltage, mixed frequency activity, the epoch is scored as Stage 1.

The beauty of this manual is that it enables everyone to say that "this epoch is REM sleep, this epoch is Stage 2, this epoch is Stage 4, this epoch is wakefulness . . ." and so on.

There are many implications underlying what become arbitrary decisions about stages, but such peripheral problems usually develop when temporal quantification is involved. Thus, it is true that an epoch containing eye movements and sleep spindles both, may be scored Stage 2, but it is obviously true that this epoch is not pure Stage 2. If transitions in sleep, and we will say more about this later, can occur at rates greater than once every thirty seconds, then it is obvious that the scoring is not ultimately precise.

A similar scoring manual[3] has recently been published for the scoring of sleep stages in infants. This manual was more difficult to prepare because the criteria and the actual descriptive phenomenology of sleep in newborn infants is much more complicated than in human adults.

Investigators have worked on similar standardization in other animals, but very little progress has been made. Ursin[282] has proposed a two–stage division for NREM sleep in cats. Adey, Kado and Rhodes[1] have described sleep stages in the chimpanzee and Weitzman et al.[294] have described sleep stages and sleep cycles in the monkey, but precise criteria have not been widely accepted. Kales et al.[177] and Kahn and his colleagues[157] have described sleep in the elderly and it is clear that there are differences, particularly in that the Stage 4 criteria would not apply in the elderly. Whether these problems of precise definitions and quantification will be resolved in the same way that they have been resolved in the past, or whether new ways of processing this kind of data will simply take over and obviate the need in this area remains to be seen.

Limitations of the Two State Notion of Sleep

Although development of the concept of two kinds of sleep was a major advance, it was inevitably carried too far. In some way, the notion of two kinds of sleep was transmogrified so that these states became things in their own right. People began to assume, a priori, that what was true for one state absolutely could not be true for the other. For example, since dreaming is clearly associated with REM sleep, dreaming cannot be associated with NREM sleep. Or, if serotonin is the neurotransmitter for NREM sleep, it cannot play a role in REM sleep. Jouvet[150,151] has, in a sense, recognized and avoided this conceptual error in proposing that serotonin plays a priming role for the onset of REM sleep. Of course, REM sleep and NREM sleep represent the same brain doing two somewhat different things. Thus, the notion of mutual exclusivity

is almost as if people regarded a car that is moving and the same car standing still as two entirely different and unrelated entities.

In addition to such problems for biochemical approaches, the notion of two totally different states of being definitely affected approaches to the problems of sleep function. Because the phenomenological aspects of REM and NREM sleep seemed so divergent, researchers felt that their functions ought to be equally divergent. This kind of mythology grew up where we assumed the selective loss of NREM sleep would lead to sleepiness, whereas the selective loss of REM sleep would lead to excitation and hyperarousal. Because sleep loss in total sleep deprivation is around 75 percent NREM sleep, we assumed the overt consequences of total sleep loss primarily reflected the loss of NREM sleep. We further assumed that REM sleep loss contributed some excitation and thus diluted the effect of sleep deprivation. Accordingly, if the baseline sleep in some animal were hypothetically characterized by 50 percent REM sleep and 50 percent NREM sleep, total sleep deprivation would have essentially no effect on waking behavior because the two opposite consequences would cancel each other. Further, we could assume that if an animal had only NREM sleep, it would be extremely vulnerable to total sleep loss since the only effect would be depression of function and sleepiness.

An attempt to test this latter supposition was made by sleep depriving adult chickens in our laboratory. Adult chickens have only NREM sleep. We observed that chickens did appear to succumb to total sleep loss somewhat more quickly than mammals, e.g., rats and cats. However, we felt that the findings were really the result of anatomical considerations: i.e., the chicken, having only two feet, could not walk a treadmill or remain physically active as long as most mammals that have four feet.

At this point, we would like to mention two observations that will exemplify a host of findings that do not support the extremes to which the "two kinds of sleep" position has been carried. The first is an as yet unpublished* study by Paul Naitoh and Lavern Johnson who totally sleep deprived subjects for two full days and then deprived selectively of REM or NREM Stage 4 during the recovery period. They found that regardless of the procedure the recovery function proceeded at the same rate, probably being dependent *only* on total amount of sleep time.

The second is the casual but very startling observation that the sleepiness of a narcoleptic patient, which is in no way distinguishable from the drowsiness of someone who has suffered prolonged sleep loss, can be reversed if he has ten to twenty minutes of pure REM sleep (the characteristic sleep onset REM period of the narcoleptic patient). In other words, there is no cortical synchronization, no spindles, just the furious rapid eye movements, twitches, and implied neuronal "storm" of REM sleep. Yet, the tiredness and sleepiness is reversed, as it would be by ten to twenty minutes of NREM sleep—a normal nap.

We mention these things not to suggest that the old theorists who felt that REM and NREM were really manifestations of a unitary process were right, but merely to suggest that there is much more to the problem of two kinds of sleep than meets the eye. There are a great many things going on, some of which are common to *both* of the defined states of sleep and some of which are not.

Interspecific Generality of the Two States of Sleep

In addition to the move toward more rigorous analysis of human sleep, another great push in the last decade was a far reaching phylogenic description of sleep.† Such re-

search probed the evolutionary and interspecific generality of sleep behavior. One striking finding from this large body of data is the widespread interspecific similarity of mammalian sleep. It is now accepted that in most mammals and many avian species polygraphically defined wakefulness, NREM sleep and REM sleep always appear and are at least qualitatively and sequentially comparable across species. Of course much more descriptive and experimental work exists and will continue on various quantitative sleep differences[2,213,283] between species.

Ontogenic Studies of Sleep

In another vein, cutting across phylogeny, a vast developmental description of sleep has come into being.‡ One major theme of such investigations was that the electrophysiological and behavioral variables, which in adult organisms help to distinguish among the states of sleep, were of inconsistent value in determining behavioral states in young organisms. For example, adult human slow–wave sleep (Stages 3 and 4) is characterized by high voltage, slow (delta) EEG patterns, regular respiration, and tonically moderate EMG activity. In infants these variables often bear very different and inconsistent interrelationships. One may see, for example, delta activity with irregular respiration and irregular but low EMG activity. Such disassociated patterns in common sleep variables necessitate handling infant sleep records in a different manner than that used for adults.[3] The way sleep in young humans is scored may be regarded as using what we call a process view of sleep. (We will deal more extensively with this process view in another section.) While adult sleep is defined by constantly recurring patterns in many physiological processes, developmental sleep researchers recognize that patterns may not consistently appear in infancy. The adult patterns develop from very different and inconsistent constellations seen in young organisms. Consequently, in studying infant sleep, physi-

---

* See references 2, 57, 190, 236, and 258.

† These data have now begun to appear since our first writing. Lubin A., Moses, J., Johnson, L., and Naitoh, P. The recuperative effects of REM sleep and stage 4 sleep on human performance after complete sleep loss: Experiment 1. Psychophysiology, 11(2): 133–146, 1974. And Johnson, L., Naitoh, P., Moses, J., and Lubin, A. Interaction of REM deprivation and stage 4 deprivation with total sleep loss: Experiment 2. Psychophysiol. 11(2): 147–159, 1974.

‡ See references 3, 27, 82, 156, 234, 261, 263, 167, and 166.

ological variables are studied concurrently but regarded as independent processes. The relative importance of each index is established by the investigator, depending on the questions he wishes to ask.

❲ The Process View of Sleep

The foregoing material provides an appropriate introduction to a consideration of what we may call a process view of sleep. While of heuristic value, we have seen that the notion of state and, in particular, two sleep states does have certain limitations. Today many workers would agree that sleep states are really the outward manifestations of a number of discrete processes that are going on simultaneously but with as yet unspecified degrees of independence. The beginning of this systems concept of sleep could probably be dated to the Lyon Conference on the Neurophysiology of the States of Sleep in 1963 when Prof. Guiseppe Moruzzi[224] made some extemporaneous remarks (duly recorded and transcribed) to the effect that it would be helpful in describing REM sleep to distinguish between phasic (short–lasting) and tonic (long–lasting) activities. Thus, although REM sleep was generally considered as a single "something," Moruzzi's suggestion formally recognized the fact that there were at least two attributes of REM periods that could be dealt with more or less independently. The further development of this line of thought has led to a relatively new point of view that is best set forth by a consideration of REM sleep.

Independent Processes in REM Sleep

Full–blown REM sleep is defined in most mammalian species when we can note the simultaneous occurrence of at least three distinct classes of events. Perhaps the most essential and characteristic process of REM sleep is an actively induced, tonic, nonreciprocal motor inhibition. The most widely used and convenient indicator of this inhibitory process

is a continuous recording of the electromyogram, or EMG. Suppression of EMG activity is highly correlated with the onset of REM sleep (see Figure 8–3). EMG suppression is

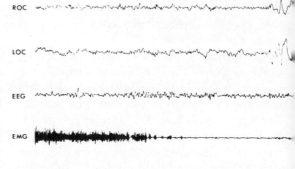

Figure 8–3. This figure illustrates the transition from Stage 2 sleep to REM sleep. Note that the EMG suppression precedes the appearance of rapid eye movements by several seconds.
Derivations: ROC—monopolarelectrooculogram from right outer canthus; monopolarelectrooculogram from LOC: left outer canthus.
EEG—monopolar electroencephalogram derived from C_3/A_2;
EMG—electromyogram from placements over digastric muscle.

also highly correlated with other indicators of active motor inhibition, for example, suppression of electrically induced reflexes[137] and a number of measures as studied by Pompeiano and his associates[245,346] in cats. According to Pompeiano, during REM sleep there is a tonic hyperpolarization of alpha motor neurons; and if the cataplectic attack in narcoleptic patients is representative of the effectiveness of this inhibitory process[77] (see also section on "Tonic Motor Inhibition and Cataplexy-Narcolepsy") REM sleep is a time of profound motor paralysis in which tendon reflexes cannot be elicited and in which voluntary movement is totally impossible. In cats, the presence of motor inhibition during REM sleep is also confirmed by an extreme flaccidity.

There is a dream that has been experienced by most people. It is the dream of trying to run, usually to escape some great danger, and being completely unable to move, or of moving slowly, with great difficulty as if one's limbs were weighted with lead. It is quite likely that this dream represents a breakthrough into dreaming consciousness of an awareness of the true neurophysiological condition, much as a narcoleptic is aware that he cannot move during an attack of sleep paralysis.

The second process is central nervous system (CNS) arousal or activation. It is a well-known fact that in many respects, the brain in REM sleep appears to be aroused or awake.[57, 63,66] We must, therefore, postulate some sort of nonspecific arousal process or system that operates more or less tonically during REM periods. It is still a matter of great puzzlement whether the observed CNS arousal is true wakefulness or a totally different process that merely resembles wakefulness in terms of most of the nonspecific measures of CNS activity levels such as brain temperature, EEG activation, cerebral blood flow, and so forth. Certain differences between wakefulness and REM sleep could, of course, be quantitative. Thus, atropine might block EEG activation[295] during waking behavior but not during REM sleep at one dose, but would block EEG activation in both states at a higher dose. Early studies[196,197] suggested different pathways by showing that lesions in the reticular formation brought about prolonged EEG synchronization in wakefulness, yet, when REM periods occurred, normal EEG activation was seen. This is not so clear in humans because the EEG patterns in REM sleep do not resemble patterns seen during the waking state. However, there is still some controversy about just where the REM sleep EEG actually belongs from a conceptual point of view. Is the REM sleep EEG a combination of activated patterns plus superimposed saw-tooth slow rhythms, or is it really a different spectrum more analogous to NREM Stage 1? The subjective descriptions by narcoleptic patients of the transition from unequivocal wakefulness directly into REM sleep[77] lead us to feel that perhaps REM arousal is truly the same arousal process as in wakefulness. If the narcoleptic patient is interacting verbally with a bedside observer, the transition appears to be a gradual pre-empting of the waking sensorium by internally generated sensory input. Thus, the narcoleptic on the verge of full-blown REM sleep, with certain aspects of this state—namely, EMG suppression and rapid eye movements—already established, is still clearly awake in terms of the usual definitions of wakefulness.

The third process characteristic of REM sleep is called *phasic activity*. At the present time, there is no widely accepted definition of this activity. The underlying neurophysiology is far from clear, and different investigators will think of different things when the term is used. In its most global definition, phasic activity merely refers to short-lasting events. The exact time limits for this definition have not been specified nor would it be practically useful to do so. Generally we are thinking of phenomena lasting for a second or less. These events may, of course, occur in bursts. The most important aspect of this phasic activity derives from the assumption that phasic activity is generated exclusively from *within* the brain.

What are some examples of phasic activity? The most dramatic and the first to be observed was, of course, rapid eye motility. The rapid jerks of the eyeballs are binocularly synchronous and occur in bursts or singly and in all directions and sizes of arc. This activity has been described in the cat and numerous other mammals as well as the human adult and infant.

Other things we can mention are muscle twitches,[11] sudden changes in pupil diameter,[20] sharp fluctuations in penile tumescence,[96] cardiovascular irregularities,[14,107] and phasic, middle-ear contractions.[81] The latter were uniquely studied in the cat until recently when Pessah et al.[235] published their beautifully thorough observations demonstrating middle-ear muscle activity in human REM periods.

Finally, the most intriguing and widely studied phasic events are the discrete bursts of high amplitude, biphasic sharp waves in the electrical recordings from the pons, oculomotor nuclei, lateral geniculate nuclei, and visual cortices of the cat (the PGO wave).[30, 31,154,227] Many investigators have speculated that these PGO waves represent the primary phasic event in that they may be the electrical sign of the basic trigger of other phasic events, e.g., eye movements, middle–ear muscle contractions, and so on. Figure 8–4 illustrates a typical example of PGO activity. Certainly, if there were a generator for PGO waves, this generator might stimulate many areas of the brain where a potential change resembling a PGO wave could not be recorded. This is suggested by unit studies that show in almost every area of the brain phasic bursts of firing which seem to be correlated fairly well with PGO waves. Thus, it is important to know whether or not every other phasic event is uniformly linked in time to the occurrence of PGO waves. Another problem is whether or not PGO waves and the underlying neurophysiological events are unique to REM sleep, since there are waves in the lateral geniculate that appear to be merely a response to eye movements in the waking state. Data of Brooks and Gershon[32] raise the question of whether such eye movement potentials have the same anatomical substrate as the REM–PGO wave. Recent studies addressing this issue include a careful description of the temporal relationship between eye movements and geniculate waves[264] and some demonstrations from thalamic stimulation that eye movement potentials are elicitable in any state, but that REM–PGO waves have a longer latency and can only be elicited during REM sleep and periods of NREM sleep that immediately precede REM sleep.[231]

At the present time, clear relationships have been described in the cat between PGO waves and a variety of peripheral events such as eye movements, limb twitches, and, most recently, phasic contractions of middle–ear muscles[260] in the cat. However, the relationships among these peripheral activities are not entirely clear. In addition, there are events that really lie between "phasic" (one hundred to one thousand msec.) as exemplified by the PGO wave, and tonic as exemplified by the duration of the REM period itself. Thus, the original description of middle–ear muscle activity by Dewson et al.[81] was mainly of contractions lasting several seconds that were not necessarily related to rapid eye movements. Roffwarg et al.[260] noted these longer contractions but referred to them as "tonic" and also not necessarily related to PGO waves. We will consider this problem again in relation to "psychophysiological correlations and dreaming."

It is important to emphasize here that there is little cross–species data to affirm (1) the

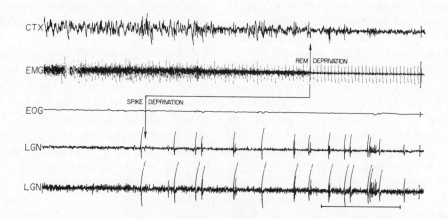

Figure 8–4. A comparison of "spike" deprivation and REM deprivation. In the latter procedure, the cat would have been aroused at the exact onset of the REM period (B) signaled by EMG suppression and EEG activation. If the cat had been undergoing spike deprivation, the arousal would have been accomplished a little earlier (A) immediately after the first PGO spike. In this example, such an arousal would have deprived the cat of thirteen NREM PGO spikes in addition to those occurring in the REM period, and twenty-six seconds of NREM sleep.

apparent "pacemaker" properties of the feline PGO wave vis–à–vis other phasic events and (2) the generality of the distribution of the feline PGO wave in sleep. Nevertheless, we all assume that there is some phasic generator in all the many mammalian and avian species who have REM sleep characterized by other phasic events such as muscle twitches and eye movements. Figure 8–5 presents a highly idealized conception of such a generator. In this conception, PGO waves represent a low threshold response. Whether or not any particular response occurs would be a complex function of the moment–to–moment excitability of the responding structure and the stimulus output it receives from the generator. The generator itself could be exceedingly simple with a rhythmic constant output, or exceedingly complex with its output varying in terms of intensity, duration, direction (to which particular structure), timing, and sequence. Given the postulated brain–stem origins of such activity, we may ask the question, is there some structure or area in which such a complex function could be housed? The desire to look at this activity in association with dreaming in humans has led to a search for some sort of PGO analogue in humans. There are three important candidates. The first is the phasic–integrated muscle potential (PIP) de-

scribed by Rechtschaffen, Michel, and Metz,[254] who observed that discharge in the eye muscle was always associated with PGO waves in the cat and decided to look at this activity in the human. Second, the phasic EMG suppression described by Pivik and Dement,[243] which is apparently analogous to the phasic inhibition described by Pompeiano,[245,246] can be seen only during NREM sleep in humans because it is observed against the tonically active EMG background. It has been confirmed by H–reflex studies that such phasic inhibition is short lasting but generalized. Third, there are EEG events that may be related to phasic activity. The saw-tooth waves of REM sleep could be human cortical or scalp derivations of phasic electrical activity, and the so–called K–complex, seen more frequently in NREM sleep, may represent a kind of response to some spontaneously occurring internal event. We will say more about this later.

Independent Processes in NREM Sleep

What about NREM sleep? Most people think of NREM sleep as slow waves and spindles in the EEG (see Figure 8–2), and further feel that these imply deactivation of the cortex. However, we might ask the question, what is the absolutely essential difference between being awake and being asleep (NREM sleep)? In our opinion, after considerable reflection, the salient feature of wakefulness is the environmental engagement of the organism. It sees, hears, and responds to the world around it either behaviorally or perceptually. The onset of sleep (normally NREM sleep) always entails the cessation of the above perceptual activities. There is a fairly discrete point somewhere in the transition from wakefulness to sleep where the organism essentially, though perhaps not in every detail, stops perceiving its environment. It becomes in one instant blind, deaf, dumb, and numb. The important point, and of this we are quite certain, is that the moment of perceptual shutdown is *not* the moment at which slow waves and spindles appear. Therefore, the significance of spindles and slow waves in the EEG

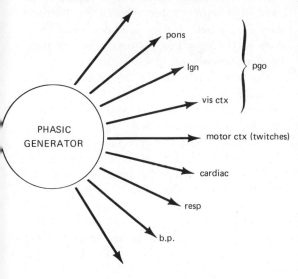

Figure 8–5.   Diagrammatic representation of the phasic event generator.

may not be crucial to the onset of sleep, convenient though they may be as signs of NREM sleep.

The moment of sleep (i.e., the cessation of perception) is apparently quite abrupt. While there may be important predisposing changes leading up to it, and consequences of its occurrence leading away from it, the point of sleep onset itself seems relatively easy to determine within a second or two. For example, suppose we ask an individual to sit with his eyes taped open and to make a motor response when a light flash is presented. At some point he will not respond. The moment of sleep is best defined by such a point of perceptual disengagement. We have recently used this technique to demonstrate pathological lapses in patients complaining of excessive sleepiness.[237] Immediately after such a failure the EEG patterns can still show waking patterns, such as alpha rhythm. Thus, we could conceivably abolish slow waves and spindles without abolishing the process of perceptual disengagement. Accordingly, we must acknowledge that it is not clear if slow waves and spindles are processes that really begin at the point of response inhibition and only build up enough to appear in the EEG a few minutes later or are entirely separate and perhaps redundant processes. But until proven otherwise, we must think of slow waves and spindles as meaningful although often belated signs of a central inhibitory state. However, aside from the kind of behavioral study we have mentioned, even the more sophisticated neurophysiological techniques, such as unit activities studies, have not shown changes in firing patterns that are commensurate with the vast functional differences among states. It may be, however, that such studies compare unit activity at the onset of sleep (i.e., after perceptual changes but before the conventional signs such as slow waves and spindles) with the sleep stage a few minutes later when slow waves and spindles have appeared.

In our opinion, the best sign of the exact moment of sleep appears to be the breakdown of the ability to maintain visual fixation, which is usually signaled by the appearance of a slow drifting of the eyes.[100,101] If the transi-

tion is prolonged, it is typical to see rhythmic, to-and-fro, slow, horizontal movements that resemble a sinewave when recorded by conventional polygraphic electrooculographic methods. According to other investigators, pupillary myosis in dim light may also be such a precise sign,[188] although others[302] have suggested that relative myosis is a sign of "drowsiness" in the waking state.

Another possible alteration in NREM sleep that could, by stretching a point, be called an independent process has to do with memory mechanisms. It seems reasonably clear, from the work of Portnoff et al.[247] and the unpublished results of Kamiya and his colleagues, that sleep either erases short–term memories or that long-term memory mechanisms do not operate in NREM sleep. These changes could possibly be invoked to account for the blackouts or amnesic episodes that are often experienced by narcoleptics.

Dissociative Aspects of Normal Sleep

As we have shown, it is possible to take the phenomenology of normal sleep and conceptually divide it into independent processes. However, the real test is whether these processes can truly be dissociated from one another on a temporal basis. This is crucial to the issue of whether states are entirely different things or whether they are mere manifestations of the simultaneous occurrence of independent processes.

The best illustration of the process view in normal sleep is phasic activity. Phasic activity, as exemplified by the PGO spike in the cat, is not limited to REM sleep. PGO spikes typically occur in NREM sleep. Thus, what occurs in, is true for, REM sleep also occurs in, is true for, NREM sleep. The most characteristic time in NREM sleep when PGO spikes appear is about ten to thirty seconds prior to the onset of the REM period (see Figure 8–4). To illustrate how absolute this is, we looked at the beginning of more than two thousand REM periods distributed among sleep periods of about thirty cats in our laboratory and failed to find, in normal intact animals, a single instance where REM sleep (as defined by EEG activation closely followed by EMG suppression and eye movements) ever occurred before at least a few PGO waves (usually ten to thirty) were discharged in the preceding NREM interval. Phasic activity in the form of PGO waves is actually far more distributed throughout NREM sleep than most people realize and more than we have already described.

Although absolutely characteristic of REM periods in the cat, it is also true that phasic activity in the form of PGO waves may be present in more than 50 percent of the total amount of NREM sleep, at least in some cats. In addition, intervals of NREM sleep in the cat in which there are absolutely no PGO waves at all are relatively brief, for the most part no longer than two or three minutes. Discharge rate of PGO spikes during REM periods varies from cat to cat, ranging from about forty per minute to more than one hundred. The discharge rate during epochs of NREM sleep is highly variable, although well below the rates seen during REM periods. The total number of PGO spikes per day in the cat has been estimated to vary between ten thousand and twenty thousand. Approximately 15 percent of this total typically occurs in NREM sleep as defined by slow waves and spindles in the EEG and the presence of tonic electrical activity in the neck muscles. Most of the other phasic activities tend to be less prominent in NREM sleep, but the truth of the matter is that we have not looked at them closely. Thus, there may be occasional rapid eye movements in NREM sleep, occasional fluctuations in heart rate, penile tumescence, and so on, but we have simply not emphasized these findings.

In human subjects, there is also plentiful evidence that phasic activity is widely disseminated throughout NREM sleep. For example, Rechtschaffen and Chernik[250] have reported an almost continual discharge of phasic–integrated muscle potentials or "PIPs" [255,256,257] during NREM periods as well as REM periods. Pivik and Dement[243] have reported a similar distribution and intensity for phasic EMG suppressions. Finally, K–complexes, if they represent phasic activity, are also distributed throughout much of NREM sleep.

If we look at tonic EMG suppression, we find that it, too, can precede the onset of the REM period, often by a minute or more. Thus, we can have intervals of NREM sleep that are characterized by what is usually considered the sine qua non of REM sleep. In one of the early studies of long–term REM sleep deprivation, we observed that the gap between EMG suppression and EEG activation (NREM Stage 2 to REM patterns) underwent a steady enlargement.[61] Penile tumescence, which appears to be a consistent concomitant of REM periods in humans and monkeys,[96,82] has been reported to occur in NREM sleep in humans if REM sleep is prevented from occurring.[81]

(Conclusions

The upshot of this section's discussion is that we can conceptualize individual processes existing within or as part of the two states of sleep. In REM sleep, we can speak of motor inhibition, CNS arousal, and phasic activity. Obviously, this list is arbitrary; there are other processes, too. In NREM sleep, we can speak of the control of cortical rhythms, higher processing or inhibition of sensory input, and perhaps control of long–term memory processes or consolidation. Throughout the remainder of this chapter we will see many of the implications and ramifications of the notion that sleep comprises many temporally linked processes.

(Phasic Activity and the Selective Deprivation of REM Sleep

With the realization that there were two kinds of sleep came the realization that total sleep deprivation might be an approach that confounded the effects of two entirely different deficits. Accordingly, the first attempt was made to study the effect of selective deprivation of REM sleep by arousing subjects at the onset of REM periods. The experiments produced some anecdotal findings from the subjects in the area of behavioral disturbance, but, more important, there was a marked "rebound" in REM sleep time in the all-night sleep recordings immediately after the nights of REM sleep deprivation.[58]

These results suggested that there might be a specific "need" for REM sleep, the rebound on recovery nights representing a "compensation," and, because of this need, it was further suggested that prolonged REM sleep loss might lead inevitably to some psychological dysfunction or even more serious organic impairment if carried on long enough. The actual temporal organization of the physiological concomitants of REM sleep (EMG suppression closely followed by EEG activation and rapid eye movements) made it relatively easy to carry out deprivation experiments by awakening organisms at the precise onset of each successive REM period, or by placing them in special situations where the motor inhibition of a developing REM period led to an arousing consequence.[71] Thus, the state of REM sleep could be sharply, almost surgically eliminated while leaving NREM sleep essentially intact, and the effects of this "extirpation" could be systematically observed with the hope of clarifying what normal REM periods accomplished for the organism.

A sort of philosophical underpinning or justification for this kind of experiment was that the processes of evolution and natural selection would not have allowed this "thing" (REM sleep), with its unique physiology and neuroanatomical substrate, to achieve universal distribution among most mammals of all ages unless it held some very important advantage or vital function. An initial offshoot of the very first attempt to understand the function of REM sleep was the hypothesis that REM sleep (dream) deprivation might lead to insanity, a formulation markedly influenced by psychoanalytic theories about the psychology of the dream process and metaphorical organization of the psyche.[95] In the early 1960s, probably because of the absence of a biochemical knowledge as well as the above

zeitgeist, there was a premature reification of the so-called hydraulic model of REM sleep, with its associated metaphorical constructs of REM pressure, REM reservoir, compensatory rebound, REM quota, and so forth. However, in recent years, there has been an explosive increase in knowledge about CNS metabolic processes. It is therefore no longer appropriate to explain REM deprivation–compensation in metaphorical terms. The REM rebound is a very real and intriguing response and must have a biochemical mechanism.

The Stanford University Sleep Laboratory has been in the forefront of the struggle to understand REM sleep, at least in terms of man-, cat-, and rat-hours devoted to selective REM–deprivation studies.* A number of experiments undertaken by the Stanford group were essentially open-ended, i.e., the end point was not defined in advance. Rather, organisms were to be selectively deprived of REM sleep until clear-cut effects were seen. It was confidently expected in the beginning of these efforts that if the procedure were carried on long enough it would be life threatening, and that prior to this terminal eventuality, serious derangements of behavior would be observed. A number of spectacularly long (up to seventy consecutive days) deprivation experiments were carried out in laboratory animals.

As early as 1965, we were forced to conclude, despite the dramatic and highly consistent alterations in recovery sleep (enormous REM rebounds) that REM periods in the adult animal did not serve a vital function, and that the organism could probably live indefinitely without them. This conclusion was published in several places (see 66, 67) including Volume III of the first edition this *Handbook* in 1966. "These results strongly suggest that REM sleep does not perform a vital function in the adult cat."[64]

The possibility that there might still be some harmful effect of REM sleep loss in susceptible individuals was tested by REM-depriving schizophrenic patients.[288] In human studies, chronic administration of monoamine

* See references 45, 61, 63, 65, 66, 68, 69, 70, 71, 90, and 122.

oxidase inhibitors was found to completely suppress REM sleep[232,233] and when administered for many months with periodic testing of the REM suppression did not produce adverse psychological effects.[297] In some instances, REM sleep was completely suppressed for as long as a year. The overall results in animals and man indicate that REM sleep deprivation per se is not harmful and support the conclusion reached by Vogel[288] that REM suppression does not lead to psychosis. In a roughly similar vein are the findings of Kales et al.[164,173] in their sleep studies of long–term barbiturate addiction. To be sure, withdrawal from any of these REM suppressive drugs, particularly after prolonged usage, is likely to be fraught with difficulties, but the absence of discernible REM periods for a year or more would seem to eliminate in a most conclusive manner the possibility that these periods in themselves serve a vital function, or that their prolonged absence would play a role in the genesis of psychotic disturbances. It is important to emphasize this point very strongly because it is our impression that aphorisms such as "dreams preserve sanity" and "loss of dreaming may lead to insanity" are still very much preserved in the collective psychiatric consciousness.

There remains one problem to solve in this area however. All of the work cited earlier was done from the point of view of regarding REM sleep as a thing that could, in fact, be extirpated. Our discussion of the so–called process view of sleep should suggest that this concept of REM deprivation might be questioned. For a variety of reasons, we have turned our attention toward phasic activity to illuminate the function of sleep. The basic assumption to be tested is that the function of REM sleep is to permit the efficient discharge of phasic events (PGO spikes). It is difficult to justify this assumption in neurophysiological or biochemical terms, but it is equally hard at the present level of knowledge to refute it on these terms.

If we recall that nearly 15 percent of the total number of PGO spikes are discharged in NREM sleep and that every REM period is preceded by NREM–PGO spike discharge,

we can see that REM sleep deprivation per se cannot solve the problem. In the first place, as REM sleep deprivation proceeds, there is the well–known effect of an increasing number of REM periods that must be interrupted. Since a finite number of PGO spikes occur before each arousal, it is obvious that the total number can become very large. Secondly, there is evidence that the "intensity" of PGO spike discharge increases in *both* REM and NREM sleep as a function of prior REM deprivation.[68] Thus, at some point, the daily count of NREM–PGO spikes would presumably equal the total number discharged during REM periods in a typical baseline day. In other words, if the function of REM sleep was somehow involved in phasic activity, the function would be *totally* fulfilled in NREM sleep. At this hypothetical point, no further deprivation effect would accumulate even if the selective deprivation of REM periods were continued indefinitely.

These arguments led to a painstaking series of experiments that essentially consisted of making the REM deprivation arousal a little earlier so that the NREM– (or pre–REM–) PGO spikes would also be prevented along with all those normally occurring within REM periods.

This procedure is illustrated in Figure 8–4. A glance at the illustration shows that if the animal is aroused at the precise moment indicated by the left arrow a more effective "spike deprivation" is accomplished than if he is aroused at the onset of the REM period (right arrow). Several cats were deprived in this manner for two consecutive days. In addition, the same cats served as their own controls by undergoing a "standard" REM deprivation procedure for an identical amount of time. The latter procedure produced the usual result in terms of a REM rebound and increased number of REM periods. The spike deprivation procedure, which was essentially conventional REM deprivation plus the elimination of additional NREM–PGO spikes, produced a picture that was identical to a longer period of REM deprivation. In other words, there were larger REM rebounds. These results are illustrated in Figure 8–6. They clearly, albeit in-

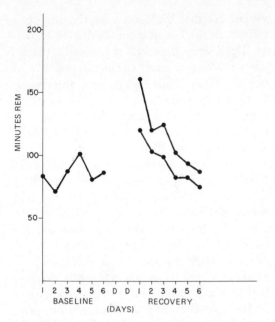

Figure 8–6. The results of classical REM sleep deprivation versus spike deprivation in one representative cat. The minutes of REM sleep per day on an eight-hour schedule (baseline) are plotted on the left. The upper curve on the right shows the daily REM times immediately after two days of spike deprivation (D), and the lower curve is after two days of REM deprivation.

directly, support the hypothesis that the essential ingredient of REM periods is phasic activity.

The point of all this discussion is that conclusive tests of whether or not there is a need for REM sleep have not yet been done. While the "PGO spike hypothesis" may seem a little far-fetched (i.e., what useful function do PGO spikes perform?) it is still a possibility that must be ruled out before we can conclude there is no need for REM sleep or any of its processes. The same consideration applies to the long–term administrations of powerful REM suppressant drugs, e.g., monoamine–oxidase inhibitors (MAOIs), since careful monitoring in cats has not been done to see if there has been a buildup of phasic activity (PGO spike) discharge in NREM sleep. In short–term studies of MAOI in cats, there appears to be a complete suppression of PGO spike activity, but most observations have been casual at best, and only of a few days duration. Finally, there is still the difficult

question of whether absence of the PGO waves per se means that the phasic activity function is not being discharged. This latter is further considered in the section on "Phasic Activity and a Theory of Psychosis."

(Tonic Motor Inhibition and Narcolepsy with Cataplexy

It has been noted that motor inhibition is an important process associated with REM sleep. We will see that the syndrome of narcolepsy with cataplexy may be regarded as a disorder involving abnormal occurrences of this and other REM sleep components.

Narcolepsy is always characterized by recurring episodes of daytime sleep. Such sleep episodes may be related to fatigue, boredom, monotony, or drug ingestion, but are most characteristic of the illness when they occur in inappropriate situations. Cataplexy is often involved in narcolepsy. Cataplexy is defined by a rapid loss of voluntary muscle control leading to partial muscle weakness or a complete body collapse. The cataplectic episodes are usually quite short, lasting only one to ten seconds and rarely as long as one minute. Cataplectic attacks are characteristically precipitated by sudden strong emotion, most typically laughter and anger, although being startled, fear, and other emotions may be involved. Cataplexy may also occur without any precipitating emotion on rare occasions.

The mechanism of this generalized motor inhibition is not clear. Pompeiano and his co-workers[112,245,246] have shown, however, that the tonic inhibition of REM sleep descends from the brain stem to the spinal cord in the ventral halves of the lateral fasciculi. Rostrally, there is evidence that the locus coeruleus is involved in REM sleep inhibition,[152] and caudally the lumbar spinal cord has been implicated.[223] Such inhibition may involve cholinergic mechanisms since from a behavioral and global point of view generalized motor inhibition can be produced by focal injection of cholinomimetic drugs into the pontine reticular formation.[51,111,214] Similar nonreciprocal inhibition can also be produced by electrical stimulation of areas such as the orbital cortex[265] and the ventromedial medulla[205] in the lightly anesthetized cat. However, most individuals who are investigating these phenomena assume that the medullary inhibitory area of Magoun and Rhines is some sort of final common inhibitory pathway.

Other manifestations of the narcolepsy–cataplexy syndrome are the so–called auxiliary symptoms: sleep paralysis, hypnogogic hallucinations, and disrupted nocturnal sleep. Sleep paralysis consists of episodes of paralysis occurring at sleep onset or at the end of a sleep period. Patients report that they maintain consciousness during these episodes. Although the episodes are not precipitated by emotion, they are often associated with great anxiety generated by the helplessness, which usually persists for several minutes. Hypnogogic hallucinations are intense and vivid, often frightening hallucinations occurring at the onset of sleep. Finally, narcoleptic patients may experience multiple arousals and frightening dreams during the night.

Thus, just as we conceive of motor inhibition and endogenous sensory input (presumably heralded by phasic activity) as REM sleep processes, we can also conceive of narcolepsy–cataplexy as a disorder involving the uncoupling or disassociation of such processes from the normal wakefulness–sleep cycle.*

(Phasic Events and the Psychophysiology of Dreaming

An area of sleep research that has certainly received both theoretical and practical implementation by the notion of independent processes within sleep is the psychophysiology of dreaming. This area is concerned with the physiological activities that correlate with (a)

* Since our first writing, we have begun studies on dogs apparently afflicted with narcolepsy-cataplexy. Such efforts may disclose much concerning the neurological deficit underlying the syndrome. See Mitler, M., Boysen, B., Campbell, L. and Dement, W. Narcolepsy-cataplexy in a female dog. *Exp. Neurol.* (in press) for an account of this work.

the presence or absence of dreaming in humans and with (b) specific elements of dream content within the overall dream episode. The ultimate goal is to understand the special CNS events that are specifically involved in the genesis of complex hallucinatory experiences during sleep and, by implication, hallucinations that occur abnormally during wakefulness.

In the beginning, this seemed to be a relatively simple problem. The discovery of REM sleep and the early work that showed a startlingly high incidence of dream recall when subjects were aroused from REM sleep periods and a contrastingly low incidence from NREM periods (see 275) seemed to settle the issue. The terms, REM sleep and dreaming sleep, were treated as being exactly synonymous, and it seemed that further investigations of the "unique" neurophysiology of the REM state would lead eventually to a description of the brain processes giving rise to the remarkable hallucinatory experiences of dreaming. The concept of a sharply differentiated physiological substrate underlying the two basic sleep states reinforced these expectations.

Unfortunately, the conceptual identity of REM sleep and dreaming was soon undermined by a steady flow of results that continued to show that a substantial amount of dream recall could be elicited from NREM sleep arousals. An attempt was made to develop definitions based on quality and quantity of dream recall so that, although one could not say that mental activity was not totally absent in NREM sleep, one could say that it was quantitatively different from that which occurred in REM periods.

However, when investigators looked at the discriminability of REM and NREM reports,[221] it was clear that many NREM reports could not be discriminated from REM reports defined as "full–blown" dream recall. This was particularly true when the reports were elicited from sleep onset NREM.[103,104] [287] In other words, it appeared that intense, complicated, bizarre, emotional, hallucinatory experiences could occur at the onset of sleep as well as occasionally in other NREM stages.

This situation posed a dilemma for those who were interested in the neurophysiological substrate of dreaming and hallucinations; but a way out of the dilemma suggested itself when it was realized that certain events thought to be ineluctably linked to REM sleep[31] also occurred in NREM sleep. These events were the PGO waves or phasic activity. Their typical occurrence in the NREM sleep just prior to REM periods is illustrated in Figure 8–4, but the waves or spikes also occur in a widely disseminated fashion throughout NREM intervals.

It was almost inevitable that the PGO spike should become the focus of attention when investigators began to look for a single "marker" that could account for dreaming in both REM and NREM sleep. In terms of looking for more specific events *within* REM periods, the suggestion was made quite early[61,62] that the dream was experienced as "real" and the major problem would be to find the neural events that were effectively substituting for sensory input. The brain–stem generation of PGO spikes as described by Brooks and Bizzi[31] and Jouvet,[149] and the apparent distribution of this activity along the visual–oculo-motor pathways[210,211,227] definitely suggested a quasi–sensory function. Furthermore, these studies clearly showed that the rapid eye movements in the cat were precisely related to PGO spikes, and it was already known that arousals at the very moment when eye movements were being executed within REM periods frequently provided the very best recall of dreaming. Thus, a major shift in viewpoint occurred in the area of dream psychophysiology that suggested that phasic activity would be a much better predictor of dream recall and, hence, a better correlate of dreaming than REM periods. Taking individual rapid eye movements as phasic events, Molinari and Foulkes[217] have carried out an elegant study that compares tonic (REM periods) and phasic events as dream correlates. All of these considerations have subsequently guided what might be called the search for the perfect indicator of dreaming.

It is obvious that phasic activity (short-lasting events) can be conceptualized *within* REM periods in essentially all mammals including humans since the rapid eye movements themselves are phasic events. There is also no problem in identifying phasic activity in NREM sleep in animals where cortical and subcortical recordings can reveal PGO spikes or bursts of unit discharge. The big problem is to find a phasic event that satisfactorily cuts across sleep states in the human. It should also bear some analogous relationship to the feline PGO waves. K–complexes in the EEG certainly qualify as phasic events, but they do not occur in the EEG of REM sleep. Parenthetically, Pivik and his colleagues[244] have studied the possible relationship of K–complexes and NREM dream recall. They found no simple relationship. Body movements, respiratory changes, heart–rate changes and other relatively nonspecific physiological variables have been examined from this point of view.

The search for a really useful indicator of the presence of phasic activity in the human, particularly during NREM sleep has turned up three promising candidates. The first was described by Pivik and Dement.[243] It is essentially seen as a brief (two hundred to five hundred msec.) suppression of the tonic EMG activity in NREM sleep (see Figure 8–7). Utilizing electrically induced reflex activity, Pivik and Dement were able to show that the phasic EMG suppressions were coincident with active motor inhibitory influences. Similar phasic EMG suppressions were found to occur in the cat during NREM sleep and were often coincident with a NREM–PGO spike (also Figure 8–7). Because of the latter relationship, it seemed reasonable to postulate that the phasic EMG suppressions represented a human analogue of the phasic inhibitory process described in cats by Pompeiano.[245,246] Although not usually detectable in REM periods because of the absence of the tonic EMG background, on the rare occasions that this background is *not* totally suppressed plentiful phasic EMG suppressions are easily seen *within* REM periods most commonly in connection with rapid eye movements.

The relationship of phasic EMG suppres-

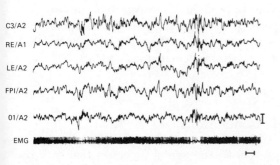

Figure 8–7. This figure shows phasic (short–lasting) EMG suppression occurring in Stage 3 NREM sleep. Note that a K complex (C_3/A_2) occurs simultaneously with the phasic muscle suppression.
Derivations: all EEG placements use the standard ten-twenty system;
  RE/A_1—right eye recorded from right outer canthus;
  LE/A_2—left eye recorded from left outer canthus;
EMG—recorded from placements over diagastric muscles.
Calibrations: horizontal one second; vertical fifty μv.

sions in NREM sleep to recall of mental content was tested by Pivik.[241] Significant results were not obtained. Parenthetically, another relationship has been discovered that elevates the status of EMG suppressions beyond the level of laboratory curiosity. Guilleminault et al.[118] have shown that the motor discharge in *nocturnal myoclonus* frequently follows phasic EMG suppression.

The second phasic indicator is the phasic integrated potential or PIP reported by Rechtschaffen et al.[255] in 1970. These discharges are recorded from ordinary disc electrodes placed near the eye, but the authors were not certain exactly which muscles were involved. However, they felt that the PIPs were exact homologues of similar discharges recorded in the cat that were, in turn, precisely related to PGO spike discharge in both REM and NREM sleep.[211] The human PIPs have the advantage of being easily seen in both REM and NREM sleep. In the former state, they are clearly related to rapid eye move-

ments although they also appear (as do PGO spikes in the cat) in the absence of ocular deviations. They are distributed throughout NREM sleep, although the discharge rate is clearly higher immediately preceding REM periods than immediately after.

A series of reports by Rechtschaffen and his colleagues[250,256,257,289] explicated relationships of periorbital PIPs to mental activity in both REM and NREM sleep. These studies also developed a new concept about phasic activity and dreaming, which will probably be very important in guiding future investigations. Four arousal conditions were described by the authors: (1) a "tonic" condition that was characterized by a brief (several seconds) burst of periorbital EMG activity without PIPs; (2) a phasic condition characterized by periorbital PIPs without tonic periorbital EMG activity; (3) a phasic–tonic condition when both of the foregoing were present; and (4) a control condition in which there has been no PIPs or tonic activity for at least one minute. Hundreds of arousals were carried out in these exhaustive studies. The responses were rated in terms of presence or absence of recall of mental content, amount of recall in content reports, and amount of distortion, implausibility, and bizarreness in these reports.

In NREM sleep, the presence or absence of PIPs did *not* predict the presence or absence of mental content. The latter was, however, significantly predicted by the tonic periorbital activity. PIPs alone were not correlated with an increased probability of obtaining mental content over the control condition. However, if content was present, PIPs were correlated with experiences judged to be bizarre. Similar relationships obtained in REM periods although the tonic condition was not recordable, ostensibly because of the REM associated motor inhibition. We may infer that it exists because tonic potentials have been recorded directly from the inferior rectus muscle during REM sleep in humans.

These studies are extremely relevant to the psychophysiology of dreaming, and, once again, they have introduced a further refinement in conceptual organization of sleep physiology. Thus, there appears to be a process involving sustained activity of a few seconds duration during which thoughts, associations, vague images, etc., are raised to hallucinatory intensity. The correlate of this process is what the Rechtschaffen group call "tonic EMG activity." It is important to avoid confusion when a clear distinction is made between this process which lasts only a few seconds, and the use of the word tonic to describe changes that are sustained throughout the entirety of the REM period as described in the previous section.

A second process, which is indicated by PGO spikes in the cat and PIPs in the human, seems to represent neural events that contribute to distortion and bizarreness by loosening and disrupting associative connections. Thus, phasic activity per se does not appear to be an indicator of the presence of dreaming, although it is clearly implicated in the overall dream process. This refinement contributed by the Rechtschaffen group makes it possible to understand how activity that seems so characteristic of REM periods and, by implication, so important to dreaming does not predict NREM dream recall.

Finally, there is a very interesting report by Pessah and Roffwarg[235] describing middle ear muscle activity during sleep in human subjects. This activity parallels the occurrence of other phasic events, notably rapid eye movements, but represents a refreshing departure from the visual system that has been so intensively studied. In the cat,[260] there is an almost one-to-one correlation between PGO spikes and phasic discharge in the tensor tympani. This is true in both REM and NREM sleep. However, it is clear from studies of the cat, particularly those of Dewson et al.,[81] that a similar dichotomy probably exists for middle ear muscle activity, i.e., very brief phasic discharges versus somewhat longer (several seconds) contractions. The tonic contractions were not necessarily related to rapid eye movements[81] or PGO spikes.[260] In human subjects, the recording technique utilizing acoustic impedance and AC amplifiers does not lend itself to this type of differentiation.

The most fascinating aspect of this work is perhaps the data suggesting a relationship to dream imagery in the auditory sphere (Roffwarg, personal communication).

Conclusions

Obviously, the neural processes that give rise to sights, sounds, feelings, and thoughts during sleep are very complex. It would seem that this complexity is infinitely beyond the information carrying capacities of PGO spikes. Even the recognition of additional activities beyond the punctate PGO waves or PIPs (i.e., Rechtschaffen's periorbital tonic discharge) falls far short of the presumed complexity. However, it is quite possible that there is a single indicator that "turns on," independent of REM or NREM sleep, when dreaming is present, and that it has little to do with specific hallucinatory percepts. Accepting the Rechtschaffen group's results at face value, the indicator does not appear to be phasic events that are analogous to PGO spikes. A better candidate would appear to be the tonic periorbital potentials. However, at the present time, these EMG discharges lack specificity in terms of attempting to identify some underlying unique neural events. It seems clear that "events of intermediate duration" and phasic events are more likely to coexist in REM periods. In NREM periods, it is obvious that the dream process can occur (tonic potentials) without concurrent phasic activity. In this instance, the associated experiences are presumably coherent and rational or at least more so than we are accustomed to expecting in typical dreams. It may even be that the sleeping subject does not label the experiences as dreams. If the "intermediate" tonic potentials are absent in NREM sleep, suggesting the absence of dreaming, phasic activity may do nothing unless it actually arouses the individual. If ongoing hallucinatory activity is present, the phasic discharge derails it, disrupts it, etc., and thus may contribute those qualities which we find most characteristic of the average dream. This whole formulation is based on minimal evidence, but, as will be seen, it accounts for certain behavioral correlates of PGO spike discharge in wakefulness better than any yet proposed.

Psychophysiology of Dream Content— the "Scanning" Hypothesis

In addition to indicators of the presence or absence of dreaming that will satisfactorily account for the relative incidences of dream recall in REM and NREM sleep, there is a concern about indicators which will "predict" specific content. For example, if there was a high heart rate in a REM period one might expect to elicit a frightening or exciting or nightmarish dream upon awakening the subject.

Most of the work in this specific area has focused around one controversial, empirical finding, namely, that a direct relationship exists between the rapid eye movements and hallucinated visual images of REM dreams. The correlation of specific items of content or emotion with other peripheral measures has been suggested but not extensively investigated. Much of the latter work is reviewed in a paper by Roffwarg[259] in which he also discusses and dispenses with a number of issues he feels are "irrelevant" to the eye movement dream relationship in human adults such as occurrence of rapid eye movements in newborn infants, decorticate humans and animals, the nonspecificity of certain neural events during REM periods, etc.

The basic procedure in investigations on eye movement mentation relationships involves arousing subjects during REM periods with the arousal specifically related to a temporal sequence of rapid eye movements measured with horizontal and vertical eye leads. This electro–oculogram (EOG) gives a precise record of the temporal sequence of eye movements leading up to the arousal. An interrogator, who awakens the subject, asks questions about the dream experience and from the dreamer's answers attempts to predict the sequence of eye movements leading up to the awakening. Actually, a detailed prediction is impossible unless the implied eye movement sequence is very characteristic. Thus, if the dream imagery is all in the vertical plane, the interrogator might predict eye movements only on the vertical plane and this could be ascertained from the EOG. On the other hand, the kind of activity that is associated with a few seconds of frantic looking around in all directions is impossible to dissect and describe with any accuracy at all simply because of its intensity and complexity.

Alternative procedures involve (a) attempting to match a limited number of EOG tracings with their associated dream narratives, say five of each, and (b) limiting the prediction to the final eye movement that immediately precedes the awakening.

In the early phase of correlating eye movement patterns and dream content, there were several reports that supported such a relationship,* culminating in the very positive report of Roffwarg and his colleagues.[262]

A number of years passed before the relationship was specifically tested by other investigators. Moskowitz and Berger,[226] utilizing a matching procedure, found that their results were not significantly better than chance. Jacobs and his colleagues,[144,145] using DC EOG techniques, also found no relationship. Finally, Krippner et al.[191] added negative data from a single subject. Thus, the original optimistic and potentially biased reports were not confirmed.

The most recent study by Bussel et al.[36] adopted a number of control procedures that helped to clarify the issues. It is clear that the sheer difficulty of obtaining dream recall of sufficient detail and accuracy so as to permit a correct prediction is a major source of error. Any forgetting or inaccurate reporting will make a correct prediction impossible. Bussel et al. conclusively exposed this error source by carrying out their study using EOGs and recall from wakefulness as well as REM sleep. They showed that the ability of an interrogator to predict the direction of the last eye movement based on recall of visual imagery and gaze fixation from REM arousals was minimally accurate, but significantly better than

* See references 18, 19, 74, 78, and 239.

chance, given a large number of data points. *Further, the level of accuracy and significance was exactly the same in the waking trials!* Thus, it is clear that any study that purports to test this relationship with all its inherent difficulties must be based on a large amount of data. It is our opinion that there will be continued attempts to work on this problem in the years to come, and that the evidence favoring a relationship will begin to mount.

In spite of the relatively few studies, the possibility of a relationship is more than a laboratory curiosity. It is an important issue on two counts. In the first place, the establishment of such a relationship would allow judgment as to whether the dream actually occurred as sensed by the dreamer. Although dreaming is widely reported, the certainty of its occurrence is in doubt. Even the correlation between eye movements and the dream report would not be absolute proof, but the principle of parsimony would allow no other conclusion if we awaken a sleeping subject and he claimed that he was watching a ball thrown up and down, and, prior to the arousal, we had recorded up–and–down eye movement deflections. Secondly, a lack of correlation between neurophysiologically determined events such as eye movements and the dream experience would seriously undermine the axiom that events in the mind have physical and potentially measurable counterparts in the brain soma.

❲ Dreams

The basic unity underlying much of what is described under this heading is the use of polygraphic monitoring of sleep to define sleep states and the utilization of this information for anatomical, physiological, pharmacological, biochemical, and, in particular, psychological correlation. In general, research in this field is called sleep *and* dream research. Thus, it seems worthwhile to discuss dreams briefly and to ask what has been learned about dreaming as a result of laboratory sleep research.

In the twenty-plus years since the discovery of REM sleep, a number of quantitative aspects of the occurrence of dreaming have been clarified. Certainly there is much more dreaming per se than pre–REM investigators thought. We now know something about the time course of the dream; and we have much more data on the content and characteristics of typical dreams and dreams in a variety of personality types and pathological subjects; and we know something of the effects of pre-sleep and ongoing stimuli on these variables. However, much of this work was conducted in the late 1950s and early 1960s. After that it would seem that the dream subsection of modern sleep and dream research "attained a plateau from which it seems steadily more difficult to reach higher ground." This opinion, which is in some ways as shattering to the smugness of current sleep research as the statement that "the emperor has no clothes," was made by Foulkes in a remarkable position paper[102] delivered at the 1973 meeting of the Association for the Psychophysiological Study of Sleep (APSS). As Rechtschaffen cautioned a number of years ago, "if we do not keep our attention on the psychology of the dream, we might find out a lot of the biology without knowing very well what it is the biology of."[248]

Foulkes addressed himself to such questions as "what do dreams mean?" and "why do we dream what we do?" and "why are dreams the way they are?" and so on. And he concludes that almost no progress has been made since Freud's monumental efforts to answer these questions. In his book, *The Interpretation of Dreams*,[106] Freud propounded both a theory of dream formation and a method of dream interpretation. It was Foulkes's thesis, unchallenged by any of his discussants[102] that either the modern techniques of sleep research have not enabled investigators to confirm or refute Freud's theories or that ingenious investigators have not pursued these questions with tenacious vigor. The situation appears to be one in which those who use the technique of dream interpretation remain unconcerned with its ultimate validity and continue to confuse meaning and causality while those who carry the banner of science and research cannot or will not devise direct experimental tests of psychoanalytic theories about dreaming.

With the exception of certain investigators who have utilized content analysis with outstandingly productive results,* money, talent, and dedication are relatively absent in the areas outlined by Foulkes.

Although, the content findings can be quite interesting—e.g., women dream more often of strangers than do men and so on—again, the important questions about dreaming are not addressed. That is, there must be a set of rules for determining dream content that can be "discovered."

It seems possible that a carefully systematic study of the effects of external stimuli on dream content might reveal some of the rules by which one set of psychic percepts are transformed into another set of dream percepts. In a recent study by Augustyn et al.,[7] characteristic auditory stimuli were presented during REM sleep. It is of interest that the transformations and incorporations of these stimuli into dream content were about half visual and half auditory. Why did the sound of a locomotive whistle produce the image of a train in some dreams and only the sound of a train in others? It is not unthinkable that there is some reason for these differences, some explanation to be found.

Moreover, to what extent will physiological state, e.g., hunger, thirst, stress, determine dream content? This aspect has been studied with equivocal results,† but the studies have been only preliminary and far from systematic.

Finally, innumerable studies of REM sleep deprivation have demonstrated a so-called physiological need for REM sleep (i.e., REM rebound), and investigators, assuming the identity of REM sleep and dreaming, have postulated a similar need for dreaming.[37,38,39] But little attention has been directed to simply the psychological need or excuse for dreaming. What, if anything, do dreams do for us in and of themselves, regardless of their physiological correlates? This question and those

asked by Foulkes[102] are the kinds of problems that should generate more investigation in the future.

It seems obvious that much future work is needed to establish and clarify the role of the psychological side of dreams and the psychic economy of the organism.[59] The dream must regain its status as a psychological event, while at the same time retaining its position as a neurophysiological process.

([Selective REM Sleep Deprivation and Schizophrenia

As was noted earlier, an almost inevitable consequence of selective REM sleep deprivation is a usually substantial REM sleep increase, above baseline levels in the immediate post-deprivation (recovery) period. In the non-drug technique, which utilizes continual instrumental interruptions of REM periods at their beginning, the size or degree of the rebound is a function of the duration of the deprivation period. Thus, for extended periods of deprivation in healthy animals, the REM rebound certainly seems to be an inevitable response. By interrupting REM periods, some sort of biochemical-metabolic-physiologic process is set into motion that drastically alters the REM–NREM ratio in favor of REM sleep.

We do not recall any instance in a normal cat or rat[71,83,222] where a REM rebound failed to appear after two or more days of REM sleep deprivation. In addition, substantial REM rebounds appear after certain drugs that suppress REM sleep are withdrawn such as amphetamines, monoamine–oxidase inhibitors, and barbiturates. Certain exceptions have been noted. If REM sleep is substantially reduced in the cat by diphenylhydantoin[47] or by electroconvulsive shock,[45] no rebound appears. Finally, on certain occasions, the development of a febrile illness has been observed to interfere with an expected REMS rebound.

It must be emphasized, however, that the rebound is never a linear function. Dement et al.[68] have summarized their extensive REM

---

* See references 125, 189, 197, 285, and 286.
    † See references 10, 26, 28, 78, 230, 238, 296, and 73.

deprivation studies in animals and have reported that there appears to be a limit to the size of this rebound in two ways: the REM percentage in their studies was rarely above 70 percent even during a lengthy, *ad libitum* sleep period; and in cats, at least, after twenty-five to thirty consecutive days of deprivation, no further increases in recovery function could be detected. Such lengthy periods of REM sleep deprivation have not been done with humans, but in several cases,[61,63,165] subjects were REM sleep deprived as completely as possible for ten to fifteen consecutive nights and monitored during the day to rule out napping. In these subjects there were spectacular shifts in the structure of sleep to allow for a great increase in total REM sleep time and REM sleep percentage.

There is, however, some problem when relatively brief durations of selective REM sleep deprivation are carried out in human subjects —"normal human volunteers." In the first study of REM deprivation,[58] there was a questionable response in one subject, who was REM deprived for four nights, although he was not monitored during the day. The size of the rebound varies considerably in human subjects, but a number of nonspecific factors usually play a role. For example, there is the structure of human sleep with widely spaced REM periods such that if the morning awakening occurs a little prematurely or after a long NREM period, the REM percent is artifactually reduced. In addition, humans generally experience a certain amount of NREM sleep reduction that tends to interfere with the expression of REM sleep. It was felt by Dement[63] that these problems would have little effect when REM sleep deprivation periods were extended beyond the usual two to five nights and the evidence to date, which is minimal to be sure, suggests that this is true. However, such lengthy durations are difficult to accomplish in psychiatrically disturbed subjects and, therefore, data in these subjects must be compared to data in normal humans who have undergone short durations of REM sleep deprivation. It is in this area that some question arises, i.e., will all "normal" humans show a rebound in REM sleep following deprivation, or are there some apparently normal individuals who lack this attribute or capacity? Cartwright et al.[40] feel that a group of "noncompensators" exists with distinguishable personality traits on the basis of failing to rebound after three nights of deprivation. In addition to those mentioned above, possible artifactual causes of rebound failure are sleeping during the day, improper deprivation procedure, covert drug ingestion (for example, neo–synephrine nose drops), and failure to carry out recovery monitoring long enough. With regard to the latter, there is clear evidence that a rebound can be delayed.[69] As a test of the ultimate validity, one of the Cartwright noncompensators was REM deprived a second time by the Stanford group[303] with twenty-four-hour monitoring and prolonged recovery studies. The rebound failure was confirmed, but the patient was apparently an ambulatory schizophrenic.

All during the decade when speculation was rife that REM sleep deprivation might play a role in the pathogenesis of the psychotic state, there was a feeling that the REM deprivation technique ought to be applied to schizophrenic patients as a crucial test of this notion, the expectation being that such a procedure would drastically worsen their condition. It was indeed this expectation, not to mention the substantial complexities of such an experiment, that probably caused many investigators to hesitate. Nonetheless, the first reports by Azumi et al.[9] and Zarcone et al.[305] of REM sleep deprivation in schizophrenics appeared in 1967. The former group selectively REM deprived three "chronic schizophrenics" for five consecutive nights. Two of the three patients did not experience a rebound. The latter group has carried out extensive studies of this phenomenon.[304,306,307] In their overall program, they selectively REM deprived actively ill schizophrenics, remitted schizophrenics, and nonschizophrenics for two nights; and in one actively ill patient, REM deprivation was carried on for eight nights with the aid of nighttime amphetamines. This group attempted to reduce some of the confounding variables by keeping phenothiazine medications absolutely constant throughout the period of study and by carefully delineating the clinical state of the patient population. The observations focused on two groups of chronic schizophrenics with evidence of deterioration in occupational and social functioning. The patients in one group were experiencing active symptomotology, hallucinations, thought disorders, bizarre motor activity, and affective abnormalities. The continuing symptomotology was accepted by these patients and seemed to explain their situation and seemed, in a way, to communicate their anxiety. The second group of schizophrenics was as clinically differentiated from the first as possible, consisting essentially of patients with no active symptomatology whatsoever. All patients were subjected to two consecutive nights of selective REM sleep deprivation with prior baseline and subsequent recovery recordings. A major consideration in these studies was the fact that one patient was actually in both groups as a result of clinical change, and thereby served as his own control. The latter particularly applies to the possibility of a coincidence between some genetic failure in the mechanism subserving the REM rebound and the schizophrenic state. Nine patients were studied in the activity ill group, and eight failed to show a postdeprivation rise in total REM sleep time (REM rebound). The ninth showed a small rebound that was not nearly as great as that seen during remission. Over an entire five–night recovery period, they averaged only 5 percent makeup of the REM time lost on the two deprivation nights. One patient, a hebephrenic who constantly hallucinated, was REM deprived for an extended period of eight consecutive nights and he also failed to show the usual compensatory REM rebound. On the other hand, the patients in remission, including the one who had been studied while actively ill, all showed substantial rebounds averaging over 200 percent makeup following deprivation. Normal controls and nonschizophrenic control patients, while showing considerable variability, averaged a 50 to 60 percent REM sleep makeup.

The studies of the acutely ill patients appeared to be in marked contrast to the report of Vogel and Traub[288] and to the study of De Barros.[12] The former investigators carried out the REM deprivation procedure with five chronic schizophrenics for seven nights by awakenings and by administration of nighttime phenobarbital and amphetamines. Four of these patients were taking phenothiazines and all patients had an increase in REM sleep above baseline levels in the postdeprivation recovery period. De Barros carried out the REM deprivation for three nights each in six chronic schizophrenics and reported that all six experienced a "REM rebound."

The whole question of REM rebound in acute schizophrenic subjects was further investigated by Gillin and Wyatt.[114] These investigators have concluded that actively ill schizophrenic patients do indeed fail to have a normal REM rebound following deprivation of REM sleep. They did not study patients in remission. Their studies were exceedingly careful and represent very strong support.

Without making interpretive comments on this phenomena, we believe the failure of REM rebound is a valid concomitant of schizophrenia in at least the acute phase, and, because of this, it is in some way related to the active psychotic process. If the relation to the clinical state, i.e., normal or excessive rebound when the psychotic process was in abeyance, was confirmed it could be a very meaningful correlate. Certainly, in view of the difficulty of achieving some satisfactory pathogenic explanation of schizophrenia, this phenomenon warrants further investigation. Gillin and Wyatt present an extensive discussion of their findings in this area and in other areas relating to a general theory, which will be discussed in the succeeding section.

One of the early interpretations made by Zarcone et al. to account for the rebound failure was based on a somewhat metaphorical notion of a phasic activity quota either being discharged in REM sleep or building up. It was speculated that phasic activity was being discharged in the waking state in the "actively ill" patients and therefore nothing "built up" to instigate the REM rebound. The process view of sleep says nothing about any kind of quota. However, if it is the reduction in phasic activity that is implicated in the REM deprivation recovery phenomenon, certainly the phasic activity could be discharged at other times. One of the ways of accounting for the limit to the REM deprivation effect is that eventually as much phasic activity is occurring in NREM sleep as originally occurred in REM periods. There is obviously a strong resistance to such a disassociation. Otherwise, there could be no REM deprivation effect since phasic activity would immediately shift to NREM sleep.

◖ Phasic Events and a Theory of Psychosis

It is not easy to generate enthusiasm or even interest about a theory of psychosis in these days that have seen so many prior proposals. One of the most recent is a hypothesis put forth by Stein[276] that involves the endogenous production of 6-hydroxydopamine in schizophrenics. Behavioral effects in humans have obviously not been studied, but Stein feels that certain behavioral effects in rats are analogous to pathological processes in schizophrenics.

The theory that will be discussed in this section has one unique aspect. It is based on the notion expressed by many theorists that dreams represent nonpathological psychotic activities. Such activities are nonpathological because all of us dream and because what we do in our dreams is safely sequestered in the minds of our paralyzed bodies. This view further holds that the mechanisms underlying the dream state and the dream experience must also be involved in the psychotic activities considered by most to be pathological. The notion that dreams and psychoses are related has had many proponents. For example, we have the statement, "We ourselves, in fact, can experience in dreams almost all the phenomena to be met with in insane asylums", which is attributed to Wilhelm Wundt. Hughlings Jackson said, "Find out about dreams and you will find out about insanity."[140] The pursuance of this general notion is based upon an abiding faith that somehow the psychotic state and REM sleep–dream processes are related.

The various theoretical convolutions and ramifications of this notion have been considered at length in at least two papers,[70,79] and we will remain concerned here as much as possible only with the empirical facts.

The basic tenet of this theory or hypothesis is that psychosis represents some aspect of the dream process intruding into the waking state. Such an intrusion would not have to be the experience of full–blown hallucinatory dream images in wakefulness, although it could at times. We already know that the dream process, insofar as it is related to sleep mechanisms, is complex and involves at least several independent systems. Thus, the disorganization of the psychotic state could be produced by the intrusion of only one of those systems.

The PGO spike was actually discovered by Jouvet and his colleagues,[149] who were the first to undertake brain–stem recordings during REM sleep in the cat. The Lyon investigators were also the first to show that the PGO waves could be entirely dissociated from normal REM periods. Matsumoto and Jouvet[206] found that REM periods in the cat were abolished by high doses of reserpine, but that PGO spikes were continuously discharged throughout the interval of REM suppression. Although the reserpinized state was clearly not wakefulness, it was clearly not REM sleep. A more impressive demonstration, however, came from this group when Delorme et al.[56] showed that administration of the serotonin depletor, parachlorophenylalanine, was followed by a release of PGO spikes in what was both behaviorally and polygraphically an apparently normal waking state. Similar findings for reserpine have been reported by Brooks[30, 33,34] and by Monachon et al.[218] The observations of the Stanford group on PCPA administration were focused on a detailed account of the behavioral correlates of waking PGO spikes and a careful description of the changes in sleep states and PGO spike distribution as the treatment progressed.* Both of

* See references 49, 50, 76, 79, 89, 91, 92, 215, 308, and 88.

these areas gave information that could be effectively related to observations in human subjects and patients.

Repeated direct simultaneous scrutiny of both behavior and subcortical EEG has made it absolutely clear that the occurrence of a PGO spike during wakefulness in the PCPA treated animal, or, better yet a burst of spikes, is associated with a behavioral response in the complete absence of any external sensory event. There is some remaining controversy about whether or not these behavioral responses in the cat could be said to resemble full–blown hallucinatory experiences. Probably not. They appear to be more appropriately described as intrusions and disruptions of the ongoing perceptual–behavioral stream. The affected cat does appear, when left to his own devices, almost continually preoccupied with these internal disturbances; and in this regard, he is uncannily reminiscent of the preoccupied psychotic. Occasionally, there is a

brief, wild, agitation that seems to correlate with a very intense burst of spike activity, but, on the whole, the behavior of the cat is much more of an orienting, searching, distracted, repeatedly disrupted kind of behavior. Often, it is as if someone was pounding or knocking on the wall of the cage, and the cat was searching for the source of the disturbance. Other behavioral disturbances have been reported in PCPA treated animals,[86,278,279] but are still somewhat controversial. The key principle is that the cat's behavior during PCPA administration is no longer totally determined by the events in the real world, and it is no longer a series of completely "rational" responses to events in the real world. Something continually intrudes and that something appears to be the phasic event of REM sleep.

The sleep changes associated with chronic PCPA treatment in the cat are also worth noting. There is a transient insomnia that usually develops on the third day of PCPA treatment

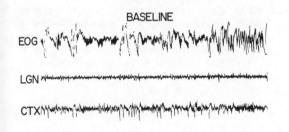
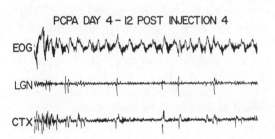

Figure 8–8.   Emergence of REM–type PGO waves into wakefulness following four days of PCPA treatment.

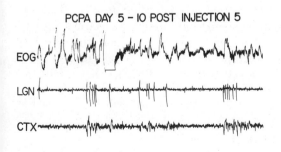
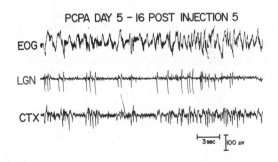

Figure 8–9.   The development of more dense waking PGO activity late in chronic PCPA treatment.

and lasts three or four days. Then, there is a return of considerable amounts of both REM and NREM sleep. A major difference between normal sleep and PCPA sleep is that the number of PGO spikes during PCPA–REM periods is greatly reduced while the overall number during NREM periods is greatly increased. The major overall effect appears to be a kind of dissemination or complete lack of regulation of the spike activity so that it is discharged with approximately equal intensity in all behavioral states. This intensity is somewhat lower than in the normal cat where most of the PGO spike activity is concentrated in REM periods.

A final pertinent observation in these PCPA treated animals involves REM sleep deprivation. All changes can be quickly reversed by administration of 5-hydroxytryptophan (5-HTP). In the chronically PCPA treated cat, REM sleep deprivation does not appear to elicit a rebound. This is illustrated in Figure 8–10. On the other hand, if REM deprivation is carried out in the cat, and PCPA is given only during the recovery period, the REM rebound is greatly enhanced until the full–blown PCPA effect is evident. The parallel of this rebound failure in the PCPA cat and the diminished or absent response to selective REM deprivation in acute schizophrenics discussed in the last section is obvious.

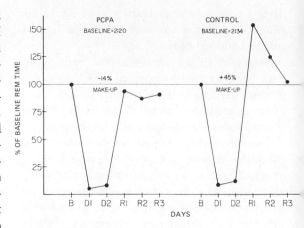

Figure 8–10. Rebound failure in a cat chronically treated with p–chlorophenylalanine (PCPA). The daily REM time values in this cat during the two deprivation periods are expressed in percent of the baseline REM sleep time. Since there is usually a small reduction in the daily REM time after an animal has been stabilized on PCPA, 100 percent of baseline actually represents a different value in the PCPA condition versus the control condition. These values are indicated on the graph in hours and minutes. As can be seen, although this cat was averaging two hours, twenty minutes of REM sleep per day on a twelve-to-twelve schedule (twelve hours on treadmill—twelve hours in recording cage) in the PCPA condition, two days of deprivation resulted in no makeup at all. The REM rebound following the similar period of deprivation prior to the administration of PCPA was of normal size.

Neurochemical Regulation and Basis of the PGO Spike

There seems to be broad agreement that serotonergic neurons are involved in the regulation of phasic activity. This regulation appears to be inhibitory. Certainly, a primary effect of the inhibition of serotonin synthesis is the correlated reduction of serotonin in all brain areas and the emergence of waking PGO spikes. Lesions in the raphe nuclei that destroy substantial numbers of serotonergic neurons lead to exactly the same dual effect.[151] In the case of PCPA, the effects are reversed by small amounts of 5–HTP; in the case of lesions, they are not.

Further aspects of the neurophysiology of PGO regulation were described by McGinty

and Harper* who measured firing in raphe units in relation to PGO waves. These units continued to fire at all times in wakefulness and NREM sleep. They became quiescent when NRE–MPGO waves appeared and remained so throughout the following REM sleep period. Unpublished results by Jacobs and Dement† indicated that electrical stimulation of the raphe nuclei had the effect of blocking PGO waves in normal cats.

Jouvet and his colleagues have felt that

* A discussion of these findings can be found in: McGinty, D., Harper, R., and Fairbanks, M., "Neuronal unit activity and the control of sleep states," *Adv. Sleep Res.* 1, (1974), 173–216.

† These data are now published: Jacobs, B., Asher, R., and Dement, W. "Electophysiological and behavioral effects of electrical stimulation of the raphe nuclei in cats," *Physiol. Behav.* 11, (1973), 243–252.

PGO waves are catecholaminergic.[150,151] Their major evidence is that lesions in and around clusters of catecholaminergic cell bodies tend to be followed by a reduction or disappearance of PGO waves. In addition, alphamethyl–Dopa, which is metabolized to the false transmitter alphamethylnoradrenaline, rapidly and effectively suppresses PGO spike activity.

The most damaging evidence against this notion are the several studies[187] with alphamethylparatyrosine (AMPT) which selectively inhibits the tyroside hydroxylase and leads to a depletion of noradrenaline and dopamine. This compound is nephrotoxic, however. In an effort to overcome this nephrotoxic effect, Henriksen and Dement administered AMPT to cats by intravenous drip in a dosage calculated to be supramaximal and saw that there was a modest increase in the amount of slow wave sleep and, more importantly, an increase in the amount of REM sleep. Thus, it is very difficult to attribute the PGO discharge to catecholaminergic neurons. Furthermore, Haefely and his colleagues[120] have elaborated an hypothesis that catecholamines are actually involved in the inhibition of PGO spike activity.

The Stanford group has pointed out that REM sleep is acutely susceptible to disruption by pharmacologic intervention in the normal animal. Thus, it is difficult to study the neurochemical basis of any single component. If a drug treatment blocked tonic muscle inhibition, produced nausea or discomfort, or raised the arousal level, it would probably block the occurrence of REM sleep, and therefore, secondarily, it would also block the appearance of PGO waves. Given the opportunity of producing a dissociation of PGO waves from REM sleep by PCPA treatment, this phasic activity can then be studied without concern about other REM components. Thus, Jacobs et al.[141] have studied waking PGO waves following PCPA treatment after administering the following presumptive receptor blockers: pimozide, a dopamine receptor blocker; phentolamine and phenoxybenzamine, alpha–adrenergic blockers; propranolol, a beta–adrenergic blocker; and atropine, a cholinergic blocker. The results were dramatically un-

equivocal. None of the four catecholamine receptor blockers had a significant effect on the PGO wave discharge. On the other hand, atropine, in very low doses in chronic PCPA cats totally blocked the occurrence of PGO waves and the effect could be partially reversed by eserine. Henriksen et al. administered atropine to REM deprived normal cats and found that bursts of PGO waves were blocked while REM periods per se and muscular twitching were not.

Interest in a postulated relationship between PGO waves and hallucinations stimulated electrographic observations on cats treated with hallucinogenic drugs. It might be expected that the administration of hallucinogenic compounds would be accompanied by a discharge of PGO waves in wakefulness, particularly if hallucinatory behavior ensued. This does not appear to be the case. Henriksen et al.[131] have administered hallucinogenic doses of LSD and, following the lead of Jones,[148] have also given tropolone, a catechol–o–methyl transferase inhibitor, to cats. Full–blown hallucinatory behavior was easily produced, but in no case was this behavior accompanied by clear–cut discharge of typical PGO spikes. These data may not support the alleged role of PGO spikes in hallucinatory conditions, but neither do they completely disallow it. In the Jones preparation, PGO spikes were not precisely coincident with hallucinatory behavior, but they did appear in wakefulness immediately after the abnormal behavior had subsided.

Parallel Studies in Humans

PCPA has been given to human subjects by Wyatt et al.[299] These authors felt that it did not produce the appearance of severe behavioral abnormalities or hallucinations. Boelkins[25] carefully observed the behavior of three monkeys given PCPA in a quasi–natural environment. He did not report hallucinations or maniacal behavior. On the other hand, he did observe certain inappropriate responses as well as substantial depression.

It is well–known that phenothiazines have

an ameliorative effect in psychotic, nonde-pressed humans. Cohen et al.[46] have recently reported that chlorpromazine administered to the PCPA cat at the height of the PCPA effect with insomnia and waking spikes will imme-diately reinstitute sleep and suppress PGO spikes.

A consistent effect of PCPA in the cat is a change in the REM–NREM ratio of PGO spike intensity. In other words, the intensity goes down in REM sleep and up in NREM sleep as compared to baseline. Wyatt et al.[300] have examined this ratio in human subjects receiving PCPA using PIP discharge as the in-dicator of phasic activity. They found a com-parable change in the REM–NREM–PIP ratio.

If one assumes that some part of the psy-chotic process is due to faulty regulation of phasic events, this is tantamount to assuming that a serotonin defect exists. This suggests that a test of the overall hypothesis would be treatment of psychotic humans with a com-pound that might offset this defect. In just such a trial, Wyatt has shown modest im-provement in schizophrenic patients given 5-hydroxytryptophane.[298,301]

Finally, a very exciting preliminary report has appeared by Watson et al.[290] to the effect that the periorbital phasic integrated poten-tials (PIPs) show a definite relationship to the psychotic process in acute schizophrenics. During the initial and most severe phase of the psychosis in two acute schizophrenic pa-tients, PIP activity in NREM sleep was greatly increased while activity in REM sleep was somewhat decreased.

A puzzling but consistent finding in chroni-cally treated PCPA cats, who show substantial amounts of REM sleep in twenty-four-hour continuous polygraphic monitoring, is that se-lective deprivation of this REM sleep does not induce the typical REM rebound.[66,79] Such deprivation was accomplished by interrupting each REM period by hand awakenings just as EMG suppression begins. In the preceding section, we have discussed similar failures to find rebound after REM sleep deprivation in acute schizophrenics. The parallel is obvious.

Interpretive Remarks

As we have said earlier, the basic tenet of the theory under consideration is that psycho-sis represents some aspect of the dream pro-cess intruding into the waking state. We have speculated elsewhere that what intrudes is phasic activity, or whatever is analogous in humans to the feline PGO spike. If this is as-sumed, then we may postulate some defect in serotonin metabolism or function, assuming further that serotonin has the same phasic event regulatory function in humans that it appears to have in cats. The animal model or analogue of this hypothesis is the chronically treated PCPA cat. When we look at schizo-phrenics for parallels to the findings in the PCPA cat, we find a sufficient number to keep the hypothesis viable.

There are two sources of confusion, how-ever, that should be considered. The first has to do with overly simple notions about the consequences of dream processes intruding into wakefulness; the second has to do with overly simple notions about the neurophysiol-ogy of these dream processes. With regard to the former, we have repeatedly emphasized that overt behavioral manifestations of sero-tonin depletion and PGO spike release, though definitely present, are minimal. It is clear that a PGO spike does not make a cat "see" a non-existent mouse. Rather, if anything, the cat is relatively calm but preoccupied, internally dis-tracted from a smooth interaction with the environment. A misunderstanding of these findings and the consequent erroneous ex-pectations may have beclouded observations of humans and monkeys receiving PCPA treat-ment. Investigators might have seen changes in behavior had they been looking for less dramatic manifestations than full–blown maniacal hallucinations. In addition to the possibility that it is only part of the dream process rather than the whole dream that in-trudes, there is also a complication having to do with the possible consequences of com-bining, or attempting to combine, waking and dreaming functions. We know that PGO spike generation in the brain stem gives rise to responses in the lateral geniculate nucleus[21] during REM sleep. Of course, during sleep there is a great reduction in retinal input. There is no data to tell us what happens when retinal and brain–stem inputs "collide" at the lateral geniculate receptors.

With regard to the second source of confusion, there is a tendency to regard the PGO spike as the sine qua non of dreaming and hallucinations. We can already introduce two qualifications. The first is drawn from the Rechtschaffen experiments described in the section on "Phasic Activity and the Psychophysiology of Dreaming." If one assumes that the PIP is the human analogue of the PGO spike, it is reasonably clear that PGO spikes are not the generators of dream and hallucinatory imagery. Another process or other processes seem to be more crucial. The only clue to the latter is the "tonic periorbital EMG discharge." The problem with this indicator is that it is essentially nonspecific. Tonic upsurges in periorbital EMG can be individualized in sleep, but not in wakefulness where EMG levels are normally quite high. This leaves the PGO spike or phasic activity process with only a disruptive role. The question we cannot answer at the present time with any assurance is whether both of these processes or just phasic activity are released into the waking state by serotonin depletion. The behavior of the PCPA cat would suggest that it is just phasic activity. Even so, we can assume that such intrusive jolts to the entire brain would, by themselves, have very serious consequences for the human stream of consciousness. A second qualification has to do with the significance of the actual PGO wave as an electrical, potential change. In this regard, it is merely a response—an electrical sign of underlying cellular events. Referring back to Figure 8–5, we can conceive of a "generator" that initiates all phasic activity from muscular twitches to bursts of unit discharge in the hippocampus. In certain areas of the brain for purely structural reasons, relatively synchronous bursts of discharge in a pool of units give rise to a PGO spike. The

point is that if we do not see PGO spikes, it does not prove the absence of phasic activity. Such a point receives experimental support from the work of Henriksen et al.[130] who gave atropine to cats deprived of REM sleep for five consecutive days. They found that periods of atonia with concurrent prolonged EMG suppression continued to appear, although atropine blocked cortical desynchronization. During these atonic periods, there were typical phasic events such as muscular twitches, rapid eye movements, and even single PGO waves. However, atropine blocked the bursts of PGO waves characteristically associated with eye movement bursts in normal cats. Thus, in this instance, it was demonstrated that phasic activity can occur in the absence of its electrical sign (PGO spike). Given this possibility, we may reconsider the work with hallucinogenic preparations in the cat[131,148] wherein it was noted that induced hallucinatory behavior was not accompanied by PGO spike discharge. We may make two interpretations: (a) that the PCPA–induced behavioral abnormalities, associated with PGO spikes in the waking state, are fundamentally different neurophysiologically from whatever events give rise to the behavior in cats treated with tropolone plus L–DOPA and other known hallucinogens; or (b) phasic activity was indeed released by these compounds, although PGO waves per se were not. Parenthetically, there is plentiful evidence that these hallucinogenic pharmacological manipulations do effect serotonin metabolism.

❨ Conclusions

We have tried to summarize and explicate findings that implicate sleep mechanism in the pathogenesis of psychotic behavior. At least one basic biochemical defect is postulated that is in the serotonin system. Evidence for the serotonin hypothesis independent of sleep is summarized by Gillin and Wyatt.[114] The sleep studies essentially deal with the mediating mechanisms and attempt to explain why a serotonin defect might produce the puzzling manifestations of a schizophrenic psychosis rather than something else. Thus, whatever else it might do in the CNS, serotonin is assumed to regulate the phasic activity of REM sleep and prevent its release in the waking state. A breakdown in this function is postulated to result in phasic discharge in wakefulness and NREM sleep. This, in turn, produces behavioral abnormality, increased manifestations of NREM disturbance, and, somehow, a failure to produce the usual response to selective deprivation of REM sleep.

⟮ Biochemistry and Cellular Neurophysiology

It is clearly beyond the scope of this chapter to review the voluminous cellular neurophysiological and biochemical literature that deals with sleep. Furthermore, these two disciplines utilize technical refinements that are sometimes difficult for outsiders to readily comprehend. Nonetheless, they represent the points at which understanding of brain mechanisms has been pushed the farthest and is most replicable and precise. To the extent that sleep mechanisms are biochemical and neurophysiological, it is therefore appropriate to indicate some current trends and well–established findings in these areas. Our additional purpose is to highlight several of the developments that seem most relevant to psychiatry. We have, in previous sections, alluded to some of the most crucial biochemical and neurophysiological issues in sleep research, but the interested reader should consult one or more of the following reviews[150,151,186] as well as the BIS summary, *Neuronal Activity in Sleep* by Hobson and McCarley.[135]

Suspicions that something "wet" or biochemical as opposed to "dry" or electrophysiological[266] was involved in sleep certainly dates at least as far back as Pieron's[239] search for some blood–born hypnotoxin.

It is now generally accepted that neural circuits control wakefulness, NREM, and REM sleep, and also that electrophysiological studies of such circuits have not yet yielded the best explanation of control processes. However, this may soon change since many exciting findings are now coming from single unit work. To date, though, most progress has come from studying the neurochemistry of the monoamines and sleep. This is true partly because much is known about the biosynthesis of these compounds and because better techniques of localization and estimating turnover are available.

In terms of putative neural transmitters, acetylcholine has certainly received a great deal of early research attention (see[132]). However, it is probable that work with this tertiary amine did not receive the recognition it should have vis–à–vis monoamines because anatomical localization with histofluorescent techniques is currently possible only for serotonin and the catecholamines.

Modern biochemistry of sleep may be said to have begun with Jouvet's observations on the reserpinized cat.[150,151] Jouvet found that depletion of monoamines led to the disappearance of the states of sleep. He found that this effect was reversed by both 5–hydroxtryptphan, a precursor of serotonin, and by L–DOPA, the precursor of dopamine and noradrenalin. Jouvet suspected that serotonin had something to do with NREM sleep and catecholamines with REM sleep. At that time Swedish investigators were developing histofluorescent techniques that led to the localization of serotonergic and catecholaminergic cells and their projections. It was then that Jouvet developed the serotonin hypothesis of NREM sleep on the basis of raphe lesion and neuropharmacological experiments; other studies had already implicated catecholamines, the pons, and nucleus locus coeruleus as crucial for REM sleep. Jouvet and his colleagues observed the effects of specific attacks upon serotonergic neurons. They achieved pharmacological specificity with acute administration of the serotonin depletor, parachlorophenylalanine (PCPA), and anatomical specificity with stereotaxic lesions. Both of these attacks led to insomnia or a great reduction in total sleep time and the emergence of PGO activity in the waking state. Our laboratory focused on chronic PCPA administration.

These data have been reported elsewhere.[76] Very briefly, we found that PCPA reduced serotonin concentrations in all parts of the brain (0 to 10 percent of controls) by the fifth PCPA–treatment day. During the first twenty-four hours after the beginning of PCPA administration, REM time generally stayed the same or increased. NREM was slightly reduced. Near the end of the third day, total sleep dropped precipitously and often reached zero for limited periods. Minima were generally seen on the fifth day of PCPA treatment. After two or three days of very low values, a marked recovery in total sleep time began, reaching approximately 70 percent of the baseline values even during continued administration of PCPA.

One of the clearest findings was the emergence of PGO activity throughout NREM and the waking state. Such activity could be seen at each point in the pons–geniculate–occipital–cortex circuit. As this activity appeared in the waking state, the overall rate of spike discharge began to drop in REM sleep. Accompanying PGO waves in the waking state were behavioral effects, such as orienting behavior that occurred during bursts of PGO waves. Such behavior occasionally assumed the organization and the intensity of an hallucinatory episode. These observations led to the hypothesis that serotonin regulated REM sleep's endogenous sensory stimulation and that some defect in such a regulation mechanism is associated with psychotic behavior. Several clinical studies have lent some support to this notion by showing some reciprocity between REM sleep and the severity of psychotic symptoms.[304,306] (See[114] for a review.)

However, it must be noted that the PCPA serotonin–sleep literature does indeed have ample examples of negative and/or hard-to-reconcile findings.[134,253,300]

Unit Activity during Sleep

The study of single brain cells in animals while they go through wakefulness–sleep cycles has become a popular tool to further investigate neurophysiological differences with respect to wakefulness, NREM sleep, and REM sleep.[*]

In one sense these studies confirm the qualitative differences between NREM and REM sleep. In general, unit studies have demonstrated that many cells have slower discharge rates during NREM sleep compared with wakefulness and REM sleep. However, some cells that have relatively slow firing rates during wakefulness may increase discharge rate during NREM sleep. In REM sleep, most cells have high firing rates, often equal to or greater than wakefulness rates. Firing usually occurs in bursts during REM sleep and these bursts are often in temporal association with other short–lasting phenomena (phasic events) such as rapid-eye movements and fasciculation of skeletal musculature. However, neurons in the amygdala and the dorsal raphe nucleus have been shown to depart from this pattern; these cells slow their firing rates during REM sleep.[142,143]

In another sense, unit data also point to the difficulties inherent in regarding NREM and REM sleep as distinct, mutually exclusive states. First, it is possible to experimentally dissociate EEG characteristics from behavior.[295] Harper[126] has shown that unit activity slows to NREM sleep rates during atropine-induced EEG synchronization and during the immobility response induced by inversion and restraint. These data are noteworthy since they demonstrate that when behavioral sleep is dissociated experimentally from EEG patterns or from locomotor inactivity some electrophysiological indices (unit firing rates) follow sleep patterns and others (say, eye movements) follow wakefulness patterns.

These kinds of observations have led investigators of unit activity to pursue more and more precise temporal relationships between unit firing patterns and macroscopic components of sleep states.[244,284]

This trend in unit research will undoubtedly continue. Many workers are probing brain–stem areas in search of direct associations between sleep processes and unit activity patterns. However, in order to comprehend at the

[*] See references 15, 126, 136, 142, 185, and 207; for a review see 143.

unit level the complex changes in state, such as the transition from NREM to REM sleep, it would seem that even more elaborate techniques are required. For example, the finding that certain pontine neurons fire in bursts before and during REM sleep, rapid eye movements[284] is exciting but problematic since these neurons may also fire in bursts during wakefulness and with waking eye movements. (D. McGinty, S. Henriksen, personal communications.) Such an interpretive dilemma may be amenable to a systems approach that would regard these pontine neurons as members of a component that operates in one mode during wakefulness and another mode during REM sleep. The logical strategy, then, is to simultaneously search for neuronal firing patterns that could characterize a switching mechanism to place pontine neurons related to eye movements in either the wakefulness or the REM sleep mode. Such an approach may require simultaneous recordings in two or more areas as well as a detailed analysis of any interstate differences in the temporal relationships between unit activity and eye movement.

❪ The Importance of Circadian Rhythms for Sleep Research

We have noted that up to about 1960, sleep was considered by most researchers to be a unitary state. Anything that was true of a part of sleep was assumed to be true for all of sleep, allowing for some quantitative variation. We have also pointed out some of the pervasive consequences of the discovery that sleep was, in a most far–reaching and fundamental way, at least two entirely different things. At one stroke, nearly all of the opinions about sleep were invalidated. At best, most of the conclusions had to be applied exclusively to NREM sleep and, at worst, entire categories of physiological study had to be reexamined.

A major point of this chapter is that, analogous to early sleep researchers facing the conceptual ramifications associated with the discovery of REM sleep, sleep researchers will now have to deal with the implications of circadian rhythms for sleep. It is possible that all prior theorizing and conceptualizing about sleep has been very misleading and narrow, because it has left out factors of daily oscillation. The early model for sleep studies was what might be called a "contingency model" or a "recovery model," that is, things happened because other things had happened. Sleep was thought to be a product of fatigue or so many minutes of prior wakefulness, regardless of time, day or night. This viewpoint left us with certain puzzling variabilities to account for. Because of these variabilities and methodological problems, the recovery model could not really be pursued to its extrapolated end. Nevertheless sleepiness was still thought to be the consequence of prolonged wakefulness.

Such early notions of sleep as recovery were first challenged by the jet–lag studies that simply pointed out that times of sleepiness and wakefulness certainly shifted complexly in adaptation to new time zones. The recovery model also had difficulty in accounting for the data that REM sleep periods might have some relation to clock time.[115] Furthermore Mitler et al.[216] presented data that directly challenged the recovery model by showing that, like the well–known, activity–inactivity rhythm, wakefulness–sleep also appears to be under the control of an internal circadian oscillator.

Recently, there has been increased interest in combining techniques of circadian rhythm research with those of sleep research to better assess the influence of daily cycles on sleep.[208] Webb and his coworkers[291] have led in recording sleep at different times of the day and pointing out that there is a kind of programming or tendency for REM sleep to be favored at certain times, slow wave to be favored at certain times, and so on. Such data come from looking at sleep samples in morning, afternoon, and evening. In another vein, Crowley and his coworkers[52,53] have begun to examine several variables over a twenty-four-hour period in order to begin understanding how sleep interrelates with other daily biological cycles. Such multi-variate studies are very significant since they not only combine circadian rhythm and sleep approaches, but they also adopt a process view in that components of behavioral state, such as temperature, body motility, and eye movement, are examined as separate oscillators.

To better understand the significance of combined circadian rhythm and sleep studies, it may be useful to give a cursory review of some concepts and terminology of circadian rhythms of special relevance to sleep.

It is clear that at any point in a twenty-four-hour period, we could examine an individual with respect to many biological and electrophysiological variables such as urine volume, body temperature, electroencephalogram, and even physical posture. We now use whole constellations of such variables to diagnose illness and to determine behavioral states. However, it is important to remember two facts when interpreting such data. First, each variable we choose to examine changes in amplitude over any extended period, and usually reaches a peak at the same time each day. Second, not all variables peak at the same time; there are intervals between peaks of some variables. Under most normal circumstances such intervals will be of constant duration over a number of days. Thus, each variable oscillates in a measureable phase relationship to all other variables, and, in most cases, phase relationships are constant over days.

Consider the three idealized daily rhythms (X, Y, and Z) shown in Figure 8-11. Curves like these can be obtained by taking measures of, say, urine volume, blood–sugar concentration and body temperature every fifteen minutes or so for ninety-six consecutive hours. To make amplitude compatible, we have plotted standard scores for each variable. Note, too, that the data are double–plotted so that forty-eight-hour records can be seen by scanning horizontally, and trends over days can be seen by scanning vertically. The peaks and troughs for each curve occur at approximately the same point each day, as if the variables had their oscillations synchronized to some external environmental signal. When curves look like this day after day, the subject is considered to be entrained to the cycle of his envi-

HIGHLY STYLIZED REPRESENTATION OF
DAILY RHYTHMS OF 3 VARIABLES

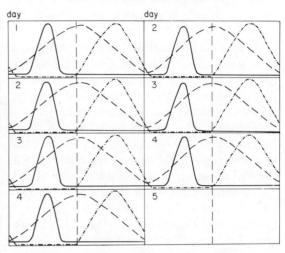

Figure 8–11. This figure presents a double plot of three variables: X (solid line), Y (dashed line), and Z (dotted and dashed line). Day–to–day cycles can best be seen by scanning horizontally; trends over several days can best be seen by scanning vertically. The values are standardized to allow plotting on the same scale.

ronment. Under entrainment, phase relationships among variables are quite constant over days.

Next we must consider what happens if an individual is removed from his normal environment so that he has no information about the time of day. This is difficult to achieve because only so many cues can be withheld from the subject. One strategy is to place a subject in a cave along with all the materials he needs for life. Under such constant conditions, it has been repeatedly shown that any species will maintain periodicities in most variables. The period of each variable will be about twenty-four hours; often the periods are slightly longer, say twenty-five hours; occasionally periods of twenty-two or twenty-three hours have been observed. These periodicities or rhythms manifested under constant environmental conditions have been termed circadian rhythms from the Latin word *circa* (around) and *dies* (day).[121,122,123,124] These rhythms are significant since they suggest that biological systems show oscillations that can occur independently of environmental signals. When an individual presents such independent rhythms in constant conditions, he is said to be free running.

If we look at variable Y in a subject who is free running, we may see a twenty-five-hour period (illustrated in Figure 8–12). In other words, after twenty-four hours, he will not have completed his full circadian cycle. In twenty-four days he will have lost a full day according to this physiological clock. Yet, if we return temporal cues to his environment, he will reentrain to a twenty-four-hour schedule. Another subject may show a different free-running period, say twenty-three hours (illustrated in Figure 8–13). Thus, in twenty-four days, he will gain a full day.

This discussion underscores the fact that each variable we study oscillates with a period of around twenty-four hours and usually oscillates in relationship to our daily behavior. Under constant conditions such entrained cycling can disappear and be replaced by circadian cycling. The plasticity of daily cycles is further evidenced by the many studies demonstrating that variables can entrain to artificial environmental periods ranging from about twenty-two to about twenty-six hours.

Up to now, we have been speaking about free running in one dimension. It is easy to assume mistakenly that curves for variables X and Z would look like curves for variable Y. Such an assumption ignores our second point. We said that under most normal circumstances each variable oscillates with a specifiable phase relationship to all other variables. What happens under constant conditions when we study more than one variable? Here, the time–gain or time–loss story may very quickly become complicated since variables can change phase relationships in free–run conditions. Under constant conditions, oscillators can become uncoupled. Such uncoupling of variables has been called internal desynchronization[5] and is graphically represented in Figure 8–14.

Now we should ask if we can consider sleep a single oscillator. Probably we cannot. Sleep and wakefulness are states. As such, they are constellations of values in many variables. We

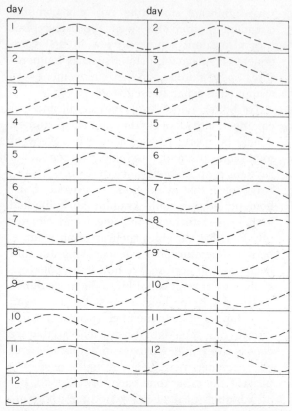

Figure 8–12. Double plot of entrainment through day five followed by free running with a period longer than twenty-four hours in variable Y. Dashed vertical lines denote twelve noon.

conceive of sleep as low responsiveness to stimuli, recumbent posture, low and falling body temperature, electroencephalographic synchronization, etc. Sleep specialists agree on the necessary and sufficient portions of the sleep constellation. However, we are just beginning to understand what other portions of the sleep constellation predispose to the emergence and maintenance of sleep. In the entrained human, many oscillating variables must form a stereotypical pattern prior to sleep onset.

Now consider what would happen if we alter the individual's environment so that everyone around him is predisposed to sleep several hours earlier than he is. Such circumstances frequently arise. For example, if we jet a subject to a different time zone, seven hours later we will produce the well–known, jet–lag syndrome. He arrives at, say, 11 P.M., local

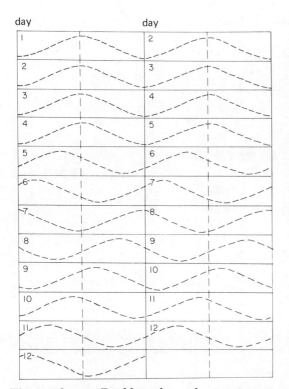

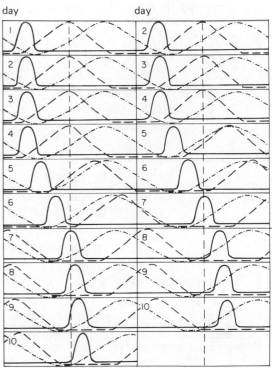

Figure 8–13. Double plot of entrainment through day five followed by free running with a period shorter than twenty-four hours in variable Y. Dashed vertical lines denote twelve noon.

Figure 8–14. Double plot of entrainment followed by free running in variables X, Y, and Z. Note that during the free–run period, phase relationships are different from those of the first five days. Dashed vertical lines denote twelve noon.

time—bedtime. Yet he cannot sleep and is restless all night. Moreover, the next day he will be fatigued and frequently predisposed to sleep. The subject may attribute this fatigue to lack of sleep during the night, but required duties may not allow him to sleep during the day. This temporary condition distinctly resembles insomnia. Several days are necessary to reentrain sleep time to the new environmental cycle, but one may need *weeks* to resynchronize relevant physiological oscillators to their approximate former phase relationships.[293] Thus, phase relationships change not only under free–running circumstances, but also when environmental cues have been abruptly shifted with respect to physiological time, since variables can show different rates of reentrainment.

Fortunately reentrainment does occur, making jet–lag disruptions reversible phenomena. But suppose there are certain individuals who cannot remain entrained to any twenty-four-hour schedule. Perhaps one or more physio-

logical processes operate on a natural frequency too short or too long to ever remain firmly entrained to a twenty-four-hour period. Or perhaps due to some low sensitivity to social or environmental cues, he cannot entrain to existing time cues. What might such a person complain of? One guess would be chronic insomnia. The patient may show inconstant phase relationships among various variables. Let's examine the consequences of such inconstant relationships. At different times from day to day, the patient may be physiologically predisposed to some condition that *approximates* normal sleep. Occasionally predisposition to sleep might coincide with common sleep times; then the patient's complaints of insomnia would subside. At other times predisposition to sleep may occur at inappropriate times of day; then the patient might complain of nighttime insomnia, daytime fatigue, and being ineffective at work. Finally, the phase relationships among certain oscillators

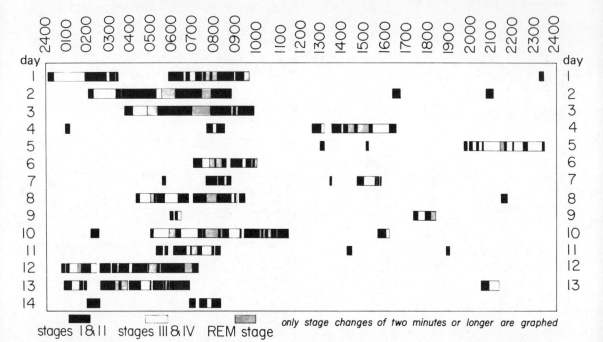

Figure 8–15. Periods of Stage 1 or 2 sleep, Stage 3 or 4 sleep, and REM sleep plotted by time of occurrence over fourteen consecutive days in a patient who complained of insomnia. Note long periods without sleep and the inconsistent structure of the sleep periods. These data suggest that sleep may be free running and that the cycles which predispose to sleep may be internally desynchronized.

may preclude sleep completely; it may be days before sleep is again possible.

This reasoning has led us to a condition that closely parallels the symptoms frequently observed in insomnia. We have plotted for several days the sleep of an insomniac in Figure 8–15. During this test the patient was allowed to sleep whenever he wished. For over thirty hours we saw no sleep. At other times sleep onset occurred successively later, day after day, reminiscent of free running. But the staging structure and amount of sleep varied throughout the test. We may conclude that predisposition to sleep varies in two ways. First, predisposition slides in time, reflected by changing sleep–onset times. Second, it changes in effectiveness, reflected by varying structure and quantity of sleep. These data support the notion that sleep is not a single oscillator but a state whose occurrence may depend on the phase relationships of other variables that oscillate in time.

Observations like these have convinced us that circadian rhythms and their relation to functional problems of sleep should be a major new research area. Very little is known now about such relationships except that sleep is favored at certain phases of the circadian oscillation. In addition to our insomnia data, a recent study in our laboratory[72] suggests that circadian programming of sleep stages may override the conventional contingency notion that, for example, REM sleep can only occur after a certain amount of slow wave sleep. In this study, one subject lived on a ninety-minute cycle (thirty minutes of sleep and sixty minutes of wakefulness) for six days. The limited sleep period obviated the normal occurrence of REM sleep. Yet, although the subject obtained approximately five hours of sleep per twenty-four hours, REM sleep occurred during sixteen of the sleep periods. In fact, many sleep onset REM periods were seen. It is interesting to note that this simple alteration of scheduling produced sleep onset REM periods quite easily as opposed to the heroic methods of REM sleep deprivation or pharmacological manipulation utilized in the past. However, at present, we can only guess at the many consequences to sleep sequencing when phase relationships are radically altered or when the organism is free running.

Finally, it is probable that in addition to restructuring theoretical and clinical issues in sleep, circadian rhythms will have profound implications for the areas of sleep deprivation and the biochemistry of sleep. First, in the last twenty years virtually hundreds of people have been studied before and after total sleep deprivation, partial sleep deprivation, and selective sleep deprivation. In general, data indicated that after deprivation, Stage 4 is greatly favored while REM sleep is depressed. In a careful analysis of these findings researchers have noted that after a deprivation period people tended to go to bed earlier in the day. Thus, any configuration of postdeprivation sleep was probably very much a function of the time of day rather than deprivation per se. In short, after a period of deprivation recovery sleep may look very different if it begins during normal waking hours as opposed to normal sleeping hours. In the latter case, recovery sleep shows fewer changes in structure. Thus, time of recovery sleep can account for much individual variability in the structure of recovery sleep. Second, it is usually assumed that sleep–wakefulness is biochemically controlled. We will have to explain eventually why there are well–known large circadian changes in level and turnover of biogenic amines, but very small changes in these variables as a function of state.[271]

⟨ Sleep Disorders

In the review[64] that appeared in the first edition of the *American Handbook of Psychiatry*, Volume III, we discussed the "chicken or the egg" problem of mental illness and sleep. In other words, is a sleep disturbance a symptom of mental illness or is it a cause, either directly or indirectly as a precipitating stress? This question has not been entirely resolved in the last decade, although material presented earlier in a previous section suggests that sleep loss per se will not necessarily lead to serious mental, emotional, or physical breakdown. In addition, this point of view is supported by observations of volunteers who stayed awake for *more* than two hundred consecutive hours.[119,176,147]

In Volume III, we stated that "it is virtually axiomatic that a disturbance of the mind can manifest itself in the sleeping state as well as the waking state. In fact, the former state is often the more sensitive barometer of psychic turbulence."[64] This remains the case whether or not one assumes that the sleep disturbance is the cause of the psychiatric disorder or vice versa. Psychiatric causes of insomnia are generally thought to be anxiety, depression, or the agitation of acute psychotic episodes. Yet the question persists as to whether these are the causes or only the correlates of the sleep disturbance. Further, if a patient who complains of insomnia is found, for example, to be depressed, can we then assume that there is no other cause of the insomnia?

Although the clinical aspects of sleep are covered elsewhere in this volume, we feel that some additional discussion of sleep disturbance as a symptom is appropriate to this chapter. Such discussion can serve two purposes. The first of these is to illustrate the point that sleep studies are often too limited in their scope to be effective clinical tools. The second involves the consideration of an approach to the patient who complains of insomnia.

In a recent survey of several hundred practicing physicians, we found that psychiatrists and internists saw a great majority of patients complaining of insomnia. It was clear that this complaint is considered an essentially psychiatric and by implication "emotional" or "psychological" problem by the medical community. We should, of course, remind our reader that sleep disturbance also includes complaints of hypersomnia, but our survey indicated that, in general, hypersomnia is considered a neurological problem. (Occasionally, however, there is a question of the association of hypersomnia and depression.)

The sleep laboratory approach to clinical sleep problems has been most vigorously advocated and pursued by Kales and his group who have made contributions in the area of insomnia,[158,161,170] drug dependency,[164,173] sleeping pill effectiveness,* sleepwalking,† as well as a variety of medically related conditions such as duodenal ulcer,[4] asthma,[160,172] hypothyroidism,[163] etc. Others have also contributed in this area.‡ If the psychiatrist is concerned about the complaint of insomnia on a routine basis, he should have some notion of the evolving differential diagnosis in this area; he should also have some developing list of causes and of the techniques of evaluation as well as of treatment.

The situation is analogous to the complaint of a chronic headache: if the psychiatrist is confronted with such a patient, he will want to ascertain, either on his own or by checking the appropriate referral procedures, that certain well–known organic causes, such as brain tumor or hypertension, are not implicated. By the same token, it is very important to recognize that insomnia requires similar evaluation. At this point, rather than presenting an exhaustive description, we will consider several examples of the conditions that proper evaluation can identify. Thus, we hope to demonstrate that when a psychiatrist is confronted with a patient who complains of chronic insomnia, he cannot assume that anxiety and/or depression are his only concerns, or that the referring general physician, if one is in the picture, has ruled out all organic causes.

Sleep Apnea–Insomnia Syndrome

Sleep apnea–insomnia was first described by Guilleminault et al.[116,117] in 1972. Sleep apnea had been recognized prior to this discovery, but had been described almost exclusively in patients complaining of hypersom-

nia§ and accasionally in narcolepsy[116,195,269] and in other medical conditions.[193] Sleep apnea–insomnia was first observed in a man who had complained of insomnia for nearly twenty years and who had sought both medical and psychiatric help for his condition. The remarkable aspect of the discovery of sleep apnea in this patient was the fact that, although he had several all–night sleep recordings using the standard sleep monitoring techniques (i.e., EEG, EOG, EMG) and although an objective sleep disturbance was duly noted, the recordings failed to implicate the true nature of the man's condition—that his respiration ceased during sleep. Appraisal of sleep apnea was made only after respiration gauges were added to the sleep recording parameters in order to investigate the claims of the patient's wife that he snored excessively.

Because of this discovery, measures of respiration (either mercury stain gauges placed on thorax or abdomen, thermistors taped near the nose or mouth, or both) are routinely included in all–night sleep recordings of insomniac patients at the Stanford University Sleep Disorders Clinic. In approximately fifty patients complaining of insomnia who have had all–night sleep recordings with respiratory measurements since the discovery of sleep apnea–insomnia, this syndrome has been identified in five patients (10 percent). While this is an extremely preliminary figure, Hauri has confirmed the presence of sleep apnea in three of his insomniac patients (personal communication).

The etiology of sleep apnea is not clearly understood at the present time, but three types of pathologic apneas during sleep have been described.[84,109,110,281] The first type is peripheral or obstructive apnea, thought to be due primarily to an obstruction of the airway caused by large adenoids, large tonsils, collapse of the pharyngeal muscles, thyroid goiter, etc. Obstructive apnea is typical of the Pickwickian syndrome. Central or diaphragmatic apnea involves a cessation of diaphragmatic movements during sleep. Thirdly, mixed

---

* See references 159, 162, 171, 173, 175, and 179.
† See references 166, 168, 169, 174, and 178.
‡ See references 80, 180, 183, 184, 249, 252, 128,

129, 233, and 309.
§ See references 44, 133, 194, 200, 203, 280, and 281.

apnea is characterized by a diaphragmatic apneic component followed by an obstructive apnea.

The sleep apnea–insomnia syndrome seems to involve primarily the diaphragmatic type of apnea. Figure 8–16 shows a recording of this condition. In general, we have found that insomniacs who have sleep apnea have little or no difficulty falling asleep, but complain of many lengthy nighttime awakenings, early morning awakening, and daytime fatigue. In addition, a history of nightly periodic snoring frequently suggests the diagnosis.

Most conventional treatments, whether they involve psychotherapy or chemotherapy, are ineffective in sleep apnea–insomnia. In fact, there is great danger in prescribing drugs that are respiratory depressants. Finally, it has been shown in other of the sleep apnea syndromes that cor pulmonale, cardiac failure, pulmonary artery, systemic hyperpressure, and other serious cardiovascular difficulties

may arise,* and there is no reason to believe that such complications will not result in sleep apnea–insomnia as well.

Restless Legs Syndrome and Nocturnal Myoclonus

Restless legs syndrome, characterized by deep paresthesis and limb movements occurring during extended muscular rest and when falling asleep,[85] and nocturnal myoclonus—intense muscle jerks that occur primarily in the legs at sleep onset and throughout the sleep period—[277] are often associated and may induce severe insomnia.[201] Furthermore, the severity of the illness may often lead to the development of depression and suicidal ideation in these patients.[42] Here, then, is the case of an insomniac in whom depression can be diagnosed, but whose insomnia (and indi-

* See references 43, 98, 99, 116, 192, 204, and 209.

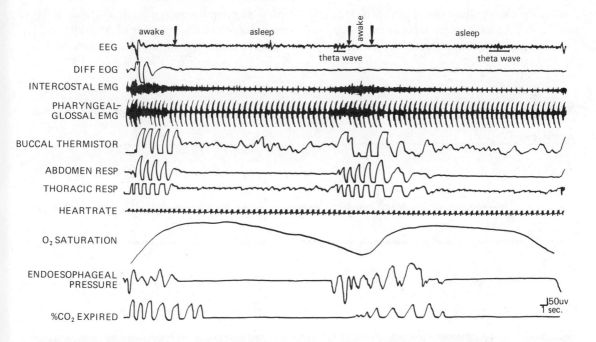

Figure 8–16. Polygraphic recording of sleep apnea episode recorded in a patient complaining of insomnia. Note that the EEG tracing shows periods of wakefulness when the patient breathes. When sleep ensues, breathing again ceases.

rectly depression) stem from a neurologic disorder.

In general, one can obtain a very good indication of nocturnal myoclonus from the history of the patient, but polygraphic sleep recording with the usual sleep parameters, as well as various limb muscles, is necessary to make the diagnosis. We have performed such recording on one patient who complained of both restless legs and nocturnal myoclonus, a seventy–year–old woman who had a thirty-two-year history of insomnia. A remarkable feature of her recording was the fact that the myoclonic jerks in her legs often coincided with short EMG suppressions recorded from the digastric muscle (see Figure 8–17). Pivik and Dement[243] have also recorded similar short–lasting EMG suppressions during sleep and have hypothesized that the EMG suppressions might be an indication of phasic events during NREM sleep. It is possible, then, that the myoclonic jerks of nocturnal myoclonus represent an abnormal response to phasic event discharges that occur in NREM sleep.

Restless legs syndrome has been treated with some success with tocopherol, vitamin E.[8] Our patient has reported relief with 5-hydroxytryptophan, which we have utilized on an experimental basis.

Pseudoinsomnia

When certain obvious factors have been ruled out, such as sleep apnea, drug dependency, and nocturnal myoclonus, one is left with a very large question mark with regard to patients who complain of insomnia. These patients have been evaluated by a number of workers. Kales, in particular, emphasized significant elevations in MMPI scales.[158] However, the question we ask is, what is really going on in the sleep of such patients? To answer this question, we have routinely conducted all–night sleep recordings utilizing standard parameters as well as respiratory and other variables on all insomniac patients who are referred to us. Thus we have studied a heterogeneous population rather than a highly selected group.

To date, we have evaluated approximately fifty patients with *no* obvious cause of their insomnia. We have looked at objectively recorded sleep parameters, such as total sleep times, sleep latency, number of arousals, etc., as well as a number of subjective assessments

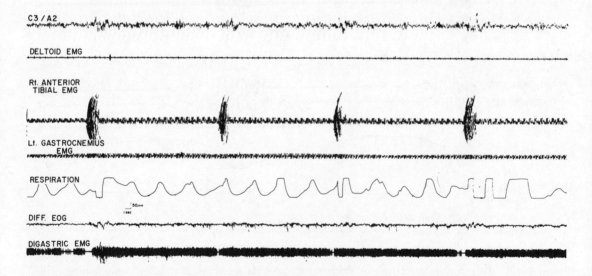

Figure 8–17. Nocturnal Myoclonus. Note the violent phasic EMG activity in the anterior tibialis associated with K-complexes in the EEG and with phasic suppressions of digastric EMG activity. Such twitches are disruptive of sleep and can lead to insomnia.

of the complaint both before and after the sleep laboratory experience. In Figure 8–18, we present a histogram in which each bar represents a mean sleep latency of four or more nights in the laboratory, rank ordered from longest to shortest. It can be seen that a number of patients, but by no means all, have sleep latencies that must be regarded as normal. Further, many of these latencies are under thirty minutes, which we use as a kind of rule-of-thumb cutoff for abnormal sleep latency. All of the patients complained that sleep onset was delayed and many complained that it took them "hours" to fall asleep.

Figure 8–19 is a similar description of total sleep time. Here again, there is a wide variation in this parameter in spite of the fact that all of the patients complained that they only slept a few hours at night even during their laboratory experience. The mean for the entire group was approximately six and one half hours, which is not abnormal when the mean age of the group is considered.

An obvious consideration, which has not been aggressively emphasized by others, is that an understanding of insomnia will surely require looking at more than these obvious factors. That is, in patients who fall asleep immediately and sleep adequately long periods without significant interruptions, we must look elsewhere for the cause of their complaint. "Elsewhere" may be in more subtle physiological measures, such as heart rate, body temperature, and other parameters as originally described by Monroe;[219] or it may be in more subtle dysfunctions of perception of sleep; or in the use of of the complaint as a symptom when the patient is anxious and/or

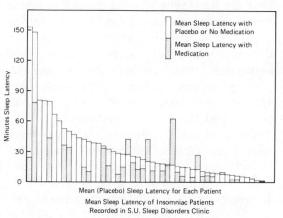

Mean Sleep Latency of Insomniac Patients
Recorded in S.U. Sleep Disorders Clinic

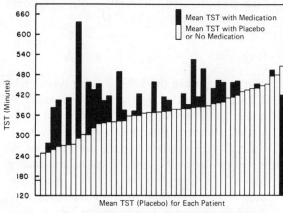

Mean Total Sleep Time of Insomniac Patients Recorded in
Stanford University Sleep Disorders Clinic

Figure 8–18. This figure is a rank order histogram showing the average sleep latencies of fifty insomniac patients recorded at the Stanford University Sleep Disorders Clinic for at least two consecutive nights with no medication or placebo (white bars). Certain patients were also recorded on at least two nights when the hypnotic medication (stipled bars), either Dalmane, fifteen mg or thirty mg; Sinequan, fifty mg; or GP41299 (an experimental hypnotic), one hundred mg.

It is interesting to note that although all patients complained of sleep latencies longer than sixty minutes, in only seven patients was this complaint confirmed! Only eleven patients had sleep latencies between thirty and sixty minutes. The majority of patients fell asleep in less than thirty minutes on placebo in spite of the fact that they had complained of severe difficulty falling asleep.

Figure 8–19. This figure is a rank order histogram of TST on placebo or no medication nights (white bar) and medication (black bar) nights in the same patients shown in Figure 8–18.

Although all patients complained of less than six hours sleep, this complaint was confirmed in only twenty-one patients on placebo nights. Of the remainder, fourteen had mean TST between six and seven hours and the rest had a mean TST over seven hours. Thus, again, the complaint was not reflected by the sleep recording.

Another interesting finding illustrated by this figure is the effect of sleeping medications on TST. The efficacy of the medication seems to be less as the subjects sleep longer on placebo nights. In other words, the longer an insomniac sleeps, the less likely he is to be significantly helped in terms of increased TST by hypnotic medications.

depressed; and, finally, it is clear that such patients should also be evaluated from the point of view of circadian rhythms. Every good judgment cries out that it is a heterogeneous group.

Night Terrors

A final mention should be made of a disorder that is very dramatic, but probably not overly fraught with psychological significance. This is the night terror or pavor nocturnus. Work in this area has been done by Fisher et al.,[93,94] Broughton,[35] Gastaut,[108] and others. This disturbance appears to involve some physiological–biological defect. According to Fisher,[94] there is no detectable premonitory sign of the abrupt onset of the night terror. We wonder if it is not precipitated by a burst of phasic activity arising in NREM sleep. Fisher has treated the night terror syndrome effectively with diazepam.[97]

Implications for Sleep Research

With regard to the field of sleep research, it is clear that, after two decades or more in which basic research and experimental approaches to the sleep mechanisms have certainly been the predominant concern, an interest in sleep disorders is emerging that is basically independent of medical specialties, such as neurology, internal medicine, or even its foster parent psychiatry, but which combines all of these areas. The classical sleep complaints of insomnia, hypersomnia, sleepwalking, bedwetting, and so on are the concern of the psychiatric sleep specialist or of anyone who is interested in the clinical aspects of sleep. In view of the fact that most clinical sleep research has been conducted under a psychiatric umbrella, it seems reasonable that the evaluation and treatment of sleep disorders as a clinical subspecialty should be regarded as a subspecialty of psychiatry. This appears to be the best option, in spite of the fact that such clearly organic problems as sleep apnea, hypersomnia, narcolepsy, and so on are involved. In a recent paper delivered at

the Association for the Psychophysiological Study of Sleep, Dement made the point that it is economically mandatory to combine sleep disorders under one specialty because of the tremendous investment required to provide monitoring equipment, twenty-four-hour coverage, and an adequate number of bedrooms to handle sleep–disorders patients. It is therefore very impractical to have a psychiatric–clinical sleep laboratory for insomnia and a duplication of this facility for what are traditionally regarded as neurological complaints.

It is also clear that we must begin to be wary of the limitations of the so-called "standard sleep recording."[251] In patients with sleep apnea or nocturnal myoclonus, the standard sleep recording is inadequate both for description and for diagnosis. It also seems obvious that total sleep time, sleep latency, and other traditional measures are not the parameters that will effectively define the psychological and physiological discomfort that is experienced by insomniacs. In terms of examining the sleep of the insomniac patient, the surface has only been scratched. Body movements, muscle tension, cardiac and respiratory factors, gastric motility—all these areas need thorough investigation and comparison with the normal population.

The final point, which will surely receive greater emphasis in the future, however disconcerting it may be, is that sleep is not necessarily a blessing greatly to be desired and to be sought at any cost. Sleep may instead constitute a subtle life–threatening imbalance: to accomplish the metamorphosis from the waking state to sleep may be a much more difficult adjustment than we have heretofore realized. For example, when we are confronted with a sleep apneic patient, we tend to ask the question, why do some people stop breathing when they fall asleep? It is more appropriate, knowing that the respiratory control systems are heavily dependent upon activity in the reticular formation, to ask: how do people continue to breathe when they fall asleep? This point is emphasized in a study by Lugaresi et al.,[202] in which they document a variety of imbalances and instabilities in autonomic parameters during sleep, particularly respiration. The transition from wakefulness to sleep may be especially vulnerable. A similar behavioral instability is evident when one examines heart rate: a small movement in the waking state will barely accelerate the heart rate; yet a similar small movement during NREM sleep will produce an enormous change.

All of these considerations will become the concern of the well–trained psychiatrist of the future, and it is certainly time to get some of these items into the psychiatric residency program.

(Instrumentation and Data Analysis

In this section, we would like to touch on two areas that will undoubtedly figure importantly in the future of sleep research.

First are the many advances in automatic processing of polygraphic data. As the scope of sleep observations extends in time among species and into odd locations like the moon, the sky lab, and perhaps Mars, it becomes necessary to process more and more data. Further, in addition to the classical measurement of EEG, EOG, and EMG, we have become much more interested in recording other variables when possible. In the human this includes blood pressure, cardiac functions, and respiration. In animals additional variables include primarily unit data, biochemical data by push–pull cannulae and reflex facilitation. The most important advance is use of the computer in a manner analogous to the human scorer. Systems have been developed by Itil,[138,139] by the Florida group,[273,274] and by others[146] that will perform this task. To date, while computers perform much more rapidly, they are not really able to match the flexibility and accuracy of human scorers. However, one implication is that the standards, presumably more consistent, that are used in computer scoring will in some way shape our future concepts of sleep. The computer may also be used to look at other events

in the sleep period in ways analogous to that which obviated the drudgery of looking at evoked potentials. There are now programs for counting K–complexes, eye movements, and PGO spikes. Advanced techniques of pattern recognition, masking techniques, and so forth may apply in recognizing patterns of discharge, phasic activity units, and other electrophysiological phenomena. We have just begun to utilize advanced methods of data processing in this area, but we expect great advances in the future. This may also include fairly radical departures in looking at the data. An example of this is the Stanford Slowgram[272] and a similar approach developed by Johnson et al.[146] in terms of delta cycles. The point is that instead of looking at the amount of Stage 4, we measure the decay in amplitude, the rate of rise, and so on. All of this can be done almost totally by a computer at the end of the night and written out. Figure 8–20 illustrates a Stanford Slowgram.

Second, many advances should be made in the next few years in the general area of experimental design and statistical analysis of data from sleep experiments. Early work on sleep was difficult enough without being concerned with such factors as seasonal change between the beginning and the end of the data–gathering period, the statistically appropriate number of variables to be analyzed from one set of subjects, and the best combination of measures to use in asking experimental questions.

Today, however, since most sleep recording routines are firmly established and most investigators have automated data reduction capabilities, more attention can be given to design and statistics. For example, it is now quite possible to do a two–or–three–condition study lasting as long as five or six weeks with humans. The study could involve recording over fifty variates per night, and the study could be designed to make all nights comparable by, for example, letting the subjects sleep at home on weekends, allowing Monday to serve as a laboratory adaptation night, and having Tuesday and Thursday be study nights. Seasonal change could be assessed by doing

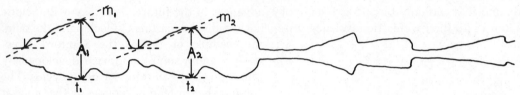

Figure 8–20. (Top) Cortical EEG of a male subject, age twenty-four, recorded on a compressed time scale during a night's sleep.
(Bottom) Diagramatic representation of sleep–EEG. m_1, m_2, . . . , are midpoints of the maximum amplitude plateau in that particular cycle.

two or more comparable runs at different times of the year. As Lubin (personal communication) has suggested, experimental conditions can easily be differentiated by using the statistical technique of discriminant analysis and then assessing the significance of any differences by another technique called multivariate analysis of variance. The dividends of such statistical treatment should far outweigh the costs of conducting the long and elaborately designed study. First, if the data are organized so that nights are comparable and seasonal factors are assessable, then the investigator need not guess as to what variates to look at: discriminant analysis will tell him precisely. Further, the investigator need not worry about performing many independent statistical tests on different but nonindependent variates from the same subjects: multivariate analysis of variance automatically accounts for nonindependence. Thus, very precise answers may be obtained from large and complicated data matrices if the data is simply organized appropriately. Such new design and analysis procedures should improve all aspects of sleep research from patient evaluation to determining hypnotic effectiveness.

❬ Conclusion

In the early part of this century, while sleep may well have been a pressing concern to many, laboratory research was extremely meager and almost totally uninvolved with human problems. The discovery of REM sleep, coming as it did at what retrospectively seems like the zenith of the psychoanalytic movement (with its insistence on the practical and theoretical importance of the dream) was to inaugurate an explosive increase in sleep research much of which was carried out by psychiatrists or in psychiatry departments and generously supported by the National Institute of Mental Health. However, other specialists were soon attracted into the sleep research field and over the past decade they have accomplished a great deal in a wide variety of highly sophisticated areas. There is a great deal of work that is directly relevant to traditional psychiatric problems. However, there is now a great deal of knowledge that is directly and almost exclusively relevant to sleep and sleep pathologies, and, by implication, to whoever is primarily responsible for these areas. It is our feeling that basic and clinical sleep research need to be presented in a unified manner. We do not feel that the sleepy person belongs to a neurologist and a sleepless person to a psychiatrist. We feel that one of these disciplines should either assume overall responsibility at least for the sleep pathologies or that the biochemistry, physiology, and pathology of sleep should be a discipline unto itself. In his preface to Volume III of the first edition of the *Handbook*, Silvano Arieti remarked: "Perhaps no other field of human endeavor is so encompassing and difficult to define as that of psychiatry." Within such nebulous and fuzzy boundaries, surely the field of sleep research can be easily and fully accommodated.

The area continues to grow and new information is accumulating at a frightening rate. However, the old problems are still with us. Do we really need to sleep? Why does REM sleep exist? What is insomnia? Why do we dream (exactly) what we do? These are fascinating and frustrating problems. We can safely estimate that a young sleep researcher will be well-occupied throughout his entire career. However, we must be aware of the concrete solutions that have been achieved. The anatomical localization of sleep mechanisms, an enormous increase in physiological understanding, a rational approach to pharmacology, a great clarification of pathophysiology in a variety of sleep disorders, and, finally, a number of promising leads in unraveling the role of sleep processes in mental illness.

All of this should be taught by someone in an integrated fashion. Here again, who will assume the responsibility? There is at least a hint in the very fact that so much space is devoted to the topic in this *Handbook*. It should be said that the foregoing material has only touched the highlights, and not all of those either. Reviews or overviews with similar goals will have more difficult problems in the future. Further, it is clear that many of the areas we touched upon are just beginning, and will soon be epicenters of intense scientific activity. If there were any surprises in this chapter, there will surely be many more in the future. This is the kernel of a final thought. It is hoped that each section will have been viewed as a guidepost of the present, pointing out future trends in research and clinical application, and that the interested student will see more clearly how sleep and dream research may be interwoven with his own career.

❨ Bibliography

1. ADEY, W., R. KADO, and J. RHODES. "Sleep: Cortical and Subcortical Recordings in the Chimpanzee," *Science*, 141 (1963), 932–933.

2. ALLISON, T. and H. VAN TWYVER. "The Evolution of Sleep," *Natrl. His.*, 79 (1970), 56–65.

3. ANDERS, T., R. EMDE, and A. PARMELEE, eds., *A Manual of Standardized Terminology, Techniques, and Criteria for Scoring of States of Sleep and Wakefulness in Newborn Infants*. Los Angeles: BRI Publications, 1971.

4. ARMSTRONG, R., D. BURNAP, A. JACOBSON et al. "Dreams and Gastric Secretions in Duodenal Ulcer Patients," *New Physician*, 14 (1965), 241–243.

5. ASCHOFF, J. "Desynchronization and Resynchronization of Human Circadian Rhythms," *Aerosp. Med.*, 40 (1969), 844–849.

6. ASERINSKY, E. and N. KLEITMAN. "Regularly Occurring Periods of Eye Motility and Concomitant Phenomena During Sleep," *Science*, 118 (1953), 273–274.

7. AUGUSTYN, D., A. GEBALLE, J. JENEST et al. "The Effect of Familiar Sounds on Dream Content," *Stanford Quarterly Review*, Winter (1972), 10–19.

8. AYRES, S. and R. MIHAN. "Leg Cramps (Systremma) and 'Restless Legs' Syndrome. Response to Vitamin E," *Calif. Med.*, 111 (1969), 87–91.

9. AZUMI, K., S. TAKAHASHI, K. TAKAHASHI et al. "The Effects of Dream Deprivation on Chronic Schizophrenics and Normal Adults—A Comparative Study," *Folia Psychiatr. Neurol. Jap.*, 21 (1967), 205–225.

10. BAEKELAND, F., D. KOULACK, and R. LASKY. "Effects of a Stressful Presleep Experience

on Electroencephalograph-recorded Sleep," *Psychophysiology*, 4 (1968), 436–443.

11. BALDRIDGE, B., R. WHITMAN, and M. KRAMER. "The Concurrence of Fine Muscle Activity and Rapid Eye Movements During Sleep," *Psychosom. Med.*, 27 (1965), 19–26.

12. BARROS, F., DE. "Analise dos Diferentes Ciclos Electroencefalograficos de Sono de Seis Esquizofrenicos Cronicos. Correlacoes Poligraficas. (Electrodermograma e Electromiograma)," *Actas Luso Esp. Neurol. Psiquiatr.*, 28 (1969), 215–238.

13. BAUST, W., G. BERLUCCHI, and G. MoRUZZI. "Changes in the Auditory Input During Arousal in Cats with Tenotomized Middle Ear Muscles," *Arch. Ital. Biol.*, 102 (1964), 675–685.

14. BAUST, W. and B. BOHNERT. "The Regulation of Heart Rate During Sleep," *Exp. Brain Res.*, 7 (1969), 169–180.

15. BENOIT, O. "Spontaneous Repetitive Discharge of Thalamic Units During Sleep in Cats," *Psychophysiology*, 7 (1970), 310–311.

16. BERGER, H. "Ueber das Elektroenkephalogramm des Menschen," *J. Psychol. Neurol.*, 40 (1930), 160–179.

17. BERGER, R. "Tonus of Extrinsic Laryngeal Muscles During Sleep and Dreaming," *Science*, 134 (1961), 840.

18. BERGER, R., P. OLLEY, and I. OSWALD. "The EEG, Eye Movements and Dreams of the Blind," *Q. J. Exp. Physiol.*, 14 (1962), 183–186.

19. BERGER, R. and I. OSWALD. "Eye Movements During Active and Passive Dreams," *Science*, 137 (1962), 601.

20. BERLUCCHI, G., G. MORUZZI, G. SALVI et al. "Pupil Behavior and Ocular Movements During Synchronized and Desynchronized Sleep," *Arch. Ital. Biol.*, 102 (1964), 230–245.

21. BIZZI, E. and D. BROOKS. "Functional Connections Between Pontine Reticular Formation and Lateral Geniculate Nucleus During Deep Sleep," *Arch. Ital. Biol.*, 101 (1963), 666–680.

22. BLAKE, H. "Brain Potentials and Depth of Sleep," *Am. J. Physiol.*, 119 (1937), 273–274.

23. BLAKE, H. and R. GERARD. "Brain Potential During Sleep," *Am. J. Physiol.*, 119 (1937), 692–703.

24. BLAKE, H., R. GERARD, and N. KLEITMAN. "Factors Influencing Brain Potentials During Sleep," *J. Neurophysiol.*, 2 (1939), 48–60.

25. BOELKINS, C. "Effects of Para–chlorophenylalanine on the Behavior of Monkeys," in J. Barchas and E. Usdin, eds., *Serotonin and Behavior*, pp. 357–364. New York: Academic Press, 1973.

26. BOKERT, E. "The Effects of Thirst and a Related Auditory Stimulus on Dream Reports." 5th Annual Meeting of the Association for the Psychophysiological Study of Sleep, Washington, March, 1965.

27. BOWE-ANDERS, C., J. ADRIEN, and H. ROFFWARG. "The Ontogenesis of PGO Waves in the Kitten." *Sleep Res.*, 1 (1972), 82.

28. BREGER, L., I. HUNTER, and R. LANE. "The Effect of Stress on Dreams," *Psychol. Issues*, 7 (1971), 1–213.

29. BREMER, F. "Introductory Remarks," in M. Chase, ed., *Perspectives in the Brain Sciences*, Vol. 1, *The Sleeping Brain*, p. xiii, Los Angeles: Brain Res. Inst., 1972.

30. BROOKS, D. "Localization of the Lateral Geniculate Nucleus Monophasic Waves Associated with Paradoxical Sleep in the Cat," *Electroencephalogr. Clin. Neurophysiol.*, 23 (1967), 123–135.

31. BROOKS, D. and E. BIZZI. "Brain Stem Electrical Activity During Deep Sleep," *Arch. Ital. Biol.*, 101 (1963), 648–665.

32. BROOKS, D. and M. GERSHON. "Eye Movement Potentials," *Brain Res.*, 27 (1971), 223–239.

33. ———. "An Analysis of the Effect of Reserpine Upon Ponto–geniculo–occipital Wave Activity in the Cat," *Neuropharmacology*, 11 (1972), 499–510.

34. BROOKS, D., M. GERSHON, and R. SIMON. "Brain Stem Serotonin Depletion and Ponto–geniculo–occipital Wave Activity in the Cat Treated with Reserpine," *Neuropharmacology*, 11 (1972), 511–520.

35. BROUGHTON, R. "Sleep Disorders: Disorders of Arousal?," *Science*, 159 (1968) 1070–1078.

36. BUSSEL, J., W. DEMENT, and T. PIVIK. "The Eye Movement–imagery Relationship in REM Sleep and Waking," *Sleep Res.*, 1 (1972), 100.

37. CARTWRIGHT, R. "*Dreams, Reality, and Fantasy*," in J. Fisher and L. Breger, eds., *The Meaning of Dreams—Recent Insights from the Laboratory*. Calif. Ment. Health Res. Symp., No. 3, 1969.

38. ———. "REM and NREM Mentation in Normal and Schizophrenic Persons," *Sleep Res.*, 1 (1972), 101.

39. CARTWRIGHT, R. and L. MONROE. "Relation of Dreaming and REM Sleep—The Effects of REM Deprivation Under Two Conditions," *J. Pers. Soc. Psychol.*, 10 (1968), 69–74.

40. CARTWRIGHT, R., L. MONROE, and C. PALMER. "Individual Differences in Response to REM Deprivation," *Arch. Gen. Psychiatry*, 16 (1967), 297–303.

41. CHASE, M., ed., *Perspectives in the Brain Sciences*, Vol. 1, *The Sleeping Brain*. Los Angeles: Brain Res. Inst., 1972.

42. COCCAGNA, G. and E. LUGARESI. "Insomnia in the Restless Legs Syndrome," in H. Gastaut, E. Lugaresi, G. Berti-Ceroni et al., eds., *The Abnormalities of Sleep in Man*, pp. 139–144. Bologna: Gaggi, 1968.

43. COCCAGNA, G. M. MANTOVANI, F. BRIGNAMI et al. "Continuous Recordings of the Pulmonary and Systemic Arterial Pressure During Sleep in Syndromes of Hypernomnia with Periodic Breathing," *Bull. Physiopathol. Respir.*, 8 (1972), 1159–1172.

44. COCCAGNA, G., A. PETRELLA, G. BERTI-CERONI et al. "Polygraphic Contribution to Hypersomnia and Respiratory Troubles in Pickwickian Syndrome," in H. Gastaut, E. Lugaresi, G. Berti-Ceroni et al., eds., *The Abnormalities of Sleep in Man*, pp. 215–221. Bologna: Gaggi, 1968.

45. COHEN, H. and W. DEMENT. "Sleep: Suppression of Rapid Eye Movement Phase in Cat after Electroconvulsive Shock," *Science*, 154 (1966), 396–398.

46. COHEN, H., W. DEMENT, and J. BARCHAS. "Effects of Chlorpromazine on Sleep in Cats Pretreated with Parachlorophenylalanine," *Brain Res.*, 53 (1973), 363–371.

47. COHEN, H., R. DUNCAN, and W. DEMENT. "The Effect of Diphenylhydentoin on Sleep in the Cat," *Electroencephalogr. Clin. Neurophysiol.*, 24 (1968), 401–408.

48. COLEMAN, P., F. GRAY, and K. WATANABE. "EEG Amplitude and Reaction Time During Sleep," *J. Appl. Physiol.*, 14 (1959), 397–400.

49. CONNOR, R., J. STOLK, J. BARCHAS et al. "The Effect of Parachlorophenylalanine (PCPA) on Shock-induced Fighting Behavior in Rats," *Physiol. Behav.*, 5 (1970), 1221–1224.

50. CONNOR, R., J. STOLK, J. BARCHAS et al. "Parachlorophenylalanine and Habituation to Repetitive Auditory Startle Stimuli in Rats," *Physiol. Behav.*, 5 (1970), 1215–1219.

51. CORDEAU, J., A. MOREAU, A. BEAULNES et al. "EEG and Behavioral Cycles Following Microinjections of Acetycholine and Adrenaline in the Brain Stem of Cats," *Arch. Ital. Biol.*, 101 (1963), 30–47.

52. CROWLEY, T., F. HALBERG, D. KRIPKE et al. "Individual Variation in Circadian Rhythms of Sleep, EEG, Temperature and Activity Among Monkeys: Implications for Regulatory Mechanisms," in M. Menaker, ed., *Biochronometry*. Washington: Natl. Acad. Sci., 1971, pp. 30–53.

53. CROWLEY, T., D. KRIPKE, F. HALBERG et al. "Circadian Rhythms of Macaca Mulatta: Sleep, EEG, Body and Eye Movement, and Temperature," *Primates* 13(2) (1972), 149–168.

54. DAVIS, H., P. DAVIS, A. LOOMIS et al. "Human Brain Potentials During the Onset of Sleep," *J. Neurophysiol.*, 1 (1938), 24–38.

55. DAVIS, H., P. DAVIS, A. LOOMIS et al. "Electrical Reactions of Human Brain to Auditory Stimulation During Sleep," *J. Neurophysiol.*, 2 (1939), 500–514.

56. DELORME, F., J. FROMENT, and M. JOUVET. "Suppression du sommeil par la p-chloromethamphetamine et la p-chlorophenylalanine." *Comptes Rendus des Séances de la Société de Biologie et Ses Fibiales*, 160 (1966), 2347–2351.

57. DEMENT, W. "The Occurrence of Low Voltage, Fast Electroencephalogram Patterns During Behavioral Sleep in the Cat." *Electroencephalogr. Clin. Neurophysiol.*, 10 (1958), 291–296.

58. ———. "The Effect of Dream Deprivation," *Science*, 131 (1960), 1705–1707.

59. ———. "Experimental Dream Studies," in J. H. Masserman, ed., *Science and Psychoanalysis*, Vol. 7, *Development and Research*, pp. 129–162. New York: Grune & Stratton, 1964.

60. ———. "Eye Movements During Sleep," in M. Bender, ed., *The Oculomotor System*, pp. 366–416. New York: Harper and Row, 1964.

61. ———. "An Essay on Dreams: The Role of Physiology in Understanding Their Nature," in *New Directions in Psychology II*,

pp. 135–257. New York: Holt, Rinehart & Winston, 1965.

62. ———. "Perception During Sleep," in J. Zubin, ed., *The Psychopathology of Perception*, pp. 247–270. New York: Grune and Stratton, 1965.

63. ———. "Studies on the Function of Rapid Eye Movement (paradoxical) Sleep in Human Subjects," in M. Jouvet, ed., *Aspects Anatomofonctionnels de la Physiologie du Sommeil*, pp. 571–611. Paris: CNRS, 1965.

64. ———. "Psychophysiology of Sleep and Dreams," in S. Arieti, ed., *American Handbook of Psychiatry*, Vol. 3, 1st ed. pp. 290–332. New York: Basic Books, 1966.

65. ———. "Possible Physiological Determinants of a Possible Dream-Intensity Cycle," *J. Exp. Neurol.*, 4 (1967), 38–55.

66. ———. "The Biological Role of REM Sleep (circa 1969)," in A. Kales, ed., *Sleep, Physiology and Pathology*, Philadelphia: Lippincott, 1969.

67. ———. *Some Must Watch While Some Must Sleep*. Stanford: Stanford Alumni Assoc., 1972.

68. DEMENT, W., J. FERGUSON, H. COHEN et al. "Nonchemical Methods and Data Using a Biochemical Model: The REM Quanta," in A. Mandell, ed., *Methods and Strategy in Human Psychochemical Research*, pp. 275–325. New York: Academic Press, 1969.

69. DEMENT, W., S. GREENBERG, and R. KLEIN. "The Effect of Partial REM Sleep Deprivation and Delayed Recovery," *J. Psychiatr. Res.*, 4 (1966), 141–152.

70. DEMENT, W., C. HALPER, T. PIVIK et al. "Hallucinations and Dreaming," in D. Hamburg, ed., *Perception and Its Disorders*, pp. 335–359. Baltimore: Williams & Wilkins, 1970.

71. DEMENT, W., P. HENRY, H. COHEN et al. "Studies on the Effect of REM Deprivation in Humans and in Animals," in S. Kety, E. Evarts and H. Williams, eds., *Sleep and Altered States of Consciousness*, pp. 456–468. Baltimore: Williams & Wilkins, 1967.

72. DEMENT, W., J. KELLEY, E. LAUGHLIN et al. "Life on the 'The Basic Rest–Activity Cycle'," *Psychophysiology*, 9 (1972), 132.

73. DEMENT, W., E. KAHN, and H. ROFFWARG. "The Influence of the Laboratory Situation on the Dreams of the Experimental Sub-

ject," *J. Nerv. Ment. Dis.*, 140 (1965) 119–131.

74. DEMENT, W. and N. KLEITMAN. "The Relation of Eye Movements During Sleep to Dream Activity: An Objective Method of the Study of Dreaming," *J. Exp. Psychol.*, 53 (1957), 339–346.

75. ———. "Cyclic Variations in EEG During Sleep and Their Relation to Eye Movements, Body Mobility, and Dreaming," *Electroencephalogr. Clin. Neurophysiol.*, 9 (1957), 673–690.

76. DEMENT, W., M. MITLER, and S. HENRIKSEN. "Sleep Changes During Chronic Administration of Parachlorophenylalanine," *Rev. Can. Biol.*, 31 (1972), 239–246.

77. DEMENT, W. and A. RECHTSCHAFFEN. "Narcolepsy: Polygraphic Aspects, Experimental and Theoretical Considerations," in H. Gastaut, E. Lugaresi, G. BertiCeroni et al., eds., *The Abnormalities of Sleep in Man*, pp. 147–164. Bologna: Aulo Gaggi Editore, 1968.

78. DEMENT, W. and E. WOLPERT. "The Relation of Eye Movements, Body Motility, and External Stimuli to Dream Content," *J. Exp. Psychol.*, 55 (1958), 543–553.

79. DEMENT, W., V. ZARCONE, J. FERGUSON et al. "Some Parallel Findings in Schizophrenic Patients and Serotonin-Depleted Cats," in S. Sankar, ed., *Schizophrenia: Current Concepts and Research*, pp. 775–811. New York: PJD Pub., 1969.

80. DEMENT, W., P. ZARCONE, E. HODDES et al. "Sleep Laboratory and Clinical Studies with Flurazepam (Dalmane)," in S. Garattini and L. Randall, eds., *Proc. Int. Sym. Benzodiazepines*, pp. 599–611. New York, Raven Press, 1973.

81. DEWSON, J., W. DEMENT, and F. SIMMONS. "Middle Ear Muscle Activity in Cats During Sleep," *Exp. Neurol.*, 12 (1965), 1–8.

82. DREYFUS–BRISAC, C. "Sleep Ontogenesis in Early Human Prematurity from Twenty-four to Twenty-seven Weeks of Conceptual Age," *Dev. Psychobiol.*, 1 (1968), 162–169.

83. DUNCAN, R., P. HENRY, V. KARADZIC et al. "Manipulations of the Sleep–Wakefulness Cycle in the Rat: A Longitudinal Study," *Psychophysiology*, 4 (1968), 379.

84. DURON, B., C. TASSINARI, and H. GASTAUT. "Analyse spirographique et électromyographique de la respiration au cours du sommeil controlé par l'EEG chez l'homme

normal," *Rev. Neurol.*, 115 (1966), 562–574.

85. EKBOM, K. A. "Restless Legs Syndrome," *Neurology*, 10 (1960), 868–873.

86. ENGELMAN, K., W. LOVENBERG, and A. SJOERDSMA. "Inhibition of Serotonin Synthesise by Parachlorophenylalanine in Patients with the Carcinoid Syndrome," *N. Eng. J. Med.*, 277 (1967), 1103–1109.

87. EVARTS, E. V. "Effects of Sleep and Waking on Spontaneous and Evoked Discharge of Single Units in Visual Cortex," *Fed. Proc.: Fed. Am. Soc. Exp. Biol.*, 19 (1960), 828–837.

88. FERGUSON, J., H. COHEN, J. BARCHAS et al. "Sleep and Wakefulness: A Closer Look." Presented at Fed. Am. Soc. Exp. Bio., Sym. on "Neurohumoral Aspects of Sleep and Wakefulness." Atlantic City, 1969.

89. FERGUSON, J., H. COHEN, S. HENRIKSEN et al. "The Effect of Chronic Administration of PCPA on Sleep in the Cat," *Psychophysiology*, 6 (1969), 220–221.

90. FERGUSON, J. and W. DEMENT. "Changes in the Intensity of REM Sleep with Deprivation," *Psychophysiology*, 4 (1968), 380–381.

91. FERGUSON, J., S. HENRIKSEN, H. COHEN et al. "The Effect of Chronic Administration of Para–Chlorophenylalanine on the Behavior of Cats," *Psychophysiology*, 6 (1969), 221.

92. FERGUSON, J., S. HENRIKSEN, H. COHEN et al. " 'Hypersexuality' and Behavioral Changes in Cats Caused by Administration of P–chlorophenylalanine," *Science*, 168 (1970), 499–501.

93. FISHER, C., J. BYRNE, A. EDWARDS et al. "A Psychophysiological Study of Nightmares," *J. Am. Psychoanal. Assoc.*, 18 (1970), 747–782.

94. ———. "REM and NREM Nightmares," in E. Hartmann, ed., *Sleep and Dreaming*. Boston: Little, Brown, *Int. Psychiat. Clin.*, 7, (1970), 183–187.

95. FISHER, C. and W. DEMENT. "Studies on the Psychopathology of Sleep and Dreams," *Am. J. Psychiatry*, 119 (1963), 1160–1168.

96. FISHER, C., J. GROSS, and J. ZUCH. "Cycle of Penile Erection Synchronous with Dreaming (REM) Sleep," *Arch. of Gen. Psychiatry*, 12 (1965), 29–45.

97. FISHER, C., E. KAHN, A. EDWARDS et al. "A Psychophysiological Study of Nightmares and Night Terrors," *Arch. Gen. Psychiatry*, 28 (1973), 252–262.

98. FISHMAN, A. "The Syndrome of Chronic Alveolar Hypoventilation," *Bull. Physiopathol. Respir.*, 8 (1972), 971–980.

99. FISHMAN, A., R. GOLDRING, and G. TURINO. "General Alveolar Hypoventilation: A Syndrome of Respiratory and Cardiac Failure in Patients with Normal Lungs," *Q. J. Med.*, 35 (1966), 261–274.

100. FOULKES, D. "Dream Reports from Different Stages of Sleep," *J. Abnorm. Psychol.*, 65 (1962), 14–25.

101. ———. "Nonrapid Eye Movement Mentation," *Exp. Neurol. Sup.*, 4 (1967), 28–38.

102. ———. "What Do We Know About Dreams—And How Did We Learn It?" Paper and Discussion. 13th Annu. Meet. Assoc. Psychophysiolog. Study of Sleep. *Conference Report* #32, pp. 57–72. Los Angeles: Brain Information Service, U.C.L.A., 1973.

103. FOULKES, D., P. SPEAR, and J. SYMONDS. "Individual Differences in Mental Activity at Sleep Onset," *J. Abnorm. Psychol.*, 71 (1966) 280–286.

104. FOULKES, D. and G. VOGEL. "Mental Activity at Sleep Onset," *J. Abnorm. Psychol.*, 70 (1965), 231–243.

105. FREEMON, F. *Sleep Research, A Critical Review*. Illinois: Charles C. Thomas, 1972.

106. FREUD, S. *The Interpretation of Dreams*. J. Strachey, transl. New York: Basic Books, 1955.

107. GASSEL, M., B. GHELARDUCCI, P. MARCHIAFAVA et al. "Phasic Changes in Blood Pressure and Heart Rate during the Rapid Eye Movement Episodes of Desynchronized Sleep in Unrestrained Cats," *Arch. Ital. Biol.*, 102 (1964), 530–544.

108. GASTAUT, H. and R. BROUGHTON. "A Clinical and Polygraphic Study of Episodic Phenomena During Sleep," *Recent Ad. Biolog. Psychiatry*, 7 (1964), 197–221.

109. GASTAUT, H., B. DURON, J. PAPY et al. "Étude polygraphique comparative du cycle nychtemerique chez les narcoleptiques, les Pickwickiens, les obèses et les insuffisants respiratoires," *Rev. Neurol.*, 115 (1966), 456–462.

110. GASTAUT, H., C. TASSINARI, and B. DURON. "Étude polygraphique des manifestation épisodiques (hypniques et respiratoires) diurnes et nocturnes du syndrome de Pick-

wick," *Rev. Neurol.*, 112 (1965), 573–579.

111. GEORGE, R., W. HASLETT, and D. JENDEN. "A Cholinergic Mechanism in the Brain Stem Reticular Formation: Induction of Paradoxical Sleep," *Int. J. Neuropharmacol.*, 3 (1964), 541–552.

112. GIAQUINTO, S., O. POMPEIANO, and I. SOMOGYI. "Descending Inhibitory Influences on Spinal Reflexes During Natural Sleep," *Arch. Ital. Biol.*, 102 (1964), 282–307.

113. GIBBS, F. and E. GIBBS. *Atlas of Electroencephalography. I. Methodology and Normal Controls.* Cambridge: Addison-Wesley, 1950.

114. GILLIN, J. and R. WYATT. "Schizophrenia: Perchance a Dream?", *Biol. Psychiatry*, in press.

115. GLOBUS, G., R. GARDNER, and T. WILLIAMS. "Relation of Sleep Onset to Rapid Eye Movement Sleep," *Arch. Gen. Psychiatry*, 21 (1969), 151–154.

116. GUILLEMINAULT, C., F. ELDRIDGE, and W. DEMENT. "Narcolepsy, Insomnia and Sleep Apneas," *Bulletin de Physio-pathol. Respir.*, 8 (1972), 1127–1138.

117. ———. "Insomnia with Sleep Apnea: a New Syndrome," *Science*, 181 (1973), 856–858.

118. GUILLEMINAULT, C., S. HENRIKSEN, R. WILSON et al. "Noctural Myoclonus and Phasic Events," *Sleep Res.*, 2 (1973), 151.

119. GULEVICH, G., W. DEMENT, and L. JOHNSON. "Psychiatric and EEG Observations on a Case of Prolonged (264 Hours) Wakefulness," *Arch. Gen. Psychiatry*, 15 (1966), 29–35.

120. HAEFELY, W., M. JALFRE, and M. MONACHON. "Drug–Induced PGO Waves: A Neurolpharmacological Method for Evaluating Agents Which Interact with Central Norepinephrine (NE) and Serotonin (5HT) Neurons and Receptors." Paper. 5th Int. Cong. Pharmacol. San Francisco, 1972.

121. HALBERG, F. "Some Physiological and Clinical Aspects of Twenty-four-Hour Periodicity," *Lancet*, 73 (1953), 20.

122. ———. "Physiologic 24-Hour Periodicity: General and Procedural Considerations with Reference to the Adrenal Cycle," *Z. Vit.-Hor.*, 10 (1959), 225–296.

123. ———. "Temporal Coordination of Physiologic Function." Symp. Quant. Biol., Long Island Biol. Assoc., New York, 1960.

124. ———. "Chronobiology," *Annu. Rev. Physiol.*, 31 (1969), 675–725.

125. HALL, C. and R. VAN DE CASTLE. *The Content Analysis of Dreams.* New York: Appleton–Century–Crofts, 1966.

126. HARPER, R. "Activity of Single Neurons During Sleep and Altered States of Consciousness," *Psychophysiology*, 7 (1971), 312.

127. HARTMANN, E., T. BRIDWELL, and J. SCHILDKRAUT. "Alpha–methylparatyrosine and Sleep in the Rat," *Psychopharmacologia*, 21 (1971), 157–164.

128. HAURI, P. "Clinical Use of the Sleep Laboratory," *Sleep Res.*, 2 (1972), 154.

129. HELD, R., B. SCHWARTZ, and H. FISCHGOLD. "Fausse insomnie; étude psychoanalytique et electroencephalographique," *Presse Med.*, 67 (1959), 141–143.

130. HENRIKSEN, S., B. JACOBS, and W. DEMENT. "Dependence of REM sleep PGO Waves on Cholinergic Mechanism," *Brain Res.*, 48 (1972), 412–416.

131. ———. "LSD–25 Induced 'Hallucinatory' Behavior in Cats—Relationship to REM PGO Wave," *Sleep Res.*, 1 (1972), 36.

132. HERNANDEZ–PEON, R. "A Neurophysiologic Model of Dreams and Hallucinations," *J. Nerv. Ment. Dis.*, 141 (1965), 623–650.

133. HISHIKAWA, Y., E. FURUYA, H. WAKAMATSU et al. "A Polygraphic Study of Hypersomnia with Periodic Breathing and Primary Alveolar Hypoventilation," *Bull. Physiopathol. Respir.*, 8 (1972), 1139–1151.

134. HOBSON, J. "Sleep: Biochemical Aspects," *N. Engl. J. Med.*, 281 (1969), 1468–1470.

135. HOBSON, J. and R. McCARLEY, eds., *Neuronal Activity in Sleep—An Annotated Bibliography.* Los Angeles: UCLA Brain Information Service.

136. ———. "Cortical Unit Activity in Sleep and Waking," *Electroencephalogr. Clin. Neurophysiol.*, 30 (1971), 91–112.

137. HODES, R. and W. DEMENT. "Depression of Electrically Induced Reflexes ('H–Reflexes') in Man During Low Voltage EEG 'Sleep'," *Electroencephalogr. Clin. Neurophysiol.*, 17 (1964), 617–629.

138. ITIL, T. "Automatic Classification of Sleep Stages and the Discrimination of Vigilance Changes Using Digital Computer Methods," *Agressologie*, 10 (1969) 603–610.

139. ———. "Digital Computer Analysis of the Electroencephalogram During Rapid Eye

Movement Sleep State in Man," *J. Nerv. Ment. Dis.*, 150 (1970), 201–208.

140. JACKSON, J. *Selected Writings*, vol. 2, ed., J. Taylor. New York: Basic Books, 1958.

141. JACOBS, B., S. HENRIKSEN, and W. DEMENT. "Neurochemical Bases of the PGO Wave," *Brain Res.*, 48 (1972), 406–411.

142. JACOBS, B. and D. MCGINTY. "Amygdala Unit Activity During Sleep and Waking," *Exp. Neurol.*, 33 (1971), 1–15.

143. JACOBS, B., D. MCGINTY, and R. HARPER. "Brain Single Unit Activity During Sleep —Wakefulness: A Review," in M. Phillips, ed., *Brain Unit Activity During Behavior*, pp. 165–178. Iowa City: University of Iowa Press, 1973.

144. JACOBS, L., M. FELDMAN, and M. BENDER. "Eye Movements During Sleep," *Arch. Neurol.*, 25 (1971), 212–217.

145. ———. "Eye Movements During Sleep. 1. The Pattern in the Normal Human," *Arch. Gen. Neurol.*, 25 (1971), 151–159.

146. JOHNSON, L., A. LUBIN, P. NAITOH et al. "Spectral Analysis of the EEG of Dominant and Non–Dominant Alpha Subjects During Waking and Sleeping," *Electroencephalogr. Clin. Neurophysiol.*, 26 (1969), 361–370.

147. JOHNSON, L., E. SLYE, and W. DEMENT. "Electroencephalographic and Autonomic Activity During and After Prolonged Sleep Deprivation," *Psychosom. Med.*, 27 (1965), 415–423.

148. JONES, B. "The Respective Involvement of Noradrenaline and Its Dexaminated Metabolites in Waking and Paradoxical Sleep," *Brain Res.*, 41 (1972), 199–204.

149. JOUVET, M. "Recherches sur les structures nerveuses et les mécanismes responsables des différentes phases du sommeil physiologique," *Arch. Ital. Biol.*, 100 (1962), 125–206.

150. ———. "Biogenic Amines and the Stages of Sleep," *Science*, 163 (1969), 32–41.

151. ———. "The Role of Monoamines and Acetylcholine–Containing Neurons in the Regulation of the Sleep–Waking Cycle," *Ergeb. Physiol.*, 64 (1972), 116–307.

152. JOUVET, M. and F. DELORME. "Locus coeruleus et sommeil paradoxal," *Comptes Rendus des Séances de la Société de Biologie et de Ses Filiales*, 159 (1965), 895–899.

153. JOUVET, M. and F. MICHEL. "Corrélations électromyographiques du sommeil chez le chat décortiqué et mésencéphalique chronique," *Comptes Rendus des Séances de la Société de Biologie et des Ses Filiales*, 153 (1959), 422–425.

154. ———. "Sur les voies nerveuses responsables de l'activité rapide corticale au cours du sommeil physiologique chez le chat (Phase Paradoxale)," *J. Physiol.*, 52 (1960), 130–131.

155. JOUVET, M., F. MICHEL, and J. COURJON. "Sur un stade d'activité électrique cérébrale rapide au cours du sommeil physiologique," *Comptes Rendus Séances de la Société de Biologie et de Ses Filiales*, 153 (1959), 1024–1028.

156. JOUVET–MOUNIER, D., L. ASTIC, and D. LACOTE. "Ontogenesis of the States of Sleep in Rat, Cat, and Guinea Pig During the First Postnatal Month," *Dev. Psychobiol.*, 2 (1970), 216–239.

157. KAHN, E., C. FISHER, and L. LIEBERMAN. "Sleep Characteristics of the Human Aged Female," *Compr. Psychiatry*, 11 (1970), 274–278.

158. KALES, A. "Psychophysiological Studies of Insomnia," *Ann. Intern. Med.*, 71 (1969), 625–629.

159. KALES, A., C. ALLEN, M. SCHARF et al. "Hypnotic Drugs and Their Effectiveness. All–night EEG Studies of Insomniac Subjects," *Arch. Gen. Psychiatry*, 23 (1970), 226–232.

160. KALES, A., G. BEALL, G. BAJOR et al. "Sleep Studies in Asthmatic Adults: Relationship of Attacks to Sleep Stage and Time of Night," *J. Allergy Clin. Immunol.*, 41 (1968), 164–173.

161. KALES, A. and R. BERGER. "Psychopathology of Sleep," in G. Costello, ed., *Symptoms of Psychopathology. A Handbook*. New York: Wiley, 1970.

162. KALES, A. and G. CARY. "Treating Insomnia," in E. Robins, ed., "Psychiatry—1971," pp. 55–56. *Medical World News Suppl.*, 1971.

163. KALES, A., G. HEUSER, A. JACOBSON et al. "All night Sleep Studies in Hypothyroid Patients Before and After Treatment," *J. Clin. Endocrinol. Metab.*, 27 (1967), 1593–1599.

164. KALES, A., G. HEUSER, J. KALES, et al. "Drug Dependency. Investigations of Stimulants and Depressants," *Ann. Intern. Med.*, 70 (1969), 591–614.

165. KALES, A., F. HODEMAKER, A. JACOBSON et al. "Dream Deprivation: An Experimental Reappraisal," *Nature*, 204 (1964), 1337–1338.

166. KALES, A. and A. JACOBSON. "Clinical and Electrophysiological Studies of Somnabulism," in H. Gastaut, E. Lugaresi, G. Berti-Ceroni et al., eds., *The Abnormalities of Sleep in Man*. Bologna: Gaggi, 1968, pp. 295–302.

167. KALES, A., A. JACOBSON, J. KALES et al. "All Night EEG Sleep Measurements in Young Adults," *Psychonomic Sci.*, 7 (1967), 67–68.

168. KALES, A., A. JACOBSON, T. KUN et al. "Somnambulism: Further All–night EEG Studies," *Electroencephalogr. Clin. Neurophysiol.*, 21 (1966), 410.

169. KALES, A., A. JACOBSON, M. PAULSON et al. "Somnambulism: Psychophysiological Correlates. 1. All-night EEG Studies," *Arch. Gen. Psychiatry*, 14 (1966), 586–594.

170. KALES, A. and J. KALES. "Evaluation Diagnosis and Treatment of Clinical Conditions Related to Sleep," *JAMA*, 213 (1970), 2229–2235.

171. KALES, A., J. KALES, M. SCHARF et al. "Hypnotics and Altered Sleep–Dream Patterns. 2. All–night EEG Studies of Chloral Hydrate, Flurazepam, and Methaqualone," *Arch. Gen. Psychiatry*, 23 (1970), 219–225.

172. KALES. A., J. KALES, R. SLY et al. "Sleep Patterns of Asthmatic Children: All–night Electroencephalographic Studies," *J. Allergy Clin. Immunol.*, 46 (1970), 300–308.

173. KALES, A., E. MALMSTROM, M. SCHARF et al. "Psychophysiological and Biochemical Changes Following Use and Withdrawal of Hypnotics," in A. Kales, ed., *Sleep—Physiology and Pathology*, pp. 331–343. Philadelphia: Lippincott, 1969.

174. KALES, A., M. PAULSON, A. JACOBSON et al. "Somnambulism: Psychophysiological Correlates. 2. Psychiatric Interviews, Psychological Testing, and Discussion," *Arch. Gen. Psychiatry*, 14 (1966), 595–604.

175. KALES, A., T. PRESTON, T. TAN et al. "Hypnotics and Altered Sleep–Dream Patterns. 1. All-night EEG Studies of Glutethimide, Methyprylon, and Pentobarbital," *Arch. Gen. Psychiatry*, 23 (1970), 211–218.

176. KALES, A., T. TAN, E. KOLLAR et al. "Sleep Patterns Following 205 Hours of Sleep Deprivation," *Psychonomic Med.*, 32 (1970), 189–200.

177. KALES, A., T. WILSON, J. KALES et al. "Measurements of All-night Sleep in Normal Elderly Persons: Effects of Aging," *J. Am. Geriatr. Soc.*, 15 (1967), 405–415.

178. KALES, J., A. JACOBSON and A. KALES. "Sleep Disorders in Children," *Progress in Clinical Psychology*, 8 (1968), 63–73.

179. KALES, J., T. TAN, C. SWEARINGEN et al. "Are Over-the-Counter Sleep Medications Effective. All-Night EEG Studies," *Curr. Ther. Res.*, 13 (1971), 143–151.

180. KARACAN, I. "Insomnia: All Nights Are Not The Same." 5th World Cong. Psychiatry. November, 1971.

181. KARACAN, I. and D. GOODENOUGH. "REM Deprivation in Relation to Evection Cycle During Sleep in Adults." 6th Annu. Meet. Assoc. Psychophysiol. Study of Sleep. March, 1966.

182. KARACAN, I. and F. SNYDER. "Erection Cycle During Sleep in Mucaca Mulatta (Preliminary Report)." 6th Annu. Assoc. Psychophysiolog. Study of Sleep. March, 1966.

183. KARACAN, I. and R. WILLIAMS. "Insomnia: Old Wine in a New Bottle," *Psychiatric Q.*, 45 (1971), 274–288.

184. KARACAN, I., R. WILLIAMS, P. SALIS et al. "New Approaches to the Evaluation and Treatment of Insomnia (Preliminary Results)," *Psychosomatics*, 12 (1971), 81–88.

185. KASAMATSU, T. "Maintained and Evoked Unit Activity in the Mesencephalic Reticular Formation of the Freely Behaving Cat," *Exp. Neurol.*, 28 (1970), 450–470.

186. KING, C. "The Pharmacology of Rapid Eye Movement Sleep," *Adv. Pharmacol. Chemother.*, 9 (1971), 1–91.

187. KING, C. and R. JEWETT. "The Effects of Alpha–methyltyrosine on Sleep and Brain Norepinepherine in Cats," *J. Pharamacol. Exp. Ther.*, 177 (1971), 188–195.

188. KLEITMAN, N. *Sleep and Wakefulness*. Chicago: University of Chicago Press, 1963.

189. KRAMER, M. "Manifest Dream Content in Normal and Psychopathologic States," *Arch. Gen. Psychiatry*, 22 (1970), 149–159.

190. KRIPKE, D., M. REITE, G. PEGRAM et al. "Nocturnal Sleep in Rhesus Monkeys," *Electroencephalogr. Clin. Neurophysiol.*, 24 (1968), 582–586.

191. KRIPPNER, S., M. CAVALLO, and R. KEENAN.

"Content Analysis Approach to Visual Scanning Theory in Dreams," *Percept. Mot. Skills*, 34(1) (1972), 41–42.

192. KUHLO, W. and E. DOLL. "Pulmonary Hypertension and the Effect of Tracheotomy in a Case of Pickwickian Syndrome," *Bull. Physiopathol. Respir.*, 8 (1972), 1205–1216.

193. KUMASHIRO, H., M. SATO, J. HIRATO et al. "Sleep Apneas and Sleep Regulating Mechanism," *Folia Psychiatr. Neurol. Jap.*, 25 (1971), 41–49.

194. KURTZ, D., J. BAPST–REITER, R. FLETTO et al. "Les formes de transition du syndrome pickwickien," *Bull. Physiopathol. Respir.*, 8 (1972), 1115–1125.

195. KURTZ, D., J. MEUNIER–CARUS, J. BAPST–REITER et al. "Problemes Nosologiques Poses Par Certaines Formes D'Hypersomnie," *Rev. Electroencephalogr. Neurophysiol.*, 1 (1971), 227–230.

196. LINDSLEY, D., J. BOWDEN, and H. MAGOUN. "Effect Upon the EEG of Acute Injury to the Brain Stem Activating System," *Electroencephalography and Clinical Neurophysiology*, 1 (1949), 475–486.

197. LINDSLEY, D., L. SCHREINER, W. KNOWLES et al. "Behavorial and EEG Changes Following Chronic Brain Stem Lesions in the Cat," *Electroencephalogr. Clin. Neurophysiol.*, 2 (1950), 483–498.

198. LONSDORFER, J., J. MEUNIER–CARUS, E. LAMPERT–BENIGNUS et al. "Aspects hemodynamiques et respiratoires du syndrome pickwickien," *Bull. Physiopathol. Respir.*, 8 (1972), 1181–1192.

199. LOOMIS, A., E. HARVEY, and G. HOBART. "Cerebral States During Sleep as Studied by Human Brain Potentials," *J. Exp. Psychol.*, 21 (1937), 127–144.

200. LUGARESI, E., G. COCCAGNA, and G. BERTI-CERONI. "Syndrome de Pickwick et Syndrome d'Hypoventilation Alveolaire Primaire," *Acta Neurol. Belg.*, 68 (1968), 15–25.

201. ———. "Restless Legs Syndrome and Nocturnal Myoclonus," in H. Gastaut, E. Lugaresi, G. Berti-Ceroni, and G. Coccagna, eds., *The Abnormalities of Sleep in Man*, pp. 285–294. Bologna: Gaggi, 1968.

202. LUGARESI, E., G. COCCAGNA, M. MANTOVANI et al. "Some Periodic Phenomena Arising During Drowiness and Sleep in Man," *Electroencephalogr. Clin. Neuro-*

physiol., 32 (1972), 701–705.

203. LUGARESI, E., G. COCCAGNA, A. PETRELLA et al. "Il Disturbo Del Sonno E Del Respito Nella Sindrome Pickwickiana," *Sist. Nerv.*, 20 (1968), 38–50.

204. LUKE, M., A. MEHRIZI, G. FOLGER, JR. et al. "Chronic Nasopharyngeal Obstruction as Cause of Cardiomegaly, Corpulmonale, and Pulmonary Edema," *Pediatrics*, 37 (1966), 762–768.

205. MAGOUN, H. and R. RHINES. "An Inhibitory Mechanism in the Bulbar Reticular Formation," *J. Neurophysiol.*, 9 (1946), 165–171.

206. MATSUMOTO, J. and M. JOUVET. "Effects de reserpine, DOPA et 5HTP sur les deux états du sommeil," *Comptes Rendus des Séances de la Société de Biologie et ses Filiales*, 158 (1964), 2137–2140.

207. McCARLEY, R. and J. HOBSON. "Single Neuron Activity in Cat Gigantocellular Tegmental Field: Selectivity of Discharge in Desynchronized Sleep," *Science*, 174 (1971), 1250–1252.

208. McNEW, J., R. BURSON, T. HOSHIZAKI et al. "Sleep-wake Cycle of an Unrestrained Isolated Chimpanzee Under Entrained and Free–running Conditions," *Aerosp. Med.*, 43 (1972), 155–161.

209. MENASHE, V., C. FARREHI, and M. MILLER. "Hypoventilation and Cor Pulmonale Due to Chronic Upper Airway Obstruction," *J. Pediatr.*, 67 (1965), 198–203.

210. MICHEL, F., M. JEANNEROD, J. MOURET et al. "Sur les mécanismes de l'activité de pointes au niveau du système visuel au cours de la phase paradoxale du sommeil," *Comptes Rendus des Séances de la Société de Biologie et Ses Filiales*, 158 (1964), 103–106.

211. MICHEL, F., A. RECHTSCHAFFEN, and P. VIMONT-VICARY. "Activité électrique des muscles oculaires extrinseques au cours du cycle veille–sommeil," *Comptes Rendus des Séances de la Société de Biologie et Ses Filiales*, 158 (1964), 106–109.

212. MIKITEN, T., P. NIEBYL, and C. HENDLEY. "EEG Desynchronization of Behavioral Sleep Associated with Spike Discharges from the Thalamus of the Cat," *Fed. Proc.*, 20 (1961), 327.

213. MITLER, M., H. COHEN, J. GRATTAN et al. "Sleep and Serotonin in Two Inbred Strains of Mice (*M. musculus*)," *Sleep Res.*, 1 (1972), 69.

214. Mitler, M. and W. Dement. "Cataplectic-like Behavior in Cats After Micro-injections of Carbachol in the Pontine Reticular Formation," *Brain Res.*, 68 (1974), 335–343.

215. Mitler, M., B. Morden, S. Levine et al. "The Effects of Parachlorophenylalanine on Mating Behavior of Male Rats," *Physiol. Beh.*, 8 (1972), 1147–1150.

216. Mitler, M., P. Sokolove, C. Pittendrigh et al. "Activity–inactivity and Wakefulness–sleep Rhythms in the Hamster Under Three Lighting Conditions," *Sleep Res.*, 2 (1973), 189.

217. Molinari, S. and D. Foulkes. "Tonic and Phasic Events During Sleep: Psychological Correlates and Implications," *Percept Mot. Skills*, 29 (1969), 343–368.

218. Monachon, M., M. Jalfre, and W. Haefely. "A Modulating Effect of Chlordiazepoxide on Drug–induced PGO Spikes in the Cat," in S. Garattini, E. Mussini, and L. Randall, eds., *The Benzodiazepines*, pp. 513–529. New York: Raven Press, 1973.

219. Monroe, L. "Psychological and Physiological Differences Between Good and Poor Sleepers," *J. Abnorm. Psychol.*, 72 (1967), 255–264.

220. ———. "Inter–rater Reliability and the Role of Experience in Scoring EEG Sleep Records: Phase I," *Psychophysiology*, 5 (1969), 376–384.

221. Monroe, L., A. Rechtschaffen, D. Foulkes et al. "Discriminability of REM and NREM Reports," *J. Pers. Soc. Psychol.*, 2 (1965), 246–250.

222. Morden, B., G. Mitchell, and W. Dement. "Selective REM Sleep Deprivation and Compensation Phenomena in the Rat," *Brain Res.*, 5 (1967), 339–349.

223. Morrison, A. and R. Bowker. "A Lumbar Source of Cervical and Forelimb Inhibition During Sleep," *Psychophysiology*, 9 (1972), 103.

224. Moruzzi, G. Quoted in M. Jouvet, ed., *Aspects anotomo-fonctionnels de la physiologie du sommeil*, pp. 638–640. Paris: Centre National de la Recherche Scientifique, 1965.

225. Moruzzi, G. and H. Magoun. "Brain Stem Reticular Formation and Activation of the EEG," *Electroencephalogr. Clin. Neurophysiol.*, 1 (1949), 455–473.

226. Moskowitz, E. and R. Berger. "Rapid Eye Movements and Dream Imagery: Are They Related?" *Nature*, 224 (1969), 613–614.

227. Mouret, J., M. Jeannerod, and M. Jouvet. "L'activité électrique du systèm visuel au cours de la phase paradoxale du sommeil chez le chat," *J. Physiol.*, 55 (1963), 305–306.

228. Mouret, J., B. Renaud, P. Quenin et al. "Monoamines et régulation de la vigilance. Apport et interprétation biochimique des données polygraphiques," in P. Girard and P. Courteaux, eds., *Les Médiateurs Chimiques*, pp. 139–155. Paris: Masson, 1972.

229. Offenkrantz, W. and E. Wolpert. "The Detection of Dreaming in a Congenitally Blind Subject," *J. Nerv. Ment. Dis.*, 136 (1963), 88–90.

230. O'Neill, C. "A Cross-cultural Study of Hunger and Thirst Motivation Manifested in Dreams, *Hum. Dev.*, 8 (1965), 181–193.

231. Orem, J., S. Henriksen, and W. Dement. "Do Eye Movement Potentials and REM PGO Waves Involve Independent Neural Systems?" *Sleep Res.*, 2 (1973), 41.

232. Oswald, I. "Sleep Mechanisms: Recent Advances," *Proc. R. Soc. Med.*, 55 (1962), 910–912.

233. ———. "Insomnia", in H. Gastaut, E. Lugaresi, G. Berti-Ceroni et al., eds., *The Abnormalities of Man*. Proc. 15th Eur. Meet. Electroencephalogr., Bologna, 1968.

234. Parmelee, A., H. Schultz, and M. Disbrow. "Sleep Patterns of the Newborn," *Pediatrics*, 58 (1961), 241–250.

235. Pessah, M. and H. Roffwarg. "Spontaneous Middle Ear Muscle Activity in Man: A Rapid Eye Movement Sleep Phenomenon," *Science*, 178 (1972), 773–776.

236. Peyrethon, J. "*Sommeil et évolution. étude polygraphique des états de sommeil chez les poisson et les reptiles.*" Lyon: J. Tixier & Fils, 1968.

237. Phillips, R., C. Guilleminault, and W. Dement. "A Study on Hypersomnia," *Sleep Res.*, 2, (1973), 161.

238. Pierce, C., J. Mathis, B. Lester et al. "Dreams of Food During Sleep Experiments," *Psychosomatics*, 5 (1964), 374–377.

239. Pieron, H. "Le problème physiologique du sommeil," Paris: Masson, 1913.

240. Pietrusky, F. "Das Verhalten der Augen im Schlafe," *Klin. Monatsbl. Augenheilkd.*, 68 (1922), 355–360.

241. Pivik, R. "Mental Activity and Phasic

Events During Sleep." Ph.D. thesis, Stanford University, 1970.

242. PIVIK, R., J. HOBSON, and R. McCARLEY. "Eye Movement Associated Rate Changes in Neural Activity During Desynchronized Sleep: A Comparison of Brain Stem Regions," *Sleep Res.*, 2, (1973), 35.

243. PIVIK, T. and W. DEMENT. "Phasic Changes in Muscular and Reflex Activity During NREM Sleep," *Exp. Neurol.*, 27 (1970), 115–124.

244. PIVIK, T., C. HALPER, and W. DEMENT. "Phasic Events and Mentation During Sleep," *Psychophysiology*, 6 (1969), 215.

245. POMPEIANO, O. "Supraspinal Control Reflexes During Sleep and Wakefulness," in M. Jouvet, ed., *Aspects Anatomo–Fonctionnels de la Physiologie du Sommeil*, pp. 309–395. Paris: Centre National de la Recherche Scientifique, 1965.

246. ———. "Mechanisms of Sensory Integration During Sleep," *Prog. Physiol. Psychol.*, 3 (1970), 1–179.

247. PORTNOFF, G., F. BAEKLAND, D. GOODENOUGH et al. "Retention of Verbal Materials Perceived Immediately Prior to Onset of Non–REM Sleep," *Percept. Mot. Skills*, 22 (1966), 751–758.

248. RECHTSCHAFFEN, A. In the discussion of W. Dement's paper, "Experimental Dream Studies," in J. Masserman, ed., *Science and Psychoanalysis*, vol. 7, *Development and Research*, pp. 129–184. New York: Grune & Stratton, 1964.

249. ———. "Polygraphic Aspects of Insomnia," in H. Gastaut, E. Lugaresi, G. Berti-Ceroni et al., eds., *The Abnormalities of Sleep in Man*. Proc. 15th Eur. Meet. Electroencephalogr., pp. 109–125. Bologna: Gaggi, 1968.

250. RECHTSCHAFFEN, A. and D. CHERNIK. "The Effect of REM Deprivation on Periorbital Spike Activity in NREM Sleep," *Psychophysiology*, 9 (1972) 128.

251. RECHTSCHAFFEN, A. and A. KALES, eds., *A Manual of Standardized Terminology Techniques, and Scoring System for Sleep Stages of Human Subjects*. Washington: U.S. Government Printing Office, 1968.

252. RECHTSCHAFFEN, A. and L. MONROE. "Laboratory Studies of Insomnia," in A. Kales, ed., *Sleep—Physiology and Pathology*, pp. 158–169. Philadelphia: Lippincott, 1969.

253. RECHTSCHAFFEN, A., R. LOVELL, D. FRIED-

MAN et al. "The Effect Parachlorophenylalanine on Sleep in the Rat: Some Implications for the Serotonin—Sleep Hypothesis," in J. Barchas and E. Usdin, eds., *Serotonin and Behavior*, pp. 401–418. New York: Academic Press, 1973.

254. RECHTSCHAFFEN, A., F. MICHEL, and J. METZ. "Relationship Between Extra–ocular and PGO Activity in the Cat," *Psychophysiology*, 9 (1972), 128.

255. RECHTSCHAFFEN, A., S. MOLINARI, R. WATSON et al. "Extra–ocular Potentials: A Possible Indicator of PGO Activity in the Human," *Psychophysiology*, 7 (1970), 336.

256. RECHTSCHAFFEN, A., R. WATSON, M. WINCOR et al. "Orbital Phenomena and Mental Activity in NREM Sleep," *Psychophysiology*, 9 (1972), 128.

257. ———. "The Relationship of Phasic and Tonic Periorbital EMG Activity to NREM Mentation," *Sleep Research*, 1 (1972), 114.

258. REITE, M., J. RHODES, E. KAVAN et al. "Normal Sleep Patterns in Macaque Monkey," *Arch. Neurol.*, 12 (1965), 133–144.

259. ROFFWARG, H. "Relevancies and Irrelevancies Concerning a Proposed Association Between Rapid Eye Movements and the Visual Imagery of the Dream," in *Oculomotor System and Brain Functions*. Smolenice, Czechoslovakia: Slovakian Acad. Sci., forthcoming.

260. ROFFWARG, H., J. ADRIEN, C. BOWIE-ANDERS et al. "The Place of Middle Ear Muscle Activity in the Neurophysiology of the REM State," *Sleep Res.*, 2 (1973), 36.

261. ROFFWARG, H., W. DEMENT, and C. FISHER. "Preliminary Observations of the Sleep–dream Patterns in Neonates, Infants, Children, and Adults," in E. Harms, ed., *Problems of Sleep and Dream in Children*, Int. Ser. Monographs Child Psychiatry, Vol. 2, pp. 60–72. Oxford: Pergamon Press, 1964.

262. ROFFWARG, H., W. DEMENT, J. MUZIO et al. "Dream Imagery: Relationship to Rapid Eye Movements of Sleep," *Arch. Gen. Psychiatry*, 7 (1962), 235–258.

263. ROFFWARG, H., J. MUZIO, and W. DEMENT. "The Ontogenetic Development of the Sleep–dream Cycle in the Human," *Science*, 152 (1966), 604–619.

264. SAKAI, K. "Lateral Geniculate and Visual Cortex Waves With Eye Movements in

Waking and Sleeping Cats," Paper presented at the 13th Ann. Meet. Assoc. Psychophysiol. Study of Sleep. San Diego, 1973.

265. SAUERLAND, E., T. KNAUSS, Y. NAKAMURA et al. "Inhibition of Monosynaptic and Polysynaptic Reflexes and Muscle Tone by Electrical Stimulation of the Cerebral Cortex," *Exp. Neurol.*, 17 (1967), 159–171.

266. SCHMITT, F. "Macro–molecular Specificity and Biological Memory," in F. Schmitt, ed., *Macro–molecular Specificity and Biological Memory*, pp. 1–6. Cambridge: MIT Press, 1962.

267. SCHWARTZ, B. "EEG et mouvements oculaires dans le sommeil de nuit," *Electroencephalogr. Clin. Neurophysiol.*, 14 (1962), 126–128.

268. SHIMAZONO, Y., T. HORIE, Y. YANAGISAWA et al. "The Correlation of the Rhythmic Waves of the Hippocampus with the Behaviors of Dogs," *Neurol. Med. Chir.*, 2 (1960), 82–88.

269. SIEKER, H., A. HEYMAN, and R. BIRCHFIELD. "The Effects of Natural Sleep and Hypersomnolent States on Respiratory Function," *Ann. Intern. Med.*, 52 (1960), 500–516.

270. SIMON, C. and W. EMMONS. "The EEG, Consciousness, and Sleep," *Science*, 124 (1956), 1066–1069.

271. SINHA, A., S. HENRIKSEN, W. DEMENT et al. "Cat Brain Amine Content During Sleep," *Am. J. Physiol.*, 224 (1973), 381–383.

272. SINHA, A., H. SMYTHE, V. ZARCONE et al. "Human Sleepelectroencephalogram: A Damped Oscillatory Phenomenon," *J. Theor. Biol.*, 35 (1972), 387–393.

273. SMITH, J., M. CRONIN, and I. KARACAN. "A Multichannel Hybrid System for Rapid Eye Movement Detection (REM Detection)," *Comput. Biomed. Res.*, 4 (1971), 275–290.

274. SMITH, J. and I. KARACAN. "EEG Sleep Stage Scoring by an Automatic Hybrid System," *Electroencephalogr. Clin. Neurophysiol.*, 31 (1971), 231–239.

275. SNYDER, F. and J. SCOTT. "The Psychophysiology of Sleep," in N. Greenfield and R. Sternbach, eds., *Handbook of Psychophysiology*, pp. 645–708. New York: Holt, Rinehart, & Winston. 1972.

276. STEIN, L. and C. WISE. "Possible Etiology of Schizophrenia: Progressive Damage to the Noradrenergic Reward System by 6-Hydroxydopamine," *Science*, 171 (1971) 1032–1036.

277. SYMONDS, C. "Nocturnal Myoclonus," *J. Neurol., Neurosurg. Psychiatry*, 16 (1953), 116–121.

278. TAGLIAMONTE, A., P. TAGLIAMONTE, G. GESSA et al. "Compulsive Sexual Activity Induced by P-chlorophenylalanine in Normal and Pinealectomized Male Rats," *Science*, 166 (1969), 1433–1435.

279. TAGLIAMONTE, P., A. TAGLIAMONTE, S. STERN et al. "Inhibition of Sexual Behavior in Male Rats by a Monoamine Oxidase Inhibitor (MAOI): Reversal of This Effect by P-chlorophenylalanine (PCPA)," *Clin. Res.*, 18 (1970), 671.

280. TAMMELING, G., E. BLOKZI, S. BOONSTRA et al. "Micrognathia, Hypersomnia and Periodic Breathing," *Bull. Physiopathol. Respir.*, 8 (1972), 1229–1238.

281. TASSINARI, C., B. DALLA BERNARDINA, F. CIRIGNOTTA et al. "Apnoeic Periods and the Respiratory Related Arousal Patterns During Sleep in the Pickwickian Syndrome: A Polygraphic Study," *Bull. Physiopathol. Respir.*, 8 (1972), 1087–1102.

282. URSIN, R. "The Two Stages of Slow Wave Sleep in the Cat and Their Relation to REM Sleep," *Brain Res.*, 11 (1968), 347–356.

283. VALATX, J., R. BUGAT, and M. JOUVET. "Genetic Studies of Sleep in Mice," *Nature*, 238 (1972), 226–227.

284. VALLEALA, P. "The Temporal Relation of Unit Discharge in Visual Cortex and Activity of the Extraocular Muscles During Sleep," *Arch. Ital. Biol.*, 105 (1967), 1–14.

285. VAN DE CASTLE, R. "Animal Figures in Dreams: Age, Sex, and Cultural Differences," *Am. Psychol.*, 21 (1966), 623.

286. ———. *The Psychology of Dreaming*. New York: Gen. Learn. Press, 1971.

287. VOGEL, G., B. BARROWCLOUGH, and A. GRESLER. "Limited Discriminability of REM and Sleep Onset Reports and Its Psychiatric Implications," *Arch. Gen. Psychiatry*, 26 (1972), 449–455.

288. VOGEL, G. and A. TRAUB. "REM Deprivation. I. The Effect on Schizophrenic Patients," *Arch. Gen. Psychiatry*, 18 (1968), 287–300.

289. WATSON, R. "Mental Correlates of Periorbital PIPs During REM Sleep," *Sleep Res.*, 1 (1972), 116.

290. WATSON, R., K. LIEBMANN, and S. WATSON.

"Periorbital Phasic Integrated Potentials in Acute Schizophrenics," *Sleep Res.*, 2 (1973), 134.

291. WEBB, W. "Twenty-four-hour Sleep Cycling," in A. Kales, ed., *Sleep—Physiology and Pathology*, pp. 53–65. Philadelphia: Lippincott, 1969.

292. ———. Ed., *Sleep: An Active Process—Research and Commentary*. Glenview, Ill.: Scott, Foresman, 1973.

293. WEITZMAN, E., D. KRIPKE, D. GOLD-MACHER et al. "Acute Reversal of the Sleep–waking Cycle in Man," *Arch. Neurol.*, 22 (1970), 483–489.

294. WEITZMAN, E., D. KRIPKE, C. POLLAK et al. "Cyclic Activity in Sleep of Macaca Mulatta," *Arch. Neurol.*, 12 (1965), 463–467.

295. WIKLER, A. "Pharmacologic Dissociation of Behavior and EEG 'Sleep Patterns' in Dogs: Morphine, N-allylnormorphine, and Atropine," *Proc. Soc. Exp. Biol. Med.*, 79 (1952), 261–265.

296. WITKIN, H. "Presleep Experiences and Dreams," in J. Fisher and L. Breger, eds., *The Meaning of Dreams: Recent Insights from the Laboratory*, pp. 1–37. Calif. Dep. Ment. Hyg., Res. Sym. No. 3, 1969.

297. WYATT, R. "The Serotonin-Catecholamine-Dream Bicycle: A Clinical Study," *Biol. Psychiatry*, 5 (1972), 33–64.

298. WYATT, R., T. CHASE, K. ENGELMAN et al. "Reversal of Parachlorophenylalanine (PCPA) REM Suppression in Man by 5-Hydroxytryptophan (5HTP)," *Psychophysiology*, 7 (1970), 318–319.

299. WYATT, R., K. ENGELMAN, D. KUPFER et al. "Effects of Para-chlorophenylalanine on Sleep in Man," *Electroencephalogr. Clin. Neurophysiol.*, 27 (1969), 529–532.

300. WYATT, R., J. GILLIN, R. GREEN et al. "Measurement of Phasic Integrated Potentials (PIP) During Treatment with Parachlorophenylalanine (PCPA)," *Psychophysiology*, 9 (1972), 127.

301. WYATT, R., T. VAUGHAN, M. GALANTER et al. "Behavioral Changes of Chronic Schizophrenic Patients Given L-5-hydroxy-tryptophan," *Science*, 177 (1972), 1124–1126.

302. YOSS, R., N. MOYER, and R. HOLLENHORST. "Pupil Size and Spontaneous Pupillary Waves Associated with Alertness, Drowsiness and Sleep," *Neurology*, 20 (1970), 545–554.

303. ZARCONE, V., K. AZUMI, A. DE LA PENA et al. "Individual Differences in Response to REM Deprivation," *Psychophysiology*, 6 (1969), 239.

304. ZARCONE, V., G. GULEVICH, T. PIVIK et al. "REM Deprivation and Schizophrenia," *Biol. Psychiatry*, 1 (1969), 179–184.

305. ———. "Schizophrenia and Partial REM Sleep Deprivation." Paper presented 7th Annu. Meet. Assoc. Psychophysiol. Study of Sleep. April, 1967.

306. ———. "Partial REM Phase Deprivation and Schizophrenia," *Arch. Gen. Psychiatry*, 18 (1968), 194–202.

307. ZARCONE, V., A. KALES, M. SCHARF et al. "The Effect of Chronic Oral Ingestion of 5-Hydroxytryptophan (5HTP) on Behavior and Sleep Physiology in Two Schizophrenic Children," *N. Engl. J. Med.*, submitted for publication.

308. ZITRIN, A., F. BEACH, J. BARCHAS et al. "Sexual Behavior of Male Cats After Administration of Parachlorophenylalanine," *Science*, 170 (1970) 868–869.

309. ZUNG, W. "Insomnia and Disordered Sleep," *Int. Psychiatry Clin.*, 7 (1970), 123–146.

CHAPTER 9

SCIENTIFIC CONCEPTS AND THE NATURE OF CONSCIOUS EXPERIENCE

Frederic G. Worden

The ability of purely physical processes to account for all externally observable details of behavior means, among other things, that no aspect of another person's activity—tone of voice, facial expression, appearance of the eyes, or any of the other cues by which we judge what is 'in his mind' —can provide proof that he experiences the kind of awareness that we call consciousness. By the same token, every detail of the past and future history of mankind would be the same if consciousness were completely nonexistent, just so long as the physical laws of nature were kept unchanged.

Dean Wooldridge,
Mechanical Man [P. 134][50]

Introduction*

THE NATURE of conscious experience is the most conspicuously perplexing enigma that challenges the mind of man. There has been an explosion of new information about the brain, especially in the last three decades, about its molecular and cellular machinery, its neural circuitry, and its complexly organized hierarchies of systems. What does this new information tell us about conscious experience? Wooldridge, as quoted above, states the extreme of one position clearly and forcefully. The evidence and logic supporting it is available in three of his books.[48,49,50] These books provide a panoramic view of the interface between the sciences and the mystery of life, including the nature of man. As their titles suggest, they document the concept, accepted explicitly or implicitly by many scientists, that life and man himself are to be understood as machinery, subject only to the "physical" laws of nature as currently defined and, therefore, in no

* I am indebted to colleagues and friends for suggestions, and especially to Rodolfo and Gillian Llinas, whose critique of the manuscript was so telling that it inspired me to make significant revisions. Responsibility for the final version is, of course, mine.

way influenced by phenomena like conscious experience, which are currently relegated to a "nonphysical" status. Borrowing from Wooldridge, I shall henceforth refer to this as the "mechanical-man" concept. The question of whether this is the most tenable scientific view of conscious experience will be approached first by examining weaknesses in the mechanical-man concept. Alternative concepts will then be considered, especially with regard to framing questions that seem important for a science of conscious experience. Finally, examples from current neuroscience research will be used to illustrate certain approaches that bear on these questions. The goal is to use new knowledge to reformulate old questions and to discover new ones about relationships between scientific knowledge and conscious experience, and how both might be integrated into a new conceptual model, encompassing both "objective" and "subjective" realities. Unlike the mechanical-man concept the approach here assumes that no scientific position about consciousness is yet established, and that science itself, especially its logical and conceptual structure, must be seen as part of the problem rather than as merely the tool to use for understanding conscious experience. Science develops from, and is part of, conscious experience, and one can find in science, reflected as in a mirror, properties of the human mind that express themselves in all human thought. To recognize this clarifies the need for a new scientific frame of reference taking into account characteristics of conscious experience that have influenced the development of science.

(Science, Common Sense, and Subjective Experience

The notion that "mankind" would be no different without consciousness seems outrageous to common sense. So do many scientifically established models of reality, but these are accepted because they are supported by compelling evidence. This is the case, for example, with regard to the conflict between common sense and certain concepts of relativity theory. The dimensions of a meter stick do not depend on its velocity under conditions of common experience on earth, but the concept that its length *is* a function of its velocity under uncommon conditions (i.e., *not* ordinary experience) is accepted as a valid model of reality. For the mechanical-man concept, however, it should be noted that the problem is complicated by the fact that it is not just common sense but especially subjective experience that is outraged by the notion that consciousness has no function. For each individual human, the power of "mind over matter" is confirmed by the daily experience of volitional activity, even down to such trivial and frivolous actions as lifting a little finger. This subjective experience is private and inaccessible to confirmation by outside observers, but disturbances in the ability to initiate volitional activity are easily recognized through behavioral observations as a serious deviation from normal. If "common sense" is taken to mean knowledge gained via the sensory system and subject to consensual validation, then the subjective sense of conscious control of mind and body might be termed "common experience," to suggest knowledge that is directly accessible only to the individual subject. To evaluate the mechanical-man concept it is necessary to consider not only common sense and scientific evidence, but also the evidence of common subjective experience, and how these domains of knowledge can be brought into a unifying frame of reference. These are epistemological quicksands where many have struggled, and I shall confine myself to only a few points, hoping thereby to avoid the risk of getting bogged down. The comments here extend and develop some thoughts about scientific and subjective reality that are presented in an earlier paper, "Questions About Man's Attempt To Understand Himself."[51]

(Mechanical Man Has Some Problems

There are both factual and logical problems in the mechanical-man concept. If it be stipulated that "purely physical" processes account for *all* externally observable behavior, then it is tautological to argue that, ipso facto, externally observable behavior cannot be evidence of processes that are not "purely physical" (i.e., consciousness). Furthermore, as a matter of fact, observable behavior remains a mystery to science that cannot explain the initiation of even the most simple voluntary action. Considerable progress has been made toward understanding the neurophysiology of sensory systems and of motor systems, but almost nothing is known about how sensory inputs and ongoing brain activities culminate in the generation of those patterns of efferent activity that mediate behavior.[11]

It is a non sequitur to conclude from the fact that awareness is not externally observable and not part of the current scientific understanding of the "physical" laws of nature that, therefore, it has no biological function. The argument depends upon accepting the premise that nothing about reality remains to be discovered that is not already within the scope of scientific observation. To accept this means that, by definition, subjective experience springs from and is, inherently, "nonreality."

To argue that mankind would be the same without consciousness, provided the physical laws of nature are kept unchanged, is either a self-contradictory or a metaphysical assertion. Insofar as conscious experience is taken to be an emergent property of some unknown level of brain functioning, it would contradict the "laws of nature" to postulate the same functional machinery without this emergent property, whether or not consciousness plays an influential role in human behavior.

On the other hand, the assertion that consciousness has no function cannot be empirically tested because there is no way to abolish it without modifying any other aspect of brain function. This would require postulating that consciousness is not an aspect of any level of brain function, but is rather a disembodied and supernatural phenomenon. Thus, the question of its function would be subject to metaphysical or philosophical evaluation, but

not to refutation or confirmation on an observational basis, even in principle.

Wooldridge[50] places consciousness in the domain of science on the ground that it is an effect caused by physical processes in the brain:

In short, according to this thesis the evidence for the operation of physical cause and effect in conscious phenomena is convincing and therefore consciousness, in the mid-twentieth century, is finally ready to make the same transition from metaphysics to physics that was set in motion for the other functions of the body in the early 1600's. [P. 162]

It seems to me that conscious experience remains assigned to metaphysics, because science models reality exclusively in terms of objects and cannot explain how some objects, like the brain, are also subjects of experience. To rescue conscious experience from metaphysics will require new scientific models of reality that correct for the distortion of the subjectively imposed dichotomy between the observer and the observed, upon which rests the whole structure of present-day science.

The concept of man as a machine that cannot be influenced by consciousness interferes in no way with the pursuit of further scientific knowledge about "purely physical" (i.e., nonmental) processes. At the same time, it may preclude progress toward a better understanding of conscious experience because it perpetuates without question the dichotomy mental versus physical, and rejects the possibility that the gap between them is only a hiatus in man's current understanding, rather than an irreconcilable difference between mental and physical realities.

If the mechanical-man hypothesis cannot be tested empirically, is there some other basis on which it can be evaluated? Popper[30] suggests a useful approach:

In other words every *rational* theory, no matter whether scientific or philosophical, is rational in so far as it tries to solve *certain problems*. A theory is comprehensible and reasonable only in its relation to a given *problem-situation*, and it can

be rationally discussed only by discussing this relation.

Now if we look upon a theory as a proposed
solution to a set of problems, then the theory immediately lends itself to critical discussion—even
if it is non-empirical and irrefutable. For we can
now ask questions such as, Does it solve the problem? Does it solve it better than other theories?
Has it perhaps merely shifted the problem? Is the
solution simple? Is it fruitful? Does it perhaps
contradict other philosophical theories needed for
solving other problems? [P. 199]

If we adopt this pragmatic approach suggested by Popper, it appears that two old and
important problems are solved by the concept
of mechanical man: How can mental phenomena influence physical processes? How
can self-determination (free will) be reconciled with causal determinism? Historically,
these questions have proven so endlessly in-
scrutable as to suggest that they are not properly framed to permit progress toward understanding the problems, whatever they are, that
give rise to them. This suggests that it might
be important to evaluate not just putative
answers, but also the validity of the questions
themselves.

(Can Mind Influence Matter?

The scientific method approaches reality on
the basis of information reaching the mind via
the sensory systems. In this approach, science
has taken conscious awareness as the "given"
for two reasons: (1) Awareness arrives directly at the mind, without benefit of the sensory systems (i.e., it is experienced not observed), and science has found no way to
inspect it via the sensory systems. (2) Subjective experience (perception and cognition) is
the basis on which the scientist carries out his
efforts to discover new knowledge. The observing process itself is accessible in subjective
experience only as an infinitely regressive "I"
that feels itself to be inherently separated
from whatever is being observed. This quality
of conscious experience leads to a model of

"reality" in which no interaction is possible
across the dichotomy between "mental" and
"physical."

In the era of modern neurophysiology,
Sherrington has stated the problem eloquently,
and struggled with it in detail, especially in
the Gifford lectures given in 1937–38.[35] He
cites Eddington's account, contrasting the
difference between the perceptible qualities of
his table and his elbow and the scientific
understanding of them in which they are conceived to be electric charges and fields of force
in space. Sherrington[35] goes on to illustrate
how science uses the concept of energy to explain the perceptible world.

The width of applicability of this concept 'energy' bears witness to its analytic depth. It unites
all sensible structure and brings it into a form of
doing. By it the atom, the rose we cultivate, and
the dog our companion are alike describable.
Within the descriptive competence of this unification comes our whole perceptible world, what it is
and what it does. [P. 235]

Elsewhere[51] I have discussed the fact that
scientific explanations depend upon a logic of
cause and effect that treats objects, even if
they are alive and subject to experience, as if
they were objects without subjective experience and influenced only by impersonal
"causes." The system of explanatory logic that
tries to deal with living subjects as subjects is
humanistic logic, in which meanings, rather
than causes, are invoked as explanatory principles.[21,18] Meanings, unlike causes, cannot
be observed but are experienced directly, and
so humanistic explanations of subjective behavior have to rest upon inferences derived by
one subject from projective identifications
with another subject. The power of the scientific system lies in the fact that it gives a more
reliable and useful picture of the perceptible
world than does the projective method underlying the animistic approach to the outer
world. The notion that rain depends upon a
friendly person in the sky does not lead to
effective attempts to predict, let alone influence, the weather. On the other hand, unreliable as it may be, the only successful approach

to understanding the "inner world" of other living subjects is the method of projective identification that takes observable behavior (facial expression, tone of voice, acting, etc.) and uses it to support an inference answering the question, If I were behaving that way, how would I be feeling? That this method works is illustrated by the success with which people transact the complexities of their relationships with each other; the fallibility of the method is illuminated by the problems that so richly characterize human affairs.

Sherrington is correct to say that science can use the energy concept to describe the dog, but incorrect when he says it can describe "the dog our companion," because "companion" is a subjectively experienced meaning to which the logic of science is blind.

On the problem of object and subject, as it pertains to the brain, Sherrington wrote:[35]

Physiology has got so far therefore as examining the electrical activity in a 'mental' part of the brain when activity there is in normal progress. But has it brought us to the 'mind'? It has brought us to the brain as a telephone-exchange. All the exchange consists of is switches. What we wanted really of the brain was the subscribers using the exchange. The subscribers with their thoughts, their desires, their anticipations, their motives, their anxieties, their rejoicings. If it is for mind that we are searching the brain, then we are supposing the brain to be much more than a telephone-exchange. We are supposing it a telephone-exchange along with the subscribers as well. Does our admirably delicate electrical exploration vouchsafe us any word about them? Its finger is ultra-sensitive, but energy is all that it can feel. And is the mind in any strict sense energy? [P. 222]

Despite this dilemma, Sherrington[35] refused to reject subjective evidence that the "mental" can influence the "physical" as is clear in this passage:

Mind, always, as we know it, finite and individual, is individually insulated and devoid of direct liaison with other minds. These latter too are individual and each one finite and insulated. By means of the brain, liaison as it is between mind and energy, the finite mind obtains indirect liaison with other finite minds around it. Energy is the medium of this the indirect, but sole, liaison be-

tween mind and mind. The isolation of finite mind from finite mind is thus overcome, indirectly and by energy. Speech, to instance a detail, illustrates this indirect liaison by means of energy between finite mind and finite mind. [P. 206]

The role attributed by Sherrington to mind depends on a relationship to energy that Sherrington, and science, cannot explain. The mechanical man solves this issue by asserting that consciousness has no role, and therefore there is nothing to explain. It postulates that the subjective evidence that mind can influence matter is an artifact of the limited view of brain mechanisms provided by conscious awareness.

An alternative view would be that consciousness is an emergent property of certain unknown levels of brain function, and that it can influence other, known levels of brain function, and that failure to understand how it does so is an artifact of limitations in the scientific view of reality. Implicit in this assertion is the premise that the current scientifically achieved model of reality can be modified to correct for this artifact, and to make understandable how consciousness and physical energy are related.

◖ Can Self-Determination Override Causal Determinism?

Subjective evidence in support of the concept of free will and personal responsibility is difficult to reconcile with the deterministic cause-and-effect logic of science. Man has struggled with this issue for centuries, invoking explanations at a variety of levels ranging from theology and metaphysics to empiricism and behaviorism. The concept of mechanical man solves this by asserting that free will is, like the influence of mind on brain processes, merely an artifact of subjective experience and that all aspects of human life are, therefore, causally predetermined. Wooldridge[50] states this as follows:

In the context of a completely physical biology, free will poses no problem—it simply doesn't exist. Obviously, it cannot, if conscious personality is no more than a derived, passive property of certain states of organization and electrochemical activity of the neurons. On this basis our thoughts and actions must be as rigidly controlled by the operation of inexorable physical law among the material particles of the universe as is the movement of wind and wave. [P. 183]

At a recent conference reported in the book *Brain and Conscious Experience*,[9] Sperry[37] commented on causal predetermination as follows:

In other words, behavioral science tells us that there is no reason to think that any of us here today had any real choice to be anywhere else, nor even to believe in principle that our presence here was not already in the cards, so to speak, five, ten or fifteen years ago. I do not like or feel comfortable about this kind of thinking any more than you do, but so far I have not found any satisfactory way around it. [P. 304]

In order to reconcile the breadth of freedom of choice that man appears to have with the logic of causal determinism, Sperry[37] goes on to suggest:

If one were assigned the task of trying to design and build the perfect free will model—let us say the perfect all-wise decision-making machine to top all competitor's decision-making machines—consider the possibility that instead of trying to *free* the machinery from causal contact, it might be better perhaps to aim at the opposite: that is, to try to incorporate into the model the potential value of *universal causal contact*; in other words, contact with all related information in proper proportion—past, present, and future.

It is clear that the human brain has come a long way in evolution in exactly this direction when you consider what goes on between its input and output in the process of making a decisive response. [P. 305]

We do not yet have a scientific knowledge of machines having "universal causal contact," but if the brain is such a system, to understand the constraints under which it functions will clearly require modification of the concept of causal determinism. Such modification might eliminate the apparent conflict between self-determination and causal determinism, and thereby provide an alternative solution to that of the mechanical-man concept.

The Question of Machine "Intelligence"

Machines have been built that "observe" and "recognize" patterns, that retrieve from a store of "memory," that "play" checkers and chess, that "learn" from experience, and that otherwise display what is called machine "intelligence." The words in quotation marks ordinarily imply conscious experience and their use in reference to machines tends to reinforce the analogy between machine performance and human thinking. From this analogy an extrapolation is made to future machines that will have conscious experience. For example, Wooldridge[50] writes:

Indeed our thesis requires that we keep an open mind as to the possibility that among the wires and transistors of existing electronic computers, there already flickers the dim glimmering of the same kind of personal awareness as that which has become, for man, his most precious possession. [P. 174]

The possibility that present-day computer performance justifies the hope of building machines capable of conscious experience is important because it is cited as evidence in favor of the concept that the living brain is merely a complex machine. In a classic paper, Turing[42] points out that the question, "Can machines think?" is too meaningless to discuss, and he proposes alternative ways of formulating it. He lists objections to the idea of an intelligent machine and provides answers for each. A more recent review of many of the same issues[17] suggests that the strongest argument against the practicability of an intelligent machine is the fact that the brain has so many components. Curiously, Turing did not even include this argument in his article. He suggested that one of the strong arguments against the possibility of a thinking machine is based upon the phenomena of extrasensory perception! Other reviews of progress in the computer and brain sciences are available in the volume *Computers and Brains*.[33]

Three considerations seem important to me for the question of whether present day machine performance suggests that someday conscious, intelligent machines can be built. The first is the question of whether machine performance does, in some rudimentary way, resemble brain performance. The second is the question of whether a design can even be imagined for a machine with as many components as the living brain. The third issue concerns problems that might arise in the attempt to build an extraordinarily complex machine of nonliving components.

I believe that the use of anthropomorphic language has seriously blurred the distinction between machine performance and human performance. Benson,[3] reporting a conference on artificial intelligence, describes examples of this type of misuse of language, and comments: "There is a twofold danger in such linguistic abuse—for man's conception of himself, and for his understanding of the capabilities of machines." Weizenbaum,[46] writing on the dangers of allowing the "technological metaphor" to dominate our thinking, comments:

Computer science, particularly its artificial intelligence branch, coughed. Perhaps the press has unduly amplified that cough—but it is only a cough nevertheless. I cannot help but think that the eagerness to believe that man's whole nature has suddenly been exposed by that cough, and that it has been shown to be a clockwork, is a symptom of something terribly wrong.

What is wrong, I think, is that we have permitted technological metaphors, what Mumford calls the 'myth of the machine', and technique itself to so thoroughly pervade our thought processes that we have finally abdicated to technology the very duty to formulate questions. [P. 611]

One factor in this abuse is the manifestly incorrect reasoning that, if two outputs are equivalent, then the processes leading to those outputs must be equivalent. This logical error is compounded by an observational error wherein part of the output of the human brain is taken as the whole of the output. For example, a machine is said to be playing chess if it can generate a series of moves that will win a chess game or, at least, look like a well-planned game. It should be obvious that similarity in the type of moves generated does not imply that the processes in the machine are similar to the processes going on in man. For the human being, playing any game is enjoyable by reason of many different levels of conscious and unconscious meanings attached to the pieces and to the procedures of the game. The motivational and emotional significance of these meanings derives from analogical and metaphorical associations linking various aspects of the game with such human dramas as war, sex, family relationships, and other patterns of personal experience. These motivational factors are separate from those logical considerations required for the analysis of the positions and values of the various chess pieces, and the choice of the next move. It is the interaction of these nonlogical conscious and unconscious processes with the logical ones that contributes to the style of play, whether careless, careful, aggressive, plodding, imaginative, or subtle. If chess consisted solely of the unfeeling logical analysis of contingency trees, it is doubtful that humans would play, and certainly it would be a chore more than a game. It is instructive to try to imagine a method of play that might reduce human performance to that of a machine. One may think of a giant list, computer printed, of unequivocal instructions for every contingency possible in a chess game. For each move by his opponent, the human player would flip to the appropriate page and execute the indicated move. Actually, even in these circumstances, the thoughts and feelings of the human would enliven the procedure in a most unmachinelike fashion, including perhaps even playful or spiteful deviations from instructions.

Another way of putting this argument is to suggest that future machines may be constructed that can produce outputs equivalent to certain aspects of human thinking, but there is not yet any evidence that the means of producing the outputs will include conscious awareness. Production of a sentence in a natural language is not evidence that a computer, or a parrot, is using the same type of conscious systems as a man speaking the same words.

Presumably the design of the human brain has some importance for the problem of designing a thinking machine. Unfortunately, it is not yet clear even how many components there are in the human brain. In discussing the component argument, Good[17] cites figures for neurons (five billion) and synapses (one thousand million million, or 10^{15}) in the gray matter of the cerebral cortex, but available evidence suggests that, far from being restricted to the cortex, neural activities subserving conscious experience are spread throughout most, if not all, of the cortical-subcortical interacting systems of the brain. There are substantially more than ten billion neurons in these systems, and each neuron is in intimate functional relationships with large numbers of glial cells that may well be as influential for brain function as the neurons themselves. Thus, at the level of cells, it is reasonable to postulate a ball-park figure of at least fifty billion components in the brain (5×10^{10}).

This estimate is a serious oversimplification because it is now clear that each neuron is an exceedingly complex computer within itself, and that it therefore should not be regarded as an elemental component of the brain. The neuronal membrane carries an array of complex molecular machinery that mediates transactions between the cell membrane and other elements (e.g., nucleus) of the neuron, and between one neuron and other neurons, and between the neuron and the rest of the body, as via substances (e.g., hormones) circulating in the blood. How many of these molecular machines exist in one brain is not clear, but work on the acetylcholine receptor in torpedo fish[19] and on neuromuscular junctions in rat diaphragm[13] yields estimates on the order of 10^4 receptor molecules per square micron of the motor end plate. Available data[6] suggest a similar density for receptor molecules in post synaptic membranes of the central nervous system. Many different types of specific molecular receptor mechanisms have already been identified, but we do not know how many more remain to be discovered. It is therefore not possible to guess how many such molecular receptors are arrayed on an individual neuron, but assuming 5×10^{10} neurons per brain, there would be at least 10^{20} molecular receptors arrayed on their surfaces.

It is already clear that these receptors mediate extremely sophisticated recognition tasks and produce powerful amplification effects. For example, the cyclic adenosine monophosphate (AMP) system acts as the intracellular mediator of a wide variety of cellular responses to triggers (e.g., hormone molecules) that activate specific molecular receptors on the cell membrane.[32] The staggering number of such molecular machines, and the still undiscovered processes that they may mediate, suggests a far more difficult goal for machine mimicry than does a model of the brain that takes the neuron as its basic element.

The organization of brain components into hierarchical systems is complex beyond any imaginable machine, and even with progress in microcircuitry there is no forseeable prospect of a machine involving such myriad systems of components. The possibility exists that a conscious thinking machine might be constructed with fewer components than the human brain, but until more is known about conscious experience, it seems fruitless to try to guess how many less components might be needed.

The third, and to me the most important consideration, is the problem of constructing such a machine from nonliving components. If it is to have anything of the order of complexity of the human brain, the use of nonliving elements will introduce serious problems. For example, in ontogenesis the living cells of the human brain proliferate, differentiate, and literally connect themselves up in specific circuitry on the basis of genetic information contained in DNA molecules interacting with fields, gradients, and other physical and chemical factors operative during brain development.[10] Since neurons may have as many as one hundred thousand dendrites and since each dendrite has many thousands of synaptic connections with other neurons, the task of attempting to wire the circuitry of such a system out of dead elements would require a technology so radically new as to stagger the imagination.

Secondly, during brain function each living element, however small, continuously adjusts itself in relationship to hierarchical systems acting at organizational levels above and below it. These include housekeeping systems that maintain the nutrition and metabolism of the cells, as well as information-processing features such as the regulation of changes in excitability thresholds, the influence of current and past experience on response patterns of individual cells, and other processes still little understood or unknown.

The maintenance of the human brain also depends on the fact that its living elements continuously replenish themselves. For example, the protein constituents of neurons change as a result of a balance maintained between the degradation of proteins and the synthesis of new proteins.[36] This ongoing turnover and renewal of brain substances would not, of course, be available in the machine.

Reviewing the turnover of proteins in living cells, Schimke[34] points out that all of the cellular proteins turn over, that the turnover rates are heterogeneous (the half life of proteins ranges from less than one hour to many days) and that both the processes of synthesis and of degradation are subject to complex regulatory mechanisms. Variables influencing protein turnover include substrate concentration, nutrition, and genetic and developmental factors. In neurons, substances synthesized in the cell body are delivered by axoplasmic flow[1] to nerve terminals. Furthermore, the triggering of electrical activity (action potentials) is an important factor influencing chemical processes[2,4,15,16] and morphological features[31] in the neuron. It is clear from these facts that a dynamic potential for plastic change in the cell, on both a short and a long-term basis, is provided through the diversity of these mechanisms for regulating the turnover of cellular substances. In systems having great levels of complexity, such a potential might be critically important for normal function.

It should be noted, also, that the properties of living systems reflect principles, as yet undiscovered, that are not active in nonliving elements; these principles may well be crucial for the emergence of conscious experience. In other words, it is not possible to explain life on the basis of physics and chemistry. With regard to progress in the application of physics and chemistry to biology, Bohr[6] wrote:

In this promising development we have to do with a very important and, according to its character, hardly limited extension of the application of purely physical and chemical ideas to biological problems, and since quantum mechanics appears as a rational generalization of classical physics, the whole approach may be termed mechanistic. The question, however, is in what sense such progress has removed the foundation for the application of so-called finalistic arguments in biology. Here we must realize that description and comprehension of the closed quantum phenomena exhibit no feature indicating that an organization of atoms is able to adapt itself to the surroundings in the way we witness in the maintenance and evolution of living organisms. [P. 100]

In summary, the main point to be emphasized is that the performance of electronic computers provides a rational basis for hoping that future machines may be capable of complex tasks now performed only by humans, perhaps even the translation of one natural language into another, the writing of poetry, or the formulation of new hypotheses significant for research progress. At the same time, there is no rational basis whatsoever for thinking that present-day computers produce their output by processes that represent a step, however rudimentary, toward conscious intelligence as displayed by the living human brain. The complexity of electronic computers, the use of anthropomorphic labels for machine performance, and the failure to appreciate that human intelligence is necessary to design, build, program, and recognize the output of the computer, all of these factors have encouraged the belief that present-day electronic machines are a step toward the eventual development of a machine capable of conscious experience. The slide rule is clearly a tool of human intelligence, but no one assumes that its use for calculation means that it is showing intelligent behavior. Even if the movements of a slide rule were automated by machinery that could be programmed for long sequences of calculations, with optical scanners to read the products, magnetic tape to accumulate the results, and perhaps an audio system to read aloud intermediate and final stages of the calculation, it seems unlikely that intelligence would be attributed to the system because the key element, the slide rule, is so simple a device. Replacement of the slide rule, however, by solid state microcircuitry, might encourage some to believe that in some mysterious manner the performance of the machine amounted to a small step toward conscious experience.

One may ask what difference it makes whether future machines are conscious or not so long as they accomplish sophisticated tasks now possible only for intelligent humans. One difference is that, no matter how complexly elaborated, nonconscious machines will function only as passive extensions of human intelligence, no different in principle from a slide rule. That is, such machines, in the absence of interaction with human intelligence, would grind out their products, or grind to a halt, their successes unrecognized and unused, and their failures unnoticed and unmourned. One might object that the same could be said for the human being, but this would not be relevant to the question of the fate of nonconscious machines writing poetry or composing music in the absence of interaction with conscious human intelligence. Indeed, it may be that the emergence of conscious experience in human evolutionary development was contingent on the inherently social nature of man; this suggests that a conscious machine might require "social relations" with other conscious machines, or with man.

Another difference that consciousness might make for a machine depends upon the question of how conscious experience contributes to brain function. In particular, are there information processing tasks that simply cannot be accomplished without conscious experience? If so, then machines without the property of conscious experience could not perform such tasks.

❪ The Observer and the Observed in Science

The mechanical-man concept attempts to reconcile conscious experience with the materialistic view of reality constructed by science. This mechanistic and materialistic view, as applied so successfully in Newtonian mechanics, draws a sharp dichotomy between the observer, taken for granted, and the observed, taken as an object for study. It seems curious that the first definitive effort to include the observer in scientific explanations was made in physics, presumably the most "objective" discipline, rather than in psychology, for which the problem of subjectivity might seem more relevant. Physics was forced to make the observer an integral part of its description of nature when it attempted to account for the behavior of atomic particles. A truly revolutionary event for epistemology was Planck's discovery of the universal quantum of action. Of it, Bohr[6] writes:

This discovery revealed in atomic processes a feature of wholeness quite foreign to the mechanical conception of nature, and made it evident that the classical physical theories are idealizations valid only in the description of phenomena in the analysis of which all actions are sufficiently large to permit the neglect of the quantum. While this condition is amply fulfilled in phenomena on the ordinary scale, we meet in atomic phenomena regularities of quite a new kind, defying deterministic pictorial description. [P. 71]

Even the Einstein correction of the Newtonian view to take account of subjective bias, as for observers traveling at close to the speed of light, did not imperil the dichotomy between nature and the observer that underlies the materialistic model of reality. Only with the development of quantum mechanics was the whole conceptual structure of scientific knowledge brought into question as described by Heisenberg:[20]

For the materialistic world view, it is important only that the possibility remains of taking these smallest constituents of the atoms as the final objective reality. On this foundation rested the coherent world view of the nineteenth and early twentieth centuries. . . .

It has turned out that the hoped-for objective reality of the elementary particles represents too rough a simplification of the true state of affairs and must yield to much more abstract conceptions. When we wish to picture to ourselves the nature of the existence of the elementary particles, we may no longer ignore the physical processes by which we obtain information about them. When we are observing objects of our daily experience the physical process transmitting the observation of course plays only a secondary role. However, for the smallest building blocks of matter every process of observation causes a major disturbance; it turns out that we can no longer talk of the behavior of the particle apart from the process of observation. In consequence, we are finally led to believe that the laws of nature which we formulate mathematically in quantum theory deal no longer with the particles themselves but with our knowledge of the elementary particles. . . . [P. 99]

The conception of the objective reality of the elementary particles has thus evaporated in a curious way, not into the fog of some new, obscure, or not yet understood reality concept, but into the transparent clarity of a mathematics that represents no longer the behavior of the elementary particles but rather our knowledge of this behavior. [P. 100]

The role of the observer in the structure of scientific knowledge is, of course, not restricted to quantum theory, but underlies the question of all human knowledge, as emphasized by Wigner:[47]

The principal argument against materialism is not that illustrated in the last two sections: that it is incompatible with quantum theory. The principal argument is that thought processes and consciousness are the primary concepts, that our knowledge of the external world is the content of our consciousness and that consciousness, therefore, cannot be denied. On the contrary, logically, the external world could be denied—though it is not very practical to do so. [P. 290]

The rejection of materialism and causal determination in quantum theory does not invalidate all scientific knowledge gained within the framework of these doctrines, any more than Einstein's theories invalidate Newtonian physics. In both cases, limitations are discov-

ered beyond which an older conceptual system has to be supplemented by a newer frame of reference. The history of science documents the reluctance with which scientists, like other human beings, recognize the need for shifting to a new frame of reference.

Scientific research in many domains of knowledge has indeed time and again proved the necessity of abandoning or remoulding points of view which, because of their fruitfulness and apparently unrestricted applicability, were regarded as indispensable for rational explanation. [P. 67][6]

Although the classical materialistic doctrine has certainly been fruitful, it should be noted that scientific progress with it has been limited to the explication of systems that are simple to the point of triviality by comparison with the brain. Indeed, the hope that life processes, including brain function, could be explained in the reductionistic, cause-and-effect logic applicable to simple mechanisms suggests that the appeal of classical materialistic doctrine may include nonrational factors as powerful, or more powerful, than rational considerations. For example, the concept of causality appears in human conscious experience as a fundamental principle of nature, even though it is a characteristic of thought itself rather than of the world outside the mind. As Mach[24] said:

There is no cause nor effect in nature; nature has but an individual existence; nature simply *is*. Recurrence of like cases in which A is always connected with B, that is, like results under like circumstances, that is again, the essence of the connection of cause and effect, exist but in the abstraction which we perform for the purpose of mentally reproducing the facts. [P. 1788]

In discussing the danger to clear thinking from the misuse of terms of language, Weiss[43] speculates on the historical emergence of the concept of "cause":

I shall not dwell on its historical roots; they are I would submit, deeply embedded in man's extrapolation to nature of his own spontaneity in willing an act. Presumably, primitive man then went on to populate the universe in his imagination with 'actors' after his own image. Sophisticated man simply reversed the process by invoking 'primary causes' which he then let be followed in linear ascending series, domino-fashion, by secondary, tertiary, etc., causes, confident or persuaded that ultimately the causal chain will 'explain' man's own spontaneity, which had served him as the model for the whole argument in the first place. [P. 927]

The peculiar power of the logic of causality may be due to the fact that it is presented to us without conscious effort, and with the subjective quality of seeming to be independent of the unreliability of thinking. That is, it masquerades as something to be thought about, rather than as a way of thinking.

Much of the authority of the ideas of cause and effect is due to the fact that they are developed instinctively and involuntarily, and that we are distinctly sensible of having personally contributed nothing to their formation. We may, indeed, say that our sense of causality is not acquired by the individual, but has been perfected in the development of the race. [P. 1789][24]

Insofar as the logic of causal determinism is modelled after voluntary action, the problem of reconciling free will with it can be seen to be a particularly poignant and circular paradox.

There are, of course, also rational reasons for the appeal of the classical materialistic doctrine. Methodologically, simple systems can be studied more easily than complex ones. It is technically feasible to record from one neuron, or even several neurons simultaneously, but there is little prospect of recording from, say, ten thousand neurons. Furthermore, the logic of causality is adequate for explaining the behavior of a neuron artificially isolated from the system in which it functions, but completely new conceptual tools will have to be developed to comprehend the behavior of large populations of neurons. It follows that all scientific knowledge of the brain takes the form of information about artificially isolated and identified subsystems within it, seen as mechanisms obeying the principles of rather direct causality. According to the logic of science, no matter at what level of brain organization it is applied, the subsystem under study is conceptualized as an object, so that conscious experience always remains a built-in will-o'-the-wisp. For example, no matter where one goes in the brain, sensory neurophysiology always sees an objective system that registers inputs in neural "codes," and transforms them into neural outputs. The question is never addressed of how these neural processes culminate in, or are read out as, a subjectively experienced percept (e.g., a visual or a sound image). To leave the observer out of a science of clockworks is a useful artifice of the mind, but to leave the observer out of a science of the brain is to see nothing but clockworks while overlooking that sentience, without which clocks are a meaningless absurdity.

The fact that the brain is an observing system is probably a better reason for modifying materialism than the difficulty of trying to describe atomic particles without reference to the observing process. Clearly progress depends upon recognizing the limitations of the doctrines of classical materialism and causality, and replacing these models of reality with new concepts that bring so-called "objective" and "subjective" knowledge together in a unifying theory.

(Requirements for a Science of Conscious Experience

If we postulate that conscious experience is an emergent property of certain levels of brain organization and that it plays an important role in brain function, what kind of questions have to be answered to develop a scientific understanding of it? Perhaps more importantly, what kind of questions do *not* have to be answered? For example, it is important to recognize that science need not explain what consciousness is, how it is produced, nor even how its effects are brought about. Science does not explain what gravitational force is, how it is created by, or generated from, mass, nor how the effects of gravity can act across vast reaches of space. The laws of gravity take gravitational force for granted, as a fundamental property, and restrict themselves merely to defining those lawful relationships existing between mass and gravitational force. In a similar fashion, a science of conscious experience can begin by describing precisely what kinds of systems have the property of awareness, what conditions within these systems are necessary and sufficient for the emergence of this property, what aspects of brain systems are influenced by the conscious property, and what lawful relationships exist between the quality of consciousness and the nature of the effects it has on the brain.

In this light, conscious experience is an enigma only insofar as science cannot yet define either the systems having this property or those influenced by it. This is not surprising since, as we have seen, science has so far been methodologically and conceptually limited to simple systems perceived as objects, whereas those living systems capable of being subjects are exceedingly complex.

It would be fruitless, not to say irrational, to suggest methodological or conceptual developments that will lead to a science of systems complex enough to have conscious awareness. Hard work and new discoveries are required for this progress to occur. It does seem worthwhile, however, to make a few comments about certain properties of the hierarchical organization of living systems. For a more thorough introduction to the topic, readers are referred to publications by Koestler,[22] Polanyi,[29] Weiss,[45] and Szentagothai and Arbib.[41]

By definition, a system is said to be hierarchically organized if, at each level of its organization, properties emerge that cannot be understood or predicted on the basis of information at the next lower level of organization. This, of course, precludes the hope that, by accumulating enough information about artificially isolated subsystems of the brain, a position can be reached where it can all be added together to yield an understanding of the whole brain. The concept of "boundary conditions"[29] defines relationships between different levels of organization. For example, the performance of an electronic computer in solving a mathematical problem cannot be understood on the basis of the physics of its

solid-state devices, nor even on the basis of the diagram of its circuitry, but only at the level of the program defining the sequence of steps in the computation. Each of these levels of organization provides boundary conditions within which the principles at the next lower level are allowed to operate. That is, the circuit design is not determined by the laws of physics, nor does it change the laws of physics, it merely provides a harness within which the laws of physics contribute to the function of the machine. Similarly, the software program is a boundary condition not explained by the circuit diagram, but providing limits within which the circuitry functions.

A further property of unique importance for living systems, distinguishing them from all machines and other nonliving systems, is that the elements of which they are composed "cooperate" to preserve the configuration of structure and behavior of the system. Weiss[45] writes:

The notion of 'cooperation' is, of course, a useful and excusable relapse into the analytic mental artifact of 'independence'; it really means that subunits, which always have been interrelated just *somehow*, now seem to follow a common pattern —some *integral guidance*. If outside their systemic domain they displayed a high degree of freedom, this freedom has within the assembled state become severely restricted by restraints that can only be described in reference to all the members of the group. At every instant, the behavior of any one component unit is affected in unique fashion by the behavior of all the others, which to an outside observer, of course, gives the impression as if they all had a common aim—stability— and knew how to attain it. Whenever one group of components of the system deviates fortuitously, or is made to deviate, from its standard course too far in one direction, the rest automatically change course in the reverse direction so as to counteract the distortion of the pattern of the whole. But, one may ask, how do they come to know what happens everywhere and anywhere in their crowd and how do they manage to react appropriately? [P. 14]

This remarkable capacity for the whole to recover from distortions through the redeployment of subunits characterizes every level of living hierarchical systems—from those within cells to those at the level of multicellular organisms functioning as whole animals.

Another problem is directly related to the need for science to advance from simple mechanisms to complex systems. This is the question of how the breadth and diversity of brain systems are integrated into the unitary quality so characteristic of conscious awareness. In part, at least, this problem is an artifact of the analytical approach that investigates artificially isolated subsystems of the brain, and as science progresses to higher levels of brain organization it may discover systems having a more unified functional quality, reflecting the convergence of many subsystems. It is a possibility, perhaps highly probable, that this convergence will involve communicational processes that transcend the structural and functional limits of brain circuitry as represented by transmission of action potentials over the system of axons, synapses, and dendrites. At any rate, it is clear that only a fraction of total brain activity is represented within the focus of attention at any moment, and that the contents of this fraction change from moment to moment so that, over time, many, but by no means all, brain activities can gain conscious representation. It is further clear that information defined at the level of brain physiology is translated and transformed through conscious representation into information defined at the level of the whole organism. That is, the frame of reference changes from what kind of inputs make a difference for the output of one or another brain system to the question of what environmental circumstances confront the adaptive behavioral resources of the animal. This requires the selection and synthesis of information from many different brain systems in order to reconstruct, on the basis of past experience and the current sensory input from the external and internal (bodily state) worlds, an integrated representation or model of the whole organism and its relationships in time and space to meaningful objects in the environment. Sherrington[35] contrasted the limited and mechanical adaptive value of a protective reflex with the flexibility introduced by conscious awareness:

A mental event, pain, superadded to a reflex, the protective reflex, seems here to reinforce and amplify the physical act. The local reflex itself affords its limited protection and relief, e.g., by holding the part taut and quiet. But the 'pain' through the mind can enjoin keeping the whole body motionless though tense. In ourselves, social and sophisticated, it may provoke the train of action of 'calling in' the doctor. In short, under the rubric 'pain' we meet mind moving matter to help mind in mind's distress. [P. 225]

It is not yet possible to guess how the transform from brain to conscious levels of information occurs, but there is no compelling reason to believe that the flexibility with which conscious awareness selectively and shiftingly integrates the outputs of so many brain processes depends upon the same connectionistic circuitry that mediates transactions between different areas of the brain. Indeed, the importance of action potentials and circuitry may have been greatly exaggerated by the adventitious fact that neurons are easier to find with the exploring electrode if they fire an action potential. For example, recent advances in the study of retinal physiology reveal that nonspike, slow potential processing of information is important in retinal circuitry from the receptor to the ganglion cell.[8] This discovery was facilitated by the fact that the retinal elements are more accessible to investigations than are brain cells, but since the retina is embryologically formed as an extension of the brain, these results suggest the possibility that nonaction potential processes may play a much more important role in the brain than has been suspected previously.

Certain requirements for a science of conscious experience have been suggested. Can science ever meet these requirements? Two considerations are critical. The first is that conscious awareness is private, so that its presence in other persons or in animals is only an inference. In principle, this problem will be resolved when the effects of conscious influences on brain systems have been discovered and specified. Consciousness would then be as observable as gravitational force, at least in principle. In the meantime, experimentation can proceed on the basis of assuming that other persons and higher animals are, indeed, as subject to conscious experience as the investigator himself.

The second consideration seems more ominous to me. The need to investigate more complex systems may require methods that become increasingly incompatible with life. Only future research can reveal how much of a hindrance to progress this will come to be.

❨ Brain Research and Conscious Experience

As we have seen, the classical frame of reference of science is mechanistic, and the explanatory logic of science deals with objects but cannot deal with subjects. In this section, a few examples will be given to illustrate the kind of problems faced by investigators attempting to deal with conscious experience in experimental programs.

Penfield has used electrical stimulation to examine mind-brain relationships in more than one thousand conscious human patients undergoing craniotomy under local anesthesia.[27,28] He suggests[25] that conscious attentive states "program" the developing brain:

Each man 'programs' his own brain by focusing and altering his attention, especially in childhood. In a sense, each individual mind is creating the brain mechanisms, establishing the brain connections that are functional. He does this by the selection of things to which he attends. It is easier to think of it during the earlier years of childhood. The child is establishing the functional pattern of connections. If the brain is tested later by electrical stimulation, it becomes evident that he has done one thing in one part of his cortex and another thing in another. In a sense, the child's mind is stepping in and creating the machinery of the brain. [P. 248]

With electrical testing of the waking brain, Penfield[26,27,28] has identified a system of "interpretive cortex," the electrical stimulation of which evokes a stream of conscious experience. This may take two forms:[26]

Either he is aware of a sudden alteration in his interpretation of present experience (what he sees and hears seems suddenly familiar, or strange, or frightening, or coming closer or going away, etc.), or, he has a sudden 'flashback', an awareness of some previous experience.

Although he is still aware of where he is, an earlier experience comes to him and the stream of that former consciousness moves forward again in full detail as it did in some previous period of time. . . .

The sudden interpretation of the present and the flashback of the past are evidently parts of a scanning mechanism that normally enables an individual to compare present experience with similar past experience automatically. [P. 221]

If the neural activities evoked by this type of electrical stimulation could be defined, it would be a considerable step toward identifying the type of functional brain systems having the property of conscious awareness. Unfortunately, stimulation at a cortical point induces widespread cortical and subcortical activities, so that defining them would require animal experiments; but in these, reports of the evoked conscious experience would not be available.

Another type of observation reported by Penfield[26] involves blocking of the speech mechanism by electrical stimulation of the cortex without impairing the patient's capacity for perception and reasoning. During electrical stimulation of the posterior speech area, a patient remained silent when shown a picture of a butterfly, which he knew he was supposed to name aloud.

After withdrawal of the electrode, he exclaimed as though with relief: "Now I can talk, butterfly!" Then he added, "I couldn't get that word butterfly" and then I tried to get the word "moth."

The speech mechanism had failed when called upon. To his surprise, he found himself aphasic. If he had not tried to speak, he would not have known that he was aphasic. [P. 230]

In this instance, a visual stimulus evokes a nonverbal percept of a butterfly, and an intention by the patient to label the percept with a word. On the basis of extensive experience with circumscribed cortical excisions, Penfield concludes that this nonverbal idea of a butterfly, and the intention to name it, arise from diencephalic centers. "The initiating demand arriving at the speech area must come from the diencephalon, whether it is an idea calling for a word or a word calling for the idea."[26]

The fact that the idea of a butterfly arises through a neural system separate from that subserving the word by which the idea is labelled is, of course, a long way from understanding the functional neural systems that have the property of being aware of the idea and of the word; but, at the same time, such observations are a beginning.

In another type of research, the central mechanisms mediating voluntary movement are being investigated with new experimental methods for recording from conscious animals making reflex movements, stimulus-triggered movements and spontaneously initiated movements.[11] For example, Evarts[12] describes a monkey fitted with devices for immobilizing the head so that microelectrode recordings from pyramidal tract neurons can be made while the animal grasps a handle and makes certain movements in response to visual stimuli. Through standard operant conditioning techniques, the animal can be trained to make very complex movements, holding the handle in a certain position, or exerting a certain force, or pushing or pulling it. A microelectrode is lowered through motor cortex, while electrical stimuli are applied via implanted electrodes to the medullary pyramidal tract, so that cortical pyramidal tract neurons can be identified by the fact that antidromic spikes are evoked.

Important features of this experimental paradigm are that the responses of one neuron can be recorded during many repetitions of the same motor act, and many different neurons can be recorded during very similar motor movements. Comparisons can be made between neurons in the precentral motor cortex and those in the postcentral cortex, as well as between neuronal response during 'spontaneous' as contrasted with stimulus-triggered movements. During tasks of the 'reaction-time' type, time intervals can be measured between visual stimulus and motor-cortical response, and between motor cortex and the movement measured electromyographically. It can be determined whether a particular neuron's response is temporally locked to the stimulus or to the motor response, and whether the pattern of its response differs as a function of the type movement (e.g., some neurons respond differently when the monkey pulls the lever than when he pushes, etc.).

In experiments of this kind, the possibility exists for observing differences in neural mechanisms as a function of variables such as attention, intention, and learning, so that even though only isolated mechanisms are observed, each of these mechanistically seen subsystems represents a glimpse of part of the complex systems having the conscious properties characteristic of the waking brain. For example, Fetz and Finocchio[14] report that the relationship between activity in a precentral cortical cell and a motor response can be disassociated through the use of operant conditioning techniques. A precentral cell, activity of which had been correlated with a specific muscle response, began to fire in bursts without its correlated electromyographic response after a period of training in which reinforcement was contingent on activity in that cortical cell with simultaneous suppression of all muscle activity. In other words, the monkey learned to disrupt the physiological correlation between a particular cortical motor neuron and a specific muscle response. It seems probable that this flexibility is dependent upon the fact that one cortical cell, seen in relative isolation, is but a small component in the complex cellular systems underlying motor activity.

A final example of the experimental approach to conscious experience is the study of human subjects in whom the main communication systems between the two cerebral hemispheres (corpus callosum, anterior commissure, hippocampal commissure, and massa intermedia) have been surgically interrupted. Sperry[37,38] and his group have been studying such "split brain" animals and humans for some years, using techniques whereby stimulus inputs, whether visual or tactile, reach one cerebral hemisphere but not the other. For example, for both eyes, a stimulus in the left half field, presented tachistoscopically to prevent scanning eye movements, reaches only the right hemisphere, whereas a stimulus in the right half field reaches only the left hemisphere. In right-handed persons, the dominant (left) hemisphere can express itself in speaking, but the minor (right) hemisphere, is mute. By the use of nonverbal testing procedures, the mute hemisphere can report on its experiences much as an aphasic patient can. For example, a tactile form presented, out of sight, to the left hand, can be selected from a set of different forms by the left hand, but not by the right hand. Questioning reveals that the dominant left hemisphere doesn't know what form the left hand, controlled by the right hemisphere, has identified.

Two parallel tasks can be accomplished simultaneously, without interference, and with no awareness in one hemisphere of what the other hemisphere is doing. If the number "5" is flashed in the left half field simultaneously with a "7" in the right half field, the two hands, out of sight, can retrieve the corresponding tactile forms simultaneously, a "5" by the left hand, and a "7" by the right hand. If questioned, the subject will be able to identify only the "7" picked up by the right hand on the basis of information in the left (speaking) hemisphere.

Complementary specialization of each of the hemispheres for particular types of information processing (e.g., recognition of faces, unfamiliar forms, etc.) was investigated by using "chimeric" stimuli that result in simultaneous parallel processing of two different inputs.[23] These stimuli are made up of two different half pictures, split vertically down the middle. For example, a chimeric "face" is made up of the left half of one person's face adjoined to the right half of another person's face. For the split-brain subject, each half face is filled in by a process of "perceptual completion," so that one hemisphere perceives one face while the other hemisphere sees the other face. When questioned, the subjects were unaware of anything peculiar about the stimuli, even though with nonverbal responding (pointing to a set of pictures from which the chimeric picture had been constructed) it was clear that each hemisphere had recognized a different face.

Sperry concludes from these results that there are two separate spheres of conscious awareness running in parallel in each of the two hemispheres, particularly with regard to visual, tactile, and auditory information processing. Certain aspects of consciousness (e.g., sleep–wakefulness, hunger) are mediated by brainstem mechanisms that affect both hemispheres.

The inference that the minor (mute) hemisphere subserves conscious awareness is supported not only by the kind of information processing of which it is capable (e.g., facial recognition, pattern recognition) but also by evidence that it responds emotionally. Sperry[38] writes:

The minor hemisphere also seems to demonstrate appropriate emotional reactions, as for example, when a pin-up shot of a nude is interjected by surprise into a series of neutral or nonemotional stimuli being flashed to right and left visual fields at random. The subject under these conditions will characteristically say that he or she saw nothing, just a white light, as regularly happens for stimuli projected into the left field. However, one may then notice an inner grin beginning to spread over the subject's features which then lingers and carries over through the next couple of trials or so. It may also cause blushing and giggling and affect the tone of voice coming from the major side. If one then asks the subject what he is grinning about, the reply suggests that the talking hemisphere has no idea what it was that turned him on. He may say something like, 'That's some machine you have there!' or 'Wowee—that light!' Apparently the emotional tone alone gets across to the speaking hemisphere as if the cognitive aspect could not be articulated through the brainstem. [P. 319]

These results are not congruent with the traditional view that only unitary persons have conscious experience. For the split-brain person, choices made on the basis of information available only to one hemisphere are unknown to the other hemisphere, suggesting that each hemisphere is an adequate neural substrate for conscious awareness.

On the basis of his research with animals and humans, Sperry[39] has postulated that conscious processes play a causal role in brain function. In response to questions by Bindra,[5]

Sperry[40] further clarifies some of the issues involved in such a postulated functional role for conscious experience, differentiating his concept from dualistic notions, psychoneural interactionism, the theory that subjective phenomena are "identical" with neural activity, and the gestalt concept of parallelistic isomorphism.

It seems obvious from these few examples that as neuroscience research has begun to approach conscious experience more directly, it is increasingly handicapped by the analytical and mechanistic approach. As methods for approaching conscious phenomena in physiological experiments are improved, conceptual developments will become increasingly necessary. History suggests that this necessity will be the mother of invention, and that conceptualizations will be developed in the neurosciences that encompass more and more complex systems, including those having conscious awareness as an emergent property.

(Concluding Remarks

The materialistic and mechanistic frame of reference, of nineteenth- and early twentieth-century science, has been examined with reference to the problem of conscious experience. It is emphasized that science itself is a product of conscious experience, and that the dichotomy between the observer and the observed that characterizes conscious experience has been impressed upon the classical materialistic model of reality, thereby consigning conscious experience to nonreality by excluding it from scientific reality. Logical and factual weaknesses in the mechanistic concept of man and conscious experience are reviewed, and a critique is given of the analogy between electronic computers and brains, especially insofar as it holds that machine performance is already a primitive step toward machines with conscious awareness. Some conceptual requirements for a science of conscious experience are suggested, especially the need to discover the relationships existing between complex hierarchically organized brain systems and the

property of conscious awareness. The logic of cause and effect that treats living subjects as if they were only objects analytically dissected into artificially isolated simple mechanisms is contrasted with the conceptual requirements for understanding those extraordinarily complex, living systems that manifest conscious awareness. Examples from neuroscience research are given to illustrate how, as investigators become more directly concerned with conscious phenomena, the inadequacies of the classical materialistic doctrine are increasingly troublesome, giving rise to the search for better conceptual systems.

(Bibliography

1. BARONDES, S. H. "Axoplasmic Transport," in F. O. Schmitt, T. Melnechuk, G. C. Quarton et al., eds., *Neurosciences Research Symposium Summaries*, pp. 191–299. Cambridge: MIT Press, 1969.
2. BASS, L. and W. J. MOORE. "A Proteolytic Memory Element Based on the Integrating Function of the Neuron," *Brain Res.*, 33 (1971), 451–462.
3. BENSON, I. "Machines That Mimic Thought," *N. Scient. Sci. J.*, 51 (1971), 525–528.
4. BERRY, R. W. "Ribonucleic Acid Metabolism of a Single Neuron: Correlation with Electrical Activity," *Science*, 166 (1969), 1021–1023.
5. BINDRA, D. "The Problem of Subjective Experience: Puzzlement on Reading R. W. Sperry's 'A Modified Concept of Consciousness,'" *Psychol. Rev.*, 77 (1970), 581–584.
6. BOHR, N. *Atomic Physics and Human Knowledge.* New York: Science Editions, 1961.
7. DE ROBERTIS, E. "Molecular Biology of Synaptic Receptors," *Science*, 171 (1971), 963–971.
8. DOWLING, J. E. and F. S. WERBLIN. "Synaptic Organization of the Vertebrate Retina," in T. Shipley and J. E. Dowling, eds., *Visual Processes in Vertebrates.* Vis. Res. Suppl. No. 3. Oxford: Pergamon, 1971.
9. ECCLES, J. C. *Brain and Conscious Experience.* New York: Springer-Verlag, 1966.
10. EDDS, M. V., D. S. BARKELEY, and D. M. FAMBROUGH. "Genesis of Neuronal Pat-

terns," *Neurosci. Res. Program Bull.*, 10 (1972), 253–367.

11. EVARTS, E. V., E. BIZZI, R. E. BURKE et al. "Central Control of Movement," *Neurosci. Res. Program Bull.*, 9 (1971), 1–170.

12. EVARTS, E. V. "Central Processing of Sensory Input Leading to Motor Output," in F. O. Schmitt and F. G. Worden, eds., *The Neurosciences: Third Study Program.* Cambridge: M.I.T. Press, 1974.

13. FAMBROUGH, D. M. and H. C. HARTZELL. "Acetylcholine Receptors: Number and Distribution at Neuromuscular Junctions in Rat Diaphragm," *Science*, 176 (1972), 189–191.

14. FETZ, E. G. and D. V. FINOCCHIO. "Operant Conditioning of Isolated Activity in Specific Muscles and Precentral Cells," *Brain Res.*, 40 (1972), 19–23.

15. GISIGER, V. "Triggering of RNA Synthesis by Acetylcholine Stimulation of the Postsynaptic Membrane in a Mammalian Sympathetic Ganglion," *Brain Res.*, 33 (1971), 139–146.

16. GISIGER, V. and A-C GAIDE-HUGUENIN. "Effect of Preganglionic Stimulation Upon RNA Synthesis in the Isolated Sympathetic Ganglion of the Rat," *Prog. Brain Res.*, 31 (1969), 125–129.

17. GOOD, I. J. "Human and Machine Intelligence: Comparisons and Contrasts," *Impact Sci. Soc.*, 21 (1971), 305–322.

18. GUNTRIP, H. "The Concept of Psychodynamic Science," *Int. J. Psychoanal.*, 48 (1967), 32–43.

19. HAMMES, G. G., P. B. MOLINOFF, and F. E. BLOCM. "Receptor Biophysics and Biochemistry," *Neurosci. Res. Program Bull.*, 11 (1973), 161–294.

20. HEISENBERG, W. "The Representation of Nature in Contemporary Physics," *Daedalus*, 87 (1958), 95–108.

21. HOME, H. J. M. "The Concept of Mind," *Int. J. Psychoanal.*, 47 (1966), 42–49.

22. KOESTLER, A. *The Ghost in the Machine.* New York: Macmillan, 1967.

23. LEVY, J., C. TREVARTHEN, and R. W. SPERRY. "Perception of Bilateral Chimeric Figures Following Hemispheric Deconnexion," *Brain*, 95 (1972), 61–78.

24. MACH, E. "The Economy of Science," in James R. Newman, ed., *The World of Mathematics*, Vol. 3, pp. 1787–1797. New York: Simon & Schuster, 1956.

25. PENFIELD, W. "Comments in Discussion," in John C. Eccles, ed., *Brain and Conscious Experience*, p. 248. New York: Springer-Verlag, 1966.

26. ———. "Speech, Perception, and the Uncommitted Cortex," in J. C. Eccles, ed., *Brain and Conscious Experience*, pp. 217–237. New York: Springer-Verlag, 1966.

27. ———. "Epilepsy, Neurophysiology, and Some Brain Mechanisms Related to Consciousness," in H. H. Jasper, A. A. Ward, and A. Pope, eds., *Basic Mechanisms of the Epilepsies*, pp. 791–805. Boston: Little, Brown, 1969.

28. PENFIELD, W. and P. PEROT. "The Brain's Record of Auditory and Visual Experience," *Brain*, 86 (1963), 595–696.

29. POLANYI, M. "Life's Irreducible Structure," *Science*, 160 (1968), 1308–1312.

30. POPPER, K. R. *Conjectures and Refutations: The Growth of Scientific Knowledge.* New York: Harper Torch Books. Harper and Row, 1968.

31. PYSH, J. J. and R. G. WILEY. "Morphologic Alterations of Synapses in Electrically Stimulated Superior Cervical Ganglia of the Cat," *Science*, 176 (1972), 191–193.

32. RALL, T. W. and A. G. GILMAN. "The Role of Cyclic AMP in the Nervous System," *Neurosci. Res. Program Bull.*, 8 (1970), 221–323.

33. SCHADE, J. P. and J. SMITH. eds. *Computers and Brains.* Progress in Brain Research, Vol. 33, New York: Elsevier, 1970.

34. SCHIMKE, R. T. "Principles Underlying the Regulation of Synthesis and Degradation of Proteins in Animal Tissues," in F. O. Schmitt and F. G. Worden, eds., *The Neurosciences: Third Study Program*, pp. 813–825. Cambridge: MIT Press, 1974.

35. SHERRINGTON, C. *Man On His Nature*, 2nd ed. London: Cambridge University Press, 1953.

36. SINGER, S. J. and L. J. ROTHFIELD. "Synthesis and Turnover of Cell Membranes," *Neurosci. Res. Program Bull.*, 11 (1973), 1–86.

37. SPERRY, R. W. "Brain Bisection and Mechanisms of Consciousness," in J. C. Eccles, ed., *Brain and Conscious Experience*, pp. 298–313. New York: Springer-Verlag, 1966.

38. ———. "Mental Unity Following Surgical Disconnection of the Cerebral Hemispheres," in *The Harvey Lectures, Series 62*, pp. 293–323. New York: Academic, 1968.

39. ———. "A Modified Concept of Consciousness," *Psychol. Rev.*, 76 (1969), 532–536.

40. ———. "An Objective Approach to Subjective Experience: Further Explanation of a Hypothesis," *Psychol. Rev.*, 77 (1970), 585–590.

41. SZENTAGOTHAI, J. and M. A. ARBIB. "Conceptual Models of Neural Organization," *Neurosci. Res. Program Bull.*, 12 (1974), 305–510.

42. TURING, A. M. "Can A Machine Think?," in James R. Newman, ed., *The World of Mathematics*, Vol. 4, pp. 2099–2123. New York: Simon & Schuster, 1956.

43. WEISS, P. A. "Depolarization: Pointers to Conceptual Disarmament," *Stud. Gen.*, 23 (1970), 925–940.

44. ———. *Hierarchically Organized Systems in Theory and Practice*. New York: Hafner, 1971.

45. ———. "The Basic Concept of Hierarchic Systems," in P. Weiss, ed., *Hierarchically Organized Systems in Theory and Practice*, pp. 1–43. New York: Hafner, 1971.

46. WEIZENBAUM, J. "On the Impact of the Computer on Society," *Science*, 176 (1972), 609–614.

47. WIGNER, E. P. "Remarks on the Mind-Body Problem," in I. J. Good, ed., *The Scientist Speculates*, pp. 284–302. New York: Basic Books, 1962.

48. WOOLDRIDGE, D. E. *The Machinery of the Brain*. New York: McGraw-Hill, 1963.

49. ———. *The Machinery of Life*. New York: McGraw-Hill, 1966.

50. ———. *Mechanical Man, The Physical Basis of Intelligent Life*. New York: McGraw-Hill, 1968.

51. WORDEN, F. G. "Questions About Man's Attempt To Understand Himself," in Robert R. Holt and Emanuel Peterfreund, eds., *Psychoanalysis and Contemporary Science*, Vol. 1, pp. 38–59. New York: Macmillan, 1972.

CHAPTER 10

SELF-EVALUATIONS OF COMPETENCE AND WORTH IN ADULTHOOD*

Chad Gordon, Charles M. Gaitz, and Judith Scott

❲ Theoretical Orientation and Objectives

PREVIOUS THEORY and research on personal self-evaluation has generally focused on an extremely general and abstract dimension, usually termed self-esteem. The ambiguity of this global concept has led to very little solid research establishing sizable and dependable relationships between self-evaluation and important social-structural circumstances, attitudinal correlates, or consequences

* This research was partially supported by NIMH Grant No. MH 15708. Computer services were provided by the Common Research Computer Facility, Texas Medical Center, Houston, Texas, supported by USPHS Grant No. RR 00524, and the Institute of Computer Sciences, Baylor College of Medicine, Houston, supported by NIH Grant No. RR 00259.

for subsequent conduct. Even where some more specific aspect of self-evaluation (such as "competence" or "self-acceptance") has been tapped in an empirical study, the researcher often simply equates this particular dimension with general "self-esteem." Thus the literature now contains apparently discrepant and contradictory findings, relating diverse versions of "self-esteem" to important social and individual variables, especially regarding the development of self-esteem over the course of the life cycle.

Our purpose here is to offer a more differentiated theoretical approach to self-evaluation, in which four qualitatively different dimensions are distinguished: competence, self-determination, unity, and moral worth. We will then turn to analysis of empirical evidence from a recent survey to show how two of these evaluative dimensions (competence and moral worth) have quite different patterns of relation to life-cycle stage. Finally, we will attempt to show the differential impact on the senses of competence and moral worth of three of the social-structural parameters that have most often been suggested as crucial to all forms of self-conception development over the life cycle: sex, ethnic group, and socio-economic status.

Background

Self-esteem (defined as the most global and general evaluative dimension of self-conception) has been a continuing element of major importance throughout the development of the philosophy of consciousness, humanistic psychology, and the symbolic interactionist branch of sociology. William James, James Baldwin, and George Herbert Mead brought philosophical perspectives to the early study of reflexive evaluation.[17] Adler,[1] Horney,[19] Fromm,[8] Rogers,[35] Sarbin,[40] Sullivan,[43] Maslow,[27] and Coopersmith[4] are among the strongest of the psychological contributors. Sociological analysis more and more frequently in recent years has dealt with the relation of self-esteem to social structure and social interaction.[*]

Regardless of theoretical persuasion, the essential element in each of these conceptualizations is that individuals develop a generalized and pervasive evaluative self-assessment, abstracted from the indefinitely large number of "identity fragments" concerning any of the person's self-conceived characteristics, attributes, memberships, identifications, roles, values, beliefs, abilities, problems, goals, etc.

[*] See references 41, 36, 37, 9, 10, 12, and 15.

Many of these more concrete aspects of self-conception have been discussed and analyzed in other writings.[10,12]

As an alternative approach, however, four "systemic senses of self" have been proposed[10,11,12] as *intermediate in level of generality* between the particular identity fragments and the most global form, self-esteem. In brief, Gordon proposed that a distinct dimension of self-evaluation corresponds to each of the "system problems" that every person (as a functioning system) must face.[30,31,32,33] Further, Gordon has asserted that each of these four "systemic senses of self" is engendered, supported, and maintained by one of four distinct forms of social reward. Specifically, it is argued that the sense of *competence* is nurtured by social approval for valued performance; the sense of *self-determination* is engendered and maintained by social responsiveness and direct consummatory gratification; the sense of *unity* derives from social acceptance; and the sense of *moral worth* emerges from expressions of respect in relation to generalized cultural-value ethics.[13,14] Thus the theoretical orientation guiding this analysis assumes the correspondence as shown in the table below. This theoretical approach formulates an individual's level of global self-esteem as largely determined by his particular current positions on these more specific dimensions, combined with the relative weight he assigns to each.

Hypothesized Determinants of the Various Self-Evaluations

Theory and research on the development of self-conceptions have generally focused on direct interactive rewards *or* on social-structural circumstances. Such elements as family composition, ethnic group, socioeconomic status, occupational situation, or condition as a la-

SYSTEM PROBLEM	SYSTEMIC SENSE OF SELF	INTERACTIVE SYMBOLIC REWARD
Adaptation	COMPETENCE	Approval
Goal-attainment	SELF-DETERMINATION	Response/Gratification
Integration	UNITY	Acceptance
Pattern maintenance	MORAL WORTH	Respect

beled "deviant" are presumed to shape and control the pattern of interactive rewards, and at only one particular stage in the life cycle.[17] Childhood has received much more attention than has adolescence and socialization to particular occupations, while self-conception changes in middle age and old age have received least attention of all.[28] The books by Bühler,[3] Erikson[7] and Lidz[25] are preeminent among the very few that attempt to deal with the different stages of the life cycle. Even these comprehensive works presume to characterize developmental patterns typical only of contemporary, urban, white middle- or upper-middle-class Americans. Gordon's recent effort at integration and social-psychological reformulation of these and other authors' ideas on life-cyle stages[14] is no exception to this restricted perspective (see Table 10–1).

Present Objective

Our primary goal is to ascertain the unique and combined effects on selected dimensions of self-evaluation of three major structural characteristics (sex, ethnic group, and socioeconomic status) in combination with life-cycle stage. No research has yet been conducted on the immensely complicated interconnections of social characteristics and life-cycle stage as these operate through explicitly measured interactive sanctions to raise or lower self-evaluations among an adequate sample of persons. A study of the relation of leisure and mental health, done in Houston, Texas, in 1969, was designed to provide representative sampling with regard to sex, ethnic group, and occupational status as well as age. The survey interview measured two of the four systemic senses of self-outlined above: competence and moral worth.

Thus, the specific objective of the present analysis is to portray the levels of sensed moral worth and several forms of sensed competence in groups currently at different stages in the life cycle. In addition, the unique and combined impact of sex, ethnic group, socioeconomic status and life-cycle stage in determining the level of each aspect of self-evaluation will be assessed. Before offering detailed

rationales and hypotheses, the Houston study will be described.

(The Leisure Mental-Health and Life-Cycle Survey

A structured interview concerning leisure activities, value preferences, social attitudes, and various aspects of mental health was administered to a sample of adults in Houston, Texas, during the period of November 1969 to February 1970. The interview guide and sampling plan were designed by Dr. Sally Hacker, a sociologist trained by the Committee on Human Development at the University of Chicago and now teaching at Drake University. The National Opinion Research Center recruited and trained the interviewers, pretested the interview guide, selected the sample, supervised the field work, coded the interviews, and processed the data to the point of providing initial frequency distributions.

Study Design

The sample included 1,441 persons and was stratified according to sex, ethnicity, family occupational status level, and age group. The latter three dimensions require elaboration.

Ethnicity. Respondents were drawn from Houston's three major ethnic groups—Anglo, black, and Mexican American. It should be noted that interviewers were matched with respondents as regards ethnicity, an important procedure that is frequently advocated but rarely accomplished.[20]

Family occupational status level. After the interviewers had obtained information from the respondent concerning the current and previous occupations of all working members of the family, the family itself was designated as being of "lower" or "higher" occupational status. Occupations requiring little formal training were defined as "lower status," and generally included operative, semiskilled, laboring, and service jobs. Skilled crafts, clerical, sales, professional, and managerial occupations were generally defined as "higher status," depending upon the specific nature of the work. It should be noted that this procedure provided enough "higher-status" cases for analysis in the minority samples, but had the effect of overrepresenting "lower-status" Anglo respondents in comparison to what would have been found in a strictly random sample of Houston adults. This overrepresentation of lower-status families among the Anglos was increased by matching Anglo neighborhoods as closely as possible to minority neighborhoods on the basis of socioeconomic indicators from the 1960 census.

TABLE 10–1. Stage Developmental Model of the Ideal-Typical Life Cycle in Contemporary, Urban, Middle-Class America—Giving Approximate Ages, the Most Significant Other Persons, and the Major Dilemmas of Value-Theme Differentiation and Integration

LIFE-CYCLE STAGE	APPROXIMATE AGES	MOST SIGNIFICANT OTHERS	MAJOR DILEMMA OF VALUE-THEME DIFFERENTIATION AND INTEGRATION *Security/Challenge*
1. Infancy	0–12 months	mother	Affective gratification/ sensorimotor experiencing
2. Early childhood	1–2 years	mother, father	Compliance/self-control
3. Oedipal period	3–5 years	father, mother, siblings, playmates	Expressivity/instrumentality
4. Later childhood	6–11 years	parents, same sex peers, teachers	Peer relationships/ evaluated abilities
5. Early adolescence	12–15 years	parents, same sex peers, opposite sex peers, teachers	Acceptance/achievement
6. Later adolescence	16–20 years	same sex peers, opposite sex peers, parents, teachers, loved one, wife or husband	Intimacy/autonomy
7. Young adulthood	21–29 years	loved one, husband or wife, children, employers, friends	Connection/self-determination
8. Early maturity	30–44 years	wife or husband, children, superiors, colleagues, friends, parents	Stability/accomplishment
9. Full maturity	45 to retirement age	wife or husband, children, colleagues, friends, younger associates	Dignity/control
10. Old age	Retirement age to death	remaining family, long-term friends, neighbors	Meaningful integration/autonomy

Age group and life–cycle stage. Approximately two hundred forty respondents were chosen for each of six age groups (20 to 29, 30 to 39, 40 to 54, 55 to 64, 65 to 74, 75 to 94 years). This procedure obviously resulted in an overrepresentation of people in older age groups, but it had the benefit of providing enough cases to permit analysis of the life situations of these persons, which were of great theoretical and humane interest. For purposes of analysis, these six age groups were collapsed into five categories more closely approximating the life-cycle stages proposed by one of the present authors:[14]

AGE GROUP	LIFE-CYCLE STAGE	NUMBER OF RESPONDENTS
20–29	7. Young adult	248
30–44	8. Early maturity	308
45–64	9. Full maturity	425
65–74	10. Old age	242
75–94	11. Very old age	218
	Total sample	1,441

These chronologically defined groups are taken to represent (in at least a rough way) the periods of (7) job and family connection establishment, (8) occupational and child-raising accomplishment, (9) occupational leveling off and empty nest period, (10) the role-relinquishment period, and (11) the period of physical decline. More detailed treatment should use these sociological-stage positions directly rather than using the less complex but also less valid approach through chronological age.[29]

Taken together, the four dimensions (sex, ethnicity, status level, and age group) yielded seventy-two cells, each containing about twenty respondents. While the quotas were fully met for the Anglo and black samples, Mexican-Americans are slightly underrepresented because of difficulties in locating a sufficient number of older, higher-status Mexican-Americans.

After census tracts were drawn on the basis of ethnicity and indicators of socioeconomic status, block sampling was used to locate individuals within the quota requirements. The total sample of 1,441 persons is not intended to represent Houston as a whole nor all of contemporary urban America. It does, however, adequately represent each of the seventy-two cells of the design, and has the important advantage of providing sufficient cases in all of the empirically sparse but theoretically interesting cells. This claimed representativeness is of course only within the context of Houston, but this city itself typifies the kind of dynamic and rapidly changing urban center in which questions of leisure and psychological well-being are becoming quite pressing.

Self-Evaluation Dimensions

The study included a wide range of relatively specific self-evaluation dimensions. The following measures were included:

1. Leisure competence index
2. Work skills self-rating
3. Self-rated intelligence
4. Self-satisfaction rating

Leisure Competence Index

One major segment of the study had to do with a broad range of activities in the home or in leisure pursuits outside the home and away from the regular course of work. Specific interview items enabled the respondent to rate his skill regarding seventeen different leisure activities.[18] The scale included the responses: "not good," "average," and "good," which were evaluated numerically from one for the least competent-appearing answer to three for the most competent answer, and then combined into a *leisure-competence index* by the indicator-mean procedure.[14,15] Using this procedure the mean of the scores of the seventeen indicators was computed and then multiplied by ten, rounded to remove decimal fractions, and then reduced by ten so as to produce a final range of scores between zero and twenty. Where any of the seventeen indicators were unanswered, the averaging procedure simply increased slightly the proportional contribution of the other indicators. A minimum of twelve of the seventeen indicators, however, was required for a respondent to have a leisure-competence score. The resulting score is taken as a measure of competence in the sphere of *personal expressivity* (our definition of leisure).[16]

The seventeen competence items and their part-whole correlations with the leisure-competence index were:

.58 Skill at understanding and discussing local or national problems.

.57 Skill at trip planning—making reservations, buying tickets, figuring route, etc.

.57 Skill at sports for someone your age.

.56 Skill at leading or speaking out at clubs or organizations.

.55 Skill at being a good follower, getting work done, encouraging others in clubs and organizations.

.52 Skill in camping, fishing, hiking, or any outing in the country or at the beach.

.50 Knowledge about art or music.

.50 Skill at drawing, singing, playing an instrument.

.48 Skill at talking with people, being sociable.

.48 Skill at dancing.

.47 Knowledge about players, performers, or teams in the world of sports.

.38 Skill at sewing, mending, decorating, fixing, building, or working in the yard.

.38 Skill at cooking, baking, barbecuing for family or friends. (Intended as a measure of "party" or "gourmet" cooking expressivity.)

.37 Skill at being a drinking companion.

.31 Skill at housework.

.27 Skill at managing the needs of your family.

.24 Skill at finding satisfying things to do when alone.

Work Skills Self-Rating

The respondent was also asked to rate himself on work skills by the question: "In terms of getting or holding a job now, would you say your work or job skills are excellent, good, fair, or poor?" This single item is taken to represent *instrumental competence*. The overall distribution for the sample was:

work skills rating

26% excellent
33% good
20% fair
21% poor
100%

(1,419) (Twenty-two gave no answer to this interview question.)

Self-Rated Intelligence

The respondents rated their general intelligence on a four-point scale, ranging from "not very high" through "about average" and "pretty high" to "very high." The following distribution resulted:

self-rated intelligence

7% very high
12% pretty high
71% about average
10% not very high
100%

(1,426) (Fifteen gave no answer to this question.)

Self-Satisfaction Rating—A Weak Version of "Moral Worth"

Finally, the interview contained the question: "*How do you feel about yourself as a person*—pretty good, just okay, could be better, or not so good?" Although quite vague and indirect, this item is the only one in the interview that is at all concerned with the dimension of moral worth (being "good" rather than "good at" something). The distribution of responses to this admittedly slim moral-worth item was:

self-satisfaction rating

47% pretty good
23% just okay
28% could be better
2% not so good
100%

(1,440) (One respondent gave no answer.)

The responses to each of the single-item measures were assigned the numerical value 1, 2, 3 or 4, with the most favorable-to-self response receiving the highest value, and the same was done with the quartile groups on the leisure-competence index. Our analyses were carried out on the correlations of these four-point scales with each other and with the independent variables.

We used the logic of four-way analysis of variance on the dependent variables, even though it is explicitly recognized that these scales do not meet the assumption of an equal interval between any pair of adjacent points. Any measurement error introduced by the restricted score range and by unequal intervals tends to *understate* magnitudes of relationship

and inferred probabilities in the statistical analyses that follow, and are thus conservative in nature. We can assume that improved measurement of the variables would produce results at least as strong as the present ones. The power and parsimony of these multivariate procedures are simply felt to outweigh doubts about the measurement levels.

The interested reader will find information on the construct validation of our measures in the Technical Appendix to this chapter.

Inspection of the intercorrelations of these four scores (presented at the bottom of Table 10–2 reveals that they are tapping quite dis-

TABLE 10–2.   **Correlations of Four Self-Evaluations with Mental-Health Measures and with Each Other**

MENTAL-HEALTH MEASURES	LEISURE COMPETENCE INDEX	SELF-RATED INTELLIGENCE	SELF-RATED WORK SKILLS	SENSE OF SELF-SATISFACTION
Positive Affect Score	.32***	.10***	.07**	.03
Negative Affect Score	−.10***	−.08**	−.14***	−.22***
Twenty-two Item Symptom Score	−.23***	−.15***	−.24***	−.28***
Anxiety Items Score	−.17***	−.13***	−.18***	−.28***
Depressed Items Score	−.22***	−.10***	−.25***	−.16***
Somatic Items Score	−.12***	−.04	−.12***	−.16***
Self-rated Happiness	.22***	.13***	.18***	.24***
Self-evaluation Intercorrelations:				
Leisure Competence	1.00	.41***	.37***	.15***
Self-rated Intelligence	.41***	1.00	.21***	.16***
Work Skills	.37***	.21***	1.00	.11***
Self-satisfaction	.15***	.16***	.11***	1.00
Average Intercorrelation	.31	.26	.23	.14

NOTE: See Technical Appendix for discussion of the mental-health measures and of our construct validation procedures.

Three asterisks indicate statistical significance beyond the .001 level, two asterisks indicate significance beyond the .01 level and one asterisk designates the .05 level of confidence that a given correlation was not produced by chance sampling fluctuation from a population in which there is actually a zero correlation between the variables. It should be noted that samples as large as ours (1,441) will show these levels of "statistical significance" on correlations yielding very little predictive or explanatory power.

tinct and different facets of self-evaluation. The leisure-competence index shows the strongest relationships to the others, especially with the other forms of competence ($+.41$ with self-rated intelligence and $+.37$ with work skills). Self-satisfaction has a consistent positive but very weak relation to the forms of competence ($+.11$ with work skills, $+.15$ with leisure competence and $+.16$ with self-rated intelligence). We will report our findings at first for the four self-conceptions separately, and then will focus on a combined instrumental/expressive competence measure as contrasted with the self-satisfaction dimension.

❰ Hypotheses

For each of the dependent variables (leisure-competence index, work-skills rating, self-rated intelligence, and sense of self-satisfaction), specific predictions can be made in relation to life-cycle stage and each of the social-structural variables (sex, ethnicity, and occupational status). However, the major thrust of the present paper is directed to analysis of the unique and combined impact of life-cycle stage and the other three independent variables when they are simultaneously brought into relation with each of the self-evaluations in turn.

The necessity and wisdom of this combined and interactive approach was demonstrated by one of the very few studies that related age to some form of self-evaluation, and simultaneously took into account additional factors that theoretically should condition the relationship. Kaplan and Pokorny[22] reviewed a number of studies that had indicated a negative association between age and "self-derogation" (suggested as stemming in part from lessened feelings of role inadequacy as burdensome roles are relinquished). Other studies showed no relationship between age and self-derogation, while still others found a *positive* pattern of association. Using the Rosenberg[36] self-attitude items, Kaplan and Pokorny demonstrated that the older respondents (sixty or above) evidenced *less* self-

derogation than did younger respondents in a survey of five hundred adults living in Houston, but *only if* the respondents were free from one or more of the following disturbing influences:

Aging was observed to be associated with lower self-derogation where the Ss: (1) reported no recent life experiences requiring behavioral adaptation; (2) reported no disparity between their current and hoped for standard of living; (3) reported that as children they were not afraid of being left alone; and (4) were living with their spouses in independent households. However, for Ss characterized by the complementary circumstances, either no relationship between self-attitude and aging was observed or there was a nonsignificant tendency for the older Ss to be more self-derogatory than the younger Ss. [Pp. 248–249][22]

Thus we gain further support for the general prediction that the direction and strength of any relationship between age and self-evaluation will be conditional upon the life circumstances of the persons, especially as these circumstances effect the flows of social rewards.

Furthermore, although Kaplan and Pokorny followed Rosenberg in using a single general dimension of self-evaluation, close inspection of their data suggests that age will be differently related to different *aspects* of self-evaluation. In particular, those aspects reflecting sensed *competence* are expected to be less favorable among the older respondents (especially p. 224 and Table 1).[22]

Thus, beyond the general hypothesis that life-cycle stage and each of the three social characteristics will be appreciably related to each of the self-evaluations, we will test the following more specific hypotheses derived from the above considerations and from our previous theoretical work:[14,18]

1. *Life cycle stage* and *sex* will be the most important predictors of self-evaluations that have strong physiological components (leisure competence and work skills); the general form of the relation between age and these forms of competence will be negative, and males will score higher than females.

2. *Occupational status* and *ethnic group* will have greater impact than life-cycle stage and sex in the areas of self-rated intelligence and self-satisfaction.
3. Life-cycle stage will generally relate more strongly than will sex to the various dimensions of self-evaluation.

Each of these hypothesized relations is derived from the fundamental idea that the various aspects of self-evaluation are engendered, maintained, and increased or decreased according to the flows of particular interactive sanctions from significant others, while these reward flows are in turn structured by the role relations associated with gender, ethnicity, socioeconomic status and, especially, the shifting matrix of stage in the life cycle.

(Findings and Interpretations

Overall Age Trends

Before testing our three specific hypotheses, we must demonstrate that, in fact, the different aspects of self-evaluation do have distinct patterns of difference and trend among the groups at different stages in the life cycle.

Figure 10–1 displays the mean scores on each of the four self-evaluations for the five life-cycle stages. It should be clearly noted that these are age comparisons of *different cohorts* of persons assessed at the *same time, not changes* in given individuals as they move through their life cycles. Longitudinal data would, of course, be necessary for an adequate test of theory concerning how social-structural factors relate to changes or "development" in self-evaluation. Comparative cohort analysis of cross-sectional data from a single survey provides only a weak approximation to the inference of change over time. However, we can use these data to test hypotheses such as ours concerning life-cycle-stage differences (rather than change in given individuals). This form of comparative analysis does not require the assumption that older cohorts were (when young) similar to those now young.

The data supports our general hypothesis

that life-cycle stage will be a very important predictor of those self-evaluations having implicit physiological components. Two self-evaluations are distinctly less favorable among the older groups: leisure competence correlates $-.34$*** with life-cycle stage (numerically represented by the digits 1–5), and self-rated, work-skills goodness correlates $-.29$***. The over-sixty-five respondents (and especially those over seventy-five) much more frequently report poor physical health than do the younger respondents; consequently, less favorable leisure-competence and work-skills self-assessment among the older respondents very likely reflect the impact of functional impairment related to physical condition. The other two self-evaluations show essentially no appreciable relation to life-cycle stage: satisfaction correlates $+.08$** with age, self-rated intelligence stands at $-.04$. The fact that two self-evaluations show negative associations with age while two others show small but positive association with age supports our contention that aspects of self-conception should be

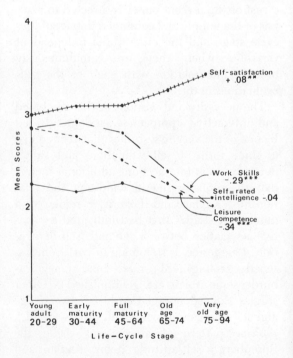

Figure 10–1. Four Dimensions of Self-Evaluation by Life-cycle Stage

measured and analyzed separately, rather than being combined into a single dimension labeled "self-esteem." This idea is given further support by the following analyses, which demonstrate that the different self-evaluation dimensions are rather differently related to the social-structural characteristics.

Testing Hypothesis 1

Our first specific hypothesis asserted that life-cycle stage and sex would be stronger predictors of leisure and work-skill competence than would ethnic group and occupational status. In addition to the above-mentioned idea about physiological impairment and age, this assertion was based on the ideas that women in our society (and especially older women) often have been socialized to think that the ability to support themselves economically is not a prime component of their major roles. Further, women had probably not been socialized to high objective levels of either work-skill competence or leisure competence. In short, we felt that women have very generally been socialized more for

social-emotional concerns than for competence (even in leisure activity), and would not feel that competence was vital to their sense of personal worth.

Examination of our data generally supports our argument regarding the importance of life-cycle stage and sex, especially regarding self-rated work skills. Both life-cycle stage and sex are significantly and moderately strongly related to both leisure competence and work skills. Just as predicted, life-cycle stage is significantly and appreciably negatively related both to work-skills goodness ($-.29***$) and leisure competence ($-.34***$). What was not anticipated, however, was the fact that in relation to leisure competence, ethnic group and occupational status were more important than was sex. Veblen's assertion[44] that socioeconomic status and leisure competence are related seems to be valid, even far below the leisure class. Here are the rank orderings of the independent variables, with strength of predictive power assessed by the unique percentage of the variance in the dependent variable associated with each independent variable ($***$ p = < .001):

WORK-SKILLS GOODNESS	%	LEISURE COMPETENCE	%
Life-cycle stage	10.5***	Life-cycle stage	9.6***
Sex	5.5***	Ethnic group	4.9***
Occupational status	3.5***	Occupational status	3.3***
Ethnic group	3.0***	Sex	3.0***
Total variance "explained" (including numerous small interaction effects)	28%	Total variance "explained"	25%

The less-than-predicted importance of sex in shaping the level of self-reported leisure competence suggests that women *are* expected to be competent in expressive activity (leisure),

while less demands are made on women for instrumental competence.

As predicted by hypothesis 1, life-cycle stage and sex contribute the most explanatory power for work-skill ratings; this data is presented graphically in Figure 10–2. The male–female curves are almost identical in shape, with males showing a consistently higher level of reported work skills across all life-cycle stages.

predictors for leisure competence are life-cycle stage and ethnicity. For all ethnic groups, there is a lower average leisure-competence score for each successive life-cycle stage.

The same relative position between ethnic groups is maintained across all life-cycle

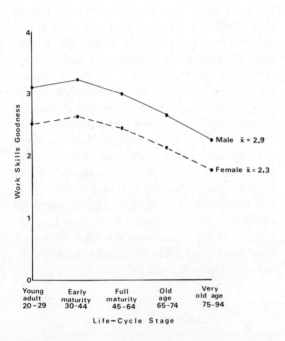

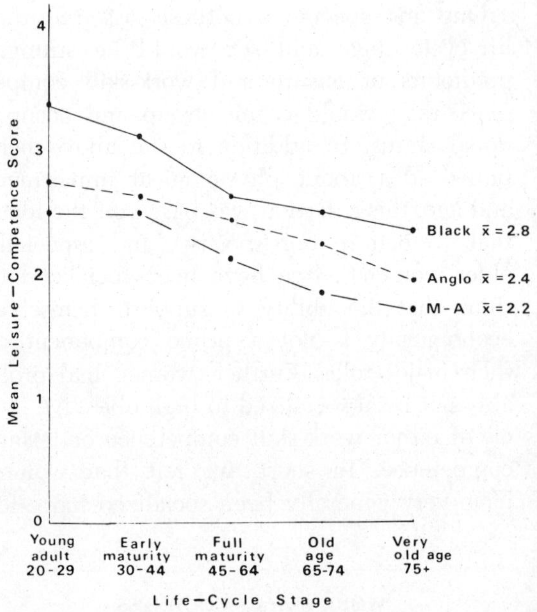

Figure 10–2. Work Skill Goodness of Life-cycle Stage and Sex

Figure 10–3. Leisure Competence by Life-cycle Stage and Ethnic Group

These data seem consistent with socialization to male–female roles, and probably represent a realistic appraisal by each group. For both men and women, those over sixty-five, and especially those over seventy-five, rate their work skills lower on the average than do the younger respondents. Continued employment is very rare among these aged respondents, and the combined effect of the symbolic act of retirement, the unavoidable comparisons with younger persons and an actual decline in functional capacity associated with physical impairment may account for much of the gap in self-rated work-skills.

As Figure 10–3 reveals, the two strongest

stages: Blacks consistently rank themselves the highest on leisure competence (x = 2.8), followed by Anglos (x = 2.4), and then by the Mexican-Americans (x = 2.2). This pattern might be a result of several factors. First, the sample selection procedures produced a set of Anglos who are relatively low in education, occupation, and income (in comparison with Houston's total Anglo population), while black and Mexican-American samples more often included "successes." Second, recent efforts to engender ethnic pride among blacks may be an important factor in producing their high scores. Third, a high score may be a reflection of compensatory overstatement.

Fourth, of necessity, black lower-class and working-class cultures have long stressed competence in expressive leisure activities since instrumental work success was so thoroughly blocked.[6,26]

Thus, on the basis of these findings we may conclude that (as predicted) life-cycle stage, sex, ethnicity, and occupational status level are all related to self-rated leisure and work-skills competence. Second, age is *negatively* related to both of these competence self-evaluations. Finally, while age is of primary importance in relation to both of these performance self-evaluations, sex is one of the top two variables only for work-skill competence.

Testing Hypothesis 2

Our second specific hypothesis stated that occupational status and ethnic-group member-ship will have greater impact in the areas of self-rated intelligence and self-satisfaction than will life-cycle stage and sex. Since these areas involve less overt physical components and less specific sex-role socialization than was the case in the performance realm, occupational position (as a broad indicator of socio-economic status) and ethnicity should be more influential in shaping the levels of these particular self-evaluations.

Examination of the data partially supports this hypothesis. Ethnicity contributes to both ratings, but occupational status is influential only for self-rated intelligence. Life-cycle stage and sex are not important in predicting either self-rated intelligence or self-satisfaction. Here are the rank orderings of the independent variables, and the percent of the variance in the dependent variable associated with each independent variable:

SELF-RATED INTELLIGENCE	%	SELF-SATISFACTION	%
Occupational status	2.4***	Ethnic group	2.6***
Ethnic group	2.4***	Life-cycle stage	.6*
Life-cycle stage	.4	Sex	.3*
Sex	.3*	Occupational status	.1
Total variance "explained" (including numerous small interaction effects)	11%	Total Variance "explained"	.8%

The total "explained variance" figures for self-rated intelligence and for self-satisfaction are considerably lower than for leisure and work-skill competence. Following our practice of structuring the discussion around the two most important independent variables, Figures 10–4 and 10–5 present ethnic and occu-pational-skill-group means in relation to self-rated intelligence, and ethnic-group and life-cycle-stage means for self-satisfaction. Several points are worth noting in these data. The phenomena of blacks reporting somewhat more favorable self-evaluations than do other ethnic groups is seen in relation to both self-rated intelligence and self-satisfaction. These data reinforce the idea of successful attempts to develop pride among blacks. Anglos are third in self-satisfaction ratings in all of the five life-cycle stages and second in self-rated intelligence. This finding supports the idea that the Anglos in our sample may be suffer-ing a sense of relative deprivation in relation to the wider reference group of Houston Anglos. Another important feature is the lack of any downward trend among the life stages in self-satisfaction rankings; in fact, there is a very slight upward trend (+.08**, see Figure 10–2). The lack of importance of life-cycle stages to self-rated intelligence supports the earlier argument: if active physical perfor-

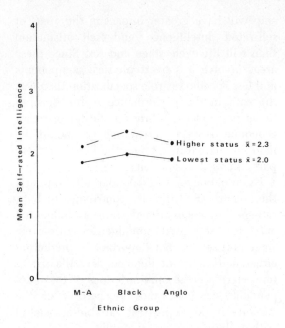

Figure 10–4. Self-Rated Intelligence by Occupational Status and Ethnic Group

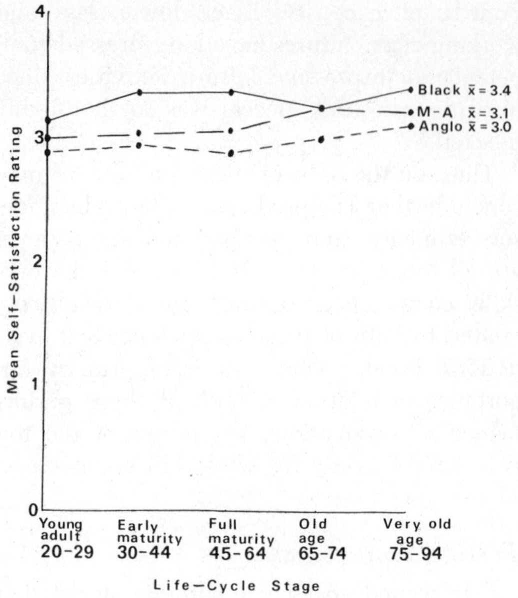

Figure 10–5. Self-Satisfaction by Ethnic Group and Life-cycle Stage

mance is not directly involved in the aspect of self-evaluation being rated, age is not a crucial factor.

We may conclude that regarding self-rated intelligence, occupational status and ethnic group are the most important determinants, thus partially confirming our second hypothesis. Regarding self-satisfaction, however, ethnic group is most important—as predicted —while occupational status is unrelated.

tence and work-skills competence and slightly stronger regarding self-rated intellectual ability and self-satisfaction. Thus, all four outcomes were in the predicted direction, but large differences were found for two of the four self-evaluations we are considering. This differential relation of sex to the two pairs of self-evaluations probably is a reflection of the fact that our culture has not mandated performance competence for females, but still expects them to be "good" and at least moderately intelligent.

Testing Hypothesis 3

Our third specific hypothesis asserted that life-cycle stage will generally relate more strongly to the various dimensions of self-evaluation than will sex. The data already presented support this hypothesis. Life-cycle stage was found to be appreciably more important than sex in predicting leisure compe-

Life-cycle Stage and Performance Competence

In the preceding analysis we have presented data for each of four aspects of self-evaluation as related to life-cycle stage, sex, occupational status, and ethnicity. Following such an analysis, we arrive at a logical justification to combine two aspects of self-conception (work-skills competence and leisure competence) into one index of performance competence. Both of these represent self-ratings of abilities necessary in performing instrumental and expressive activities. Weighting the two performance components equally and then averaging, a performance-competence index score (with a possible range from 0–30) was assigned to each respondent.

Figure 10–6 displays the average performance-competence scores for the respondents classified into groups defined by the combination of ethnicity, sex, and life-cycle stage. Occupational-status comparisons were ignored in this figure so that the patterns would not be blurred by too much detail; for numerical analysis, however, the status comparison was preserved.

Life-cycle stage. The general finding is quite clear and strong: *the older the person, the lower the self-rated performance competence.* At the extremes this pattern is very pronounced; older Mexican-American women averaged about 4.0 on our 0–30 scale, while young adult black males scored more than six times higher (24.1). The age trends were generally quite similar across the sex and ethnic-group comparisons: young adults (twenty to twenty-nine) and those in early maturity (thirty to forty-four) scored quite high on this measure of self-conceived performance-competence. Those in full maturity (forty-five to sixty-four) scored distinctly lower, and those in the two older age groups (sixty-five to seventy-four, seventy-five to ninety-four) scored very much lower (except for the very old black males). Without regard to sex, ethnic group, or occupational status, the mean performance-competence scores from youngest to oldest life-cycle stages were 18.8, 18.8, 16.2, 12.8, and 9.7. Even after introducing the other three factors, life-cycle stage still was associated with 14.4 percent of the variance in performance-competence self-evaluation. In almost every instance, the greatest difference can be observed between those fully mature and those over sixty-five, or be-

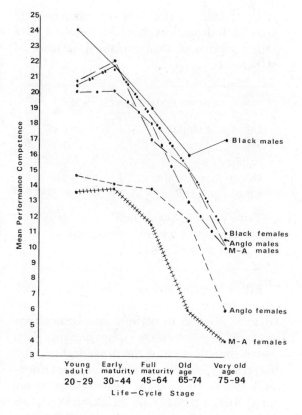

Figure 10–6. Performance Competence by Sex, Ethnic Group, and Life-cycle Stage

tween the old and very old. This pattern of results provides empirical support for the sociological generalization that *role loss* in old age (such as retirement, widowhood, loss of friends and relatives through death and residence relocation, withdrawal from active organizational participation, and invalidism) produces great personal stress and reduced life satisfaction.*

A four-way analysis of variance in the performance-competence scores using life-cycle

* See references 14, 38, 39, 28, and 34.

stage, ethnicity, sex, and occupational-skill level as independent variables resulted in a rather substantial total explained variance of 36 percent:

LEISURE COMPETENCE INDEX

Life-cycle stage	14.4%***
Sex	6.0%***
Ethnicity	5.7%***
Occupational status	5.0%***
Ethnic and status	.9%***
Total variance "explained" (including various small interaction effects)	36%

Ethnic groups and sex. The only appreciable interaction among the independent variables in relation to performance competence occurred between ethnic groups and sex. Even before introduction of the other factors, ethnic group showed a clear relation to performance evaluation (Mexican-Americans averaged 12.9, Anglos = 14.4, and blacks = 18.3), accounting for a unique 5.7 percent of the variance. Sex was also significantly related to performance competence (females averaged 12.9, males = 17.6), accounting for an additional 6.0 percent of the variance. In particular, the Mexican-American females and the Anglo females scored very low—the other ethnic/sex groups were much closer together in height of score pattern.

Black males and females scored consistently higher than all other groups, with the one exception of Anglo males in early maturity (thirty to forty-four) matching the score level of black females and scoring slightly higher than black males. Black females in early maturity (thirty to forty-four) scored higher in performance competence than every group except the young black males. This seems to be rather striking evidence of the impact of women in a particular subculture assuming responsible instrumental roles and frequently functioning as heads of households. These black women scored at levels comparable to the three male groups and well above the two other female groups. In contrast, the Anglo

females show much lower performance-competence levels, and the Mexican-American women (traditionally confined to the home and supported in decision-making dependency) score below every other group at every stage in the life cycle.

⟨ Conclusions and Prospects

This analysis has used a differentiated approach to self-evaluation in order to attempt resolution of an apparent contradiction in the literature concerning the relation of global "self-esteem" to age or stage in the life cycle. One previous approach[22] has made progress toward this resolution through tracing out the social circumstances under which this general relation seems to be positive, negative, or flat. The present paper builds upon this "conditional relationship" strategy, but then goes on to distinguish "performance competence" self-evaluations from forms of "self-acceptance" evaluation, following the logic of one of the author's previous theoretical work.[10,11,12] Both general and specific hypotheses were formulated predicting different relations of age or life-cycle stage to competence self-evaluation as compared to self-acceptance, and regarding the relations of each form of self-evaluation to sex, ethnic group, and socioeconomic status.

Empirical data from the Houston Leisure and Mental Health Study were used to test these hypotheses and to develop a first-approximation estimate of the relative and combined effects of sex, ethnicity, socioeconomic status, and age group on each of the four distinct self-evaluations.

The results of this double-differentiation analysis strategy were quite clear:

1. Leisure competence, work-skills competence (and a recombined performance-competence index) were negatively related to age in our sample, and stood in complex relation with the other "conditioning" independent variables. Together, the four independent variables "explained" a relatively high proportion of the variance in the competence self-evaluations.

2. As predicted, however, the self-acceptance (moral-worth) measure was more weakly and *positively* related to age, while self-rated intelligence showed no correlation with age at all. Again, specific unique and combined effects were discovered when the social-structural variables were taken into account, but the total explanatory power was much lower regarding self-acceptance and self-rated intelligence than was the case for the two forms of competence.

These findings demonstrated the importance of differentiating subdimensions of self-evaluation, and demand further analysis of the impact on the different self-evaluations of particular social events[21,22] and of life-cycle stage (marriage, parenthood, divorce, empty nest, retirement, widowhood, invalidism, etc.), all nested within the macrosocial-structural parameters.

❐ Technical Appendix

Construct Validation of Four Dimensions of Self-Evaluation

Construct validation was shown by Cronbach and Meehl in their pioneering article[5] to be the essential feature in any attempt to validate a particular measurement procedure regarding a theoretically interesting but nonobservable property. Other forms of validation, such as known-groups discrimination, prediction of a criterion outcome, and the naively popular "face validity" assessment, are desirable but often impossible alternatives in dealing with self-conceptions,[12] since it is logically impossible to define an overt criterion for dimensions of self-conception against which a particular operational procedure could be validated. The most important assessment remains the way in which the scores (derived from the operationalization procedure), actually relate to scores on *other* theoretically relevant variables. Mental functioning is theoretically relevant. Data collected in the Houston survey provided several measures of mental health, and we chose to use some of these measures to validate the construct of the four

dimensions of self-evaluation. We examined the relationship of these dimensions with the Affect Balance Scale, the Twenty-two Item Symptom Report Scale, and a self-report by the respondent of happiness.

Affect Balance Scale. Bradburn[2] developed the Affect Balance Scale with which to tap a respondent's affective state at a particular time. Bradburn clearly sets out the principle that positive affect and negative affect are distinct entities rather than opposite poles of the same dimension. This assertion is borne out in our sample, in which the positive-affect and negative-affect scores are completely uncorrelated ($-.01$).

All four measured dimensions of self-evaluation show the expected direction of positive correlation with high positive–affect scores and negative relation with the negative–affect scores. The low levels of correlation, however, show that the dimensions of self-evaluation we have tapped are by no means simple, internalized views of the respondent's happiness with the state of affairs of the world in general.

The strength of the correlations with positive-affect range from $+.32$ with leisure competence to an essentially zero relationship with self-satisfaction ($+.03$), suggesting a close relationship of positive feelings to social participation, as Bradburn suggests.[2] The relationships between the four self-evaluation dimensions and negative-affect score are somewhat stronger than their relations with the positive-affect score, the strongest associations being with the variables of work skills ($-.14$) and self-satisfaction ($-.22$). The closer connection of self-conception to negative rather than positive affect probably stems from the American cultural prescription that a cheerful presentation of self is most socially desirable.

Twenty-two Item Symptom Report. Langner and his colleagues[23,24] developed a scale based on predominantly psychosomatic- and neurotic-symptom reports by the respondent. These include a number of physiological symptoms, such as frequent headaches, heart beating hard, poor appetite, shortness of breath, etc., and an approximately equal number of more clearly psychological items, such as reports of being the "worrying type," being nervous often, being restless, feeling that nothing goes right, and wondering about the worthwhileness of activities. This type of symptom report scale is very similar to the psychosomatic or "nervousness" scales developed in the American soldier research during World War II[42] and forms of symptom reports used more recently by Morris Rosenberg in his attempt to validate his direct self-esteem scale.[36] Rosenberg has shown that in his sample of some 5,000 high school students, a rather straightforward self-esteem scale correlated approximately −.44 with psychosomatic symptom reports (using the Epsilon measure calculated from Rosenberg's Table 3). Our finding of consistent negative correlations ranging from −.15 for self-rated intelligence to −.28 for sense of self-satisfaction is rather convincing evidence that our measures are in fact tapping important psychological dimensions, since these relations are predicted by many forms of theory. A study by Kaplan and Pokorny[21] showing an association of similar magnitude and direction between an anxiety symptom report and self-derogation offers additional basis for these claims.

Symptom factor scores. A factor analysis of the twenty-two symptoms indicated three major factors: anxiety, depression, and somatic complaints. A score was created by weighting the most important symptoms of each factor by the factor loading of that item, and then taking a rounded mean score of these products. Each respondent thus received a weighted score for each of the three specific symptom groups in addition to the total twenty-two symptom score.

The correlations of these scores with the four self-conceptions (Figure 10–2) confirm again, by direction and magnitude, the validity of the measurements as variables relevant to mental functioning. The depression-symptom syndrome has the strongest negative associations with self-rated leisure and work competence (−.22, −.25). The anxiety-symptom syndrome relates most strongly to self-satisfaction (−.28). The somatic symptoms show the weakest associations of the three symptom groups.

Self-rating of happiness. The respondents were asked to rate their happiness by the question: "All things considered, how happy would you say you are right now—very happy, pretty happy, or not too happy?" Again, the correlations with the four measured aspects of self-conception are not large, but are all in the predicted direction (+.13 to +.24).

This diverse range of predicted correlations (with negative-affect, positive-affect, twenty-two-item symptom scale, anxiety, depression, somatic-symptoms, and level of self-rated happiness) forms a fairly persuasive picture of the construct validity of the four measured dimensions of self-conception.

⟮ Bibliography

1. ADLER, A. *The Practice and Theory of Individual Psychology.* New York: Harcourt, 1927.
2. BRADBURN, N. *The Structure of Psychological Well-Being.* Chicago: Aldine, 1969.
3. BÜHLER, C. and F. MASSARIK, eds. *The Course of Human Life, A Study of Goals in the Humanistic Perspective.* New York: Springer, 1968.
4. COOPERSMITH, S. *The Antecedents of Self-Esteem.* San Francisco: W. H. Freeman, 1967.
5. CRONBACH, L. J. and P. S. MEEHL. "Construct Validity in Psychological Tests," *Psychol. Bull.,* 52 (1955), 281–302.
6. ELKINS, S. M. *Slavery.* Chicago: University of Chicago Press, 1959.
7. ERIKSON, E. "Identity and the Life Cycle," *Psychol. Issues,* 1 (1959), 50–100.
8. FROMM, E. *Man for Himself.* New York: Holt, Rinehart and Winston, 1947.
9. GORDON, C. "Self-Conceptions and Social Achievement." Ph.D. thesis. Ann Arbor: University Microfilms, 1963.
10. ———. "Self-Conceptions: Configurations of Content," in C. Gordon and K. J. Gergen, eds., *The Self in Social Interaction,* pp. 115–136. New York: Wiley, 1968.
11. ———. "Systemic Senses of Self," *Sociol. Inquiry,* 38 (1968), 161–178.
12. ———. "Self-Conceptions Methodologies," *J. Nerv. Ment. Dis.,* 148 (1969), 328–364.
13. ———. "Review of *The Antecedents of Self-*

Esteem by S. Coopersmith," *Psychiatry*, 33 (1970), 282–286.

14. ———. "Role and Value Development Across the Life Cycle," in J. Jackson, ed., *Studies in Sociological Theory IV; Role*, London: pp. 65–105. Cambridge University Press, 1971.

15. ———. *Looking Ahead: Self-Conception, Race and Family Factors as Determinants of Adolescent Achievement Orientations*. Washington: Am. Sociol. Assoc., Rose Monograph Series, 1972.

16. GORDON, C. and C. M. GAITZ. "Leisure and Mental Health Late in the Life Cycle," *Psychiatr. Ann.*, 2 (1972), 38–68.

17. GORDON, C. and K. J. GERGEN, eds., *The Self in Social Interaction*, Vol. 1. New York: Wiley, 1968.

18. GORDON, C., J. SCOTT, and C. M. GAITZ. "Leisure Activities and Mental Health, With Some Sex Role and Life Cycle Consideration." Submitted for publication.

19. HORNEY, K. *Our Inner Conflicts*. New York: Norton, 1945.

20. HYMAN, H. H. *Interviewing in Social Research*. Chicago: University of Chicago Press, 1954.

21. KAPLAN, H. B. and A. D. POKORNY. "Self-Derogation and Psychosocial Adjustment," *J. Nerv. Ment. Dis.*, 149 (1969), 421–434.

22. ———. "Aging and Self-Attitude: A Conditional Relationship," *Aging Hum. Dev.*, 1 (1970), 241–250.

23. LANGNER, T. S. "A Twenty-two Item Screening Score of Psychiatric Symptoms Indicating Impairment," *J. Health Soc. Behav.*, 3 (1962), 269–276.

24. LANGNER, T. S. and S. T. MICHAEL. *Life Stress and Mental Health*. New York: Free Press, 1963.

25. LIDZ, T. *The Person: His Development Throughout the Life Cycle*. New York: Basic Books, 1968.

26. LIEBOW, E. *Tally's Corner*. Boston: Little, Brown, 1966.

27. MASLOW, A. H. *Motivation and Personality*. New York: Harper and Brothers, 1954.

28. NEUGARTEN, B. L., ed. *Middle Age and Aging*. Chicago: University of Chicago Press, 1968.

29. ———. "Grow Old Along With Me! The Best Is Yet To Be," *Psychol. Today*, 5 (1971), 45–48; 79; 81.

30. PARSONS, T. *Toward a General Theory of Action*. Cambridge: Harvard University Press, 1951.

31. ———. *The Social System*. New York: Free Press, 1951.

32. ———. "An Approach to Psychological Theory in Terms of the Theory of Action," in S. Koch, ed., *Psychology: The Study of a Science*, Vol. 3, pp. 612–711. New York: McGraw-Hill, 1959.

33. ———. "The Position of Identity in the General Theory of Action," in C. Gordon, and K. J. Gergen, eds., *The Self in Social Interaction*, pp. 11–24. Vol. 1. New York: Wiley, 1968.

34. RILEY, M. W. and A. FONER. *Aging and Society*, Vol. 1. New York: Russell Sage Foundation, 1968.

35. ROGERS, C. *Client-centered Therapy: Its Current Practice, Implications, and Theory*. Boston: Houghton, 1951.

36. ROSENBERG, M. *Society and the Adolescent Self-Image*. Princeton: Princeton University Press, 1965.

37. ———. *Negro Self-esteem*. Washington: Am. Sociol. Assoc., Rose Monograph Series, 1972.

38. ROSOW, I. *Social Integration of the Aged*. New York: Free Press, 1967.

39. ———. "The Social Context of the Aging Self," *Gerontologist*, 13 (1973), 82–87.

40. SARBIN, T. R. "A Preface to a Psychological Analysis of Self," in C. Gordon and K. J. Gergen, eds., *The Self in Social Interaction*, Vol. 1. pp. 179–188. New York: Wiley, 1968.

41. SHIBUTANI, T. *Society and Personality*, Englewood Cliffs, N.J.: Prentice-Hall, 1961.

42. STAR, S. "The Screening of Psychoneurotics in the Army: Technical Development of Tests," in S. A. Stauffer, ed., *Measurement and Prediction*. Princeton: Princeton University Press, 1950.

43. SULLIVAN, H. S. *The Interpersonal Theory of Psychiatry*. New York: Norton, 1953.

44. VEBLEN, T. (1899) *The Theory of the Leisure Class*. New York: Mentor Books, 1953.

CHAPTER 11

CREATIVITY AND ITS CULTIVATION: RELATION TO PSYCHOPATHOLOGY AND MENTAL HEALTH

Silvano Arieti

THE INTERCONNECTIONS and possibilities of cross-fertilizations between modern psychiatry and other disciplines are rapidly increasing. Recently a new area, the study of creativity, was added to this long list, especially in relation to psychopathology, mental health, and school psychiatry.

At first glance, any linking of creativity with psychopathology might appear unwarranted, for the creative process is not pathological but something to be desired and encouraged. But similar linkings have occurred in the history of medicine. For instance, general pathology has been of great help in understanding the physiology of the normal organism.

Creativity is an important part of the study of man and can be approached in many ways.

This chapter will deal with some aspects of this subject that are related to psychiatry.

Many authors have recently studied creativity from other points of view and have defined the creative process in various ways for instance, Ghiselin,[20] Anderson,[1] Stein and Heinze,[33] Hammer,[22] Taylor and Barron,[34] Getzels and Jackson,[19] Gruber, Terrell and Wertheimer,[21] Eiduson,[12] and Koestler.[23]

By the term "creative process" the present author means a special process by which man tries to transcend in a desirable form the usual ways of feeling, understanding, relating, and doing (Arieti[4,7,8]; see also Von Bertalanffy[35]).

Although there is a fundamental difference between the infrahuman animal that has a limited number of responses and the symbol-making human being, man, too, tends to act and relate in fixed ways. Whether his way of coping with any situation occurs immediately after the stimulus or whether it follows a complicated set of symbols and choices, man tends to use the repertory of activities provided by his usual psychological faculties or by ways that have become the common style of his culture. If his activities are mediated by cognitive processes, they generally follow what, in Freudian psychoanalysis, has been called the secondary process or, in more general parlance, Aristotelian or ordinary logical thinking.

The creative process allows man to liberate himself from the fetters of these secondary-process responses. But creativity is not simply originality and freedom. It is much more than that; it also imposes restrictions. First of all, although it uses methods other than the secondary process, it must not be in disagreement with the secondary process. Otherwise, the result would be bizarre, not creative. Secondly, it must attain an additional aim: a desirable enlargement of human experience— either aesthetic pleasure, as in art, or usefulness, understanding, and predictability, as in science. In this second respect, creativity may be seen in a dual role: at the same time that it enlarges the universe by adding or uncovering new dimensions, it also enriches man, who will be able to experience inwardly these new dimensions.

Thirdly, the creative process tends to fulfill a longing or a search for a new object or for a state of experience or of existence that is not easily found or easily attainable. Especially in aesthetic creativity, the work often represents not only the new object but this longing, this indefinite search, this sustained, yet never completed effort with its conscious or unconscious motivation.

❲ Previous Psychiatric or Psychoanalytic Interpretations

In 1864, the Italian psychiatrist Cesare Lombroso wrote an essay on "Genius and Insanity,"* which was followed by many books on the same subject. Lombroso tried to prove that such geniuses as Cellini, Goethe, Vico, Tasso, Newton, Rousseau, Comte, Ampère, and many others had experienced attacks of insanity: specifically, such psychiatric conditions as delusional and hallucinatory syndromes, depressions, and manic states. Although Lombroso reported several cases of creative men who, according to indisputable evidence, had had attacks of psychosis, in other cases it was difficult to tell whether they had suffered from real psychoses or from what other authors would call peculiarities of character and temperament. Moreover, Lombroso dealt only with the negative qualities of great men. He did not deal with the positive qualities or with the processes that transform psychopathology into creative activity. In his last books, Lombroso expressed the opinion that the quality of being a genius is associated with epilepsy. The peculiarities of these geniuses would be explained as epileptic equivalents. He felt that being a genius may be the expression of a "degenerative psychosis."

For several decades Lombroso's works enjoyed a great popularity in Europe, but finally their lack of scientific basis, absence of clear-cut definitions of genius and of insanity, and the inability to prove the veracity of anecdotal reports made even Lombroso's own pupils skeptical about his work. Lombroso's contributions, however, will retain historical importance, for they represent one of the first and most prolonged attempts to find connections between psychopathology and creativity.

We must wait for the advent of the psychoanalytic school for a new and more rewarding approach to the problem of creativity. According to Freud, creativity originates in man's conflicts, which stem from fundamental biological drives.[14] The urge to create is seen as an attempt to find a solution to these conflicts.

Just as the child attains wish fulfillment or some control over reality through play and games, in which he generally impersonates an

* For a scholarly review of Lombroso's life and work see Mora.[27] The data about Lombroso, presented in this chapter, are to a large extent taken from Mora's article.

important adult—a political leader, an army general, a movie star, a parent, etc.—so the creative person produces a work of art in which he can realize his daydreams. However, Freud adds, we are often ashamed of our daydreams, just as we are of drives that give rise to nocturnal dreams. In our nocturnal dreams the censorship diminishes the shame by making the manifest aspect of the dream very different from its meaning. Freud gives a similar interpretation for the aesthetic transformation of the original daydream: ". . . The essential *ars poetica* lies in the technique by which our feeling of repulsion is overcome. . . . The writer softens the egotistical character of the daydream by changes and disguises, and he bribes us by the offer of a purely formal, that is, aesthetic, pleasure in the presentation of his fantasies."[14]

According to Freud, childhood experiences are very important in accounting for the content of the creative product. Thus, it is not an accident that in a famous painting by Leonardo da Vinci the Virgin Mary and St. Anna both appear with the infant Jesus, in contrast to the usual representation of the holy family in Italian painting.[17] Leonardo had the unconscious need to reproduce a childhood experience. He was raised by two mothers: his real mother, a peasant woman, and his father's legal wife, in whose home Leonardo grew up.

According to Freud, the role of sexuality in creativity is always prominent.[17] He traces the creative person's desire to know the unknown back to the child's sexual curiosity, which begins with the third year of life. In Freud's opinion the child's interest in sex has three possible outcomes. The first is energetic repression, favored by educational and religious inhibitions. The second, a transformation of psychological mechanisms, occurs when sexual investigation is not totally repressed but is dealt with by thought processes or by compulsive defenses. This transformation takes place when the intellectual development is sufficiently strong. In the third case, "the most rare and most perfect type," sexual curiosity is sublimated into that curiosity which leads to creativity.

These brief remarks are sufficient to illustrate that Freud was mainly concerned with the importance and relevance of motivation in creativity, not with the essence of creativity itself. Unconscious motivation is indeed a very important subject, but it does not include the various aspects of the problem of creativity. We want to determine why and how a few gifted men are able to transform their motivations and their personal experiences into creative products.

Within the theoretical framework of the Freudian school, Kris[24] is, perhaps, the most prominent author who has studied creativity not exclusively from the point of view of unconscious motivation. Kris must be given credit for stressing the importance of the primary process in the formal mechanisms of creativity. The primary and secondary processes were described by Freud in Chapter 7 of *The Interpretation of Dreams*;[18] but he connected these concepts to the problem of unconscious motivation, not to the formal aspects of creativity. By primary process, Freud meant a special type of organization that governs unconscious processes.[15,18] It is characterized, from a cognitive point of view, by the phenomena of displacement, condensation, and substitution. From the point of view of the libido theory, it is characterized by easy discharge or easy shifting of libidinal charge. Kris considered the use of the primary process in creativity as a "regression in the service of the ego."[24] In other words, in the creative work the creative person uses such processes as condensation and substitution. This would take place in the preconscious system.

Still in the framework of the Freudian school, Kubie[26] adds support to Kris's idea that creativity is a product of the preconscious and not of the unconscious, as had previously been assumed by some psychoanalysts.

Jung has also made a significant contribution to the problem of creativity, especially in reference to the aesthetic process.[28] Jung believed that the creative process, at least when it pertains to art, may occur in two modes: the psychological and the visionary.

In the psychological mode, the content of the creative product is drawn from the realm of human consciousness. Although the vast and rich realm of human experience, in its relation to such things as love, family, environment, society, crime, or human destiny in general, usually appears in the content of the work of art, this mode of creativity "nowhere transcends the bounds of psychological intelligibility. . . . Everything that it embraces belongs to the realm of the understanding."[28] The psychological mode requires submitting the material to a direct, conscious, and purposeful aim.

It is the visionary mode that concerns Jung more than anything else. In this second mode, the content does not originate from the lessons of life but from the depths of time. It reproduces primordial experiences that surpass understanding. These experiences may be many-sided, demonic, grotesque. They come from the collective unconscious—that part of the psyche which is the depository of experiences that have occurred repeatedly over the course of a large number of generations. These deposits are the archetypes.

In the visionary mode, the method is again different. The creative person is at the mercy of the reemerging content. He is in a passive situation. "The work brings with it its own form." The creative person is more conscious of an "alien" will or intention beyond his comprehension. In the visionary mode, the creative process consists in an *unconscious animation of the archetype*.

(**The Primary Process**

Jung is correct in pointing out that a great work of art is not the exclusive result of life experience or of the usual ways of thinking but also of primordial processes. However, the present author believes that these primordial processes do not come from the collective unconscious and have little to do with the content of the product of creativity. He believes, as Kris does, that these processes consist of primary-process mechanisms described by Freud. These mechanisms deal with the cognitive forms of the creative process, not with its content.

As we have already mentioned, although Freud discovered the primary process, he did not pursue the study of the cognitive mechanisms of the primary process and therefore could not sufficiently apply his discovery to the understanding of creativity. On the other hand, Kris, who understood the relevance of the study of the primary process in relation to creativity, did not show how, in the different forms of creativity, the primary process must integrate with the mechanisms of the secondary process.

In my opinion it is from an appropriate matching of secondary-process mechanisms with those of the primary process that the creative process emerges. I have proposed the use of the expression *tertiary process* for this special combination.[7,8] In a certain number of creative processes the matching is not exclusively between primary- and secondary-process mechanisms but also between faulty or archaic and normal mechanisms, all of which belong to the secondary process. For these combinations, too, the designation tertiary process will be retained.

In the different areas of creativity specific modes can be recognized by virtue of which these mechanisms integrate so that innovation emerges. In the course of this chapter we shall illustrate some of these modalities.

The relations between the primary process and the creative process are many. Such extremely important topics as the image, imagery, the endocept, and the phenomena of a dualism were discussed at length in my book, *The Intrapsychic Self*,[8] and will receive further elaboration in a book now in preparation.[11] Also, for reference to painting see my article on "Schizophrenic Art and Relation to Modern Art."[9] Limitations of space demand that I focus on only one of the relations between the primary process and the creative. For this purpose, I have chosen one of the most basic and far reaching: identification based upon similarity. Some attention will also be paid to other mechanisms; such as putting the concept into words (verbalization), making it concrete (concretization), and its attempted transformation into a perception (perceptualization).

For the sake of clarity and continuity let me summarize some things I have said about the primary process in my work on schizophrenia.*

The seriously ill schizophrenic, although living in a state of utter confusion, tries to recapture some understanding and to give organization to his fragmented universe. This organization is to a large extent reached by connecting things that have similar parts in common. Many patients force themselves to see similarities everywhere. In their relentless search for similarities they see strange coincidences, that is, similar elements occurring in two or more instances at the same time or at brief intervals. By considering these similarities as identities they attempt to find some clarity in the confusion of the world, a solution for the big jigsaw puzzle.

A red-haired young woman in a postpartum schizoprhenic phychosis developed an infection in one of her fingers. The terminal phalanx was swollen and red. She told the writer several times, "This finger is me." Pointing to it she said, "This is my red and rotten head." She did not mean that her finger was a symbolic representation of herself, but, in a way incomprehensible to use, it was really herself—or a actual duplicate of herself. Another patient believed that the two men she loved in her life were actually the same person, although one lived in Mexico City and the other in New York. In fact, both of them played the guitar and both of them loved her. Another example that the author often quotes is that of a patient who thought she was the Virgin Mary. Asked why, she replied, "I am a virgin; I am the Virgin Mary."

Many patients at this stage of regression indulge in an orgy of identifications. The patient tries to find glimpses of regularities in the midst of the confusion in which he lives. He tends to register identical segments of experience and to build up systems of regularity upon them. Not only does he experience an increased immediate grasping of similarity, but he responds to such similarities as if they were identities. If we want a logical formulation for this disorder we could say with Von

Domarus that, "Whereas the normal person accepts identity only upon the basis of identical subjects, the schizophrenic, when he thinks in a typical schizophrenic way, accepts identity based on identical predicates."[36] In other words, in the primary-process type of organization, similarity becomes identity. In Aristotelian logic, only like subjects are identified. The subjects are fixed; therefore, only a limited number of deductions are possible. In paleologic thinking the predicates lead to the identification. Since the predicates of the same subject are numerous, the deduction reached by this type of thinking is not easy to predict. The choice of the predicate that will lead to the identification is psychodynamically determined by conscious or unconscious motivational trends.

This cognitive organization of the primary process is susceptible to different interpretations that actually refer to the same phenomena. We may, for instance, state that the primary process organizes classes or categories that differ from those of secondary-process thinking. In secondary-process thinking, a class is a collection of objects to which a concept applies. For instance, Washington, Lincoln, Roosevelt, Jefferson, et al. form a class to which the concept "President of the United States" applies. In paleologic or primary-process thinking, a class is a collection of objects that have a predicate or part in common (for instance, the state of being virgin) and that, therefore, become identical or equivalent. The formulation of a primary (process) class is often an unconscious mechanism. Whereas the members of a secondary (process) class are recognized as being similar (and it is actually on their similarity that their classification is based) the members of a primary class are freely interchanged: for instance, the patient becomes the Virgin Mary.

Another characteristic of the paleologic organization is the change in the significance of words. The words lose part of their connotation. That is, they may not refer to a class any more, but the verbalization, that is, the word as a phonetic entity, independent of its meaning, acquires prominence. Other primary-process mechanisms may take place after atten-

* See references 2, 5, 6, 8, and 10. Also, Vol. 3, Chap. 24.

tion has been focused on verbalization. In many expressions of patients who think paleologically, two or more objects or concepts are identified because they can be represented by the same word. The verbal symbol thus becomes the identifying predicate. This leads to what seems to be plays on words. For instance, a patient who was asked to define "life" started to define *Life* magazine. An Italian patient, whose name was Stella, thought she was a fallen star. Another patient thought she was black like the night. Her name was Laila, which means night in Hebrew. An American patient, whose name was Marcia, thought she was a rotten person. In Italian, a language she knew well because she had spent her childhood in Italy, the word *marcia* means rotten.

Homonymy and similarity of words are also used in other more complicated forms of paleologic thinking in order to obtain identification or to give plausibility to thoughts that are determined not by logic but by otherwise unsustainable motivations. As an example from pathology, I shall quote a patient whom I examined during the second world war.[5] During the examination, she told me that the next time the Japanese attacked the Americans it would be at Diamond Harbor or Gold Harbor. When she was asked why, she replied: "The first time they attacked at Pearl Harbor; now they will attack at Diamond Harbor or at Sapphire Harbor." "Do you think that the Japanese attacked Pearl Harbor because of its name?" I asked. "No, no," she replied. "It was a happy coincidence." Note the inappropriateness of the adjective happy. It was a happy coincidence for her, because she could prove thereby the alleged validity of her present paleologic thinking. Her train of thought was stimulated by the word "Pearl," which aroused associations with precious stones. Another primary-process mechanism, common to dreams and schizophrenia, is the concretization of the concept. In schizophrenia concepts that cannot be endured by the patient as long as he uses them at an abstract level are translated into concrete representations. For instance, a patient had the delusion that his wife was poisoning his food. He had a gustatory hallucination that made him taste the poison in the food. In this case, the patient was actually experiencing a general situation in which he felt his wife was "poisoning" his life. Another patient had an olfactory hallucination. He smelled a "bad odor" emanating from his body. He was actually concerned, at an abstract level, with his character. He felt he had a stinking personality. In dreams also, thoughts are transformed into concrete perceptual media, predominantly visual.

(Wit

Freud first developed his concepts about the primary process in his studies on dreams, and later he applied them to his studies of psychoneurotic symptoms. He opened a direct path to the understanding of the creative process with his book on the psychology of wit. Freud[16] became interested in the problem of wit when he noticed that certain dreams resembled jokes, especially when they were interpreted. He did not disregard this apparently accidental similarity, and on studying the problem he discovered numerous analogies between wit and dreams. In wit, as in dreams, Freud focused his attention on the unconscious motivation of the joke—a very important point indeed. However, he made a rather hasty analysis of the formal mechanisms of the joke.

Let us examine some examples of jokes quoted by Freud. One of them is a famous witticism of the poet Heine, who, in talking about a lady, said, "This woman is like the Venus de Milo in many ways. Like her, she is extremely old, has no teeth, and has spots on the yellow surface of her body." Freud believed that the technique of this joke consists of "representation through the opposite." Ugliness is made to agree with the most beautiful. I believe that trying to identify a subject with its opposite reinforces the effect of the joke, but that the fundamental factor in this joke is the possibility of identifying two apparently unidentifiable subjects. Heine wanted to say of a particular woman that she was ugly. The artistic method he resorted to was indeed unpredictable and bizarre: he identified the ugly woman with the most beautiful—the Venus de Milo. How could this logically impossible identification be made? By abandoning Aristotelian logic and reverting to the paleologic of the primary process, like the logic of the schizophrenic. The woman and the statue of Venus are identical because they have some predicates or parts in common: namely, being old, having no teeth, and having spots on the yellow surface of their bodies.

Here is another example from Freud, a joke that was very common at the time of the Dreyfus trial, the French Jew unjustly accused of treason by the French Army: "That girl reminds me of Dreyfus. The Army does not believe in her innocence." Freud believed that the technique of this joke is mainly that of ambiguity, but it is obvious that here again an improbable identification is made. Dreyfus and the girl are identified because they have a common predicate, "innocence not believed in by the Army." The predicate is common to both subjects only as the same verbalization is applied to two different concepts. In fact, in the case of Dreyfus, innocence means "state of not being guilty of treason"; in the case of the girl it means "lack of sexual experience." Also the word "army" has a different slant in the two cases. In the case of Dreyfus, it means "general staff"; in the case of the girl, it means "group of men," with emphasis on their being male. We see, thus, how identity based only upon a similarity of a part or a predicate is an important formal component of jokes. However, as I have written in much greater detail elsewhere,[4] the cognitive mechanisms of witticisms are more complicated in some cases.

Let us examine another joke, this time not from Freud.

A woman sues a man by whom she claims she has been raped. The plaintiff and the defendant are in front of the judge. The judge looks at both of them and sees that the woman is tall and stout, the man short and thin. With some astonishment he asks the woman, "Is this the man who raped you? How did he do it?"

The woman answers, "He pushed me against a wall and he raped me."

"How is it possible?" asks the perplexed judge. "You are so tall and he is so short!"

"Well," says the woman, "I bent my knees a little bit!"

The woman is logical. If she bends her knees, the sexual act is possible. In the attempt to use logic in self-defense, however, she accuses herself, because the bending of the knees implies her willingness to be a partner and automatically excludes the act of rape. Though in this case no paleologic is involved, it is still the logical mechanism that is the basis of the joke—a logical mechanism that is used by the woman in self-defense and which, on the contrary, turns out to be a self-accusation.

This example shows that in some jokes faulty cognitive mechanisms, which technically belong to the secondary process, are used instead of primary-process mechanisms. These faulty mechanisms consist at times of correct logical processes that are based on false premises; at other times, of logical ways of thinking that implicitly invalidate the allegation made or prove only an inconsequential issue. These faulty mechanisms are used not only in jokes but also in the rationalizations of normal as well as psychoneurotic and psychotic persons who want to defend an allegation, a hostile attitude, or a desire.

We must clarify a specific point in order to avoid conveying a wrong impression. It has not been suggested here that the witty character of the joke is due simply to the use of primary process paleologic or to faulty logic. More than that is necessary. Let us examine again the Dreyfus joke and let us assume that the girl who was identified with Dreyfus was Jewish. If a person had said, "This girl has something in common with Dreyfus; she is Jewish," this would have been a logically correct statement but platitudinous. It would have been a statement made with the application of a secondary-process mechanism. Let us assume that a schizophrenic patient had said, "This girl is Dreyfus: she is Jewish." This would be a paleologic, primary-process identification because of a common predicate (being Jewish). This statement would be delusional but not witty.

Thus, it is not the use of primary-process paleologic or of faulty logic that confers the witty character to the joke. In my opinion, *one perceives a stimulus as witty when he is set to react to logic and then realizes that he is, instead, reacting to paleologic or to faulty logic.*

The listener is temporarily deceived because he first apprehends the intellectual process of the joke as logical. A fraction of a second later, however, he realizes that the intellectual process is not logical at all, and he laughs. The listener discovers that he is not reacting to logic but either to paleologic or to faulty logic. Logic, faulty logic, and paleologic may be very similar and, when they are associated as they are in the joke, may deceive us as do identical twins. It is just a fleeting deception, however. As soon as we become aware of it, we laugh. If we know that we are going to listen to a joke, we prepare ourselves to be temporarily deceived.

In the creation of a joke, the creative process is thus based on the following factors: (1) Primary-process mechanisms, or cognitive mechanisms that are usually discarded because of faults, become available to the creative person. (2) Out of those primary-process and/or faulty cognitive mechanisms which have become available, the creative person is able to select those which give the fleeting impression of being valid secondary-process mechanisms. The witty or comic response on the part of the listener occurs when there is recognition of logic-paleologic discordance.* The listener recognizes that what seemed a logical process is instead a primary or paleologic process, and he laughs. The creative process of wit consists in putting together the primary- and secondary-process mechanisms and automatically comparing them. It is the comparison that reveals the discordance and provokes laughter.

* If faulty logic is used instead of paleologic, then there will be a logic-faulty logic discordance. In the following discussion, we shall take into consideration only logic versus paleologic and secondary process versus primary, because these seem the most typical and most frequent combinations in creativity. However, the same notions could be repeated for logic versus faulty logic and secondary versus faulty secondary process.

It is possible now to understand why most paleologic expressions of the schizophrenic are bizarre but not witty. The language of the schizophrenic is often so remote from reality that no similarity or possibility of confusion with logic is left. Only when such confusion is possible for the listener are expressions witty. Occasionally they are; as a matter of fact, I owe the origins of my interest in the psychology of creativity to some witty expressions of schizophrenic patients. For instance, a patient whom I examined many years ago had the habit of oiling her body. Asked why she would do so, she replied, "The human body is a machine and has to be lubricated." The word "machine," applied in a figurative sense to the human body, had led to the identification with man-made machines.

The creative process as we have described it is not involved in what this patient said. She did not know that what she was saying was witty. She meant literally what she said. Her delusional remark is witty only for us. In this case we, not the patient, create the joke, because we recognize her illogicality in her apparent logicality.

It is from the appropriate matching of a secondary-process mechanism with a primary-process mechanism that a tertiary process emerges and a primitive or faulty form of cognition is transformed into an innovation. In the different fields of creativity there are specific ways in which the secondary process is matched with the primary process so that innovation emerges. We have seen that, in wit, the specific method consists of pairing similar logical and paleological mechanisms and in recognizing the logic-paleologic discordance. We shall now consider the specific modalities that are used in the arts and sciences.

From Puns to Parables

In such products of creativity as puns, proverbs, parables, and even in some commercial advertisements, expressions are used in which there is no logic-paleologic discordance, but the contrary: namely, paleologic reinforcement. Here paleologic actually strengthens logic. The result is not humor but great verbal effectiveness.

These expressions may be compared to those rare dreams whose manifest content coincides with the latent, or to those neurotic manifestations which coincide with the demands of reality. A beautiful example of paleologic reinforcement is found in Benjamin Franklin's historical statement, "We must all hang together, or assuredly we shall all hang separately." This sentence has great vigor and effect because it follows both logic and paleologic. It has practically no comic effect because the meaning is not sustained by paleologic alone. Franklin wanted to convey the message, "We must remain united," but he did not use this ordinary phrase. He said instead something like this, "One way or another we're going to hang; so, let's hang together rather than separately." But to "hang together" means to remain united, and "hang separately" means to be executed on the gallows. In a fleeting preconscious moment all the meanings of the words "to hang" are identified. When they are recognized as being different, the artistic effect is experienced.

We may take another example that has been considered with veneration throughout the centuries: In the Gospels it is written that people who wanted to confuse Jesus asked him whether it was proper to pay taxes to Caesar. Jesus requested that money be shown to him and then asked whose image was on the coin. They replied, "Caesar's." Jesus then said, "Render therefore unto Caesar the things that are Caesar's, and to God the things that are God's." The Gospels say that the people were astonished at such an unexpected answer, just as an increasing number of people have been throughout the centuries.

Jesus' answer is enigmatic and has been interpreted in many ways. And yet we immediately perceive its great vigor and we sense that it conveys a great meaning. Why is this so? It is difficult to examine Jesus' sentence from an exclusively formal, strictly literal and concrete point of view, because as soon as we hear it we become inundated by its various and deep abstract meanings. Nevertheless, it seems that if we make an effort we can recognize in this sentence a concrete and literal basis, as we do in parables in general. The image on the coin was Caesar's only as it represented the likeness of Caesar, not because it belonged to Caesar. In other words, only the image was Caesar's, not the ownership of the coin. Therefore, if we take this sentence in an extremely literal, concrete sense, Jesus would be wrong; he based his statement only on a play of words, on the fact that the expression "Caesar's" would paleologically acquire the meaning "being the property of Caesar." The coin, then, would have to be given back (rendered) to Caesar, its rightful owner. But taxes would have to be paid even if the coins did not show the image of Caesar, and, as a matter of fact, some Roman coins did not show Caesar's image or name.

Why, then, does the story not appear humorous, in spite of having a partially paleologic foundation? The expression reinforced the important message that Jesus wanted to convey to the people: that money *did* belong to Caesar, not in a literal but a metaphorical, sense. Money meant material things. It belonged more to Caesar and to the materialistic world of Rome than to the spiritual world of Jerusalem. Jesus' followers should not be concerned with such things but only with the "things which are God's and must be rendered to God." Jesus was trying to placate the discontent of the people by showing, in an unusual, unpredictable way, that it was acceptable to pay the unfair tribute to Caesar. With his words he did not show a pro-Roman attitude, nor did he come out against payment of taxes. This would have been a rebellious position. At the same time, in a new and highly artistic way, he supported the old Hebrew religious tradition that stressed the antithesis between God and Moloch. Moloch is a contemptuous word for king, a king being interested in temporal, earthly values only. In this parable, Caesar is Moloch.

In this example we can see the fusion or contemporaneous occurrence of several levels of meaning. Had Jesus resorted just to a play on words, his remarks would have been witty but not epoch-making. Had he tried to mitigate the sorrow of discontented taxpayers, his intent would have been a noble one but not a revelation. Jesus wanted to reveal what, for him, was a highest truth. This revelation was made not through a scientific demonstration but through paleologic reinforcement. Paleologic reinforcement is the opposite of logic-paleologic discordance. It does not pertain to the comic but to the general realm of art and, occasionally, of science as demonstrated hereafter.

(Poetry

The poet, too, is looking for a similarity that will reinforce his theme. This occurs in that creative process called the metaphor. Aristotle wrote, "The greatest thing by far is to be a master of metaphor; it is the one thing that cannot be learnt from others; and it is also a sign of genius, since a good metaphor implies an intuitive perception of the similarity in dissimilar." (*Poetics*, 1459a)

Poetry, of course, is not based exclusively on metaphor, but metaphorical language is one of its fundamental components. Let us take as an example Blake's beautiful poem "The Sick Rose":

> *O Rose, thou art sick!*
> *The invisible worm*
> *That flies in the night,*
> *In the howling storm,*
>
> *Has found out thy bed*
> *Of crimson joy;*
> *And his dark secret love*
> *Does thy life destroy.*

Ostensibly the poem is about a beautiful flower that has been invaded and is being destroyed by an ugly worm. But there are many more levels of metaphorical meaning. What comes easily to mind is that the rose stands for a beautiful woman and that the worm stands for a fatal illness that soon will destroy her. In fact, the poet addresses the rose as a person. He says, "thou art sick!" Such comparisons between flowers and women, and worms and illnesses, occur not only in poetry but also in dreams and in schizophrenic ideation.

We have seen how in psychopathologic conditions and in dreams common predicates lead to metamorphosis: that is, to identifications with what, to normal or waking people, seem dissimilar subjects. In poetry there is no *metamorphosis*, but *metaphor*. The poet knows that the rose is not a woman, but he feels the woman is like a rose.

In order to compare the sick flower to the sick woman, the poet has accessibility to the formation of a primary class that was described at the beginning of this chapter as consisting of equivalent or interchangeable members. Now, is a primary class involved in the making of a poetic metaphor? Yes and no.

The poet does not *actually* substitute the sick rose for the sick woman. The sick rose is not the sick woman; but in the sick rose he sees the sick woman. In schizophrenia, the interchangeability or displacement is complete instead of partial: for instance, in the example in which the patient becomes the Virgin Mary. In the schizophrenic, the primary class of virgin women was an unconscious class.

In poetry, the displacement—for instance, from the woman to the rose—is conscious. The poet wants to react to the sick woman as he would to a sick rose. Whereas in psychopathologic conditions and in dreams the displacement is from the real object to the symbolic, in poetry it is from the symbolic object (the rose) to the real (the woman). The difference is deeper than that. Let us take Blake's poem again. As we have already mentioned, the rose does not *replace* the woman (as the Virgin Mary replaces the patient, who is no longer the patient but who has undergone the delusional metamorphosis of becoming the Virgin Mary). In the poem we see the woman in the rose. The woman and the rose are fused; but it is not that bizarre fusion that we see in schizophrenic drawings and delusions. The woman and the rose, though fused, retain their individuality. The retention of their individuality permits a comparison, yet does not lead to identification. How is this possible? It is possible because by putting the sick rose and the sick woman together, we become at least partially *conscious* of a class: the class of "beautiful life destroyed by illness." As a matter of fact, it is enough for the human cognitive faculties to be aware of only two members of a class to become aware of the whole class.

But is this class primary or secondary? Both, and, in a certain way, neither. In the act of being created, the class is primary. Finding common predicates among different subjects, and identifying by virtue of these common predicates is a primary-process mechanism. The primary process tends to remain primary: the rose and the woman tend to interchange or to remain together; but as the concept of the class "beautiful life destroyed by illness" emerges, their fusion does not become, so to speak, consummated. They remain distinct. However, the level of secondary class is not reached completely in the poem, or does not remain independent from the primary-process origin. The poet does not deal on a cognitive level with "beauty destroyed by illness." Only the student of art may translate the poem into a secondary-level content. The poem itself oscillates between a primary level and a secondary level, which is inferred. Here is, thus, an important difference between art and psychopathology: *whereas in the psychopathologic use of the primary process there is no consciousness of abstraction* (as a matter of fact, the power of abstraction is impaired and has to find concrete channels) *in art the use of the primary process does not eliminate the abstract. On the contrary, it is through the medium of the primary process that the abstract concept emerges.*

A physician would not compare a woman to a rose in order to clarify the outcome of a fatal illness or in order to lead to the formation of a new class. Why does a poet need a rose invaded by a worm to tell us that fatal sickness in a beautiful woman is a horrible thing? Why does he need to resort to his unusual accessibility to primary classes?

The poet discovers that things abound in similarities. New similarities take on new meanings because each recognized similarity is a concept and implies the formation of a new class. One of the main ways of expanding knowledge that the aesthetic fields have in common with science, as we shall show below,

is the formation of new classes or categories.

Let us remember what happens in jokes: the joke is based on the eventual recognition that logic and paleologic are not identical but only similar. The recognition of the logic-paleologic discordance leads to the comic reaction. In some puns and parables there is more agreement than disagreement between the logic and the paleologic. In poetry, there is agreement between paleologic and logic. Paleologic actually reinforces logic.

Art, indeed, is founded to a great extent on *paleologic reinforcement.* At the same time that the work of art elicits the abstract concept, it sustains itself upon the paleologic reinforcement, or identification with a concrete example. There is almost a perfect welding of the abstract concept with the concrete example, of the replaced object with its metaphor. The concrete object of the metaphor is not only a symbol, it is a participant in producing the effect. In paleologic mechanisms, as used by the schizophrenic, the object that is replaced or symbolized fades away (at least from consciousness) or it is replaced by its symbol. In our example the virgin patient disappears and is replaced by the Virgin Mary. In dreams, too, what is symbolized is no longer present. For instance, in a dream a gorilla may stand for one's father. The image of the father is completely absent, and only psychoanalytic work can recapture it. In art the replaced object fades away also, but not entirely. It fades away only in its concrete essence; its presence is felt in its absence. The woman is not mentioned in Blake's poem, but her presence is felt. She exists in the artistic assumption. At the same time that the work of art eliminates her, she is there as a rose. Symbolism and reality hold hands.

There are other factors to be considered in the study of the metaphor. In a brief poetic passage we may find only one metaphor, but in highly artistic works more than one metaphor is combined. Let us reexamine Blake's poem. We have seen that the rose stands for a beautiful woman who is sick and that we are, so to speak, invited to pity the fate of this woman. In some respects, this is a recurring theme in literature. It is simple to think of an ailing woman named after the flowers she liked so much: *la dame aux camelias* of French literature. We can also think of heroines in Italian operas: in *La Bohème*, Mimi is not a sick flower but a sick maker of artificial flowers. Her beauty is compared to the crimson beauty of dawn and of sunset. Something vaguely associated with this image is also found in Dante. In the first of the dreams reported in his early book *La Vita Nuova*, he describes how Beatrice appeared to him in the arms of a male figure, Eros or Love. Beatrice is partially covered by a red cloth. The whole scene takes place in a cloud, red as fire. Dante knows that Beatrice is going to die because of something Love has made her eat.

In Blake's poem, however, many other metaphorical meanings are suggested. As in Dante's dream, the invader is a male (*his* dark secret love). The bed of crimson joy conveys the image of femininity and sexuality, from the point of view of a male (crimson are the cheeks, lips, and, perhaps, the vagina of the woman). The rose becomes more female, the worm more male. Accessory predicates that lead to more identification increase the artistic value, just as they do in jokes.

But there is much more in the poem. The invisible worm that flies in the night, in the howling storm, which with his secret love invades the bed of crimson joy and destroys life, may suggest an evil-producing sexuality, a sadistic passion, a "dark" love, not something appropriate for crimson joy.

At this level of understanding the poem would represent a drama between two people, woman and man, the battle of the sexes. But the poem can be interpreted at a much more abstract level where it represents beauty and evil that must, but cannot, coexist in the same universe, for, in the end, evil often destroys beauty. The worm may represent the seed of spiritual decay. And yet the worm may even appear not so evil in its evil, because it is capable of loving and it is only that love which leads to destruction. The worm, too, wants to flee from the "howling storm," that is, from the horrible and tempestuous world; but, inasmuch as it is part of that world, it will end by producing evil.

We could find other levels of meaning. The rose and the woman appear like sisters, in the sense in which Francis of Assisi saw the brotherhood and sisterhood in the disparate existences of the universe. The new class or "family," to which the rose and the woman belong, reasserts the universal encounter with life, love, sorrow, decay, and death. We enter, thus, into an indefinite realm of symbolism, for the classes of symbolized objects accrue by a sequence of paleologic analogies that are like more and more windows, more and more doors, opening into unguessed aspects of reality, into unpredicted worlds. In the great work of art we can seek and find more and more analogic expansions. Thus, though the new object has been found, the longing and the search continue. The finiteness of the new object contrasts with the indeterminacy of the search. And yet the search itself becomes part of the newly created work, of the new unity, an aesthetic entity that in its totality appears for the first time in the universe. This is occasionally referred to as the unfinished statement of the work of art.

We are ready to appreciate new aesthetic unities. All of us respond to phonetically beautiful words and to their rhythm; we pity beautiful women who become sick and die; we are concerned with evil that destroys beauty; we are receptive to the sensuous beauty of flowers and have some distaste for earthy worms. Everything was ready for the fitting of all these elements together, but somebody had to make them click. Blake did this by harmoniously blending primary and secondary processes, as in a symphony, never heard before, of unsuspected predicates. The synthesis Blake achieved can easily be communicated and shared. The originality of the new unity contrasts with the response to such a unity, which is almost a general one.

Can then a poetic fusion of primary and secondary processses be compared to a discovery? In a certain way, yes; but only to a special type. An aesthetic discovery may not make us know things that we did not know before. However, it creates a new affective experience.

Schizophrenic language and dreams, too,

have different meanings and different levels of cognition. However, in psychopathological conditions these different meanings are discordant; furthermore, often they do not coexist but replace one another. That is, the dreamer and the talking schozophrenic are aware only of what they see in the dream or of what they say at a manifest level. They need the therapist to recapture all or many of the meanings. If there is a unity, it is in the atmospheric feeling or in a sort of primitive affective gestalt. Although the schizophrenic experience is also a new experience, it is actually a reduction to a concrete level, a restriction, not an enlargement, unless some new understanding or the recapturing of the abstract meaning is obtained through recovery or therapy.

At times the artist has a capacity for imagery almost to the extent that the dreamer has, or that capacity for "orgies of identification" that the schizophrenic has. He is able, however, to use them in unpredictable syntheses that become works of art. Victor Hugo, in his poems, compares the stars in multiple and, to the average person, inconceivable ways: to diamonds, other jewels, golden clouds, golden pebbles, lamps, lighted temples, flowers of eternal summer, silvery lilies, eyes of the night, vague eyes of the twilight, embers of the sky, holes in a huge ceiling, bees that fly in the sky, drops of Adam's blood, and even to the colored spots on the tail of the peacock.

Another characteristic that literary men, especially poets, and people using primary-process thinking have in common, is the use of homonymy or similarity of words, as I have already mentioned. I shall start with a classic example from Shakespeare.

In Shakespeare's *Othello*, Othello is a black man, a Moor. Actually, in the original Italian story, written by Giovanni Battista Giraldi Cintio, from which Shakespeare took the plot, Othello was a white man, a Venetian patrician who was a lieutenant in Cyprus in the year 1508. Giraldi's story gives no names, but historical documents indicate that the episodes reported by Giraldi Cintio really took place and that the family name of this lieutenant

was *Moro. Moro*, in Italian, means Negro or Moor, but in the case of this lieutenant, Moro was his last name, which had no reference whatever to his race or color. It could be that Shakespeare mistook a family name for a name referring to the color of the person involved. I am more inclined to believe that such coincidence stimulated Shakespeare's mental associations. Shakespeare may have had the inspiration that if Othello were really a Moro (Moor) or Negro, the story would have an uncommon artistic twist and the contrast with the fair, "divine" Desdemona would be accentuated. A real pun was made of the name *Moro*.

Similar puns, quasi-puns, and strange plays on words are common in literature and especially in poetry. A typical one is from Petrarch, who in a great variety of ways plays on the word *Laura*, the name of the woman he loved.

*L'aura che 'l verde lauro e l'aureo crine
soavemente sospirando move. . . .*

Here the name Laura is felt and heard in three different words (*l'aura*—the zephyr; *lauro*—the laurel; *l'aureo crine*—the golden hair).

Dante too resorts to plays on words that, at first impression, are reminiscent of schizophrenic cognition. In *La Vita Nuova*, a book consisting of poems and poetic prose, he wrote that once he saw Beatrice walking on the street, *preceded* by her girlfriend, Giovanna, who was once the beloved of Dante's friend and fellow poet Cavalcanti. Dante wrote that Giovanna, because of her beauty, was often called *Primavera*, which in Italian means spring. Dante then makes a peculiar play on words. *Primavera* signifies for him *prima verrà*, which in Italian means "she will come first, before." (That is, before or preceding Beatrice while walking.) But a second play on words is even more revealing. The real name of Beatrice's friend is Giovanna (the feminine of Giovanni or John in English). Dante then compared her to John the Baptist who *came before* or *preceded* the coming of Christ.

The underlying, unconscious motivation appearing several times in Dante's works resides in his wish to identify Beatrice, whom he occasionally calls the daughter of God, to Jesus Christ. He wants to make this identification not only in order to glorify the object of his love, in real life a woman named Beatrice, but in order to transform his profane or earthly love into a sacred or divine love.

Dante must resort to the ambiguity of primary-process thinking in order to make this identification possible. But he knows that this way of thinking, which he follows, is not logical. He knows that if people believed that he accepted these ideas as true they would consider him insane, but he manages to pass the reality test by using a trick made available by his secondary-process mechanism. He says that he does not really believe in these ideas. He writes "it seemed that Love spoke in my heart" and said those things. He tells the reader that this is fantasy, but there seems to be little doubt that he would like to believe part at least of this fantasy. As a matter of fact, the whole *La Vita Nuova* and *The Divine Comedy* are suffused with a mysticism that is not just part of an aesthetic technique. This mysticism is a special type of reality for the poet: I would say not just the reality of a wish, but the real reality.

Some recovering schizophrenics retain a greater accessibility to the primary process than normal persons and are, nevertheless, in a position to use the secondary process. Reports of such cases are rare because the examiner has to see these patients during a special transitional stage that lasts a very short time and is easily missed if not looked for. These reports are extremely important. More than anything else, they disclose the double role that the primary process can play in illness and creativity.

Let me quote a thirteen-year-old, schizophrenic girl, who was admitted to the hospital following a rather acute psychotic episode. During this episode she experienced hallucinations, delusions, and ideas of reference. In a routine mental examination three days later, she was asked to "explain the difference between character and reputation." She replied: "Reputation is stamped on and can never be erased. Your reputation is a bed; and when you get in, you can't get out of it. Character is like a bedspread which can be taken off, or character is like dirt on a sheet which, if you wash it, can be removed." The patient was asked to define the word despair. She answered: "Despair is like a wall covered with thick grease, and a person is trying to climb up this wall by digging his fingers in. Down below is a deep, bottomless pit. Up at the top of the wall on the ceiling is a big, black spider. I have been in this deep pit during the past year, but now I am climbing up a rope, trying to get out of it."

These definitions of character, reputation, and despair are not those that we would read in a dictionary. They have a great deal to do with the life experiences of the patient, and they are representations of concepts by means of visual images as they occur in dreams and in other functions where the primary process prevails. They are examples of what we have called perceptualization of the concept.

I want to mention briefly another patient, a poetess who experienced occasionally quasi-schizophrenic episodes. They were elusive in nature; often it was difficult to determine whether or not she was in a psychotic state. At times her poems resembled almost schizophrenic word salad; at other times they had a genuine beauty. They were, nevertheless, always difficult to understand, like many examples of contemporary poetry. At the beginning of her treatment, she used to speak of human beings as worms. She also wrote poems in which people were represented as worms. There would not have been any difficulty in accepting such ideas at a metaphorical level, except for the fact that she insisted that people were really worms. It was impossible to determine whether this statement was made in a metaphorical sense or not. There was a flavor of literalness on her remarks. Even if she meant "worms" metaphorically, there was a resolute attachment to this metaphor, as if it literally represented reality. Her expressions seemed to belong to an intermediate, hard-to-delineate stage between metamorphosis and metaphor. As her condition improved, she wrote poems in which the metaphorical meaning of the word worm could no longer be doubted.*

❮ Science

In a by-now-classic work on creativity, the great French mathematician Poincaré described the moments of creative illumination that he experienced.[29] In the morning, following a sleepless night spent working on a mathematical problem without finding the looked-for result, he got on a bus. At the moment he put his foot on the step, the idea came to him, apparently without any conscious effort, that the transformation he had used to define the Fuchsian functions were identical with those of non-Euclidian geometry. This sudden illumination was a breakthrough leading to great expansion in the field of mathematics.

Poincaré described his subjective experiences extremely well, but he did not stress the fact that his creative insight consisted of seeing an *identity* between two previously reputed dissimilar transformations: the Fuchsian and the non-Euclidian. During the previous night, and for fourteen days prior to that night, Poincaré had accumulated facts. But accumulation of data is not creativity; many people are able to accumulate facts. The creative leap occurs when observed facts are correlated; that is, when by perceiving a heretofore unsuspected identity, a conjunctive path or a new order is discovered.

We could multiply endlessly the instances where great discoveries were made by the act of perceiving an identity among two or more things that had seemed dissimilar or unrelated. Newton observed an apple falling from a tree and saw a common quality in the apple attracted by the earth and the motions of heavenly bodies. Newton perceived the similarity between two forces, that which caused an apple to fall to the earth and that which retains the moon in its orbit. He validated this

* For other examples of poetry in schizophrenia see Arieti[8, 10] and a fine article by Forrest.[13]

insight by comparing the rate of falling bodies on the earth with the rate at which the moon deviated from the straight line that it would have followed had the earth not existed.

Darwin saw a similarity between Malthus's theories and the life of the jungle, and this association led him to conceive his theory of evolution. Freud saw formal similarities between dreams and jokes, and this observation opened the path to the study of the creative process, although he did not become aware of the possibility of this new development.

Of course, the observation of similarity is not enough. For instance, the transformations used by Poincaré and those of non-Euclidian geometry are not in every respect identical. An apple is dissimilar in size, origin, and chemical structure from the moon, and yet Newton saw a similarity. In what way are the moon and the apple similar? What does their partial identity consist of? Of being members of a class of bodies subjected to gravitation. Thus, at the same time that Newton saw the similarity between the apple and the moon, *a new class was formed* to which an indefinite number of members could be added. The new object for which he was searching, and which he found, was a class.

The discovery of this class revealed a new way of looking at the universe, because each member of the class came to be recognized as having similar properties. Is this new class a primary class as we have described it at the beginning of this paper? Obviously not. It differs on many counts.

First, when Newton perceived the identical element, he did not respond to the stimulus but to the class. Had he been a regressed schizophrenic, after seeing a similarity between the moon and the apple he could have paleologically identified the moon with the apple and could have thought that the moon could be eaten like an apple; or thought it could be sucked like the maternal breast, as Renée, a by-now-famous schizophrenic patient reported by Sechehaye, did during a stage of her illness.[32]

Second, Newton's creativity consisted in seeing a common property in the moon and the apple, and in not identifying them but in seeing them as members of a new class. An increased ability to see similarities, which is a property of the primary process, is here connected with a concept and the tertiary process emerges. The secondary class loses all its original connections with the primary process. However, although the new class is very well-defined, the search is not ended. The understanding of the Newtonian system is a prerequisite to the eventual opening of the Einsteinian world of classes.

(Some Conclusions About Formal Mechanisms in Creativity

We could at this point, as a sort of summary, state that in wit an ostensibly secondary class is recognized as primary. In poetic metaphor, a primary and a secondary class reinforce one another; in science, what originated as a primary class proves to be a secondary class.

If we look at the three basic processes, primary, secondary, and tertiary, we can conclude that an important common characteristic of them all resides in the ability to differentiate similarities from manifold experience.

Similarity indicates that there is some kind of recurrence and, therefore, regularity in the universe. It is from these segments of regularity that the human mind plunges into the understanding of the cosmos. In psychopathology, normality, and creativity, the ability to register similarity is the common guiding principle—a tiny and tremulous light with which to pierce the secret of universal night! It is on the varying responses to similarity that the ultimate rise or the ultimate fall of man depends. We can represent these variations by resorting to imagery: for the primary process, all that glitters is gold. It will be the labor of the secondary process to discover that all that glitters is not gold. The tertiary process will do at least one of two things: either it will bestow the glitter of the gold to other substances to beautify them artistically or it will create a new class of glittering objects.

(The Cultivation of Creativity

It is well known that creative people appear in particularly large numbers in certain periods of history in given geographical areas. This uneven distribution seems to indicate that special environmental circumstances and not exclusively biological factors determine the occurrence of creativity. It is enough to think of four major examples—the classic Greek period, the Italian Renaissance, the group of people who conceived the American revolution and gave the world a new concept of man, the contributions of the Jewish people since the nineteenth century—to realize that creativity does not occur at random, but is enhanced by environmental factors.

Kroeber[25] states that "inasmuch as even the people possessing higher civilization have produced cultural products of value only intermittently, during relatively small fractions of their time span, it follows that more individuals born with the endowment of genius have been inhibited by the cultural situations into which they were born than have been developed by other cultural situations." He also states that "genetics leaves only an infinitesimal possibility for the racial stock occupying England to have given birth to no geniuses at all between 1450 and 1550 and a whole series of geniuses in literature, music, science, philosophy, and politics between 1550 and 1650. Similarly with the Germany of 1550–1650 and 1700–1800, respectively, and innumerable other instances in history." If Kroeber is correct in his conclusions, we must accept that the possibility for the development of a large number of creative people always exists in certain populations. We may add that, in addition to general sociohistorical factors, special personal factors and attitudes acquired from early childhood through the whole period of adolescence are important in actualizing a potentiality toward creativity.

It is to be expected that educators and sociologists will resort more and more to child and adolescent psychiatry, school psychology, school psychiatry, and mental hygiene in their efforts to accumulate that body of knowledge which, once applied, could promote creativity and remove inhibiting factors. There is also the possibility, as it will appear from what follows, that some characteristics or habits that have so far been considered unhealthy or undesirable may be recognized as favorable to creativity. The reverse may also be true.

Studies made independently by several authors have determined that highly intelligent persons are not necessarily highly creative (Getzels and Jackson,[19] Hammer[22]). Although creative people are intelligent persons, an exceptionally high IQ is not a prerequisite for creativity. On the contrary, it may inhibit the inner resources of the individual because of too rigid self-criticism or too quick learning of what the cultural environment has to offer. We must add that a great ability to deduce according to the laws of logic and mathematics makes for disciplined thinkers, but not necessarily for creative people.

The science of promoting creativity is in the initial stages. The author can suggest only rudimentary and tentative notions, deduced from his psychoanalytic-psychotherapeutic treatment of a relatively large number of creative people. These notions have to be confirmed or disproved by much more evidence than is available now. Statistical data are difficult to find because standards are lacking. In fact it is an arduous task to get agreement on a definition of that particular cognitive gift which is creativity.

Two things now seem established:

1) An inclination toward creativity must be fostered in childhood and/or adolescence, even if it is not revealed until much later in life.

2) As a whole, American culture has not enhanced creativity. The psychiatrist Jurgen Ruesch[31] has pointed out that, in proportion to her population, Switzerland has a much larger number of Nobel Prize winners than the United States.

American culture, following perhaps the attitude toward work and the acquisitive spirit of the early pioneers, has placed greater value on doing than on creating, especially when what is created is artistic or theoretical. Americans are predominantly a nation of doers, and as doers they are generally very efficient, both in technology and productivity. Now it is time to reexamine our methods of fostering creativity just as we reexamined our teaching methods after Sputnik.

In the present chapter we have seen how the use of primitive forms of cognition is a prerequisite for many forms of creativity. We certainly do not advocate a fostering of psychopathology for the enhancement of creativity. Some people have tried to do so pharmacologically, by means of alcohol, opium derivatives, and, more recently, by lysergic acid diethylamide. These are methods that a psychiatrist cannot recommend: in addition to the danger of addiction, their value as promoters of creativity is more than doubtful. If it is true that they facilitate the reemergence of the primary process, they impair the use of the secondary process, and we have seen that creativity (or the tertiary process) emerges only by a harmonious matching of the two processes.

Instead of resorting to toxic procedures, we must consider, and possibly recommend, special attitudes, habits, and environmental conditions. The first condition to be considered is *aloneness*. Aloneness may be viewed as a partial sensory deprivation. To a much smaller degree it tends to reproduce what the experimentally induced sensory deprivation brings about. The solitary individual is not constantly and directly exposed to the conventional stimulations supplied by society. He has more possibility of listening to his inner self, to come in contact with his inner resources and with some manifestations of the primary process. Unfortunately, being alone is not advocated in our modern forms of educating adolescents. On the contrary, gregariousness and popularity are held in high esteem. The emphasis today is on "togetherness" and on what Riesman calls "other-directedness."[30] Calling a person an introvert has become a derogatory remark.

Aloneness should not be confused with painful loneliness or with withdrawal or constant solitude. It should only mean being able periodically to remain alone for a few hours. Aloneness, as we have characterized it, should be recommended not only as a preparation for a life of creativity, but also as a state of being when creative work is in process. At the present time, emphasis is on teamwork, especially in scientific research. It is highly doubtful that an original idea can come from a team, although teamwork is often useful for expanding and applying an original idea and, more than anything else, for developing the technology by which an original idea is applied for practical purposes.

In art, teamwork is almost unthinkable, although occasionally resorted to in second-rate work. One cannot even theoretically imagine such classics as *The Divine Comedy*, Michelangelo's statue of Moses, Shakespeare's *Macbeth*, or Beethoven's Ninth Symphony being created by more than one person.

In science, too, great discoveries and inventions have been made by single individuals. When more than one individual has made the same discovery or invention, the innovating ideas were arrived at independently (for instance, Newton and Leibnitz in the case of the calculus and Wallace and Darwin with respect to evolution).

A second condition that seems to promote creativity is in direct opposition to the present spirit of American culture: *inactivity*.

By inactivity, of course, we do not mean schizophrenic withdrawal or catatonic immobility, or excessive loafing, but taking time off to do nothing so far as a critical observer can see. If a person must always fix his attention on external work, he limits the possibility of developing his inner resources. Here again American upbringing pursues the opposite approach: high school and college students are encouraged to work during summer vacations. Any kind of manual labor is considered valuable in building the character of the future adult citizen. As a general rule, it is commendable to encourage youngsters to work. It promotes a sense of responsibility and of good citizenship. However, people with creative tendencies should, whenever possible, be given relatively long stretches of time for thinking and feeling about other things than work.

What we have just said about youngsters could, with some modifications, be said about adults who have already shown creative tendencies. Too much in the way of routine stifles mental activity and creativity. Moreover, even a creative career that has already started should be allowed to proceed at its own pace, which may be very slow, irregular, and intermittent.

The third characteristic is *daydreaming*. Daydreaming is often discouraged as unrealistic or, at least, as enlarging the gap between the individual's ambitions and capacities. Often it is discouraged because it is thought to promote a vicarious fantasy life that slows up the implementing of realistic and approved-of behavior. Although it is true that excessive daydreaming may have these characteristics, it is equally true that daydreaming is a source of fantasy life that may open up unforeseeable, new paths of growth and discovery to the individual. It is in daydreams that the individual permits himself to stray from the usual paths and go on little excursions into irrational worlds. Daydreaming affords human beings relief from the everyday conventions of society.

Remembrance and inner replaying of past traumatic conflicts is another important condition. It is generally assumed that once a person has overcome a psychological conflict or the effects of an early trauma, he should try to forget them. Forgetting in these cases requires an act of suppression, not of repression.

Some creative people recognize this belief is wrong, but they themselves fall into another error. They believe that the neurotic conflict is a prerequisite for creativity. At times they are reluctant to undergo psychotherapy or psychoanalytic therapy because they are afraid that if they lost their conflicts they would also lose the motivation and need to create. We must remember that conflicts *always* exist in the psyche of man. It is our job to distinguish between nontraumatic conflicts and traumatic or neurotic conflicts. Nontraumatic conflicts need not concern us here. But the creative person's traumatic or neurotic conflicts should be resolved, though not ignored after their solution. If these conflicts are not dealt with, they will continue being too deeply felt and too personal. The creative person will not be able to transcend his own subjective involvement and his work will lack universal significance or general resonance. The resolved or almost-resolved conflict, on the other hand can be viewed both with a sense of familiarity and as from distance by the creative person and thus be more easily transformed into a work of art or a scientific theory or discovery.

Another requirement for the creative person is even more difficult to accept: *gullibility.* This word is used here to mean the willingness to accept, at least temporarily or until proved wrong, that there are certain underlying orderly arrangements in everything outside us and inside us. Creativity often implies the discovery of these underlying orderly arrangements more than the inventing of new things. Connected with this special gullibility is the naive regard for similarities to be differentiated from the manifold of the universe. In preceding sections of this chapter we have discussed the importance of recognizing similarities.

The alleged discovery of underlying arrangements may, of course, be part also of paranoiac-paranoid ideation, and the acceptance of a similarity as a fact having significance may be part of schizophrenic thinking in general. However, the creative person does not accept such insights or seeming insights indiscriminately. He is gullible only to the extent of not discarding them a priori as nonsense. In fact, he goes a step further: he becomes more attuned to what seem to him truths. However, his final acceptance or rejection must depend on his secondary-process mechanisms.

Alertness and *discipline* are two other conditions necessary to creativity. Although they are also necessary prerequisites for productivity in general, they take on a particular aspect in creativity. Many would-be creative persons, especially in the artistic fields, like to believe that only such qualities as imagination, inspiration, intuition, and talent are important. They are reluctant to submit themselves to the rigor of learning techniques, discipline, logical thinking on the pretext that all these things would stultify their creativity. They ignore the fact that even such people as Giotto, Leonardo, Freud, and Einstein had teachers.

A humorous remark, which has by now become commonplace but in which there is a great deal of metaphorical truth, is that creativity is 10 percent inspiration and 90 percent perspiration. The personal traits and attitudes we have mentioned can, and should, be encouraged in our educational systems as well as in our daily lives.

The characteristics so briefly sketched, as well as others to be discovered in future studies, facilitate new combinations of primary and secondary processes that lead to the tertiary process. By this statement we do not mean that a process of creativity is just a "recombination" of already existing elements. The process and works of creativity are not just recombinations. From a new combination unexpected, at times completely new, entities come into being. In the midst of all these factors, the results of genetics, of history, and of chance man emerges as the unifier of motivation, knowledge, choice, and inexplicable subjectivity.

As we have already mentioned, there are also important social factors which bring about cultural combinations that facilitate creativity. The author of this chapter can only briefly allude to them, as he is not a historian or a sociologist. The Italian Renaissance emerged in an environment of relative freedom and prosperity as a kind of amalgam of the rediscovered classic Greco-Roman culture and the medieval Christian culture. The elements that precipitated the American revolution were a combination of English philosophy, values and traditions and the new adventurous, enterprising, and individualistic spirit of the American colonists. The notable achievements of Swiss citizens may partially be ascribed to the meeting and cross-fertilization of three different cultures. The recent achievements of the Jewish people, culminating in the appearance of such persons as Freud and Einstein, can be ascribed, in part, to the meeting of the old Hebrew culture with the rest of Western civilization.

The United States of America is in a privileged position today by virtue of its many cultural minorities living in what is basically an Anglo-Saxon culture. If a mingling of all the minorities rather than an assimilation into the predominant culture is permitted, then the most favorable conditions possible for creativity will arise. That is, if in addition, the necessary educational facilities are provided and special care is taken of the promising individual.

(Bibliography

1. ANDERSON, H. H., ed., *Creativity and Its Cultivation*. New York: Harper & Bros., 1959.
2. ARIETI, SILVANO. "Special Logic of Schizophrenic and Other Types of Autistic Thought," *Psychiatry*, 11 (1948), 325–338.
3. ———. "Primitive Intellectual Mechanisms in Psychopathological Conditions. Study of the Archaic Ego," *Am. J. Psychother.*, 4 (1950), 4–15.
4. ———. "New Views on the Psychology and Psychopathology of Wit and of the Comic," *Psychiatry*, 13 (1950), 43–62.
5. ———. *Interpretation of Schizophrenia*. New York: Robert Brunner, 1955.
6. ———. "The Microgeny of Thought and Perception: A Psychiatric Contribution," *Arch. Gen. Psychiatry*, 6 (1962), 454–468.
7. ———. "The Rise of Creativity: From Primary to Tertiary Process," *Cont. Psychoanal.*, 1 (1964), 51–68.
8. ———. *The Intrapsychic Self. Feeling, Cognition and Creativity in Health and Mental Illness*. New York: Basic Books, 1967.
9. ———. "Schizophrenic Art and Relation to Modern Art," *J. Am. Acad. Psychoanal.*, 1 (1973), 333–365.
10. ———. *Interpretation of Schizophrenia*. Revised 2nd ed. New York: Basic Books, 1974.
11. ———. *Creativity*. (tentative title). New York: Basic Books, forthcoming.
12. EIDUSON, B. T. *Scientists; Their Psychological World*. New York: Basic Books, 1962.
13. FORREST, D. V. "Poiesis and the Language of Schizophrenia," *Psychiatry*, 28 (1965), 1–18.
14. FREUD, SIGMUND. "The Relation of the Poet to Day-Dreaming" (1908), in B. Nelson, ed., *Freud on Creativity and the Unconscious*, pp. 44–54. New York: Harper & Bros., 1958.
15. ———. "The Unconscious" (1915), in *Collected Papers*, Vol. 4, pp. 98–136. New York: Basic Books, 1959.
16. ———. *Wit and Its Relation to the Unconscious* (1916), in *The Basic Writings of Sigmund Freud*, pp. 633–803. New York: Modern Library, 1938.
17. ———. *Leonardo Da Vinci: A Study in Psychosexuality*. New York: Random House, 1947.
18. ———. *The Interpretation of Dreams*. James Strachey, transl. New York: Basic Books, 1960.
19. GETZELS, J. W. and P. W. JACKSON. *Creativity and Intelligence. Explorations with Gifted Children*. New York: Wiley, 1962.
20. GHISELIN, B. *The Creative Process*. Berkeley: University of California Press, 1952.
21. GRUBER, H. E., G. TERRELL, and M. WERTHEIMER. *Contemporary Approaches to Creative Thinking*. New York: Atherton, 1962.
22. HAMMER, E. F. *Creativity*. New York: Random House, 1961.
23. KOESTLER, A. *The Act of Creation*. New York: Macmillan, 1964.
24. KRIS, ERNST. *Psychoanalytic Explorations in Art*. New York: International Universities Press, 1952.
25. KROEBER, ALFRED L. *Configurations of Culture Growth*. Berkeley: University of California Press, 1944.
26. KUBIE, LAWRENCE S. *Neurotic Distortion of the Creative Process*. Lawrence: University of Kansas Press, 1958.
27. MORA, G. "One Hundred Years from Lombroso's First Essay, 'Genius and Insanity,' " *Am. J. Psychiatry*, 121 (1964), 562–571.
28. PHILIPSON, M. *Outline of Jungian Aesthetics*. Evanston: Northwestern University Press, 1963.
29. POINCARÉ, HENRI. "Mathematical Creation," pp. 383–394, in *The Foundation of Science*. Lancaster, Pa.: The Science Press, 1946.
30. RIESMAN, DAVID, NATHAN GLAZER, and R. DENNEY. *The Lonely Crowd*. New Haven: Yale University Press, 1950.
31. RUESCH, JURGEN. "The Trouble with Psychiatric Research," *Arch. Neurol. Psychiatry*, 77 (1957), 93–107.

32. SECHEHAYE, M. A. *Symbolic Realization.* New York: International Universities Press, 1951.

33. STEIN, M. I. and S. J. HEINZE. *Creativity and the Individual. Summary of Selected Literature in Psychology and Psychiatry.* Glencoe, Ill.: The Free Press, 1960.

34. TAYLOR, G. W. and F. BARRON, eds., *Scientific Creativity: Its Recognition and Development.* New York: Wiley, 1963.

35. VON BERTALANFFY, LUDWIG. "The Mind-Body Problem: A New View," *Psychosom. Med.,* 24 (1964), 29–45.

36. VON DOMARUS, E. "The Specific Laws of Logic in Schizophrenia," in J. S. Kasanin, ed., *Language and Thought in Schizophrenia: Collected Papers,* pp. 104–114. Berkeley: University of California Press, 1944.

CHAPTER 12

THE RELEVANCE OF GENERAL SYSTEMS THEORY TO PSYCHIATRY

Roy R. Grinker, Sr.

(**Introduction**

THE RELATIONSHIP of systems theory to psychiatry is appropriate for consideration at this time despite at least two decades of neglect and even resistance.[9] Obstructions against bringing the two together are somewhat surprising in view of their historical origins and similar modern fate. The general laws of biological systems and their universal applicability were understood by the now-extinct naturalists in the early part of the twentieth century. Psychiatry beginning during the age of reason in the eighteenth century as a derivative of philosophy by way of psychology also began with holistic approaches. Unfortunately, biological sciences fragmented into smaller and smaller units or disciplines that became increasingly reductionistic, and

psychiatry fragmented into schools representing its parts.

Paul Weiss[42,92] expressed this succinctly: "In breaking down the Universe into smaller systems, into the society, the group, the organism, the cells, the cellular parts, and so forth, we dissect the system: that is we sever relations, and then we try awkwardly and clumsily to restore those relations systematically but frequently very inadequately." Again Paul Weiss: "If we had come down from the universe gradually through the hierarchy of systems to the atoms, we would be much better off. Instead we now have to resynthesize the conceptual bonds between those parts which we have cut in the first place."

Increasing attempts are now being made to develop unifying theories for all sciences, particularly the biological and others applicable to human behavior. It is as if systems analysis is searching for fitting empirical data and methods by which to test its basic concepts, and the extended and fragmented field of psychiatry is searching for appropriate general theory. The question of relevance of systems analysis for psychiatry is one example of modern dynamic or process thinkings which involves pluralistic[1] or multifactorial[4] approaches.

(Systems Theory

DERIVATION

As supernatural and philosophical "holism" gave way to modern science, increasingly detailed and isolated bits of information were elicited from investigations of living and nonliving structures and functions. This corresponds to what Weiss termed "breaking down the universe into smaller systems." Physicochemical processes were expected eventually to explain life and all its attributes by so-called reductionists, as contrasted with the humanistic broad approaches by social scientists.

Academic psychology became patterned within the reductionistic framework as it imitated the hard sciences by utilizing the stimulus-response paradigm of reflex activity. Life processes were viewed as being in a natural state of rest or equilibrium disturbed only by powerful drives utilized in the service of survival or in response to extraneous stimuli. This equilibrium theory viewed life processes as primarily *reactive* and man was viewed as a robot.[11,24]

Against this early twentieth-century tide a small coterie of naturalists working on experimental animals developed a series of process propositions on which many of our current concepts are based.[21,54] Briefly stated they are: hypothetical whole living organisms function not simply as sums of their parts but subserve new emergent functions; organisms mature by differentiation of primary undifferentiated structure-functions; living boundary

structures are semipermeable and permit control of input and output; substructures of whole organisms exist in gradients under central control or regulation; final common pathways[56] carry many processes from divergent internal sources to achieve near-identical actions; living organisms maintain homeostasis within a healthy range under conditions of moderate stress.

These and other paradigms derived from the biological, psychological, and social sciences produced isolated and sometimes disparate bits of information. How do laboratory and behavioral researches dovetail and how do regulations at various levels of organization interdigitate? These questions within the general climate of philosophic appraisal of relevance led to the quest for theories concerned with the unity of science and especially of human behavior.[10]

DEFINITION OF "SYSTEMS"

Systems have been defined with the use of many sets of words, but their basic meanings are almost identical. Clearly one must differentiate between living and nonliving systems, the latter being closed, with minimal or at least very slow exchange with their environments. The former are actively engaged in transactions with their environments as open systems. In fact, living systems can only exist by virtue of such exchanges.

The emergence and expansion of behavioral and social sciences, the abandonment of the reactive robot psychology applied to man, and the sterility of the reductionistic approaches to man stimulated multidisciplinary research oriented toward understanding total behavior and its component parts. Failure to reduce all behavior to a common basis and sterility of an encyclopedic accumulation of knowledge led to efforts at synthesis of total systems[19] or, in other words, a unified theory of human behavior.[42]

General systems may be defined succinctly as, for example, "a set of objects together with relationship between the objects and between their attributes";[97] a complex of components in mutual interaction;[8] a goal-setting principle variably operating by an "interplay of code-terminates";[16] "a regulated set of relations" with degrees of stability, change and meaning;[89] or "a broad vision of a totally integrated field composed of many part functions and transactions, each of which constitutes the focus of a wide variety of scientific disciplines";[47] or, finally, "it is only recently that the term System has been emerging as a symbol for a key concept indicating a trend toward unified theory. To achieve such a step there are required at least three major advances: (1) to define organization, structural and functional wholeness and its relation to its parts and its environment; (2) to define basic principles applicable to the analysis of all systems of inquiry and (3) to define operations, in terms of procedures used, by which these definitions may be acquired."[42]

Finally a more elegant definition has been furnished by Boulding.[12]

General systems theory is a name which has come into use to describe a level of theoretical model building which lies somewhere between the highly generalized constructions of pure mathematics and the specific theories of the specialized disciplines. The objectives of general systems theory can be set out with varying degrees of ambition and confidence. At a low level of ambition but with a high degree of confidence it aims to point out similarities in the theoretical constructions of different disciplines, where these exist, and to develop theoretical models having application to at least two different fields of study. At a higher level of ambition, but with perhaps a lower degree of confidence it hopes to develop something like a "spectrum" of theories—a system of systems which may perform the function of a 'gestalt' in the theoretical construction. Such 'gestalts' in special fields have been of great value in directing research towards the gaps which they reveal.

As a conceptual system in itself general systems theory can be treated by attempting to formulate its functional wholeness, its internal structure-function and the manner in which it leads to operational definitions. In a more practical way Ruesch[42,77] states that the observer characteristics, the coding characteristics, the form of information exchanges and empirical applications are necessary attributes of systems.

General system theory is what may be called a metatheory that is a conceptual overarching global theory which embraces several limited theories. These are the parts of the total system. These theoretical parts may be grouped according to Spiegel[83] into *constitutional*, which includes the internal structure–function of the system, *integrative*, which functions to relate the parts to the whole and prevent their disintegration or fragmentation, and *determinants* that describe the function of the system in relation to other external systems.

It is not possible to enumerate the many subtheories or sub-subtheories since these are chosen according to taste, discipline, and available operations. But for the purposes of delineating parts of general systems theory that later will be considered relevant to psychiatry I shall briefly describe theories related to (1) ontogeny, (2) differentiation and de-differentiation, (3) regulation and homeostasis, (4) hierarchies, isomorphism and boundaries, (5) communications of information by transactions, and (6) growth, creativity, and evolution.

ONTOGENY

Systems do not develop de novo because they and their parts have a past that remains part of their present even though partially obscured. A process of maturation and development characterizes both living and conceptual systems. For the latter, social-historical processes, changing value systems, and ethics contribute to conceptual shifts whether we speak of social changes or scientific ethics.

The developmental processes within living systems are more obvious although still not clearly understood. The science of genetics has been furthered by increased understanding of the genetic code incorporated in DNA and its transmission by RNA. Both aberrant and healthy genetic and experiential factors form the background of subsequent behavior at all levels of the organism from infancy to old age. Biogenetics and behavioral genetics are species and individual specific and constitute a system with only limited independence of environmental stimuli and conditions that are necessary to release the inherent or innate.

An appreciation of the ontogenic system must include isolating not only the factors concerned with growth but also critical periods during which a jump step is made across a boundary, after which different forms of development are possible. Within this system, phases of the individual life cycle of health and illness from birth to death have their own structure, function, susceptibilities, coping mechanisms, and predominate types of degradation.

DIFFERENTIATION AND DEDIFFERENTIATION

Parts of systems come into focus by a process of *differentiation* from an undifferentiated whole.[21,54] These parts may be enumerated in various ways, depending upon the position of the observer and the resolving power of the observer's instruments. Here we may limit our view to that of the human intrapersonal system beyond the physicochemical substrate of elementary particles, atoms and molecules, and the individual cells. Then we would include the confluence of cells into individual organs and organ systems, the communicating systems of hormones, enzymes and the nervous system, the psychological system that extends beyond structure–function,[54] and the social and cultural systems learned or incorporated within psychological functions. Obviously many more and finer subdivisions or subsystems may be included.

Each differentiated part subserves special functions in relation to each other and the whole by some form of regulation. In this sense they function in cooperation but are also in conflict or antagonism. These vectors of synthesis and fragmentation usually function adequately through opposing systems of enzymes and antagonists, nervous facilitation and inhibition, negative and positive feedback and by quantitative and temporal gradients. In the psychological sense drive impulses and external or incorporated social restrictions reach a level of accommodation.

Probably the processes of *dedifferentiation* begin very early. To quote an ancient saying: "The first tottering steps of the child are toward the grave." We are less concerned with this inevitable slow process of aging than with the various stress stimuli that evoke greater degrees of responses ending in physical disease or psychological disintegration.

From a single subsystem, which strain may cause to disintegrate functionally, to all subsystems and eventually to a total response, stress responses progressively spread and increase. The result is a multiplicity of circular and corrective processes between subsystems that are oriented toward stabilizing the organism and maintaining its integration. A breakdown between boundaries and an intensification of activity occur only when the strain becomes too severe. Likewise, the pattern of behavior partially resumes its primitive infantile functions when the several subsystems that have been fractionated out of the whole are no longer able to handle the stress. At first, stress stimuli facilitate defenses, but when continued and increased, they disrupt and ultimately result in dedifferentiation. When the differentiated systems are under critical strain, the whole takes over and earlier patterns return.

Whether the organism reacts as a primitive whole before differentiation, or has been reduced by excessive stress to a dedifferentiated whole, the somatic and psychic systems are in a constant state of transaction with each other. Concomitant somatic and psychological action patterns probably occur only as the result either of lasting traumatic impressions made upon a total system before differentiation or of current stress forcing regression to that state.[34,42]

REGULATION AND HOMEOSTASIS

As parts of a system become differentiated they do not separate as in primary fission. Instead they constitute parts of a system characterized by a totality of elements held together by some form of central *regulation* that maintains integration or in other words functions against disintegration. In embryonic phases such a regulator functions to integrate the differentiating parts in proper temporal sequence. Within the functioning organism local feedback circuits maintain homeostatic balance directed to a great extent by the pituitary or master gland. The central nervous system regulates somatosensory activities in many ways but essentially in starting and stopping action, and relinquishing further control to lower levels. In psychological terms, ego functions maintain a balance among the pressures of needs, desires, and adaptive behavior.

Sometimes subsystems get out of control and the whole system decays. In other cases the regulator may be congenitally weak or crippled by drugs, disease, or fatigue. An example of the latter is the syndrome of ego depletion.[50] The soldier's experiences after a war destroy or weaken the compromises he has made between drives and reality and between their opposing trends. As a result of a breakdown of such psychological regulation the soldier regresses to apparently more immature coping attempts that cannot be successful in adult life.

It is not implied that functions of subsystems, their regulation or whole system, are rigidly and exactly programmed. There is a wide range of successful *homeostatic* functions that are wider in the young, narrower in the old. Failure results from exceeding these ranges.

HIERARCHIES, BOUNDARIES AND ISOMORPHISM

Hierarchies do not impose values on levels or subsystems in nonliving physicochemical processes, but they do in living foci such as cell, organ, psyche, society, and culture. All are essential for life that culminates in cultural levels developed by human symbolic evolution. Hierarchies may be defined in an evolutionary sense in that each level is necessary for the development of the next succeeding, higher in the sense of greater degrees of complexity and more flexible, organization. Levels of organization are related to their evolution in time.

Since subsystems are functionally interrelated, we may agree with Wilson[93] that the span of a system is "the number of subsystems into which it may be partitioned." It is also axiomatic that interactions *among* subsystems or systems are weaker than *within* subsystems or systems.

Living systems have *boundaries* that, in contrast with nonliving systems, are semipermeable, permitting substances and information to proceed in either direction. Von Bertalanffy[8] uses the term *isomorphism* to denote identity of the basic laws of function characteristic of each level of organization or of each subsystem. There is probably some validity at an abstract level to this concept, but by virtue of organization there is a subordination of lower to higher levels and a specialization at each individual level. As Rapaport[76] exemplifies, at the individual level there is a wide range of metabolic activity as contrasted with natural selection at the level of population. Each kind of behavior serves varying degrees of adaptation, not always adequate.

Hierarchies are dependent on higher levels maintaining a regulatory dampening control over lower levels, but as higher levels weaken they release from inhibition the functional independence of lower levels. This corresponds to the Jacksonian[56] concept of evolution and dissolution of functional levels of the nervous system. Also von Bertalanffy's equifinality, meaning that similar action may be expressed independent of the primary source or state of the exciting agent, is similar to Jackson's final common pathway.

INFORMATION AND COMMUNICATION

Theories of *communication* until recently have been reductionistic in depicting energy exchange as the basic process. There is no doubt that in living somatic systems this is largely correct. When, however, we proceed to the psychological system, although its fuel is dependent on energy furnished by the soma, its processes are conducted by means of communication of information.[5] These may be described by a variety of vocabularies, such as those of mathematics, logic, linguistics, etc., but they incorporate values that have symbolic meaning for the more evolved species.

Information in open systems corresponds to negative entropy in that it organizes and consolidates the chaos of multiple stimuli into meaningful data. In other words, organisms do organize and counteract the degradation of life. No longer is the mechanical view of man passively incorporating mass for transformation into energy possible nor is vitalism tenable.

Man especially seeks goals, as an active personality system, for more than the gratification of his biological needs. He also searches for new goals. But what are the linkages among subsystems and systems except in informational processes? These have only become possible because man has created, uses, and modifies *symbolic systems* that are the bases for his more complex, flexibly adaptive, creative acts. An erudite somewhat philosophic discourse on language behavior is in Bateson.[3]

Symbolic systems are not linear nor are linear explanations valid in cause-and-effect explanations. Instead we use the concept of *transactional* communication in which reverberating, corrective, circular systems of behavior at all levels are possible.

EVOLUTION, GROWTH AND CREATIVITY

Systems have evolved. They are born, they develop and decay. Their position in this cycle of events is not always easy to determine. Dynamically, as organistic complexity evolved, systems became subsystems of larger systems, environments become part of expanding systems from cell to cosmos. In contrast, as systems decay they break up so that their subsystems became free and separately functioning systems.

The function of a system should be viewed in relation to other whole systems as, for example, the personality system in relation to society and culture or one social system to another. Herein lies purpose or teleology: "Teleology is a lady without whom no biologist can live. Yet he is ashamed to show himself with her in public."[14]

Abstractions, concepts, and theories are useful tools, not facts of "real nature." They organize experiences but do not describe their real essence. Experience with empirical phenomenon is the real test of knowing. Since techniques vary with each system, operations cannot be described by generalizations. From the use of objective models, general systems theory may be graphically demonstrated for

public scrutiny.[28] One such model and its applicability to psychiatry will be stated later.

CRITIQUE

Theories serve heuristic purposes and are never meant to endure should they be shown to be internally inconsistent and fruitless in generating testable hypothesis. A theory of systems should do more than furnish satisfaction for believers as if it were a religion. General systems theory has had its share of criticism especially because it has introduced a new language, applicable to its role as a metatheory, highly abstract and far removed from empirical data. One critic says, "So what? It only establishes analogies among levels of organization or a number of systems and contributes no real progress." Yet analogies are indeed significant sources from which to create new approaches to problem areas; one only has to listen to multidisciplinary conferences to hear etiological "hunches." Symbolic thought is indeed analogical thinking for the most part and one of its creations has been the analogue computer.[23]

General systems theory has no methodology as do no other theories, but it does establish a paradigm or outline a way of thinking of relationships, of parts and wholes, and of inputs and outputs. Furthermore, if adequately demonstrated by one of several models, it enables the observer or experimenter to identify his position among a vast number of variables. Although isomorphism has been accentuated as a characteristic of living systems, it in no way denies that individual processes, levels, hierarchies, or subsystems in addition to common properties also have specific functions and lawful regularities differing from each other.

General systems theory should not be confused with data or used as their substantiation, as we have experienced interminably in psychoanalytic publications in which the language of theory and data form a confusing mixture. Instead theory orients the observer toward a search for empirical relevancies on which the theory depends for its continued existence. These should include "resolution levels" or time as permanent, relatively permanent, or temporary. The laws of regularity may be absolute, relative, or local.

Nevertheless, a valid criticism against general systems theory is its premature mathematization indulged in by several theorists, turning away those who cannot understand such language or who consider it as yet too abstract or who erroneously misplace confidence in formulae instead of searching for empirical data.

There are two ways of dealing with complex, or multivariate, problems. One is to introduce arbitrary simplifications so that we can use the techniques of analysis that may be available. This is the mathematical approach. The other is to accept the complexity as an irreducible element in the situation and search for a structure or pattern that will enable us to examine it as a whole. This is the systematic approach.[5]

A critique that involves a serious problem for a general systems or a unitary theory is the question of how subjective experiences are explained. This concerns its relation to psychoanalysis, studied especially by M. F. Basch in unpublished material entitled: "Psychoanalysis and the Resolution of the Mind–Body Paradox." He states that analogies enhance and deepen comprehension but are not explanations. The essence of general systems theory is not mathematization, the language of relationships, but the reordering of relations by transformation of nondiscursive or presentational symbolism (primary process) expressed through art, music, rituals, dreams, and metaphors into verbal discursive symbols. The subjective or presentational symbols are concerned with meaning and values that are qualitative rather than quantitative in their transformation into denotative language. In the psychoanalytic process much is lost although publicly accepted information is gained.

(Applicability of General Systems Theory—Social Sciences

The word "general" implies applicability to all human living systems and their environments and products (anthropology, sociology, cul- ture, religion, education, political science, legal systems, etc.). Such abstract systems as mathematics, logic, philosophy, etc. are included and finally, more practically, systems theory is applied to business, management, and corporate structures. Not all of the postulates of general systems theory are applied to each of these areas because some are not appropriate, but at least efforts are now directed toward systematic analysis of each. To consider all of these would require multiauthored encyclopedias. Since our major interest concerns relevance to psychiatry, to be discussed in a later section, only certain aspects of the *social sciences* closely related to psychiatry will be briefly considered here.

Although the systems of symbols will be discussed later it is essential to understand that man is a symbol-creating animal whose behavior is thereby less directed by signs. Representative symbols are continually being created and transmitted by tradition as the genes of culture.[26] Toman[88] points out that even in chemical memory feedback may develop jump steps, one at a time, that become permanently differentiated experiences and accrete to the organism's structure rather than simply reproducing it. At a higher level, social systems have developed and are continually changing in accelerated fashion. But Toda[87] points to the inefficiency of a fast moving, extremely energized society that needs a lessening in its positive feedbacks in order to develop more stability lest civilization breaks down.

Emerson elaborates:[25]

Symbolization is a sort of evolutionary trigger that profoundly differentiated humans and which lead to an integration in time with all the other humans. We are integrated in time with the cultural system. Now this integration in time also includes the organic, the physiological and the individual systems. Remember that the genes and the gene patterns in any organism, plant or animal, are a product of a long process of selective adjustment through millions of years. Any given individual organism at the moment is a product of its past. It is what it is because of past events that affected its ancestors and selected its ancestors and gave direction to the process of evolution. All living organisms are decidedly integrated with past evolutionary sequences. We are partly what we are because we had fish ancestors adjusted to a marine environment. But the mechanism of integration in time becomes vastly different with the advent of the symbolic systems in cultural evolution.

My other point is that in spite of the change in the mechanisms of integration between an organism and a group, in spite of the changes that involve innate behavior contrasted to learned behavior, in spite of the changes involved in individual learning as contrasted to symbolic learning which integrates us with a society to which we belong, in spite of all these actual differences, the direction still has similarity. Every one of these systems is moving toward a higher degree of division of labor between parts of a whole; every one of them is evolving a greater system of integration of parts; every one of them is moving toward an increase in homeostasis.

The leading theoretical proponents in sociology are Talcott Parsons and his colleagues.[70,71,72,73] Social systems do not identify individuals, but they deal with egos and alter egos characterized by action and reaction (transaction) while playing social roles within specific situations (environments). Culture is a complex, symbolically meaningful system arising out of social transactions and embodied in them. Parsons describes two classes of systems of action—personalities and social systems, related to each other by learning processes of internalization in personality and institutionalization in the social and cultural systems.[37] Parsons states that social systems and personality systems are not only interdependent, but they also interpenetrate, creating boundary problems as one attempts to translate meaning from one to another.[73] It is, therefore, extremely difficult to pinpoint cooperation and conformity to norms, conflict, competition, and deviation.[16]

Parsons clearly states that there is a plurality of systems in the field of human behavior, and he believes that these may be arranged in hierarchies, in contrast to Spiegel who states: "The structural-functional interdependence of all parts of the field makes statements describing dominance or hierarchical relations of one part of the field over another essentially meaningless."[83] But evolutionary development of organizational complexities requires regulation

of smaller systems or subsystems; hence the concept of levels and hierarchies is probably valid.

If we concede that the environment of a system becomes part of it only as we move up in the hierarchy, then by adding the biological to Parsons's four basic action systems we have, in addition, behaving organisms, personality, social, and cultural systems (the latter two separate). It is not coincidental that somatic muscular contractions appear first in biological embryogenesis, followed by sensory controls and modifiers. Thus, all systems are primarily action systems (i.e., behaving systems).

Emerson says: "I maintain that human society is moving definitely toward increased homeostasis and I equate homeostasis with progress."[25] Thus homeostasis for Emerson is not only a unifying principle applicable to all forms of living organization but a broad principle as well, encompassing not only stability but growth, evolution, social organization, increasing complexity, and optimum variability. It has survival value if one applies homeostasis to "multiple systems and multiple compromises, both in time and contemporaneously, and between levels."[25]

The scientific principle of homeostasis assists in the resolution of many controversies and dilemmas. It relates the individual to the group, divergence to convergence, competition to cooperation, isolation to integration, independence to dependence, conflict to harmony, life to death, regression to progress, conservativism to creativity, organic evolution to social evolution, psychology to biology, emotion to intelligence, the conscious to the unconscious, science to ethics and esthetics, reality to value, and means to ends. It is both a mechanism and a trend of life processes. It indicates the gaps in our knowledge and understanding, and it directs future investigations.[25]

Sociologists ignore the physical properties of the component parts of society, their origins and ontogenic properties. Action is not concerned with the internal structure of processes of the organism, but with the organism as a unit in a set of relationships. A good example is embodied in role theory where individual persons are omitted as units and replaced by roles that they play in various situations under various conditions at different times. The richness of personality depends on the number and variety of internalized social roles appropriate to multiple situations—and not rigidly organized for a supposedly expectable environment. Self-identity is attained when multiple identifications have permitted durable satisfactory object relations and society recognizes the subject as a person.[39]

Wallerstein and Smelser,[91] in discussing the articulation of sociology with psychoanalysis, speak of general principles applicable to any bridging process. They indicate the particular problems, determinants, hypotheses, and research methods of each discipline, and the need for realistic complementarity between the two. They specify the need to evaluate costs and benefits of articulations, the consequences of comparing multiple levels, and the value differences that essentially differentiate behaviors.

Laura Thompson enumerates the conditions necessary for an adequate theory of culture and then states:[86]

A human local community-in-environment is not primarily an inorganic, physico-chemical system, nor is it primarily a system of human relations (i.e., a societal system). It is an organic organization of or structure-function web-of-life composed of diverse species or kinds of animals, microorganisms, plants and human groups, in the content of inorganic nature. Seen all-of-a-piece human community is an integral part of a larger organic whole or complex web-of-life, and its existence and welfare depend on the existence of the welfare of the larger whole in environmental context.

Definition of Psychiatry

Before considering the relevance of general systems theory to psychiatry, we should define psychiatry as clearly as possible in order to know its component parts and its extent, and to differentiate psychiatry as a medical-clinical specialty from psychiatry as a science. Especially is this true since the entire field is rapidly evolving, extending, and developing interfaces with increasing numbers of other specialties and systems. Unfortunately as

Shepherd states:[80] "During the past 14 years, I would maintain that the expanding role of the psychiatrist has far outstripped the gains in established knowledge."

But psychiatry is a specific science only as it is concerned with a particular system of verbal, gestural, and behavioral communications characterizing observant–subject (patient) transactions. It is in addition a conglomerate of many sciences involved in the study of human behavior, including biological, psychological, and social sciences. Since man is a biopsychosocial creature, psychiatry must include these sciences as part of the total system characterized by whatever variables are in focus at the time. Likewise the applications of these parts and the total system have become so extended that psychiatrists have been likened to pioneer riders searching for fences that bound their territories.[40]

Finally, the scientific approach to clinical psychiatry, according to Offer and Freedman, is approximately only three decades old and clinical research psychiatrists are indeed few in number.[67] Nevertheless, it will be demonstrated that a general systems approach to clinical psychiatry is not only feasible but it is also productive, and that practice, reflection, investigation, and communication are the parts of a functional system characterizing a clinical investigator.

According to Mora[65] many histories of psychiatry have been written from a variety of new points. In his paper the reader will find an excellent bibliography. There seems to be no question that psychiatry, by any name used during the ages and representing man's attitude toward his fellow men with emotional distress, expresses the social and cultural philosophies of the time. Despite the movement of professional psychiatry into medicine and science, it still is heavily burdened by philosophies that shape psychiatry into their molds (existentialism, Freudian metapsychology).

Modern medicine seriously began to include psychiatry as a specialty in the nineteenth century in its concern with organic diseases of the brain. Specific cellular changes described by pathologists were presumed to be caused by diseases of the mind. Neighboring disciplines such as psychology with its brass-instrument techniques and later with its stimulus-response-robot concept of human mentality helped little. Beginning with the twentieth century, psychoanalysis offered etiological paradigms that turned out to be explanations of meaning never sufficiently proven.

It seems as if psychiatry, really psychiatrists, was divided into one group composed of therapists, including psychotherapists, somato-therapists or sociotherapists,[84] and another group involved in research conducted by scientific psychiatrists. This is not to assume that the latter works in the laboratory and the former in the clinic. Both are to some degree therapists and investigators. But as far as the public and the vast majority of physicians are concerned, psychiatry conforms to the medical definition of a specialty devoted to the diagnosis, treatment, and the prevention of mental illness. Psychiatric investigators used their essentially unipolar training and experience in special techniques, such as biochemistry, pathology, physiology, etc., with little reference to other techniques, developing thereby many small subspecialities.

After World War II the focus of concern transcended the individual, a process continuing with rapid acceleration as a product of the times. Disciplines began to form multidisciplinary research groups, which were not really woven together but operated within a relatively broad or nonexistent unified framework with great difficulty.[60] It was then, in the 1950s, that models were developed, and even though they only approximated reality and had but a brief life, they did create testable hypotheses.[98]

Sometime in the latter part of the 1950s research and clinical psychiatrists became self-conscious when they suddenly discovered that psychiatry was an integral part of the vast field of behavioral sciences.[28] Their focus could no longer scotomatize larger areas of behavior such as the biological, psychological, social, or economic. Ideas of unified, or systems, theory seem to furnish answers in their concepts of openness, communications, transactions, homeostasis, and isomorphism (see Ruesch, reference[42]). Thus, on the one hand

clinical psychiatry began to participate in social action under increased political freedom,[52] and on the other hand research psychiatry absorbed field theories.

In separating the practice of clinical psychiatry from psychiatry as a science, we are dealing with a weak dichotomy. Clinical psychiatry can be approached scientifically, and the sciences that form the system of scientific psychiatry are ultimately concerned with deviations in human behavior that require clinical contact and expertise in eliciting behavioral, cognitive, and affective data. The data of the basic sciences and those at the psychological level supplement each other. Unfortunately, life histories of patients reveal considerable diversity and general principles are difficult to abstract. In other words, it is difficult to separate what is individual and incidental from what is general and essential, thus making a system of classification extremely difficult (nomothetic and ideographic).

Menninger, Mayman, and Pruyser[62] have developed a systems approach to psychiatric entities as a substitute for our inadequate nosological classification. Their four principles include (1) individual–environmental interaction producing adjustment or adaptation,(2) organization by homeostatic mechanisms serving balance, (3) regulation and control according to the theory of ego or boundary functions, (4) motivation or instinct theory. They then describe a unitary theory of illness (instead of classification) related to coping reactions to stress. These are five orders of dysfunction or dyscontrol of aggression. They include: (1) mild nervous tension, (2) neuroses, (3) naked aggression, (4) psychoses, (5) rupture and complete decompensation.

The application of general systems or unitary theory to much of clinical psychiatry is difficult. In an extraordinarily lucid paper, Spiegel sketches the theoretical propositions involving the transactional field and how those are applied to a study of families of various ethnic characteristics. Spiegel comments:[83] "Evidently it is difficult almost by definition to keep the larger field of transactions in view when conducting clinical studies of diagnostic entities." This is correct. In our study of the Borderline Syndrome,[51] although we devoted a chapter to "Society, Culture and the Borderline," we could only make general statements since we were unable to obtain significant data other than from the behavior of the subjects under study. Other clinical studies have suffered from the same deficiencies.[49]

Once unitary theories were understood and accepted (sadly after about twenty-five years) psychiatry experienced expansionary trends. Today it is involved in health and in all the problems of human life from cell to cosmos as well as in all the progressive and destructive things that man has created in his environment. Man has begun to recognize that he is more than a mechanical reactive organism: he has evolved, grown, acts and creates, although he is still burdened by attributes unsuited to the modern world (unrealistic anxieties); and general biology has broadened its scientific vistas by including man as a psychological being.[24]

The extension of psychiatry does not require the abandonment of any theory, or in our terms subtheory, but instead a redefinition to involve more inclusive, larger theories of systems. For example, Schildkraut and Kety[78] state that biochemical abnormalities are not necessarily genetic or constitutional, because early experiences may cause enduring biochemical changes. A multifactorial, theoretical framework is necessary.

Caws states:[19]

The most useful conception of the unity of science seems to me to lie somewhere in the middle of the triangle defined by the reductive, synthetic, and encyclopedic conceptions. Where reduction can be done usefully, it should be done; where isomorphisms can be found they should be found; and where disciplinary barriers to communication can be broken down, they should be broken down. What I have been chiefly criticizing here is an a priori approach to this problem, the assumption that there must be isomorphisms, the assumption that every science must fit into some rational order of the sciences. What I should wish to substitute for this is an empirical approach—not the claim that isomorphisms are necessary, but the recognition that they are possible, and the resolve

to search for them wherever they occur. If a direct bridge is thus built between physics and biology, or between crystal growth and population movement, it is not because there *had to be* a bridge but because there *happens to be* one which somebody had the sense to exploit.

Where there is no bridge or at least bridging language, analogy is still possible and stimulating. For example, we may analogize social institutionalization with psychological internalization. Emerson[25] analogizes the gene with the symbols of culture and Parsons[73] the human incest taboo with sex differentiation at the organic level.

Interdigitation of "Systems" and "Psychiatry"

A theory's greatest value is that it leads to operations suitable for the testing of derived hypotheses. Such heuristic values may not be apparent at first. General systems theories enable the investigator to have confidence that there are some natural laws of isomorphism and insofunctionalism, and that research can discover both one's position as an observer with respect to evolution, birth, growth, stability, and death as well as their effects on the observed. The theory enables us to wander through forests of the unknown with some confidence that there are pathways to be found. An example of such confidence in 1959 the editor of the then new *Archives of General Psychiatry* wrote the following editorial for the first number:

We publish contributions from all disciplines, whether morphological, physiological, biochemical, endocrinological, psychosomatic, psychological, psychiatric, child–psychiatric, psychoanalytical, sociological, or anthropological, that are related to the study of the behavior of man in health and illness. We attempt to implement the concept that man's behavior cannot in our day be viewed profitably from a narrow frame of reference. Instead, it requires a broad vision of a totally integrated field composed of many part functions and transactions, each of which constitutes the focus of a wide variety of scientific disciplines. Eventually, a unified science, or systems theory, of behavior may emerge.[44]

This section includes personal, among other, examples of the uses of general systems theory for various psychiatric activities—one cannot say purely clinical or purely research, basic or applied, therapeutic or denotative.[69] Although many writers have discussed the theory, few have applied it to research in psychiatry.

PSYCHOTHERAPY AND PSYCHOANALYSIS

Psychotherapy has many shapes, each constituting a "school." There is little reason to enumerate or define them all (psychoanalysis, dynamic psychotherapy, and other individual psychotherapies, group, family, community therapies, etc.). I shall now present one form in which I have consciously attempted to utilize parts of general systems theory: field, role, transaction, and information.[48]

In this *transactional approach* the setting or field of operations must be known not as a fixed state but as an ever changing matrix which affects the persons involved and is altered by them. The behavior of each participant can be viewed as portrayed through explicit instrumental social roles and by implicit roles expressing affective or emotionally meaningful messages. Through these rapidly changing roles within slowly moving fields, information is exchanged by means of verbal, nonverbal, and paralingual communications. Finally the cyclical reverberating influence of one on the other, back to the first, and back again, eventually reaches closure when information becomes repetitive and explicit role-complementarity has been achieved. At this point the implicit meaning of the transaction is communicated, and a new focus of communication is opened up.

The transactional approach is operational; it requires an understanding of the tactics of skilled relationships. Its underlying basic theories involve field-role, and communication theories. It restricts the use of psychodynamic theory to the understanding of underlying motivations, conflicts, and defenses without the confusing use of modified psychoanalytic techniques.

The transactional approach furthers the understanding of human beings in relationships with one or more other persons. Thus, it is a means for understanding social workers in relationship to colleagues, to staff, to members of other disciplines in the psychiatric teams, and primarily to patients, but this approach as we have used it is applicable to the understanding of persons in trouble by all therapists of any discipline. It is essentially the most adequate frame of reference from which to understand what people try to say in any relationship, especially when the role relationship is structured as that between the need-requesting client or patient and the helping social worker or therapist.[48]

Wallerstein's[90] highly perceptive critique of the transactional approach to psychotherapy correctly defines that one who has for so long been involved in psychoanalytic theory and its practical applications could not easily or completely reject its ingrained influences. Wallerstein transposes the language of the old to that of the new when applied to psychotherapeutic technics. Such transpositions have been frequently used to deny that anything new or different has been created. This is at least partially true as far as the core theory is involved but decidedly in error where the operational procedures are concerned. By adding field, transactional, and communication theories, the system even though maintaining some of the original Freudian core theories becomes a different system. This can be witnessed in the behaviors of many younger psychoanalysts who by thinking and applying systems theory have achieved a much more powerful tool in their therapeutic endeavors.

Others have also criticized psychoanalytic theory, important here only in relation to systems.[58] For example, Farrell[27] states that psychoanalysis is not a unified theory and as such is not refutable. Its parts, such as those related to instincts or dynamics, development, psychic structures, economics, or defense and symptom formation, are not related to each other in transactions to indicate a general system.[44] Charny and Carroll also state that efforts to bring psychoanalytic science into relationship with the larger scientific scene have not been promising. They state:[20]

Because the (general systems) theory calls for precise specification of the relationship of each level of organization to the next (vertical), as well as intralevel specification (horizontal), it provides a useful approach to behavioral and biological problems not easily dealt with in conventional physical theory. Specifically, it provides a rationale for the application of general systems theory to the study of psychoanalysis, for it allows for the ordering of complex data without implying direct causality; rather, this hypothesis carries with it the implication of simultaneous multiple causation inherent in the psychoanalytic notion of over-determination, or in Waelder's principle of multiple function.

Gill[32] has attempted to equate psychoanalytic structural theory with a theory of systems involving modes of function (process) and modes of organization (structure). Indeed, there are indications that some more scientific psychoanalysts have utilized some aspects of general systems theory in their writings. Among the most erudite is Frenkel-Brunswik[29] who wrote about psychoanalysis and the unity of science; Colby[23] has done considerable research on psychoanalysis and information theory. Sullivan[85] groped in this direction when he considered schizophrenia as a human process. Pumpian-Mindlin[75] attempted to relate psychoanalysis to biological and social sciences, and Beres[7] considered an ego system of structure function in psychoanalysis. Finally, Anna Freud[30] defined openness and multifactorial process in growth and development, in health and illness, and in therapeutic success and failure as hypotheses essential for the testing of psychoanalytic theory by a variety of methods.

Peterfreund[74] attempts to relate psychoanalysis to information and systems theory. This provocative monograph is introduced by Bernard Rubinstein's prefatory statement: "Theoretical psychological models cannot be devoid of neurophysiological meaning." In the monograph, psychoanalysis is considered a segment of natural phenomenon, meaning part of a larger system. Nevertheless, psychoanalysts have tried to force the world of biology, physiology, and evolutionary time into a world the center of which is the mind of man. As we have read many times, beginning with Sherrington,[81] "psychic energy" has no relation to physical energy. Instead it is a quality of information.[2] Psychoanalysis still deals with conflict, and linear causes and effects, since it has permitted little cross-fertilization.[61]

"It is possible to construct statements that, though necessarily either true or false, cannot be proved or disproved within the limits of the system itself. In order to demonstrate that such statements are necessarily true or false, we must construct a richer system that will provide the elements requisite for the proof."[5] Attempts can be made, however, to interdigitate general systems theory with some aspects or parts of psychoanalytic theory, though not all, especially since psychoanalysis is still a hodgepodge of unrelated concepts, old and new, good and bad, productive and handicapping. For example, topological theory identifies symbolic systems (unconscious, preconscious, and conscious) in terms of their positions in relation to conscious awareness. How these develop and transact may be summarized as follows:[45]

(1) The symbolic system has developed from a system of signs by an evolutionary jump-step, resulting in preconscious and conscious process as distinctly (?) human phenomena. (2) There are ontological phases of learning from body signs to visual imagery to primitive symbols to creative thinking, but the flow of information among these phases persists in all directions throughout life. (3) There are flexible transactional operations among these parts so that all are involved in all forms of thinking. (4) All the phases or parts of the symbolic system are in transactional relationship with reality and inner experiences. (5) A disintegration of optimum or effective relations among parts of the symbolic systems may lead to breaking off of transactions (repression), and thereby to distorted thinking and behavior or to temporary acceleration of creativity.

In a forthcoming monograph entitled "Systems of Psychic Functioning and their Psychoanalytic Conceptualization," John Gedo and Arnold Goldberg[31] attempt to investigate the hierarchical interrelationships of "models of the mind" or systems of function. "By arranging the various psychoanalytical models and delineating the appropriate function of each to explain various systems or modes of psychic life, a supraordinate model may be constructed and used on a flexible basis as the situation demands." They emphasize a sequence reflecting the succession of developmental phases through a chronologically organized scheme. Their overall plan is to describe the existing psychoanalytic models of the mind, to define their range of relevance, to delineate further models implicit in accepted theory, and to select and correlate the lines of development used for important nosological distinction into an overall hierarchical model under which all the described subsystems may be subsumed.

In discussing psychosocial aspects of disease Cleghorn states:[22]

As a paradigm for mental functioning, psychoanalysis was enormously stimulating. As a paradigm for mental disease, it is less apt. It has had a vast impact on social, anthropological and literary studies, which cannot concern us here. Perhaps its most pervasive, if unobtrusive, influence has been in the social attitude to illness. Here, of course, it shares with other social influences the responsibility for the re-emergence of humanism in the consideration of social ills and the psychosocial aspects of disease. The key concept is the meaning to the patient, which may include threat, loss, gain or insignificance.

According to most social scientists the family is a small system serving to protect and educate the young. It is not surprising that family studies in the best of hands should be oriented toward the understanding of the families' role in the production of deviance in one or more of the progeny, especially in their aberrant forms of communication;[94,95,82,64] and the same holds true for therapy of disturbed youngsters whose problems lead one to family therapy. Minuchin[63] applies general systems theory to the treatment of the family with what he calls an "ecological framework." Group therapy has become widespread, and we look forward to its codification in terms of systems theory.

HEALTH AND ILLNESS AND EDUCATION

Only recently have psychiatrists paid attention to what is normal or healthy. According to Offer and Sabshin,[68] there are several frames of reference from which to view normality: normality as an ideal fiction, normality as optimal integration, normality as adapta-

tion within context. This is in contrast to Yahoda[96] who writes about "positive mental health."

There are many other partial definitions of health. Buhler[15] writes about four basic life tendencies on which personal fulfillment is dependent: need satisfaction, upholding of internal order, adaptation, and creativity. Zubin[98] indicates that transcultural psychiatry may help to discriminate the culture-free from the culture-fair factors in health and illness.

In using systems approach Grinker[34] stressed the relationship between soma and psyche in maturation and development and applied it to concepts of so-called psychosomatic diseases. Included was a blueprint for research on how early experiences become imprinted on both psyche and soma, reappearing as related defects in both, in the process of dedifferentiation. In later research on a group of healthy young males termed "homoclites," Grinker[39,47] developed a number of variables within the total transactional field that contribute to mental health. These include among many others: physical health, average intelligence, adequate affection and communication in the family, fair discipline, early-work experiences, sound ideals and goal-seeking rather than goal-changing. The end result contributed to adaptation within a specified environment. Bowlby[13] also utilized a systems approach as he discussed the ontogeny of human attachment, dependency, and detachment from maternal figures.

The health–illness systems cannot be separated to define health and illness, each in absolute terms. Health is dependent on factors such as age, culture, and social attitudes, internal compensations, defenses, coping, etc.[41] In general, health is maintained when strains affecting one part of the biopsychological system is compensated for or counteracted in some way by other parts. Even a new relationship or dysequilibrium of the parts caused by stress may eventuate in an adequate adaptation.[50]

In general, the health–illness system involving body and mind extends from the genetic to the sociocultural and encompasses development and decline.[59] This includes birth, infancy, childhood, adolescence, young adulthood, maturity, aging, dying, and death. Each phase has its characteristic internal processes, its specific stresses and capacities for defense, coping and reconstitution. Each and the whole have their interfaces with specific sociocultural environments, their ecosystems. This concept transcends disciplinary lines; it combines knowledge of laboratory procedures, life in pairs, families, groups, and the larger society. It is concerned with phases of stability, stress–responses, and despair.[79]

Stages in the life cycle considered as a system may be viewed in several ways. For example, in one manner we may view the subsystems of ontogeny, including genetics (bioamines), family (communications), experience (trauma), as parts of ontogeny all leading to health or illness as well as degrees of susceptibility to the latter and coping devices for the former.

In another manner the stages can be enumerated as follows: (1) the relatively undifferentiated neonate; (2) the phases of differentiation or learning through imprinting, reinforcement, imitation, identification, etc; (3) the phase of specific personality, psychosomatic, and coping development; (4) the phase of health, including proneness to disease; (5) the phase of disease; (6) the phase of chronic illness; and (7) the phase of dying and death.

Each phase has its genic, environmental, and experiential components, and to a point not yet understood, spontaneous movement and shifts due to intervention may occur. Corresponding to general systems theory, the principle of isomorphism of each level may be assumed. It is important for research and for the practical goals of therapy to incorporate phases of the individual life cycle into our educational processes in universities and medical schools.[46]

From another point of view Greenblatt[33] has recently considered education and action in management as a multiplicity of systems. For psychiatric administration there has been little concern, although it is increasing in importance because of the multiple functions all psychiatrists must serve. He states:

When the resident becomes a Ward Chief or Senior Resident he is in a more complex world—the world of patient groups; of environmental systems, both physical and social; and of administrative systems of the hospital, which he begins to appreciate for the first time. He is also in the interface system between the hospital and community; the system of professional organizations to which he and other professionals belong; and the university system, if he is in training in an academic environment and especially if he has professional ambitions.

Everything that Greenblatt states about residents applies to all psychiatrists to greater or lesser degree, and systems approaches seem the only solution to what is an "impossible profession."

COMMUNITY PSYCHIATRY

Currently psychiatry more than any health–illness system has become involved in the community, not only because of the need to furnish services to the indigent and working poor but also because of the vast amount of federal money available and the pressures from these funding agencies. More important than these reasons is the fact that after World War II the importance of the individual declined, and the focus turned on the convergence of man in groups within a social environment as part of a larger social movement. This necessitated attempts to link the disciplines of psychiatry with those of psychology, sociology, and anthropology (see Ruesch[42]). In fact, vigorous attempts are being made to substitute a social model of psychiatry for the medical model that will depict psychiatric disturbances as social disabilities leading to more or less permanent exclusion of the individual from his group.

Extravagant claims have been made for community psychiatry without sound processes of evaluation, except in rare instances. Kellam and Branch[57] indicate that currently community psychiatry is a nonsystem in an experimental area where mental health is poorly defined except as internal well-being and appropriate adaptation. They state:

In our view intervention should be intimately related to the processes which occur in social contexts in the community. Thus the targets of intervention are not restricted to individuals or families as in the case of the clinic setting. On the contrary, any aspect of the social field-processes related to the individual's sense of well-being can be subject to intervention. In school the classroom is a major social field and the teacher, the peer group, the family, the administration of the school, or even the curriculum can receive the attention of the intervention process.

Such a social system view of intervention requires, however, more than mental health skills. Other health, education, and welfare workers, who are under increasing duress because of the general failure to meet human needs, may also ascribe to such a view. Indeed our own experience, based on systematic studies and clinical impressions, raises the question as to whether our focus ought to be on mental health as a speciality or on an integrated human service system that seeks to approach mental health through institutional processes which are more consciously and purposefully concerned with the breadth of human need.

If we subtract the utopian concept of "primary prevention" from the *Community Mental Health Movement*, then it becomes simply a complicated organizational process by which the delivery of mental-health services is improved. Two basic changes can be effected: (1) the medically indigent will receive appropriate services within their own communities, and (2) all the resources within and near the community will be available without delay or bureaucratic obstacles. Thus community mental health becomes a system of services containing parts, having appropriate linkages, under unitary supraordinate organization with interfaces, to other social welfare systems.[66] It needs no modification of systems theory, but it requires money, manpower, and political structure, and competent management. Its effectiveness is as yet not proven, but requires extensive well-planned evaluations. Hansell states:[53] "The formulation of a mental health service network as a system is an acknowledgement of the related facts that the human personality is a system, that society can be understood as a system, and that the casualty management network is a subsystem of that society."

Social Psychiatry on the other hand is a rudimentary scientific hybrid, not clearly defined since it represents the combination of two fields. One deals with aberrant, internal psychological processes and deviant behavior classified as diseases, the other deals with aggregates of people characterized by specific functional structures, values, and moral philosophies. The combination of any two disciplines such as implied in social psychiatry, biochemistry, psychophysiology, etc. is fraught with difficulties and resultant errors. As pointed out by Wallerstein and Smelser, unless there is a complementary articulation between disciplines a low rate of predictability ensues.[91]

It seems evident that social life structures opportunities for individual, instinctual gratification, but it also frustrates them by demanding many renunciations. The concept of balance between these polarities characterizes unitary thinking, although the empirical phenomena indicate that one or the other polarity has dominated at various times in the history of each society. Society provides ego ideals, ideologies, and social roles for personality development, but the social structure is developed and is maintained by a variety of personality conglomerates.

It then may be assumed that, out of this matrix, factors promoting types of health and/or illness have great significance no matter how strong biogenetic defects may be. Psychiatric problems arise out of a social matrix and in turn alter that matrix with the same reciprocity that articulates personality with society. The relevance of social psychiatry in the development and persistence of deviant feeling, thinking, and behavior is what concerns us. If we know the what and how of this influence, it may be possible consciously to prevent or even change those social and cultural factors that most significantly facilitate psychiatric problems and thus become a part of a system of health services and of primary prevention. From a practical standpoint, the operations of so-called community psychiatry should be based on the characteristics of multiple subsystems within a community-mental-health center and on the transactions among various systems within special communities such as social agencies, police, courts, schools, churches, etc.[53]

AFFECTS, STRESS AND COPING

Experiences related in *Men Under Stress* as well as the results of other researches indicated that emotional specificity in the production of psychosomatic disturbances is rare. Indeed, after much time, energy, and work we began to understand that a variety of stress stimuli could produce specific responses in individuals. The theory of response specificity was thus developed and, perforce, had to include the wide number of subsystems that preceded and contributed to classes of responses, including experience, coping mechanisms, and personality characteristics.[36]

We developed systems of quantification of affects: at first, anxiety and, then, depression and anger, as well as defenses against emotional responses. To translate this conceptual position, it became necessary to develop a multidisciplinary team and to utilize general systems theory. The latter as related to anxiety on which we concentrated first is as follows:

As the determinant of a system, anxiety maintains components or processes of organization involving total behavior in the social environment, cognitive and connative functioning, and physiological actions, all of which are adaptive under conditions in which anxiety exists, for as long as it remains. The total system is involved with the environment in that external influences or internal disturbances acting on the anxiety system may augment its component activities or stimulate behavior of the organism to remove itself safely from the dangerous stimulus to which it is highly sensitive, or to attach in attempting to destroy the danger. Thus, even if interest is centered on anxiety as an organization, with its multiplicity of component parts, transactions that involve environmental parameters are ever present. The total social and interpersonal setting in which the observed subject lives and moves should, therefore, be taken into account, either by recording its changes or controlling its constancy as much as possible. We could define the component parts or sub-systems of anxiety according to our own choice of variables hoping from the biological point of view to measure activities as close as possible to the central nervous system and the hormonal systems. These choices were dependent on the available methods and the available experienced personnel. Within the system we hoped to stimulate in turn various sub-systems but in reality concentrated on stirring up anxiety, anger, depression and defenses in different experiments.[36]

SCHIZOPHRENIA RESEARCH

Investigations of this most mysterious scourge of mankind have produced thousands of papers from biogenetics to sociology. Each scientific group offers something different in the form of etiological theory, but we cannot even be sure that the sample of patients each studies is identical or even similar. This points up that although we freely use the term schizophrenia, we do not know the *what* of the disease.

For example, Macfie Campbell,[17] commenting on the increased frequency of this diagnosis as long ago as 1935, stated that dementia precox (schizophrenia) is not a disease but a Greek letter society: "The conditions for admission are obscure, inclusion and exclusion vary from year to year and place to place, and the Board of Directors is not known."

A research program on schizophrenia is therefore an excellent focus on which to exemplify the application of general systems theory and an area from which to derive a theoretical model.[2,55]

Schizophrenia is probably a polyvalent outcome of several variables comprising a system or organization that represents a form of functional adaptation. The form is only fixed as an end product, since individuals show a high degree of variability and since the forms differ as indicated in the high degree of variability between individuals.

There is not sufficient evidence to determine whether the primary defect is within *a part of* a developing or functioning psychobiological system or in the *organizational processes* ordinarily successfully integrating the parts. These roughly may be biological (biogenetic, etc.) psychological (childhood experiences, etc.) or environmental (stress stimuli, etc.). What can be assumed is the requirement that experimental challenges evoke the vulnerabilities within the parts of the whole system and that spontaneous or life challenges are necessary to move a schizotaxic individual to overt schizophrenia and possibly eventually into a psychosis.

We recognize that even though we may on theoretical grounds consider the propositions that the schizophrenic is primarily characterized by a disorder of proprioceptive and autonomic feedback, or that the schizophrenic is adapting to a primary unique quality of anxiety, or to a defect in attention and memory, or to a deficient capacity in internal information searching, or to a deficiency in central nervous system and/or endocrine functions, some adequate linkings or bridgings are necessary in a general systems approach.[18]

A scheme or model for the representation of variables to be considered in a study of schizophrenia is appropriate. To be emphasized is the transactional nature of such a model. Attribution of cause and the role of conflict are omitted. The model would assume the form of a cylinder with the height representing levels or hierarchical placement of items. The cylinder would indicate the relationship of the parts within three component columns. The first would represent somatic variables such a physiological, biochemical, enzymatic, cardiovascular, central nervous system, drives, and regulatory and control systems pertaining to these variables. In the psychological column, there would be such psychological systems as memory, perception-motor behavior, cognition in general, superego functions, and the regulatory and controlling systems relevant to these variables. Under the column of environmental aspects, there would be the various kinds of stimuli that impinge upon the organism, the various stresses and strains and human objects available for relationships. This scheme does not state anything *specific* about the relationship between and within the columns, but it does assume that there is some kind of a functional relationship between and among all three of these columns. Thus, variations would occur and, therefore, one could not ascribe a specific cause to any one of the three columns. Behavioral scientists have attempted to conceptual-

ize the variations by naming them "psycho-somatic," "psychosocial," "psychodynamic," "medical-social," and so on. These terms seem to beg the question concerning the nature of the "interact," and that such interaction gives rise to behavior. It may be more accurate to look upon the contingent variations as giving rise to *experience*, which becomes associated with behavior that has particular meanings.

The manifestation of each of these variables must be observed in transaction. It may be quite beyond our grasp to observe more than two of these three variables in a transactional field at any one time, plus the observer. Therefore, one should always include the psychological variables and observe the variations of the two others. We would thus be observing one ego function in one particular steady state or at one particular point or time, and we would observe the effects of that variable on another dependent variable at the same time. It would be a methodological error to attempt comparisons across temporal zones. Thus, it would be a mistake to relate a particular kind of heart-rate pattern of today with poor mothering twenty years ago.

The model of the cylinder permits one to move in two directions: from trait to trait in the psychological field, or across time within the psychological field, thus giving a longitudinal cast to a study. In such an instance, we would be observing the changing nature of specific functions over time. The depth of the cylinder gives the model the dimension of differentiation; the center would be the point of maximal differentiation. Thus, plotting the schizophrenic's behavior over a lifetime, it would be understandable that in later years the schizophrenic patient would show a greater independence from drive functions or even from his environment, which would give the appearance of the "burned-out schizophrenic."

The cylinder is thus in the form of a periodic table, indicating to us those variables which would be important to study. We recognize that these subsystems are only concepts, empirically not at all dependent, and we can view them as conceptually isolated. Such conceptual isolation, however, does not relieve one from the task of recognizing the effects of other variables on a particular one under scrutiny. It is therefore important that we attempt to keep constant or under control the variations occurring in other subsystems. The scheme makes no provision for causation, for explanation, for purpose.

To recapitulate, we should ask ourselves several general questions, a few of which are outlined. What is the nature of the deficit or of the regressive dedifferentiation? What parts of the total biopsychosocial system are most involved or most vulnerable? Is the deficiency in some general organizational process? What are the appropriate stress stimuli and their meaning for survival? What and when are the earliest indicators of differences? How do we separate the essential primary process from its secondary elaborations or adaptations? Is anxiety as a quality an inherent or experimental difference? Can response specificity to ordinary challenges, artifically induced stress-stimuli or historical data be determined? Does the schizophrenic reveal a different level of arousal potentiality? These and many other questions become important in clinical research programs oriented toward studying "process" rather than "content," and they are the basis of selection from the wide variety of individual projects focusing on parts of the total system.

Concluding Remarks

The essential components of general systems theory have been outlined as a meta-theory. Many years of resistance were influenced by the fact that psychiatry for a long time was only a medical speciality and dominated by psychoanalysis, which had its own umbrella called metapsychology. When scientific or research psychiatry became part of the behavioral sciences, a general theory was needed to counteract the parochialism of its contributory sciences. On the other side of the coin, the Society for General Systems Theory and its journal *General Systems* was a mixed bag. Few authors were actually doing research —they philosophized and many of them prematurely resolved dilemmas by mathematical equations, in a language poorly understood by the empirical investigator.

Gradually, more and more psychiatrists became interested and organized their own special groups, hoping to communicate in a common language consonant and not disjunctive with their own biological, psychological, and social models. They were tired of senseless controversy about who knows *the* cause; they became convinced of multicausality and reciprocal relations rather than linearity of cause and effect. As a result, the probabilities of a systems approach were enhanced. This is not to assume that any scientist could cover the entire field, but he could feel more comfortable knowing where he was, instead of endlessly riding around in search of boundaries.

Psychiatrists began to recognize that systems and subsystems constituting hierarchies, bounded by permeable borders encasing reverberating transactions, had structure functions and integrative processes. But more than that, they realized that a system functions in relation to other systems. In fact, the proof or validation of a system's functions cannot come from within, but depends on its "purpose" in relation to another system. This respectable teleology gives meaning to human research that, admitted or not, is the goal of science rather than its being simply a game that we enjoy playing.

Following the outline, systems approach to the social sciences accentuated human symbolic functions that are the essence of humanity—individual, group, or society. It is deviation in development, disturbance in integration, and failure to react conservatively to human or inanimate environmental-disturbing stimuli that constitute the essence of disease.

Next, the relevance to psychiatry was considered by exemplifying a few problems with which the author has been involved, for which systems theory could operationally assist in answering. These included psychotherapy and psychoanalysis; health, illness, and education; community and social psychiatry; affect, stress, and coping; and schizophrenia. In not one example can the entire systems theory be applied, but some parts of it are readily available and profitable. In the future psychiatrists can anticipate more and more use of operational research based on general systems theory, which will enhance our knowledge of causes and courses of and therapies for psychological disturbances.

⟨ Bibliography

1. ARIETI, S. "The Present Status of Psychiatric Theory," *Am. J. Psychiatry*, 124 (1968), 619–629.
2. ARTISS, K. L. *The Symptom as Communication in Schizophrenia*. New York: Grune & Stratton, 1959.
3. BATESON, G. "The Message of Reinforcement," in J. Akin, A. Goldberg, G. Myers et al., eds., *Language Behavior*. New York: Monton, 1971.
4. BELLAK, L. *Schizophrenia*. New York: Logos Press, 1958.
5. BENNETT, J. G. "Total Man: An Essay in the Systematics of Human Nature," *Systematics*, 1 (1964), 282–310.
6. BENTLY, A. F. *Inquiry into Inquiries*. Boston: Beacon, 1954.
7. BERES, D. "Structure and Function in Psychoanalysis," *Int. J. Psychoanal.*, 46 (1965), 53–63.
8. BERTALANFFY, L. VON. "General Systems Theory: A Critical Review," *Yearbook Soc. Gen. Sys. Theory*, 7 (1962), 1–21.
9. ———. "General System Theory and Psychiatry," in S. Arieti, ed., *American Handbook of Psychiatry*, Vol. 3, 1st ed., pp. 705–721. New York: Basic Books, 1966.
10. ———. "General Theory of Systems: Application to Psychology," *Soc. Sci. Inf.*, 6 (1967), 125–136.
11. ———. *Robots, Men and Minds*. New York: Braziller, 1967.
12. BOULDING, K. "General Systems Theory: The Skeleton of Science," *Gen. Sys.*, 1 (1956), 11.
13. BOWLBY, J. *Attachment and Loss*. Vol. 1. New York: Basic Books, 1969.
14. BRUECKE, C. VON. Quoted in W. Cannon: *The Way of an Investigator: A Scientist's Experience in Medical Research*. New York: Norton, 1945.
15. BÜHLER, C. and F. MASSERIK. *The Course of Human Life*. New York: Springer, 1968.
16. BUCKLEY, W. *Modern Systems Research for the Behavioral Scientist*. Chicago: Aldine, 1968.
17. CAMPBELL, C. M. *Destiny and Disease in Mental Disorders*. New York: Norton, 1937.
18. CANCRO, R. *The Schizophrenic Reactions*. New York: Bruner-Mazel, 1970.
19. CAWS, P. "Science and System: On the Unity and Diversity of Scientific Theory," *Gen. Sys.*, 13 (1968), 3–20.
20. CHARNY, E. J. and E. J. CARROL. "General Systems Theory and Psychoanalysis," *Psychoanal. Q.*, 35 (1966), 377–387.
21. CHILD, C. M. *Patterns and Problems of Development*. Chicago: University of Chicago Press, 1941.
22. CLEGHORN, R. A. "The Shaping of Psychiatry by Science and Humanism," *Can. Ment. Assoc. J.*, 103 (1970), 933–941.
23. COLBY, K. M. "Research in Psychoanalytic Information Theory," *Am. Sci.*, 49 (1961), 358–369.
24. DUBOS, R. "Humanistic Biology," *Am. Sci.*, 53 (1965), 4–19.
25. EMERSON, A. E. "Dynamic Homeostasis: A Unifying Principle in Organic, Social and Ethical Evolution," *Scientific Monthly*, 78 (1954), 67–85.
26. ———. "Homeostasis and Comparison of Systems," in R. R. Grinker, Sr., ed., *Toward a Unified Theory of Human Behavior*, pp. 147–163. New York: Basic Books, 1967.
27. FARRELL, B. A. "Can Psychoanalysis Be Refuted?" *Inquiry*, 1 (1961), 16–36.
28. FINCH, J. R. "A Further Extension of General Systems Theory for Psychiatry," *Gen. Sys.*, 12 (1967), 103–105.
29. FRENKEL-BRUNSWIK, E. "Psychoanalysis and the Unity of Science," *Proc. Am. Acad. Arts Sci.*, 80 (1952), 80–271.
30. FREUD, A. *Normality and Pathology in Childhood*. New York: International Universities Press, 1965.
31. GEDO, J. and A. GOLDBERG. Personal communication.
32. GILL, M. "Topography and Systems in Psychoanalytic Theory," *Psychol. Issues*, (1963), Monograph No. 3.
33. GREENBLATT, M. "The Elongated Shadow," *Compr. Psychiatry*, 12 (1971), 293–303.
34. GRINKER, R. R., SR. *Psychosomatic Research*. New York: Norton, 1953.

35. ———. "Psychosomatic Approach to Anxiety," *Am. J. Psychiatry*, 113 (1956), 443.

36. ———. "A Theoretical and Experimental Approach to Problems of Anxiety," *Arch. Neurol. Psychiatry*, 76 (1956), 420–431.

37. ———. "On Identification," *Int. J. Psychoanal.*, 38 (1957), 379.

38. ———. "A Transactional Model for Psychotherapy," in M. E. Stein, ed., *Contemporary Psychotherapies*. New York: Free Press, 1961.

39. ———. "A Dynamic Study of the 'Homoclite'," *Sci. Psychoanal.*, 5 (1963), 115–134.

40. ———. "Psychiatry Rides Madly in All Directions," *Arch. Gen. Psychiatry*, 10 (1964), 228–237.

41. ———. "Normality Viewed as a System," *Arch. Gen. Psychiatry*, 17 (1967), 320–324.

42. ———. *Toward a Unified Theory of Human Behavior*, 2nd ed. New York: Basic Books, 1967.

43. ———. "Conceptual Progress in Psychoanalysis," in J. Marmor, ed., *Modern Psychoanalysis*, pp. 19–33. New York: Basic Books, 1968.

44. ———. "An Editors Farewell," *Arch. Gen. Psychiatry*, 21 (1969), 641–645.

45. ———. "Symbolism and General Systems Theory," in W. Gray, Duhl and Rizzo, eds., *General Systems Theory and Psychiatry*. Boston: Little, Brown, 1969.

46. ———. "Biochemical Education as a System," *Arch. Gen. Psychiatry*, 24 (1971), 290–298.

47. GRINKER, R. R., SR., R. R. GRINKER, JR., and J. TIMBERLAKE. "Mentally Healthy Young Males (Homoclites)," *Arch. Gen. Psychiatry*, 6 (1962), 405–453.

48. GRINKER, R. R., SR., J. MACGREGOR, K. SELAN et al. *Psychiatric Social Work: A Transactional Case Book*. New York: Basic Books, 1961.

49. GRINKER, R. R., SR., J. MILLER, M. SABSHIN et al. *The Phenomena of Depressions*. New York: Hoeber, 1961.

50. GRINKER, R. R., SR. and J. P. SPIEGEL. *Men Under Stress*. New York: Blakiston, 1945.

51. GRINKER, R. R., SR., B. WERBLE and R. C. DRYE. *The Borderline Syndrome*. New York: Basic Books, 1968.

52. HAMBURG, D. A. *Psychiatry as a Behavioral Science*. Englewood Cliffs, N.J.: Prentice-Hall, 1970.

53. HANSELL, N. "Patient Predicament and Clinical Service: A System," *Arch. Gen. Psychiatry*, 17 (1967), 204–210.

54. HERRICK, C. J. *George Ellet Coghill—Naturalist and Philosopher*. Chicago: University of Chicago Press, 1949.

55. HESTON, L. L. "Psychiatric Disorders in Foster Home Reared Children of Schizophrenic Mothers," *British Journal Psychiatry*, 112 (1966), 489.

56. JACKSON, H. "Croonian Lectures on Evolution and Dissolution of the Nervous System," *British Medical Journal* (1884), 591.

57. KELLAM, S. G. and J. D. BRANCH. "Strategies in Urban Community Mental Health," in S. Golann, and C. Eisdorfer, eds., *Handbook of Community Psychology*. New York: Appleton, 1971.

58. LEITES, N. *The New Ego*. New York: Science House, 1971.

59. LIDZ, T. *The Person: His Development Throughout the Life-Cycle*. New York: Basic Books, 1968.

60. LUSZKI, M. N. *Interdisciplinary Team Research, Methods and Problems*. New York: New York University Press, 1958.

61. MARCUS, R. L. "The Nature of Instinct and the Physical Basis of Libido," *Gen. Sys.*, 7 (1962), 133–157.

62. MENNINGER, K., M. Mayman, and P. Pruyser. *The Vital Balance*. New York: Viking, 1963.

63. MINUCHIN, S. "Reconceptualization of Adolescent Dynamics from the Family Point of View," in D. Offer and J. F. Masterson, eds., *Teaching and Learning Adolescent Psychiatry*. Springfield: Thomas, 1971.

64. MISCHLER, E. G. and HERTZIG. "Family Interaction Patterns and Schizophrenia," in J. Romano, ed., *The Origins of Schizophrenia*, pp. 121–131. Amsterdam: Excerpta Medica Press, 1967.

65. MORA, G. "The History of Psychiatry: A Cultural and Bibliographical Survey," *Int. J. Psychiatry*, 2 (1966), 335–356.

66. NEWBROUGH, J. R. *Community Mental Health: Individual Adjustment or Social Planning*. Bethesda, Md.: NIMH, 1964.

67. OFFER, D., D. FREEDMAN, and J. OFFER. "The Psychiatrist as Researcher," in D. Offer and D. X. Freedman, eds., *Modern Psychiatry and Clinical Research*, pp, 208–234. New York: Basic Books, 1972.

68. OFFER, D., and M. Sabshin. *Normality: Theoretical and Clinical Concepts of Men-*

tal Health. New York: Basic Books, 1966.

69. OFFER, J. L. "Summaries of Research Undertaken by Roy R. Grinker, Sr.," in D. Offer and D. X. Freedman, eds., *Modern Psychiatry and Clinical Research*, pp. 235–289. New York: Basic Books, 1972.

70. PARSONS, T. *The Social System*. New York: Free Press, 1951.

71. ———. "Some Comments on the State of the General Theory of Action," *Am. Sociol. Rev.*, 18 (1953), 618.

72. ———. "The Social System: A General Theory of Action," in R. R. Grinker, Sr., ed., *Toward a Unified Theory of Human Behavior*, pp. 55–69. New York: Basic Books, 1956.

73. ———. "Field Theory and Systems Theory: With Special Reference to the Relations Between Psychobiological and Social Systems," in D. Offer and D. X. Freedman, eds., *Modern Psychiatry and Clinical Research*, pp. 3–16. New York: Basic Books, 1972.

74. PETERFREUND, E. "Information, Systems and Psychoanalysis," *New York Psychological Issues* Vol. 3. New York: Int. Universities, 1963.

75. PUMPIAN-MINDLIN, E. "The Position of Psychoanalysis in Relation to the Biological and Social Sciences," in E. Pumpian-Mindlin ed., *Psychoanalysis as Science*, pp. 125–158. Stanford: Stanford University Press, 1952.

76. RAPAPORT, A. "Remarks on General Systems Theory," *General Systems*, 8 (1963), 123–125.

77. RUESCH, J. and G. BATESON. *Communication: The Social Matrix of Psychiatry*. New York: Norton, 1968.

78. SCHILDKRAUT, J. J. and S. S. KETY. "Biogenic Amines and Emotion," *Science*, 156 (1967), 21–30.

79. SCHWEBEL, M. *Behavioral Sciences and Human Survival*. Palo Alto: Science & Behavior Books, 1965.

80. SHEPHERD, M. "A Critical Appraisal of Contemporary Psychiatry," *Contemp. Psychiatry*, 12 (1971), 302–321.

81. SHERRINGTON, C. *Man on His Nature*. Cambridge: Cambridge University Press, 1940.

82. SINGER, M. "Family Transactions and Schizophrenia: I. Recent Research Findings," in J. Romano, ed., *The Origins of Schizophrenia*. Amsterdam: Excerpta Medica Press, 1967.

83. SPIEGEL, J. P. "Transactional Theory and Social Change," in D. Offer and D. X. Freedman, eds., *Modern Psychiatry and Clinical Research*, pp. 17–29. New York: Basic Books, 1972.

84. STRAUSS, A., L. SCHATZMAN, R. BUCKER et al. *Psychiatric Ideologies and Institutions*. New York: Free Press, 1964.

85. SULLIVAN, H. S. *Schizophrenia as a Human Process*. New York: Norton, 1962.

86. THOMPSON, L. "The Societal System, Culture and the Community," in R. R. Grinker, Sr., ed., *Toward a Unified Theory of Human Behavior*, pp. 70–82. New York: Basic Books, 1956.

87. TODA, M. "Possible Roles of Psychology in the Very Distant Society," *Gen. Sys.*, 15 (1970), 105–108.

88. TOMAN, J. E. P. "Stability *vs* Adaptation: Some Speculations on the Evolution of Dynamic Reciprocating Mechanisms," in R. R. Grinker, Sr., ed., *Toward a Unified Theory of Human Behavior*, pp. 247–263. New York: Basic Books, 1956.

89. VICKERS, G. "A Classification of Systems," *Gen. Sys.*, 15 (1970), 3–6.

90. WALLERSTEIN, R. S. "Transactional Psychotherapy," in D. Offer and D. X. Freedman, eds., *Modern Psychiatry and Clinical Research*, pp. 120–135. New York: Basic Books, 1972.

91. WALLERSTEIN, R. and N. SMELSER. "Psychoanalysis and Sociology," *Int. J. Psychoanal.*, 50 (1969), 693–716.

92. WEISS, P. *Principles of Development*. New York: Holt, 1939.

93. WILSON, D. "Forms of Hierarchy: A Selected Bibliography," *Gen. Sys.*, 14 (1969), 3.

94. WYNNE, L. and M. T. SINGER. "Thought Disorder and Family Relations of Schizophrenics," *Arch. Gen. Psychiatry*, 9 (1963), 191–198.

95. WYNNE, L. C. "Family Transactions and Schizophrenia: II. Conceptual Considerations for a Research Strategy," in J. Romano, ed., *The Origins of Schizophrenia*, pp. 165–179. Amsterdam: Excerpta Medica Press, 1967.

96. YAHODA, M. *Current Concepts of Positive Mental Health*. New York: Basic Books, 1959.

97. YOUNG, O. R. "A Survey of General Systems Theory," *Gen. Sys.*, 9 (1964), 61–80.

98. ZUBIN, J. "On the Powers of Models," *J. Pers.*, 20 (1952), 430–439.

PART TWO

---

*The Development
of Behavior*

CHAPTER 13

POVERTY, SOCIAL DEPRECIATION, AND CHILD DEVELOPMENT*

Leon Eisenberg and Felton J. Earls

(Introduction

THERE IS by now a large literature on the association between poverty, social depreciation, and distortions of child development. This is not to suggest that our understanding is complete nor that the available data are altogether consistent. Nothing could be farther from the truth. However, more is needed than simply the generation of additional empirical studies; lack of conceptual clarity precludes the use of "data" for the resolutions of the apparent contradictions that beset the field. Further to the point, political ideology leads to a refusal to accept certain

* To the memory of Professor Herbert G. Birch (1918–1973) whose scientific life was dedicated to the understanding and amelioration of those factors that interfere with the optimal development of every child and whose work, both conceptual and empirical, provided much of the groundwork of this chapter.

"facts" and to prefer particular "explanations" for the facts that are accepted as valid.

In this chapter we shall attempt to set forth the alternative ways of viewing the findings that are evident wherever the so-called disadvantaged child has been studied. We shall not undertake an exhaustive review of literature and a point by point contrast of the available studies; reference will be made to comprehensive reviews and to particularly incisive studies and critiques. We hope to stimulate thoughtful consideration of the issues central to the effects of poverty and social depreciation. We make no pretense at neutrality. But we are less concerned with persuading the reader to accept our view than to make him aware of the reasoning that underlies current viewpoints.

We emphasize, at the outset, what we shall recall at the conclusion: it does not take research to prove that children should not be permitted to go hungry, cold, unloved, and unschooled.[22] Even if these misfortunes had no long-term consequences, the immediate suffering they generate is sufficient to indict any society for tolerating them, especially one so wealthy as our own. It is a political, not a scientific, question as to why we permit such conditions to exist in the face of our announced commitment to human welfare.[26] And it becomes an ethical imperative for the psychiatrist as citizen to use his professional position to reduce this suffering, even as he undertakes studies to better understand those conditions which will permit the optimal development of each child's potential. For, what confronts us is not the (unsolved) problem of what is best, but the unambiguous problem of infants and children who lack the minimum for normal growth. To meet the latter challenge, what is missing is not information but moral commitment.

❲ Methods and Data Interpretation

Social class and ethnic differences in test performance on a wide variety of school-related measures have been reported in many countries during the more than seventy years since psychometric measurement was introduced. In general, there is a strong correlation between test performance and social class; even with class "controlled," white children score better than black children, urban children than rural children, Northern children than Southern children. Similar findings have been reported in other Western countries when factors such as social class and minority status have been examined.[45] Further, these test differences are not a passing phenomenon of childhood, but are registered in similar fashion when adult populations are compared. The issue is not whether such differences exist; they clearly do, as thousands of empirical studies attest. The important debate concerns the inferences that may reasonably be drawn from these data. But before we turn to that debate, the central concern of this chapter, it is necessary to begin

by addressing problems of definition and methodology.

Intelligence Tests

A wide variety of measures has been employed in such studies. One broad category purports to measure "intelligence"; another more modestly acknowledges that it measures "achievement." Although intelligence tests had earlier origins, the basic design for them was provided by Alfred Binet and Théodore Simon who undertook, at the request of French educational authorities, to determine the characteristics that differentiated slow from normal learners. They attempted to sample a wide variety of classroom-related behavior that seemed, on the face of it, to be what most people would consider intelligent behavior. The extraordinary success of their method led to a reification of the intelligence the test was measuring. To both the lay public and most professional psychologists, conventional belief holds that intelligence is something the child is "born with" in contrast to achievement that is taken to represent the accomplishment resulting from the application of that intelligence. It seems rarely to have troubled theorists that there is no way of measuring this intelligence at birth because of the limited behavioral repertoire of the newborn; indeed, there is no obvious behavioral difference between the anencephalic infant and the normal neonate. The lack of correlation between infant developmental tests (which attempt to carry the same principles of testing into infancy) and the standard tests for childhood intelligence creates additional difficulties for the proposition.[38] The first age at which we can measure differences that correlate respectably with later childhood performance is in the third year of life. Surely, by then, the child has been influenced significantly by experience. If developmental tests truly measure infant intelligence, then we must assume that infants differ relatively little from each other; indeed, the very same groups of black and white infants who will differ significantly when they are three show no significant differences when they are forty weeks of age.

Alternatively, we can conclude that we have no way of measuring what may be "real" differences in intelligence before the third year but must assume their existence. Parenthetically, it should be noted that these statements do not apply to neurologically impaired infants whose markedly delayed development does foreshadow later test deficiency.[43] But these are only a very small fraction of the total population and display observable indices of central nervous system damage. The difficulty in assuming that there are innate differences, even if we are not clever enough to measure them, is that by the time differences become ascertainable, the child has been exposed to some years of differential experience within the family and the community. We are not arguing that there are no biological differences underlying variations in intelligent behavior but rather pointing to the great difficulty of disentangling genetic from experiential factors when the differences we wish to understand occur precisely in the context of differential experience.[50] The problem is quite different when we examine individual differences in test behavior within a population of children of nearly identical social class. But that is another matter.

It is an ironic footnote to history, if not a depressing one, that Binet himself wrote in 1911:

. . . Some recent philosophers appear to have given their consent to the deplorable verdict that the intelligence of the individual is a fixed quantity . . . we must protest and act against this brutal pessimism . . . a child's mind is like a field for which an expert farmer has advised a change in the method of cultivation, with the result that in place of desert land, we now have a harvest. It is in this particular sense, the one which is significant, that we say that the intelligence of children may be increased. One increases that which constitutes the intelligence of the school child; namely, the capacity to learn, to improve with instruction . . . [*Les idées moderne sur les enfants*]

A second try at teasing out experiential effects has been the attempt to design "culture-free" or "culture-fair" tests. Here, the test constructor endeavors to exclude items that can-

not be answered by the child simply because he has had no exposure to them just as one would draw no conclusions from the failure of a child who speaks English to answer questions in French. As an example, one subtest of intelligence is the ability to reason by analogy. The child is asked to answer a question such as: a book is to an author as a symphony is to a ———? He is then offered five choices, one of which is the word composer. The same question can be rephrased: a hammer is to a carpenter as a wrench is to a ———? This time the set of alternatives includes the word plumber. When the results from these two questions are compared in children of two social classes, the gap between lower- and middle-class children is less on the second question than it is on the first because of the limited likelihood that a lower-class child will have heard such words as symphony and composer. The first form of the question requires a larger vocabulary as well as reasoning. The difficulty in this test design lies in our incomplete knowledge of the differences in life experience and of the extent to which such factors as vocabulary, examination "set," and motivation rather than intelligence are influencing performance. Lower-class children are less familiar with academic "games" and less concerned with doing well on them. All too often, the child responds so as to terminate the testing experience rather than to do well. Let us cite one clinical experience. In the course of carrying out comparative testing in two schools of different social class, we were struck by the frequency of calls from anguished middle-class parents whose children came home to report that they had tested poorly in school; we had not a single call of complaint from the parents of lower-class children. Whether this was because the lower-class child did not trouble to tell his parents about testing or whether his parents were less concerned with what he did report, we cannot say. What remains important is the difference in how salient this behavior was in the context of the family. In general, culture-free or culture-fair tests show fewer differences between social classes, but they do not obliterate them. One can either conclude that the tests are not as culture fair as they profess to be or that class differences remain even when culture is "factored out" of the test situation.

Achievement Tests

In contrast, achievement tests are less concerned with the differentiation of the innate from the acquired, but the contention is that they measure variations in the skills the child possesses. Problems in test construction in this area are of another order. The prototype is the reading test.[23] The child is given a passage of variable length, of more or less complex syntax, and of restricted or varied vocabulary. He is then asked to answer questions based on the passage. One immediate problem is whether the answers to the questions require comprehension of the paragraph or can be deduced from the questions themselves. One of our colleagues (Arthur Applebee) has demonstrated that a respectable performance can be attained by children and adults given the questions without the preceding paragraph; the questions and multiple-choice answers are sufficiently interrelated that an intelligent person can deduce the probable answer from the nature of the question. A second problem in reading tests is that they depend, to a degree greater than recognized, on the language skills the child possesses *before* he begins to learn to read. The magnitude of the task he faces depends on the discrepancy between his native dialect and the standard language that comprises the reading test. For example, Mexican Indian children who are required to learn to read in Spanish at the same time that they are learning Spanish do poorly. If they are first taught to read from primers in the native language, they can then transfer their reading skills more readily to tests in Spanish. Nonetheless, if one asks whether a child can read proficiently in the language that is taken as the standard, the fact remains that he performs less well than does his advantaged age-mate. What differs is the explanation that one would offer for this deficit and the remedies that one would propose to diminish the deficit.[23]

Differences, Real or Spurious?

In a variety of ways, we have been asking whether the manifest differences in scores are "real" or "spurious." That is, to what extent are they artifacts of test administration and/or construction? There are inconsistencies in the literature. Some evidence suggests that the race of the tester may have differential effects on the performance of black subjects; that is, black college students, given a group test by a white test administrator, will perform less well than if the examiner is black. These effects have been more difficult to detect in younger subjects; in some studies, they have been trivial. Other test conditions clearly do influence performance. Preschool children of lower social class will score better on such tests, as the Binet, if given experience with items similar to those used in the test itself; if encouraged to try when they might have simply given up; if required not to answer immediately but to think before replying; and if supported by a warm and sympathetic tester. Obviously, there are also idiosyncratic, individual factors that will depress performance: physical illness, excessive anxiety, distracting noise and other stimuli, and the like. Depending upon test demands, these effects can vary considerably. In a study of our own, black children were given an auditory-discrimination test. To our surprise, their performance was as poor as that of hard-of-hearing children, although they had normal audiograms! In the test employed, the Wepman Auditory Discrimination test, the child is asked to respond "same" or "different" to a pair of words that are either identical or differ in a single vowel or consonant. It occurred to us that either the children were simply not attending to the task or were so uninterested in "doing well" on the test that they gave any answer that would get it over with. When the study was repeated with an alternate form of the Wepman and with the examiner using sternness or encouragement (depending on her assessment of what would be appropriate for the individual child) there was a striking reduction in the number of "erroneous" responses. Thus, we were able to demonstrate that the children had the "ability" to respond correctly under *altered test conditions*; yet we still must recognize that under standard conditions, the performance was subpar. Our assessment of a very large literature on this question is that, although conditions of test administration do account for some of the social-class difference, they do not account for all of it.

The matter of test construction is more complex. We have all seen young adults who have failed arithmetic, but who can lay bets, calculate odds, and play crap with much greater dexterity and rapidity than many of us who have done well in formal courses in probability statistics. In nonliterate cultures, adults may be able to tally large assemblies of familiar objects with impressive speed despite limited ability to count novel objects. Indeed, in some cultures, the system of numeration varies with the class of object to be counted.[13] The same Guatemalan Indian child who is able to weave intricate geometric designs on a rug may be unable to match solid forms on a Seguin formboard. As a final example, the same person who fails to solve a Porteus maze may be able to track a wild animal through the bush or find his way from one distant location to another.

Differences or Deficits?

The question we are now asking is whether we are measuring differences (just as some people have blue eyes and others brown) or deficits (as some see and others are blind). This becomes peculiarly germane in the assessment of linguistic competence. A lower-class, preschool child may demonstrate developmental immaturity on a test of syntax in standard English when compared with the competence of his middle-class age mate. That "deficiency" is important if it is going to be necessary for him to communicate to others in standard English. But the implications are rather different if it can be demonstrated that he has syntactical equivalents in his own dialect. That is, one would anticipate restriction

in the finer discriminations of thought itself (if thought is shaped by language) when linguistic competence is deficient. If, on the other hand, the language possessed by the child is just as powerful though different, then there should be no impairment in thinking. There is a growing body of evidence that there are different but equivalent grammatical forms in black English.[19] What appears to be a deficit in linguistic competence is a deficit in standard English but not in language competence.

Thus, quite apart from the debate about the "innateness" of intelligence, there are problems inherent in the attempt to measure intelligence by particular problem-solving skills. Most psychologists believe that there is a general intelligence, the so-called g factor; many also believe that there are specific abilities that correlate only moderately with this general factor; fewer today would argue for a series of discrete abilities that show little intercorrelation. One does not have to believe that a Mozart is solely the product of his environment to acknowledge that he could not have written symphonies had he been born into a society without the musical heritage in which he was imbedded. Under such circumstances, would Mozart still have had the same musical genius even if it were unable to be developed or would the precursors of that genius simply have atrophied? If a society provides the opportunity to refine hunting skills but not mathematical skills, can some quantitative measurement of the skills the individual has give us a clue to what he might have shown in some other area? In the instances chosen, probably not, since one might expect a low order of correlation between hunting and mathematical abilities. Does solving the problems of survival in an inhospitable arctic environment predict how well an Eskimo might have done in the differential calculus? Closer to home, do the skills acquired for survival on the street in the slums of the inner city give us any measure of what that child might have done in academic subjects had he been born into a middle-class environment? The answer is unknown. The point of this exercise is to caution against the assumption that what is being measured in standard tests of intelligence is adequate to comprehend all of what falls under the rubric of intelligent or effective adaptive behavior. The only thing that I.Q. tests predict reasonably well is success in school; success in school, however, is not a very effective predictor of success in vocational tasks, except insofar as it provides a credential necessary for entrance into a particular occupation.[3]

Population Differences Versus Individual Differences

If, for the moment, we acknowledge that test differences on measured performance are real in the context of this society, it is necessary to emphasize one important caution. Such differences are differences between population means. The distributions for the two populations (whether they be black and white or rich and poor) show a very considerable overlap. Thus, a substantial number of the disadvantaged population will display performances that exceed the mean of the advantaged population. In short, whatever statements may be warranted in population comparisons, they do *not* justify any *a priori* conclusions about individuals. The fact that a child performs poorly on a given test may be a moderately accurate predictor of his performance in a classroom. The fact that a child is black or that a child is poor, however, does not warrant a prediction as to whether his performance is above or below the norm. Unhappily, psychological stereotyping is such that the demographic characteristic is often taken as though it were a reasonable basis for prediction; the child may be assigned to one or another classroom as though his performance had actually been measured. Such evidence as we have suggests that assignment to a slow moving class and expectation by a teacher that a child will be a slow learner are likely to lead him to perform as the relevant social group expects him to. When he fails to learn, this may be taken as support for the original prediction; there will be a cumulative effect over time that will tend to further separate those assigned to better and worse classes.[24]

Permanent or Reversible?

Let us suppose that we are dealing with deficits and that they are real. We then must consider whether they are permanent or reversible. Obviously, even temporary deficits are not desirable; they become far more ominous if they are irreversible. A scientific decision on this question must be taken with full foreknowledge of its consequences. Resources being finite, no one will support their expenditure to treat the untreatable. Unfortunately, moreover, the judgment that a deficit is irreversible and the consequent failure to try to remedy it will, ipso facto, guarantee that it will be permanent. We would therefore contend that such a conclusion should be accepted only on the basis of solid evidence lest we cripple children permanently by the very formulation of a prognosis.

Educational theorists have long held that the younger the child, the more malleable he is and that the impact of early influences on character and intelligence is likely to be far more enduring than those of later years. This has been reinforced by metaphors drawn from embryology.[25,50] For example, there is a short interval in embryologic life when the extrusion of the optic cup induces in the overlying ectoderm the formation of a crystalline lens. Exposure of ectoderm to the optic cup, earlier or later than that critical period, shows no such induction. Animal behaviorists suggested an analogue to the phenomenon of this critical period when ethologists reported "imprinting." In certain birds and in certain ungulates, the newborn will become attached to an artificial object that it will follow as it would have otherwise followed its mother. Moreover, the consequence of the distortion in social development induced by this pattern will lead to difficulties in the display of species appropriate sexual behavior when the bird is an adult. However, these phenomena are restricted to a limited number of species; in general, the longer the period of dependency of the young on the adult of the species, the greater the time periods in which such crucial learning can occur and the more modifiable it is by subsequent experience.

It is more usual to find references in current literature to "sensitive periods" than to critical periods. This change in terminology reflects a growing recognition that there may be developmental epochs in which a skill is most rapidly and efficiently acquired, but that the time limits are greater and the differences in efficiency of acquisition are relative rather than absolute. Moreover, many of the studies that emphasize the critical or sensitive period fail to take into account the relationship between the permanence of the effect and the organism's subsequent life experience.[50] For example, Harry Harlow's motherless monkeys were not only motherless but also were confined to an environment devoid of peers or other adults. The clinical psychiatric literature, much influenced by these animal models, has stressed the permanence of the traumatic effects of early deprivation. What has been overlooked in these studies has been the persistence of the deprivation. There are growing numbers of case reports of youngsters rescued from early deprivation and placed in good homes under expert care; such youngsters function remarkably well (i.e., in relatively normal fashion) even though we have no way of determining whether their performance might have been even better, had they not suffered the early misfortune. The most remarkable cases reported are the children described a quarter of a century ago by Anna Freud, children who had survived the horrors of the concentration camp at Theresienstadt. Although detailed information obviously could not be obtained, these children had experienced inadequate, inconsistent, and minimal mothering; what was most striking about them was their fierce loyalty to one another. Under the expert care of Miss Freud's workers in a group home, these children were successfully placed in foster homes over the next several years. Unpublished information on them as young adults provides remarkable testimony to the resilience of the human spirit—and to

the skills and compassion of the Hampstead Group. As young adults, all but one are relatively well-adjusted members of society and that one functions at a better than marginal level!

Our main thrust in this section has been to emphasize the unjustifiability of conclusions that either intelligence or achievement cannot be modified by suitable therapeutic intervention even in the later years of childhood and adolescence. Military experience with marginal draftees in World War II indicates what can be done to improve the performance of young adults when a real effort is made. We do not suggest that all deficits are correctable; we do maintain that it would be premature as well as unethical to conclude that educational deficits are irreversible until the best effort we are capable of has been directed to their correction. All too often, brief trials of inadequate therapies are offered to socially handicapped children; results are meager and frequently transient; instead of concluding that we have failed them, as we have, we judge the children to be failures.

Do the Differences Have Consequences?

The final way of viewing the test discrepancies, whether they be differences or deficits, permanent or reversible, is to ask whether they are "consequential." That is, what do they portend for current as well as later levels of behavioral function? We do know that I.Q. scores correlate with school grades at about a value of 0.6; in other words, I.Q. level "accounts" for about 36 percent of the variance in school grades. Clearly, even this leaves the greatest amount of the variance unexplained. The question remains: how much of the apparent correlation flows from the "I.Q." and how much from the fact that the same class and ethnic factors continue to operate on the child so as to maintain the relationship between I.Q. and grades? We suggest that the same cluster of elements that operate within the context of his family to bring the child to school with a borderline I.Q. acts to determine the school he goes to, the way he is treated at school, the way his family views his school work, the kind of experience he has after school, and the expectations others set for him. Thus, the apparent consistency of performance is not "intrinsic" to the child's nature but rather results from the set of external variables that continue to operate upon him. Furthermore, the association between dropping out of school and subsequent limited occupational attainment may reflect the lack of job opportunities as much as the lack of occupational skills. Black, high-school graduates are more likely to be unemployed than white, high-school graduates with similar academic records. The same applies, with even greater force, to white and black high-school dropouts. Since the high-school dropout is not able to demonstrate such skills as he may have in jobs where a diploma is a requirement, we do not know what that youngster might have done had the job been offered him. Even if we suppose, as is likely, that his job performance might not have been as good as that of a high-school graduate, his poorer performance may reflect inadequate work habits, motivational factors, and personal deportment rather than intellectual or academic deficits. The point is that each of us is imbedded in a sociocultural matrix that imposes upon us a continuity of behavior that may be mistaken for intrinsic characteristics when, in fact, the key determinants are external.[50]

We have stressed, throughout, alternative ways of viewing the abundant epidemiologic data that reveal group differences. Whatever the extent to which they are best accounted for in other ways than the conventional, the depressing facts remain: socially depreciated and financially impoverished children perform, in and out of school, at levels below the norms attained by their advantaged age mates. How is this to be explained?

❡ Explanatory Hypothesis

The explanations that have been put forth to account for these differences fall into three broad categories: genetic, biological insult, and sociocultural "deprivation." Though these explanatory hypotheses are frequently stated as though they were mutually exclusive, it is clear that interactional effects not only can occur but often are decisive. For example, the Kauai Study demonstrated that the childhood morbidity, resulting from similar pregnancy complications, was far greater among children of lower social class than those of middle class.[51] That is, not only was the likelihood of prematurity greater among lower-class births but the likelihood that the premature child would show intellectual and academic defects was far greater when those who were premature and differed in class were compared to one another. Similarly, the child who is malnourished is more likely at the same time to have parents with little education, poor health care, and so on. Further, one would expect the child, who for genetic reasons has a borderline intellectual potential, to test in the mentally defective range if he is simultaneously exposed to biological or cultural disadvantage. To put this crudely, if cultural disadvantage lowers I.Q. attainment by twenty points, the child who might have had the potential for an I.Q. of one hundred and twenty will function at a test quotient of one hundred (or within the normal range); if he might have attained ninety, he will attain seventy and thus will function at a mildly retarded level. It is, of course, not necessarily true that the absolute depression of potential score would be identical in the two instances, but the use of simplified assumptions serves to illustrate the point.

Genetic Theories

The notion that social class is explained by heredity goes back at least as far as the Greeks. In Plato's *Republic*, Socrates sets forth the myth that God has framed men differently: of gold for those with the power to command, of silver for those who are auxiliaries, and of brass and iron for those who are to be husbandmen and craftsmen. He adds that the species will be preserved in the children and that meddlesome interchange between the three classes would be mischievous. Thomas Malthus in the eighteenth century was not only concerned with the overgrowth of the population relative to the supply of food but with the large size of the families who were poor, a fact that he took as auguring deterioration of the quality of the species. In the nineteenth century Herbert Spencer was concerned that charitable measures to mitigate the struggle for survival would lead to the preservation of the imbecile at the expense of the wise. The eugenics movement, which began in America at the turn of the twentieth century, advised measures to sterilize the poor and encourage the rich to have larger families in order to avoid an otherwise inevitable decline in biological quality because of differential birthrates.[40] All took for granted that success in society was a measure of biological superiority, a comfortable assumption for those who had it made, much akin to fundamentalist religious beliefs that worldly acquisition reflects God's rewards for good works.

The same concerns are reflected in contemporary debate on the subject.[8] None of the handwringers have been troubled to explain why there has not been a decline in average I.Q. despite the long existence of this differential in the birthrate. Most of the arguments have been innocent of any consideration of population genetics. For optimal adaptation to occur in a population, a wide range of individual variance has to be maintained. Lionel Penrose has shown that in order to maintain an average population I.Q., inheritance must be derived from a wide range of individual genotypes. Genetic contributions from those functioning below average as well as those functioning at a superior level stabilize average function over time. Moreover, eugenic approaches assume we know how to identify optimal characteristics in order to breed supermen. Given the likelihood of polygenetic inheritance for intelligence, as well as the probability that individual components of intelligence may be linked to other biologic attributes that may not be desirable, artificial imposition of mating patterns could lead to disasterous results. An example from agronomy may clarify the point. Strains of wheat have been carefully selected for optimal crop production under current environmental circumstances, which include reliance on petro-chemical fertilizers. The introduction of a new pathogen or a change in climatic conditions or unavailability of oil can have drastic effects on the yield from a strain of wheat with little genetic variance. Such events have already occurred. Recently, the National Academy of Sciences has urged the necessity of maintaining, in a central repository, a "bank" of seed of the widest variety in order that we may be able to reintroduce strains resistant to some new hazard, should it appear. By analogy, were we to be able to select those with the right to reproduce in order to encourage the flourishing of some ideal type, the restricted variance would put this new "race" in grave danger of a biological calamity from some unanticipated environmental change. Diversity insures survival, just as variation serves to guarantee the uniqueness of each human being.

The development in the modern state of the belief that there is a national responsibility to mitigate the extremes of poverty has resulted in more visible "welfare" costs. The advocates of family planning, long assailed for their efforts to make contraception available to the poor, suddenly found new allies. Those opposed to welfare costs became convinced that reduction in family size might diminish the drain on the tax dollar. During the 1950s and 1960s, there were openly racist arguments for making contraception imperative or sterilization mandatory as a condition for obtaining welfare "benefits." Some welfare-rights organizations and some black nationalist groups began to oppose family-planning clinics as instruments of genocide.[17]

This is to confuse the motivation behind a program with its potential value for the population at whom it is directed. Whether or not covert racism is behind the push for family planning in poor communities, family planning itself increases the options available to minority-group families. Obstetrical evidence indicates that spacing of pregnancies diminishes the hazards to both mother and child. The need to divide meager resources among many children increases the burdens on the whole family. Mothers overwhelmed by too many young children can hardly be expected to function at their best. And the mother condemned to have child after child because contraceptives are unavailable to her is denied her human right to choice. The availability of contraception and therapeutic abortion—as a voluntary decision of each family—enhances the freedom of that family. The ecological arguments in favor of population limitation are, in fact, more appropriately directed at the haves than the have-nots.[23] Our major environmental problem is not food supply but the consumption of energy, the production of wastes, and so on, to which the affluent contribute in greater proportion than the deprived, not by design but because of the availability of resources. On a worldwide scale it is the developed nations whose population provides the greatest risks to world ecology rather than the developing or the quiescent.

None of this denies the existence of a genetic basis for elements of that complex of behavior that we regard as intelligence. What we question is the ready assumption that phenotypical population differences reflect genotypes. Since one never proves the negative hypothesis, it is of course possible that there *may* be a difference in gene distribution related to intelligence among ethnic groups. To suggest that this should be a major focus of research is evil on two grounds.[8,25] First, we simply do not have the methodology to separate nature from nurture in assessing *social* behavior. Second, it lends credence to prevailing bigotry. As noted earlier, even if we accept present test data as though they measured genotypes, the overlap among populations is so considerable that the variation is more impressive than the differences between the means. Thus, if the argument is raised that we should be concerned to identify characteristics of children that make them better able to profit from particular modes of instruction, we still face the necessity of evaluating each child *individually* to determine his suitability for a certain program rather than to classify the child by class or race. Given the intertwining of test results and prior experience, test classification itself is suspect because test-based segregation is likely to increase divergences rather than to ameliorate them.

Biologic Insult

The disadvantage to which the lower-class child is subject begins, not only before birth but before conception. Intergenerational effects of malnutrition have been demonstrated in animal experiments and are strongly supported by human data. One clear consequence of malnutrition in childhood is the stunting of growth.[31] Short mothers (less than five feet one inch) have been shown to have higher rates of fetal mortality, delivery complications, prematurity, and perinatal deaths.[1,2] In part this appears related to a difference in pelvic outlet[32] and in part to reduced reproductive efficiency. In studies with rodents, mothers starved as infants show reduced reproductive efficiency.[12,14] If they, in addition, are malnourished during pregnancy, their offspring are twice as vulnerable.

Numerous studies have demonstrated that complications of pregnancy and parturition are greater among women of lower social class, for reasons related to poor nutrition and poor health care. Pasamanick and his coworkers[43] have introduced the concept of a "continuum of reproductive casualty." Abortions and stillbirths are taken to represent the extreme result of reproductive failure. The less severely impaired child will survive, but it may have epilepsy, cerebral palsy, mental retardation, and/or behavior disorders. Premature infants (below fifteen hundred grams) have been shown to fare poorly in elementary school in contrast to their well-born peers.[35,52] As noted earlier, the child born of a complicated pregnancy is more likely to demonstrate permanent sequellae if he is raised in a lower-class home, thus demonstrating an interactional effect.[51]

The major spurt in human brain growth extends from midpregnancy well into the second postnatal year. Early, there is multiplication of neuronal cell number,[54] later glial multiplication and continuing myelination[18,20] and proliferation of dendritic connections.[27,34] Severe malnutrition during the last half of pregnancy or in the first year of life has been shown to be associated with reduction in brain cell number and with retarded intellectual performance in those children who survive.[7,16] Less severe malnutrition[42] is probably associated with less dramatic but nonetheless demonstrable academic retardation. In the studies in Jamaica[33] by Hertzig and coworkers, index cases were chosen by identifying children who had been hospitalized in early childhood for severe malnutrition. At school age these youngsters were contrasted with sibling controls and classroom controls. The children with known, severe malnutrition performed less well than their siblings, thus indicating that the decrement in performance could not be explained simply by the culture of the home. On the other hand, the sibling control group remained inferior to the classroom controls. It is likely that the siblings of children who had experienced severe and obvious malnutrition underwent chronic subnutrition, although without the acute episodes. They may also have experienced home environments less conducive to learning and thus exhibited the product of both biological and psychological malnutrition.

Malnutrition, through its depression of immunologic defense mechanisms, also renders the infant and child more vulnerable to infection.[47] Infection leads to reduced dietary intake at the very time that metabolic demand is increased. Thus, the impact of malnutrition is exacerbated. Indeed, cultural practices to reduce child feeding in the presence of infection may lead to a further decrease in intake when additional nourishment is what the child requires.

There is growing evidence that malnutrition in itself leads to central nervous system damage.[54] Moreover, malnutrition leads to apathy, unresponsiveness to the environment and, thus, loss of time and opportunity for learning, particularly when associated with hospitalization.[5] Hospitalization itself, though it may be necessary as a life-saving measure, removes the child from a familiar environment and may induce further apathy. This interlocking sequence of biological and behavioral consequences may have its impact heightened if it occurs during a sensitive period for the acquisition of particular developmental skills. It is

to engage in scholastic argument to insist on the priority of one or another factor when they occur concurrently and when they interact. It is the *complex* of malnutrition, infection, and social disadvantage that combines to produce children and adolescents markedly impaired in their adaptive capacities.

In a letter to the *Lancet* on January 6, 1973, John Dobbing wrote:

On the available evidence, may we now beg pediatricians, and more especially politicians, to accept the whole of the human brain growth spurt? From mid-pregnancy well into the second post-natal year, is a period, not only of brain vulnerability, but of opportunity actively to promote the proper growth of the human brain, by providing the best environmental conditions.

There is an additional class of biological insults to the brain that merits close attention: environmental toxins. Lead poisoning serves as a prototype.[21] Epidemiologic studies reveal differential social-class distribution. One major source of this difference is the frequency with which lead-containing, interior paints are found in dilapidated housing in the inner city; atmospheric concentrations of lead vary in different sections of the city because of traffic patterns and industrial pollution. The encephalopathy that results from acute exposure is well recognized as a major public-health hazard. More recently, there have been suggestions that continuing exposure to dosages that do not produce acute symptoms may nonetheless lead to chronic brain syndromes with manifestations such as hyperkinesis, learning disorder, and behavior problems. Housing conditions, disorganized family life, and lack of adequate supervision of young children result in an excess of cases of accidental poisoning from ingestion of other toxic substances.[41] Moreover, the same factors plus traffic conditions in the inner city put these children at greater risk of brain trauma from automobile and other accidents. Finally, the limited availability of health care and its inadequate quality subject the lower-class child to the persistence of uncorrected health deficits that impair his adaptation.

Emphasis on biologic insult to the brain

does not arouse the political passions that are stirred by genetic hypotheses; yet, it can lead to similar hopelessness about efforts to help children already damaged. While we lack therapies to restore brain integrity, sequellae can be minimized by vigorous treatment and by the provision of adequate rehabilitative measures. There remains a wide discrepancy between what we know how to do and what we actually do do for the endangered children. Handicapped children are too often condemned to levels of social function far below their capabilities because of social stigma and lack of suitable occupational opportunities (sheltered workshops and the like).

Cultural Factors

We have thus far employed "class" and "ethnicity" as if they were almost interchangeable terms. This becomes an inevitable shorthand because minority groups are disproportionately represented among the lower social classes. When attempts are made to "match" class among majority and minority groups, minority-group children continue to test at a lower level. In part, this reflects the imprecision of matching for class. Families at the same income level may not be in the same position as consumers. Housing segregation leads to higher rents for those forced to live in ghettos. Prices for staple items are not equivalent throughout the city. Supermarkets and drugstores have been shown to charge higher prices in the inner city because they have a captive population, which cannot travel as readily for shopping. Thus, disposable income is not the same for white and black families with identical earnings.

Our knowledge of the interrelationship between child-rearing practices and child development remains fragmentary.[9,37,55] Nonetheless, there are a large number of studies that indicate that lower-class families are more likely to rely on nonverbal than verbal cues, to transmit concrete rather than abstract problem-solving modes, and to be strict rather than permissive. This is thought to result in a set of attributes that are dysfunctional in school.

Contrariwise, the middle-class child is more likely to have been exposed to books, to sophisticated language, and to games with parents and siblings that encourage attention, reflectiveness rather than impulsiveness, and an awareness of language nuances. Moreover, the middle-class child will have been prepared to take school seriously (perhaps even too seriously) as a determinant of his occupational mobility.

There are important differences in family structure between blacks and whites.[4] In part, this stems from historical roots. Slave owners deliberately maintained matriarchal patterns by using the male as a salable commodity.[29] Welfare regulations tend to reinforce the same structure by making support more available when there is no father in the household. Given the lack of opportunity for employment for the black male, the family may be better off financially if he is out of the home and unemployed rather than home and unemployed. The black family, more often than the white, is an extended rather than a nuclear family, with grandmothers, collateral relatives, and even strangers providing care and support at times of family stress. Black mothers express the same hopes for their children in education and occupation as do middle-class mothers; however, the same mother who expresses the wish to see her son go on to college and become a professional conveys to him the futility of her hopes because of her own long experience with the discrepancy between dream and reality. The child's own experience reinforces this sense of futility when he or she observes how often children in the neighborhood drop out of school and are locked into the ranks of the uneducated and the unemployed.[39]

All of this has been condensed into the slogan: "the culture of poverty," an expression that implies that the poor remain poor because of the social customs that stabilize poverty-producing behavior. This runs directly contrary to G. B. Shaw's dictum that what the poor lack is money. The concept of the culture of poverty permits policy makers, teachers, and other professionals to conclude that no matter what is done to employ and educate the poor, they will remain poor.[46] But the poor exist in a structured society that requires poverty as a condition for maintaining its differential wage structure and institutionalizes stereotypes of behavior to guarantee the existence of this under class.[48] It has been suggested, for example, that schools are not failing; to the contrary, they are doing what they have been designed to do: namely, to produce that variety of competence and incompetence which will provide occupants for the occupational niches that society requires.[30]

Further, the emotional response of society to crime results in a disproportionate emphasis on the amount and kind of social deviance among the poor. Crimes like income-tax evasion, stock manipulation, and embezzlement arouse far less public condemnation than crimes against property and person. We do not suggest that either type of crime is trivial; rather, we take issue with the stereotyping of lower class morality. Public morality *is* a serious issue throughout this country at a time when railroad stockholders, corporation executives, federal judges, and elected officials including the president himself do not hesitate to enrich themselves at the expense of the public. The tax structure of our society has built into it major inequities in the burden exacted from below-median and above-median income earners.[15]

The developmental failure of poor and black children is exacerbated at adolescence. It is most evident in the high rates of school casualties at this period. During puberty the child is beginning to evaluate his environment and to develop ways of thinking about and interacting with it. Given his limited choices, the lower-class youngster has difficulty in establishing effective modes of behavior that are both satisfying and accepted by the mores of the majority culture. One of the few pathways to personal success is through sports. This has been true for successive waves of immigrants for the last century. For the vast majority, this is not an available track; failure is multidimensional with school being pivotal. Resort to personally less-satisfying and, at the same time, socially disruptive kinds of behavior is common as is attested by the population of

the jail system where poor minority group members predominate.

The systematic devaluation[10] of the person and the family of the minority-group child operates upon him so as to create a negative self-image; having been pressed to devalue himself, he acts out the stereotype of those expectations.[48] Treated as though he were "stupid", he acts stupid, that is, he fails to try to learn, he gives the first answer that comes to mind as a way of avoiding the question rather than thinking about it. He belittles school just as school denigrates him and shifts his investment to those out-of-school activities which offer some promise of success: rage against a hateful environment is transformed into self-hatred. His values become a negative image of the values of the majority culture but, nonetheless, a mirror reflection of them. Unless he is helped to develop a perspective that makes understandable the nature of his circumstances and suggests constructive modes of action to change them, he becomes what he was predicted to be; his behavior provides further "justification" for prevailing beliefs.

The most noteworthy development in grappling with this psychological problem has been the emergence of the concepts subsumed under the term: black nationalism. The positive aspects of black culture and group identity are stressed as the basis for the acquisition of a sense of personal integrity through social action. It is perhaps inevitable that a social movement, emerging to resist white stereotypes about blacks, will result in some stereotyping of whites, most obviously present in the Black Muslim movement. However disagreeable counterviolence may be, the most effective way of dealing with it is by terminating white violence against blacks.[44] More dangerous to the constructive creation of black pride is a too ready identification of black with good, thus constraining the availability of self-criticism. A sociopolitical movement can be subverted from within as well as from without; its slogans can be prated by those more concerned with self-advantage through political office than with group progress. Black studies can become an effective medium for learning how to read, but rap sessions cannot substitute for learning to read. The technical skills essential for a productive role in contemporary society will more readily be acquired by a student who believes in his people and in himself, but the concentrated, personal effort to master them remains essential. All in all, it is our view that the movement for black pride is one key to reversing the waste of human talent and the loss of human happiness that have been the terrible price of a racist society.[49]

(Future Directions

The social disadvantage of poor and minority-group children has been so thoroughly documented that there is no need for further descriptive research. We need to undertake a coordinated program of preventive and remedial measures now. We need prompt action to combat malnutrition—during pregnancy and the early years of life in particular—but throughout childhood and adolescence. We need a system of health care that will ensure delivery of health services to all Americans. First in order of priority would be pregnant women, infants, children, and adolescents. But there is no excuse for inadequate health care for the aged and the adult. Family-income-support programs should assure parents and their children an equal opportunity for lives of dignity. Good foster-care and group-care homes must be available to children whose families are disrupted. Enforcement of existing legislation can mitigate occupational discrimination if not altogether eliminate it. For these things we may need periodic checks of social indicators to measure how near we are to our goals. But it does not take research to prove that we should move forward. The problem is moral, not scientific.

We are on less certain grounds when we confront the challenge of undoing the effects of early neglect. It is not enough to label an educational program "compensatory" or "enriched." It must be demonstrated that the new program is responsive to the children's needs and, in fact, produces the desired changes in

behavior. Here research in child development must play a central role in guiding public policy.[9] What is needed is action research: the assessment of the changes that follow the introduction of experimental programs rather than merely the continued documentation of failures to satisfy traditional standards. We face, however, a major problem in persuading the public to support the long-term investment required.

Typically, educational innovation has consisted in the introduction of a new program, usually underfunded, for a brief period. Even when good results, the changes prove to be transient when the child moves from the experimental into the regular classroom. It is as if we expected a good diet at the age of five to prevent malnutrition at the age of six after dietary supplementation has been discontinued. It is necessary to impress on our national consciousness Jean Piaget's metaphor that cognitive development depends upon psychological "alimentation" *throughout* the years of childhood and adolescence. Once this principle is accepted, the challenge to educational and psychological knowledge remains formidable; namely, the systematic construction of public systems of education that will promote child development at an optimal level. Research in the school setting that assesses the characteristics of the children, the behavior of the teachers, *and* the operation of the system as an institution, will be crucial if we are to do our children justice. Present research methodology will enable us to address some of the foregoing issues, although available instruments will require further refining, and better conceptualizations are needed.

The tools of social psychiatry are the least adequate when it comes to understanding the inertia of social institutions and the ways of fostering institutional change. These problems play back onto individual development; the individual must feel himself to be to some degree the master of his own fate before he can undertake the prodigous efforts necessary to change the world outside. The complexity and the bureaucratization of our society generates apathy in the face of cumbersome and unresponsive social institutions. Even when an investigator is able to demonstrate that instructional method A produces results better than B or equal to B at less cost, there is frequently no visible consequence to the demonstration. It is published, forgotten, and perhaps rediscovered a decade later. One does not have to invoke malevolence to explain this disregard. Inertia and self-protection account for much of it. The new method may require a teacher or a principal to unlearn old ways; it may threaten professional prerogatives; it may produce more cognitive dissonance than the audience is willing to tolerate because it belies conventional wisdom. The gap between research and its application can be appreciably diminished if the consumer (the educator and the parent) is involved from the first in generating the questions to be asked, in participating in the gathering of data, and in analyzing the results. There must, in the first instance, be a willingness to recognize the inadequacy of traditional formulations. Without such a climate, data will produce no change in conviction. One has only to consider official attitudes on marijuana and pornography to recognize that systematic documentation proving that conventional attitudes have no basis in fact does not by itself shake belief.

Finally, there *is* a malevolent component in resistance to change. One does not have to be a prophet to predict that those who benefit from social injustice will fight to maintain their privileged position. Slum properties bring profitable rents to their owners. Disenfranchised voters enable those who possess the vote to control the outcome. The existence of a pool of unemployed acts as a brake on wages. Bitterly enough, the sense of superiority generated in whites, who are taught to look down on blacks, permits the exploitation of lower-class whites by political leaders who seek their own advantage.[24] It is not merely ignorance, though ignorance is present, that permits our society to tolerate the social ills we have outlined; they are perpetuated by the short-run view of self-interest. Those who challenge privilege can expect little praise. Their sustenance must come from the recognition that, in the words of Frederick Douglass, "Without struggle, there can be no progress."

(Bibliography

1. BAIRD, D. "Social Factors in Obstetrics," *Lancet*, 1 (1949), 1079–1083.
2. ———. "The Epidemiology of Prematurity," *J. Pediatr.*, 65 (1964), 909–924.
3. BERG, I. *Education and Jobs: The Great Training Robbery*. New York: Praeger, 1970.
4. BILLINGSLEY, A. *Black Families in White America*. Englewood Cliffs: Prentice-Hall, 1968.
5. BIRCH, H. G. and J. D. GUSSOW. *Disadvantaged Children: Health, Nutrition and School Failure*. New York: Harcourt Brace and World, 1970.
6. BIRCH, H. G. and A. LEFFORD. "Intersensory Development in Children," *Monogr. Soc. Res. Child Dev.*, 28 (1963), 1–48.
7. BIRCH, H. G., C. PINEIRO, E. ALCALDE et al. "Kwashiorkor in early childhood and intelligence at school age," *Pediatr. Res.*, 5 (1971), 579–585.
8. BOWLES, S. and H. GINTIS. "IQ in the U.S. Class Structure," *Soc. Policy*, 3 (1973), 65–96.
9. CALDWELL, B. "Critical Issues in Infancy and Early Child Development," *Res. Publ. Assoc. Res. Nerv. Ment. Dis.*, 51 (1972), 333–351.
10. CAMPBELL, A. *White Attitudes Toward Black People*. Ann Arbor: Litho Crafters, 1971.
11. CHASE, H. P. and H. P. MARTIN. "Undernutrition and Child Development," *N. Engl. J. Med.*, 282 (1970), 933–976.
12. CHOW, B. F., B. BLACKWELL, T. Y. HOU et al. "Maternal Nutrition and Metabolism of the Offspring: Studies in Rats and Man," *Am. J. Public Health*, 58 (1968), 668–677.
13. COLE, M., J. GAY, J. A. GLICK et al. *The Cultural Context of Learning and Thinking*. New York: Basic Books, 1971.
14. COWLEY, J. J. and R. D. GRIESEL. "The Effect on Growth and Behavior of Rehabilitating First and Second Generation Low Protein Rats," *Anim. Behav.*, 14 (1966), 506–517.
15. CORWIN, R. and S. M. MILLER. "Taxation and Its Beneficiaries," *Am. J. Orthopsychiatry*, 42 (1972), 200–214.
16. CRAVIOTO, J., E. R. DELICARDIE, and H. G. BIRCH. "Nutrition, growth, and neuroin-

tegrative development: an experimental and ecologic study," *Pediatrics*, 38 (1966), Part II, Suppl., 319–372.

17. DARETY, W. A. and C. B. CASTELLANO. "Family Planning, Race Consciousness, and the Fear of Race Genocide," *Am. J. Public Health*, 62 (1972), 1454–1459.

18. DAVISON, A. N. and J. DOBBING. "Myelination as a Vulnerable Period in Brain Development," *Br. Med. Bull.*, 22 (1966), 40–44.

19. DILLARD, J. L. *Black English*. New York: Random House, 1972.

20. DOBBING, J. "The Influence of Early Nutrition on the Development and Myelination of the Brain," *Proc. R. Soc.*, 159 (1964), 503–509.

21. Editorial. "Subclinical Lead Poisoning," *Lancet*, 1 (1973), 87.

22. EISENBERG, L. "The Sins of the Fathers: Urban Decay and Social Pathology," *Am. J. Orthopsychiatry*, 32 (1962), 5–17.

23. ———. "Neuropsychiatric Aspects of Reading Disability," *Pediatrics*, 37 (1966), 17–33.

24. ———. "Racism, Family and Society," *Ment. Hyg.*, 52 (1968), 512–520.

25. ———. "The *Human* Nature of Human Nature," *Science*, 176 (1972), 123–128.

26. ———. "Poverty, Professionalism and Politics," *Am. J. Orthopsychiatry*, 42 (1972), 748–754.

27. ELLIOT, K. and J. KNIGHT, eds. *Lipids, Malnutrition and the Developing Brain*. London: Assoc. Sci., 1972.

28. ELLISON, R., L. R. JAMES, and D. G. FOX. "The Identification of Talent Among Negro and White Students From Biographical Data," *Catalogue of Sel. Doc. in Psycho.*, 2 (1972).

29. FRAZIER, E. F. *Black Bourgeoisie*. New York: Free Press, 1957.

30. GREER, C. *The Great School Legend*. New York, Basic Books, 1972.

31. GREULICH, W. W. "Growth of Children of the Same Race Under Different Environmental Conditions", *Science*, 127 (1958), 515–516.

32. GREULICH, W. W., H. THOMS, and R. C. TWADDLE. "A Study of Pelvis Type and Its Relationship to Body Build in White Women," *J.A.M.A.*, 112 (1939), 485–492.

33. HERTZIG, M. E., H. G. BIRCH, J. TIZARD et al. "Growth Sequelae of Severe Infantile Malnutrition," *Pediatrics*, 49 (1972), 814–824.

34. JACOBSON, M. *Developmental Neurobiology*. New York: Holt, Rinehart and Winston, 1970.

35. KNOBLOCH, H., B. PASAMANICK, P. A. HARPER et al. "The Effect of Prematurity on Health and Growth," *Am. J. Public Health*, 49 (1959), 1164–1173.

36. KOHN, M. L. *Class and Conformity: A Study in Values*. Homewood, Ill.: Dorsey, 1969.

37. LESSER, G., G. FIFER, and D. CLARK. "Mental Abilities of Children from Different Social Class and Cultural Groups," *Monogr. Soc. Res. Child Dev.*, 102 (1965), 1–115.

38. LEWIS, M. and H. McGURK. "Evaluation of Infant Intelligence," *Science*, 178 (1972), 1174–1177.

39. LIEBOW, E. *Talley's Corner*. Boston: Little, Brown, 1967.

40. LUDMERER, K. M. *Genetics and American Society*. Baltimore: Johns Hopkins University Press, 1972.

41. McFARLAND, R. A. and R. C. MOORE. "Childhood Accidents and Injuries," in N. B. Talbot, J. Kagan, and L. Eisenberg, eds, *Behavioral Science in Pediatric Medicine*, pp. 350–396. Philadelphia: Saunders, 1971.

42. MYERS, M. L., S. C. O'BRIEN, J. A. MABEL et al. "A Nutrition Study of School Children in a Depressed Urban District. 1. Dietary Findings," *J. Am. Diet. Assoc.*, 53 (1968), 226–233.

43. PASAMANICK, B. and H. KNOBLOCK. "Brain Damage and Reproductive Casualty," *Amer. J. Orthopsychiatry*, 30 (1960), 298–305.

44. PIERCE, C. "Violence and Counterviolence," *Amer. J. Orthopsychiatry*, 39 (1969), 553–568.

45. RUTTER, M., J. TIZARD, and K. WHITMORE. *Education, Health and Behavior*. London: Longman, 1970.

46. RYAN, W. *Blaming the Victim*. New York: Pantheon, 1971.

47. SCRIMSHAW, N. S. and J. E. GORDON, eds. *Malnutrition, Learning, and Behavior*. Cambridge: M.I.T. Press, 1968.

48. STEIN, A. "Strategies of Failure," *Harvard Ed. Rev.*, 41 (1971), 158–204.

49. THOMAS, A. and S. SILLEN. *Racism in Psychiatry*. New York: Brunner-Mazel, 1972.

50. TOBACH, E., L. R. ARONSON, and E. SHAW. *The Biopsychology of Development.* New York: Academic, 1971.

51. WERNER, E. "Cumulative Effect of Perinatal Complications and Deprived Environment on Physical, Intellectual and Social Development of Preschool Children," *Pediatrics,* 39 (1967), 490–505.

52. WIENER, G., R. V. RIDER, W. C. OPPEL et al. "Correlates of Low Birth Weight: Psychological Status at Eight to Ten Years of Age," *Pediatr. Res.,* 2 (1968), 110–118.

53. WILLERMAN, L. "Biosocial Influences on Human Development," *Am. J. Orthopsychiatry,* 42 (1972), 452–462.

54. WINICK, M. and P. ROSSO. "The Effect of Severe Early Malnutrition in Cellular Growth of the Human Brain," *Pediat. Res.,* 3 (1969), 181–184.

55. WORTIS, H. "Child Rearing Practices in a Low Socioeconomic Group," *Pediatrics,* 32 (1963), 298–307.

CHAPTER 14

ATTACHMENT THEORY, SEPARATION ANXIETY, AND MOURNING

John Bowlby

ATTACHMENT THEORY is a way of conceptualizing the propensity of human beings to make strong affectional bonds to particular others and the many forms of emotional distress and disturbance, which include anxiety, anger, and depression, to which unwilling separation and loss give rise. As a body of theory it is concerned with the same range of phenomena as psychoanalytic object-relations theory, and it incorporates much psychoanalytic thinking. It differs from traditional psychoanalysis in adopting a number of principles that derive from the relatively new disciplines of ethology and control theory; by so doing it is enabled to dispense with concepts of psychic energy and drive and also to forge close links with cognitive psychology. In addition, the theory draws freely on data regarding human behavior and development obtained by a broad range of methods and, when appropriate, compares the findings with similar findings from studies of animals, notably nonhuman primates.

Attachment behavior is conceived as any form of behavior that results in a person attaining or retaining proximity to some other differentiated and preferred individual, usually conceived as stronger and/or wiser. As such the behavior includes following, clinging, crying, calling, greeting, smiling, and other more sophisticated forms. It is developing during the second trimester of life and is evident from six months onward when an infant shows by his behavior that he discriminates sharply between his mother-figure,* a few other familiar people, and everyone else. In the company

* Although the text often refers to "mother" and not "mother-figure," reference is always to the person who mothers the child. For most children this is also the child's natural mother.

of his mother he is cheerful, relaxed, and inclined to explore and play. When alone with strangers he is apt to become acutely distressed: he protests his mother's absence and strives to regain contact with her. These responses are at a maximum during the second and third years of life and then diminish slowly. Thenceforward, although attachment behavior is less evident in both the frequency of its occurrence and its intensity, it nonetheless persists as an important part of man's behavioral equipment, not only during later childhood but during adolescence and adult life as well. In adults it is especially evident when a person is distressed, ill, or afraid.

Attachment behavior is conceived as a class of behavior that is distinct from feeding behavior and sexual behavior and of at least an equal significance in human life. Many forms of psychiatric disturbance are attributed either to deviations that have occurred in the development of attachment behavior or, more rarely, to a failure of its development.

(History of the Concept of Attachment

For many years the phenomena to which attachment theory addresses itself have been dealt with in terms either of "dependency need"[74] or of "object relations."[27]

Until the midfifties only one view of the nature and origin of affectional bonds was prevalent, and in this matter there was agreement between psychoanalysts and learning theorists. Bonds between individuals develop, it was held, because an individual discovers that, in order to reduce certain drives, e.g., for food in infancy and for sex in adult life, another human being is necessary. This type of theory postulates two kinds of drive, primary and secondary; it categorizes food and sex as primary and "dependency" as secondary. As a result the variables postulated as relevant to an understanding of variations in the development of affectional bonds have been concerned with methods by which a child is fed and his body cared for. A practical corollary of this type of theorizing is that once a child is

old enough to feed himself and control his sphincters, he is expected to become independent.

Studies of the ill effects on personality development of deprivation of maternal care, which were first published during the thirties and forties (see review by Bowlby[11] and subsequent reviews by Ainsworth[1] and Rutter[73]), led the present writer to question the adequacy of the traditional model and to seek a new one. Early in the fifties Konrad Lorenz's work on imprinting, which had first appeared in 1935, became more generally known and offered an alternative approach. At least in some species of bird, he had found, strong bonds to a mother-figure develop during the early days of life without any reference to food and simply through the young being exposed to and becoming familiar with the figure in question. Arguing that the empirical data on the development of a human child's tie to his mother can be understood better in terms of a model derived from ethology, Bowlby in 1958 sketched the outline of a theory of attachment and introduced the term.[12] Simultaneously and independently, Harlow in the same year published the results of his first studies of infant rhesus monkeys reared on dummy mothers.[39] A young monkey, he found, will cling to a dummy that does not feed it, provided the dummy is soft and is comfortable to cling to.

During the past fifteen years the results of a number of empirical studies of human children have been published,[*] theory has been greatly amplified,[17,3] and the relationship of attachment theory to dependency theory examined.[32] New formulations regarding pathological anxiety and phobia have been advanced by Bowlby[18] and regarding mourning and its psychiatric complications by Bowlby,[14, 15,16] by Parkes,[61,64,65] and by Bowlby and Parkes.[19] Parkes has also extended the theory to cover the range of responses seen whenever a person encounters a major change in his life situation.[63]

In applying attachment theory to the elucidation of psychiatric syndromes, its advocates

* See references 69, 42, 2, 4, 5, and 8.

adopt an approach very different from that usually adopted by psychopathologists. Traditionally, psychoanalysts and others have selected for study patients diagnosed as suffering from the syndrome being investigated and have attempted thence to both reconstruct the phases of development that may have preceded the condition and to infer the causal agents that may have been responsible for it. The approach adopted by attachment theorists is the opposite.

Using as primary data how young children behave in certain defined situations, an attempt is made to describe certain early phases of personality functioning and, from them, to extrapolate forwards. In particular, the aim is to describe certain patterns of response that occur regularly in early childhood and, thence, to trace out how similar patterns of response are to be discerned in the functioning of later personality. The change in perspective is radical. It entails taking as our starting-point, not this or that symptom or syndrome that is giving trouble, but an event or experience deemed to be potentially pathogenic to the developing personality. [p. 4][17]

Although a shift in approach of this kind is still unusual in psychiatry, it occurred long ago in physiological medicine, e.g., the study of the healthy and pathological consequences of a specified infective agent.

❨ Main Features of Attachment Theory

The main features of attachment theory, in contrast to dependency theory, are as follows:

1. *Specificity* Attachment behavior is directed toward one or a few specific individuals, usually in clear order of preference. For the great majority of children the mother is the most preferred with the father, or perhaps the grandmother, next in order.

2. *Duration* An attachment endures, usually for a large part of the life cycle. Although during adolescence early attachments may attenuate and become supplemented by new ones—and in some cases are replaced by them —early attachments are not easily abandoned and they commonly persist.

3. *Engagement of emotion* Many of the most intense emotions arise during the formation, the maintenance, the disruption, and the renewal of attachment relationships; hence the term, affectional bonds. In the language of subjective experience, the formation of a bond is described as falling in love, maintaining a bond as loving someone, and losing a partner as grieving over someone. Similarly, threat of loss arouses anxiety and actual loss gives rise to sorrow; whilst each of these situations is likely to arouse anger. The unchallenged maintenance of a bond is experienced as a source of security and the renewal of a bond as a source of joy. Because intense emotion is commonly a reflection of the state of a person's affectional bonds, the psychology and psychopathology of emotion is found to be in large part the psychology and psychopathology of affectional bonds.

4. *Ontogeny* In the great majority of human infants attachment behavior to a preferred figure develops during the first nine months of life. Initially, social responses are elicited by a wide array of stimuli; during the second trimester their elicitation becomes confined to stimuli arising from one or a few familiar individuals. The more experience of social interaction an infant has with a person the more likely he is to become attached to that person, and thenceforward he prefers that figure to all others. Because from six months onward, and especially after nine months, an infant is likely to respond to a stranger with fear, the development of attachment to a new figure becomes increasingly difficult, especially after the end of the first year. If no opportunity has been given for an attachment to develop before a child's second birthday, it may never do so. Preference for the familiar and fear of the strange, two basic responses hitherto given scant attention in human psychology, play a major part in the development of attachment. The threshold for activation of attachment behavior remains low until near the end of the third year; in healthy development it rises gradually thereafter.

5. *Learning* Whereas learning to distinguish the familiar from the strange is a key process in the development of attachment, the con-

ventional rewards and punishments used by experimental psychologists play only a small part. Indeed, an attachment can develop despite repeated punishment from the attachment figure.

6. *Organization* Initially attachment behavior is mediated by responses organized on fairly simple lines. From the end of the first year, it becomes mediated by increasingly sophisticated behavioral systems, organized cybernetically and incorporating representational models of the environment and self. These systems are activated by certain conditions and terminated by others. Among activating conditions are strangeness, hunger, fatigue, and anything that frightens a child. Terminating conditions include sight or sound of mother: when attachment behavior is strongly aroused, termination may require touching or clinging to her and/or being cuddled by her. Conversely, when the mother is present or her whereabouts well-known, a child ceases to show attachment behavior and, instead, explores his environment.

7. *Parental Behavior* Complementary to attachment behavior is the caretaking behavior of parents. Not only do most parents respond to a child's approaches, but when a child strays, one of his parents usually takes action to restore mutual proximity. By so doing a parent induces a sense of security and is providing the child with a "secure" base from which he can explore. When, by contrast, a parent does not play his or her part, a child becomes distressed and sometimes angry.

8. *Biological function* Attachment behavior occurs in the young of almost all species of bird and mammal, and in a number of species it persists into and throughout adult life. Although there are many differences of detail between species, maintenance of proximity by an immature animal to a preferred adult, almost always the mother, is the rule. Since it is most unlikely that such behavior has no survival value, the question arises what that may be. Bowlby argues that by far the most likely function of attachment behavior is protection, mainly from predators.[17] He bases this view on three classes of evidence: (1) observations of many species of bird and mammal show that an isolated individual is much more likely to be seized by a predator than is one that stays bunched together with others of its kind; and what knowledge there is of hunting and gathering tribes suggests that the same is true of humans, their principal predators being leopards, wolves, and hyenas; (2) attachment behavior is elicited particularly easily and intensely in animals that, by reason of age, size, or condition, are especially vulnerable to predators; for example, the young, pregnant females, the sick; (3) attachment behavior is always elicited at high intensity in situations of alarm that are commonly stimulus situations of the kind which would occur on the approach of a possible predator. No other existing theory fits these facts.

(Reasons for Discarding Concepts of Dependence, Dependency Need, and Object Cathexis

Learning theorists are now agreed that the concept of dependence is distinct from that of attachment.[32] Dependence is not specifically related to maintenance of proximity; it is not directed toward a specific individual; it does not imply an enduring bond, nor is it necessarily associated with strong feeling. No biological function is attributed to it.

In addition to these reasons, there are value implications in the concept of dependence that are the exact opposite of those which the concept of attachment not only conveys but is intended to convey. Whereas to refer to someone as dependent tends always to be disparaging, to describe him as attached to someone can well be an expression of approval. Conversely, for a person to be detached in his personal relations is usually regarded as less than admirable. The disparaging element in the concept of dependence is held to be a fatal weakness to its clinical use.

The defects of the term "dependence" as applied to what is here termed attachment are confounded when it is combined with "need," to make "dependency need." The term "need" is ambiguous. Sometimes it refers to a psychological state, often best described as a desire; at other times it refers to what is required for individual or species survival. Since what is desired and what is required do not always match, indeed are sometimes entirely incompatible, the word can easily create confusion.

The term "object-cathexis" derives from Freud's energy theory and is inappropriate to a control-systems theory.

(Separation Anxiety

Although it has long been evident that unwilling separation or threat of separation from an attachment figure is a very common cause of anxiety, there has been the greatest reluctance to accept the evidence at its face value. The reasoning has been as follows. Realistic anxiety, it is supposed, is elicited only in conditions that are truly dangerous. Since mere separation from an attachment figure cannot be regarded as truly dangerous, anxiety over separation cannot be regarded as realistic. Hence its occurrence has to be explained in some other way. A common explanation is that anxiety over separation is a manifestation, in disguise, of anxiety that is elicited by some other situation, usually conceived as intrapsychic; and as such it is deemed neurotic.

This argument, stems from Freud's earliest work and led him to advance a succession of theories[30,78] and runs through all later psychoanalytic theorizing. It is held to be based on a false assumption; namely that, to be healthy, fear should be elicited only in conditions that are truly dangerous. Empirical observation shows a different state of affairs. It is therefore necessary to consider the matter afresh.

When approached empirically separation from an attachment figure is found to be one of a class of situations, each of which is likely to elicit fear but none of which can be regarded as intrinsically dangerous. These situations comprise, among others, darkness, sudden large changes of stimulus level including loud noises, sudden movement, strange people, and strange things. Evidence shows that animals of many species are alarmed by such situations,[47] and that this is true of human children and also of adults.[48] Furthermore, fear is especially likely to be elicited when two or more of these conditions are present simultaneously, for example, hearing a loud noise when alone in the dark.

The explanation of why individuals should so regularly respond to these situations with fear is held to be that, whilst none of the situations is intrinsically dangerous, each carries with it an *increased risk* of danger. Noise, strangeness, isolation, and for many species darkness, all these are conditions statistically associated with an increased risk of danger. Noise may presage a natural disaster—fire, flood, a landslide. To a young animal a predator is strange, it moves, and it often strikes at night; and it is far more likely to do so when the potential victim is alone.

Because to behave so promotes both survival and breeding success, the theory runs, the young of species that have survived, including man, are found to be genetically biased so to develop that they respond to the properties of noise, strangeness, sudden approach, and darkness by taking avoiding action or running away—they behave in fact as though danger were actually present. In a comparable way they respond to isolation by seeking company. Fear responses elicited by such naturally occurring clues to danger are a part of man's basic behavioral equipment. [p. 85][18]

Seen in this light anxiety over unwilling separation from an attachment figure resembles the anxiety that the general of an expeditionary force feels when communications with his base are cut or threatened.

Thus, anxiety over an unwilling separation is regarded as a normal and healthy reaction. At what intensity the reaction is to be expected turns on a very large number of variables, both organismic (e.g., age, sex, health of the individual) and environmental (e.g., presence of other fear-arousing situations, behavior of attachment figure). A great deal of normative work is required to fill out this picture before we can be confident of the limits of healthy variation. Meanwhile, a clinician is constantly confronted with patients who are exhibiting chronic anxiety over separation from an attachment figure at an intensity that appears inappropriate for the individual's age and situation. Though clinicians might agree in judging such anxiety as neurotic, they are likely to disagree about how it is to be explained.

❨ Behavior Indicative of Fear

There are three quite distinct forms of behavior commonly classified as indicative of fear. They are: (a) withdrawal from a situation; (b) freezing immobile; and (c) turning or retreating toward an attachment figure. The first is so well-known as to require no comment. The second is well-known in other species and may perhaps play a larger part in humans than is generally conceded. The third is also well-known but in almost all theorizing about fear in humans tends to be overlooked.

Which of these forms of fear behavior is elicited in an animal turns on its species, age, and sex and also on the situation. In the presence of a predator animals of certain species, e.g., plover and deer, habitually clump together; others, e.g., arboreal monkeys, tend to scatter; others again, e.g., opossum, freeze. In very many species of mammal, the young seek their mother and remain in close proximity to her. In all the species of nonhuman primate, the young cling tightly to the mother; though in their earliest weeks of life the young of a few primate species, e.g., gorilla, need assistance from the mother in doing so.

In the case of the human baby, because it is born so immature, proximity keeping when afraid is not possible until after the age of six months. As soon as motor equipment has matured, however, it becomes the usual response and remains so for many years. In adult humans proximity keeping is also common, and it is present at high intensity whenever a situation is especially alarming, as in disasters.[46]

In animals of species that habitually seek the company of others in a fear-arousing situation, the intensity with which fear is aroused is influenced in great degree by the presence or absence of a trusted companion. This has been shown experimentally for rhesus monkeys by Rowell and Hinde,[72] for human infants after the age of nine months by Morgan and Ricciuti,[57] and for children between their second and sixth birthdays by Jersild.[48] In every case the presence of a familiar companion who can be turned to greatly reduces fear responses. Common experience leaves little doubt that the same is true of older children, adolescents, and adults. Nevertheless, in a society that lays great emphasis on the development of independence, this common human tendency tends to be either overlooked or disparaged.

❨ Personality Development and Family Experience

On the basis of these findings regarding the role of trusted companions, particularly parents, in reducing the intensity of fear responses, it can be postulated that a human child who is confident that a parent will be accessible and helpful when called upon will be less prone to respond with fear to a potentially alarming situation than will one who for any reason does not have that confidence. This, together with observations made during the practice of family psychiatry, has led the present writer to advance three complementary propositions.[18] The first is that, when an individual is confident that an attachment figure will be available when called upon, that person will be much less prone to either intense or chronic fear than will an individual who has no such confidence. The second postulates that confidence in the availability of attachment figures, or a lack of it, is built up slowly during the years of immaturity—infancy, childhood, and adolescence—and that whatever expectations are developed during those years tend to persist relatively unchanged throughout the rest of life. The third postulates that the varied expectations that different individuals develop during the years of immaturity are tolerably accurate reflections of the experiences those individuals have actually had.

The first proposition is in keeping with psychoanalytic object relations theory in which a person's confidence, or lack of it, in the availability of an attachment figure is expressed in terms of his having either introjected, or failed to introject, a good object,[50,27,84] The third proposition attaches far more importance to the role of actual experience than has been common in traditional psychoanalytic theorizing; and the second proposition extends the sensitive period during which personality is conceived as undergoing major change and development from the first three or four years of life to include the next ten years or more.

The theoretical position adopted is held to be supported by evidence of several different kinds. One class of evidence derives from the many studies published during the past decade or so which seek to relate variations in the personality development of children and adolescents, found in fairly representative samples drawn from schools and colleges, to the experiences the children have had in their families.[66,37,70,59] The findings are consistent in showing that children and adolescents who are developing a healthy self-reliance, coupled with a capacity to cooperate with others and to seek advice and support when in difficulty, are those who are growing up in stable homes in which they are given much encouragement and support by their parents and are subjected to predictable and moderate discipline. The findings are consistent, too, in showing that, conversely, those who grow up lacking in self-confidence and self-esteem and who are prone to depression, anxiety, and psychosomatic symptoms, or are given to aggressive destructive behavior, are likely to come from homes that are unstable or broken, or else from those in which there is either oversevere and arbitrary discipline or neglect and indifference. Studies of samples of preschool children[6] and of one-year-olds[4] yield findings that point to the same conclusions.

(Anxious Attachment (Overdependency)

Perhaps no terms are used more frequently in clinical discussion than "dependent" and "overdependent." A child who tends to be clinging, an adolescent chary of leaving home, a wife or husband in constant contact with mother, an invalid who demands attention, all these are likely to be dubbed dependent or overdependent and always in the use of these words there is an aura of disapproval. To avoid that aura, and to draw attention to what is believed to be the true nature of the condition, the term anxious attachment is introduced.[18]

In examining the condition, we are faced with two main problems:

(a) what are the criteria that lead us to judge the behavior to lie outside healthy limits?

(b) for those cases that it is agreed lie outside normal limits, how do we account for the development of the condition?

To answer the first question requires extensive normative study of the development of attachment behavior through every phase of the life cycle, taking into account not only age and sex but the particular conditions of life to which an individual is exposed. Ignorance of normal development among medical, educational, and psychological personnel leads at present to frequent misjudgment. Individuals in danger of being criticized wrongly as "overdependent" are children who look older than they are, who are ill or fatigued, or who have to share mother with a new baby, and also adults who are occupied with young children, are ill or are recently bereaved. In all such cases attachment behavior is likely to be shown more frequently and/or more urgently than would otherwise be the case.

Answers to the second question, how do we account for the development of anxious attachment of pathological degree, are of four main kinds:

(1) theories that invoke genetic factors

(2) theories that inculpate traumata occurring during pregnancy, birth, or the early weeks of life which are held to increase the (organic) anxiety response

(3) theories that postulate that such individuals have been "spoiled" during childhood by having been given excessive gratification

(4) theories that postulate that such people have been made especially sensitive to the possibility of separation or loss of love through experiencing either actual separations or threats of abandonment during childhood.

In evaluating these theories we may note that (1) the possible role of genetic factors cannot at present be tested; (2) there is evidence[80] that mishaps during pregnancy or birth can make some children especially sensitive to environmental change during their first five years of life; (3) that the theory of spoiling, although repeatedly favored by Freud[29,30] and still frequently invoked, has received no empirical support; (4) that, by contrast, there is extensive support for the view that anxious attachment is a common consequence of a child having experienced actual separation, threats of abandonment, or combinations of the two.

Evidence in support of the theory that anxious attachment is a result of a child experiencing either actual separation or threats of separation is of two main sorts: (a) retrospective studies of samples of older individuals who are judged to be overdependent; (b) current studies of children who have recently experienced either a separation or a serious threat of abandonment.

Retrospective studies of individuals who are deemed to be overdependent show that cases fall into two unequally sized groups.[76,74,56] The majority group comprises individuals who are constantly apprehensive about the whereabouts of attachment figures. They come from unsettled homes in which they have been (and perhaps still are) subjected to one or more of the following—irritable scolding, dis-

paraging comparisons with others, quarreling parents, threats of abandonment or loss of love, changes from one mother figure to another, periods of separation with strange people in strange places. The minority group comprises individuals who do not show anxious attachment but who, in comparison to others of the same age, are less able to do things for themselves. They are found to come from stable homes but to have a mother* who tends to discourage her child from learning to do things for himself. Such a mother is commonly found to be suffering from anxious attachment herself and to be demanding, either overtly or covertly, that the child act as a caretaker to her; thereby she is inverting the normal parent–child roles. The immediate source of the trouble is found usually to lie in mother's relationship with her own mother. In such cases the child himself is not showing anxious attachment and he often welcomes release from the demands by his mother that he should mother her.

Findings from current studies strongly support those from retrospective ones.

Evidence that a young child shows intense anxiety after returning home from a period in a strange place with strange people, usually a residential nursery or hospital ward, is now well documented.[42] After an initial period of detachment, during which he fails to exhibit attachment behavior toward his mother, he commonly becomes extremely clinging and insists on accompanying his mother everywhere. Even months after his return home, by which time he may appear to have regained confidence, he may be thrown into acute anxiety by a reminder of the separation, e.g., the visit to his home of someone he knew in the separation environment or being left briefly in a place that resembles that environment. Thereupon he again becomes intensely clinging and cannot bear to let mother out of his sight.

Threats to abandon a child, either used deliberately as a disciplinary measure or ex-

---

* In some cases pathogenic patterns of relationship involve a father or grandfather but these appear to be much less common than those involving a mother and grandmother.

claimed impulsively in a fit of anger, can have a similar effect. Newson and Newson[58] give a number of examples of four-year-old children whose parents have used threats to abandon them as a means of enforcing their wishes. In some cases the threat was made convincing by the parents packing the child's clothes and walking him round the block as though they were really going to take him to a "bad boys home." In other cases anxiety can be aroused by a parent threatening not to love a child unless he is good, especially when the threat is given substance by the parent refusing to talk or have anything to do with the child for a day or more. Evidence presented by the Newsons for a sample drawn from the English midlands and by Sears, Maccoby, and Levin[74] for a sample from New England suggests that a substantial minority of young children are subjected to these threats.

Other experiences that can lead a child or adolescent to become intensely, and perhaps chronically, anxious about the availability and support he can expect from his attachment figures are when parents quarrel, threaten suicide, or attempt it. When parents quarrel, there is plainly some risk of one of them deserting the family; and not infrequently explicit threats of that kind are made. Threats by a parent to commit suicide are even more frightening. Finally, when a parent actually makes a suicide attempt, a child inevitably becomes intensely anxious. Figures from Edinburgh suggest that about 5 percent of the children growing up in the city today are exposed to attempts at suicide by one of their parents (usually the mother) by the time they reach the age of twenty.*

It is strange to find how little attention has been given to such family experiences by theorists seeking to explain the origin of intense and pathological anxiety. The reasons appear to be, first, that patients and their families often omit to give such information, or even suppress or falsify it, and, secondly, that the theoretical position of many clinicians leads

* This estimate is made by the present writer on the basis of figures made available by Norman Kreitman, Director of the M.R.C. Unit for Epidemiological Studies in Psychiatry.

them to overlook or discount such information if it is offered. As described later, situations known to cause anxious attachment are found very frequently in the families of patients diagnosed as "phobic."

⟨ Anger and Attachment: Detachment

Anxious attachment is only one of several possible responses to unwilling separation and threats of separation. Another common response is anger. It has been observed in young children during a period in a strange place with strange people[21,68,41] and also after a child's return home.[68,42] Although observation shows that such anger can be directed toward many targets, evidence suggests that it is elicited by and aimed mainly against the mother. As a result, it is typical for a child to show more or less intensely ambivalent behavior toward his mother after returning from a stay away from her. Records of how bereaved adults respond to loss of a loved relative show that outbursts of anger are very common in them also.

In the past, anger as a common and typical response to unwilling separation from the mother has been given little recognition. Because of that the origin of such anger has proved puzzling. Attempts to explain it have led to much speculative theorizing, for example, that the anger is genetically determined or is a manifestation of oral sadism or of the action of a death instinct. Once it is seen as a reaction to separation or loss, and as potentially healthy, it can be understood. Bowlby,[13,18] argues that its functions are, first, to overcome obstacles to reunion with the mother and, secondly, when directed against the mother after reunion, to discourage her from permitting another separation to occur. In other words, anger during and after an unwilling separation is a healthy component of attachment behavior.

Nevertheless, not all anger elicited in such circumstances is functional. On the contrary, when intense and prolonged it can readily lead to unfavorable consequences for the child.

Those responsible for his care during the separation become irritable that their attentions are not appreciated, while after reunion his mother, who may not understand what has elicited her child's hostility, may become intolerant and punitive. In this way vicious circles develop. The more separations that occur the more the balance of ambivalence in the child's relation to his mother shifts from predominantly positive to predominantly negative.[38] Unless the circular process is checked, the child or adolescent comes to develop a persistently hostile attitude not only to his parents but to other parental figures.

Although less well documented, it is very probable that similar and perhaps worse vicious circles can be set up when a parent repeatedly utters threats to abandon a child. Whereas some children conform anxiously to such threats, others, mainly boys, retaliate. After studying some hundred adolescent boys in a residential school for delinquents, Stott[77] reached the conclusion that in a fairly large proportion of cases parents' threats to abandon their children had played a major role in the development of a delinquent pattern of behavior.

Whenever a child who has been threatened with abandonment has to be away from his parents for any reason, e.g., hospitalization, he inevitably interprets the experience as a punishment. It is probable that combinations of threats with actual separations have especially damaging and long-lasting effects on personality development.

One of the most adverse disturbances of attachment behavior yet known is when a child has no opportunity to develop a stable attachment during the first two or three years of his life. This can occur when a child is reared in an impersonal institution, when he is moved repeatedly from one mother-figure to another, and when he is subjected to some combination of these regimes.[51,9,33,34] Cases are also on record that have developed when a child who is in course of making a normal attachment to his mother has been removed to a long stay hospital at the age of eighteen months.[10]

Such children grow up in a condition of pathological detachment and are more or less totally incapable of making stable affectional bonds with anyone. Although some are asocial, others are superficially sociable and may become plausible frauds. Such individuals are not amenable to discipline or any of the other controls to which healthy persons are sensitive, and in due course are likely to be diagnosed as psychopathic or sociopathic.[26,35]

(Phobias

Persons to whom the label "phobic" is attached fall into two main groups:[54] (a) those who respond with unusually intense fear to a specified situation, e.g., to animals of a certain species, but who in all other ways are stable and healthy personalities; (b) those who exhibit unusually intense fear in a number of situations, often difficult to specify, and who are prone also to develop bouts of fairly acute anxiety and depression that may last weeks or months. Persons in the former group are unlikely to be referred to a psychiatrist. Those in the latter, which includes cases diagnosed as school phobia and agoraphobia, belong within the broad group of psychoneuroses.

Many studies have been reported of the syndrome traditionally termed *school phobia* and nowadays more often referred to as school refusal. Such children not only refuse to attend school but express much anxiety when pressed to do so. Their nonattendance is well known to their parents, and a majority of the children remain at home during school hours. Not infrequently the condition is accompanied by, or masked by, psychosomatic symptoms of one kind or another—for example, anorexia, nausea, abdominal pain, feeling faint. Fears of many kinds are expressed—of animals, of the dark, of being bullied, of mother coming to harm, of being deserted. Occasionally a child seems to panic. Tearfulness and general misery are common. As a rule, the children are well behaved, anxious, and inhibited. Most come from intact families, have not experienced long or frequent separations from home, and have parents who express great concern about their child and his refusal to attend school. Relations between child and parents are close, sometimes to the point of suffocation. In all these respects the condition differs from truancy.[43]

With only a few exceptions workers are now agreed that the condition is to be understood, not as fear of going to school, but as anxiety about leaving home.[49,44,23,82] Reviewing the literature and his own experience Bowlby concludes that a large majority of cases of school refusal can be understood as the products of four main patterns of family interaction:[18]

Pattern A—mother, or more rarely father, is a sufferer from chronic anxiety regarding attachment figures and retains the child at home to be a companion

Pattern B—the child fears that something dreadful may happen to mother, or possibly father, while he is at school and so remains at home to prevent its happening

Pattern C—the child fears that something dreadful may happen to himself if he is away from home and so remains at home to prevent that happening

Pattern D—mother, or more rarely father, fears that something dreadful will happen to the child while he is at school and so keeps him at home.

Pattern A is the commonest and can be combined with any of the other three.

Pattern A

A mother (or father) who retains her child at home may do so deliberately and consciously or may be unaware of what she is doing and why. In all such cases the parent is found to have grown up intensely anxious about the availability of attachment figures and to be inverting the normal parent–child relationship. In effect she requires her child to act as parent whilst she herself adopts the role of child. Investigation shows that during their childhoods such mothers have been subjected to one or other of the experiences now known to lead to anxious attachment.

When, as is common, a mother is unaware that she is inverting the relationship, it may

appear to a clinician inexperienced in family psychiatry that the child is being "spoiled." Closer examination shows, however, that the reverse is the case. In seeking belated satisfaction for the loving care the mother either never had as a child or perhaps lost, she is placing a heavy burden on her child and preventing his engaging in school and play with peers.* Not only so, but it is sometimes found that a mother's relationship to her child is in fact intensely ambivalent and that she swings from genuine concern for his welfare to hostility and threats. A mother's hostile behavior toward her school-refusing child can be understood—in terms of her own psychopathology and childhood experience—as a product of one or more of at least three closely related processes:

(a) redirecting (displacing) anger, engendered initially by own mother, against the child

(b) misattributing to child the rejecting characteristics and/or the demanding characteristics of own mother, and being angry with the child accordingly

(c) modeling angry behavior toward child on the angry behavior exhibited by own mother.

Pattern B

Both Talbot[79] and Hersov[44] report that, in their series of twenty-four and fifty cases respectively, fear of some harm befalling the mother was the commonest single explanation given by the children of why they did not attend school. This finding is corroborated by many other workers. There is, however, no agreement as to how such fear arises. Among psychoanalysts it is usual to attribute it to the child's harboring unconscious hostile wishes

* Sometimes the term "symbiosis" is used to describe these suffocatingly close relationships between mother and child. The term is not happily chosen, however, since in biology it is used to denote an adaptive partnership between two organisms in which each contributes to the other's survival; whereas the relationship with which we are concerned here is certainly not to the child's advantage and often is not to the parent's either.

toward his parent and being afraid lest his wishes come true. An alternative explanation is that the fear arises from the child's actual experiences within his family. These can be of two kinds: (a) events such as mother's illness or the deaths of relatives or neighbors (see especially studies by Hersov[44] and Davidson[24]); (b) threats by the mother to desert or commit suicide (see especially studies by Talbot[79] and Weiss & Cain[83]). Of the main alternative explanations the one that invokes the child's real experiences is held by the present writer to account for an overwhelming proportion of cases. Nevertheless, in some of them a child's fears are exacerbated by the hostility he feels toward his parent. Even so, not infrequently this hostility is itself a product of the way his parent has treated him.

An examination of Freud's case of Little Hans,[28] which has been the paradigm for the psychoanalytic theory of phobia, shows that Hans's earliest symptoms were fear that his mother might vanish and fear of going out of the house with his nursemaid. Only later did he express fear that, if he went out, a horse might bite him. The case history shows that mother used various threats to discipline her small boy and that these included threats that, if he were naughty, she would go away and never return (pp. 44–45). The pattern of family interaction can therefore be regarded as comforming to Pattern B.

Patterns C and D

Patterns C and D are less common than Patterns A and B. When the patterns of interaction prevailing in the family become known, the child's unwillingness to leave home becomes easy to understand.

There is much evidence that the real events that have been going on within a patient's family, and that are frequently still going on, are often not reported either by the patient or by members of the family and that they are sometimes deliberately suppressed or falsified. Unless a clinician has a clear grasp of what patterns are likely to lie behind the symptoms, and is patient and skilled in his investigations, he can easily be misled.

When the syndrome of *agoraphobia* is examined in the light of attachment theory and family interaction it is apparent that it has much in common with school phobia. In both types of case the patient is alleged to be afraid of going into a place filled with other people; in both the patient is apt to be afraid of various other situations as well; in both the patient is prone to anxiety attacks, depression, and psychosomatic symptoms; in both the condition is precipitated often by an illness or death; in both the patient is found to be overdependent, to be the child of parents one or both of whom suffer from long-standing neurosis, and frequently also to be under the domination of an overprotective mother. Finally, a significant number of agoraphobic patients were school refusers as children.

Often an agoraphobic patient is intensely anxious, apt to panic when unable to get home quickly, and to be afraid of an extraordinarily broad range of situations. Among all the situations that may be feared, two can be identified that are feared in virtually every case and are also the most feared. These situations are, first, leaving familiar surroundings and, second, being alone, especially when out of the house.[71,54] Snaith agrees and reports that the more anxious an agoraphobic patient becomes the more intense grows his fear of leaving home and also that when a patient becomes more anxious, his fear of leaving home is magnified in intensity by a factor many times greater than is his fear of anything else.[75]

Although scrutiny of the literature (see Bowlby[18]) reveals strong presumptive evidence that behind the symptoms of patients diagnosed as agoraphobic lie patterns of family interaction similar to those found in cases labeled school phobic, so far no research study appears to have made the necessary inquiries. It is of interest, however, that Webster,[81] who draws on material obtained during the psychotherapy of a series of twenty-five female patients, concludes that in all but one case the patients' feelings of insecurity could be understood as being due in all likelihood to the way they had been and were being treated by their mothers. Of twenty-five mothers, twenty-four were believed to be dominant and overprotec-

tive. They were described as being "most solic-
itous of the daughter's welfare, rewarding her
often without good reason and rejecting or
threatening to reject her or actually telling her
she would not love her any more if she did not
behave."

Studies in which firsthand observations are
made of patients interacting with their families are urgently required. The days of relying
on hearsay evidence are past.

❲ Mourning: Healthy and Pathological

A large number of investigators have reported
a raised incidence of loss of a parent by
death or desertion during the childhoods of
patients suffering from anxiety and depression
or who have attempted suicide (see review by
Hill[45]). In addition, there is evidence that
similar symptoms can be reactions to bereave-
ments that have occurred in the more recent
past.[52,60,61,20] These studies point to the need
for an accurate understanding of the responses
to bereavement typical at different ages, of the
forms characteristic of pathological responses,
and of the factors that may result in mourning
taking a pathological course.

Studies of responses to bereavement in
fairly typical samples of adults are reported by
Lindemann,[52] Marris,[55] and Parkes.[64] Studies of responses to temporary loss of mother
are reported by Robertson,[68] and Heinicke
and Westheimer.[42] Generalizations in terms
derived from attachment theory have been attempted by Bowlby[14,15,16] and by Parkes[62,65]
who have worked together on the problem.

Four main phases of response can be recognized:

1. phase of numbness that, in adults, usually
   lasts from a few hours to a week and may
   be interrupted by outbursts of extremely
   intense distress and/or anger;
2. phase of yearning and searching for the
   lost figure, often lasting for months and
   sometimes for years;
3. phase of disorganization and despair;
4. phase of greater or less degree of reorganization.

While in the long term a bereaved person
tends to move progressively through these
phases, during the short term there is much
oscillation back and forth from one phase to
another.

Studies of widows show that following the
first phase, during which she may feel stunned,
there follows a phase during which, on the
one hand, she begins to register the reality of
her loss while, on the other, she shows evidence of disbelief that it has really occurred.
This leads to inconsistent perceptions and reactions that are as baffling to the widow herself as to those trying to help her. Whenever
she is recognizing the reality of the loss, she is
likely to be seized by pangs of intense distress
and tearfulness. Yet, only moments later, she
may be preoccupied with thoughts of her husband, often combined with a sense of his actual presence. In the latter mood she is liable
to interpret sights and sounds as indicative of
his imminent return. Footsteps at 5:00 P.M.
are perceived as her husband coming home
from work; a man in the street is taken for
him. Of 227 widows and 66 widowers, Rees
reports 39 percent as having these experiences;[67] while 14 percent of the sample experienced hallucinations or illusions of the
spouse's presence.

Attitudes to material reminders of the dead
person can vacillate between aversion to anything that may precipitate renewed pangs of
grief and treasuring all such reminders. Cultures differ in their evaluation of these contradictory responses. Whereas Western cultures
tend to regard dwelling on the past with dis-
favor, Yamomoto and his colleagues describe
how in Japan a widow is encouraged to maintain a constant sense of her dead husband's
presence.[86]

There is much other evidence to support the
view that during the second phase of mourning not only yearning but searching for the
lost figure is the rule. The anger commonly
expressed by bereaved people is regarded as a
component of the struggle to recover the lost
person. It usually takes the form of blaming
someone for having contributed to the loss as
though, by identifying the agent responsible,
the loss can be reversed. Such anger is di-

rected at any or all of three targets—the self, the dead person, and third parties. Often it is recognized by the bereaved as unfair and misplaced. In other cases it becomes an obsession. Because to blame the dead person may be unthinkable, blame may become directed persistently against the self and so give rise to pathological self-reproach.

It is believed that attachment theory enables these responses to be understood. Because in the case of spouses, and also of children and parents, attachment behavior has been long directed toward the other, and has continued so during temporary separations, the behavior persists in being thus directed even when the separation is one that cannot be reversed. As a result a bereaved person lives in two incompatible worlds—a world in which the lost figure is believed recoverable and a world in which the figure is believed to be gone forever. Given time and the company of some other person who understands the dilemma, the bereaved is likely to move slowly, if unsteadily, toward the new and dreaded view. In other circumstances a part of mental life may continue to be organized on the assumption that the dead person is still recoverable. In some cases the bereaved is aware that he entertains that expectation; in others he is wholly unaware of it. The former condition is one that appears to be common in children who have lost a parent, especially when they have had no opportunity to verify or talk about the loss,[85] and was termed by Freud[31] a split in the ego. When a bereaved person is unaware that some part of himself is still searching for the lost figure, the process responsible is usually termed repression. In either case the individual is prone to inexplicable moods of anxiety and depression and is liable to have great difficulties in his personal relationships.[25,16]

A great many variables appear to influence the course of mourning, and much further work is required before their influence is accurately known. The more numerous the roles —emotional, social, and economic—that the lost person filled in the life of the bereaved, the heavier the blow. The same is true of a loss that occurs suddenly and unexpectedly.

Both these conditions hold when a parent is lost by a child and when a husband is lost by a woman with a young family. They may also hold after the death of one of a couple who have been living isolated from others.

The more secure the attachment has been to the lost figure the more likely is the bereaved in due course to recover from the loss and also to retain a comforting sense of the lost one's presence. Conversely, the more anxious and ambivalent the attachment the more likely is mourning to become disturbed and/or pathological and for memories to be guilt-ridden. It is likely that many of the most disturbed responses to loss occur in those who during their childhoods have been subjected to periods away from their mother with strange people, to threats of being abandoned, and to combinations of these experiences.

Mourning is more likely to lead to psychiatric disturbance in those who, after the loss, have no one to care for and sympathize with them than in those who are cared for and listened to. This has long been suspected in the case of children and is supported by the recent findings of Caplan and Douglas[22] and of Birtchnell.[7] In a study of widows Maddison and Walker found that those who showed a relatively good outcome at the end of twelve months reported how they had received support from people who had made it easy for them to cry and to talk freely about their husband and his death, whereas those who showed a relatively poor outcome described how they had met with people who were intolerant of the expression of grief and anger and who insisted, instead, that the widow pull herself together.[53] Much other evidence, including that from psychotherapy, shows that when affectional bonds are strong they can be relinquished only gradually and after the expression of much yearning, anger, and sadness.

⟨ Extension of Theory

The theory outlined has still to be extended to other areas of personality organization and psychopathology. A major deficiency is an account of defensive processes. These, it is believed, can be approached in terms of mutiple, and often incompatible, representational models of both self and environment. Since representational models act as part determinants of feeling state and behavior, the postulated presence of incompatible models can help explain conflict of feeling and also behavior that has inconsistent or maladaptive consequences. Some of the more influential but less conscious of these models are believed to have been built up on the basis of past experience but, because of changes in environment and/or self, to be no longer relevant to the current situation. The model of a dead person as still alive, which often governs a large part of the feeling and behavior of someone bereaved, is a particularly clear example.

How successful attachment theory will be in providing a revised paradigm for understanding personality development and psychopathology can be discovered only by attempting to apply it to data already available and by testing predictions derived from it in new research.

❲ Application of Theory

The theory can provide a systematic basis for preventive and therapeutic measures, including many of those at present practiced which derive from one or other of the existing traditions of psychoanalytic theorizing.

In the preventive field the theory lays stress on measures that provide people of all ages with a familiar and trustworthy base from which they can operate. In the case of children and adolescents that means encouraging parents to provide them with unfailing support, especially when a child of any age is anxious or distressed. In the case of parents it means encouraging members of the community, and especially professional personnel, to recognize the indispensable and onerous role of parents, to respect that role, and to provide parents with the support necessary for them, in turn, to support their children. Other preventive measures stem from recognition that,

whenever a person is subjected to a major change in his life situation, stress is inevitable and support is required to assist him to negotiate the change (see chapters in Volume 2 of this *Handbook*).

In the clinical field, the application of attachment theory requires diagnosis to take full account of the family situation both as it is and, so far as possible, as it has been in the past. Special attention is given to psychosocial transitions to which members are being or have been subjected and to the results of any failure to negotiate them. The extent to which the symptoms of the designated patient (of whatever age) may be reflections of disturbances that occurred in the development of the attachment behavior of one or both of his parents, and that may from his birth onward have influenced the way they treat him, is considered.

When symptomatology appears intelligible in terms of the factors mentioned, treatment is directed whenever possible to all members of the family who appear to be playing a role. When treating an individual, it is borne in mind that sometimes his thoughts, mood, and behavior are more appropriate to the situation in which he finds himself than the clinician at first supposes; and, further, that when, on careful examination, thoughts, mood, and behavior are found inappropriate to the current situation, they may be found far from inappropriate to the situations to which the patient has been exposed during his childhood. Since the account that a patient is able to give during the early phases of treatment is often seriously incomplete and distorted, it is usually a skilled task to help him explore the family situations that he has found himself in, especially when they have proved painful or have, perhaps, shown his parents in a light either much less favorable or more favorable than he had supposed. The role of the psychiatrist is seen as providing the patient with a temporary attachment figure. The way the patient perceives him casts light on the representational models of attachment figures that govern the patient's perceptions and behavior. By calling the patient's attention to these models (by transference interpretations) the psychotherapist is attempting to help the patient understand those models more clearly and reconsider the extent to which they are appropriate to the person of the therapist.

(Bibliography

1. AINSWORTH, M. D. S. "The Effects of Maternal Deprivation: A Review of Findings and Controversy in the Context of Research Strategy," in *Deprivation of Maternal Care: A Reassessment of Its Ill Effects*, pp. 97–165. Public Health Papers: No. 14. Geneva: WHO, 1962.
2. ———. *Infancy in Uganda: Infant Care and the Growth of Attachment*. Baltimore: The Johns Hopkins Press, 1967.
3. ———. "Object Relations, Dependency and Attachment: A Theoretical Review of the Infant-Mother Relationship," *Child Dev.*, 40 (1969), 969–1027.
4. AINSWORTH, M. D. S., S. M. V. BELL, and D. J. STAYTON. "Individual Differences in Strange-Situation Behaviour of One-Year-Olds," in H. R. Schaffer, ed., *The Origins of Human Social Relations*, pp. 17–52. New York: Academic Press, 1971.
5. ———. "Infant-Mother Attachment and Social Development: 'Socialization' as a Product of Reciprocal Responsiveness to Signals," in M. P. M. Richards, ed., *The Integration of a Child into a Social World*, pp. 99–135. Cambridge: Cambridge University Press, 1974.
6. BAUMRIND, D. "Child Care Practices Anteceding Three Patterns of Preschool Behaviour," *Genet. Psychol. Monogr.*, 75 (1967), 43–88.
7. BIRTCHNELL, J. "Case-Register Study of Bereavement," *Proc. R. Soc. Med.*, 64 (1971), 279–282.
8. BLURTON-JONES, N., ed. *Ethological Studies of Child Behaviour*. Cambridge: Cambridge University Press, 1972.
9. BOWLBY, J. "The Influence of Early Environment in the Development of Neurosis and Neurotic Character," *Int. J. Psychoanal.*, 21 (1940), 154–178.
10. ———. "Forty-four Juvenile Thieves: Their Characters and Home Life," *Int. J. Psychoanal.*, 25 (1944), 15–52, 107–127.
11. ———. *Maternal Care and Mental Health.*

Geneva: WHO Monograph No. 2, 1951. Reprint. New York: Schocken, 1966.
12. ———. "The Nature of the Child's Tie to His Mother," *Int. J. Psychoanal.*, 39 (1958), 350–373.
13. ———. "Separation Anxiety," *Int. J. Psychoanal.*, 41 (1960), 89–113.
14. ———. "Grief and Mourning in Infancy and Early Childhood," in *The Psychoanalytic Study of the Child*, Vol. 15, pp. 9–52. New York: International Universities Press, 1960.
15. ———. "Processes of Mourning," *Int. J. Psychoanal.*, 42 (1961), 317–340.
16. ———. "Pathological Mourning and Childhood Mourning," *J. Am. Psychoanal. Assoc.*, 11 (1963), 500–541.
17. ———. *Attachment and Loss*, Vol. 1, Attachment. New York: Basic Books, 1969.
18. ———. *Attachment and Loss*, Vol. 2, Separation: Anxiety and Anger. New York: Basic Books, 1973.
19. BOWLBY, J. and C. M. PARKES. "Separation and Loss Within the Family," in E. J. Anthony and C. Koupernik, eds., *The Child in His Family*, pp. 197–216. New York: Wiley, 1970.
20. BUNCH, J. "Recent Bereavement in Relation to Suicide," *J. Psychosom. Res.*, 16 (1972), 361–366.
21. BURLINGHAM, D. and A. FREUD. The Writings of Anna Freud, Vol. 3, *Infants Without Families: Reports on the Hampstead Nurseries, 1935–1945*. New York: International Universities Press, 1973.
22. CAPLAN, M. G. and V. I. DOUGLAS. "Incidence of Parent Loss in Children with Depressed Mood," *J. Child Psychol. Psychiatry*, 10 (1969), 225–232.
23. CLYNE, M. B. *Absent: School Refusal as an Expression of Disturbed Family Relationships*. London: Tavistock, 1966.
24. DAVIDSON, S. "School Phobia as a Manifestation of Family Disturbance: Its Structure and Treatment," *J. Child Psychol. Psychiatry*, 1 (1961), 270–287.
25. DEUTSCH, H. "Absence of Grief," *Psychoanal. Q.*, 6 (1937), 12–22.
26. EARLE, A. M. and B. V. EARLE. "Early Maternal Deprivation and Later Psychiatric Illness," *Am. J. Orthopsychiatry*, 31 (1961), 181–186.
27. FAIRBAIRN, W. R. D. *Psychoanalytic Studies of the Personality*. London: Tavistock, 1952.

28. FREUD, S. (1925) "Analysis of a Phobia in a Five-Year-Old Boy," in J. Strachey, ed., *Standard Edition*, Vol. 10, pp. 5–147. London: Hogarth Press, 1955.

29. ———. (1917) "Introductory Lectures on Psycho-Analysis," Part 3, in J. Strachey, ed., *Standard Edition*, Vol. 16, p. 408. London: Hogarth Press, 1959.

30. ———. (1926) "Inhibitions, Symptoms and Anxiety," in J. Strachey, ed., *Standard Edition*, Vol. 20, pp. 77–175. London: Hogarth Press, 1959.

31. ———. (1940) "Splitting of the Ego in the Process of Defence," in J. Strachey, ed., *Standard Edition*, Vol. 23, pp. 275–278. London: Hogarth Press, 1959.

32. GEWIRTZ, J. L., ed. *Attachment and Dependency*. Washington: V. H. Winston, 1972.

33. GOLDFARB, W. "Infant Rearing and Problem Behavior," *Am. J. Orthopsychiatry*, 13 (1943), 249–265.

34. ———. "Emotional and Intellectual Consequences of Psychologic Deprivation in Infancy: A Revaluation," in P. H. Hoch and J. Zubin, eds., *Psychopathology of Childhood*, pp. 105–119. New York: Grune & Stratton, 1955.

35. GREER, S. "Study of Parental Loss in Neurotics and Psychopaths," *Arch. Gen. Psychiatry*, 11 (1964), 177–180.

36. ———. "The Relationship Between Parental Loss and Attempted Suicide: A Control Study," *Br. J. Psychiatry*, 110 (1964), 698–705.

37. GRINKER, R. R., SR. " 'Mentally Healthy' Young Males (Homoclites)," *Arch. Gen. Psychiatry*, 6 (1962), 405–453.

38. HANSBURG, H. G. *Adolescent Separation Anxiety: A Method for the Study of Adolescent Separation Problems*. Springfield, Ill.: C. C. Thomas, 1972.

39. HARLOW, H. F. "The Nature of Love," *Am. Psychol.*, 13 (1958), 673–685.

40. HARLOW, H. F. and M. K. HARLOW. "The Affectional Systems," in A. M. Schrier, H. F. Harlow, and F. Stollnitz, eds., *Behavior of Non-Human Primates*, Vol. 2, pp. 287–334. New York: Academic, 1965.

41. HEINICKE, C. "Some Affects of Separating Two-Year-Old Children from Their Parents: A Comparative Study," *Hum. Rel.*, 9 (1956), 105–176.

42. HEINICKE, C. and I. WESTHEIMER. *Brief Separations*. New York: International Universities Press, 1966.

43. HERSOV, L. A. "Persistent Non-Attendance at School," *J. Child Psychol. Psychiatry*, 1 (1960), 130–136.

44. ———. "Refusal To Go to School," *J. Child Psychol. Psychiatry*, 1 (1960), 137–145.

45. HILL, O. "Childhood Bereavement and Adult Psychiatric Disturbance," *J. Psychosom. Res.*, 16 (1972), 357–361.

46. HILL, R. and D. A. HANSEN. "Families in Disaster," in G. W. Baker and D. W. Chapman, eds., *Man and Society in Disaster*, pp. 185–221. New York: Basic Books, 1962.

47. HINDE, R. A. *Animal Behavior: A Synthesis of Ethology and Comparative Psychology*, 2nd ed. New York: McGraw-Hill, 1970.

48. JERSILD, A. T. *Child Psychology*, 3rd ed. London: Staples Press, 1947.

49. JOHNSON, A. M., E. I. FALSTEIN, S. A. SZUREK et al. "School Phobia," *Am. J. Orthopsychiatry*, 11 (1941), 702–711.

50. KLEIN, M. *Contributions to Psychoanalysis—1921–1945*. New York: Hillary, 1950.

51. LEVY, D. "Primary Affect Hunger," *Am. J. Psychiatry*, 94 (1937), 643–652.

52. LINDEMANN, E. "Symptomatology and Management of Acute Grief," *Am. J. Psychiatry*, 101 (1944), 141–149.

53. MADDISON, D. and W. L. WALKER. "Factors Affecting the Outcome of Conjugal Bereavement," *Br. J. Psychiatry*, 113 (1967), 1057–1067.

54. MARKS, I. M. *Fears and Phobias*. London: Heinemann Medical, 1969.

55. MARRIS, P. *Widows and Their Families*. London: Routledge & Kegan Paul, 1958.

56. McCORD, W., J. McCORD, and P. VERDEN. "Familial and Behavioral Correlates of Dependency in Male Children," *Child Dev.*, 33 (1962), 313–326.

57. MORGAN, G. and H. N. RICCIUTI. "Infants' Responses to Strangers During the First Year," in B. M. Foss, ed., *Determinants of Infant Behavior*, Vol. 4, pp. 253–272. London: Methuen, 1969.

58. NEWSON, J. and E. NEWSON. *Four-Years Old in an Urban Community*. Chicago: Aldine, 1968.

59. OFFER, D. *The Psychological World of the Teen-Ager: A Study of Normal Adolescent Boys*. New York: Basic Books, 1969.

60. PARKES, C. M. "Recent Bereavement as a

Cause of Mental Illness," *Br. J. Psychiatry*, 110 (1964), 198–204.

61. ———. "Bereavement and Mental Illness," *Br. J. Med. Psychol.*, 38 (1965), 1–26.

62. ———. "Separation Anxiety: An Aspect of the Search for a Lost Object," in M. H. Lader, ed., *Studies of Anxiety*, pp. 87–92. *Br. J. Psychiatry Spec. Pub.* 3, 1969.

63. ———. "Psycho-Social Transitions: A Field of Study," *Soc. Sci. Med.*, 5 (1971), 101–115.

64. ———. "The First Year of Bereavement: A Longitudinal Study of the Reactions of London Widows to the Death of Their Husbands," *Psychiatry*, 33 (1971), 444–467.

65. ———. *Bereavement: Studies of Grief in Adult Life*. New York: International Universities Press, 1972.

66. PECK, R. F. and R. J. HAVIGHURST. *The Psychology of Character Development*. New York: Wiley, 1960.

67. REES, W. D. "The Hallucinations of Widowhood," *Br. Med. J.*, 4 (1971), 37–41.

68. ROBERTSON, J. *Young Children in Hospital*, 2nd ed. London: Tavistock, 1970.

69. ROBERTSON, J. and J. ROBERTSON. *Young Children in Brief Separation*. Film series. London: Tavistock Inst. Hum. Rel., 1967–1972.

70. ROSENBERG, M. *Society and the Adolescent Self-Image*. Princeton: Princeton University Press, 1965.

71. ROTH, M. "The Phobic Anxiety Depersonalization Syndrome," *Proc. R. Soc. Med.*, 52 (1959), 587–595.

72. ROWELL, T. E. and R. A. HINDE. "Responses of Rhesus Monkeys to Mildly Stressful Situations," *Anim. Behav.*, 11 (1963), 235–243.

73. RUTTER, M. *Maternal Deprivation Reassessed*. Harmondsworth: Penguin, 1972.

74. SEARS, R. R., E. E. MACCOBY, and H. LEVIN. *Patterns of Child Rearing*. Evanston: Row, Peterson, 1957.

75. SNAITH, R. P. "A Clinical Investigation of Phobias," *Br. J. Psychiatry*, 114 (1968), 673–698.

76. STENDLER, C. B. "Possible Causes of Overdependency in Young Children," *Child Dev.*, 25 (1954), 125–146.

77. STOTT, D. H. *Delinquency and Human Nature*. Dunfermline, Fife: Carnegie U. K. Trust, 1950.

78. STRACHEY, J. "Introduction" to Freud's "Inhibitions, Symptoms and Anxiety," in J. Strachey, ed., *Standard Edition*, Vol. 20, pp. 77–86. London: Hogarth Press, 1959.

79. TALBOT, M. "Panic in School Phobia," *Am. J. Orthopsychiatry*, 27 (1957), 286–295.

80. UCKO, L. E. "A Comparative Study of Asphyxiated and Non-Asphyxiated Boys from Birth to Five Years," *Dev. Med. Child Neurol.*, 7 (1965), 643–657.

81. WEBSTER, A. S. "The Development of Phobias in Married Women," *Psychol. Monog.*, 67 (1953), No. 17.

82. WEISS, M. and A. BURKE. "A 5- to 10-year Follow-up of Hospitalized School Phobic Children and Adolescents," *Am. J. Orthopsychiatry*, 40 (1970), 672–676.

83. WEISS, M. and B. CAIN. "The Residential Treatment of Children and Adolescents with School Phobia," *Am. J. Orthopsychiatry*, 34 (1964), 103–114.

84. WINNICOTT, D. W. *The Maturational Process and the Facilitating Environment*. New York: International Universities Press, 1965.

85. WOLFENSTEIN, M. "How Is Mourning Possible?" in *The Psychoanalytic Study of the Child*, Vol. 21, pp. 93–123. New York: International Universities Press, 1966.

86. YAMOMOTO, J., K. OKONOGI, T. IWASAKI et al. "Mourning in Japan," *Am. J. Psychiatry*, 125 (1969), 1660–1665.

CHAPTER 15

EXPERIMENTAL PSYCHOPATHOLOGY IN NONHUMAN PRIMATES[*]

William T. McKinney, Jr., Stephen J. Suomi, and Harry F. Harlow

❦ Introduction

CAN MONKEYS be made as mad as men? Phrased more scientifically, can primate models be useful in understanding human psychopathology? If so, how and what

* The writing of this chapter and much of the research described was supported by Grants MH–11894, MH–18070, and MH–21892 from the National Institute of Mental Health and by RR–00167 from the National Institutes of Health to the University of Wisconsin Primate Laboratory and Regional Primate Research Center; the Grant Foundation; by Research Scientist Development Award K01–MH–47353 (Dr. McKinney); and by the Wisconsin Psychiatric Institute. The authors wish to express their appreciation to Ms. Elaine Moran, Dr. Hagop Akiskal, and Dr. Laurens Young for their critical reading of this manuscript.

are the specific behavioral, neurophysiological, and biochemical changes seen? What rehabilitation methods are effective in reversing each of the abnormal behavior syndromes? These questions now occupy the attention of several investigators and are the key queries with which this chapter will be concerned.

During the last ten years the field of experimental psychopathology in nonhuman primates has undergone considerable development. It is now possible through utilization of specific social and biological induction methods to produce syndromes of abnormal behavior that can be objectively documented and evaluated. If behavioral and biochemical studies whose findings may subsequently be applied to human beings are to be performed, ideally one should use a species as close to man as possible. From this viewpoint the great apes might be the logical choice. However, due to the scarcity and the difficulties and expense of working with large primates in a laboratory much of the work to be reviewed in this paper has utilized only rhesus monkeys as subjects. Also, the life span of monkeys is considerably compressed in comparison to man or the apes, thus facilitating longitudinal studies. However, occasional reference will be made to work employing other species because the issue of species variation, particularly with regard to social behavior, is a critical one.

The interest of most clinicians in the experimental simulation of abnormal behavioral states in nonhumans has ranged from excessive anthropomorphism to indifference to hostility to confusion. The skepticism with which much animal behavioral work has been received lies partly in the history of the field and partly in the attitude of some psychiatrists who refuse to accept animal work as relevant to human disorders. This latter school of thought has been most actively represented by Kubie[48] who states: "Thus the imitation in animals of the emotional states which attend neuroses in man is not the experimental production of the essence of neuroses itself." Kubie's contention is that behavior is only the "sign-language" of an underlying symbolic disorder that is the real core of psychopathology. He feels that animals do not have symbolic capacities and, therefore, it is not possible to produce a "true" neurotic or psychotic state in nonhumans. This position is predicated on an assumption about human psychopathology that many would disagree with, namely, that behavior is important only as an indicator of something more important that is the "real" disorder. Others would insist that observations of behavior are the only way to define disorders reliably. Also, the assumption that higher-order primates do not have symbolic capacities is open to serious question.[21,80]

However, Kubie in his criticisms did focus on an important issue in this field. Various terms have been applied far too loosely to the abnormal behavioral states created in different species. Labels such as "experimental neurosis," "phobia," "anxiety," "behavioral disorder," "chronic emotional disorder," "experimental neurasthenia," and "depression" have been utilized, often without adequate behavioral descriptions. The laxity in labeling has often alienated clinicians who fail to see the similarities between conditions used to produce abnormal behavior in many animal studies and those which are thought to predispose to human psychopathology.

Many criticisms of the field are justified as will be apparent from the historical section of this chapter. However, there is no intrinsic reason why specific forms of human psychopathology cannot be examined at an animal level. It has been pointed out by Seligman[97] and by McKinney and Bunney[60] that the difficulty in moving from a dramatic analogue to animal models has been due in large part to the lack of ground rules or criteria that might validate the model. This will be reviewed following the historical section. Subsequently, a discussion will be presented of some of the more carefully defined syndromes of abnormal behavior in primates, the conditions that produce them, and, in some cases, effective ways to reverse them. The areas to be covered will include: (a) social isolation, (b) the Harlow vertical chamber, (c) experimental "helplessness," and (d) attachment-behavior and separation studies. An approach to biochemical studies in primate models and data from recently completed studies will be outlined. Finally, a perspective on the field of experimental psychopathology in primates will be presented and possible future directions discussed.

It should be mentioned that this chapter concerns itself only with experimental-laboratory investigations and does not deal with the broad range of important field studies that are available. However, field studies and laboratory studies of primates should be viewed as complementary rather than competitive, with each having inherent advantages and limitations. Admittedly the choice of topics to be discussed is arbitrary, but hopefully they include the ones of most interest to psychiatrists.

❨ Historical Approaches

The first research on animal neuroses originated in the laboratories of Ivan P. Pavlov of Russia.[78] In 1921, he described a method for producing an "experimental neurosis" using a conditioning paradigm. A previously quiet dog, subjected to prolonged classical conditioning, became unable to distinguish between the appearance of a circle as a signal for food and an almost circular elipse as a signal for no food. He suddenly exhibited extreme and persistent agitation as evidenced by constant struggling and howling. Pavlov viewed neurosis as a chronic deviation of the higher nervous system, lasting weeks, months, or years. He felt higher nervous activity was manifested chiefly in the system of conditioned positive and negative reflexes to any stimulus and partially in the general behavior of his dogs. A neurosis in Pavlov's paradigm resulted from a collision, in time or space, of the processes of excitation and inhibition, e.g., receiving positive and negative stimuli too close together.

Gantt[20] also used conditioning paradigms to produce what he called "behavior disorders," though it seems clear that he was not able to model specific syndromes so much as to produce a variety of autonomic responses to different conditioning tasks. He produced experimental conflicts by forcing dogs to make difficult differentiations of conditioned signals and studied the effects of this type of conflict on the animal's neurophysiological functioning. He presented detailed, longitudinal histories of dogs made behaviorally abnormal by this method. Pavlov's approach was also extended and modified by Cook[10] in rats, and by Dworkin[12,13] in dogs and cats.

Liddell made the first observation of experimental neurosis using sheep as subjects. In 1927, Liddell and Bayne[54] reported what they labeled "experimental neurasthenia" in a sheep subjected to an unsignaled doubling of the number of conditioning trials per day. The animal was observed to have become very excited and agitated. Liddell and his group continued to perform experimental-neurosis research on sheep, goats, and pigs using

conditioning paradigms.[49,50,51,52,53] They presented the concept that experimental disorders in animals represented primitive, relatively undifferentiated behavioral states rather than one specific syndrome. This group also performed longitudinal studies of the effects of stressful conditioning paradigms at different developmental stages in the animal's life cycle.

Masserman[70,71] used motivational conflict situations to induce abnormal behavior first in cats and later in monkeys. Subjects were conditioned to remove food pellets from a box and subsequently, on certain trials, were subjected to a blast of air when they approached the food, thus producing a conflict between hunger and fear. He described "anxiety" in and out of the experimental situation, frequent startle reactions, "phobic" hypersensitivity, "compulsive" patterns of hiding and escape, motor disturbance (restlessness, cataleptoid immobility), regressive automatisms such as licking or preening, and marked behavioral inhibition that, when directed toward food, could lead to self-starvation. Masserman also studied a variety of methods designed to alleviate the abnormal behavior resulting from the motivational conflict induced. The greatest contribution of Masserman's work lay not in its simulation of any particular behavioral state, but in its demonstration that certain psychoanalytic principles can be made operational and tested experimentally. This was no small contribution in its time or even today.

There have been many other experimenters in this area. For instance, Hebb's[39] description of spontaneous neurosis in chimpanzees was important in terms of its relation to clinical and experimental phenomena. He described what he termed a "phobia" in one case where a chimp suddenly became afraid of large chunks of food. The other case involved naturally occurring episodic depression. Babkin[3] reported that bromides could reset the balance between excitatory and inhibitory processes thought by Pavlov and Gantt to be important in experimental neuroses. Stainbrook[104] called attention to the value of experimentally producing acute behavioral disorders in animals as a method of psychosomatic research and discussed some of the previous work done in several species.

It is not surprising that the field of experimental psychopathology in nonhumans has been of little interest to clinicians. Most of the work described in the previous section used conditioning techniques and terms whose relevance to clinical phenomena were poorly understood. Clinical terms were thrown about far too loosely to describe certain behavioral states in animals. Little attention was paid to the theoretical problems implicit in using nonhumans to study human psychopathology. In the next section this latter issue will be discussed, since it is basic to what follows in the rest of the chapter.

(Criteria for Animal Models

The basic controversy that has developed from the above work, as well as from recent data, is whether a laboratory phenomenon in animals can model a form, or forms, of psychopathology in man. The theoretical considerations regarding this general issue have been discussed by Senay,[99] McKinney and Bunney,[60] Harlow and McKinney,[32] Seligman,[97] and Mitchell.[75] The last article also contains an excellent review of abnormal behavior in primates, which readers of this chapter may find useful.

The above authors stated their criteria in different terms, but the content of what each said was very similar. Much of the work previously described in the historical section suffered from a lack of prior criteria by which the syndromes produced could be evaluated. The establishment of such criteria for animal-model research in recent years has been a major advancement and has had considerable heurestic value.

Forms of human psychopathology are not entities that can be studied at an animal level if appropriate criteria have not been previously established. The following criteria have been proposed by several workers as being useful in evaluating nonhuman experimental psychopathology research:

1. The behavioral manifestations of the syndrome being modeled should be similar to those seen in the human condition.
2. These behavioral changes should be able to be objectively detected by independent observers in different laboratories.
3. The behavioral state induced should be persistent and generalizable.
4. Etiological-inducing conditions used in animals should be similar to those present in human psychopathology.
5. Treatment modalities effective in reversing the human disorder should be effective in primates.
6. There must be sufficient reference-control data available.

While these criteria suggest needed research in the creation of models, it should also be remembered that the condition being modeled is often itself poorly defined from a behavioral standpoint. While this point can be used as a rebuttal to critics who demand more preciseness from "models" research than is currently available, it also delineates one of the potential values of animal-model research, i.e., to aid in more clearly defining human syndromes from a behavioral standpoint.

In essence what is being attempted in the creation of experimental models in primates is the production of a syndrome(s) that meets the criteria outlined above. The value of a model system in animals is that it leads itself to more direct manipulation of social and biological variables than is possible in human beings from ethical and/or practical standpoints. This is not to contend that monkeys are humans or vice versa. Obviously, there are differences, but the similarities far outweigh most differences, especially with regard to social development and affectional systems.

In other medical specialties, animals are frequently used as models for some conditions. Psychiatry does not have this tradition. Primate behavioral research has characteristically been the domain of the experimental psychologist, the ethological zoologist, and the anthropologist. Why this has been so has been discussed earlier in this chapter. As will be apparent, however, there are primate behavioral data available that provide a firm base for understanding of clinical phenomena in several areas. For example, experimental work on social isolation of nonhuman primates has documented the short- and long-term effects of insufficient social input early in development, and recent rehabilitation experiments have indicated successful therapeutic approaches. These data have considerable relevance for human psychopathology as well as for the better understanding of the effects of different rearing conditions.

(Social Isolation

The technique of social isolation involves rearing animals from birth either in total isolation chambers where they have no social contact with other monkeys or in bare wire cages where their only contact is visual and auditory.

Social isolation is only one of many different rearing conditions that are possible in a controlled laboratory setting. Harlow[30] and Sackett[88] have discussed each of these rearing conditions and their effects on the behavioral development of rhesus monkey subjects. Each method has an influence on the rapidity and/or nature of development of social behavior but, in general, all, except social isolation, can be used to rear socially normal rhesus monkeys. Social isolation early in life produces severe and persistent syndromes of abnormal behavior involving the destruction or severe disruption of the major "affectional systems" as proposed by Harlow.[24,26,27,28,29]

The mechanisms underlying the dramatic effects of social isolation are poorly understood and there are virtually no data about possible neurophysiological and/or neuroendocrinological substrates of the syndrome. Sackett[89,90] has summarized the four most frequent explanations thus:

1. Atrophy—Deprivation effects are due to physical atrophy of sensory mechanisms that were mature at birth or shortly thereafter.

2. Developmental failure and potentiation—Environments void of certain critical inputs may produce later deficits because the physiological substrate underlying a response or information processing fails to mature.

3. Learning deficits—Social-deprivation deficits are caused by a failure of the early environment to provide experiences critical for basic perceptual-motor development. A failure to integrate perceptual and motor responses early in life permanently impairs the ability to adapt to change.

4. Emergence trauma—Deficits are a function of the discrepancy between rearing and testing environments, i.e., the shock of removal from a stimulus-poor environment to a stimulus-rich one.

None of these explanations can be accepted as the chief one at present because of the absence of data. However, it is known that the emergence-trauma theory is not supportable. Experimenters have tried to alleviate the occurrence of such trauma by adapting the subjects during the isolation period to the test situation to be employed following removal from isolation. No substantial positive effects were apparent. The "adapted" isolates exhibited social behavior generally as incompetent as that of isolates denied this experience.[109]

It is also known, from recent rehabilitation experiments, that a rigid fatalistic, critical-period hypothesis is not true. With appropriate rehabilitative methods, it has been possible to reverse the social deficits that resulted from early isolation.

Social-isolation data are most extensive in rhesus monkey subjects, and these will be summarized below. However, the isolation syndrome has also been studied in dogs,[19] in pigtail monkeys,[15] and in chimpanzees.[72,73,111] The measurement techniques differed from study to study in terms of how the effects of early social isolation were documented, and also the specific techniques of isolation varied. Nevertheless, one can make a general statement that, in all species studied thus far, early social isolation has been a powerful method for inducing persistent patterns of abnormal behavior.

In rhesus monkeys, for example, subjects reared in total social isolation for the first six to twelve months of life exhibit, upon emergence from isolation, severe deficits in locomotive, exploratory, and social behavior.[22,25,33,68][69,76] The appropriate responses of grooming, play, and other social interactions are minimal in these subjects. They spend the majority of their time engaging in autisticlike self-clasping, stereotyped rocking and huddling, and self-mouthing behavior. One of these isolates is shown in Figure 15-1. Appropriate sexual responses are virtually absent among isolate-reared monkeys,[31,93] and those females artificially inseminated typically display grossly inadequate maternal behavior, characterized by indifference or brutality toward their infants. In general, aggressive behavior is either self-directed or inappropriately directed. For example, a chronologically mature social isolate will readily attack a neonate, an act rarely initiated by a socially normal monkey, or it may attack a dominant adult male, a blunder that few socially sophisticated monkeys are foolish enough to attempt. Socially isolated rhesus monkeys have also been reported to exhibit hyperphagia and polydipsia as adults.[74]

Several variables are important in the production of the isolation syndrome. The most severe effects are produced when the isolation is total, when it begins at birth, and when it lasts for a minimum of six months. Alteration of any of these factors will produce a less severe and/or a less persistent syndrome.

The isolation syndrome until recently had been considered permanent. No technique that had been tried had been successful in reversing the syndrome, including aversive conditioning-type procedures, frequent social experience with peers, and prevention of the "emergence trauma." The first successful rehabilitation of social isolates was brought about by "monkey psychiatrists," a term that refers to chronologically younger, normal monkeys who served as the therapists in the social rehabilitation study.[36,109] The specific experiment studied six-month isolates and utilized three-month-old, normal female animals as "therapists." The isolates were allowed to interact with the therapist monkeys two hours per day, three days per week as pairs (one isolate, one therapist) and two days per week in a group of four (two isolates, two therapists) in a playroom.

The isolates' initial response to both situations was to huddle in a corner, and the therapists' first response was to approach and cling to the isolates. Within a week in the home cage and two weeks in the playroom the isolates were reciprocating the clinging. Concurrently the therapists were exhibiting elementary play patterns among themselves and attempting to initiate such patterns with the isolates. Within two weeks in the home cage and a month in the playroom the isolates were reciprocating these kinds of behavior. Shortly thereafter the isolates began to initiate play behavior themselves and, correspondingly, their disturbance activity, which originally had accounted for most of their behavioral repertoire, decreased to insignificant levels. By

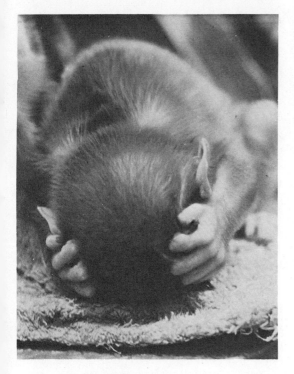

Figure 15-1. A typical isolate rhesus monkey huddling and self-clasping.

one year of age the isolates were virtually indistinguishable from the therapists in the amount of exploration, locomotion, and kinds of play behavior.

Not only have isolated monkeys responded to social-treatment methods, they have also improved on chlorpromazine. In a recent pilot study,[67] rhesus monkeys subjected to partial social isolation for the first year of life, plus other traumatic experiences involving being immobilized or seeing peers immobilized, exhibited severe patterns of abnormal behavior such as huddling, rocking, self-clasping, retreat to corners away from other animals, and self-mouthing. When they were two and a half years of age, four such subjects were started on chlorpromazine and the dosage adjusted to 7.5 mgm/kgm given once a day by intubation. Within four to eight weeks on this regimen, the "active" self-disturbance behavior such as self-mouthing, clasping, huddling, etc., had decreased significantly and a few social encounters such as play and social exploration occurred in some subjects.

These studies involving attempts to reverse the social isolation syndrome are being extended to one combining chlorpromazine plus social experience as well as the use of other drugs.

In terms of models it is still unclear what human syndrome is being represented by the isolation syndrome. Labels such as "autism," "schizophrenia," "psychoses," "depression," have been used by some professionals in describing these animals. A cautious approach to labeling is indicated at present. Certainly the behavioral parallels between these isolate monkeys and certain aspects of each of the above syndromes exist, yet several criteria for models presented earlier have not been met or even approached. One criteria that is particularly critical to keep in mind is the comparability of inducing conditions. It is difficult to hypothesize a documentable human analogy to total social isolation except for the few cases of drastic neglect of infants. Partial social isolation, on the other hand, has a clearer analogue in the limited and stereotyped social input to children present in many groups and families. There are virtually no biological data

available on isolated monkeys that might help to understand the mechanisms, and help with the definition of the syndrome. It has been said that rehabilitation studies can help the syndrome and within limits this is true. It appears that a socially induced syndrome can be improved by appropriate social therapy and by use of an antipsychotic drug. The social therapy involved gentle physical contact and nonthreatening social interactions. However, did the drug therapy involve chlorpromazine's antipsychotic properties or did it facilitate social interaction by making the subjects less fearful of each other? Or some combination of the two? Further work is necessary to clarify this issue.

In conclusion, it is known that a syndrome of abnormal behavior can be predictably produced by early social isolation. This syndrome can be well defined behaviorally, but additional investigations are critical in order to clarify the mechanisms involved and the significance of the syndrome itself as a model for human psychopathology.

⟮ Harlow Vertical Chamber*

The technique of social isolation requires six to twelve months for effective production of severe syndromes of abnormal behavior. Attempts have been made recently to create other social-deprivation methods that might produce psychopathological behavior in a much shorter period of time. Several pilot studies have been conducted at Wisconsin that indicate that confinement in an apparatus called the vertical chamber may also be capable of producing dramatic behavioral changes in rhesus monkeys.

The vertical chambers are illustrated in Figure 15–2. Essentially, they are troughs constructed of stainless steel, open at the top, with sides that slope inward to a rounded bottom that forms one-half of a cylinder. There are smaller chambers for infants and larger ones for older subjects. One inch above the bottom of both chamber types is a wire mesh

* See references 34, 38, 37, 62, and 63.

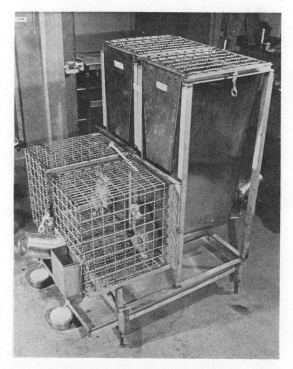

Figure 15–2. Vertical chamber apparatus with an attached living cage.

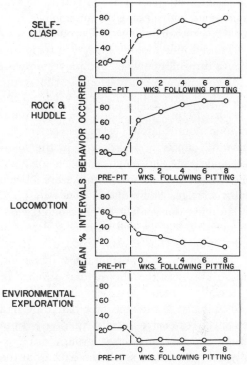

Figure 15–3. Effect of thirty days of vertical chamber confinement on selected behaviors of four rhesus monkeys (age six to thirteen months).

floor that allows waste material to drop through to the pit bottom. Holes drilled in the bottom permit urine collection while the monkey is in the chamber. The chamber is equipped with a food box and a water-bottle holder and is covered by a pyramidal top designed to discourage confined subjects from hanging from the upper part of the trough. While in the chamber a subject would have no tactual or visual contact with other monkeys. Depending on the placement of the chamber in the laboratory, he could or could not have auditory contact.

In an exploratory study, four individually reared subjects with an age range of six to thirteen months were placed in single chambers for a period of thirty days. Figure 15–3 illustrates some of the kinds of home cage behavior prior to chamber isolation and for two months following removal. It is obvious that their behavior patterns after removal from the

chamber were drastically altered, with marked increases in self-clasping, rocking, huddling, and marked decreases in locomotion and environmental exploration.

This pilot study suggested that the vertical chamber had potential for the rapid production of psychopathological behavior in monkeys. Total social isolation from birth to three months results in only transient behavioral disturbance. Also, the effectiveness of social isolation decreases even more if not initiated at or shortly after birth. In contrast, vertical chamber confinement of only thirty days duration produced disturbances even in subjects six to thirteen months old at the time of confinement. Two of the animals were able to be followed for almost a year after removal and little recovery was evident. However, additional long-term studies are necessary to assess the effects of early chambering.

In a second study four monkeys forty-five

days of age were placed in individual vertical chambers for six weeks. Upon emergence they were three months of age. Subsequently they were housed individually, but given social experience three days a week in a playroom with equal-aged monkeys. Figure 15–4 shows the animals four days following removal from the chambers. Figure 15–5 shows the same monkeys four months later. The persistence of the behavioral effects was also seen in the monkeys' home cage and playroom behavior eight months later when the animals were eleven months of age. Self-mouthing, self-clasping, and huddling dominated the chambered monkeys' activity, but were virtually nonexistent in control subjects. The reverse was true regarding locomotive and exploratory behavior. Most striking was the almost total absence of any socially directed behavior in the chambered animals despite the fact that they had been given extensive social experience from four months of age. Other groups are currently being tested to see if the data from the pilot experiment described above can be replicated.

A third study combined peer separation, to be described in a later section (p. 325), with vertical chamber confinement. Infants were paired with each other as a group of four from birth to three months, then separated from each other a total of twenty times, four days for each separation in exactly the same sequence as the multiple-infant-separation study to be discussed later. The difference in the current study was that during the separation phase the infants were housed in vertical chambers rather than individual cages. Upon reunion, the chambered monkeys showed significantly lower levels of social clinging and higher levels of self-clasping than the cage-separated monkeys. In other words, they did not reattach to each other as the animals housed in standard laboratory cages during separation did. These data are the only suggestion from the Wisconsin laboratory that it might be possible to produce Bowlby's "detachment" stage in monkeys. Mitchell[75] has also observed a phenomenon resembling detachment when infant rhesus monkeys are reunited with their mothers. In any event, it is

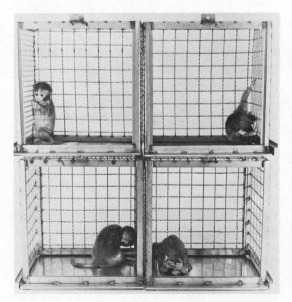

Figure 15–4. Four rhesus monkeys immediately after six weeks of vertical chamber confinement.

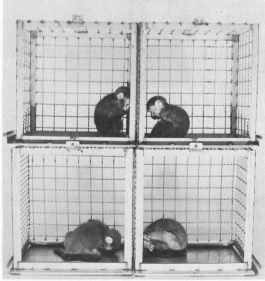

Figure 15–5. Four rhesus monkeys four months after six weeks of vertical chamber confinement.

apparent that chamber confinement coupled with separation produced effects beyond those produced by either procedure alone.

When the vertical chamber studies were extended beyond infants to juvenile-age rhesus monkeys three years old, a very different effect was observed. Such subjects when confined to vertical chambers for as long as eighty days exhibited, upon removal, significant decreases in locomotion and activity levels, and significant increases in contact clinging and passivity as illustrated in Figure 15–6. Such behavior is clearly inappropriate for three-year-old monkeys and seems more typical of monkeys at an earlier stage of development. Thus, as will also be seen in the separation studies, age or developmental stage is a critical variable in determining a subject's response to chambering.

There is considerable question as to what the behavioral changes induced by vertical-chamber confinement represent. There was an initial hope that the chambers could be used to create feelings of "helplessness and hope-

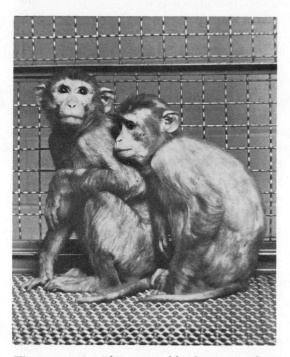

Figure 15–6. Three-year-old rhesus monkeys clinging to each other after eighty days of vertical-chamber confinement.

lessness." This may or may not prove to be the mechanism involved in this severe form of environmental deprivation. That such a state can be created in nonhumans is indicated by Seligman's work to be discussed in the next section. However, based on currently available data, the vertical chamber seems to be an effective means of producing severe and persistent psychopathology in rhesus monkeys. The roles of environmental deprivation, and such parameters as chamber shape, chamber construction, decreased mobility, duration of confinement, and prior social experience are largely unknown, and studies investigating these factors have been initiated.

(Learned Helplessness

Seligman et al.[96,97,98] use the term "learned helplessness" to describe the interference with adaptive responding produced by inescapable shock. Most of their work has been conducted with dogs, but they note that a similar phenomenon can be observed in rats, cats, dogs, fish, mice, and men.

In the paradigm used to produce learned helplessness, subjects were first given a series of sixty-four unsignaled, inescapable electric shocks. The shocks occurred randomly. Twenty-four hours later the subjects were given ten trials of signaled, escape-avoidance training. During this phase, if the subjects jumped a barrier when the conditioned stimulus was presented, they avoided shock; failure to jump led to a shock that continued until the subjects jumped the barrier.

Learned helplessness is an operational concept used to describe subjects that have had experience with uncontrollable shock and failed to initiate responses to escape shock or were much slower in making responses than naive dogs. Also, if the subject did happen to make a response that turned off shock, it had more trouble than a naive subject in learning that responding was effective. In other words, after an initial experience in which responding could not control reinforcers (uncontrollable shock) the animals ceased to respond even when responding could now control reinforcers.

Such a model for learned helplessness has been suggested as another type of animal model for certain aspects of human depression by those who would see at least reactive depression, especially the passivity components, as having its roots in loss of control over reinforcers, e.g., gratification and alleviation of suffering. In this model, experimental helplessness is cured by letting the animal make repeated responses that turn off the shock. The analogy to depression is that one of the important features in the treatment of depressed patients is changing the patient's perception of himself as hopeless to one in which he believes that he has control over his environment.

(Separation Studies

Separation experiences, i.e., object losses, are thought to precede the development of severe depression as well as other forms of psychopathology in human beings.[16,18,91] The theories that postulate the importance of separation are largely based on retrospective studies that start with a population of clinically depressed people who have undergone separation. There is little understanding of the mechanisms underlying the apparent close connection between separation and depression, though the terms "separation" and "object loss" have themselves become well-accepted phrases among clinicians. Such phrases have been used to describe many diverse states, ranging from an infant's response to separation from his mother to an adult's loss of self-esteem when certain defense mechanisms are no longer effective or when life-threatening illnesses confront him. Unfortunately, separation is becoming a greatly overused term in the sense that its usage has far outstripped our basic understanding of its meaning. Separation is certainly more than just an event and needs to be defined in terms of many parameters. If this is not done, there

exists the risk that the term will continue to be used so broadly and loosely as to become meaningless. Many variables determine a response to separation and these need identification and study before the connection between what is called separation and depression can be understood. Also, depression may not be the only response to separation, or if it is, then depression may manifest itself differently depending on many factors that almost certainly include genetic and neurochemical ones, prior experience of separations, the conditions surrounding separation, and age to mention only a few.

It is in the area of clarifying the mechanisms underlying separation that primate models have perhaps been most useful thus far. Rhesus monkeys develop strong affectional systems and form close social bonds, factors that have facilitated the study of separation and depression. It was thought initially that these bonds were so strong that they could be manipulated to produce dramatic changes in behavior. Results thus far have confirmed this initial belief.

The issue of mother–child separation, and the mechanisms underlying the disturbance it produces in the human infant, have been discussed by Bowlby.[5,6,7] In his writing concerning separation, grief, and mourning in children and infants, he outlined six theories of separation and concluded that separation anxiety results from activation of the "component instinctual response systems" that form the base of the infant's attachment. He described three stages of the human child's response to separation: protest, despair, and detachment. The protest stemmed from anxiety; the despair from grief; the detachment from defensive reactions. Bowlby's theories, based on studies of the separation reactions of human infants,[86] have provided a major portion of the theoretical underpinnings of the mother–infant separation work in primates. Also of key importance in stimulating the experimental work were the observations of Spitz[103] on hospitalized young infants, who had been separated from their mothers. This reaction he termed "anaclitic depression." Many infant monkeys undergoing maternal separation stimulate the anaclitic depressive syndromes seen in human infants.

The major separation studies to be described are outlined in Table 15-1.

(Mother–Infant Separation Studies

A number of informal separation studies were conducted at the Wisconsin Primate Laboratory in the late fifties on thirty- to ninety-day-old rhesus infants raised with their own mothers. It was noticed that separation ranging from a few hours to a few days in duration resulted in acute disturbance for both mother and infant during separation and a marked increase in maternal protectiveness following reunion. In one case the mother, after a three day separation, kept her infant literally within reach for a period of more than a month. These observations precipitated a more formal study of mother–infant separation, which was reported in 1962 by Seay, Hansen and Harlow.[94]

The technique employed in the initial sepa-

TABLE 15-1.   **Major Separation Studies in Monkeys**

INVESTIGATORS	SPECIES	TYPE OF SEPARATION	AGE OF SUBJECTS	SEPARATION TECHNIQUE	LENGTH OF SEPARATION	REACTIONS OBSERVED
Seay, Hansen, Harlow	*Macaca mulatta*	Mother–infant	6 months	Removal of infant	3 weeks	Protest Despair Recovery
Seay, Harlow	*Macaca mulatta*	Mother–infant	7 months	Removal of infant	2 weeks	Protest Despair Recovery
Jensen, Toleman	*Macaca nemestrina*	Mother–infant	6 months	Removal of infant	1 hour	Protest
Kaufman, Rosenblum	*Macaca nemestrina*	Mother–infant	5 months	Removal of mother from group-living situation	4 weeks	Agitation Depression Recovery
Kaufman, Rosenblum	*Macaca radiata*	Mother–infant	5 months	Removal of mother from group-living situation	4 weeks	Protest
Hinde	*Macaca mulatta*	Mother–infant	8 months	Removal of mother from infant's sight	6 days	Protest Depression Recovery
Suomi, Domek, Harlow	*Macaca mulatta*	Peer	3 months	Peers repetitively removed from each other and individually housed	4 days	Protest Despair Recovery Maturational Arrest
Mitchell, Abrams, Lindburg	*Macaca mulatta*	Mother–infant	2 months 3-½ mo. 5 months	Removal of infant individual housing	48 hours	Protest Despair Detachment
Preston, Baker, Seay	*Erythrocebus patas*	Mother–infant	7 months	Removal of mother/infants housed together	3 weeks	Protest Despair Recovery
McKinney, Suomi, Harlow	*Macaca mulatta*	Peer	3 years	Peers repetitively removed from each other and individually housed	14 days	Protest Recovery

rations at Wisconsin involved the use of the playpen apparatus shown in Figure 15–7. This apparatus allowed mother–infant pairs to live together in each of four corner units with a central play area that the infants, but not the mothers, could enter via an opening in each living unit. Separation was accomplished by merely closing off this opening while the infants were in the central part, so that they could not return to their mothers. Plexiglas paneling was used to permit continued visual and auditory contact, wire mesh paneling that in addition permits tactual contact, or Masonite that allowed only auditory communication.

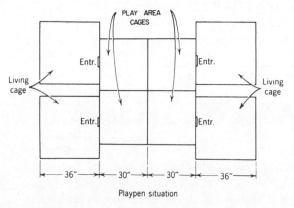

Figure 15–7. Playpen apparatus used for mother-infant separation studies.

In the original study, four infants and four mothers served as subjects. Two of the infants underwent maternal separation at 169 and 170 days of age and two at 206 and 207 days of age. The experiment was divided into three time blocks of three weeks each: preseparation period, separation period, and postseparation period. In this study Plexiglas dividers were used and thus the infants could continue to see and hear all mothers. Detailed behavioral observations were made each day. The initial reaction of all mothers and all infants after separation indicated a high degree of emotional disturbance. Immediately after separation the infants' behavior included disoriented scampering, high-pitched screeching, cooing vocalizations, and huddling up against the barrier in close proximity to their mother. The mothers displayed an increase in barking vocalizations and in threats directed toward

the experimenter, but the mothers' emotional response appeared to be both less intense and of shorter duration than that of the infants. Later during the separation period most complex forms of infant-to-infant social behavior exhibited a drastic decrease in frequency of occurrence. For instance, noncontact play was for all practical purposes obliterated. Threats, approaches, and withdrawals also decreased. During the post separation period infant–mother clinging and mother–infant cradling rose significantly and infant–mother, nonspecific contact showed a significant decrease in three of the four infants. Interestingly, one of the infants showed a significant decrease in support contact, nipple contact, and nonspecific contact during postseparation as compared to preseparation. This initial investigation demontrated that separating a rhesus monkey from its mother had striking behavioral effects, but with individual variation in terms of the nature of the response. In general, the sequence of stages seemed to parallel the "protest" and "despair" stages of Bowlby and to provide a powerful animal analogue for anaclitic depression. These stages are illustrated in Figure 15–8. It is possible that the animal that did not reattach was exhibiting something analogous to the "detachment" stage, but this was uncertain.

Another study by Seay and Harlow[95] used eight rhesus mother–infant pairs separated at about 207 days of age. In contrast to the above study, Masonite paneling was used during the separation phase and the infants were not able to see any of the mothers. Behavioral changes were similar to those already described; however, the reaction seemed more severe when the infants could see their mothers than when they could not.

Jensen and Toleman,[43] in one of the earliest separation studies, observed the short-term effects of separation of mother–infant monkey pairs (*Macaca nemestrina*) for less than one hour and found that the infants screamed almost continuously during the separation. The mothers attacked their own cages and tried to escape. On return of the infant there was a striking increase in the intensity of the mother–infant relationship. This study demonstrated

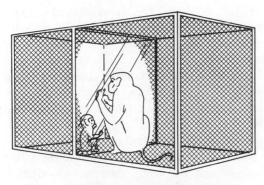

Despair stage of separation

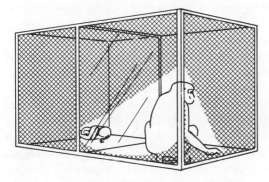

Protest stage of separation

Figure 15–8. Protest-despair reaction shown by rhesus infants following separation from mother.

that even extremely short-term separations had severe effects on both mothers and infants.

In a series of studies Kaufman and Rosenblum[44,45,87] compared the separation reactions of infant pigtail monkeys (*Macaca nemestrina*) and infant bonnet macaques (*Macaca radiata*). Their separation studies differed in several key ways from those previously described. In all their studies, subjects lived in groups consisting of several adult females, at least one adult male, and some adolescents. Separation was accomplished by removing a mother from the group, with her infant being left with the remaining members of the group. Separation from the mother in the pigtail infant study was done at age four to six months. The length of the separation was four weeks, after which the mother was brought back into the group. Reunion data were taken for three months.

Before separation bonnet groups were observed to spend long periods of time in passive contact with each other, in contrast to pigtails who did not make much physical contact except to engage in active social interactions like grooming, aggression, etc. Bonnet females even maintained their high degree of passive contact with other adult bonnets despite the birth and continued presence of their developing infants. In other words, bonnet mothers immediately returned to close contact with other females after delivery. Pigtail mothers, by contrast, were very reluctant to engage socially with others immediately following the birth of their offspring. As a result, bonnet infants spent time during the first months interacting with other adults in addition to their own mother. Pigtail infants spent almost all their time with their own mother.

During separation, i.e., removal of the mother from the group living situation, three of the four pigtail infants manifested similar reactions, which Kaufman and Rosenblum term "agitation," "depression," and "recovery." One of the four infants displayed only the first and third stage. The agitation state ("protest") was characterized by frantic searching movements, frequent cooing and loud screeching, and sporadic brief bursts of play activity. After twenty four to thirty-six hours the pattern changed. The pigtail infants sat hunched over with head down between legs, were inactive, and exhibited social withdrawal, retardation of movement, and sagging facial musculature. After five to six days the depressive phase ("despair") began to lift, and over the next twenty-four days there was recovery alternating with other depressive periods. Upon reunion of pigtail infants with their mothers, there was a reassertion of the dyadic mother–infant relationship marked by clinging by the infant, protective enclosure by the mother, and increased nipple contact ("recovery").

In contrast, when bonnet infants of comparable age had their mothers removed they exhibited nothing resembling the depression described above. It was found that there were increased interactions with other adults in the case of the bonnet macaques, and this seemed to provide adequate substitution for the mother during her absence. For example, each of the five infants in one study achieved sustained ventral-ventral contact with other adults during separation. Such contacts were never observed in the pigtail infants. In summary, the gregarious quality of group interaction in bonnets that manifested itself during the development of infants with their real mothers became even more evident when the mothers were removed.

These studies were important in terms of the different methodology used to accomplish separation, i.e., removal of the mother from a group living situation. They also highlighted the importance of cross-species studies with regard to the nature of maternal attachment, group attachment, and the effects of separation.

Hinde's group[40,41,42] focused its attention on the short- and long-term effects of short separations of rhesus macaques. The animals they studied lived in groups that consisted of a male, two to three females, and their young. Separation was accomplished by removing the mother from the infant's sight. The age of the infants at the time of the original separation was thirty to thirty-two weeks. The length of separation was six days. The infants responded to removal of the mother with behavior similar to that described above for the pigtail infants. They initially exhibited "whoo" calls and were hyperactive. Then there followed a period of "depression," including hunched posture, decreased activity, and social withdrawal. Upon reunion three of the four infants returned to the preseparation level of activity within a week, but the fourth showed less activity up to four weeks afterwards. It was also noted that the less an infant had been in contact with his mother before separation, the less clinging he displayed on return and the more quickly he returned to behavior similar to that seen before separation. This study demonstrated that the nature of the preseparation relationship affected the severity of the reaction to a six-day removal of the mother.

Several other aspects of early separation were studied by Hinde. He theorized that the length of separation was an important variable. Infants who had only a six-day separation experience displayed less depression of activity and recovered from it more rapidly than infants who had a thirteen-day separation or two separate six-day separation experiences. Hinde attempted to describe the source of individual variation among infants in terms of their reaction to separation and concluded that they resulted from differences in the nature of the mother–infant relationship itself.

These same infants were retested when they were twelve and thirty months old—that is, five months and two years after the original separation—to determine if there were any long-term consequences of the early separation experience. It was found that previously separated infants when confronted with strange objects in a strange cage were less likely to approach them than controls, particularly infants with two earlier separation experiences. Thus, the effects of a mere six-day absence from the mother were clearly discernible five months later. When tested two years later, the differences were less marked; however, the previously separated infants were significantly less active than the controls.

Mitchell et al.[75] have studied the effects of forty-eight hour separations of *Macaca mu-atta* (rhesus monkeys) infants from their mother at three different age periods: two months, three and a half months, and five months. At all ages the infants exhibited signs of protest and despair even with such a short separation period. This same group also reported that six of twenty-four infants used in their study showed signs of "detachment" when reunited with their mothers. That is, the mother would try to retrieve the infants as usual, but the infants would screech and run away before finally establishing any ventral contact despite persistent efforts of the mothers to do so.

Preston et al.[81] have extended the research on mother–infant separation to a nonmacaque species (*Erythrocebus patas*). The subjects were six infant patas monkeys who underwent separation from their mothers when they were approximately seven months of age. During the three-week separation each was individually housed, except for one hour a day when the six of them were permitted access to each other. Thus, the infants underwent maternal separation, but had the opportunity to interact with each other during the separation period.

The immediate reaction to removal of their mother was reported to include frequent and intense cooing, frantic searching about, and wide-eyed scanning of the room. The reaction was most intense during only the first half hour, though they continued with high levels of visual searching for several days. The infants also stayed in close proximity to each other and their usual behavior, e.g., play, fell to low levels immediately after removal from the mother, though the infants were reported to have remained "alert." Immediately on reunion, infant–mother nonventral gross contact and oral manipulation rose significantly. Mother–infant approaches—lip smacks and grooming—increased significantly but were short-lived. For example, four infants began peer play within fifteen minutes of their mothers' return.

Without doubt the mother–infant social relationship has received considerable attention. Mother–infant separation studies have been done many times with several species. The reactions of rhesus infants, at least, is surprisingly predictable, though there is certainly individual variation. Severance of the mother–infant bond in rhesus monkeys results in the development of a behavioral picture very similar to anaclitic depression. In some ways this may be a prototype for other depressions, and, if so, a variety of social, biochemical, and rehabilitative studies could be usefully undertaken. For example, are there any brain amine changes that occur coincident with this severe depressive syndrome? Is it reversible or preventable with antidepressants and/or tranquilizers? Are there any psychophysiological correlates? In part the usefulness of a model lies in these kinds of studies that may help elucidate the mechanisms underlying the abnormal behavioral state produced.

(Peer Separation[59,62,64,106]

The technique of peer separation has several advantages that make it a useful complement

to mother–infant separation studies. In the case of peers, one is truly manipulating affectional bonds, and the separation reaction, when it occurs, can be viewed more as an emotional reaction than a survival or adaptive response. Although mother–infant separation disrupts an affectional bond, it is complicated by the infant's dependence on the mother in terms of survival. The ensuing response upon separation has been frequently viewed as the infant's attempt at adaptation for survival. There are also certain obvious practical advantages in terms of the comparative manpower required to effect the two kinds of separations. Also, from a research standpoint there was a serious question about the effects of disrupting peer bonds. Recent studies at Wisconsin indicate that severe reactions can indeed be elicited via separation from objects other than the mother.

In the initial peer separation study, infant rhesus monkeys, reared together from birth in a large living cage but without mothers as illustrated in Figure 15–9, exhibited a very marked reaction when separated from each other at three months of age. Separation was accomplished by placing each of four subjects individually in small cages for four days, then

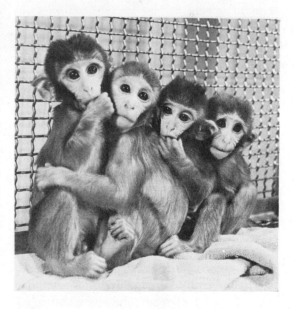

Figure 15–9. Four "together-together" peers prior to undergoing peer separations.

returning them to their home cage as a group for three days. This four-day separation, three-day reunion cycle was repeated weekly a total of twenty times, except for one six-week break between the twelfth and thirteenth separations. To each separation the animals exhibited a protest-despair reaction, with no adaptation to successive separations. High levels of infant-infant clinging characterized the seventy-two hours a week of reunion.[106]

That age is an important factor in determining the form that separation reactions take is indicated in the following peer-separation study.[64] Male rhesus monkeys three years of age were studied before, during, and after a series of four separations from equal-aged peers with which they had formed close social bonds. Each separation lasted two weeks and was followed by a one-week reunion period during which the animals were housed together as a group of four. During each separation there were significant increases in locomotion and environmental exploration and decreases in passivity. Thus, the protest stage was evident; however, there was no suggestion of a "despair" stage as reported in younger monkeys.

An overview would indicate that separation studies thus far provide the best model for certain aspects of a specific syndrome—depression. More specifically the case for a monkey analogue for human anaclitic depression seems strong in the instance of mother–infant separation. The model is becoming sufficiently well defined behaviorally so that brain-biochemical studies, psychophysiological studies, and both social- and biological-rehabilitative approaches can be tried as previously mentioned.

Great caution should be exercised however in viewing anaclitic depression as a prototype or model for all depression. That is why separation studies have recently been extended to older subjects. In contrast to the biphasic protest-despair reaction exhibited by younger monkeys upon separation, three year olds exhibit a uniphasic (protest) response without any evidence of despair. Theories about separation and depression that fail to take into consideration the age of the organism as a fac-

tor in determining response to separation are thus incomplete.

Efforts to produce a despairlike state in older subjects is continuing, and the reactions of several more age groups to separation experiences need to be determined. Also, the possible role of early separation experiences in predisposing a subject to more severe reactions to separations later in life is being pursued in monkeys.

An Approach to Biochemical Studies in Primate Models

One of the reasons for creating primate models for behavioral disorders is to be able to do direct biochemical studies. It is hoped to study rhesus monkey subjects with induced syndromes of psychopathology by directly examining the relationship between brain neurotransmitters and the abnormal behavoirs exhibited. This area of research is in its infancy and, therefore, this discussion is largely an outline of approaches now being used in primate models in order to examine the critical relationships among brain, behavior, and peripheral metabolism.

The following general approaches are proposed to illustrate how primate models might have value in our understanding of the biological substrates of abnormal behavior. They are outlined in Table 15–2.

Work in all these areas is currently underway. Despite external pressures to do so, it would have been premature to engage in biochemical studies until the behavioral aspects of primate models had been sufficiently well established, since the weakest link in most behavioral-biochemical research has been the behavioral aspect. It is also important to consider how to combine a social experiment, where animals either have to live or be tested together in groups and, simultaneously, have biological specimens collected. For instance, in several studies examining the relationship between brain biogenic amines and primate social behavior, the animals lived together in small groups. Urine collection was accom-

TABLE 15–2. **Use of Primate Models for Biological Studies**

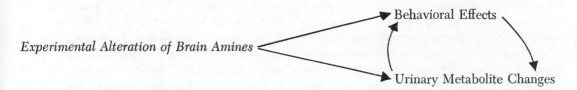

1. Reserpine
2. a methyl-paratyrosine (AMPT)
3. Para-chlorophenylalanine (PCPA)
4. 6-hydroxydopamine
5. Others

Social Induction of Syndromes of Abnormal Behavior

Techniques	*Some Possible Studies*
Social Isolation	Brain Biogenic Amine Levels and Turnover
Separation	Urinary Amine Metabolite Excretion
Vertical Chamber Confinement	Steroids (Plasma and Urine)
	Cyclic AMP
	Others

Biological Rehabilitation

Induction Techniques	*Treatment Methods*
Social Isolation	Phenothiazines
Separation	Minor Tranquilizers
Vertical Chamber Confinement	Antidepressants
Learned Helplessness	Precursors
	Lithium
	Electroshock

plished by pulling an animal from the group and putting him in a restraining chair. This technique seems less than desirable since there are considerable data that indicate severe and persistent effects on primate-group and individual social behavior following removal and reintroduction of members. If group social behavior is used as the major index of drug effect, a hopelessly confused situation ensues.

One technique recently developed involves the use of special monkey metabolism cages where subjects can live individually and have urine collected by simply changing the type of pan beneath the cage. The subjects are adapted to a specifically designed playroom where group social testing is done. At least one twenty-four-to-forty-eight hour period each week is reserved for urine collection

without social testing. Thus, a complete urine collection can be obtained while still getting meaningful group social data on the other days. This problem illustrates the difficulty of doing combined social and biological studies in nonhuman primates, yet this area is being continually developed and may prove to be a very productive area in the next several years as far as development and evaluation of primate models are concerned.

Experimental Alteration of Brain Amine Levels

This approach was suggested in 1969[60] as a method to evaluate the probable importance of biogenic amine metabolism in behavioral disorders, more specifically, depression. The methodology involves selected depletion of one or more of the biogenic amines and careful observations of the resultant behavioral changes in monkey subjects. In a broader sense this approach may permit one to learn more about the role of the monoamines—serotonin, dopamine, and norepinephrine—in the regulation of a variety of activities, e.g., appetite, temperature, sleep, alertness, motor function.

The first study using depletion techniques in monkeys involved the administration of reserpine to rhesus monkeys.[61] Over the years the reserpinized rat has been hailed as an animal model of depression. Despite many biochemical advances that have resulted from studies of rats and cats given reserpine, the suggestion that the behavioral changes seen might model depression is open to serious question. Careful behavioral measures have not usually been included in such studies, especially measures of social interaction. A comparative study in monkeys, where more extensive social data could be obtained, was thus deemed desirable. Reserpine was administered once daily for eighty-one days by nasogastric intubation in a dosage of 4 mgm/kgm to three rhesus monkeys. The subjects were tested both in their home cages and in a playroom with three control subjects who had been given a placebo by nasogastric intubation. Reserpine caused significant decreases in locomotion and visual exploration and increases in huddling and posturing. A reserpinized rhesus monkey is illustrated in Figure 15–10. The reserpine monkeys were not asleep, just extremely inactive, and would respond to social stimulation, though they would not initiate any kinds of social behavior.

Reserpine, however, is a very nonspecific drug since it reduces levels of catecholamines and indoleamines in both the brain and periphery. There are agents that are more specific and there has been some limited experience with them in primate models.

Alpha-methyl-paratyrosine (AMPT) is known to inhibit the enzyme tyrosine hydroxylase thereby blocking norepinephrine synthesis.[102] It has been given to two species of monkeys in two separate experiments.

In one study[65] four rhesus monkeys were given AMPT in a dosage of 250 mgm/kgm and their social behavior was compared with four control subjects given a placebo. Both groups were tested in their home cages and in a playroom setting where social interaction was possible. AMPT-treated monkeys became inactive as exhibited by decreased locomotion, increased passivity, increased huddling, and a decrease in all initiated social behavior. Redmond et al.[84,85] have reported similar findings in stumptail monkeys (Macaca speciosa). The latter research group has also attempted unsuccessfully to reverse the AMPT behavioral syndrome with L-Dopa or with DL,3,4-treodihydroxyphenylserine (DOPS), a compound that penetrates the blood-brain barrier and is decarboxylated directly to L-norepinephrine.[83]

On the other hand para-chlorophenylalamine (PCPA), an inhibitor of serotonin synthesis,[47] has been found by Redmond et al.,[85] as well as McKinney et al.[66] to have little or no effect on the social behavior of monkeys despite very high-dose levels (up to 800 mgm/kgm). These results contrast sharply with the reported aphrodisiac quality and the

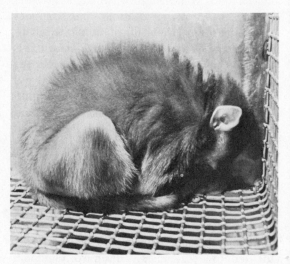

Figure 15–10.   Typical reaction of two-year-old rhesus monkey to daily reserpine (5.0 mgm/kgm) administration.

increased aggression* reported as a result of PCPA administration to rats and cats.

Both AMPT and PCPA have peripheral as well as central effects that are undesirable if one wants to study the relationship between brain amine depletion and behavior. In the spring of 1971, Wisconsin researchers, in collaboration with Drs. Breese, Prange, Howard, and Lipton of the University of North Carolina, began to study the effects of intraventricular 6-hydroxydopamine on the social behavior and on urinary amine metabolites in rhesus-monkey subjects.[8] This study was preceded by considerable work in rats concerning the neuropharmacology of 6-hydroxydopamine. This work had shown it to be a compound that selectively destroyed central noradrenergic neurons without affecting the serotonergic system or peripheral noradrenergic system when given centrally.[9] The goal has been to produce, experimentally, the defect postulated to be important in human depression, namely a central noradrenergic depletion, and to study the effect of this depletion on social behavior and on urinary metabolites. There have also been recent studies,[55,82] of the effects of 6-hydroxydopamine in three *Macaca speciosa* (stumptail) monkeys on their social behavior and on urinary metabolite excretion patterns.

Preliminary reports of the behavioral changes observed following central noradrenergic depletion with 6-hydroxydopamine in both studies consist of decreased activity, decreased alertness, and a decrease in all initiated social behaviors. A monkey given intraventricular 6-hydroxydopamine is illustrated in Figure 15–11. The preliminary nature of these findings is emphasized because the number of subjects studied is still small and there remain many problems in terms of drug toxicity that must be solved before conclusions can be drawn.

An added dimension of the 6-hydroxydopamine studies, which may prove useful, are urinary studies. Many workers have long looked for a urinary marker that would reflect human brain metabolism, since urine is the easiest body fluid to collect in humans. A vari-

* See references 2, 17, 100, 101, 105, 110, 112, and 113.

ety of metabolites including VMA, nometanephrine, and metanephrine have been shown to reflect mostly peripheral metabolism. Three-methoxy, 4-hydroxyphenylglycol (MHPG) has been postulated to be the only urinary metabolite that can be used, even in part, as a measure of brain metabolism.[56,57] In the case of the monkeys referred to in the above studies, when brain norepinephrine was depleted this change tended to be reflected in a decrease in urinary MHPG. However, there was great individual variation and large numbers of subjects will be necessary to fully document the nature of this relationship. There was no change in any of the other urinary metabolites coincident with lowered brain norepinephrine. The use of primate models represents a new approach, but one which may prove increasingly useful in elucidating the biochemical mechanisms underlying depression and, in particular, the relationship between brain and peripheral metabolism.

Socially Induced Syndromes of Psychopathology

The major social-induction techniques that are currently available are social isolation,

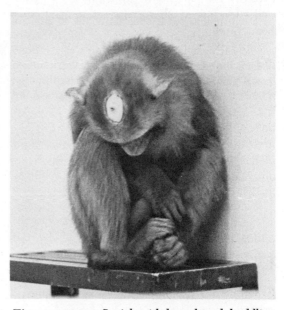

Figure 15–11. Social withdrawal and huddling posture of rhesus monkeys following intraventricular administration of 6-hydroxydopamine.

separation, and vertical-chamber confinement, all of which have been previously described in this chapter. The biochemical effects of each of these induction techniques can now be systematically studied and this research is currently underway. Included are urinary studies, plasma studies, and brain-tissue studies of monkeys who exhibit syndromes of abnormal behavior induced by social means. Steroid metabolism, catecholamine, indoleamine, and cholinergic substrates of these behavioral syndromes are being studied in an effort to relate social stress to specific biological changes.

Biological Reversal of Abnormal Behavior

In this phase of research with primate models, after a syndrome is induced, either socially or biologically, rehabilitative methods are being employed to reverse the abnormal behaviors. In this regard, a study using chlorpromazine was summarized earlier in the chapter. As far as psychopharmacology is concerned, primate models have the potential for eventually providing a better method of preclinical psychotic or antidepressant drug trials than is now available. Also important, however, are the possible implications for a better understanding of the psychopathological state being treated.

Somewhat outside the scope of this chapter, but of importance, is the recent work using monkeys to study the effects of methamphetamine[58] and "speed" usage,[14] the recent use of the chimpanzee as an animal model for alcoholism,[79] and the use of primates to study heroin addiction.[92] In these areas the primate models may also provide key breakthroughs in our understanding of the disease state being modeled.

(Perspectives

Experimental psychopathology in nonhuman primates is at the same time a new and an old field. Historically it has suffered from a too loose use of clinical terms without adequate

behavioral descriptions and the exclusive use of conditioning techniques. As a result clinicians have been uninterested in the field. This lack of interest is surely overdetermined, but hopefully it is changing somewhat as the field itself matures and psychiatrists become increasingly aware of the potential relevance of many fields of inquiry.

The major areas of interest for psychiatrists in primate models probably include the development of kinds of attachment behavior, the effects of social isolation, separation studies, the possible experimental simulation of learned helplessness, and various biological approaches being developed. It is in these areas that work has been and is being conducted that has potential clinical usefulness. Investigators may be close to developing a viable animal model for depression that may facilitate a more comprehensive understanding of this particular syndrome and enable studies to be done that are currently impossible to perform utilizing human beings. The rest of medicine has long used nonhuman primates to advance knowledge about their fields and there is no logical reason why psychiatry should not do the same.

(Bibliography

1. ANDERSON, D. D. and R. PARMENTER. "A Long-Term Study of the Experimental Neurosis in the Sheep and Dog," *Psychosom. Med. Monogr.*, 2–4 (1941), 1–150.

2. APPEL, F. C. "Just Slip This Into Her Drink," *Playboy*, Aug. (1970), 83–86.

3. BABKIN, B. P. "Experimental Neurosis in Animals and Their Treatment With Bromides," *Ed. Med. J.*, 45 (1938), 605–619.

4. BENJAMIN, L. S. "Harlow's Facts on Affects," *Voices*, 4 (1968), 49–59.

5. BOWLBY, J. "Separation Anxiety," *Int. J. Psychoanal.*, 41 (1960), 89–113.

6. ———. "Processes of Mourning," *Int. J. Psychoanal.*, 42 (1961), 317–340.

7. ———. *Attachment and Loss*, Vol. 1. New York: Basic Books, 1969.

8. BREESE, G., A. PRANGE, W. McKINNEY et al. "Behavioral and Biochemical Effects of 6-Hydroxydopamine in Rhesus Monkeys,"

Symposium on Catecholamine Metabolism and Affective Disorders. Am. Psychiatr. Assoc., May 4, 1972.

9. BREESE, G., and T. D. TRAYLOR. "Effect of 6-hydroxydopamine on Brain Norepinephrine and Dopamine: Evidence for Selective Degeneration of Catecholamine Neurons," *J. Pharmacol. Exp. Ther.*, 174 (1970), 413–420.

10. COOK, S. W. "The Production of 'Experimental Neurosis' in the White Rat," *Psychosom. Med.*, 1 (1939), 293–308.

11. CROSS, H. A. and H. F. HARLOW. "Prolonged and Progressive Effects of Partial Isolation on the Behavior of Macaque Monkeys," *J. Exp. Res. Per.*, 1 (1965), 39–49.

12. DWORKIN, S. "Conditioning Neurosis in Dog and Cat," *Psychosom. Med.*, 1 (1939), 388–396.

13. DWORKIN, S., J. BAXT, and E. DWORKIN. "Behavioral Disturbance of Vomiting and Micturition in Conditioned Cats," *Psychosom. Med.*, 4 (1942), 75–81.

14. ELLINWOOD, E. "Effect of Chronic Methamphetamine Intoxication in Rhesus Monkeys," *Biol. Psychiatry*, 3 (1971), 25–32.

15. EVANS, L. S. "Methods of Rearing and Social Interaction in *Macaque Nemestrina*," *Anim. Behav.*, 15 (1967), 263–266.

16. FENICHEL, O. *The Psychoanalytic Theory of Neurosis.* New York: Norton, 1945.

17. FERGUSON, J., S. HENDRICKSON, M. COHEN et al. "Hypersexuality and Behavioral Changes in Cats Caused by Administration of p-Chlorophenylalanine," *Science*, 168 (1970), 499–501.

18. FREUD, S. "Mourning and Melancholia," in *Collected Papers*, Vol. 4, pp. 152–172. London: Hogarth, 1950.

19. FULLER, J. L. and L. D. CLARK. "Genetic and Rx Factors Modifying the Post-Isolation Syndrome in Dogs," *J. Comp. Physiol. Psychol.*, 61 (1966), 251–257.

20. GANTT, W. H. *Experimental Basis for Neonate Behavior.* New York: Harper & Brothers, 1944.

21. GARDNER, B. T. and T. A. GARDNER. "Two-Way Communication With an Infant Chimpanzee," in A. M. Schrier and F. Stollnitz, eds., *Behavior of Nonhuman Primates*, Vol. 4, pp. 117–185. New York: Academic, 1971.

22. GRIFFIN, G. A. and H. F. HARLOW. "Effects of Three Months of Total Social Depriva-tion on Social Adjustment and Learning in the Rhesus Monkey," *Child Dev.*, 37 (1966), 533–547.

23. HAMBURG, D. A. *Psychiatry as a Behavioral Science.* Englewood Cliffs. N.J.: Prentice-Hall, 1971.

24. HARLOW, H. F. "The Nature of Love," *Am. Psychol.*, 13 (1958), 673–685.

25. ———. "Early Social Deprivation and Later Behavior in the Monkey," in A. Abrams, H. H. Garner, and J. E. P. Tomal, eds., *Unfinished Tasks in the Behavioral Sciences*, pp. 154–173. Baltimore: Williams & Wilkins, 1964.

26. ———. "Age-Mate or Peer Affectional System," in D. S. Lehrman, R. A. Hinde, and E. Shaw, eds., *Advances in the Study of Behavior*, Vol. 2, pp. 333–383. New York: Academic, 1969.

27. HARLOW, H. F. and M. K. HARLOW. "The Maternal Affectional System in Rhesus Monkeys," in H. L. Rheingold, ed., *Maternal Behavior in Mammals*, pp. 254–281. New York: Wiley, 1963.

28. ———. "Affection in Primates," *Discovery*, 27 (1966), 11–17.

29. ———. "Learning to Love," *Am. Sci.*, 54 (1966), 234–272.

30. ———. "Effects of Various Mother-Infant Relationships on Rhesus Monkey Behaviors," in B. M. Foss, ed., *Determinants of Infant Behavior IV*, pp. 15–36. London: Methuen, 1969.

31. HARLOW, H. F., M. K. HARLOW, R. O. DODSWORTH et al. "Maternal Behavior of Rhesus Monkeys Deprived of Mothering and Peer Associations in Infancy," *Proc. Am. Philos. Soc.*, 110 (1966), 58–66.

32. HARLOW, H. F. and W. T. MCKINNEY. "Nonhuman Primates and Psychoses," *J. Autism Child. Schizo.*, 1 (1971), 368–375.

33. HARLOW, H. F., G. L. ROWLAND, and G. A. GRIFFIN. "The Effect of Total Social Deprivation on the Development of Monkey Behavior," in P. Solomon and B. C. Glueck, Jr., eds., *Recent Research on Schizophrenia*, pp. 116–135. Psychiatric Research Report 19. Am. Psychiatr. Assoc., 1964.

34. HARLOW, H. F. and S. J. SUOMI. "Induced Psychopathology in Monkeys," *Eng. Sci.*, 33 (1970), 8–14.

35. ———. "Nature of Love Simplified," *Am. Psychol.*, 25 (1970), 161–168.

36. ———. "Social Recovery of Isolation-Reared Monkeys," *Proc. Natl. Acad. Sci.*, 68 (1971), 1534–1538.

37. ———. "Production of Depressive Behaviors in Young Monkeys," *J. Autism Child. Schizo.*, 1 (1971), 246–255.

38. HARLOW, H. F., S. J. SUOMI, and W. T. MCKINNEY. "Experimental Production of Depression in Monkeys," *Mainly Monkeys*, 1 (1970), 6–12.

39. HEBB, D. O. "Spontaneous Neurosis in Chimpanzees," *Psychosom. Med.*, 9 (1947), 3–19.

40. HINDE, R. A. *Animal Behavior: A Synthesis of Ethology and Comparative Psychology.* New York: McGraw-Hill, 1970.

41. HINDE, R. A. and Y. SPENCER-BOOTH. "Effects of Brief Separation From Mother on Rhesus Monkeys," *Science*, 173 (1971), 111–118.

42. HINDE, R. A., Y. SPENCER-BOOTH, and M. BRUCE. "Effects of 6-Day Maternal Deprivation on Rhesus Monkey Infants," *Nature*, 210 (1966), 1021–1023.

43. JENSEN, G. D. and C. W. TOLEMAN. "Mother-Infant Relationship in the Monkey, *Macaca Nemestrina:* The Effect of Brief Separation and Mother-Infant Specificity," *J. Comp. Physiol. Psychol.*, 55 (1962), 131–136.

44. KAUFMAN, I. C. and L. A. ROSENBLUM. "Depression in Infant Monkeys Separated From Their Mothers," *Science*, 155 (1967), 1030–1031.

45. ———. "The Reaction to Separation in Infant Monkeys: Anaclitic Depression and Conservation-Withdrawal," *Psychosom. Med.*, 29 (1967), 648–675.

46. KLÜVER, H. *Behavior Mechanisms in Monkeys.* Chicago: University of Chicago Press, 1933.

47. KOE, B. K. and A. WEISSMAN. "p-Chlorophenylalanine: A Specific Depleter of Brain Serotonin," *J. Pharmacol. Exp. Ther.*, 154 (1966), 499–516.

48. KUBIE, L. A. "The Experimental Induction of Neurotic Reactions in Man," *Yale J. Biol. Med.*, 11 (1939), 541–545.

49. LIDDELL, H. S. "The Alteration of Intestinal Processes Through the Influences of Conditioned Reflexes," *Psychosom. Med.*, 4 (1942), 390–395.

50. ———. "Conditioned Reflex Method and Experimental Neurosis," in J. M. C. V.

Hume, ed., *Personality and the Behavior Disorder*, Vol. 1, pp. 389–412. New York: Ronald Press, 1944.

51. ———. "The Experimental Neurosis," *Ann. Rev. Physiol.*, 9 (1947), 569–580.

52. ———. *Emotional Hazards in Animals and Man.* Springfield, Ill.: Charles C. Thomas, 1956.

53. LIDDELL, H. S., O. D. ANDERSON, E. KOTYUKA et al. "The Effect of Extract of Adrenal Cortex on Experimental Neurosis in Sheep," *Arch. Neurol. Psychiatry*, 34 (1935), 973–993.

54. LIDDELL, H. S. and T. L. BAYNE. "The Development of Experimental Neurasthenia in the Sheep During the Formation of Difficult Conditioned Reflexes," *Am. J. Physiol.*, 81 (1927), 494.

55. MAAS, J. W., H. DEKIRMENJIAN, D. GARVER et al. "Excretion of MHPG After Intraventricular 6-OHDA," Presented to Am. Psychiatr. Assoc., May 4, 1972.

56. MAAS, J. W., J. FAIRCETT, and H. DEKIRMENJIAN. "3-Methoxy-4-Hydroxyphenylglycol (MHPG) Excretion in Depressed States," *Arch. Gen. Psychiatry*, 19 (1968), 129–134.

57. MAAS, J. W. and D. H. LANDIS. "*In Vivo* Studies of the Metabolism of Norepinephrine in the Central Nervous System," *J. Pharmacol. Exp. Ther.*, 163 (1968), 147–171.

58. MACHIYAMA, Y., H. UTENA and M. KIKUCHI. "Behavioral Disorders in Japanese Monkeys Produced by the Long-Term Administration of Methamphetamine," *Proc. Jap. Acad.*, 46 (1970), 738–743.

59. McKINNEY, W. T. "New Models of Separation and Depression in Rhesus Monkeys," in *Separation and Depression: Research and Clinical Aspects.* Symposium at Am. Assoc. Adv. Sci. Meeting. December 1970, Forthcoming.

60. McKINNEY, W. T. and W. E. BUNNEY. "Animal Model of Depression, Review of Evidence: Implications for Research," *Arch. Gen. Psychiatry*, 21 (1969), 240–248.

61. McKINNEY, W. T., R. G. EISING, E. C. MORAN et al. "Effects of Reserpine on the Social Behavior of Rhesus Monkeys," *Dis. Nerv. Syst.*, 32 (1971), 735–741.

62. McKINNEY, W. T., S. J. SUOMI, and H. F. HARLOW. "Depression in Primates," *Am. J. Psychiatry*, 127 (1971), 1313–1320.

63. ———. "Vertical Chamber Confinement of Juvenile Age Rhesus Monkeys," *Arch. Gen. Psychiatry*, 26 (1972), 223–228.

64. ———. "Repetitive Peer Separations of Juvenile Age Rhesus Monkeys," *Arch. Gen. Psychiatry*, in press.

65. McKinney, W. T., S. J. Suomi, I. A. Mirsky et al. "Behavioral Effects of Alpha-Methyl-Para-Tyrosine in Rhesus Monkeys." In preparation.

66. ———. "Parachlorophenylalanine and Rhesus Monkeys." In preparation.

67. McKinney, W. T., L. Young, S. J. Suomi et al. "Reversing the Irreversible," Presented to Am. Psychiatr. Assoc., May 1972.

68. Mason, W. A. "The Effects of Environmental Restriction on the Social Development of Rhesus Monkeys," in C. H. Southwick, ed., *Primate Social Behavior*, pp. 161–173. Princeton: Van Nostrand, 1963.

69. Mason, W. A. and R. R. Sponholz. "Behavior of Rhesus Monkeys Raised in Isolation," *J. Psychiatr. Res.*, 1 (1963), 299–306.

70. Masserman, J. H. "Experimental Neuroses and Group Aggression," *Am. J. Orthopsychiatry*, 14 (1944), 636–643.

71. ———. *Behavior and Neurosis*. New York: Hafner, 1964.

72. Menzel, E. W., R. K. Davenport, and C. M. Rogers. "The Effects of Environmental Restriction Upon the Chimpanzee's Responsiveness to Objects," *J. Comp. Physiol. Psychol.*, 56 (1963), 78–85.

73. ———. "Effects of Environmental Restriction Upon the Chimpanzee's Responsiveness to Novel Stimulation," *J. Comp. Physiol. Psychol.*, 56 (1963), 329–334.

74. Miller, R. E., I. A. Mirsky, W. F. Carl et al. "Hyperphagia and Polydipsia in Socially Isolated Rhesus Monkeys," *Science*, 165 (1969), 1027–1028.

75. Mitchell, G. D. "Abnormal Behavior in Primates," in L. Rosenblum, ed., *Primate Behavior*, pp. 196–253. New York: Academic, 1970.

76. Mitchell, G. D. and D. L. Clark. "Long-Term Effects of Social Isolation in Non-socially Adapted Rhesus Monkeys," *J. Genet. Psychol.*, 113 (1968), 117–128.

77. Mitchell, G. D., H. F. Harlow, and G. W. Moller. "Repeated Maternal Separation in the Monkey," *Psychonom. Sci.*, 8 (1967), 197–198.

78. Pavlov, I. P. *Lectures on Conditioned Reflexes*. New York: Int. Pub., 1928.

79. Pieper, W. A., M. J. Skeen, H. M. Mc-Clure et al. "The Chimpanzee as an Animal Model for Investigating Alcoholism," *Science*, 176 (1972), 71–73.

80. Premack, D. A. "A Functional Analysis of Language," *J. Exp. Anal. Beh.*, 14 (1970), 107–125.

81. Preston, D., R. Baker, and B. Seay. "Mother-Infant Separation in the Patas Monkey," *Dev. Psychol.*, 3 (1970), 298–306.

82. Redmond, D. E., D. Garver, and J. W. Maas. "Primate Behavior and Intraventricular 6-OHDA." Presented at Am. Psychiatr. Assoc., May 4, 1972.

83. Redmond, D. E., J. W. Maas, and C. W. Graham. "The Effect of Norepinephrine Replenishment on Alpha-Methyl-p-Tyrosine Treated Monkeys." Presented at Am. Psychosom. Soc., Boston, April 1972.

84. Redmond, D. E., J. W. Maas, A. Kling et al. "Changes in Primate Social Behavior After Treatment With Alpha-Methyl-Para-Tyrosine," *Psychosom. Med.*, 33 (1971), 97–113.

85. Redmond, D. E., Jr., J. W. Maas, A. Kling et al. "Social Behavior of Monkeys Selectively Depleted of Monoamines," *Science*, 174 (1971), 428–431.

86. Robertson, J. and J. Bowlby. "Responses of Young Children to Separation From Their Mothers," *Courier du Centre International de l'Enfants*, 2 (1952), 131–142.

87. Rosenblum, L. A. and I. C. Kaufman. "Variations in Infant Development and Response to Maternal Loss in Monkeys," *Am. J. Orthopsychiatry*, 83 (1968), 418–426.

88. Sackett, G. P. "Abnormal Behavior in Laboratory Reared Rhesus Monkeys," in M. W. Fox, ed., *Abnormal Behavior in Animals*, pp. 293–331. Philadelphia: Saunders, 1968.

89. ———. "The Persistence of Abnormal Behaviour in Monkeys Following Isolation Rearing," in R. Porter, ed., *CIBA Foundation Symposium on the Role of Learning in Psychotherapy*, pp. 3–37. London: J & A Churchill, 1968.

90. ———. "Innate Mechanisms, Rearing Conditions, and a Theory of Early Experience Effects in Primates," in C. R. Carpenter,

ed., *Proceedings of U.S.-Japan Seminar on Regulatory Mechanisms in Behavioral Development*, pp. 17–53. New York: Academic, 1970.

91. SCHMALE, A. "Relation of Separation and Depression to Disease," *Psychosom. Med.*, 20 (1958), 259–277.

92. SCHUSTER, C. R., JR. "Psychological Approaches to Opiate Dependence and Self Administration by Laboratory Animals," *Fed. Proc.*, 29 (1970), 2–5.

93. SEAY, B., B. K. ALEXANDER, and H. F. HARLOW. "Maternal Behavior of Socially Deprived Rhesus Monkeys," *J. Abnorm. Psychol.*, 69 (1964), 345–354.

94. SEAY, B., E. HANSEN, and H. F. HARLOW. "Mother-Infant Separation in Monkeys," *J. Child Psychol. Psychiatry*, 3 (1962), 123–132.

95. SEAY, B. and H. F. HARLOW. "Maternal Separation in the Rhesus Monkey," *J. Nerv. Ment. Dis.*, 140 (1965), 434–441.

96. SELIGMAN, M. E. P. and D. GROVES. "Non-Transient Learned Helplessness," *Psychonom. Sci.*, 19 (1970), 191–192.

97. SELIGMAN, M. E. P. and S. F. MAIER. "Failure to Escape Traumatic Shock," *J. Exp. Psychol.*, 74 (1967), 1–9.

98. SELIGMAN, M. E. P., S. F. MAIER, and J. GEER. "The Alleviation of Learned Helplessness in the Dog," *J. Abnorm. Psychol.*, 73 (1968), 256–262.

99. SENAY, E. C. "Toward an Animal Model of Depression: A Study of Separation Behavior in Dogs," *J. Psychiatr. Res.*, 4 (1966), 65–71.

100. SHEAD, M. "The Effect of p-Chlorophenylalanine on Behavior in Rats: Relation to Brain Serotonin and 5-Hydroxyindoleacetic Acid," *Brain Res.*, 15 (1969), 524–528.

101. SHILLITO, E. E. "The Effect of p-Chlorophenylalanine on Social Interactions of Male Rats," *Br. J. Pharmacol.*, 36 (1969), 193–194.

102. SPECTOR, S., A. SJOERDSMA, and S. UDENFRIEND. "Blockade of Endogenous Norepinephrine Synthesis by Alpha-Methyl-Tyrosine, An Inhibitor of Tyrosine Hy-

droxylase," *J. Pharmacol. Exp. Ther.*, 147 (1965), 86–95.

103. SPITZ, R. A. "Anaclitic Depression: An Inquiry Into the Genesis of Psychiatric Conditions in Early Childhood," *Psychoanal. Study Child*, 2 (1946), 313–342.

104. STAINBROOK, E. "The Experimental Induction of Acute Animal Behavioral Disorders as a Method of Psychosomatic Research," *Psychosom. Med.*, 9 (1947), 256–259.

105. STOLK, J., J. BARCHAS, W. DEMENT et al. "Brain Catecholamine Metabolism Following Para-Chlorophenylalanine Treatment," *Pharmacologist*, 11 (1969), 258.

106. SUOMI, S. J., C. J. DOMEK, and H. F. HARLOW. "Effects of Repetitive Infant-Infant Separation of Young Monkeys," *J. Abnorm. Psychol.*, 76 (1970), 161–172.

107. SUOMI, S. J. and H. F. HARLOW. "Apparatus Conceptualization for Psychopathological Research in Monkeys," *Behav. Res. Meth. Instr.*, 1 (1969), 247–250.

108. SUOMI, S. J., H. F. HARLOW, and D. S. KIMBALL. "Behavioral Effects of Prolonged Partial Social Isolation in the Rhesus Monkey," *Psychol. Rep.*, 29 (1971), 1171–1177.

109. SUOMI, S. J., H. F. HARLOW, and W. T. McKINNEY. "Monkey Psychiatrists," *Am. J. Psychiatry*, 128 (1972), 927–932.

110. TAGLIAMONTE, A., P. TAGLIAMONTE, G. GESSA et al. "Compulsive Sexual Activity Induced by p-Chlorophenylalanine in Normal and Pinealectomized Male Rats," *Science*, 166 (1969), 1433–1435.

111. TURNER, C., R. K. DAVENPORT, and C. M. ROGER. "The Effect of Early Deprivation on the Social Behavior of Adolescent Chimpanzees," *Am. J. Psychiatry*, 125 (1969), 85–90.

112. WHALEN, R. E. and W. G. LUTTGE. "p-Chlorophenylalanine Methyl Ester: An Aphrodisiac?" *Science*, 169 (1970), 1000–1001.

113. ZITRIN, A., M. A. BEACH, J. D. BARCHAS et al. "Sexual Behavior of Male Cats After Administration of Parachlorophenylalanine," *Science*, 170 (1970), 868–869.

CHAPTER 16

DEVELOPMENTAL PSYCHOBIOLOGY

Seymour Levine

OVER THE last few decades biological scientists have pursued problems that overlap the boundaries of several traditional disciplines. When this interdisciplinary effort has been particularly fruitful, these interface areas themselves have become formal disciplines; for example, biophysics, neurophysiology, neuroendocrinology, psychosomatic medicine, etc. The rapid growth in research activities at the interface of psychology and biology has necessitated the formalization of a new area—psychobiology. Psychobiology is a very extensive area that includes almost all aspects of the influence of biological systems on behavior and the influence of behavior on biological systems. However, within this classification of psychobiology a number of clear subdivisions are represented, such as brain and behavior, chemical modulations of behavior, and developmental psychobiology.

This paper is concerned with some aspects of developmental psychobiology; however, developmental psychobiology is a broad area that encompasses a number of diverse ap-

proaches to the problems of determining how events that occur during critical periods in ontogenesis influence subsequent physiological and behavioral functions. Developmental psychobiologists are interested in the effects of various alterations of environmental and physiological variables in infancy on subsequent physiological function and behavior, both during development and in adulthood. An attempt at a broad review of this field would be a task of enormous proportions, eventually leading to several volumes of the magnitude of this *Handbook*. Thus, for the purposes of this chapter, we will limit our discussion to basically two phenomena that we hope will serve as examples of the field of developmental psychobiology.

The first of these is the effects of a variety of early experimental interventions, predominantly interventions of a psychological nature upon subsequent hormonal function, in particular the pituitary-adrenal system. The second will be a discussion of the effects of alterations in neonatal-hormonal environments on sexual differentiation, with particular references to sexually dimorphic behavior such as sex, aggressions, and emotions. I have taken this course chiefly because of the extensive body of information that is available and second, of course, because of my own involvement in these particular areas of investigation.

❮ Developmental Determinants of the Neuroendocrine Response to Stress

Perhaps the most labile and responsive of all hormonal systems is that associated with the hypothalamo-hypophyseal-adrenal system that results in the ultimate secretion of corticoids from the adrenal cortex. The numerous stimuli that can activate this system are so diverse as to have resulted in the concept by Hans Selye of nonspecific stress.[64] The range of environmental events that lead to the ultimate release of ACTH from the pituitary and corticoids from the adrenal vary from seemingly innocuous situations, such as placing an organism in a strange environment, to the most severe traumatic tissue damage. The essentials of the system's operation in response to stress are as follows. Information concerning the stress (coming either from external sources or from internal sources such as a change in body temperature or in the blood's composition) is received and integrated by the central nervous system (CNS) and is presumably delivered to the hypothalamus, the basal area of the brain. The hypothalamus secretes a substance called the cortiocotropin-releasing factor (CRF) that stimulates the pituitary to secrete the hormone ACTH. This in turn stimulates the cortex of the adrenal gland to increase its synthesis and secretion of hormones, particularly the glucocorticoids. In man the predominant glucocorticoid is hydrocortisone; in many lower animals, such as the rat, it is corticosterone.

The entire mechanism is controlled by a feedback system. When the glucocorticoid level in the circulating blood is elevated, the CNS, receiving the message, inhibits the process that leads to secretion of the stimulating hormone ACTH. Two experimental demonstrations have clearly verified the existence of this feedback process. If the adrenal gland is removed, the pituitary secretes abnormally high amounts of ACTH, presumably because the absence of the adrenal hormone frees it from restriction of this secretion. On the other hand, if crystals of glucocorticoid are implanted in the hypothalamus,[13] the animal's secretion of ACTH stops almost completely, just as if the adrenal cortex were releasing large quantities of the glucocorticoid. However, one of the characteristics of this system is that there are wide individual differences among organisms in response to any given stimulus. This degree of variance could indicate either that a particular stimulus has a different meaning to different organisms or that the same stimulus is responded to differentially as a function of previous events.

This section of the paper represents an attempt to specify some of the factors that contribute to the origin of individual differences in the steroid response to stress. Although there will be no attempt to elaborate a theory to account for such individual differences in stress response, there is the suggestion that such differences originate in the CNS, and that the factors we will cite have their primary action on the organization of the CNS, mediating neuroendocrinological regulation of ACTH release and subsequent steroidogenesis. The steroid response, therefore, is a reflection of the interaction of an organism with its environment. Implicit in this interaction is a perception of the environmental stimuli and integration of the perception to produce a peripheral endocrine response. For such an integrative role the CNS must be the logical candidate. Although central nervous mechanisms governing individual differences in response to stress have not yet been specifically studied, it is difficult to conceive of a peripheral system with the integrative capacity to account for such differences.

Yates and Urquhart[74] have postulated the concept of a centrally located hormonostat that regulates peripheral hormone levels. This concept suggests that there is a regulating mechanism, presumably located in the hypothalamus, that differentially responds to sensory input and peripheral hormonal concentrations to maintain a steady-state, equilibrium concentration for a given stimulus. Differences in the set of the hormonostat should, therefore, produce different peripheral responses to a given stimulus.

Regardless of the postulated central mechanisms to account for such individual differences, there is now clear evidence that major events that occur during sensitive periods of ontogenesis do indeed determine the manner in which organisms respond to a number of environmental events in adulthood. The major determinant of the organism's responsiveness with regard to pituitary-adrenal activity in adulthood appears to be the mother–infant interaction. Subsumed under this major class of environmental determinants are those studies which involve extrastimulation of the developing organism, which have been called either handling or manipulation. I believe that the major influences of extrastimulation result from an alteration of mother–infant interactions as a consequence of treating the young.

Maternal Influences

Extensive clinical and experimental data[8,22] have indicated that manipulation of mother–infant interaction leads to profound and permanent changes in the subsequent behavior of the offspring. In spite of the large amount of evidence that exists relating maternal variables to behavior, there was, until recently, remarkably little information concerning the possible relationship of maternal factors to subsequent physiological function of the offspring. During the past several years a number of laboratories have been concerned with attempting to specify those factors in the life history of the organism which affect the activity of the hypothalamo-hypophyseal-adrenal system.

In a series of studies that were designed to investigate the effects of infantile experience on the development and maturation of the neuroendocrine regulation of ACTH and adrenocortical activity, it was found[36] that handling infant rats as early as three days of age resulted in an increase in plasma corti-

costerone in the handled neonate following stress, whereas no such increase was observed in the nonhandled controls. The fact that nonhandled neonates do not respond to stress as early as three days of age is consistent with the general body of information that indicates that the neonate is generally unresponsive. However, the fact that the handled animals responded so very early in development, without what appears to be the appropriate neural and anatomical maturation for this response to occur, indicated that one of the possible mediators for the observed effects of infantile handling on the pituitary-adrenal system in the newborn was an alteration in the maternal–infant relationships, either in terms of changing maternal behavior or perhaps of modifying the physiological interactions between mother and young. Support for this hypothesis came from preliminary observations in our own laboratory where it was observed in rats that mothers of handled infants had significantly higher plasma corticosteroids than did mothers of nonhandled infants at three days. Further, a study by Young[75] indicated that lactating females showed a distinct preference on retrieval tests for warm, as opposed to cold, pups. These observations led to a series of investigations that studied the effects of various aspects of mother–infant environment on subsequent adrenocortical activity of the offspring.

Levine and Treiman[47] studied, in mice, the role of both genetic and maternal environmental determinants on adult adrenocortical function. They measured circulating plasma corticoids following a brief exposure to electric shock and reported striking differences between four inbred strains of mice. The observed differences were quantitative in terms of the amount of circulating steroids following stress, and qualitative in terms of the different time course of the stress response between different inbred strains. Thus, the DBA/2 strain showed the maximum elevation of corticosteroids approximately fifteen minutes after the base exposure to electric shock, but by the end of sixty minutes had begun to return to the normal basal levels. In contrast, the C57 BL/10 strain was still significantly elevated by the end of sixty minutes. Subsequently[71] the two strains, C57 BL/10 and DBA/2, which had been shown to differ in the steroid response to electric shock, were crossed in all four possible combinations to provide a two by two diallel cross, allowing genetic and maternal effects to be assessed. The offspring were tested under two conditions as adults, control and electric shock. The control animals were removed from their cages and rapidly sampled for corticosterone. Shocked animals were placed in the shock compartment and given an electric shock to the feet for one minute. They were then placed in a holding cage and decapitated at one of three time intervals, following the termination of shock— one minute, fifteen minutes, and sixty minutes. The data indicated that the maternal environment is a clear and important modifier of the quantitative and qualitative aspects of steroid response to electric shock. Thus, C57 BL/10 and C × D crosses, that is, hybrid mice whose mothers came from the C57 BL/10 strain, showed identical patterns of steroidogenesis following stress. In contrast, the DBA/2 and the D × C crosses, whose mothers were of the DBA/2 strain, also showed identical patterns of elevations of plasma corticosteroids. Thus, the steroid response of the hybrid animals was dependent upon the mother of the hybrid. The hybrid animals with the C mothers were identical to their parent strain, C57 BL/10 and in contrast, the hybrid offspring with D mothers were identical to their maternal strain.

Perhaps an even more dramatic series of studies demonstrating the role of maternal influences on the adult patterns of corticosteroid response to stress are those reported by Denenberg and coworkers.[14,29,30] Denenberg and coworkers have demonstrated that C57 BL/10 mice when fostered to lactating rat mothers were markedly less aggressive, less active in an open field, and preferred a rat to a mouse in a two-choice, social-preference test. Further experiments established that one of the principal variables involved in the behavior was the rat mother.

These investigators further reported[15] that when Swiss albino mice were fostered to rat mothers to study the relationship between open-field activity and corticosteroid response following exposure to the open field, it was found that rat-reared mice gave a significantly lower corticosterone response to the novel stimuli of the open field than mouse-reared mice, or rat-reared rats. The mouse reared by the rat mother showed a marked modification of its plasma corticosterone response following exposure to novelty. The rat mother could be influencing the mouse offspring either through her behavioral interactions with the pups between birth and weaning or through biochemical factors present in her milk.

In a recent experiment, in order to bypass the problems of rat milk influencing the mouse offspring, Denenberg and coworkers[16] reared mouse offspring with nonlactating adult female rats—"aunts"—together with pregnant female mice in the expectation that the rat would engage in the usual caretaking activities while the mouse would supply the milk for the young.

In one experiment, mice tended by rat aunts had a significantly lower corticosterone response to novel stimuli of being isolated for thirty minutes. In addition, the aunt-reared group was less active in the open field than the control group. In a second experiment, testing was approximately six months after weaning. Again, significant corticosterone differences were obtained with a group tended by aunts, yielding a lower value than controls. As in the first experiment, the aunt-reared group again had lower activity.

From these experiments it can be concluded that changes in adrenocortical activity and open-field behavior are brought about through behavioral mechanisms involved in the interaction between mothers and young rather than through biochemical differences in the milk of the rat and mouse mothers. These differences also appear to be permanent and profound and persist well into adulthood.

There are several further studies that also clearly indicate the maternal influence on subsequent pituitary-adrenal activity in the offspring. Denenberg and Whimbey[17] reported that in rats the offspring of mothers that had been handled in infancy were heavier at weaning than young rats of mothers that had not been handled. Further, the experience of the mother during her infancy resulted in different open-field behavior of the pups when they reached adulthood. It has been reported[35] that the offspring of mothers that had been handled in infancy show a reduced plasma steroid response to novel stimuli when compared to weaning rats of nonhandled mothers, although both groups of offspring themselves received no experimental intervention. Further, if the offspring are handled, the differences resulting from maternal differences are abolished. This can be interpreted in either of two ways: first, direct stimulation of the pups is so profound that it overrides the maternal influence or, second, handling the infant alters the maternal responses, and disturbance of the mother as a function of infantile handling tends to counteract the influence of the experience of the mother during her infancy. The work reported in this paper tends to favor the second of these interpretations.

Thus far we have discussed a variety of experiments that have resulted in a reduction of the plasma corticosterone response to stress in the offspring of both rats and mice, and mice reared with rats. Maternal influences, or the lack of maternal influences, can also lead to a significant increase in plasma corticosterone response to a variety of environmental stimuli.

Exposing a lactating female to a stressful experience results in a modification of the stress response in the offspring.[46] Lactating females were subjected to ether exposure at three, six, or nine days postpartum. An additional group of mothers was subjected to electric shock at three days following birth. The offspring of these females were not disturbed during this period. The data indicate that the offspring of females stressed while nursing showed a significantly greater elevation of plasma corticoids following exposure to novel stimuli when compared to nontreated controls. The absence of a mother during nursing in the rat also leads to a significant augmentation of the response to stress in maternally deprived rat infants.[69]

A technique has been developed for hand-rearing newborn rats. Thus rats can be separated immediately after birth and reared successfully through weaning by the use of the specific set of techniques, which have been described in detail by Thoman and Arnold.[68] This technique involves rearing the animals in an incubator in which there is a warm, moist, pulsating tube that serves as a surrogate to provide warmth and stimulate defecation in the newborn rat. The animals are tube fed at four-hour intervals until they are capable of eating solid food. A group of these hand-reared animals was tested in adulthood for their adrenocortical response to ether. Hand-reared animals showed a significant elevation in basal levels and a significantly greater increase in plasma corticosterone concentrations following stress than did mother-reared animals. Although these data tend to implicate a maternal factor, it should be noted that this procedure is a complicated one involving a large amount of stimulation in the process of hand feeding as well as different dietary conditions, in addition to the many other conditions that differ from normal rearing. Although the evidence appears to indicate that the absence of a mother results in altered pituitary-adrenal activity in adulthood, it would be difficult to specify that only removal from the mother leads to the differences observed in these experiments.

It is surprising that while there is a large and extensive literature that demonstrates the very profound influences of maternal deprivation in certain primates,[49] there has been an almost total absence of an examination of the physiological influences of these procedures on the adult monkey. One can only hope that, with the availability of better techniques for measuring circulating cortisol in the primate, these studies will soon be accomplished.

Data presented above indicate that the nature of the mother–infant environment is an important determinant of subsequent neuroendocrine regulation of ACTH. The data presented along with the extensive literature on maternal variables affecting behavior emphasize the total organismic effect of those events occurring during critical periods in development. In the mammal this critical period is intimately shared with the mother and it is not surprising, therefore, that maternal variables should affect many aspects of the total system's function.

Infantile Stimulation and Stress

Early research on the influence of infantile stimulation on behavior dealt with rats treated immediately postnatally either by simply being picked up once daily and placed in a different environment or by being given a brief electric shock once daily from the period immediately following birth until weaning at twenty-one days of age. In adulthood, when placed in a novel environment, these animals explored more freely and defecated less and when placed in avoidance-conditioning situations, they appeared to show "more adaptive behavior" by learning the avoidance conditioning significantly more rapidly.[33,40] These results also indicated no difference in the later effects between a seemingly innocuous treatment such as simply manipulating the animal or more severe procedures such as shock and shaking.[42] It was therefore concluded that the effects of infantile stimulation were a direct consequence of "stressing" the infant organism and that such stressful infantile experiences resulted in the animal's developing a capacity for being more adaptive. Implicit in this conclusion is that infantile stimulation provides a form of emotional immunization. That is, exposing an animal to stress early in ontogenesis modifies its subsequent stress response such that the emotional response is of a lesser degree, and the animal does perform in a more optimal fashion. The physiological effects of infantile stimulation tended to support this conclusion. Levine and Otis demonstrated[45] that animals that had been stimulated in infancy survived longer under a severe chronic stress of total food and water deprivation.

Other studies indicated that adrenal hypertrophy, which occurs under conditions of chronic stress, was significantly greater in nonmanipulated animals.[32] It is important to note, however, that these experiments dealt with animals placed in relatively chronic situations leading to a prolonged stress response and that these sustained responses can and

often do lead to pathological changes in the organism. Experiments based on more acute stressful conditions, both in the infant and the adult organism, tended to indicate that quite contrary to the original hypothesis, the stimulated animal was indeed more responsive to stress under some conditions. This has been demonstrated in an investigation of the effects of infantile stimulation on the acute response to a brief electric shock.[34] Adult rats subjected to a brief electric shock were sampled at various periods of time following exposure to the stimuli, and their plasma corticoids were determined. The manipulated animals showed a much more significant rise and, for the period measured, showed a more sustained increase in adrenal steroids. Further studies have demonstrated, however, that although the stimulated animals do show a more rapid elevation of plasma corticoids, thus indicating a more immediate secretion of ACTH, they do tend to return to base levels significantly sooner than do nonmanipulated animals.[26] It is clear from these data that the simple proposition that infantile stimulation reduces physiological and emotional responsiveness to stress was in error and, in fact, the animals manipulated in infancy appear to be more sensitive to their environment. On the basis of this experiment, an alternate hypothesis was developed that postulates that one of the major consequences of early stimulation may be to endow the organism with the capacity to make finer discriminations concerning the relevant aspects in the environment. The animal then is able to make responses more appropriate to demands of the environment, including appropriate responses to stress. Perhaps this is the real meaning of adaptiveness, the ability to make the appropriate discrimination in a particular situation and respond according to the demands of that situation. A more generalized response pattern, based on gross discriminations or, in fact, a lack of discrimination, appears to be characteristic of the nonmanipulated animal and leads to responses that are often inappropriate to the situation. Such responses may be viewed as maladaptive. Having thus postulated that the manipulated animals possess the capacity for more appropriate discrimination, we should then be able to predict that their responses to novel situations, where the environmental changes are not so drastic, would be much less than that of nonmanipulated animals.

In an experiment conducted by Levine et al.[41] rats were handled for the first twenty days in infancy and compared to nonhandled controls. In adulthood these animals were subdivided and tested in open field for one, two, three, or four days. Activity and defecation in the open field were recorded and, in addition, following the termination of testing, the animals were killed either immediately, five minutes afterward or fifteen minutes afterward, and plasma corticosterone was determined. Animals handled in infancy were more active in the open field on the last three test days, defecated less on all of the test days, and had a significantly lower corticosterone response on all four of the days. These data allow one to draw the conclusion that stimulation in infancy results in an animal that is less responsive to novel stimuli as measured both at the behavioral and physiological level. Thus, to reiterate, in situations where distinctly noxious stimuli are involved, the handled animal seems to be more active in terms of its pituitary-adrenal system. However, where the test situation does not inolve intense noxious stimulation, the steroid response of the handled animal is of a smaller magnitude. The nonhandled animal appears to discriminate less and reacts with a large corticosterone response regardless of the specific aspects of the test situation.

Development and Early Experience

Thus far we have been concerned predominantly with the long-term effects of variations in the environment of the neonate. The psychobiologists, however, have also investigated the developmental consequences of early environment. The results of these studies have found that the rate of development is also dependent upon variations in the infantile environment. It has been observed that stimulated organisms are heavier at weaning and maintain these weight differences through adulthood. The normal time of eye opening in nonstimulated animals is approximately fifteen to sixteen days. Stimulated rats open their eyes at about thirteen to fourteen days, and eye opening has been observed as early as twelve days of age. Following these observations of differences in the development of gross morphological characteristics, there has been a series of investigations into the effects of early stimulation on other aspects of development. In the first of these studies,[38] the maturation of the hypothalamo-hypophyseal-adrenal system was studied. Prior to the advent of appropriate measures of circulating plasma corticosterone, one response of the rat adrenal to ACTH that was used as an indicant of adrenal function was the depletion of ascorbic acid present in the adrenal. It had been demonstrated that infant rats do not respond to environmental stress with depletion of adrenal ascorbic acid until about sixteen days of age. This was true in nontreated animals. However, animals handled in infancy showed a significant adrenal, ascorbic-acid response as early as twelve days of age.

Since the maturation of the neuroendocrine regulation of ACTH is indicative of one aspect of neural development, which appeared to be accelerated as a consequence of infantile stimulation, it seemed reasonable that other aspects of neural development would also show similar acceleration. Thus myelination in the CNS has been shown to occur earlier in animals stimulated neonatally.[37] Meier demonstrated[50] an earlier onset in adult EEG patterns in Siamese kittens that had been handled. These findings would indicate that neural maturation is accelerated as a consequence of infantile stimulation. Altman et al.[1] have investigated whether handling during infancy has any effect upon the development of the brain, with particular attention to the rate and kinetics of cell proliferation and other quantifiable aspects of brain development. Rats were handled daily from day two to day eleven after birth. These animals and unhandled controls were injected on day eleven with radioactively labeled precursor of DNA and killed either six hours, three, or thirty days later. In a subsequent experiment, uninjected rats were permitted to survive until eleven, fourteen, forty-one, or one hundred and one days of age. Brain-weight measurements were taken in all animals, and the brains were compared for histology and autoradiography, and evaluated. These investigators found the following differences between the brains of handled and nonhandled animals: (1) the brains of the handled animals were consistently lighter than controls at eleven and fourteen days of age and these differences were not associated with differences in body weight; (2) planimetric measurements of sampled regions show that the brain-weight differences were correlated with areal size differences, and (3) autoradiographic cell counting indicated that cell proliferation and the formation of new microneurons were higher following injection of the radioactive precursor in the handled animals than in nonhandled rats.

Thus, in contrast to the aforementioned studies that have indicated more rapid neural development as a consequence of handling, the weight and areal measurements indicated that the brains of the handled animals were retarded in development. The autoradiographic cell counts also appeared to indicate some aspects of retarded brain development in the handled animals. In the nonhandled animals cell proliferation declined by the latter half of the second week. The cell proliferation was still brisk during this period in the handled animals, which would indicate further a delay in brain maturation. Altman interprets his data as follows:

How can this effect, the decelerated maturation of the brain, be related to the adaptive superiority displayed by handled animals in adulthood? We have postulated elsewhere that the postnatal origin of the modulatory microneurons in some brain structures may represent an opportunity for the exertion of input-regulated (behavioral) control over the finer aspects of the interconnection of neurons. This would imply that delay in the proliferation and migration of the precursors of microneurons extends the time available for the exertion of environmental modulatory influences on the organization of the brain. This hypothesis is akin to the concepts of "fetalization"[7,18] and "infantilization" postulated by writers on anthropogenesis,

which denote the retention of fetal properties after birth and excessively prolonged postnatal development, respectively, as biological characteristics of man. These evolutionary adaptations are conceived to provide longer opportunity for the exertion of environmental influences on the organization of the control mechanisms of behavior. The specific hypothesis that we are presenting here is that infantilization, which is a property shared by all altricial species, is not entirely genetically determined but is subject, during a critical period of development, to environmental influences, such as some factor (stress?) inherent in the handling procedure. [p. 19][1]

Although it is difficult at this time to reconcile those studies which report an acceleration in the maturation of certain neural systems and the study by Altman, which shows a retardation of some other neural systems, it is clear that there are definitive environmental influences on the maturation of the structure and function of the brain. These alterations in neural development and function are observed throughout the life history of the organism in alterations of behavioral and physiological processes.

❲ Hormones in Infancy

Thus far in this paper we have dealt primarily with the influence of various environmental conditions upon the subsequent neuroendocrine activity of the adult animal. However, this section of the paper deals with another experimental approach used by the developmental psychobiologist, namely, altering physiological processes during infancy and studying the influence upon subsequent development and behavior. The best example of this type of investigation comes from a now extensive series of studies that have investigated the influence of the presence or absence of specific gonadal hormones during critical periods in development on adult, sexually dimorphic behavior.

Under normal circumstances, the adult female rat becomes sexually receptive during a period in the estrous cycle when there exists the appropriate hormonal balance between estrogen and progesterone that results in ovulation. Sexual receptivity of the female rat is manifested by the presence of a lordosis response. If the female is deprived of the appropriate circulating hormones by ovariectomy, sexual receptivity is immediately abolished. However, when the appropriate hormones are replaced either in the form of chronic high doses of estrogen or small doses of estrogen followed by progesterone, sexual receptivity appears within a very short time following progesterone administration. Sexual behavior of the male involves a much more complex pattern of mounts with intromissions and ejaculation. In contrast to the cyclic pattern of receptivity exhibited by the female, the adult male is acyclic in his sexual behavior and will under normal conditions copulate as long as there is an appropriate stimulus object. Again in contrast to the female, when the male is castrated there ensues a period of time during which the male is sexually active even in the absence of circulating androgens.[31] However, eventually the male will cease normal sexual activity. But, following androgen replacement, it will resume behavior that is indistinguishable from that of the normal intact male. However, no amount of estrogen and progesterone has yet proved capable of reliably eliciting in an adult castrate male patterns of sexual behavior that are typical of the normal female. Adult castrate females administered testosterone propionate (TP) will exhibit mounting and mounts with behavioral patterns that closely resemble intromission.

It has been suggested[27,76] that gonadal hormones act on the central nervous system in different ways at two different stages of development. First, during fetal or neonatal life, sex hormones organize the sexually undifferentiated brain with regard to patterns of gonadotrophin secretion and sexual behavior. Specifically, this hypothesis states that androgens, acting on the central nervous system during critical periods in development, are responsible for the programming of male patterns of gonadotrophin secretion and sex behavior in much the same way that they determine the development of anatomical sexual characteristics. Second, during adult life gonadal hormones activate the sexually differentiated brain and elicit the responses that were programmed earlier. Third, one of the components of the process of sexual differentiation is to render the tissues that are responsive to gonadal hormones differentially sensitive in the male and the female.[44]

The evidence regarding normal patterns of sexual behavior and their dependency upon circulating hormones is consistent with the hypothesis that there are differences between the male and the female central nervous system with regard to patterns of hormone secretion and behavior. First, whereas the female is cyclic in her sexual activity, the male tends to be acyclic. Second, the female pattern of sexual receptivity is easily elicited with the appropriate regime of estrogen and progesterone replacement following castration, whereas in the male these patterns appear to be completely suppressed and cannot be elicited with doses of estrogen and progesterone that are a thousand-fold higher than those required in the female. Thus, one of the primary aspects of sexual differentiation in the rat appears to be the suppression of the capacity of the normal male to respond to estrogen and progesterone.[73]

Although the designations male and female have been used in a seemingly specific way with regard to sexual behavior, there are many experiments that cast doubt upon the validity of making behavioral distinctions between male and female rats. While normal male rats almost never exhibit any of the kinds of behavior that female rats show during estrus, lordosis cannot be called a genetically determined "female" response, since it will be shown that males castrated at birth will exhibit this behavior when administered estrogen and progesterone. As has been mentioned, normal female rats will often perform behavioral mounts and intromission patterns identical in form to those exhibited by male rats, although the quantity and temporal patterning of these responses is different. Behavioral ejaculation has been reported in genetic females.[43]

These facts, coupled with the occurrence of mounting behavior in the prepuberal play of

both sexes, make it very difficult to make rigorous behavioral distinctions between male
and female rats. One way of establishing criteria for the validation of male and female
behavior is to use as a basis the behavioral
patterns necessary for successful reproduction.
Thus, mounts and intromissions and ejaculation patterns could be termed male reproductive behavior, since these are the patterns that
animals must exhibit in order for fertilization
to take place. This, however, leaves the problem of finding some new term to describe the
mounting that is done by females. Another,
and perhaps the most satisfactory way of dealing with this problem, is to describe the behavior involved with no reference to its maleness and femaleness. Thus, a lordosis is a
given pattern of behavior without regard to
the genetic sex of the animal performing it. In
the same way, a mount is a behavior pattern
that involves a given sequence of motor acts.
Since the experiments we will describe involve
many situations in which genetic males and
females are treated with homotypical and
heterotypical hormones, the definitional problem is best handled by referring to these patterns themselves rather than to the maleness
or femaleness of a given behavior.

In 1959, Young and his colleagues[60] reported that administering testosterone to the
pregnant guinea pig resulted in the birth of
pseudohermaphroditic female offspring that
failed to respond normally to gonadal hormones in adulthood. As adults the female offspring of testosterone-treated pregnant guinea
pigs did not become receptive to males when
treated with estrogen and progesterone. They
did display an unusually high frequency of
mounting responses when administered with
testosterone. These findings were interpreted
to indicate that gonadal hormones played a
crucial role during development in a differentiation of neural tissues that mediate sexual
behavior in the adult organism.

Research on the rat also indicated that if
large amounts of TP were administered to the
newborn female rat within the first five days
of life mating behavior was abolished. However, in these experiments, mating behavior
was defined as the presence or absence of

sperm in the vagina when placed with a vigorous sexually active male.[63] In 1962, Harris
and Levine[28] injected five-day-old female rats
with a single dose of 500 μg of TP. As adults
these animals failed to exhibit lordosis when
injected with large doses of estrogen and progesterone. Goy, Phoenix, and Young[23] gave 1
mg of TP for seven consecutive days beginning on days one, ten, or twenty after birth.
Those female rats receiving injections starting
on day one and ten showed markedly decreased female sex behavior when given estrogen and progesterone in adulthood. Thus, it
appeared as though the presence of androgen
prenatally in the guinea pig and postnatally in
the rat was capable of abolishing the normal
patterns of receptivity in the female that are
elicited by estrogen and progesterone replacement. However, Barraclough and Gorski[2,3]
reported a behavioral dichotomy between female rats receiving high and low doses of TP
neonatally. Whereas females receiving 1.25
mg of TP at five days of age would not exhibit
lordosis, even when primed with estrogen and
progesterone following castration in adulthood, females receiving 10 μg of TP were consistently sexually receptive when intact and
did respond to estrogen and progesterone
after castration.

Levine and Mullins administered to independent groups of neonatal females doses of
TP ranging from 5 to 1000 μg. These females
fell into three distinct groups with regard to
their capacity to exhibit lordosis in adulthood.
Animals receiving 5 to 10 μg of TP in infancy
showed the pattern of behavior reported by
Barraclough and Gorski of continual receptivity on seven consecutive nights. Animals receiving 50 μg of testosterone tended to show
receptivity early in the testing procedure, but
toward the latter part of the test series showed
a marked drop in female sexual receptivity.
Finally, animals receiving 100 μg or above
showed very low mount-to-lordosis ratios.

It is interesting to note that although the
low-dose females were judged to be receptive,
their behavior was quite different from that
seen in normal estrous females. The darting,
hopping, and ear wiggling were almost entirely absent. The passivity of these animals

was exhibited by the nature of the lordosis. Untreated female rats will lordose when mounted by the male, but will hop away and often groom as soon as he dismounts. The TP females, however, would frequently freeze with their head near the floor and their hindquarters elevated and hold this position until the male ejaculated. When these females were judged nonreceptive, many just sat with their backs hunched while the male attempted to mount instead of exhibiting the vigorous back kicking seen in untreated nonreceptive females.

In this experiment, all females were ovariectomized and, following a two-week period, were injected with estrogen and progesterone. It is interesting to note that the lordosis to mount ratios observed with estrogen and progesterone replacement were identical to those observed during the first night of testing when intact. These results appear to be another example of the differential sensitivity of the neural tissues mediating sexual behavior and to indicate that all the circulating hormone is able to replace is that level of behavior which will normally be exhibited when the animal's own endogenous hormones are active. These data do raise many questions, however, concerning the capacity of neonatal androgen to masculinize female rats. Under all doses of androgen the ovaries are atrophied and there is no evidence of ovulation in any of the TP-treated groups. However, the low dose of TP treatment appears to produce an organism that is by no means incapable of exhibiting lordosis, albeit in many of these animals the pattern of lordosis appears to be aberrant. The data concerning neonatal androgen treatment in females tend to be ambiguous. Whereas the patterns of gonadotrophin secretion always appear to be acyclic, the effects of sexual behavior are paradoxical.

In contrast, it does appear that removal of the androgens prior to sexual differentiation uniformly leads to marked behavioral and physiological feminization of the animal. Thus, male rats that have been castrated twenty-four hours after birth appear capable of exhibiting cyclic patterns of gonadotrophin secretion that result in cyclic ovulation.[27,59]

Grady, Phoenix, and Young[24] castrated male rats on days one, five, ten, twenty, thirty and ninety after birth and administered estrogen and progesterone to these animals when they were one hundred and twenty to one hundred and fifty days of age. Animals castrated within twenty-four hours after birth displayed a lordosis response that was indistinguishable from that of normal female rats when mounted by sexually active males. Those animals which had been castrated at five days of age showed a marked reduction in lordosis, while those castrated after five days of age failed to display lordosis when mounted. This finding has been replicated by several investigators.[21,73] Whalen and Edwards[73] reported further that males that had been castrated in infancy and given 2.5 mg. of TP at the time of castration failed to exhibit the lordosis response following estrogen and progesterone in adulthood. In a similar study,[54] Mullins and Levine demonstrated that doses as low as 10 μg of TP given to the neonatal castrate at ninety-six hours after birth were also capable of suppressing lordosis in the adult male animal when given the appropriate hormonal treatment in adulthood. It should be noted that this dose of androgen given to the female does not abolish the lordosis response and, in fact, results in an animal that is continually responsive to a sexually active male.[55] It appears that even at birth the genetic male is differentially sensitive to androgen. Thus, whereas androgen given to the female does not suppress sexual receptivity, androgen given to the male deprived of its gonads at this time strikingly suppresses sexual receptivity. One possible explanation for this suppression of the lordosis response in these males is the possibility that these animals have had functioning testes present until shortly after birth. The secretions of the fetal gonads may already have sensitized the neural mechanisms that mediate the lordosis response, so that the injection of TP four days after castration resulted in the observed suppression. Further evidence of the ability of androgen present in infancy to sensitize neural mechanisms to later injections of androgen is given by Morrison and Johnson.[51] A genetically determined sensitivity to neonatal testosterone might also explain the difference observed between the males and females that received the lower doses. Since the females given the lower doses of TP did exhibit lordosis while the females with higher doses did not, it is possible that more than one injection of the smaller amounts would be necessary in order to duplicate the conditions found in the normal male. However, it should be noted that at all doses of androgen the male suppression of the lordosis response is always greater than that observed in the female.

Thus far we have focused primarily on the presence or absence of the estrogen-progesterone-induced lordosis response with little mention of those behavior patterns normally associated with the "male." Although it does appear necessary to bring these patterns of behavior into this discussion, they are confounded by many of the manipulations performed neonatally. As mentioned before, the female appears to have represented in the CNS the capacity to exhibit mounting and mounting with intromissions. Although Harris and Levine[28] reported that female rats treated with 500 μg of TP ninety-six hours after birth showed more frequent and vigorous mounting than control females, this result has not been systematically reproduced. Finally, males castrated in infancy do not develop a normal penile structure, and the cornified papillae of the penis appear to be insensitive to androgen treatments later in life.[56] It thus becomes difficult to discuss intromissions and ejaculations in organisms that have deficient penile structure.

Throughout this paper we have made the assumption that the function of gonadal hormones in infancy is to organize the CNS with regard to neuroendocrine function and patterns of behavior.

It is important to note that the concept of organization of the CNS does not necessarily imply that there are structural changes in the brain as a consequence of these gonadal hormones. In fact, it appears that one of the major influences of testosterone on the developing brain is to alter the thresholds of sensitivity to hormones in adulthood. Males that

have been castrated in infancy are now rendered sensitive to minute quantities of estrogen and progesterone and will under these treatments exhibit normal lordosis. In contrast, neonatal androgenization of the female abolishes the behavioral response to progesterone; similarly, neonatal castration makes the male rat subject to progesterone facilitation. Clemons et al.[11] have proposed that the reason female rats that have been treated with androgen do not exhibit lordosis is because they are now insensitive to progesterone treatment. There have been many studies that have also shown that thresholds of response to estrogen are clearly depressed in androgenized females.

Although the relationship between differentiation of male and female behavior patterns is still unsettled, the organizational effects of early androgen might conform to a "one anlage" model of differentiation in which a single undifferentiated mechanism in the brain of the fetus is influenced by androgen to develop in the male direction. This is analogous to the genital tubercle that differentiates either to a penis or to a clitoris, with intermediate forms but not dual structures as possible outcomes of incomplete differentiation. Alternatively, a "two anlage" model might apply, resembling the process of reproductive-tract differentiation. In this case, although the development of the male primordium usually parallels the suppression of the female primordium, both are actually retained, albeit vestigially, into adulthood, and the possibility exists of simultaneous development of both primordia. In favor of the double anlage hypothesis is the well-established fact that normal adults of both sexes can respond to heterotypical gonadal hormones by showing heterotypical sexual behavior.

Although we have focused, thus far, primarily on reproductive behavior, there have been numerous reports in the literature that have indicated that there are sex differences in nonsexual behavior.

In recent years, we have seen a growing emphasis on the physiological mechanisms regulating aggressive behavior. Aggressive behavior is generally studied in the laboratory by two principal methods. The first is the observation of spontaneous aggression that occurs frequently in laboratory mice and is usually seen when individuals are exposed to each other following a fairly long period of isolation. Spontaneous aggression is sexually dimorphic, occurring predominantly in males and rarely in females. The second laboratory method utilizes a procedure originated by Ulrich and Azrin[72] called shock-induced aggression, and is used generally in rats. Pairs of animals are placed in a small compartment and a train of electric shocks is delivered, in response to which the animals take a characteristic fighting posture, strike at each other, and usually show a full pattern of fighting behavior. This is also sexually dimorphic, as it is elicited more easily in male than in female rats.

The role of androgens in the regulation of spontaneous aggression was noted as early as 1947 by Beeman.[6] Subsequent studies have all indicated that castration usually inhibits or markedly suppresses this behavior. In contrast to castrated males, which show the full pattern of isolation-induced aggressive behavior following testosterone replacement, females do not show spontaneous or androgen-induced aggression.[70] Normally male mice did not show spontaneous aggression against females.[62] However, Mugford and Nowell[52] have shown that the tendency for male mice to attack females was increased significantly if the females were given a course of testosterone treatments.

On the basis of previous work, Mugford and Nowell[53] concluded that the change in androgenized female mice was not due directly to some pheromone that is released as a consequence of androgen, but rather that the female releases a pheromone in her urine that normally inhibits attack and that the treatment with androgen appears to suppress this urinary substance, thus changing the female's stimulus properties.

In view of the highly predictable sexual dimorphism in aggressive behavior in mice, it seems natural that the possible "organizational" role of testosterone in differentiation of aggressive behavior should receive considerable attention.

Conner and Levine[12] have demonstrated that neonatally castrated male rats show all the characteristics of the female when tested for shock-induced aggression. Castration at weaning tends to suppress aggressive behavior, but it is fully restored when testosterone is administered in adulthood. However, testosterone replacement in adulthood does not influence the aggressive behavior of neonatal castrates. Female mice given an injection of testosterone on the day of birth and then given androgen in adulthood show aggressive behavior comparable to that seen in male mice.[19] Furthermore, male mice castrated on the day of birth are less aggressive following androgen-replacement therapy in adulthood than males castrated on the tenth day of life.

Similar results have been obtained by Bronson and Desjardins.[9] These investigators have reported that single injections of testosterone were most effective in facilitating aggressive behavior in adulthood when administered to the female on the day of birth and less effective when given after that time, becoming ineffective some time between the twelfth and twenty-fourth day. Also, neonatal androgen was effective in enhancing adult aggressiveness only if it was again administered before testing. The implication of both of these studies is that early androgen treatment sensitizes appropriate neural elements to androgen encountered in adulthood. The same conclusions can be reached on the basis of studies using shock-induced aggression in rats.

More recently Edwards and Herndon[20] have shown that neonatal estrogen treatments to female mice mimic the effects of neonatal androgen, in terms of facilitating the differentiation of androgen sensitive mechanisms for adult aggressive behavior. Thus, ninety percent of the pairs of females given neonatal estrogen fought when treated with androgen in adulthood, compared to twenty-five percent of control females and one hundred percent of testosterone-treated females.

Further evidence of the control of sexually dimorphic behavior by neonatal hormone treatments comes from experiments on the learning of an avoidance response in the rat. The procedure consists usually of presenting a rat with a conditioned signal—a tone, buzzer, light, etc.—followed closely by electric shock. The animal can usually cross a barrier to another compartment to either escape further shock or avoid it by responding to the signal prior to the onset of the shock. It has been reported[39,57] that normal females tend to learn the active avoidance response more rapidly than do normal males. The Beattys[4,5] found that castrating male rats in adulthood did not influence avoidance conditioning. Testosterone injections to females in infancy, when combined with testosterone treatment in adulthood, produced rats whose avoidance behavior was masculinized in that they showed the same deficit in avoidance learning shown by males.

Further evidence of modification of sexually dimorphic behaviors comes from Pfaff and Zigmond[58] who studied yet another behavior that usually shows sex difference, namely, timidity or emotionality as exhibited by activity and defecation in an open field (a circular arena usually brightly lit). Commonly, females tend to be more active in the open field and to emerge from the home cage faster than males. Neonatally castrated male rats tend to behave more like females and neonatally androgenized females more like males in both the open-field test and tests of emergence. Similar findings have been reported by Gray and Levine[25] and by Swanson.[66,67]

In the question surrounding the problem of the cellular mechanisms of the differentiating action of androgen on the brain, certainly the first step is to characterize the physiological or biochemical differences between the brains of males and females, and this can hardly be said to have been accomplished. A promising development has emerged from the ultrastructure studies by Raisman and Field[61] on projections from the amygdala to the hypothalamus. They have found that the ratio of the number of preoptic region synapses ending on dendritic spines to those ending on dendritic shafts was significantly lower in male than in female rats.

Several laboratories have sought changes in RNA or protein synthesis in relation to androgenization. Shimada and Gorbman[65] found

evidence for synthesis of new species of RNA in the rat forebrain. Clayton, Kogura, and Kraemer[10] report that neonatal testosterone significantly affects synthesis of labeled RNA from tritiated uridine in the amygdala and preoptic areas of the female brain. Using a different autoradiographic technique, MacKinnon[48] has found changes in protein synthesis in roughly the same two regions of the mouse brain in relation to puberty and the estrous cycle. No effects of neonatal androgen on brain uptake of testosterone could be demonstrated in the female rat. Several investigators have reported lower retention of ^{3}H-estradiol in brain tissue from androgen-sterilized females, but these data do not seem to be consistent. At any rate, any differences in the uptake of hormones that may exist between males, females, and neonatally manipulated animals would seem to be rather small.

❰ Conclusions

In this paper we have attempted to do two things: first, to communicate a body of information illustrative of the very profound effects that alterations in the neonatal environment, whether they be endogenous or exogenous, have upon the subsequent function of the developing organism; second, to define an area called developmental psychobiology and to illustrate how the developmental psychobiologist proceeds to understand the nature of his universe. Developmental psychobiology is in its infancy. This is indeed a truism as it can be said of many of the areas of investigation that attempt to view the organism as a totality and to step across the traditional limitations of defined disciplines. I believe that one can only achieve a full understanding of the organism's function by viewing the organism ontogenetically.

❰ Bibliography

1. ALTMAN, J., G. D. DAS, and W. J. ANDERSON. "Effects of Infantile Handling on Morphological Development of the Rat Brain: An

Exploratory Study," *Dev. Psychobiol.*, 1 (1968), 10–20.

2. BARRACLOUGH, C. A. and R. A. GORSKI. "A Dichotomy in the Mating Behavior of Androgen-Sterilized Persistent-Estrous Rats," *Anat. Rec.*, 139 (1961), 205.

3. ———. "Studies on Mating Behaviour in the Androgen-Sterilized Female Rat in Relation to the Hypothalamic Regulation of Sexual Behaviour," *J. Endocrinol.*, 25 (1962), 175–182.

4. BEATTY, W. W. and P. A. BEATTY. "Effects of Neonatal Testosterone on the Acquisition of an Active Avoidance Response in Genotypically Female Rats," *Psychonom. Sci.*, 19 (1970), 315–316.

5. ———. "Hormonal Determinants of Sex Differences in Avoidance Behavior and Reactivity to Electric Shock in the Rat," *J. Comp. Physiol. Psychol.*, 73 (1970), 446–455.

6. BEEMAN, E. A. "The Effect of Male Hormone on Aggressive Behavior in Mice," *Physiol. Zool.*, 20 (1947), 373–405.

7. BOLK, L. *Das Problem der Menschenwerdung.* Jena: Fischer, 1926.

8. BOWLBY, J. *Maternal Care and Mental Health*, Monograph Series No. 2. Geneva: WHO, 1951.

9. BRONSON, F. H. and C. DESJARDINS. "Neonatal Androgen Administration and Adult Aggressiveness in Female Mice," *Gen. Comp. Endocrin.*, 15 (1970), 320–325.

10. CLAYTON, R. B., J. KOGURA, and H. C. KRAEMER. "Sexual Differentiation of the Brain: Effects of Testosterone on Brain RNA Metabolism in Newborn Female Rats," *Nature*, 226 (1970), 810–812.

11. CLEMENS, L. G., J. SHRYNE, and R. A. GORSKI. "Androgen and Development of Progesterone Responsiveness in Male and Female Rats," *Physiol. Behav.*, 5 (1970), 673–678.

12. CONNER, R. L. and S. LEVINE. "Hormonal Influences on Aggressive Behavior," in S. Garattini and E. B. Sigg, eds., *Aggressive Behaviour*, pp. 150–163. Amsterdam: Excerpta Medica, 1969.

13. DAVIDSON, J. M., L. E. JONES, and S. LEVINE. "Feedback Regulation of Adrenocorticotropin Secretion in 'Basal' and 'Stress' Conditions: Acute and Chronic Effects of Intrahypothalamic Corticoid Implantation," *Endocrinology*, 82 (1968), 655–663.

14. DENENBERG, V. H., G. A. HUDGENS, and M.

X. ZARROW. "Mice Reared with Rats: Modification of Behavior by Early Experience with Another Species," *Science*, 143 (1964), 380–381.

15. DENENBERG, V. H., K. M. ROSENBERG, R. PASCHKE et al. "Plasma Corticosterone Levels as a Function of Cross-Species Fostering and Species Differences," *Endocrinology*, 83 (1968), 900–902.

16. DENENBERG, V. H., K. M. ROSENBERG, R. PASCHKE et al. "Mice Reared with Rat Aunts: Effects on Plasma Corticosterone and Open Field Activity," *Nature*, 221 (1969), 73–74.

17. DENENBERG, V. H. and A. E. WHIMBEY. "Behavior of Adult Rats is Modified by the Experiences Their Mothers had as Infants," *Science*, 142 (1963), 1192–1193.

18. DOBZHANSKY, T. *Mankind Evolving.* New Haven: Yale University Press, 1962.

19. EDWARDS, D. A. "Early Androgen Stimulation and Aggressive Behavior in Male and Female Mice," *Physiol. Behav.*, 4 (1969), 333–338.

20. EDWARDS, D. A. and J. HERNDON. "Neonatal Estrogen Stimulation and Aggressive Behavior in Female Mice," *Physiol. Behav.*, 5 (1970), 993–995.

21. FEDER, H. H. and R. E. WHALEN. "Feminine Behavior in Neonatally Castrated and Estrogen-Treated Male Rats," *Science*, 147 (1965), 306–307.

22. FOSS, B. M., ed. *Determinants of Infant Behavior*, 3 vols. London: Methuen, 1959, 1961, 1963.

23. GOY, R. W., C. H. PHOENIX, and W. C. YOUNG. "A Critical Period for the Suppression of Behavioral Receptivity in Adult Female Rats by Early Treatment with Androgen," *Anat. Rec.*, 142 (1962), 307.

24. GRADY, K. L., C. H. PHOENIX, and W. C. YOUNG. "Role of the Developing Rat Testis in Differentiation of the Neural Tissues Mediating Mating Behavior," *J. Comp. Physiol. Psychol.*, 59 (1965), 176–182.

25. GRAY, J. A. and S. LEVINE. "Effect of Induced Oestrus on Emotional Behaviour in Selected Strains of Rats," *Nature*, 201 (1964), 1198–1200.

26. HALTMEYER, G. C., V. H. DENENBERG, and M. X. ZARROW. "Modification of the Plasma Corticosterone Response as a Function of Infantile Stimulation and Electric Shock Parameters," *Physiol. Behav.*, 2 (1967), 61–63.

27. HARRIS, G. W. "Sex Hormones, Brain Development and Brain Function," *Endocrinology*, 75 (1964), 627–648.

28. HARRIS, G. W., and S. LEVINE. "Sexual Differentiation of the Brain and Its Experimental Control," *J. Physiol.*, 163 (1962), 42–43.

29. HUDGENS, G. A., V. H. DENENBERG, and M. X. ZARROW. "Mice Reared with Rats: Relations between Mothers' Activity Level and Offspring's Behavior," *J. Comp. Physiol. Psychol.*, 63 (1967), 304–308.

30. ——. "Mice Reared with Rats: Effects of Preweaning and Postweaning Social Interactions upon Adult Behavior," *Behaviour*, 30 (1968), 259–274.

31. LARSSON, K. "Individual Differences in Reactivity to Androgen in Male Rats," *Physiol. Behav.*, 1 (1966), 255–258.

32. LEVINE, S. "Infantile Experience and Resistance to Physiological Stress," *Science*, 126 (1957), 405.

33. ——. "The Effects of Differential Infantile Stimulation on Emotionality at Weaning," *Can. J. Psychol.*, 13 (1959), 243–247.

34. ——. "Plasma-Free Corticosteroid Response to Electric Shock in Rats Stimulated in Infancy," *Science*, 135 (1962), 795–796.

35. ——. "Maternal and Environmental Influences on the Adrenocortical Response to Stress in Weaning Rats," *Science*, 156 (1967), 258–260.

36. ——. "Influence of Infantile Stimulation on the Response to Stress during Preweaning Development," *Dev. Psychobiol.*, 1 (1968), 67–70.

37. LEVINE, S. and M. ALPERT. "Differential Maturation of the Central Nervous System as a Function of Early Experience," *AMA Arch. Gen. Psychiatry*, 1 (1959), 403–405.

38. LEVINE, S., M. ALPERT, and G. W. LEWIS. "Differential Maturation of an Adrenal Response to Cold Stress in Rats Manipulated in Infancy," *J. Comp. Physiol. Psychol.*, 51 (1958), 774–777.

39. LEVINE, S. and P. L. BROADHURST. "Genetic and Ontogenetic Determinants of Adult Behavior in the Rat," *J. Comp. Physiol. Psychol.*, 56 (1963), 423–428.

40. LEVINE, S., J. A. CHEVALIER, and S. J. KORCHIN. "The Effects of Early Shock and Handling on Later Avoidance Learning," *J. Per.*, 24 (1956), 475–493.

41. LEVINE, S., G. C. HALTMEYER, G. G. KARAS et al. "Physiological and Behavioral Effects of Infantile Stimulation," *Physiol. Behav.*, 2 (1967), 55–59.

42. LEVINE, S. and G. W. LEWIS. "The Relative Importance of Experimenter Contact in an Effect Produced by Extra-Stimulation in Infancy," *J. Comp. Physiol. Psychol.*, 52 (1959), 368–369.

43. LEVINE, S. and R. F. MULLINS, JR. "Estrogen Administered Neonatally Affects Adult Sexual Behavior in Male and Female Rats," *Science*, 144 (1964), 185–187.

44. ——. "Sexual Differentiation and Behavior," *Excerpta Med. Int. Congr.*, 132 (1966), 925–931.

45. LEVINE, S. and L. S. OTIS. "The Effects of Handling During Pre- and Post-Weaning on the Resistance of the Albino Rat to Deprivation in Adulthood," *Can. J. Psychol.*, 12 (1958), 103–108.

46. LEVINE, S. and E. B. THOMAN. "Physiological and Behavioral Consequences of Postnatal Maternal Stress in Rats," *Physiol. Behav.*, 4 (1969), 139–142.

47. LEVINE, S. and D. M. TREIMAN. "Differential Plasma Corticosterone Response to Stress in Four Inbred Strains of Mice," *Endocrinology*, 75 (1964), 142–144.

48. MACKINNON, P. C. B. "A Comparison of Protein Synthesis in the Brains of Mice before and after Puberty," *J. Physiol.*, 210 (1970), 10–11.

49. MASON, W. A., R. K. DAVENPORT, JR., and E. W. MENZEL, JR. "Early Experience and the Social Development of Rhesus Monkeys and Chimpanzees," in G. Newton and and S. Levine, eds., *Early Experience and Behavior*, pp. 440–480. Springfield, Ill.: Charles C. Thomas, 1968.

50. MEIER, G. W. "Infantile Handling and Development in Siamese Kittens," *J. Comp. Physiol. Psychol.*, 54 (1961), 284–286.

51. MORRISON, R. L. and D. C. JOHNSON. "The Effects of Androgenization in Male Rats Castrated at Birth," *J. Endocrinol.*, 34 (1966), 117–123.

52. MUGFORD, R. A. and N. W. NOWELL. "The Aggression of Male Mice Against Androgenized Females," *Psychonom. Sci.*, 20 (1970), 191–192.

53. ——. "Pheromones and Their Effect on Aggression in Mice," *Nature*, 226 (1970), 967–968.

54. MULLINS, R. F., JR. and S. LEVINE. "Hormonal Determinants During Infancy of

Adult Sexual Behavior in the Male Rat," *Physiol. Behav.*, 3 (1968), 339–343.

55. ———. "Hormonal Determinants During Infancy of Adult Sexual Behavior in the Female Rat," *Physiol. Behav.*, 3 (1968), 333–338.

56. ———. "Differential Sensitization of Penile Tissue by Sexual Hormones in Newborn Rats," *Commun. Behav. Biol.*, 3 (1969), Part A, 1–4.

57. NAKAMURA, C. Y. and N. H. ANDERSON. "Avoidance Behavior Differences Within and Between Strains of Rats," *J. Comp. Physiol. Psychol.*, 55 (1962), 740–747.

58. PFAFF, D. W. and R. E. ZIGMOND. "Neonatal Androgen Effects on Sexual and Non-Sexual Behavior of Adult Rats Tested under Various Hormone Regimens," *Neuroendocrinology*, 7 (1971), 129–145.

59. PFEIFFER, C. A. "Sexual Differences of the Hypophyses and Their Determination by the Gonads," *Am. J. Anat.*, 58 (1936), 195–225.

60. PHOENIX, C. H., R. W. GOY, A. A. GERALL et al. "Organizing Action of Prenatally Administered Testosterone Propionate on the Tissues Mediating Mating Behavior in the Female Guinea Pig," *Endocrinology*, 65 (1959), 369–382.

61. RAISMAN, G. and P. M. FIELD. "Sexual Dimorphism in the Preoptic Area of the Rat," *Science*, 173 (1971), 731–733.

62. SCOTT, J. P. and E. FREDERICSON. "The Causes of Fighting in Mice and Rats," *Physiol. Zool.*, 24 (1951), 273–309.

63. SEGAL, S. J. and D. C. JOHNSON. "Inductive Influence of Steroid Hormones on the Neural System: Ovulation Controlling Mechanisms," *Arch. d'Anat. Microsc. Morphol., Exp.*, 48 (1959), 261–273.

64. SELYE, H. *Stress*. Montreal: Acta, 1950.

65. SHIMADA, H. and A. GORBMAN. "Long-Lasting Changes in RNA Synthesis in the Forebrains of Female Rats Treated with Testosterone Soon after Birth," *Biochem. Biophys. Res. Commun.*, 38 (1970), 423–430.

66. SWANSON, H. H. "Sex Differences in Behaviour of Hamsters in Open Field and Emergence Tests: Effects of Pre- and Post-Pubertal Gonadectomy," *Anim. Behav.*, 14 (1966), 522–529.

67. ———. "Alteration of Sex-Typical Behaviour of Hamsters in Open Field and Emergence Tests by Neonatal Administration of Androgen or Oestrogen," *Anim. Behav.*, 15 (1967), 209–216.

68. THOMAN, E. B. and W. J. ARNOLD. "Effects of Incubator Rearing with Social Deprivation on Maternal Behavior in Rats," *J. Comp. Physiol. Psychol.*, 65 (1968), 441–446.

69. THOMAN, E. B., S. LEVINE, and W. J. ARNOLD. "Effects of Maternal Deprivation and Incubator Rearing upon Adrenocortical Activity in the Adult Rat," *Dev. Psychobiol.*, 1 (1968), 21–23.

70. TOLLMAN, J. and J. A. KING. "The Effects of Testosterone Propionate on Aggression in Male and Female C57BL/10 Mice," *Br. J. Anim. Behav.*, 4 (1956), 147–149.

71. TREIMAN, D. M., D. W. FULKER, and S. LEVINE. "Interaction of Genotype and Environment as Determinants of Corticosteroid Response to Stress," *Dev. Psychobiol.*, 3 (1970), 131–140.

72. ULRICH, R. E. and N. H. AZRIN. "Reflexive Fighting in Response to Aversive Stimulation," *J. Exp. Anal. Behav.*, 5 (1962), 511–520.

73. WHALEN, R. E. and D. A. EDWARDS. "Hormonal Determinants of the Development of Masculine and Feminine Behavior in Male and Female Rats," *Anat. Rec.*, 157 (1967), 173–180.

74. YATES, F. E. and J. URQUHART. "Control of Plasma Concentrations of Adrenocortical Hormones," *Physiol. Rev.*, 42 (1962), 359–443.

75. YOUNG, R. D. "Influence of Neonatal Treatment on Maternal Behavior: A Confounding Variable," *Psychonom. Sci.*, 3 (1965), 295–296.

76. YOUNG, W. C. "The Hormones and Mating Behavior," in W. C. Young, ed., *Sex and Internal Secretions*, Vol. 2. Baltimore: Williams & Wilkins, 1961.

CHAPTER 17

PSYCHIATRIC GENETICS[*]

Seymour Kessler

THE RECENT intellectual and scientific achievements of evolutionary and molecular biology have had a profound influence on American psychiatry. New perspectives have emerged and doctrinaire approaches have yielded to interdisciplinary dialogue and research. A new generation of psychiatrists, educated in biochemistry and population biology, is beginning to explore the experimental and theoretical implications of behavior genetics research. Once resisted or ignored, the possibility of genotypic influences on human behavior now commands increasing attention in the behavorial, medical, and social sciences.

Psychiatric genetics, a subspecialty of human behavior genetics, is concerned with the genetic and environmental bases of behavioral disorder. This vast literature is rapidly expanding and no exhaustive review will be attempted here. Rather, certain areas relevant to contemporary psychiatric practice will be examined and some of the possible issues with

which future research may be concerned will be underscored. Recent reviews may be consulted for a more comprehensive bibliography of the behavioral[133,137] and psychiatric[183,208] genetics literature.

⟮ Man and Evolution

Man is a product of biological evolution. Gene variations introduced into the human gene pool by mutation are shaped, primarily by natural selection, into integrated or coadapted gene complexes that promote the various individual and species adaptations to the range of environments in which man lives. Recent studies have shown that considerable genetic variation is present in the human gene pool.[88] The Mendelian laws governing the transmission of the genetic material from parents to offspring facilitate the maintenance of this variation and ensure the biological uniqueness of virtually every individual.

Man is also a product of cultural evolution. His ability to acquire and transmit culture is among the distinctive characteristics inherent

[*] I gratefully acknowledge the suggestions offered by Drs. L. Erlenmeyer-Kimling, I. I. Gottesman, K. Kidd, and D. Rosenthal concerning various aspects of this chapter.

in man's genetic potential. Biological change over time is generally slow whereas change obtained through cultural evolution may be rapid and can transcend the limitations of both space and generations. Man has evolved and continues to evolve on both the biological and cultural levels;[47] the two are in continuous interaction. Man's biological capacities have influenced the development and direction of his cultural history. Conversely, through his patterns of mating and his technology, culture affects man's biological evolution. A persisting problem in psychiatric genetics research is the separation of cultural and biological influences on human behavioral variation.

(Genetic Determination of Behavior

Each human individual constitutes a system whose behavioral, morphological, and physiological characteristics are determined by gene-directed biological processes. The constellation of genes the individual carries, his *genotype*, exerts influences on behavior through its effects on development and on metabolic processes. The genotype, however, does not operate in a vacuum. Directly or indirectly, the intra- and intercellular milieu and other environmental factors modulate gene function. The genotype interacts with the environment to produce the *phenotype*, the visible or measurable characteristics of the individual.

Although genes are a determinant of behavior, genes do not *cause* behavior. Operationally, the genotype might be thought of as one of several variables that alter the probability that a given behavior will occur under certain environmental conditions. For example, male mice will fight each other, but some strains of mice are genotypically more predisposed to fight than others. Castrated animals of such strains are generally docile. Likewise, group-reared animals tend to be less aggressive than those reared in isolation. Thus the agonistic behavior observed between two male mice depends on many variables: the "right" geno-

type, gonadal status, previous social environment, and other biological and situational contingencies. None of these variables is a sufficient *cause* of the observed behavior, yet each plays a necessary role in determining the behavioral outcome.

One of the legacies of the nature-nuture controversy is the persisting confusion between the concepts of genotype and phenotype. The genotype of the individual is fixed at fertilization and, barring somatic mutations, persists throughout life.* Certain aspects of the phenotype, on the other hand, may change considerably, whereas, other aspects (e.g., temperament, response dispositions, etc.) may remain relatively stable over long periods of time. Inferences about the underlying genotypic determination drawn solely from the relative plasticity or stability of the phenotype may be misleading. The presence of phenotypic flexibility does not rule out the possibility of large genotypic contributions.[223] Indeed, the capacity for phenotypic change may itself be genotypically determined. On the other hand, the maintenance of relatively enduring traits could be due to nongenetic factors. For example, intermittent schedules of reinforcement are capable of maintaining behavioral responses over long periods of time. Even grossly maladaptive behavior, involving self-punitive and self-injurious responses, can be maintained by reinforcement contingencies associated with the behavior and its consequences for the organism.[12]

In the past, the tendency to associate genotypic influences on behavior with developmental determinism created misunderstanding of the goals of human behavior genetics and impeded substantive research. Some writers have implied that there are immutable states and fixed behavioral patterns blueprinted in the genome and manifested irrespective of environmental contingencies. Evidence from animal research does not support this implication.[80] Moreover, the relationship between

* Major differences exist, however, in the portion of the genome actually active at a given time during the course of life. For example, genes active in the synthesis of fetal hemoglobin (HbF), are inactive postnatally, when HbA is normally formed.

genes and behavior is far more complex and in no way analogous to the relationship between a blueprint and the structure it represents.[130] Behavior does not arise inexorably as a consequence of primary gene action; rather, it develops as a result of the joint interaction between genes and environment. The same genotype may respond differently when subjected to differential environmental treatments. The extent to which a genotype is affected phenotypically by environmental differences is a measure of the *norm of reaction* or reaction range[47] of that genotype. The reaction range of a given genotype may be relatively broad or narrow; the fact that a reaction range exists permits environmental manipulations to be used in the modification and treatment of genetically determined disorders. For example, phenylketonuria is a hereditary disorder involving a deficiency of the hepatic enzyme, phenylalanine hydroxylase; untreated individuals may be severely retarded mentally. Early dietary intervention, however, often prevents the extreme intellectual deficits associated with this disorder. The demonstration of a genotypic influence on behavior in no way implies behavioral destiny.[54]

⟨ Fundamentals of Genetics

Genes are the basic units of heredity. At fertilization, each human individual receives a complement of genes from each parent. These genes are arranged linearly along the chromosomes, normally twenty-three pairs in number. All of the cells composing the individual derive from the fertilized egg and almost all carry a full complement of chromosomes. Through the process of meiosis, during gametogenesis, sex cells are formed, each carrying normally one representative of each chromosome pair. Occasionally, errors occur and a pair of homologous chromosomes fail to separate properly. Fertilization of gametes, which are formed when such nondisjunctional events occur, may thus produce a zygote lacking a given chromosomal pair (e.g., 45,XO) or with an additional chromosome (e.g., 47,XXY).

Genes are units of deoxyribonucleic acid (DNA). The DNA molecule consists of regularly alternating chains of phosphates and deoxyribose sugar groups to which pairs of nitrogenous bases are attached. The sequence of these bases determines the functional specificity of a gene. A sequence of three successive base pairs constitutes a triplet or coding unit for one of the twenty amino acids, the building blocks of a polypeptide chain. Alterations of the sequence of base pairs due to miscopying, deletions, duplications, and the like, constitute *mutations*.

DNA acts as a template for the building of protein chains. This process involves the synthesis of a complementary chain of messenger ribonucleic acid (mRNA) that passes from the nucleus to the cytoplasm. In the cytoplasm, the mRNA chains attach themselves to ribosomes where amino acids, conveyed individually by a second species of RNA, transfer RNA (tRNA), are attached together sequentially to construct the polypeptide chain.

Genes also regulate the rates of synthesis of the enzymes that direct the metabolic events of the organism. How gene action is regulated in higher organisms is not yet understood. Gene regulatory mechanisms underlie the processes of embryological development and tissue differentiation. Elucidation of these mechanisms may have important implications for our understanding of the relationship between genes and behavior. Hormones, for example, have profound effects on cellular differentiation and function.[197] A possible hormonal influence on cellular differentiation, with long-lasting behavioral consequences, is the sexual differentiation of the central nervous system, in either a female or a male direction.[86] This early differentiation occurs during a sensitive period of development and has been shown to influence the reproductive physiology as well as the organism's later behavior as an adult.[87] The role of gene activation and/or repression in this process is likely.

Modes of Inheritance

In the first edition of the *Handbook*, Kallmann[107] provided an extensive discussion of the modes of inheritance of genes with major phenotypic effects and of the methods generally employed in psychiatric genetics research. Since behavior is produced and maintained by multiple developmental and physiological processes, each presumably directed by many genes, it is not surprising that the genetic transmission of most behavioral traits does not follow simple Mendelian modes of inheritance. Most behavioral variation is quantitative in nature.

Variation in quantitative characters is assumed to result from the joint action of many genes, each presumably with small phenotypic effect, and of environmental factors. The aim of a genetic analysis of quantitative characters is to determine the proportion of total phenotypic variation attributable to genetic causes.

Within populations, differences between individuals with respect to a given character are to varying degrees genotypic and/or environmental in origin. This phenotypic variation (V_P) generally expressed in terms of variances, is composed of a genotypic (V_G) and environmental (V_E) component; $V_P = V_G + V_E$. V_G may be further subdivided into V_A, the variance derived from the additive effects of genes and V_D, a nonadditive component, resulting from dominance. Other components of V_G representing respectively the effects of assortative or nonrandom mating and of epistasis, the interaction of genes at different loci, are sometimes present, but these will not be considered here. Estimates of the variance components may be obtained from the degree of similarity or correlation between relatives with respect to the character being studied. In practice, regression coefficients are used. A more detailed treatment of quantitative genetics may be found in Falconer.[59]

In the absence of dominance and environmental effects, the expected correlation between two relatives reflects the average number of genes they share in common. Thus, the expected correlation between a first degree relative and an index case (= proband) would be 0.5, since, on average, they share half their genes in common. For second degree relatives, who share on average one quarter of their genes in common, the expected correlation would be 0.25. The correlation between parent and offspring ($r_{p/o}$) can be shown to yield an estimate of $\frac{1}{2}V_A/V_P$ and that between sibs ($r_{s/s}$) an estimate of $(\frac{1}{2}V_A + \frac{1}{4}V_D)/V_P$.

V_A is the major cause of resemblance between relatives. If $r_{p/o}$ and $r_{s/s}$ are both about 0.5 as, for example, in the measure of total fingerprint ridge count, it suggests that most, if not all, of the variation can be accounted for simply by additive polygenic inheritance. When the correlations between first degree relatives are less than 0.5, additive variation is reduced and dominance and/or environmental contributions to V_P are increased. For example, $r_{p/o}$ and $r_{s/s}$ for systolic blood pressure are about 0.24 and 0.33 respectively.[31] The components of variance may be calculated as follows: $V_A = 2r_{p/o} = 0.48$ and $V_D = 4(r_{s/s} - r_{p/o}) = 0.36$. Thus about 84 percent of the total variation in this character appears to be genotypic in origin with V_E accounting for 16 percent of the total. The relative proportion of the phenotypic variance due to genotypic factors (V_G/V_P) defines the *degree of genetic determination*;[60] in the previous example $V_G/V_P = 84$ percent. Since the additive genetic variation is an index of the degree of resemblance between relatives, a more informative measure is V_A/V_P, which is called *heritability* and is symbolized h^2. Heritability, which represents the proportion of the phenotypic variance attributable to additive genetic variation, is of particular interest to the animal and plant breeder since it provides a measure that can be used to predict short-term gains in selective-breeding programs. In the example above $h^2 = 48$ percent.

V_E may sometimes be partitioned into subcomponents representing the between and within family environmental variation and the variation arising from ethnic and social class differences. Another source of variation arises from genotype-environment interactions, the differential responses of genotypes to different environments. For example, animals selectively bred for low error scores in a maze may, in an ordinary environment, outperform animals bred for high error scores. In an impoverished environment, however, the former may perform no better than the latter.

Two points need to be stressed. First, in the estimation of h^2 and of the components of V_P, it is assumed that heredity and environment are not correlated. This assumption may not be totally warranted since genotype and environment are often found to be correlated in studies of human behavior. For example, an individual may receive genes from his parents predisposing him to schizophrenia, but he may also be reared in a disordered family environment that in itself may promote the production of psychopathology. Under these conditions it is difficult to distinguish between genotypic contributions and environmental ones. Second, estimates of h^2 should be interpreted with caution; h^2 is a population metric that ". . . tells us only about the ratio of the *prevailing* individual genetic differences to the prevailing individual environmental differences and cannot, in general, be extrapolated to other populations or other environments."[31] For example, although the heritability of human stature is high, average height has changed substantially over the past century as a consequence of environmental changes. Thus, even where heritability measurements suggest little environmental influence, large environmental effects may be observed.

Threshold Characters

Some phenotypic characters, such as cleft lip and palate, diabetes, pyloric stenosis, talipes equinovarus, and other conditions[28] appear to share both continuous and all-or-none characteristics. The inheritance of such characters might be best understood in terms of a genetic model that includes a threshold. One such model[60] assumes that underlying the etiology of a disorder is a continuously distributed variable, *liability*, that encompasses all the endogenous and exogenous factors predisposing to the disorder; the genetic contributions are assumed to be polygenic. A point along the liability dimension marks the *threshold*, beyond which all individuals are affected. The prevalence of the disorder in the general population defines where the threshold occurs

on the liability scale. Falconer[60] provides tables by means of which the prevalence rates of a disorder among relatives of given degrees of relatedness to affected individuals may be converted into an estimate of h^2. Falconer's method has been subjected to various criticisms[3,49] and alternative threshold models have been advanced,[31,152] including one involving single genes.[32] Improvements on Falconer's method recently made by Smith[211,212] have been used to study the genetic basis of schizophrenia.[76]

Despite certain limitations, threshold genetic models have useful predictive properties; they allow the generation of hypotheses that can be tested empirically. For example, such models would predict that:

1. The risks for relatives of an affected individual would be relatively higher for rarer disorders than for more commonly occurring ones. For example, in cleft lip with or without cleft palate, which occurs in the general population at a rate of 0.1 percent, the risks for MZ twins, first, and second degree relatives are respectively, four hundred, forty, and seven times higher than that of the general population. In contrast, in congenital pyloric stenosis among males, with a general population rate of 0.5 percent, the corresponding risks are eighty, ten, and five times higher.[28]

2. The greater the number of affected individuals in a family, the higher the risk for other relatives. This is in contrast to disorders with a simple monogenic basis where the recurrence risk remains constant.

3. Assuming that the severity of a disorder is correlated with the liability above the threshold, the risk for relatives will vary directly with the severity of the disorder in the index case.

4. Where a marked difference occurs in the prevalence of a disorder in the two sexes, relatives of index cases of the less affected sex (= higher threshold) would be at proportionally greater risk than those of index cases of the sex more commonly

affected (= lower threshold). For example, stuttering among males occurs at a rate of some three to four times higher than among females. The prevalence of stuttering among fathers and brothers of a male index case are 10.2 and 15.6 percent respectively, whereas for a female index case the corresponding prevalence rates are 33.3 and 26.8 percent.[5]

Methods of Study

Family and twin studies constitute the major research methods of psychiatric genetics. In the former, the incidence of a disorder among the relatives of index cases is compared to the incidence of the disorder in the general population, or to that of a control group. Genetic models predict (1) that the incidence of the disorder will be elevated among relatives of affected individuals over that of the general population and (2) that the relative incidence of the disorder among the relatives will increase as the genetic relatedness to the index case increases.

In twin studies, comparisons of the degree of similarity are made among monozygotic (MZ) and dizygotic (DZ) groups. Since pairs of MZ twins are genetically alike whereas DZ pairs are no more alike genetically than ordinary siblings, genetic models predict that if genotypic factors are operative in the production of the disorder being studied, then co-twins of affected MZ twins will show a higher concordance or incidence of the disorder than those of affected DZ twins. Concordance rates in twin studies may be calculated on a pairwise or on a casewise (proband method) basis;[2] the latter method generally produces a higher concordance estimate than the former one. The proband method is valid when the members of a concordant twin pair are independently ascertained. Concordance rates in twin studies are also sensitive to sampling procedures. Unsystematic ascertainment and sampling among chronically affected groups, such as resident hospital populations, generally produce a bias toward higher concordance rates among MZ twin pairs than do

samples obtained from birth registers or consecutive admissions to an institution. These latter procedures presumably tap a group that is more representative of both the overall twin population and of the general population from which they are drawn.

Twin studies have been criticized in the past on two grounds: (1) possible inaccuracies in zygosity determination and (2) the possibility that MZ, but not DZ, twin pairs are subjected to systematic treatments that lead to greater intrapair similarity. The availability of multiple blood group polymorphisms, histocompatibility antigens, and dermatoglyphic techniques currently permit the objective diagnosis of zygosity with a high degree of reliability. The second problem cannot be as easily dismissed. Nevertheless, it is of interest that with respect to the major psychiatric disorders, no conclusive evidence is as yet available demonstrating a greater similarity of treatment of MZ twin pairs for environmental factors *relevant* to a given disorder.[74] However, it is generally agreed that supplementary supportive evidence from other sources is preferable to data derived from twin studies alone.

The classical family and twin methods both have difficulties in disentangling genotypic and environmental effects. Recognition of this problem has stimulated alternative lines of research that include:

1. The study of MZ twins reared apart. The number of such twin pairs has generally been too small to shed much light on the etiology of the major psychiatric disorders, although a substantial number have been studied with respect to variations in I.Q. scores.

2. The study of adopted children, born to an affected parent, but raised in homes free from psychopathology.

3. The study of discordant MZ twin pairs, to elucidate the nongenetic factors that distinguish the affected and nonaffected co-twins.

4. High-risk studies of premorbid individuals with an affected relative to elucidate the developmental and predisposing en-

vironmental factors that precipitate a given disorder.

❲ Childhood Disorders

Individual differences appear early in life. Direct observation and filmed records of neonate behavior indicate that, from the start, differences exist in the extent to which infants avail themselves of others for the purposes of seeking comfort.[123] Significant variations have been found in the frequency and duration of spontaneous crying and of sucking and mouthing activities, and in the degree to which self-comforting was sought and successfully obtained.[124,125] Individual differences among neonates also exist in the capacity to take in sensory stimuli. Measures of the frequency and duration of spontaneous visual alertness, of alertness in response to maternal ministrations, of visual pursuit of a moving object, and of responses to sounds all showed variation.[122,126] Such differences may be major determinants of how infants will experience the world around them; they may, in turn, strongly influence parental responses to the infant. Thus, individual differences at birth may have important consequences for the short- and long-range development of the individual.[123,221] Needless to say, such variation is not necessarily only genotypic in origin. Although social influences on neonatal behavioral variation are presumably minimal, pre- and perinatal influences and early life experiences cannot be ruled out as major determinants of early individual differences.

The genotypic contributions to neonatal behavioral variation have not been fully elucidated. However, it is of interest to note that significantly greater intrapair differences were found among DZ infant twin pairs than among MZ pairs in measures of mental and motor activities and of personality,[66] although the extent to which such differences persist is not clear.[22,6] Comparisons between neonates of differing ethnic background have also shown significant differences on ratings of temperament. Chinese-American newborns have been reported to be less changeable, less perturbable, to calm themselves or to be consoled more readily when upset than those of European-American backgrounds.[65] It has been suggested that some temperamental characteristics in early life may be significantly associated with behavioral disorders later in life.[64,194,222]

Mental Retardation

A genetic basis for general intelligence has been firmly established. Studies of MZ twins reared apart invariably indicate that the intrapair correlations of the IQ scores of such twin pairs are significantly higher than those of DZ twin pairs reared together.[25,55,103] Within populations, the distribution of IQ scores forms a bell-shaped curve in conformity with polygenically determined traits. However, toward the lower end of the distribution, a significantly greater number of individuals are actually observed than might be expected.[247] These can be divided into mildly (I.Q. fifty to seventy-five) and severely (I.Q. less than fifty) retarded groups. The former generally constitute part of the normal variation, representing cases of familial retardation. Siblings of such retardates have a distribution of I.Q. scores with a mean around eighty.[181] In contrast, the mean I.Q. of siblings of severe retardates is no different from that of the general population (i.e., one hundred) suggesting that most cases of severe retardation are the result of extraordinary mechanisms such as inborn errors of metabolism, chromosomal disorders, birth difficulties, and other pre- and perinatal factors. Dewey et al.[44] have suggested that approximately 114 recessive gene loci may be involved in the production of severe mental defects. This is possibly an underestimate.[138]

Among the metabolic disorders associated with mental retardation are those related to the metabolism of amino acids (e.g., phenylketonuria, *PKU*), carbohydrates (e.g., galactosemia), lipids (e.g., Tay-Sachs disease), purines (e.g., Lesch-Nyhan syndrome), metals (e.g., Wilson's disease), and steroids (e.g., adrenogenital syndrome). A review may be found in Stanbury et al.[216] Among the chromosomal disorders, autosomal anomalies are often associated with mental subnormality. The major associations with mental retardation are Klinefelter's syndrome (47,XXY) and Down's syndrome (trisomy-21).

PKU remains the prototype of an inborn error of metabolism affecting intellectual function. Although the enzymatic deficiency underlying this disorder has been known for several decades, the specific mechanisms that lead to the severe mental retardation and other behavioral features of the disorder are, as yet, unknown. Disturbance of the transport and metabolism of other amino acids,[159,220] a deficiency of serotonin,[243] and incomplete or defective myelination of the CNS,[139] possibly due to a depression in pyruvate metabolism,[21] have all been suggested as possible causes of the mental retardation associated with PKU.

With the application of large scale screening programs among newborn populations, variant forms of hyperphenylalanemia resembling classical PKU have been discovered. These include atypical, transient, persistent, and other variants among which most affected individuals appear to show normal levels of intelligence without low phenylalanine dietary treatment. This literature has been reviewed by Hsia[95] and Blaskovics and Nelson.[17] The incidence of classical PKU and persistent hyperphenylalanemia is about one in thirteen thousand[16] live births of which variants constitute one-third to one-half of the cases. Classical PKU is believed to be transmitted by a single autosomal recessive gene; the mode of inheritance of the variants has not yet been clarified. It appears that persistent hyperphenylalanemia may be due to a third or possibly a fourth recessive allele at the PKU locus or to a separate modifier gene that, in homozygous form, raises the phenylalanine level in individuals who are heterozygous at the PKU locus.[95]

Offspring born to PKU mothers and normal fathers are heterozygous at the PKU locus and would thus be expected to be intellectually normal. Nevertheless, they appear to be at particularly high risk to intellectual deficits and to various congenital anomalies.[94] Among

101 children born to twenty-nine PKU mothers, eight had PKU, twenty-two were of uncertain status and of the remainder, only three were considered to be normal.[17] Infants born of variant mothers, however, do not appear to have a higher than average risk for being retarded, suggesting that the exposure of the fetus to concentrations of phenylalanine above fifteen to twenty mg. per one hundred ml. may interfere with normal developmental processes, resulting in congenital malformations, microcephaly, and mental retardation.

In recent years, attention has begun to be paid to the psychosocial factors affecting the behavioral and intellectual concomitants of PKU. In a study of thirty PKU children, a significant decrease in IQ score and an increase in the incidence of serious behavioral pathology was found among the sixteen children who had experienced immobilization and sensory restrictions during the first three years of life.[206,242] If confirmed, such findings may have important implications for the management of affected individuals and the counseling of their families. Although behavioral deficits may owe their *origin* to an underlying metabolic abnormality, intrafamilial and other social factors appear to promote, maintain, exacerbate, or diminish the intellectual deficits and behavioral symptoms actually measured.

A recently described metabolic defect associated with behavioral dysfunction is the Lesch-Nyhan syndrome,[182,160] the symptoms of which consist of hyperuricemia, mental retardation, spastic cerebral palsy, choreoathetosis, compulsive self-mutilation, and aggressive behavior. This disorder follows an X-linked recessive mode of transmission[161] and is associated with a deficiency of hypoxanthine-guanine phosphoribosyltransferase, an enzyme involved in purine biosynthesis.[200] More than eighty cases have been described worldwide.

In a study of five children, ranging between nine and fifteen years of age, the presence of varying degrees of retardation was found.[46] Accurate assessment of the mental status of these children was difficult because of the presence of disabilities affecting speech. Nevertheless, with persistent encouragement, the children often made successful efforts to be understood and appeared eager to relate to anyone who showed an interest in them. The self-mutilative behavior of these children began before age two, often following or closely related to a traumatic episode the child had experienced. In four of the children the lips and tongue were the focus of the self-mutilative activity; finger biting appeared to develop later, before the age of five. (In other affected children severe head banging, eye gouging, and picking at open wounds has also been described.) Although most of the self-mutilation appeared to be involuntary and unpredictable, some of the children clearly used such activities for manipulation and secondary gain and in response to environmental cues. Outwardly expressed aggression often took the form of verbal and physical abuse that appeared to be purposeful. Dizmang and Cheatham[46] comment:

> [these] . . . children are in restraints much of the time and they are often intellectually far more capable of interacting with the world than their motor ability will allow. Their pinching, biting and foul language all appear to be learned behavior that is likely to get a reaction out of the people around them. It did not have the same compulsive quality that the finger and lip biting did.

Further careful observation of Lesch-Nyhan children might elucidate the factors underlying the development of the specific behavioral symptoms involved in this disorder and suggest methods of treatment, in addition to dietary and other biochemical interventions. Similar considerations are surely applicable to other metabolic and chromosomal disorders.

Learning Disorders

The high prevalence rates of learning disabilities in the general population suggest that they comprise a constellation of disorders of major significance. Indeed, they constitute a substantial fraction of the problems requiring psychiatric intervention in the preadolescent and adolescent years. The association of these disorders with scholastic underachievement and with impulsive and aggressive behavior makes affected children high-risk candidates for more severe behavioral problems later on. The costs of these disorders to the individual, his family, and to society are incalculable.

Illustrative of these disorders, minimal brain dysfunctions (MBD) and developmental dyslexia, will be discussed here. The evidence for genotypic contributions to these disorders is by no means unequivocal. Each diagnostic category appears to encompass a heterogeneous group of related disorders with multiple etiologies: environmental contingencies play a major etiological role. Nonetheless, in each, the evidence for genotypic involvement is suggestive. Each shows a decided familial concentration and, where twin studies are available, concordance rates among MZ twins generally exceed those among DZ pairs. Invariably, males are affected at higher rates than females. Investigators should keep the possibility of a genetic threshold model in mind and provide a breakdown of their data for the two sexes separately in future studies. Also, investigators should be alerted to cases of adopted children and discordant MZ twin pairs, since both would be invaluable research material for the elucidation of the etiological factors underlying these disorders.

MBD encompasses a variety of persistent behavioral problems generally marked by motor hyperactivity, excess distractibility, poorly controlled behavior, and scholastic underachievement in children whose overall intellectual ability otherwise appears adequate.[34,35] Among the disorders of childhood, MBD is believed to be the single most common one seen by child psychiatrists.[231] These disorders may occur at a prevalence rate of between 4[217] and 10 percent[96] among grade-school children; the rate among males is three or more times higher than among females. Most MBD children develop their symptoms before they enter first grade: close to half may begin to behave abnormally before age one.[217] In half[145] or more[128] of hyperactive children, the symptoms tend to diminish or disappear in later years.

Difficulty exists in the diagnosis of these disorders since hyperactivity may be associated with other behavioral problems including neurologic dysfunction, emotional disorders, and intellectual subnormality.[115] The majority of MBD children appear to have no major detectable neurological abnormalities.[217] However, an increased rate of minor or "soft" neurological signs may be present.[231]

Lopez[135] studied ten pairs of hyperkinetic twins, ranging between five and twelve years of age. All of the four MZ pairs but only one of the six DZ pairs were concordant. All of the concordant MZ pairs were males and, among the discordant DZ twins, the affected co-twin was a male in all but one instance. However, since most of the DZ group consisted of opposite-sexed pairs, no conclusion can be drawn about a genotypic etiology for hyperkinesis on the basis of these data.

The evidence for a familial concentration of MBD is scanty. A retrospective study of the parents and second-degree relatives of a group of hyperactive children revealed that a greater number of these relatives had hyperactive symptoms as children than the relatives of a matched control group.[217] However, the presence of alcoholism, sociopathy, and hysteria among the relatives of the MBD children confounded the possible contributions of genotypic factors. No large-scale attempts to separate the biological, social class, and intrafamilial environmental components of MBD have been reported. However, in a study of foster-home-reared sibs and half-sibs of MBD children it was found that about 47 percent of the full sibs exhibited repeated behavior problems, including hyperactivity, whereas only 23 percent of the half-sibs were so characterized. The greatest likelihood of receiving a diagnosis of MBD occurred in those children who had, in addition to a relatively high genetic loading, a low IQ and/or a developmental history of seizures, low birth weight, perinatal complications and congenital malformations.[195] No increased rate of chromosomal abnormalities has been found among MBD children.[229] A comprehensive discussion of the epidemiology, etiology, diagnosis and treatment of MBD has recently been published.[40]

Dyslexia is a ". . . disorder manifested by difficulty in learning to read despite conventional instruction, adequate intelligence, and sociocultural opportunity."[38] Although it was once believed that dyslexia was restricted to individuals of English-speaking nations, it now appears that this disorder may occur worldwide, including China, India, and Japan.[38] Recent estimates of the prevalence of dyslexia in the general population of Europe and of the United States range from 1 to 35 percent; the modal rate is about 10 percent, indicating that dyslexia is a problem of major magnitude.

Owen et al.[166] have recently reviewed the twin studies of dyslexia. Among a total of twelve MZ twin pairs in three separate studies, all were reported as concordant whereas only a third of the thirty-three pairs of DZ twins were concordant. Unsystematic sampling may account for the high MZ concordance rate.

Evidence for a familial concentration is summarized by Critchley.[38] Hallgren[81] found that 89 percent of 116 index cases had a positive family history of dyslexia. Most of the index cases (81 percent) were found to be members of families with one affected parent. In his study, there was no evidence of increased parental consanguinity or birth-order effects. However, youngest or last-born children have been reported to be at greater risk for dyslexia than older ones.[38] A recent study of fifty adult dyslexics showed that 34 percent had other family members with similar problems.[169]

Hallgren[81] has suggested that dyslexia may be transmitted by a single dominant gene. However, a simple dominant mode of inheritance is complicated by a disproportionate incidence of dyslexia among males; the incidence is between three to four times greater than among females. Partially this might be due to an ascertainment bias: boys with poor reading abilities may create greater disturbances in school and may be brought to the notice of teachers, parents, and reading clinics more often than girls.[227] Critchley[38] discounts this possibility because of the consistency with which the differential sex difference is found. Hallgren's data might be compatible with a threshold genetic model. In his study, male relations of a proband had a

3 6 2   THE DEVELOPMENT OF BEHAVIOR   [PT. 2]

relatively greater risk for dyslexia than female ones. Among the male probands with one affected parent, either parent was likely to be affected (thirty-five fathers and thirty-three mothers were diagnosed as dyslexic). However, among the female probands twice as many fathers (fifteen) as mothers (seven) were affected.

Childhood Psychosis

The psychotic disorders of childhood have been reviewed by Rutter[191,192] and by Rosenthal.[183] Among these disorders, those with a relatively early age of onset have tended to be distinguished from those involving regression at later ages of onset. The former group— variously called Kanner's syndrome,[109] infantile autism,[179] infantile psychosis,[178] or early childhood psychosis[71]—generally begins before the end of the second year of life, many of the children appearing withdrawn virtually from birth. These early disorders are characterized by autism, marked by aloofness and distance from other people, speech abnormalities, and ritualistic and compulsive behavior. The prevalence of childhood psychoses may be between 3.1[225] and 4.5[136] per ten thousand children; estimates for infantile autism vary from 0.7[225] to 2.1[136] per ten thousand. Males appear to be affected two to four times more often than females. Kanner[109] and others have found that first-borns are overrepresented among early onset psychotic children. However, Wing [232] has reported that in large families there may be a tendency for the affected child to appear late in the birth order. Several writers have suggested that a disproportionate number of parents of early onset psychotic children come from well-educated and higher socioeconomic groups and are cold and obsessive in personality. However, these personality characteristics have been disputed:[71] parental abnormalities, if present, might be consequences of their reactions to an abnormal child.[191,192]

Since the disorder is rare, the number of twins studied has been small; Rutter[192] provides a critical review of these data. After excluding those pairs in which major physical disabilities were present, a total of eleven out of thirteen MZ and one out of four DZ pairs has been reported to be concordant. However, among these studies, satisfactory evidence of zygosity and sufficient clinical details to substantiate the diagnosis were given for only four twin pairs (two MZ and two DZ). Among these, half of each group showed concordance, insufficient to demonstrate a genetic basis unequivocally for the disorder. On the other hand, although the rate of early onset psychosis among the siblings of affected children is low (approximately 2 percent[193]), it nevertheless appears to be between fifty and one hundred times higher than that of the general population. In general, cytogenetic studies have failed to show the presence of an increased rate of chromosomal anomalies among children with early onset psychosis.[104]

The rate of schizophrenia among the first-degree relatives of early onset psychotic children has been reported to be no higher than that of the general population.[191] In constrast, the rate of schizophrenia among the relatives of children with psychoses with later onset is as high[108] or higher[15] than that found among relatives of adult schizophrenics, suggesting that the late onset group may have a biological unity with adulthood schizophrenia,[108] whereas the early onset group constitutes a genotypically different group of disorders. Goldfarb,[71] however, has pointed out that sampling procedures might account for these apparent differences. Although only 2 percent of the parents in his study were hospitalized for psychiatric reasons, psychiatric evaluations revealed that a diagnosis of schizophrenia was applicable to 29 percent of the mothers and 13 percent of the fathers of the affected children. When the children in his study were subdivided into those with apparent neurological impairments (organic) versus those without (nonorganic) the rates of schizophrenia among the parents of the latter group were 44 and 8 percent for the mothers and fathers respectively whereas the corresponding rates among the "organic" group were 21 and 15 percent. Whether the relatively higher rate of diagnosed psychosis among the mothers of the nonorganic group represents the effects of predisposing genotypic factors is at present speculative. Also, the differential rates of psychosis in the two sexes among the parents in Goldfarb's study need to be explained. If this sex difference is confirmed, it might suggest that early onset childhood psychosis is unrelated to adult schizophrenia, since no differential sex difference among affected individuals or their parents has been shown in the latter disorder.

Clearly, the biological relationship between early and later onset forms of childhood psychosis and between the former and adult schizophrenia requires further study. Since Goldfarb's sample consisted of individuals predominantly from lower socioeconomic classes, whereas previously reported samples were generally biased in the opposite direction, greater attention to socioeconomic variables is needed, although a recent report[180] suggests that the incidence of autism is not correlated with parental social class. Also, attention needs to be paid to pre- and perinatal factors in relation to early onset childhood psychosis as several investigators have reported an association between pregnancy complications and childhood psychosis.[134,190,219]

([Adult Disorders

Alcoholism

Although precise estimates are not available, alcoholism in the United States is believed to involve between 4 to 5 percent of the general population.[188] The rate among men may be up to ten or more times higher than among women.[237] Several studies suggest that hereditary factors are operative in the etiology of alcoholism. The pertinent literature is reviewed by Rosenthal[183] and by Goodwin.[72] Invariably, the rate of alcoholism among relatives of alcoholic probands is higher than that of the general population.[4] Also, twin studies generally show that MZ pairs are more similar in their abuse of alcohol[105] and in their drinking habits[168] than

DZ pairs. However, the evidence is not unequivocal. If the social consequences of alcohol consumption are used as criteria of alcoholism, then MZ and DZ twin pairs do not appear to differ.[168] Also, in groups of individuals separated from their biological parents early in life and reared in foster homes, no significant differences in problem drinking were found between children born to alcoholic parents and children born to nonalcoholic ones.[182] In fact, none of the former children were alcoholics.

Recent studies[239] suggest that male relatives of a female proband may have a higher risk for alcoholism than those of male alcoholics. Relatives of female alcoholics also appear to show a higher prevalence of depressive disorders than those of male probands. On the other hand, the rates of schizophrenia, mental deficiency, manic-depressive illness, and epilepsy among the relatives of alcoholics do not seem to be increased above their respective rates in the general population.

In a recent study of half-sibs of sixty-nine alcoholic probands, it was reported that the presence of alcoholism in the former was strongly associated with alcoholism in the biological parent.[198] However, the significance of these findings is obscure since the rate of alcoholism among the half-sibs was as high as that among the full sibs despite the fact that the two groups share, on the average, different proportions of their genes in common with a proband. Although an X-linked mode of transmission for alcoholism has been advanced by some,[41,42] there is little supporting evidence.[234]

In the context of a clinical and pharmacological problem, genotypic influences on the development of tolerance to and physical dependence on alcohol may have an important bearing on the issue of alcohol addiction.[144,163] In this regard it has been reported that a wide range of individual differences exist in the rate of metabolism of an administered dose of alcohol.[143] Intrapair differences in the rates of alcohol elimination from blood plasma were significantly greater among healthy, nonmedicated DZ twin pairs than among MZ pairs;[228] the degree of genetic determination was estimated as 0.98, suggesting that genotypic factors might account for most of the phenotypic variation. Although different ethnic groups require a comparable quantity of alcohol per unit of body weight to reach intoxicating blood levels, some groups metabolize alcohol significantly slower than others and take longer to recover from an alcoholic debauch.[62] Wolff[241] has recently suggested that differences in autonomic nervous system responsivity to alcohol, which appear to be present at birth, may account for variations of alcoholism rates among different ethnic groups. The extent to which such differences actually contribute to the etiology of alcoholism requires further study. Current research on the biological and environmental factors involved in alcoholism is discussed in a recent publication.[201]

Criminality

The belief that heredity plays a role in the etiology of criminality is an old one. Criminality shows a familial concentration. Also, several twin studies in various countries have shown that the concordance rates for criminality among MZ twin pairs are higher than those among DZ pairs.[183] However, inadequate sampling procedures, questionable determination of zygosity, lack of double-blind assessments, and the failure to separate environmental from hereditary influences render these latter studies equivocal with respect to the demonstration of a genotypic involvement. The causes of violent behavior are complex and although age, sex, and racial differences have been documented, no convincing evidence exists to link these variations to biological and genetic differences. A comprehensive review of the pertinent literature may be found in a recent staff report to the National Commission on the Causes and Prevention of Violence.[158]

In recent years, attention has been directed to the possibility that individuals with an extra Y chromosome are liable to hyperaggressivity and criminality. It seemed reasonable to suppose that since the relative rates of violent crimes are substantially higher among males

than among females, and since males normally carry a Y chromosome, a double dose of this chromosome would increase or exaggerate those masculine characteristics which might lead an individual into conflict with the law.

The first 47,XYY male was detected in 1961.[196] He was described as a physically normal man, six feet in height, of average intelligence, and father of seven living children from two marriages. He was not a criminal; it was the presence of mongolism and other congenital anomalies among his progeny that led to his identification. Between 1961 and 1965, twelve more 47,XYY cases were found, the majority with various physical abnormalities.[10] In 1965, Jacobs and her colleagues[101] and then Price and Whatmore[175] reported on a chromosomal survey of virtually all the male patients of a maximum security state hospital located at Carstairs, Scotland. Of a total of 315 men studied, 9 (2.9 percent) were found to have a 47,XYY karyotype. Since the publication of these reports more than one hundred other 47,XYY individuals have been identified in various prisons and mental hospitals and well over fifty cases have been detected in newborn and adult population surveys, fertility clinics, and private medical practice. The literature is reviewed by Court Brown[36] and others.[117,165,202]

Jacobs et al.[101] suggested that 47,XYY males tend to be tall. In the Carstairs group, the mean height of the 47,XYY individuals was 181.2 cm. whereas that of the chromosomally normal inmates was only 170.7 cm. Since many other institutionalized 47,XYY individuals have been ascertained on the basis of height, it has been difficult to confirm the initial findings. There may be a bias on the part of the courts towards the institutionalization of tall offenders.[97] Moreover, tall institutionalized 47,XYY men may come from families with a tendency toward tallness. On the other hand, of twenty-three 47,XYY cases ascertained on a basis other than height half were at least six feet tall.[117]

The evidence for intellectual deficits associated with an extra Y chromosome is difficult to assess since most tested 47,XYY individuals were identified in institutions. Average and above average I.Q. scores have been reported in some cases.[20] Also, in studies where 47,XYY individuals were matched to chromosomally normal controls, no significant differences in mean I.Q. were found.[13,93]

In their initial report, Price and Whatmore[175] pointed out that the nine 47,XYY individuals were actually *less* openly hostile and violently aggressive than the eighteen men in a chromosomally normal control group. Although the convictions for crimes against property were proportionally the same in both groups, the 47,XYY individuals showed a significantly lower incidence of crimes of violence than did the controls (8.7 as against 21.9 percent). These findings suggest that the initial characterization of 47,XYY male as an uncontrollably aggressive psychopath was somewhat exaggerated. If these men are unusually impulsive and/or aggressive, it might be expected that a disproportionate number of 47,XYY males would be found among groups of individuals identified as hyperaggressive on personality tests and other reasonable criteria. All work based on this hypothesis, however, has shown negative findings.[43,61,230]

It has also been suggested[175] that the criminal activity of 47,XYY males begins at an early age and that a familial predisposition to criminality is absent. In the Carstairs group the mean ages at first conviction for the 47,XYY individuals and the 46,XY controls were 13.1 and 18.0 years respectively. There was only one conviction reported among the thirty-one siblings of the 47,XYY individuals, whereas 139 convictions were found among the sixty-three siblings of the control group. Kessler and Moos[117] provide a critique of this evidence. Suffice it to say that subsequent reports have confirmed neither assertion; several studies[9,78] show no differences between 47,XYY inmates and 46,XY controls with respect to age at first conviction, and it is now clear that many institutionalized 47,XYY males do come from homes that show evidence of interpersonal or psychosocial disturbance.[30,37]

With respect to a variety of physical and physiological measures, 47,XYY individuals show a broad range of expression. The evidence appears to suggest that abnormalities in these measures may occur in a fraction, but not in the majority of these males. Studies of plasma and urinary testosterone levels in 47,XYY individuals are of particular interest since androgens are associated with aggressive behavior. Elevated androgen levels might provide a potential mechanism through which the additional Y chromosome might promote behavioral changes, possibly arising or being exacerbated at the time of puberty. However, several studies[100,174,189] have shown no significant differences in testosterone levels between 47,XYY males and 46,XY fellow inmates.

A question that needs further clarification is whether or not 47,XYY individuals have a greater than average risk for criminality. The frequency of 47,XYY males in the newborn population is believed to be approximately 1.8 per one thousand[176] whereas their frequency in certain institutions may be as much as twenty times higher. It is unclear at the present time whether this elevated rate represents sampling bias, random sampling variation, or the reflection of a true predisposition to institutionalization as a consequence of having an extra Y chromosome. In the most extensive and systematic survey thus far reported, Jacobs et al.[102] examined the chromosomes of 2,538 males in a variety of penal and other corrective institutions in Scotland and found that the frequency of 47,XYY males in these institutions was not significantly different from the rate expected on the basis of the newborn incidence.* If this finding is confirmed, it would suggest that no increased risk for criminality may be attached to this chromosomal disorder.

In sum, the evidence suggesting an association between the 47,XYY karyotype and a predisposition to antisocial behavior is inconclusive at the present time. The characterization of the 47,XYY male as uncontrollably hyperaggressive has not been substantiated and, with the possible exception of a tendency to increased stature, no specific behavioral,

* Although several reports have suggested that 47,XXY males are also predisposed to criminality, they found no increase in the frequency of these individuals above that of the newborn rate.

morphological, or physiological characteristic has emerged differentiating these individuals from males with other chromosomal constitutions.

In a recent report,[199] a higher rate of mental illness and psychopathy was found among the biological relatives of a group of psychopathic adoptees than among the relatives of a matched control group. Preliminary results of another adoption study has recently appeared.[39] Further study is needed since other reports[19,182] show no clear-cut relationship between the social adjustment of adoptees and the presence of alcoholism or criminality among their biological parents.

Homosexuality

Accurate estimates of the prevalence of homosexuality are not available. Kinsey[120] reported that 37 percent of American males have homosexual experiences involving orgasm during some period of their lives; about 4 percent remain exclusively homosexual throughout their lives. Kenyon[116] suggests that homosexuality among adult females occurs at the rate of one in forty-five in England.

The literature bearing on possible genotypic contributions to homosexual behavior has been reviewed by Money[148] and others.[11,183,208] Most of the evidence derives from twin studies that generally show a higher concordance rate among MZ twin pairs than among DZ pairs.[92] However, the samples, with one exception, were small, were gathered by means of questionable sampling procedures or were otherwise biased to include mostly individuals seeking or requiring psychiatric attention. Whether such samples are representative of homosexuals in general is not known.

Evidence in a different vein, reviewed by Slater and Cowie,[208] suggests that a preponderance of brothers may be present among the sibs of male homosexuals and that homosexuals tend to be born late in the sibship to older mothers. These findings suggest that a chromosomal disorder might be involved in the etiology of homosexuality. However, attempts to find such disorders have not been fruitful. Abe

and Moran[1] have shown that the shift in maternal age is secondary to a concommitant shift in paternal age, further ruling out a chromosomal disorder associated with late maternal age as contributing to the etiology of homosexuality.

In sum, the extent to which genotypic factors are involved in the etiology of homosexual behavior is not clear. Recently, several laboratories have reported striking endocrine differences between homosexuals and nonhomosexuals. The most impressive report to date is that of Kolodny et al.[121] who studied thirty male homosexual university student volunteers and fifty heterosexual male student controls. The plasma testosterone concentrations and sperm counts among the homosexuals showed a graded decrement correlated with the degree of homosexuality, as rated on the Kinsey scale. The mean plasma testosterone concentrations of the subjects rated as Kinsey five and six (almost exclusively and exclusively homosexual) were significantly lower than that of the control group. Whether these differences are related to the pathogenesis of homosexuality or are the secondary results of a homosexual psychosocial orientation needs to be investigated. The possibility that gene-determined differences in the synthesis, transport, and metabolism of androgens may predispose some individuals toward a homosexual orientation should also be explored.

Affective Disorders

Published estimates of the prevalence of the affective disorders vary widely from country to country and at different periods of time even within a single country.[208] Estimates of manic-depressive illness in the general population range from 0.21 percent to close to 5 percent;[238] in British and Scandinavian populations an expectation of about 1 percent is a generally accepted figure.[208,245] Differences in the criteria used in the diagnosis of the affective disorders at various clinical centers probably account for the variation in prevalence rates.[79,233] Most investigators in Western countries report a relatively higher incidence of affective disorders among females than among males; the ratio of females to males in the general population, averaged over several studies, is about 1.5:1.[208]

The evidence suggesting genotypic contributions to the etiology of the affective disorders comes from twin and family studies and is summarized by Slater and Cowie[208] and others.[70,173] The average concordance rates for manic-depressive psychosis among MZ and same-sexed DZ twin pairs, in several studies, are about 68 and 23 percent respectively.[173] Estimates of the morbid risks for affective disorders among the relatives of manic-depressive probands, averaged over several studies, are shown in Table 17–1. Among the first degree relatives of affected probands the average morbid risk for affective disorders is about 14 percent, a substantial increase over the general population rate. Among second and third degree relatives, average risks are 4.8 and 3.6 percent respectively.[208]

In recent years, attempts have been made to refine the nosology of the affective disorders. Leonhard et al.[131] and subsequent workers[7,170] have suggested that depressive illness may be divided into two groups. In one (bipolar psychosis) individuals exhibit episodes of mania or hypomania and depression whereas in the other (unipolar psychosis) only episodes of depression occur. Disagreement exists as to whether these groups constitute genetically distinct entities.[183] Perris[170]

found that the morbid risks for bipolar and unipolar psychosis among the first-degree relatives of 138 bipolar probands were 16.3 and 0.8 percent respectively whereas among the relatives of 139 unipolar probands the morbid risks were 0.5 and 10.6 percent respectively for bipolar and unipolar psychoses. These data support the possibility of genetically distinct subtypes. Other workers,[6,238] however, have reported relatively high rates of unipolar psychosis among the relatives of bipolar probands, indicating that overlap of the two types of disorder exists.

The bipolar-unipolar distinction has been found to be a good one for the purpose of research into the clinical, psychophysiological, and pharmacological correlates of the affective disorders. The age of onset of bipolar psychosis tends to be earlier than that of the unipolar form,[170] and the morbid risk for affective disorder appears to be higher among the relatives of a bipolar proband than among those of a unipolar one.[6] Depressed bipolar patients have been reported to exhibit less pacing behavior, overt expressions of anger, and somatic complaints than unipolar ones.[14] In contrast to the latter, the former tend to have a lower threshold for flicker stimulation[170] and an augmenting pattern in their measured-average, evoked-cortical potentials.[22] Lithium carbonate appears to be a more effective antidepressant in bipolar patients than in unipolar

TABLE 17–1.   **Morbid Risks for Affective Disorders Among Relatives of Manic-Depressive Probands (in percent).**
(Data from Zerbin-Rüdin[245] and Slater and Cowie[208]

	NUMBER OF INVESTIGATIONS	RANGE	MEAN
Parents	9	7–23	14.3
Children	6	8–24	14.8
Sibs	10	4–23	12.9
Half-sibs	2	1–17	9.0
Nieces and Nephews	2	2–3	2.6
Grandchildren	2	1–4	2.5

ones.[24] The former, in contrast to the latter, tend to show hypomanic episodes when treated for depression with L-Dopa,[155] or with tricyclic antidepressants.[23] Red blood cell catechol O-methyltransferase(COMT) activity appears to be relatively lower among unipolar female patients than bipolar ones[48] whereas blood platelet monoamine oxidase (MAO) activity appears to be relatively lower in bipolar patients.[156] Taken together, these findings support the bipolar-unipolar dichotomy and suggest that the differentiation may be a consequence of different underlying genetic systems. Support for this hypothesis derives from data collected by Zerbin-Rüdin,[245] who carefully examined the relevant twin literature and found that concordant MZ pairs were, with only a few exceptions, similar as to subtype.

Angst[6] and Perris[171] found an increased number of affected females among the first-degree relatives of unipolar probands whereas among the relatives of bipolar probands the two sexes were equally affected. Data summarized by Winokur and his coworkers[26,27,235] suggest that a preponderance of affected female relatives may occur in families of both bipolar and unipolar female probands. These latter workers have suggested that among the relatives of female bipolar probands affected parents and children show equal proportions of females and males, but affected sisters appear to be some three times more prevalent than affected brothers. They also point out that mothers of male bipolar probands appear to be more often affected than fathers. These findings are suggestive of an X-linked dominant mode of inheritance for bipolar psychosis. In support of this hypothesis, evidence has been advanced suggesting linkage between manic-depressive disorder and the color blindness and X_g^a blood group loci.[177,240] However, the number of families involved in the linkage study was small and data of both Cadoret and Winokur[26] and other workers are not consistent with X-linkage. In two recent reports,[172,210] the distribution of secondary cases of bipolar psychosis between the maternal and paternal sides of the families of bipolar probands was found to

be more in accord with a polygenic mode of transmission rather than one involving a major gene.

Winokur and his coworkers[236] have suggested that there may be two groups of unipolar psychosis, one with a relatively early age of onset in which relatively higher morbid risks for depression occur mostly among females and the other with a relatively later age of onset in which female and male relatives of male probands share equal morbid risks for depression. Perris[172] has argued for a polygenic mode of transmission for unipolar psychosis. Another possibility that has been advanced is that the predisposition to affective disorders may have a heterogeneous genetic basis.[173] The possible association of the affective disorders with aspects of biogenic amine metabolism suggests that pharmacogenetic approaches might be worthwhile in elucidating the apparent genotypic and phenotypic heterogeneity of these disorders. Genetic variation in the metabolism of antidepressant drugs has been found.[164]

Schizophrenia

Evidence pointing to the involvement of genotypic factors in the etiology of schizophrenia has been considerably strengthened in recent years. Eleven major twin studies of schizophrenia have been carried out worldwide: all show higher rates of concordance among MZ than DZ twin pairs. In the older studies, MZ concordance rates are generally 60 percent or more whereas in those conducted after 1965, shown in Table 17–2, average MZ concordance is between 34 and 46 percent. The differences probably reflect the nature of the population studied as well as variations in sampling and statistical procedures. The older studies generally involved chronically affected resident hospital populations whereas the recent ones employed consecutive admissions or birth registers. Of the older twin studies, Kallmann's[106] is probably the best known because of the large sample (691 pairs) studied, its inordinately high age-corrected MZ concordance rate (86 percent) and the intensity of criticism it received. In

TABLE 17-2.   Concordance Rates in Recent Twin Studies of Schizophrenia (in percent).

	MZ TWINS			DZ TWINS		
	N (*pairs*)	(*a*)	(*b*)	N (*pairs*)	(*a*)	(*b*)
Kringlen[127]						
(1968) Norway	55	25–39	45	90	7–10	15
Fischer et al.[63]						
(1969) Denmark	21	24–48	56	41	10–20	26
Tienari[224]*						
(1971) Finland	19	16	35	34	3	13
Allen et al.[3]*						
(1972) U.S.A.	95	27	43	125	5	9
Gottesman and Shields[77]						
(1972) U.K.	24	42	58	33	9	12

[a] pairwise concordance
[b] proband method (from[77])
* Only male pairs studied.

their study, Gottesman and Shields[75] took account of many of the criticisms of the diagnostic and sampling procedures of the earlier twin studies. Their study was organized prospectively and consisted of a sample of consecutive admissions to a short-stay psychiatric hospital over a period of sixteen years. Both sexes were represented equally among the probands and zygosity was carefully determined. These investigators found that without age-correction 42 percent of the twenty-four MZ pairs and only 9 percent of the thirty-three same-sexed DZ twin pairs were concordant for schizophrenia. To study the effect of differential diagnostic criteria on concordance rates, summaries of the case histories of the 114 individual twins were submitted to six clinicians from three different countries representing a broad range of psychiatric orientation.[204] Each judge, blind as to diagnosis and zygosity, arrived at his own diagnostic assessment. In sum, it was found that despite individual diagnostic preferences considerable agreement existed among the judges. The consensus diagnosis yielded concordance rates similar to those found by Gottesman and Shields in their original study. Of particular

interest was the fact that neither narrow nor broad concepts of schizophrenia but rather middle-of-the-road diagnostic criteria produced the most reliable discrimination between MZ and DZ concordance rates, and hence the highest estimate of heritability.

Studies of MZ twin pairs reared apart also suggest that genotypic factors are involved in the etiology of schizophrenia. Of the seventeen such pairs compiled by Slater and Cowie,[208] eleven (65 percent) were reported to be concordant for schizophrenia. However, more than half of these pairs were not obtained in a systematic way, and, thus, discordant pairs may have been underreported.[183]

Schizophrenia shows a decided familial concentration (Table 17-3). The median morbid risk for schiozphrenia in the general population, derived from nineteen studies tabulated by Zerbin-Rüdin,[245] is about 0.8 percent. Both sexes appear to be equally at risk. Among the first-degree relatives of an affected proband, the median risk over all studies is about 8.6 percent; for second- and third-degree relatives, the risks are 2.1 and 1.7 percent respectively.[183] Thus, there is an elevation of morbid risks for schizophrenia among

TABLE 17–3.   **Estimates of Morbid Risks for Schizophrenia Among Relatives of Schizophrenic Probands (in percent). (Data from various sources.[52,183,208,246])**

Parents	4.2– 5.5
Children	9.7–13.9
Children (both parents affected)	35 –46
Sibs (all)	7.5–10.2
(neither parent affected)	6.7– 9.7
(one parent schizophrenic)	12.5–17.2
Half-sibs	3.2– 3.5
Aunts and Uncles	2.0– 3.6
Nieces and Nephews	2.2– 2.6
Grandchildren	2.8– 3.5

the relatives of probands over that of the general population, increasing as the degree of genetic relatedness to the proband increases.

The most compelling evidence for the role of genotypic factors in the etiology of schizophrenia derives from the study of adoptive children. Karlsson[111] found that among the relatives of eight schizophrenic probands who were reared by unrelated adoptive parents from the first year of life, six of the twenty-nine biologic sibs and none of the twenty-eight foster sibs were schizophrenic. In another report, Karlsson[112] discusses several other cases of affected individuals born to a schizophrenic parent but separated from them early in life. Heston[89,91] studied a group of forty-seven individuals (an experimental group) born to hospitalized schizophrenic mothers, but separated from them at birth and reared in foster homes. A control group, selected from fifty individuals who had entered the same foundling homes around the same time as the first group, was matched to the experimentals by age, sex, type of eventual placement (adoptive, foster family, or institutional) and the length of time in child-care institutions. None of the mothers of the controls had a known psychiatric disorder. Most subjects were personally interviewed and information from psychiatric, police, and social-service agencies, private physicians, friends, relatives, and other sources was also obtained.

All the subjects were about thirty-six years of age at the time of the study and were thus well into the age of risk for schizophrenia. It was found that five of the experimental group and none of the controls were diagnosed as schizophrenic. In addition, Heston found significantly lower scores on the Menninger Mental Health-Sickness Rating Scale (MHSRS) and relatively higher incidences of criminality, mental deficiency, neurotic personality disorder and sociopathic personality among the experimental group than among the controls.

A series of adoption studies have also been carried out by Kety, Rosenthal, and their coworkers in Denmark.[187] From an adoption register of the greater Copenhagen area, the names of approximately fifty-five hundred individuals were obtained who had been given up for nonfamilial adoption at an early age, between 1923 and 1947. From these records the names, addresses, and other pertinent information concerning the biological and adoptive parents were also obtained. From a psychiatric register and other sources it was possible to determine which individuals had a psychiatric history. In one study, approximately ten thousand parents of the adoptees were considered. The hospital records of the parents listed in the psychiatric register were examined independently, first by Danish psychiatrists and then by the American collaborators. If diagnostic agreement was reached, the child given up for adoption by that parent became an index case. From the remaining adoptees, a group of controls was selected, none of whose biological parents had a psychiatric history. The control and index adoptees were matched for age, sex, age at transfer to the adoptive family, and socioeconomic status of the adopting family. In this way, seventy-six index and sixty-seven control adoptees, with a mean age of thirty-three years, were collected for study.[184,186] Each received a psychiatric interview, carried out so that the interviewer was blind as to whether a given individual belonged to the index or control groups. Of the index parents, fifty were mothers and twenty-six were fathers; only ten of the parents had their first psychiatric admission antedating the birth of the index child. It was found that twenty-four (31.6 percent) of the index and twelve (17.8 percent) of the control children had a schizophrenic-spectrum diagnosis;* the difference between the two groups is statistically significant. The relative severity of the psychiatric diagnoses was greater among the index cases than among the controls. The three cases with diagnoses of chronic schizophrenia were all index cases.

In a second study,[118] the rates of schizophrenic disorders among the biological and adoptive relatives of a group of index and control adoptees were determined. Among the parents, sibs, and half-sibs of thirty-three affected index cases thirteen out of one hundred and fifty of the biological but only two out of seventy-four of the adoptive relatives had a schizophrenic-spectrum disorder, whereas among the relatives of thirty-three matched controls three of one hundred fifty-six biological and three of eighty-three adoptive relatives were found affected. Thus, although there was no significant difference in the prevalence of schizophrenic disorders among the adoptive relatives of the two groups, the rate of these disorders among the biological relatives of the index cases was significantly higher than that among the controls. Taken together with the twin and family studies, these data strongly suggest that genotypic factors play a role in the development of schizophrenia.

No widespread agreement exists as to the mode of inheritance of the genes that predispose to schizophrenia. Recent theories include major gene, polygenic, and various mixed or heterogeneity models. Following Kallmann's[106] earlier arguments, Hurst[98] has recently defended a single locus recessive model. Kidd and Cavalli-Sforza[119] have suggested that available family data are compatible with a single recessive having a gene frequency of about 10 percent and a threshold such that 50 percent or more of the homozygous recessives would be affected. Slater,[207,208]

on the other hand, has advanced a model involving a partially dominant gene with a frequency of about 3 percent and with a manifestation rate in the heterozygote of 13 percent. According to this model, most schizophrenics would be heterozygotes. Karlsson[113] has suggested a two-factor model involving a dominant principal gene with a frequency of about 7 percent and a secondary dominant with a frequency between 20 and 30 percent. Other investigators favor a polygenic mode of inheritance.[50,162] A polygenic threshold model has been advanced by Gottesman and Shields[76] who, following Falconer[60] and Smith,[211,212] have calculated the heritability of the liability to schizophrenia to be about 85 percent.[76]

Several heterogeneity models have been advanced;[58,146,147,246] these consider the possibility that schizophrenia constitutes a collection of heterogeneous disorders with differing genotypic etiologies. Genetic heterogeneity may arise as a result of the effects of genes or blocks of genes at different loci or the presence of multiple alleles at a common locus. Morton and his coworkers[44,150,151] have shown that for heterogeneous disorders like limbgirdle muscular dystrophy, deaf-mutism, and severe mental defect estimates of the proportion of all cases resulting from major gene effects can be calculated. These workers distinguish two etiological groups, a high-risk group in which the recurrence risk for sibs of affected individuals is appreciable due to the segregation of fully penetrant recessive genes, and a low-risk group of sporadic cases due to mutations, phenocopies (environmentally induced mimics of a genetic disorder) and polygenic complexes in which recurrence risks for sibs are small. For severe mental defect, 88 percent of the cases were found to belong to the sporadic group; the remainder were attributed to a minimum of twenty-two contributory recessive loci.[44] A modified version of this model might be applicable to schizophrenia.[77] However, adequate empirical tests for heterogeneity models of schizophrenia have not yet been developed. It is of interest to note that genetic heterogeneity has become an increasingly common finding in human genetics research.[33]

---

* The schizophrenic-spectrum disorders are described by Kety et al.[118] They include chronic or process, acute and borderline or psychoneurotic schizophrenia, and severely schizoid or inadequate personality.

Arguments for and against the monogenic and polygenic models for schizophrenia are discussed by several writers.[76,110,208] Major gene theories generally require auxiliary assumptions of reduced penetrance to account for the inadequate fit of family and twin data to Mendelian expectations, and selective advantages to account for the maintenance of the disorder over time in the face of the reduced reproductive rate of affected individuals.[58,209] Heston[90] attempted to bypass the difficulty of reduced penetrance by postulating that schizoid disorders and schizophrenia are alternative expressions of a single dominant gene. However, there is poor clinical consensus over what constitutes a schizoid disorder. Moreover, even when the frequency of both disorders is taken into account, the observed rates for all degrees of relationship to an affected individual are consistently lower than those expected on the basis of a fully penetrant, single dominant gene.

To account for the apparent maintenance of the genes predisposing to schizophrenia over time, some workers have suggested that heterozygotes enjoy selective advantages that lead to the maintenance of a balanced polymorphism.[99] Moran[149] has suggested that a reproductive advantage of about 10 percent in nonschizophrenic heterozygotes would be needed to maintain a balanced polymorphism. Several investigators have discussed possible sources of such advantages. Huxley et al.[99] have suggested that schizophrenics may be resistant to surgical shocks and to infections. However, with the possible exception of an increased resistance to viral infections,[29] the evidence is largely unsubstantiated. Erlenmeyer-Kimling[53] found that during the first year of life, infants born to schizophrenics have a lower mortality rate than same-sexed infants in the general population. Female offspring of a schizophrenic parent were found to have a significantly lower mortality rate during the period from birth to age fifteen than did females of the general population. If confirmed, these findings would provide some support for the possibility that the genes associated with schizophrenia confer sufficient compensatory advantages on their carriers to maintain a balanced polymorphism. Bodmer[18] has suggested that a polymorphism could be maintained through a higher relative reproductive rate among the unaffected relatives of schizophrenics. Study of the marriage and fertility trends in schizophrenic patients admitted to state hospitals in New York State revealed that over the past few decades the reproductive disadvantages of schizophrenics have declined.[57,58] Of particular interest is the fact that the reproductive rate of nonaffected sisters of schizophrenics increased, during a twenty-year period, to 140 percent that of the general population rate. Relevant to these findings are suggestions[45,89,114] that nonschizophrenic relatives of affected individuals may be predisposed to creativity, giftedness, resourcefulness, and other desirable behavioral characteristics. If these attributes are associated with the increased fertility of relatives of schizophrenics, it would suggest that the possible long-range dysgenic trends attending changes in the fertility of schizophrenics might be offset by the increase in frequency of adaptive attributes in other individuals.[18]

Polygenic models obviate the necessity of postulating the balanced polymorphism and/or reduced penetrance required by monogenic models. Available family data appear to support a polygenic model. Edwards[49] has shown that the incidence of a polygenically inherited disorder in first-degree relatives of probands would approximate the square root of the general population incidence. If the incidence of schizophrenia in the general population is 0.8 percent, then it would be expected that approximately 9 percent of the first-degree relatives of probands would be affected. This accords closely to the median morbid risk for this group of relatives (see Table 17-3). Support for a polygenic threshold model is provided by the relationship between the morbid risks in relatives and the severity of the disorder in the proband. If it is assumed that severely affected individuals carry a greater number of the relevant predisposing genes than more mildly affected persons, it would be expected that the prevalence of schizophrenia among relatives of the former would be higher than that among the latter. Although in one family study no strong relationship was found between measures of severity and the presence of a family history of schizophrenia,[56] in several twin studies the severity of the illness in MZ probands has been found to be associated with the concordance rate in the co-twins.[73] Also, pertinent to the relationship between high risk and severity are data showing that the morbid risk for sibs of affected individuals increases substantially if one parent is also affected (Table 17–3). On the basis of a simple single gene model, the risk for subsequent sibs would be expected to remain constant. However, recently advanced major gene models[51,208] account for the increase in risk about as well as a polygenic threshold model does.

In sum, available data derived from family and twin studies of schizophrenia can be fitted to multiple models of genetic transmission. Recent attempts to discriminate between different modes of inheritance in schizophrenia[77,119] and in other disorders without an obvious Mendelian pattern of transmission[152,213] suggest that this problem has no easy solution. The one point on which there is agreement is that both genotypic and environmental factors are involved in the development of schizophrenia.

Recent years have seen an increasing interest in MZ twins discordant for schizophrenia. The elucidation of the life-history differences and the biological and psychological variables that differentiate the affected and nonaffected members of MZ twin pairs would contribute to our understanding of the genotype-environment interactions involved in the precipitation of schizophrenia. Such studies might define which variables require greater attention in future research and suggest strategies of intervention that might prevent the development of illness in vulnerable individuals.[68] Stabenau and Pollin[214] have suggested that, in contrast to the nonschizophrenic co-twin, the affected one was more likely to have been weaker, shorter, and lighter at birth, and to have experienced birth complications such as neonatal asphyxia. As a child, CNS illness was also likely. Behaviorally, the affected twin was

reported to have been more submissive, sensitive, serious, obedient, dependent, stubborn, and neurotic as a child than the nonschizophrenic co-twin. The schizophrenic twin also tended to be strongly identified with the psychologically less healthy parent who had a more global cognitive style than did the other parent.[153] Other intrapair comparisons suggest that schizophrenic twins have more abnormal neurological signs,[154] a higher lactate/pyruvate ratio and higher titers of antirabbit heterophile hemagglutinin than their nonschizophrenic co-twins.[215] On the other hand, no significant differences were found in serum S_{19} macroglobulin levels or in the urinary excretion of 3,4-dimethoxyphenylethylamine (DMPEA) in discordant MZ pairs.[215] Some of the issues that need to be explored in discordancy research are the applicability of detected differences to concordant twins and to nontwin schizophrenic groups;[203] whether the differences are present prior to the onset of illness or develop as a consequence of the psychopathology; the specificity of the differences to schizophrenia; and the effects of systematic manipulations of life experiences, as, for example, through psychiatric attention, on co-twin differences. Some of the intrapair differences detected in discordancy research have not always been found among concordant twin pairs or singletons.[203]

Another important research strategy adopted in recent years is the so-called high-risk approach in which individuals predisposed to schizophrenia and their families are studied prospectively in order to elucidate the biological and psychological factors that precede the onset of schizophrenia and contribute to its precipitation. Wynne[244] has provided a provocative discussion of the various strategies employed in high-risk research. Mednick and his coworkers[140,141,142] pioneered such studies in Denmark; at least eleven other high-risk studies are currently ongoing worldwide.[69] Mednick is studying a group of 207 high-risk children born to chronically and severely schizophrenic mothers matched to a group of 104 (low-risk) controls for age, sex, social class, and other variables. Since the onset of the study in 1962, twenty of the high-risk group have suffered psychiatric breakdown. Each breakdown subject was then matched with a low-risk control. Comparisons of these with another unaffected high-risk subject and three groups have suggested that the mothers of the sick group were more severely schizophrenic and hospitalized earlier than those of the unaffected high-risk children, that the sick children have suffered one or more serious pregnancy or birth complications, and had been considerably more aggressive and disruptive in school than the children of the other groups. Galvanic skin responses (GSR) and responses on a word-association test also appeared to differentiate the sick group from the others. A preliminary report of another ongoing high-risk study being conducted by Anthony[8] has also recently appeared.

❲ Future Avenues of Research

One of the central issues in psychiatric research is the relation between life stresses and behavioral dysfunction. Clinical and experimental observations suggest that differential susceptibility to illness might be a consequence of how different individuals adapt and respond to stress. Presumably, numerous genotypic and environmental factors contribute to such individual variation. One of the promising lines of research in this area involves studies focused on the intervening hormonal substrates of behavior. Stress affects multiple endocrine systems. Conversely, hormones influence CNS function. Genetic variation affecting the synthesis and metabolism of the andrenocortical[82] and thyroid hormones[85] has been identified. It is conceivable that certain individuals carrying gene defects affecting these endocrine systems may, when subjected to sustained major stress situations, produce deficient or excessive amounts of these hormones or their metabolites, with concomitant adverse effects on CNS functioning.[84] Investigation of the interdigitation of genes, hormones, and behavior may have important implications for psychiatry and psychosomatic medicine.[83]

With the increased use of drugs in the treatment of behavioral disorders, psychopharmacogenetic research opportunities have become available. Suggestions have been made that relatives of depressive patients tend to respond to the same class of antidepressant drug, either MAO inhibitors or tricyclic compounds, in the same way as the proband.[167] No similarity of response was found when antidepressants of different groups were used. In the treatment of schizophrenics with phenothiazines, the risk of extrapyramidal side effects appears to be increased in patients with a positive family history of Parkinson's disease.[157] These and similar findings[164] need to be explored further. The study of genetically determined differences in the response of individuals to drugs that alter mood and behavior may elucidate some of the biochemical mechanisms underlying behavioral disorders and may contribute to the identification of distinct clinical subgroups among the major psychoses.

Stronger collaborative interactions are needed between biochemists and psychiatric geneticists. Too often biochemical research into behavioral disorder begins by assuming the presence of a genetic etiology, but then proceeds to ignore the implications of that assumption in the specific research carried out. A behavioral-biochemical correlation due to a common genetic cause should show predictable patterns of transmission among relatives of an affected individual. Thus, segregation studies should reveal which correlations continue to hold and which break down among relatives of probands.[205] The former situation would suggest that a common genetic basis is present whereas the latter would show that no genetic relationship exists between the biochemical variable being studied and the behavior. For example, although the protein factor identified by the L/P ratio has been found in greater concentrations in the plasma of schizophrenics than in that of normal people,[67] study of the families of schizophrenics showed that the correlation between schizophrenic symptomatology and high L/P ratio disappears.[218] Thus, whatever is being measured by the L/P ratio probably has little or no etiological relationship to schizophrenia.

Until recently, the history of psychiatric genetics has been marked by an overriding concern with nature-nurture issues, which had as their focus the demonstration of a genotypic influence on behavioral characters and on determining morbid risks and patterns of inheritance. There is a growing awareness of the need to shift the primary focus of psychiatric genetics research to the problem of genotype-environment interactions. Developmental studies should receive strong encouragement. Too little is known about the ontogeny of behavioral dysfunction in children with inborn errors of metabolism and chromosomal disorders. Studies are needed to elucidate the reaction range of a particular genotype or karyotype in differing environments. With respect to the major psychoses, the high-risk strategy has emerged as the approach with the greatest potential of clarifying the complex interplay of genotypic, biochemical, physiological, psychological, and social factors that promote or prevent behavioral disorder in predisposed individuals. Once illness is present, it is virtually impossible to tease apart the etiological variables from those which arise as consequences of the illness. Thus, the prospective, longitudinal study of premorbid individuals, preferably in conjunction with an adoption strategy, is long overdue as a central methodology of psychiatric genetics. In the face of the major contributions of experiential factors to human behavior, such research approaches may yield considerably more appropriate data for genetic analysis than that provided by classical human genetics methodology.

The increasing use of adoption studies in psychiatric genetics research suggests that greater attention needs to be paid to the psychology and sociology of adoption.[244] Adoption may involve something more than an ordinary parent–child relationship. The intriguing possibility advanced by Rosenthal[185] and others that adoption may have ameliorative consequences for the adopted individual needs further exploration. In the adoption study of schizophrenia carried out in Denmark, only 0.3 percent of the total group of fifty-five hundred adoptees were classified as chronic or process schizophrenia.[186] This rate, the lowest ever reported in a Scandinavian population, may be due to several factors. One possibility is that adoptive rearing may contribute to the reduced expression of psychopathology. The fact that the rate of hospitalized schizophrenia (1.3 percent) among the adoptees born to a schizophrenic parent was lower than that reported for offspring of schizophrenics generally is consistent with this possibility.

The rapid advances in scientific technology, particularly those related to prenatal diagnosis and to chromosome identification and mapping, will presumably have important implications for psychiatric genetics as well as for medical practice generally. Taken together with available techniques of manipulating behavior through behavioral and pharmacological means and the future possibilities of modifying behavior through genetic engineering,[129] the potential of controlling and directing man's behavioral evolution is becoming an increasing reality. To what extent and to what ends should human behavior be manipulated? Underlying these questions are important ethical and philosophical issues concerning the nature of man and the meaning of his existence. Is man beyond freedom, dignity, choice, and responsibility, or are these attributes the core of his existence? Whatever answers eventually emerge, it is clear that both the biological and sociocultural bases of human behavior will need to be taken into account.

◖ Bibliography

1. ABE, K. and P. A. P. MORAN. "Parental Age of Homosexuals," *Br. J. Psychiatry*, 115 (1969), 313–317.
2. ALLEN, G., B. HARVALD, and J. SHIELDS. "Measures of Twin Concordance," *Acta Genet. Statist. Med.*, 17 (1967), 475–481.
3. ALLEN, M. G., S. COHEN, and W. POLLIN. "Schizophrenia in Veteran Twins: A Diagnostic Review," *Am. J. Psychiatry*, 128 (1972), 939–945.
4. ÅMARK, C. "A Study in Alcoholism," *Acta Psychiatr. Neurol. Scand. Suppl.*, 70 (1951), 1–283.

5. ANDREWS, G. and M. HARRIS. *The Syndrome of Stuttering.* London: Heinemann, 1964.

6. ANGST, J. *Zur Ätiologie und Nosologie Endogener Depressiver Psychosen.* Berlin: Springer, 1966.

7. ANGST, J. and C. PERRIS. "The Nosology of Endogenous Depression. Comparison of the Results of Two Studies," *Int. J. Ment. Health*, 1 (1972), 145–158.

8. ANTHONY, E. J. "A Clinical and Experimental Study of High-Risk Children and Their Schizophrenic Parents," in A. R. Kaplan, ed., *Genetic Factors in "Schizophrenia,"* pp. 380–406. Springfield: Charles C. Thomas, 1972.

9. BAKER, D., M. A. TELFER, C. E. RICHARDSON et al. "Chromosome Errors in Men with Antisocial Behavior," *JAMA*, 214 (1970), 869–878.

10. BALODIMOS, M. C., H. LISCO, I. IRWIN et al. "XYY Karyotype in a Case of Familial Hypogonadism," *J. Clin. Endocrinol. Metabol.*, 26 (1966), 443–452.

11. BANCROFT, J. H. J. "Homosexuality in the Male," *Br. J. Hosp. Med.*, 3 (1970), 168–181.

12. BANDURA, A. *Principles of Behavior Modification.* New York: Holt, Rinehart and Winston, 1969.

13. BARTLETT, D. J., W. P. HURLEY, C. R. BRAND et al. "Chromosomes of Male Patients in a Security Prison," *Nature*, 219 (1968), 351–354.

14. BEIGEL, A. and D. L. MURPHY. "Unipolar and Bipolar Affective Illness," *Arch. Gen. Psychiatry*, 24 (1971), 215–220.

15. BENDER, L. "Childhood Schizophrenia," *Psychiatr. Q.*, 27 (1953), 663–681.

16. BERMAN. J. L., G. C. CUNNINGHAM, R. W. DAY et al. "Causes for High Phenylalanine With Normal Tyrosine in Newborn Screening Programs," *Am. J. Dis. Child.*, 117 (1969), 54–65.

17. BLASKOVICS, M. E. and T. L. NELSON. "Phenyketonuria and its Variations—A Review of Recent Developments," *Calif. Med.*, 115 (1971), 42–57.

18. BODMER, W. F. "Demographic Approaches to the Measurement of Differential Selection in Human Populations," *Proc. Natl. Acad. Sci.*, 59 (1968), 690–699.

19. BOHMAN. M. "A Comparative Study of Adopted Children, Foster Children and Children in Their Biological Environment Born After Undesired Pregnancies," *Acta Paediatr. Scand. Suppl.* 221, 1971.

20. BORGAONKAR, D. S., J. L. MURDOCH, V. A. McKUSICK et al. "The YY Syndrome," *Lancet*, 2 (1968), 461–462.

21. BOWDEN, J. A. and C. L. McARTHUR III. "Possible Biochemical Model for Phenylketonuria," *Nature*, 235 (1972), 230.

22. BUCHSBAUM, M., F. K. GOODWIN, D. L. MURPHY et al. "Average Evoked Responses in Affective Disorders," *Am. J. Psychiatry*, 128 (1971), 19–25.

23. BUNNEY, W. E., JR., H. K. H. BRODIE, D. L. MURPHY et al. "Psychopharmacological Differentiation Between Two Subgroups of Depressed Patients," *Proc. 78th Annu. Con. Am. Psychol. Assoc.*, (1970), 829–833.

24. BUNNEY, W. E., JR., F. K. GOODWIN, J. M. DAVIS et al. "A Behavioral-Biochemical Study of Lithium Treatment," *Am. J. Psychiatry*, 125 (1968), 499–512.

25. BURT, C. "The Genetic Determination of Differences in Intelligence: A Study of Monozygotic Twins Reared Together and Apart," *Br. J. Psychol.*, 57 (1966), 137–153.

26. CADORET, R. J. and G. WINOKUR. "Genetic Principles in the Classification of Affective Illnesses," *Int. J. Ment. Health*, 1 (1972), 159–175.

27. CADORET, R. J., G. WINOKUR, and P. J. CLAYTON. "Family History Studies: VII. Manic Depressive Disease versus Depressive Disease," *Br. J. Psychiatry*, 116 (1970), 625–635.

28. CARTER, C. O. "Genetics of Common Disorders," *Br. Med. Bull.*, 25 (1969), 52–57.

29. CARTER, M., and C. A. H. WATTS. "Possible Biological Advantages Among Schizophrenics' Relatives," *Br. J. Psychiatry*, 118 (1971), 453–460.

30. CASEY, M. D. "The Family and Behavioural History of Patients with Chromosome Abnormality in the Special Hospitals of Rampton and Moss Side," in D. J. West, ed., *Criminological Implications of Chromosome Abnormalities*, pp. 49–60. Cambridge: Cropwood Round-Table Conference, 1969.

31. CAVALLI-SFORZA, L. L. and W. F. BODMER. *The Genetics of Human Populations.* San Francisco: W. H. Freeman, 1971.

32. CAVALLI-SFORZA, L. L. and K. K. KIDD. "Considerations on Genetic Models of

Schizophrenia," *Neurosci. Res. Program Bull.*, 10 (1972), 406–419.

33. CHILDS, B. and V. M. DER KALOUSTIAN. "Genetic Heterogeneity," *N. Engl. J. Med.*, 279 (1968), 1205–1212; 1267–1274.

34. CLEMENTS, S. D. "Minimal Brain Dysfunction in Children," *U. S. Public Health Service Pub.*, 1415, 1966.

35. CLEMMENS, R. L. and K. GLASER. "Specific Learning Disabilities. I. Medical Aspects," *Clin. Pediatr.*, 6 (1967), 481–486.

36. COURT BROWN, W. M. "Males with an XYY Sex Chromosome Complement," *J. Med. Genet.*, 5 (1968), 341–359.

37. COURT BROWN, W. M., W. H. PRICE, and P. A. JACOBS. "Further Information on the Identity of 47,XYY Males," *Br. Med. J.*, 2 (1968), 325–328.

38. CRITCHLEY, M. *The Dyslexic Child*. London: Heinemann, 1970.

39. CROWE, R. R. "The Adopted Offspring of Women Criminal Offenders," *Arch. Gen. Psychiatry*, 27 (1972), 600–603.

40. CRUZ, F. F. DE LA, B. H. FOX, and R. H. ROBERTS. "Minimal Brain Dysfunction," *Ann. N.Y. Acad Sci.*, 205 (1972), 1–396.

41. CRUZ-COKE, R. "Genetic Aspects of Alcoholism," in Y. Israel and J. Mardones, eds., *Biological Basis of Alcoholism*, pp. 335–363. New York: Wiley, 1971.

42. CRUZ-COKE, R. and A. VARELA. "Inheritance of Alcoholism," *Lancet*, 2 (1966), 1282.

43. DAVIS, J. D., B. J. McGEE, J. EMPSON et al. "XYY and Crime," *Lancet*, 2 (1970), 1086.

44. DEWEY, W. J., I. BARRAI, N. E. MORTON et al. "Recessive Genes in Severe Mental Defect," *Am. J. Hum. Genet.*, 17 (1965), 237–256.

45. DEYKIN, E. Y., G. L. KLERMAN, and D. J. ARMOR. "The Relatives of Schizophrenic Patients: Clinical Judgements of Potential Emotional Resourcefulness," *Am. J. Orthopsychiatry*, 36 (1966), 518–528.

46. DIZMANG, L. H. and C. F. CHEATHAM. "The Lesch-Nyhan Syndrome," *Am. J. Psychiatry*, 127 (1970), 671–677.

47. DOBZHANSKY, T. *Mankind Evolving*. New Haven: Yale University Press, 1962.

48. DUNNER, D. L., C. K. COHN, E. S. GERSHON et al. "Differential Catechol-O-Methyltransferase Activity in Unipolar and Bipolar Affective Illness," *Arch. Gen. Psychiatry*, 25 (1971), 348–353.

49. EDWARDS, J. H. "Familial Predisposition in Man," *Br. Med. Bull.*, 25 (1969), 58–64.

50. ———. "The Genetical Basis of Schizophrenia," in A. R. Kaplan, ed., *Genetic Factors in "Schizophrenia*," pp. 310–314. Springfield: Charles C. Thomas, 1972.

51. ELSTON, R. C. and M. A. CAMPBELL. "Schizophrenia: Evidence for the Major Gene Hypothesis," *Behav. Genet.*, 1 (1970), 3–10.

52. ERLENMEYER-KIMLING L. "Studies on the Offspring of Two Schizophrenic Parents," in D. Rosenthal and S. S. Kety, eds., *The Transmission of Schizophrenia*, pp. 65–83. Oxford: Pergamon, 1968.

53. ———. "Mortality Rates in the Offspring of Schizophrenic Parents and a Physiological Advantage Hypothesis," *Nature*, 220 (1968), 798–800.

54. ———. "Genetics, Interaction, and Mental Illness: Setting the Problem," *Int. J. Ment. Health*, 1 (1972), 5–9.

55. ERLENMEYER-KIMLING, L. and L. F. JARVIK. "Genetics and Intelligence: A Review," *Science*, 142 (1963), 1477–1478.

56. ERLENMEYER-KIMLING, L. and S. NICOL. "Comparison of Hospitalization Measures in Schizophrenic Patients with and without a Family History of Schizophrenia," *Br. J. Psychiatry*, 115 (1969), 321–334.

57. ERLENMEYER-KIMLING, L., S. NICOL, J. D. RAINER et al. "Changes in Fertility Rates of Schizophrenic Patients in New York State," *Am. J. Psychiatry*, 125 (1969), 916–927.

58. ERLENMEYER-KIMLING, L. and W. PARADOWSKI. "Selection and Schizophrenia," *Am. Nat.*, 100 (1966), 651–665.

59. FALCONER, D. S. *Introduction to Quantitative Genetics*. Edinburgh: Oliver & Boyd, 1960.

60. ———. "The Inheritance of Liability to Certain Diseases, Estimated from the Incidence Among Relatives," *Ann. Hum. Genet.*, 29 (1965), 51–76.

61. FALEK, A., R. CRADDICK, and J. COLLUM. "An Attempt to Identify Prisoners with an XYY Chromosome Complement by Psychiatric and Psychological Means," *J. Nerv. Ment. Dis.*, 150 (1970), 165–170.

62. FENNA, D., L. MIX, O. SCHAEFER et al. "Ethanol Metabolism in Various Racial Groups," *Can. Med. Assoc. J.*, 105 (1971), 472–475.

63. FISCHER, M., B. HARVALD, and M. HAUGE. "A Danish Twin Study of Schizophrenia," *Br. J. Psychiatry*, 115 (1969), 981–990.

64. FISH, B., T. SHAPIRO, F. HALPERN et al. "The Prediction of Schizophrenia in Infancy: III. A Ten-Year Follow-Up Report of Neurological and Psychological Development," *Am. J. Psychiatry*, 121 (1965), 768–775.

65. FREEDMAN, D. G. "An Evolutionary Approach to Research on the Life Cycle," *Hum. Dev.*, 14 (1971), 87–99.

66. FREEDMAN, D. G. and B. KELLER. "Inheritance of Behavior in Infants," *Science*, 140 (1963), 196–198.

67. FROHMAN, C. E., G. TOURNEY, P. G. S. BECKETT et al. "Biochemical Identification of Schizophrenia," *Arch. Gen. Psychiatry*, 4 (1961), 404–412.

68. GARMEZY, N. "Vulnerability Research and the Issue of Primary Prevention," *Am. J. Orthopsychiatry*, 41 (1971), 101–116.

69. ———. "Models of Etiology for the Study of Children at Risk for Schizophrenia," in M. Roff, L. N. Robins, and M. Pollack, eds., *Life History Research in Psychopathology*, Vol. 2, pp. 9–23. Minneapolis: University of Minnesota Press, 1972.

70. GERSHON, E. S., D. L. DUNNER, and F. K. GOODWIN. "Toward a Biology of Affective Disorders," *Arch. Gen. Psychiatry*, 25 (1971), 1–15.

71. GOLDFARB, W. "The Subclassification of Psychotic Children: Application to a Study of Longitudinal Change," in D. Rosenthal and S. S. Kety, eds., *The Transmission of Schizophrenia*, pp. 333–343. Oxford: Pergamon, 1968.

72. GOODWIN, D. W. "Is Alcoholism Hereditary?" *Arch. Gen. Psychiatry*, 25 (1971), 545–549.

73. GOTTESMAN, I. I. "Severity/Concordance and Diagnostic Refinement in the Maudsley-Bethlem Schizophrenic Twin Study," in D. Rosenthal and S. S. Kety, eds., *The Transmission of Schizophrenia*, pp. 37–48. Oxford: Pergamon, 1968.

74. GOTTESMAN, I. I. and J. SHIELDS. "Contributions of Twin Studies to Perspectives on Schizophrenia," in B. A. Maher, ed., *Progress in Experimental Personality Research*, Vol. 3, pp. 1–84. New York: Academic, 1966.

75. ———. "Schizophrenia in Twins: 16 Years' Consecutive Admissions to a Psychiatric Clinic," *Br. J. Psychiatry*, 112 (1966), 809–818.

76. ———. "A Polygenic Theory of Schizophrenia," *Proc. Natl. Acad. Sci.*, 58 (1967), 199–205.

77. ———. *Schizophrenia and Genetics—A Twin Study Vantage Point*. New York: Academic, 1972.

78. GRIFFITHS, A. W., B. W. RICHARDS, J. ZAREMBA et al. "Psychological and Sociological Investigation of XYY Prisoners," *Nature*, 227 (1970), 290–292.

79. GURLAND, B. J., J. L. FLEISS, J. E. COOPER et al. "Cross-National Study of Diagnosis of the Mental Disorders: Some Comparisons of Diagnostic Criteria from the First Investigation," *Am. J. Psychiatry Suppl.* 125 (1969), 30–39.

80. HAILMAN, J. P. "How an Instinct is Learned," *Sci. Am.*, 221 (1969), 98–106.

81. HALLGREN, B. "Specific Dyslexia," *Acta Psychiatr. Neurol. Suppl.* 65 (1950), 1–287.

82. HAMBURG, D. A. "Genetics of Adrenocortical Hormone Metabolism in Relation to Psychological Stress," in J. Hirsch, ed., *Behavior—Genetic Analysis*, pp. 154–175. New York: McGraw-Hill, 1967.

83. ———, ed. *Psychiatry as a Behavioral Science*. Englewood Cliffs: Prentice-Hall, 1970.

84. HAMBURG, D. A. and S. KESSLER. "A Behavioural-Endocrine-Genetic Approach to Stress Problems," in S. G. Spickett, ed., *Endocrine Genetics*, pp. 249–266. London: Cambridge University Press, 1967.

85. HAMBURG, D. A. and D. T. LUNDE. "Relation of Behavioral, Genetic and Neuroendocrine Factors to Thyroid Function," in J. N. Spuhler, ed., *Genetic Diversity and Human Behavior*, pp. 135–170. Chicago: Aldine, 1967.

86. HARRIS, G. W. "Sex Hormones, Brain Development and Brain Function," *Endocrinology*, 75 (1964), 627–648.

87. HARRIS, G. W. and S. LEVINE. "Sexual Differentiation of the Brain and Its Experimental Control," *J. Physiol.*, 181 (1965), 379–400.

88. HARRIS, H. "Enzyme Variation in Man: Some General Aspects," in J. F. Crow and J. V. Neel, eds., *Proc. 3rd Int. Congr. Hum. Genet.*, pp. 207–214. Baltimore: Johns Hopkins Press, 1967.

89. HESTON, L. L. "Psychiatric Disorders in Foster Home Reared Children of Schizophrenic Mothers," *Br. J. Psychiatry*, 112 (1966), 819–825.

90. ———. "The Genetics of Schizophrenia and Schizoid Disease," *Science*, 167 (1970), 249–256.

91. HESTON, L. L. and D. DENNEY. "Interactions Between Early Life Experience and Biological Factors in Schizophrenia," in D. Rosenthal and S. S. Kety, eds., *The Transmission of Schizophrenia*, pp. 363–376. Oxford: Pergamon, 1968.

92. HESTON, L. L. and J. SHIELDS. "Homosexuality in Twins," *Arch. Gen. Psychiatry*, 18 (1968), 149–160.

93. HOPE, K., A. E. PHILIP, and J. M. LOUGHRAN. "Psychological Characteristics Associated with XYY Sex-Chromosome Complement in a State Mental Hospital," *Br. J. Psychiatry*, 113 (1967), 495–498.

94. HOWELL, R. R. and R. E. STEVENSON. "The Offspring of Phenylketonuric Women," *Soc. Biol., Suppl.* 18 (1971), S19–S29.

95. HSIA, D. Y. Y. "Phenylketonuria and Its Variants," in A. G. Steinberg and A. G. Bearn, eds., *Progress in Medical Genetics*, Vol. 7, pp. 29–68. New York: Grune & Stratton, 1970.

96. HUESSY, H. R. "Study of the Prevalence and Therapy of the Choreatiform Syndrome or Hyperkinesis in Rural Vermont," *Acta Paedopsychiatr.*, 34 (1967), 130–135.

97. HUNTER, H. "YY Chromosomes and Klinefelter's Syndrome," *Lancet*, 1 (1966), 984.

98. HURST, L. A. "Hypothesis of a Single-Locus Recessive Genotype for Schizophrenia," in A. R. Kaplan, ed., *Genetic Factors in "Schizophrenia,"* pp. 219–245. Springfield: Charles C. Thomas, 1972.

99. HUXLEY, J., E. MAYR, H. OSMOND et al. "Schizophrenia as a Genetic Morphism," *Nature*, 204 (1964), 220–221.

100. ISMAIL, A. A. A., R. A. HARKNESS, K. E. KIRKHAM et al. "Effect of Abnormal Sex-Chromosome Complements on Urinary Testosterone Levels," *Lancet*, 1 (1968), 220–222.

101. JACOBS, P. A., M. BRUNTON, M. M. MELVILLE et al. "Aggressive Behaviour, Mental Sub-normality, and the XYY Male," *Nature*, 208 (1965), 1351–1352.

102. JACOBS, P. A., W. H. PRICE, S. RICHMOND et al. "Chromosome Surveys in Penal Institutions and Approved Schools," *J. Med. Genet.*, 8 (1971), 49–58.

103. JENSEN, A. R. "IQ's of Identical Twins Reared Apart," *Behav. Genet.*, 1 (1970), 133–146.

104. JUDD, L. L. and A. J. MANDELL. "Chromosome Studies in Early Infantile Autism," *Arch. Gen. Psychiatry*, 18 (1968), 450–457.

105. KAIJ, L. *Alcoholism in Twins: Studies on the Etiology and Sequels of Abuse of Alcohol.* Stockholm: Almquist & Wiksell, 1960.

106. KALLMANN, F. J. "The Genetic Theory of Schizophrenia: An Analysis of 691 Schizophrenic Twin Index Families," *Am. J. Psychiatry*, 103 (1946), 309–322.

107. ———. "The Genetics of Mental Illness," in S. Arieti, ed., *American Handbook of Psychiatry*, Vol. 1, 1st ed., pp. 175–196. New York: Basic Books, 1959.

108. KALLMANN, F. J. and B. ROTH. "Genetic Aspects of Preadolescent Schizophrenia," *Am. J. Psychiatry*, 112 (1956), 599–606.

109. KANNER, L. "Autistic Disturbances of Affective Contact," *Nerv. Child*, 2 (1943), 217–250.

110. KAPLAN, A. R., ed. *Genetic Factors in "Schizophrenia."* Springfield: Charles C. Thomas, 1972.

111. KARLSSON, J. *The Biologic Basis of Schizophrenia.* Springfield: Charles C. Thomas, 1966.

112. KARLSSON, J. L. "The Rate of Schizophrenia in Foster-Reared Close Relatives of Schizophrenic Index Cases," *Biol. Psychiatry*, 2 (1970), 285–290.

113. ———. "A Double Dominant Genetic Mechanism for Schizophrenia," *Hereditas*, 65 (1970), 261–268.

114. ———. "Genetic Association of Giftedness and Creativity with Schizophrenia," *Hereditas*, 66 (1970), 177–182.

115. KENNY, T. J., R. L. CLEMMENS, B. W. HUDSON et al. "Characteristics of Children Referred Because of Hyperactivity," *J. Pediatr.*, 79 (1971), 618–622.

116. KENYON, F. E. "Homosexuality in the Female," *Br. J. Hosp. Med.*, 3 (1970), 183–206.

117. KESSLER, S. and R. H. MOOS. "The XYY Karyotype and Criminality: A Review," *J. Psychiatr. Res.*, 7 (1970), 153–170.

118. KETY, S. S., D. ROSENTHAL, P. H. WENDER et al. "The Types and Prevalence of Mental Illness in the Biological and Adoptive Families of Adopted Schizophrenics", in D. Rosenthal and S. S. Kety, eds., *The Transmission of Schizophrenia*, pp. 345–362. Oxford: Pergamon, 1968.

119. KIDD, K. K. and L. L. CAVALLI-SFORZA. "An Analysis of the Genetics of Schizophrenia." *Soc. Biol.*, 20 (1973), 254–265.

120. KINSEY, A. C., W. B. POMEROY, and C. E. MARTIN. *Sexual Behavior in the Human Male.* Philadelphia: W. B. Saunders, 1948.

121. KOLODNY, R. C., W. H. MASTERS, J. HENDRYX et al. "Plasma Testosterone and Semen Analysis in Male Homosexuals," *N. Engl. J. Med.*, 285 (1971), 1170–1174.

122. KORNER, A. F. "Visual Alertness in Neonates: Individual Differences and Their Correlates," *Percept. Mot. Skills*, 31 (1970), 499–509.

123. ———. "Individual Differences at Birth: Implications for Early Experience and Later Development," *Am. J. Orthopsychiatry*, 41 (1971), 608–619.

124. KORNER, A. F., B. CHUCK, and S. DONTCHOS. "Organismic Determinants of Spontaneous Oral Behavior in Neonates," *Child Dev.*, 39 (1968), 1145–1157.

125. KORNER, A. F. and H. C. KRAEMER. "Individual Differences of Spontaneous Oral Behavior in Neonates," in J. F. Bosma, ed., *Third Symposium on Oral Sensation and Perception: The Mouth of the Infant*, pp. 335–346. Springfield: Charles C. Thomas, 1972.

126. KORNER, A. F. and E. B. THOMAN. "Visual Alertness in Neonates as Evoked by Maternal Care," *J. Exp. Child Psychol.*, 10 (1970), 67–78.

127. KRINGLEN, E. "An Epidemiological-Clinical Twin Study on Schizophrenia," in D. Rosenthal and S. S. Kety, eds., *The Transmission of Schizophrenia*, pp. 49–63. Oxford: Pergamon, 1968.

128. LAUFER, M. W., E. DENHOFF, and G. SOLOMONS. "Hyperkinetic Impulse Disorder in Children's Behavior Problems," *Psychosom. Med.*, 19 (1957), 38–49.

129. LEDERBERG, J. "Experimental Genetics and Human Evolution," *Am. Nat.*, 100 (1966), 519–531.

130. LEHRMAN, D. S. "Semantic and Conceptual Issues in the Nature-Nurture Problem," in L. R. Aronson, E. Tobach, D. S. Lehrman et al., eds., *Development and Evolution of Behavior*, pp. 17–52. San Francisco: W. H. Freeman, 1970.

131. LEONHARD, K., I. KORFF, and H. SCHULZ. "Die Temperamente in den Familien der monopolaren und bipolaren phasischen Psychosen," *Psychiatr. Neurol.*, 143 (1962), 416–434.

132. LESCH, M. and W. L. NYHAN. "A Familial Disorder of Uric Acid Metabolism and Central Nervous System Function," *Am. J. Med.*, 36 (1964), 561–570.

133. LINDZEY, G., J. LOEHLIN, M. MANOSEVITZ et al. "Behavioral Genetics," *Annu. Rev. Psychol.*, 22 (1971), 39–94.

134. LOBASCHER, M. E., P. E. KINGERLEE, and S. S. GUBBAY. "Childhood Autism: An Investigation of Aetiological Factors in Twenty-Five Cases," *Br. J. Psychiatry*, 117 (1970), 525–529.

135. LOPEZ, R. E. "Hyperactivity in Twins," *Can. Psychiatr. Assoc. J.*, 10 (1965), 421–426.

136. LOTTER, V. "Epidemiology of Autistic Conditions in Young Children," *Soc. Psychiatry*, 1 (1966), 124–137.

137. McCLEARN, G. E. "Behavioral Genetics," *Annu. Rev. Genet.*, 4 (1970), 437–468.

138. McKUSICK, V. A. *Mendelian Inheritance in Man*, 3rd ed. Baltimore: Johns Hopkins Press, 1971.

139. MALAMUD, N. "Neuropathology of Phenylketonuria," *J. Neuropathol. Exp. Neurol.*, 25 (1966), 254–268.

140. MEDNICK, S. A. and T. F. McNEIL. "Current Methodology in Research on the Etiology of Schizophrenia. Serious Difficulties Which Suggest the Use of the High-Risk Group Method," *Psychol. Bull.*, 70 (1968), 681–693.

141. MEDNICK, S. A. and F. SCHULSINGER. "A Longitudinal Study of Children with a High Risk for Schizophrenia: A Preliminary Report," in S. G. Vandenberg, ed., *Methods and Goals in Human Behavior Genetics*, pp. 255–295. New York: Academic, 1965.

142. ———. "Some Premorbid Characteristics Related to Breakdown in Children with Schizophrenic Mothers," in D. Rosenthal and S. S. Kety, eds., *The Transmission of Schizophrenia*, pp. 267–291. Oxford: Pergamon, 1968.

143. MENDELSON, J. H. "Ethanol-1-C^{14} Metabolism in Alcoholics and Nonalcoholics," *Science*, 159 (1968), 319–320.

144. ———. "Biological Concomitants of Alcoholism," *N. Engl. J. Med.*, 283 (1970), 24–32; 71–81.

145. MENDELSON, W., N. JOHNSON, and M. A.

STEWART. "Hyperactive Children as Teenagers: A Follow-up Study," *J. Nerv. Ment. Dis.*, 153 (1971), 273–279.

146. MITSUDA, H. "The Clinico-Genetic Study of Schizophrenia," *Int. J. Ment. Health*, 1 (1972), 76–92.

147. ———. "Heterogeneity of Schizophrenia," in A. R. Kaplan, ed., *Genetic Factors in "Schizophrenia,"* pp. 276–293. Springfield: Charles C. Thomas, 1972.

148. MONEY, J. "Sexual Dimorphism and Homosexual Gender Identity," *Psychol. Bull.*, 74 (1970), 425–440.

149. MORAN, P. A. P. "Theoretical Considerations on Schizophrenia Genetics," in A. R. Kaplan, ed., *Genetic Factors in "Schizophrenia,"* pp. 294–309. Springfield: Charles C. Thomas, 1972.

150. MORTON, N. E. "Segregation and Linkage," in W. J. Burdette, ed., *Methodology in Human Genetics*, pp. 17–47. San Francisco: Holden-Day, 1962.

151. ———. "The Detection of Major Genes Under Additive Continuous Variation," *Am. J. Hum. Genet.*, 19 (1967), 23–34.

152. MORTON, N. E., S. YEE, R. C. ELSTON et al. "Discontinuity and Quasi-Continuity: Alternative Hypotheses of Multifactorial Inheritance," *Clin. Genet.*, 1 (1970), 81–94.

153. MOSHER, L. R., W. POLLIN, and J. R. STABENAU. "Families with Identical Twins Discordant for Schizophrenia: Some Relationships between Identification, Thinking Styles, Psychopathology and Dominance-Submissiveness," *Br. J. Psychiatry*, 118 (1971), 29–42.

154. ———. "Identical Twins Discordant for Schizophrenia," *Arch. Gen. Psychiatry*, 24 (1971), 422–430.

155. MURPHY, D. L., H. K. H. BRODIE, F. K. GOODWIN et al. "Regular Induction of Hypomania by L-Dopa in 'Bipolar' Manic-Depressive Patients," *Nature*, 229 (1971), 135–136.

156. MURPHY, D. L. and R. WEISS. "Reduced Monoamine Oxidase Activity in Blood Platelets from Bipolar Depressed Patients," *Am. J. Psychiatry*, 128 (1972), 1351–1357.

157. MYRIANTHOPOULOS, N. C., F. N. WALDROP, and B. L. VINCENT. "A Repeat Study of Hereditary Predisposition in Drug-Induced Parkinsonism," *Excerp. Med. Int. Congr. Series*, 175 (1967), 486–491.

158. NATIONAL COMMISSION ON THE CAUSES AND PREVENTION OF VIOLENCE. *Crimes of Violence*, Vol. 12. A Staff Report, 1969.

159. NEAME, K. D. "Phenylalanine as Inhibitor of Transport of Amino-Acids in Brain," *Nature*, 192 (1961), 173–174.

160. NYHAN, W. L. "Behavioral Phenotypes in Organic Genetic Disease," *Pediatr. Res.*, 6 (1972), 1–9.

161. NYHAN, W. L., J. PESEK, L. SWEETMAN et al. "Genetics of an X-Linked Disorder of Uric Acid Metabolism and Cerebral Function," *Pediatr. Res.*, 1 (1967), 5–13.

162. ODEGARD, O. "The Multifactorial Theory of Inheritance in Predisposition to Schizophrenia," in A. R. Kaplan, ed., *Genetic Factors in "Schizophrenia,"* pp. 256–275. Springfield: Charles C. Thomas, 1972.

163. OMENN, G. S., and A. G. MOTULSKY. "A Biochemical and Genetic Approach to Alcoholism," *Ann. N. Y. Acad. Sci.*, 197 (1972), 16–23.

164. ———. "Psycho-Pharmacogenetics," in A. R. Kaplan, ed., *Human Behavior Genetics*. Springfield: Charles C. Thomas, Forthcoming.

165. OWEN, D. R. "The 47, XYY Male: A Review," *Psychol. Bull.*, 78 (1972), 209–233.

166. OWEN, F. W., P. A. ADAMS, T. FORREST et al. *Learning Disorders in Children: Sibling Studies*. Monogr. Soc. Res. Child Dev., Serial No. 144, Vol. 36. Chicago: University of Chicago Press, 1971.

167. PARE, C. M. B. and J. W. MACK. "Differentiation of Two Genetically Specific Types of Depression by the Response to Antidepressant Drugs," *J. Med. Genet.*, 8 (1971), 306–309.

168. PARTANEN, J., K. BRUNN, and T. MARKKANEN. *Inheritance of Drinking Behavior: A Study on Intelligence, Personality, and Use of Alcohol of Adult Twins*. Finn. Found. Alcohol Stud. 14. Stockholm: Almquist & Wiksell, 1966.

169. PERLO, V. P. and E. T. RAK. "Developmental Dyslexia in Adults," *Neurology*, 21 (1971), 1231–1235.

170. PERRIS, C. "A Study of Bipolar (Manic-Depressive) and Unipolar Recurrent Depressive Psychoses," *Acta Psychiatr. Scand. Suppl.* 194 (1966), 1–188.

171. ———. "Genetic Transmission of Depressive Psychoses," *Acta Psychiatr. Scand. Suppl.* 203 (1968), 45–52.

172. ———. "Abnormality on Paternal and Maternal Sides: Observations in Bipolar (Manic-Depressive) and Unipolar Depressive Psychoses," *Br. J. Psychiatry*, 118 (1971), 207–210.

173. PRICE, J. S. "Genetic and Phylogenetic Aspects of Mood Variation," *Int. J. Ment. Health*, 1 (1972), 124–144.

174. PRICE, W. H. and H. J. VAN DER MOLEN. "Plasma Testosterone Levels in Males with the 47,XYY Karyotype," *J. Endocrinol*, 47 (1970), 117–122.

175. PRICE, W. H. and P. B. WHATMORE. "Behaviour Disorders and Pattern of Crime Among XYY Males Identified at a Maximum Security Hospital," *Br. Med. J.*, 1 (1967), 533–536.

176. RATCLIFFE, S. G., M. M. MELVILLE, and A. L. STEWART. "Chromosome Studies on 3,500 Newborn Male Infants," *Lancet*, 1 (1970), 121–122.

177. REICH, T., P. J. CLAYTON, and G. WINOKUR. "Family History Studies: V. The Genetics of Mania," *Am. J. Psychiatry*, 125 (1969), 1358–1368.

178. REISER, D. E. "Psychosis of Infancy and Early Childhood, as Manifested by Children with Atypical Development," *N. Engl. J. Med.*, 269 (1963), 790–798; 844–850.

179. RIMLAND, B. *Infantile Autism*. New York: Appleton-Century-Crofts, 1964.

180. RITVO, E. R., D. CANTWELL, E. JOHNSON et al. "Social Class Factors in Autism," *J. Autism Child. Schizo.*, 1 (1971), 297–310.

181. ROBERTS, J. A. F. "The Genetics of Mental Deficiency," *Eugen. Rev.*, 44 (1952), 71–83.

182. ROE, A. "The Adult Adjustment of Children of Alcoholic Parents Raised in Foster-Homes," *Q. J. Stud. Alcohol*, 5 (1944), 378–393.

183. ROSENTHAL, D. *Genetic Theory and Abnormal Behavior*. New York: McGraw-Hill, 1970.

184. ———. "Two Adoption Studies of Heredity in the Schizophrenic Disorders," in M. Bleuler and J. Angst, eds., *The Origin of Schizophrenia*. Berne: Hans Huber, 1971.

185. ———. "A Program of Research on Heredity in Schizophrenia," *Behav. Sci.*, 16 (1971), 191–201.

186. ———. "Three Adoption Studies of Heredity in the Schizophrenic Disorders," *Int. J. Ment. Health*, 1 (1972), 63–75.

187. ROSENTHAL, D. and S. S. KETY. *The Transmission of Schizophrenia*. Oxford: Pergamon, 1968.

188. RUBIN, E. and C. S. LEIBER. "Alcoholism, Alcohol, and Drugs," *Science*, 172 (1971), 1097–1102.

189. RUDD, B. T., O. M. GALAL, and M. D. CASEY. "Testosterone Excretion Rates in Normal Males and Males with an XYY Complement," *J. Med. Genet.*, 5 (1968), 286–288.

190. RUTT, C. N. and D. R. OFFORD. "Prenatal and Perinatal Complications in Childhood Schizophrenics and Their Siblings," *J. Nerv. Ment. Dis.*, 152 (1971), 324–331.

191. RUTTER, M. "Psychotic Disorders in Early Childhood," in A. Coppen and A. Walk, eds., *Recent Developments in Schizophrenia*, pp. 133–158. *Br. J. Psychiatry*, Spec. Pub., 1, 1967.

192. ———. "Concepts of Autism: A Review of Research," *J. Child Psychol. Psychiatry*, 9 (1968), 1–25.

193. RUTTER, M. L. and L. BARTAK. "Causes of Infantile Autism: Some Considerations from Recent Research," *J. Autism Child. Schizo.*, 1 (1971), 20–32.

194. RUTTER, M., H. G. BIRCH, A. THOMAS et al. "Temperamental Characteristics in Infancy and the Later Development of Behavioural Disorders," *Br. J. Psychiatry*, 110 (1964), 651–661.

195. SAFER, D. J. "A Familiar Factor in Minimal Brain Dysfunction," *Behav. Genet.*, 3 (1973), 175–186.

196. SANDBERG, A. A., G. F. KOEPF, T. ISHIHARA et al. "An XYY Male," *Lancet*, 2 (1961), 40–52.

197. SCHIMKE, R. T. "Hormone Regulation of Gene Expression," in F. Clarke-Fraser and V. A. McKusick, eds., *Proc. 3rd Int. Conf. Congen. Malform.*, pp. 60–71. *Excerp. Med. Int. Congr. Series*, 204. Amsterdam: Excerp. Med. Found., 1970.

198. SCHUKIT, M. A., D. A. GOODWIN, and G. WINOKUR. "A Study of Alcoholism in Half Siblings," *Am. J. Psychiatry*, 128 (1972), 1132–1136.

199. SCHULSINGER, F. "Psychopathy: Heredity and Environment," *Int. J. Ment. Health*, 1 (1972), 190–206.

200. SEEGMILLER, J. E., F. M. ROSENBLOOM,

and W. N. KELLEY. "Enzyme Defect Associated with a Sex-Linked Human Neurological Disorder and Excessive Purine Synthesis," *Science*, 155 (1967), 1682–1684.

201. SEIXAS, F. A., G. S. OMENN, E. D. BURK et al. "Nature and Nurture in Alcoholism," *Ann. N.Y. Acad. Sci.*, 197 (1972), 1–229.
202. SHAH, S. A. "Report on the XYY Chromosomal Abnormality," *Pub. Health Serv. Pub.* 2103, 1970.
203. SHIELDS, J. "Summary of the Genetic Evidence," in D. Rosenthal and S. S. Kety, eds., *The Transmission of Schizophrenia*, pp. 95–126. Oxford: Pergamon, 1968.
204. SHIELDS, J. and I. I. GOTTESMAN. "Cross-National Diagnosis and the Heritability of Schizophrenia." Symposium: The Transmission of Schizophrenia. 5th World Congr. Psychiatry. Mexico City, 1971.
205. SHIRE, J. G. M. "Genes, Hormones and Behavioural Variation," in J. M. Thoday and A. S. Parkes, eds., *Genetic and Environmental Influences on Behaviour*, pp. 194–205. New York: Plenum, 1968.
206. SIBINGA, M. S., C. J. FRIEDMAN, I. M. STEISEL et al. "The Effect of Immobilization and Sensory Restriction on Children with Phenylketonuria," *Pediatr. Res.*, 2 (1968), 371–377.
207. SLATER, E. "The Case for a Major Partially Dominant Gene." In A. R. Kaplan, ed., *Genetic Factors in "Schizophrenia,"* pp. 173–180. Springfield: Charles C. Thomas, 1972.
208. SLATER, E. and V. COWIE. *The Genetics of Mental Disorders*. London: Oxford University Press, 1971.
209. SLATER, E., E. H. HARE, and J. S. PRICE. "Marriage and Fertility of Psychiatric Patients Compared with National Data," *Social Biol.*, Suppl. 18 (1971), 560–573.
210. SLATER, E., J. MAXWELL, and J. S. PRICE. "Distribution of Ancestral Secondary Cases in Bipolar Affective Disorders," *Br. J. Psychiatry*, 118 (1971), 215–218.
211. SMITH, C. "Heritability of Liability and Concordance in Monozygous Twins," *Ann. Hum. Genet.*, 34 (1970), 85–91.
212. ———. "Recurrence Risks for Multifactorial Inheritance," *Am. J. Hum. Genet.*, 23 (1971), 578–588.
213. ———. "Discriminating Between Different Modes of Inheritance in Genetic Diseases," *Clin. Genet.*, 2 (1971), 303–314.
214. STABENAU, J. R. and W. POLLIN. "Early

Characteristics of Monozygotic Twins Discordant for Schizophrenia," *Arch. Gen. Psychiatry*, 17 (1967), 723–734.
215. STABENAU, J. R., W. POLLIN, L. R. MOSHER et al. "Study of Monozygotic Twins Discordant for Schizophrenia," *Arch Gen. Psychiatry*, 20 (1969), 145–158.
216. STANBURY, J. B., J. B. WYNGAARDEN, and D. S. FREDRICKSON. *The Metabolic Basis of Inherited Disease*. New York: McGraw-Hill, 1966.
217. STEWART, M. A., F. N. PITTS, A. G. CRAIG et al. "The Hyperactive Child Syndrome," *Am. J. Orthopsychiatry*, 36 (1966), 861–867.
218. SULLIVAN, T. M., C. E. FROHMAN, P. G. BECKETT et al. "Clinical and Biochemical Studies of Families of Schizophrenic Patients," *Am. J. Psychiatry*, 123 (1967), 947–952.
219. TAFT, L. and W. GOLDFARB. "Prenatal and Perinatal Factors in Childhood Schizophrenia," *Dev. Med. Child Neurol.*, 6 (1964), 32–43.
220. TASHIAN, R. E. "Inhibition of Brain Glutamic Acid Decarboxylase by Phenylalanine, Valine, and Leucine Derivatives: A Suggestion Concerning the Etiology of the Neurological Defect in Phenylketonuria and Branched-Chain Ketonuria," *Metabolism*, 10 (1961), 393–402.
221. THOMAS, A., S. CHESS, H. G. BIRCH et al. *Behavioral Individuality in Early Childhood*. New York: New York University Press, 1963.
222. THOMAS, A., S. CHESS, and H. C. BIRCH. *Temperament and Behavior Disorders in Children*. New York: New York University Press, 1968.
223. THOMPSON, W. R. "Genetics and Social Behavior," in D. C. Glass, ed., *Biology and Behavior—Genetics*, pp. 79–101. New York: Rockefeller University Press & Russell Sage Found., 1968.
224. TIENARI, P. "Schizophrenia and Monozygotic Twins," *Psychiatr. Fennica*, (1971), 97–104.
225. TREFFERT, D. A. "Epidemiology of Infantile Autism," *Arch. Gen. Psychiatry*, 22 (1970), 431–438.
226. VANDENBERG, S. G., R. E. STAFFORD, and A. M. BROWN. "The Louisville Twin Study," in S. G. Vandenberg, ed., *Progress in Human Behavior Genetics*, pp. 153–

204. Baltimore: Johns Hopkins Press, 1968.

227. VERNON, M. D. *Backwardness in Reading. A Study in Its Nature and Origin.* Cambridge: Cambridge University Press, 1957.

228. VESELL, E. S., J. G. PAGE, and G. T. PASSANANTI. "Genetic and Environmental Factors Affecting Ethanol Metabolism in Man," *Clin. Pharmacol. Ther.*, 12 (1971), 192–201.

229. WARREN, R. J., W. A. KARDUCK, S. BUSSARATID et al. "The Hyperactive Child Syndrome," *Arch. Gen. Psychiatry*, 24 (1971), 161–162.

230. WELCH, J. P., D. S. BORGOANKAR, and H. M. HERR. "Psychopathy, Mental Deficiency, Aggressiveness and the XYY Syndrome," *Nature*, 214 (1967), 500–501.

231. WENDER, P. H. *Minimal Brain Dysfunction in Children.* New York: Wiley, 1971.

232. WING, J. K. "Diagnosis, Epidemiology, Aetiology," in J. K. Wing, ed., *Childhood Autism: Clinical, Educational and Social Aspects*, pp. 3–49. London: Pergamon, 1966.

233. ———. "International Comparisons in the Study of the Functional Psychoses," *Br. Med. Bull.*, 27 (1971), 77–81.

234. WINOKUR, G. "X-borne Recessive Genes in Alcoholism," *Lancet*, 2 (1967), 466.

235. ———. "Genetic Findings and Methodological Considerations in Manic Depressive Disease," *Br. J. Psychiatry*, 117 (1970), 267–274.

236. WINOKUR, G., R. CADORET, J. DORZAB et al. "Depressive Disease," *Arch. Gen. Psychiatry*, 24 (1971), 135–144.

237. WINOKUR, G. and P. J. CLAYTON. "Family History Studies IV. Comparison of Male and Female Alcoholics," *Q. J. Stud. Alcohol*, 29 (1968), 885–891.

238. WINOKUR, G., P. J. CLAYTON, and T. REICH. *Manic Depressive Illness.* St. Louis: C. V. Mosby, 1969.

239. WINOKUR, G., T. REICH, J. RIMMER et al. "Alcoholism—III. Diagnosis and Familial Psychiatric Illness in 259 Alcoholic Probands." *Arch. Gen. Psychiatry*, 23 (1970), 104–111.

240. WINOKUR, G. and V. L. TANNA. "Possible Role of X-Linked Dominant Factor in Manic-Depressive Disease," *Dis. Nerv. Sys.*, 30 (1969), 89–94.

241. WOLFF, P. H. "Ethnic Differences in Alcohol Sensitivity," *Science*, 175 (1972), 449–450.

242. WOOD, A. C., JR., C. J. FRIEDMAN, and I. M. STIESEL. "Psychosocial Factors in Phenylketonuria," *Am. J. Orthopsychiatry*, 37 (1967), 671–679.

243. WOOLEY, D. W. and T. VAN DER HOEVEN. "Prevention of Mental Defect of Phenylketonuria with Serotonin Congeners such as Melatonin or Hydroxytryptophan," *Science*, 144 (1964), 1593–1594.

244. WYNNE, L. C. "Family Research on the Pathogenesis of Schizophrenia," in *Problems of Psychosis*, pp. 401–412. Amsterdam: Excerp. Med. Int. Congr., Series 194, 1971.

245. ZERBIN-RÜDIN, E. "Endogene Psychosen," in P. E. Becker, ed., *Humangenetik, ein Kurzes Handbuch in fünf Bänden*, Vol. 2, pp. 446–577. Stuttgart: Goerg Thiem, 1967.

246. ———. "Genetic Research and the Theory of Schizophrenia," *Int. J. Ment. Health*, 1 (1972), 42–62.

247. ZIGLER, E. "Familial Mental Retardation: A Continuing Dilemma," *Science*, 155 (1967), 292–298.

CHAPTER 18

SOCIAL CHANGE AND THE PROBLEMS OF YOUTH

Beatrix A. Hamburg

(Introduction

CHANGE is not a new phenomenon for man. Over the span of evolutionary time, natural selection has favored structural and behavioral attributes that enhance man's adaptability to environmental and social change. In fact, it might be said that man's ability systematically to effect significant changes in his environment is the salient difference between man and other creatures. Increasingly over the years man lives in a man-made environment. It may give some perspective to realize that man's evolutionary history has been characterized by rapid change as compared, for example, to social insects who have remained static for fifty million years. There is evidence that man, as a distinct primate, has existed and has been evolving for two to three million years, although primates have existed for over fifty million years. Our own species, *Homo sapiens*, has existed for only about forty thousand years.[94] Within that time man has radiated to all parts of the world and has shown a remarkable ability to adapt both to the most diverse kinds of ecological niches and to drastic environmental changes within a given niche. Man's ability to influence his environment depends on adaptations of brain, motor function, and behavior that enable him not simply to make tools but to use them in combinations and to store them for future use; that is to say, to command a mastery of technology. There also has been the unique and powerful advantage of a command of spoken and, later, of written language.

The current view that technological change is a new and troublesome phenomenon may rest on our *historical* perspective. It is true that thousands of years passed in which simple tools changed scarcely at all and all of the main features of the hunting and gathering societies were remarkably stable. The advent of agriculture was eight or nine thousand years ago. It is believed that its worldwide adoption, in effective form, required several thousand years. The Industrial Revolution took place about two centuries ago. Although the full impact of the technological advances on a worldwide basis has not yet been fully attained, the Western world has had an industrial society for only several generations or about a century. The "postindustrial" society is largely in its formative stages and even in the most advanced countries was initiated within the past twenty years.

It can be noted in this brief resume that the fact of change has been constant in man's history, but the rate of change has been rapidly accelerating. This rate phenomenon is highly salient in one's perception of change and the ability to cope. We have moved from rates of change on an evolutionary scale of millions of years to the spread of agriculture in thousands of years, to changes in the industrial Revolution that took a couple of hundred years and now, in the postindustrial society, sweeping changes seem to be occurring from one generation to the next.

The question may be raised as to whether this current rate of change may be challenging the limits of genetically determined behavioral adaptation in a species in which the period of immaturity and learning is as prolonged as it is in man. It would appear, in a perhaps analogous vein, that man in affluent cultures has reached some other genetic limits, for example, genetically determined limits to height and maturational development. Tanner[84] has evidence that the secular trends toward increase in height and decreasing age of menarche have shown a tendency to flatten out in the past couple of generations of affluent Western populations.

Contemporary rapid social change has been invoked widely as an explanation for problems of youth. However, from earliest recorded time there has always been an awareness of reckless, erratic, irritating, and often rebellious behavior of adolescents.

They have high aspirations: for they have never yet been humiliated by the experience of life, but are unacquainted with the limiting force of circumstances. . . . Again, in their actions they prefer honor to expediency. . . . If the young commit a fault, it is always on the side of excess and exaggeration. . . . They regard themselves as omniscient

and are positive in their assertions; that is, in fact, the reason of their carrying everything too far. [pp. 18–19][46]

This quotation from Aristotle has a very contemporary flavor. The kinds of behavior that reflect the developmental status of the young person are, at times, interpreted as evidence of a "generation gap." There is a need to examine whether the problems of the youth of the past decade are, in fact, merely the most recent version of perennial "growing pains" or whether they instead represent a major discontinuity with the cultural institutions of the past century, i.e., a true generation gap. If the latter is so, it would suggest that our cultural institutions are no longer adequate to the task of socializing children for their adult tasks and challenges. This paper will attempt to look at these issues.

Social Change and the Problems of Contemporary Youth

There is no doubt that throughout the world[88] youth rebellion was a dominant theme and major concern of the 1960s. In some cases it meant violent confrontations over social issues. In other instances, there was great concern about the alienated, often drug-abusing, dropouts from society. Many have viewed this generation with despair. A few have seen these kinds of behavior as evidence of social progress.[4,68,74] In any case, on all sides there is a strongly felt need to relate the behavior of these young people to the social scene and to social change. Clearly, this turbulent decade is an important study in its own right. This paper will focus on the American youth of the sixties, but it will attempt at the same time to reappraise the relation of the individual family and society as well as look at the complex interplay of forces that determine the behavior of adolescents and young adults in any era.

There is a need to define the variables that are believed to be significant in contributing to the behavioral outcomes at adolescence. In any attempt to understand ongoing social change one must consider the forces and mechanisms of change, and also the nature of their impact in terms of magnitude of effect, quality, direction, and rapidity of change. The variables to be discussed are:

1. *Cultural institutions* of the past century especially as modified by advances in technology.
2. *Specific social context of the parental generation* as it affects their child-rearing goals and practices. It should be noted that cultural subgroups will have somewhat different patterns of socialization (culture transmission) in any given era.
3. *Contemporary youth.* Analysis of current social institutions with particular emphasis on drastically new developments that are likely to shift values and change social institutions. Some attention will be paid to the range of new solutions and their differential impacts across the generations and within the generation of contemporary youth.

(Cultural Institutions: Trends of the Twentieth Century

Culture may be defined as the system of social institutions, ideologies, and values that characterize a particular social domain in its adaptation to the environment. It is also implicit in the concept that these traditions and beliefs are systematically transmitted to succeeding generations. Culture is a dynamic concept and it is assumed that none but the simplest society has a single, static, all-embracing structure.

Any factor inducing significant environmental or social change will inevitably lead to a state of disequilibrium in at least one sector of the social system. In the twentieth century it is generally believed that advances in technology have played the major role in initiating social changes. Under the stress of change, the coping styles of individuals in a society will reflect the patterns of socialization that characterized their upbringing.

Behavioral responses cannot be exclusively predicted in terms of the nature of the stimulus or specific innovation. There is a continual interaction and interdependence of behavioral response and the technologies. There are those who believe that the major challenge currently facing man is to use scientific knowledge to guide processes and directions of technological change in the future. There is the belief that the rate of change will continue to accelerate and that in addition to coping with the current technological changes related to the physical sciences, we are now on the edge of a biological revolution whose impact may be even more dramatic in terms of the implications for man's future.[6,48,49] The hope is that we will be able to mobilize "creative" behavioral responses rather than eliciting a preponderance of either passive or violent responses that seemed to characterize the sixties.

Socialization is typically viewed as the shaping of the behavior of children by parents and by other significant adults. It is also true that the behavior and the values of young persons affect parents and significant adults and can, in turn, play a significant role in shaping adult behavior. Indeed, this may be a major primate social technique for adaptation to environmental change. There would appear to be an innate age differential in the preference for novelty.[56,58] When buttressed by a secure relationship with significant adults, children and juvenile primates exhibit a strong attractive for novel stimuli. Under these circumstances they will actively enjoy the exploration of novel aspects of the environment and new kinds of behavior are typically introduced into primate groups as a result of these juvenile "experiments." This socialization of adult primates by the juveniles has been well described in Japan by Itani[43] and Tsumori.[87] In contemporary America it is clear that new styles in clothing, hair, and music have been initially espoused by youth and later adopted into the general culture. This may also be true for certain basic-value orientations. For example, many adults report that their children were of significant influence in changing their attitudes about the war in Vietnam.

It is customary to divide this century into ten-year segments, the twenties, the thirties, the fifties, etc. This is probably related mainly to the practices of the federal census. In any case, there are evocative images that have been associated with these decades and it is useful to continue to use them for purposes of our discussion of the major technological and social trends of this century.

The Turn of the Century—1900s

In 1900, the United States was a predominantly rural nation. At that time, two out of three Americans lived on farms or in small towns.[1] There were stable communities with a network of social supports. The patriarchal family, with a large number of children and closely related extended family members, was the social unit. The salience of the father as a direct provider, earning a living for the family in clearly visible job roles, was still the norm. The father's work was still within range of the home, so that his presence was quite tangible through the day. The eroding effect of machine technology on the integrity of the family was just beginning to appear. The later outcomes of this development will be further discussed in relation to contemporary society.

Significantly, the U. S. Steel Corporation was organized in 1900. Steel was then, and continues in developing countries to be, a major symbol of economic progress. Steel had general utility as a basic construction material but little meaning, as such, to individuals or families. U. S. Steel dominated the economy for the next three decades.

The total population of the U. S. in 1900 was seventy-six million people. The gross national product was roughly $20 billion. There were no motor vehicles, no radios or television sets. Telephones were rare (six per one thousand of the population). Only 6.4 percent of young Americans completed high school.[89] Profitable economic participation in society was just beginning to be dependent on higher education. Values were stable and were transmitted to the young with certainty. America was seen as a land of opportunity where hard work would be rewarded with material success. Sex roles were sharply delineated and

were generally accepted as valid. Only a few women even questioned their lack of voting rights. It was a male- and youth-oriented culture. It has also been characterized as an era of "rugged individualism."

Persons born in 1900 are now in their seventies. Some are still serving on or just retiring as chairmen of the boards of major corporations, chairmen of influential Senate committees, heads of labor unions, and members of boards of regents of major universities. Their decisions are still influencing the contemporary scene. These are the elder statesmen of today and the grandfathers of today's youth.

The Parental Generation—1920s

In the late 1920s, one generation later, the parents of today's youth were born. At that time steel was superseded by automobiles as the dominant industry and General Motors emerged as the major company. Unlike steel, automobiles had a highly salient impact on individuals and families. It enormously increased their mobility, privacy, and, probably, their sexual freedom. The negative impacts of this technological advance were not confronted until the following generation, and they constitute an important contemporary problem. Only now are questions being raised about the extensive, costly, unattractive, street-and-road systems. Only now are the problems of parking, traffic congestion, air pollution, and auto junkyards beginning to be attacked. By the mid 1920s there were about eight million automobiles in America, and the population naively enjoyed them, oblivious of the potential for destructiveness to man and the environment.

Charles Lindberg made his dramatic solo flight across the Atlantic Ocean in May, 1927. This event received worldwide attention and it was a great stimulus for aviation. But air travel was still a hobby, not a means of transportation nor a force for shrinking the size of the world.

In 1920–1930, the population was continuing its shift away from the South and Midwest. Urban centers along both East and West coasts were becoming prominent. In the 1930s only about half of the population was still residing in rural settings.[90] There was a notable migration of agricultural workers of all colors and ethnicity due to increasing automation of the farm. John Steinbeck[80] movingly wrote about the migrant workers in 1940 in *The Grapes of Wrath.* A large and less visible sector of this displaced group moved to urban slums where they settled into a "culture of poverty."[51] It was still largely true, however, that even in big cities there tended to be cohesive neighborhoods where people felt linked to each other and acted as a network of support, interpersonal modeling, and controls for each other. Information and values acquired by youth were largely filtered through the cohesive group of parents and neighborhood.[8] There was certainty about values and a national pride related to America's participation in World War I and to our worldwide industrial leadership.

Most persons born in the 1920s experienced the depression of the thirties in their early years and participated in World War II as young adults, some as soldiers, others as war workers in industry at home. Rationing and shortages of food, commodities, and services were felt by most.

The spirit of this generation has been poignantly conveyed by Vice Admiral James F. Calvert,[12] Superintendent of the U. S. Naval Academy.

The most vivid memory of my childhood is being told by my mother that my father was, as we used to say in those days, "laid off." Like all ten year old boys I thought my father was the brightest, most capable man I had ever known. If he could not make a living, how would I ever hope to do so? . . . We worried about having enough to eat during the depression . . . and then later as we were getting started in our professions all of us went away to war. It (the war) took us and scattered us throughout the world. When we came back in 1945 and 1946 we were a different breed . . . We wanted stability and affluence. We wanted the privileges, the quiet, the stability for our children that we never had. We worked hard to give it to them.

Indeed, that generation built more schools, hospitals, and libraries than all other previous American generations combined. The biomedical professions made striking inroads on disease. The material prosperity and leisure time in the American people showed similar gains.

The beliefs and values of this generation were chiefly derived from their parents. Pride in family and nation was fostered and, for the most part, deeply held. This generation was fortified by these beliefs as well as by the toughness that was bred into them through coping with war and depression. Memories of the deprivations of the depression give salience to the value of seeking security and the acquisition of material possessions for themselves and their children. This value has paved the way for the "affluent society." There was confidence in the productiveness of America to satisfy the material and social needs of the total population. A strong current of idealism about the importance of equality in our pluralistic society was also prominent. These latter two values were to be the basis of the "revolution of rising expectations"[32] that has come to characterize value systems of the current generation very strongly.

The Nineteenth Amendment, giving the vote to women, was passed in 1920. Although this was a notable event and climaxed the efforts of a dedicated band of feminists, it did not usher in a new era for women. There was simply a liberalization of the institution of voting. Actually, women at that time usually voted in accordance with their husband's preferences and showed virtually no independence in political thinking. No restructuring of social institutions occurred nor was there significant alteration in society's view of woman's traditional role of homemaker and mother.

In 1920 the population of America was 106 million persons. The gross national product was $88 billion. There were now sixteen million telephones or roughly 139 per one thousand of population.[90] There were eight million motor vehicles, and one and a half million radio sets, but no television as yet.

The persons born in this decade are now near their fifties, constitute the "establishment" and are the parents of contemporary youth.

Contemporary Scene—1970s

Today's youth was born in the 1950s. In 1950, the population of America was 151 million. Thirty-four percent of young Americans completed high school. The gross national product was $285 billion. There were fifty-six million motor vehicles. Forty-five million families owned radio sets. There were fifty million telephones, or 312 per one thousand population. Transcontinental television was first broadcast September, 1951. By 1953, there were nearly twenty-one million families who owned TV sets. By 1955, there were thirty-four million sets in use. The growth in popularity has been phenomenal. Today TV sets are in virtually every home in America. This is the first TV generation.[89]

The affluence of America, as indicated in the gross national product, was reflected in the rise in the standard of living, i.e., acquisition of material possessions, and also in a mass movement of the affluent out of the cities and into the suburbs. These suburbs have tended to be characterized by isolation, age, race, educational and socioeconomic homogeneity. The necessity for the husband to commute into the city tended to significantly diminish his role as husband and, particularly, as father. Mothers living in these suburbs have had far less support from family and community than their mothers or grandmothers. The burdens on these mothers have been enormous and only recently is there appreciation of the difficulties of raising children single-handedly in a residential ghetto, cut off from the main currents of the larger community.

Benjamin Spock[79] published a popular, inexpensive book, Baby and Child Care. When it was reprinted in paperback, this volume became the handbook, almost "bible," by which this generation of children was raised—at least in middle-class families. Parents were encouraged to be permissive and child-centered. The burdened and insecure mothers were eager to rely on this benign expert. There was a parallel shift in the advice given in Infant Care, a handbook issued by the U. S. Children's Bureau that was the other popular "authority" on child rearing. In the successive editions of Infant Care between 1914 and 1951, Wolfenstein[97] charted a shift from the strict, authoritarian approaches to childrearing in the twenties to a permissive approach by 1950. Children were given more freedom for self-determination. There were also conscious efforts at early independence training. There may have been some maternal reaction to their own early experiences because these permissive parents themselves had been raised in the "Watsonian" era of the 1920s and early thirties when rigid schedules were the accepted practice.

On the industrial scene there was a dramatic development in the technology of information processing through computer systems. IBM now has the same dominating and salient position that General Motors and U. S. Steel occupied in earlier eras. This was the beginning of the postindustrial or "technetronic" era. The implications of computer technology for increasing diversity and rates of change in all spheres of life are just beginning to be appreciated.

The launching of Sputnik by Russia in 1957 had a profound impact on the American educational system. There was a sharp shift in emphasis away from the humanities to scientific technology. The traditional format and regimentation of schools remained the same, however.

❴ The Parental Generation: Child-Rearing Practices and Goals

Throughout history in most societies, the nuclear family has been the basic social unit within which care of the young has been rooted and where cultural traditions, beliefs, and values have been transmitted from generation to generation.

The nuclear family exists as a unit but is also an integral part of the total social structure. It has membership in the wider kinship network of the extended family, subcultural groups of religion, ethnicity or social class, the local community, the nation and, in recent times, the "world community." The nuclear family tends to orient the developing child to the various elements of this social fabric in roughly the same sequence of ever-widening groups just cited.

From time to time there has been the suggestion that this traditional role of the family has been so depreciated and diminished that the "family is dead."[15] There is general agreement that this demise has been prematurely reported, but it will be worthwhile to examine the reasons for concern[44] about the strength and viability of the social institution of the family, particularly since this concern had been loudly voiced in relation to the families in the generation now under scrutiny, that is to say, the parents of contemporary youth. We will be discussing individuals who started their families in the late 1940s and the early 1950s.

Generation Gap

Before examining some of the details of changes in the social climate that have had significant impact on the social institution of the families of the fifties, it is worth reexamining the concept of the generation gap.[26] This concept refers to an alleged sharp discontinuity between the practices, aspirations, and values of parent and child. Such a discontinuity would proclaim that the traditional role of the family as a transmitter of culture had failed. In the literature and the press this "gap" has been discussed chiefly in relation to elite youth who express vocal, often violent rejection of prevailing adult values and roles. They appear to be disaffected from all aspects of the society. However, careful study of this alienated group has shown that while these young people may be rejecting traditional American values, they are generally expressing the values of their own parents.[4,53,29] Even for them there is, in fact, no generation gap. When adolescents of the middle and lower classes are studied, there are comparable findings of an absence of a generation gap. "The bulk of the

students in the survey studies[65,22] come from the nonprofessional 'white collar' and 'blue collar' families who are moderately affluent and are traditional in their orientation.[13] They and their children tend to expect a continuity of generations in terms of values and occupational niches. There is a mutual expectation of conformity and very little early striving towards autonomy. By and large these individuals live in stable communities and the children respect and wish to emulate their parents. Religious values and affiliation tend to be stronger than in the surrounding classes."[36] Douvan and Gold[23] have observed that "'rebellious youth' and 'the conflict between generations' are phrases that ring; but so far as we can tell, it is not the ring of truth they carry so much as the beguiling but misleading tone of drama."

Later on in the discussion of contemporary youth, it will be important to discuss the "*intragenerational*" gaps, that is, the several distinct contemporary youth cohorts who feel themselves in conflict with others of their own age in achieving their specific goals. At the present, it is sufficient to underscore the fact that in a pluralistic society American families are continuing, by and large, to transmit basic value patterns to their children without any sharp discontinuities.[38]

This does not imply, by any means, that the observed behavior of young people is necessarily in total conformity with that of the adults. Careful studies[27,70,7] have shown that adolescents do tend to conform to the basic values of parents and are usually more influenced by parents than peers in making long-term or otherwise significant decisions. They tend, however, to be autonomous in their decisions, or heavily influenced by peers with respect to matters of personal style such as hair, dress, music, and hobbies, and they are heavily influenced by peers in issues pertaining to peer relations. In the terminology of Merton and Rossi,[59] the parents are used as the comparative-reference group, or the group that is salient in making value judgments, while peers are used as the normative-reference group, or the group that is emulated and supplies norms of overt behavioral styles.

Structural Characteristics of the Families of the 1950s

Although the value orientation of each parental generation had its roots in the preceding generation, the particular version of these values has been significantly shaped by interactions with the technology and cultural influences impinging on individuals in their formative years. It is therefore worthwhile to try to understand the social context into which contemporary youth was born. Also, an effort will be made to understand the composite of influences that was affecting their parents in their childrearing period and influencing their socialization practices. An American value handed down from generation to generation has been the belief in the importance of the individual, coupled with the conviction that hard work would be rewarded with success. There has also been a commitment to goals of material and social progress. These are value patterns which imply an active adaptation to environmental and social conditions. It also implies a belief in society as an evolving and developing rather than a static entity. Therefore, for most of these parents, there has been a positive evaluation of change both in terms of technological advances and social mobility. This does not imply a uniform acceptance of change in different spheres or all sectors of the population. It is not a positive valuation of change for its own sake.

Shrinking of the Family

The families of the fifties were functionally much smaller than those of prior generations, despite the fact that they were often not smaller in terms of the numbers of children. The parents of the fifties had been born and raised in the depression when their parents were aware of the problems and burdens of caring for a large number of children, and the birthrate in their era was at an all-time low. In contrast, when they grew up, to become parents, they participated in the post World War II "baby boom" that raised the birthrate dramatically. The implications of this dramatic demographic shift will be explored in the discussion of the contemporary scene, particularly in relation to college population.[73]

There was, however, constriction of the family of the fifties through the loss of the extended family and, thereby, a diminution of the number of total persons, particularly adults, in the intimate orbit of the child. Mobile, uprooted nuclear families were out of regular contact with grandparents, aunts, uncles, cousins, etc. The age range and variety of role models were greatly constricted by this loss of extended family. There was also a tendency to have children in close succession so that the age spread of the children was narrow and there was, therefore, less opportunity to use siblings over a range of ages as foils, models, or parent surrogates.

In middle-class families servants who were quasi-members of the family and intimate parts of the household had usually disappeared. They had been replaced by labor-saving machines and had themselves been attracted away by jobs in industry.

The net result was a small nuclear family in which the emotional intensity among the members was heightened, but the repertory of actors to fill the needed range of roles was sharply diminished. The effects of the shrinking of the family were compounded by mobility and urbanization. These families were in need of nonfamilial supports.

Structural Isolation

The small nuclear family was now an urban or suburban phenomenon. Neither suburb nor city in any way duplicated the richness of the social network of the stable small towns of the prior generations. This has been documented by systematic research on the daily life of children growing up in a small town as compared with the lives of children in a modern city or suburb.[98] Small-town children from their earliest days onward interact with a substantially greater number of adults in different walks of life.[8] In contrast to urban and suburban children, small-town children are more likely to be active participants in the adult settings they enter. In cities there are large numbers of impersonal contacts with strangers perhaps enhancing a sense of alienation. Inadvertently, urban children were increasingly isolated in society and cut off from the supports, models, and constraints of meaningful personal adult models. The role of TV and age-segregated peer groups in filling this vacuum will be discussed later.

Decline in Parental Authority

The decline of patriarchy as a function of industrialization was mentioned previously. As Galdston stated:[30]

It removed man from field, workshop and home and harnessed him to the factory machine. It took over the vital domestic operations of the woman, so that she no longer spun, wove, sewed, baked, preserved and otherwise served her husband and children in the multitude of ways that had made her so essential to their life and well-being. It disorganized the intra-familial relations and dependencies of husband and wife, parents and children. The concept of "fatherhood" lost its power. . . . The deterioration process is now irreversible.

Other factors have also contributed to the decline of patriarchy. An important element has been the increase in the number of working mothers.[64] In 1948, 13 percent of mothers with children under six years of age were in the labor force. By 1969, this figure had nearly tripled and over 30 percent of such mothers were working. In 1948, 31 percent of mothers with children over the age of six years were working. By 1969, 51 percent of such mothers were employed.[95]

In families where the mothers were full-time housewives, they tended to take a more subservient role and ascribe decision making and authority to the husband. In homes where wives were working, they tended to take a more decisive and authoritative stance with respect to all family decisions, including child-rearing values and practices.[5,42] These mothess found support in *Infant Care* and Spock both for emphasis on independence training in their children for its own sake and as a help to them in lessening child-care responsibilities. The actual care of their children was, of course, increasingly delegated and, depending on the socioeconomic group, the child often spent considerable time in front of the TV set or with baby-sitters rather than with an actively participating parent. There were also a substantial number of women who were not working but had vocational aspirations. Many of these dissatisfied women, although full-time mothers, were found to have child-rearing difficulties.[90]

Paternal Deprivation

For a long time there has been great concern about the deleterious effects on children of maternal deprivation. There is just beginning to be general appreciation of the impact, particularly on boys, of paternal deprivation. Paternal deprivation is widespread and increasing. As was previously mentioned, in large part it represents an insidious by-product of urban, technological society.

For the affluent, this decline in the role of the father was related to time demands of the job, commuting, social and community obligations: the things one has to do to get ahead. For the poor, it was often the demands of having to work long hours for low wages, or even to hold two jobs, that claimed parents at mealtimes, evenings, and even weekends. Among the poor, fatherless families are prevalent.[39]

While the effects on girls of this trend toward paternal deprivation is not explicit, cross-sex identity has been thought to be significant.[11,16] On the other hand, substantial evidence points to the positive effects on boys of the presence, attention, and support of their fathers. Grinker and his colleagues[35] emphasized the history of strong identification with father and father figures in the cluster of conditions found in his sample of emotionally healthy college freshman males. Similarly, Rosenberg[72] has found a strong correlation with parental interest (same sex in particular) and high self-esteem.

Studies from both the United States and Norway[57,40,62] confirm the negative impact of a father's absence on the development of the male. Several lines of evidence support the concept that parental interest, guidelines, and support, particularly of the same sex parent, offer the most effective child-rearing context. It has been noted that where these are weak, or fathers missing, the adolescent males often tend to adopt styles of exaggerated masculinity including hyperindependence, high risk-taking, and aggressive behavior.[61,77] In adolescents, if there is a lack of firm guidance and availability of the same sex parent as a model and coping resource, an urgent need exists for the individual to uncritically seek peer support and adopt the badges of peer group conformity, regardless of the potential risk of antisocial outcomes.[24]

Independence Training of Children

Children of the fifties were socialized for independence rather than the obedience training of the turn of the century. Children were encouraged in exploratory and assertive behavior. This served to increase their sense of efficacy. It was very useful to the household, and the mother in particular, when children could take responsibility for self-care and household chores. Also, it increased the child's awareness of his own desires and goals. In the context of the democratic ideals of the parents and the emerging pattern of mothers, whether employed or not, who wished to more fully express themselves, there were the beginnings of a modification from the "child-centered" family to the value of personal happiness and self-fulfillment for all of the members.[81,96] The implications will be discussed further with respect to contemporary youth and their views of family structure.

Delegation of Parental Authority

In the 1900s, the family was a largely self-sustaining social unit. One important reason why values could so easily be transmitted to children by the parents was the fact that information, and evaluations, were filtered by the parents, relatives, and close friends. Children had very little direct access to informa-

tion before the advent of TV and the development of the mass media.[75] Educational and recreational activities were all family-centered and family-directed.

In contrast to this earlier pattern, the parents of the 1950s, for the reasons discussed, had far greater need for extrafamilial support than any preceding generation. In response to this, old institutions such as the schools have been given new responsibilities for the non-academic education of children: dress codes, sex education, drug education, etc. Schools have responded to perceived paternal deprivation by an effort to increase the number of male teachers, particularly in the early grades. In addition, there has been the emergence of many new formal and informal organizations to meet familial needs in spheres such as child care, health needs, special education, social needs, and recreation. The range of influences upon the child has been greatly extended as outside supports were employed. For the disadvantaged, the welfare bureaucracy deals with virtually all sectors of their family functioning. In general, the family has taken on a new role as the mediator between its members and external organizations. Each of these organizations can and often does function in defining and transmitting values. Furthermore, the parents are no longer seen by the child as being in major control of the resources that are of importance to him.

Concomitant with this development, although perhaps not the cause, there has been the rise of age segregation in the society. The most notable examples are the "retirement communities" and the "youth culture." Much more will be said of the youth culture in the following section.

In summary, by midcentury the shift in America from a predominantly rural nation to a predominantly urbanized and industrialized nation was well established.[60] In the 1950s, the impact of this shift in family structure, value systems, and role relationship within the family was clearly evident and affecting, in turn, the socialization of contemporary youth. In general, the effects of shrinking family size, isolation, and the decline of parental authority have been most strongly felt and pervasively exhibited in a bipolar distribution, that is, in the upper and upper-middle classes, on the one hand, and in the lowest socioeconomic groups on the other. "Middle America" continues to show a relatively high percentage of families with traditional structures, values, and roles. There are some changes in these families and when they occur they are in the same direction, if not to the same extent, as in the highest and lowest classes.

(Contemporary Youth

During the sixties the traditional American accent on youth turned into a national preoccupation with the student protesters and the

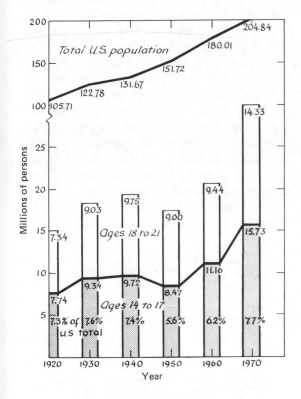

Figure 18–1. Numbers of early and later adolescents in the United States over the past fifty years. Source: U.S. Census (1971:5,8).

hippies. There was confusion, alarm, and, at times, anger over their behavior. The idealized images of youth that had been profitably fostered by the advertising industry were rudely shattered.

Another striking change occurred in the sixties, which received less publicity. This was the dramatic increase in the total youth population in that decade. Youth became important in our contemporary society because of sheer numbers.

Figure 18–1 relates the total number of adolescents to the total population of America over the past fifty years. It is clear that both of these populations have nearly doubled in this time span. Whereas the total population has shown a steady, slow increase in growth, the major increment in youth population has occurred in the past decade, the 1960s. Prior to 1960, the adolescent population was fairly stable for several decades, averaging around eighteen million with a moderate dip in 1950 to seventeen million, reflecting the lowered birthrate during the depression years of the 1930s. The postwar baby boom is reflected in the increase in youth population in the sixties when there were thirty million adolescents. Increases in the percentages of adolescents in the population have shifted the median age downward, despite the medical advances that have increased longevity. Figure 18–2 shows this effect in a graph of the median ages of the population for the past sixty years. The most youthful population reported was in 1910 when the median age was just over twenty-four years of age. The median age rose steadily to a high in 1950 of over thirty years. With the youth-population explosion of the past ten years, the median age has steadily dropped and is currently at 27.6. The same graph also projects population trends, assuming four different reproductive rates from zero population growth to 3.1 children per female. All of these predict a secular trend toward an increased median age of the population. Several years ago the most accurate predictor was thought to be the 2.45 children per female figure, and this series projects a steep rise in median age to nearly thirty-three years by the

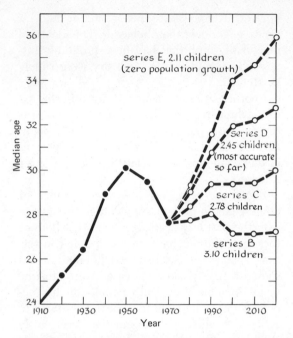

Median age

series E, 2.11 children
(zero population growth)

Series D
2.45 children
(most accurate
so far)

series C
2.78 children

series B
3.10 children

Year

Figure 18–2. Actual and predicted median ages for the total United States population, 1910 to 2020. Source: U.S. Census, 1971: Table 2; 1970: Table 2.

women of childbearing age. The average rate reported for the first eight months of 1971 was 2.2. This drop is especially notable because the number of women of childbearing age is at a record high. This recent 2.2 figure is the lowest since the mid-depression years when the rate was roughly the same. The highest rate was in 1957 when the post World War II baby boom peaked with a rate of 3.8. Over the past three generations there has been a generational swing of the pendulum from bust to boom and now, apparently, back to bust again. Some persons are already beginning to speak of a projected "birth dearth." Some of the contemporary conditions and attitudes that may be influencing the fertility rate will be discussed shortly.

In any case, at the present time the youth population is at a peak and is a potent factor affecting every aspect of American society. In general, it has led to massive demands for public services from a group of minimally economically productive citizens. In particular, there has been a notable strain on the educational system. Businessmen, on the other hand, have seen advantages in the consumer potential of this large pool of young people.

The extent of the youth explosion in the decade of the sixties can be seen in the following figures. In 1960, youth (14–24 years) comprised 15 percent of the total population as compared to 20 percent of the total population in 1971. The absolute numbers of youth in 1960 was 27.1 million persons, in 1970, 41.6 million persons. A demographic breakdown[91] of this group shows the following:

year 2020. There is, however, interesting data on the actual current birthrates.

Reports from the National Fertility Study, the Census Bureau, and the National Center for Health Statistics, as reported in the *New York Times* by Rosenthal,[73] show that there has been a recent dramatic drop in the birthrate average number of children born to

	1960	1970
Total Youth (14–24 years)	27.1 million	41.6 million
Enrolled in college		
Total	4.6 million	7.4 million
White	4.3 million	6.8 million
Negro	234,000	522,000
Other	72,000	132,000
Employed		10.8 million
Unemployed		1.3 million
Armed Forces		1.9 million

Several things are worth noting at this point. First, the tremendous jump in college enrollment during the sixties. Secondly, the fact that currently the total working population of youth exceeds the college-attending population of youth by three million. Relatively little attention has been given to this large employed group of young people. Both popular and professional writers have concerned themselves predominantly with college youth.

Youth and Universities

It is clear that college attendance has rising salience in our society. In an increasingly technological world of specialized knowledge, increasingly higher levels of education are required to accomplish many necessary tasks. It is also widely believed by all sectors of the population that lifetime earning potential is positively correlated with level of education. Rightly or wrongly, typical figures show the college graduate is earning roughly $100,000 more over his working life than the high-school graduate and, of course, earning hundreds of thousands more than the dropout.[47] The college degree elevates social as well as economic status. This outcome is prized in its own right by those seeking social mobility. Even if the income-education figures should be disproved, nevertheless some would continue to value college education just as highly as a passport to interesting, fulfilling kinds of careers. For others, the universities are seen as being at the center of society now that innovative and technological development is so highly dependent on professional expertise. For them the "knowledge industry" has become the major growth industry in America. This dependence on the university is seen in governmental as well as business spheres. It is well-known that each President relies heavily on panels of university experts to help interpret events and shape decisions. Roosevelt was both envied and derided for his "Brain Trust." The key role of Harvard professor, Henry Kissinger, in the Nixon administration is well-known. Finally, in the sixties attendance at college was a sanctuary for many young men who for either personal or ideological reasons did not wish to serve in the war in Vietnam. College men were draft exempt until 1971 when the nation turned to a national lottery that had no education exemptions.

For a variety of reasons, therefore, the college and university population was at a record high in the sixties. Some social planners who were aware of the post World War II baby boom, had forecast the problems of overcrowding and inadequate facilities that would confront colleges and universities when those boom babies grew up, but, for some reason, little action was taken on the basis of these predictions, and most colleges and universities were unprepared for the unprecedented arrival of so many new students. What was not foreseen was the potential for emotional reactions on the part of the students as a function of crowding of strangers, the confusion resulting from intimate contact with widely disparate groups, the competition for scarce resources (preferred classes, dormitory assignments, professorial time, etc.), and the frustrations brought on by inevitable bureaucratic failures of an overtaxed system.[37] Although it has had little attention as a contributing factor to the student unrest and general turmoil of campuses of the sixties, it does seem likely that sheer numbers played a nontrivial role.

In each of the past three generations there have been significant changes in American colleges. There have been changes in the demographic characteristics of the student population, in the instrumentality of a college education, and in the perception of the role of the university in the society as a whole.

In the early decades of the twentieth century, a university education was generally reserved for the elite. The university was perceived as a remote ivory tower, and, in many ways, it was. College was the final polishing process in creating young gentlemen whose careers and destiny had largely been predetermined by social status and family connections. It was used to broaden one's contacts with appropriate persons of the same class and often to find suitable marital partners. The college stood in loco parentis and continued to support the traditional values of the family. Academic demands and expectations were not rigorous. Getting into the right club or fraternity, proms, and football weekends was of greater importance to many students, than academic achievement. The students though often frivolous in their behavior, were basically quite conservative in their political views and values.

With the growth of the technological society, the role of education as a passport to career success became increasingly important. By the 1950s students were well aware of the practical importance of getting a college education and there was emphasis on competition for grades. In general, the students of the fifties were eager to achieve and task-oriented. They were quiet, serious, and worked as hard at their studies as they would later work at their jobs. They were neither frivolous nor protesting. Sometimes they were called "the silent generation." Some of their more liberal professors deplored the "passivity" of these depression-reared, post World War II era students. The college had become a serious challenge to the individual. His success in life was perceived as less correlated with the status of his family of origin and more a function of his own efforts. College was no longer largely a province of the elite but a realistic pathway for upward social mobility for many students. More middle-class whites were in attendance and now some working-class students. There were also considerable numbers of women.[21]

The students of the sixties and contemporary students were born in an era of affluence and the welfare state. By the time of their birth in the fifties, the Roosevelt New Deal programs had become an accepted American way of life. Embedded in these programs was the value mentioned earlier: of the right of all members of the pluralistic society to equal rights and the opportunity to share in material success (realization of the American dream). As was also mentioned previously, throughout their childhood these individuals had been socialized increasingly to see extrafamilial organizations as in control of important resources. In particular, they had lived with the conviction that the federal government bore a heavy responsibility for the welfare and well-being of all citizens.[67] These youths were more vehement in expressing the value of America as a land of opportunity for all than their parents. They were in the vanguard of the civil-rights movement.

Again, there was a class difference in the espousal of these liberal values. The small southern and midwestern colleges, particularly those with strong religious orientations, were much more conservative and traditional. They were not yet ready, for example, to support actively the Negro civil-rights movement of the sixties in the vocal and militant style of the students at elite colleges. However, it was true that most students, regardless of background, did share the same ideals of equality in the sixties, regardless of their degree of militancy.[31] At all of the colleges these less active students constituted a large pool of recruits for crisis and polarized situations, and it was often surprising to see how many students shared the aims and goals of the militants even when they did not support the militant tactics. When their violence was met by establishment counterviolence, the vast majority of student support was with the fellow-student radical.

The student-protest movement in America in the sixties was spearheaded and largely implemented by students in the elite schools. There was particular impetus for the movement in those schools where a tradition of liberalism existed among a small group of the faculty, and where the students received substantial adult support and guidance. The best examples of this were the University of California at Berkeley and the University of Wisconsin. Lipset[52] has pointed out that the radical-liberal history at Wisconsin goes back before World War I to when "the strength of Progressive and Socialist politics in the state contributed to the University's aura." Similarly, Berkeley's history as one of the most liberal-left universities dates from the turn of the century and has been continuous. For example, at midcentury (1949–1950) Berkeley was the only major university to amass solid faculty support for an effective revolt against the McCarthy inspired loyalty oath that was designed to weed out Communists and Communist sympathizers from university communities.

It is probably not surprising that the first major student confrontations occurred at these institutions. At Berkeley in 1963, there were sit-ins to obtain equal-employment rights for Negroes. Many of the students were directly involved in the formation of the Free Speech Movement which received nationwide publicity under the leadership of Mario Savio the following year. At Berkeley there were experienced, dedicated, and well-organized groups to draw from in forming a radical group.

It was not true that they did not trust anyone over thirty. Such veteran, elderly radicals as Herbert Marcuse provided the intellectual capital for much of the ideology of the militant youth.

The spread of the student-protest movement to schools without this kind of supporting infrastructure may be in part credited to the media and TV and to the quick, easy mobility of modern transportation. Student protests received prominent, instant TV coverage that reinforced the protesters and showed sympathizers "where the action was" in case they wanted to join in.

Even in a brief review of the forces influencing students of the sixties attention must be paid to the role of the civil-rights movement. As was noted above, sit-ins to obtain equal employment for Negroes was the issue around which the nucleus of students coalesced and it became the base for the Free Speech Movement. A great many Berkeley students had had a significant prior involvement in the civil-rights movement in the South. The civil-rights movement was a paradigm for the growth of the student-protest movements in many other colleges as well.

To review, in the 1950s there had been increasingly explicit application to the Negro of prevailing values of democracy, equality, and opportunity for all. This was particularly espoused by the affluent, college-educated upper- and upper-middle-class individuals. The legitimacy of the cause of the Negro was proclaimed with the landmark Supreme Court decisions of 1952 and 1954, pertaining to restaurant desegregation and school desegrega-

tion respectively. In the late fifties and early sixties thousands of white college students went south for personal involvement in the "cause." Many were brutalized, a significant few were killed. For almost all of them there was the stirring of real political consciousness and a moral indignation at the society that for so long had condoned the legalized segregation of the South. It was the training ground for learning tactics of confrontation and for heightening the sense of righteousness.

While the students were learning about their political power in the civil-rights movement, they also experienced a sense of failure. Some small successes were achieved in opening doors for Negroes that had been previously closed, but full equality for the Negro was certainly far from becoming a reality. They learned to use an issue with moral overtones as an attack upon the whole system of government. They learned that the civil rights of attackers are strongly defended, even when they violently assault, if the cause is deemed righteous. Later they learned that even a small minority can effectively shut down an idealistic and vulnerable institution such as a university that is loath to use force to protect itself.

When the full impact of the Vietnam War became apparent to the militant students, they had a prepared rhetoric, righteous stance, tactics, and organization with which to protest. In this issue, as in the civil-rights movement they had adult leadership and the large pool of less militant but highly sympathetic fellow students. Again, there was a very small but significant revolutionary radical group who were less concerned with Vietnam and more interested in using that issue as a wedge to attack the entire system.

The student-protest movement of the sixties has been of great interest and there are a number of detailed and fascinating studies that describe and interpret these events in rich detail.[21,25,74] I only wish to use this occasion to trace the continuity of values from the prior generation and show how the context of the contemporary scene influenced the explosive behavior of a particular group of student leaders.

Another factor that entered into the explosive mixture was the change in the demo-graphic characteristics of the college popula-tion. Colleges were increasingly liberal in their admission policies. The student body was more widely representative than ever before. Not only were there more students in colleges of the sixties, but there were more kinds of students, including minorities.

Black-Student Movement

It was noted earlier that the population of black students in college doubled in the six-ties. Just as the civil-rights movement had played a crucial role in creating the white-protest movement, it played an even more significant role in developing the black-protest movement. The failure of the white students' crusade on behalf of civil rights in the late fifties and early sixties was disillusioning for them and raised questions in their minds about the hypocrisy of the system. Of course, it was the blacks, directly affected and limited by policies of segregation, who had the most bitter reaction, and the rise of black-protest movement was directly related to this. The substitution of the terminology black for Negro was a product of this movement. It was related to fostering a sense of black pride and new identity.

A key black group that grew directly out of the Civil Rights Movement was the SNCC (Student Non-Violent Coordinating Commit-tee). It was formed by a group of black col-lege students in 1960 in Raleigh, North Caro-lina. SNCC was started in the nonviolent tradition of Martin Luther King and it initially used the tactics devised and practiced by him. The course of the black-protest movement can almost be charted by the vicissitudes of SNCC. There was an initial period of great popularity and support for the SNCC. In the course of the decade SNCC moved orthogon-ally to a position of espousal of extremely vio-lent rhetoric and tactics. As its positions and actions became more and more violent and extreme, support began to dwindle, particu-larly since the extremist tacts were found to be counterproductive in terms of achievement of realistic goals. In the last couple of years of its

existence, the membership of SNCC declined to a tiny core of dedicated revolutionaries who had virtually no credibility with the general public. The organization was finally dissolved in 1972.

The sharp increase in the numbers of black college students was due to deliberate policies of liberal universities, aimed at rapidly in-creasing the percentage of black students with access to higher education. They established preferential admission policies and generous scholarship aid for black students. Most of these black student recruits to the universities came from black ghettos. For many of them, the freedom, equality, and affluence of univer-sity life was unsettling and often guilt-provok-ing. They felt a strong need to prove that they still identified with the deprivations of the ghetto world and to demonstrate to those back home that they would use the forum of the university to attack racism in American soci-ety. In a sense, many of them felt an obliga-tion to make their activities on campus a paradigm of the revolution they wished to achieve for blacks in the larger society. There was, therefore, an emphasis on "black power." This was expressed in "non-negotiable" de-mands and a push for significant areas of total control by blacks, i.e., black studies programs, black dormitories, choice of black faculty and administrators.

Paradoxically, in the sixties the university was probably the most liberal and democratic institution in American society with respect to the blacks and, at the same time, it was the target of the greatest destructiveness and vio-lence. The academic traditions of tolerance, personal freedom, and a great reluctance to resort to counterviolence, even in its own de-fense, made it a vulnerable target for initial, easy successes in the campaigns of the attack-ing black students.

The height of violence in the black-student movement perhaps came when Cornell black students armed themselves with rifles to de-fend their seizure of the Student Union build-ing. In this episode, despite some sympathy for the initial grievance that triggered the events, the excessive nature of the response caused a loss of both black and white support.

This general response to extremist militancy had its counterpart outside the university in the responses to the Black Panther movement. The Black Panthers are now in eclipse and black-student protestors are still militant but more constructively goal-oriented, and there has been a sharp decline in violent tactics.

Young blacks are an important component of the *intragenerational* gap. They have now learned that their interests are not served by the elite white revolutionaries who had exploited black issues in the early sixties. Neither do they identify with the hippies, who, often from a position of affluence, reject the material values of American society. Finally, they are in a struggle, both on campus and off, with blue-collar youth, for status, housing opportunities, and, ultimately, jobs. Both of these latter groups want very much to obtain a share of the goods and services that are attractively displayed to them by the mass media. The young blacks have their own vision of America, and they are struggling to achieve it. They are not basically opposed to the system. They are angry and frustrated by their inability to participate fully in its benefits. They are eager to promote social change.

Blue-Collar Youth

It is worthwhile recalling again that working-class youth represents by far the bulk of the young people in America. Looking at the demographic breakdown previously cited, there are fourteen million young people of appropriate age who are not in college as compared to 7.4 million who are enrolled. It is true, however, that beginning in the sixties, colleges increasingly have come to represent a broader cross-section of the population. The percentages of women, minorities, and blue-collar youths have sharply escalated due to the mutual aspirations of universities and those target populations. This means that a significantly high percentage of college students come from working-class backgrounds at the present time.

Actually, the two student cohorts previously described represent very small minorities. A Harris Poll in 1968 estimated that there were one hundred thousand student activists or roughly 2 percent of the existing total population. The enrollment of blacks at that time was 234,000 or roughly 4 percent of the total. Even with the steady, calculated rise in black enrollments, the 1970 figure was only 522,000 out of a total of 7.4 million.

It is clear that the student activists and black-student protestors were differentially responding to the forces of social change and were themselves significant agents of further change in both planned and unplanned ways. The preponderance of blue-collar college youth were less subject to sharp impacts of social change. This was due to the buffering effects of their traditional families and to the extensions of these conservative values in their schools, which have served to buttress the familial values.[76] To put it another way, throughout their lives they lived within rather narrow confines both with respect to school and to family and were reared not to question the system. When the doors of college were opened to these children, they sought entrance to use the instrumentality of a college degree to attain vocational and, ultimately, consumer goals. Studies of student subcultures made by Lewis[50] revealed that roughly one-half of the student population sampled, came from blue-collar backgrounds and that 48.6 percent expressed consumer-vocational goals as their major motivation in attending college. Further analysis of his data revealed that only one-fifth of this group saw college as a means of expanding intellectual horizons. They were very interested in obtaining a degree. (Interestingly, the students in the nonconformist subculture were minimally interested in obtaining a degree and very high in intellectual motivation.) For technological reasons, paths to upward occupational mobility have been significantly linked to higher education. This educational ceiling on mobility has meant, therefore, that among blue-collar youth those who do not attend college experience an effective decline in their opportunities. In the noncollege blue-collar youth group this has lead to intense competition and, at times, overt hostility to the minority youths who are striving for the same occupational niches.[78]

For the blue-collar college youth there was a significant lack of political activism. They were in the "silent majority." However, despite their lack of militancy it was true that many of them did sympathize with some of the avowed goals of the student protestors. For example, some of them were concerned about injustices suffered by blacks and a great many were opposed to the war in Vietnam.[31] In general, they supported the student protestors when police counterviolence or disciplinary action was involved.

In contrast to the college blue-collar youths, a sector of noncollege working-class youths has been much more militant. Again, as with other young militants, they have often received support from their parents and other adult reference persons when their violence was directed against perceived incursions by minorities. At times these blue-collar youths have been instigators of ugly incidents involving reprisals when attempts were made to integrate housing or a union, or to bus school children for school integration. Significantly, many working-class young men are now attracted to jobs as policemen.[55] It seems to be concretization of their desire to "restore law and order," at times used to defend bigotry. Among noncollege working-class youth there is deep antagonism, not only to the minorities whose strivings are an economic threat but to student protestors and hippies as well. At times these three sets of peer contemporaries are seen by them as flaunting their deeply held value of hard work as the road to achievement. Blacks and other minorities are often seen as being given unfair unearned advantages in a kind of reverse discrimination. They envy and resent the elite young people who use the sanctuary of the university to attack the establishment and system that they value. They equally resent the hippies who flaunt the work ethic. It was surprising to some, but understandable in the light of this discussion, to learn that in 1968, the polls of Gallup, Harris, and Yankelovich revealed that 25 percent of young voters, at all educational levels, preferred George Wallace as their candidate. In looking at the twenty-five million new voters who were eligible to cast their first ballots in

the Nixon–McGovern election in 1972, Roberts[71] found marked differences between college and working youth. Only 22 percent of the blue-collar youth described themselves as liberal whereas 43 percent of the students did. At this writing, the details of the youth vote in the recent Nixon–McGovern election have not been carefully analyzed, but the preliminary scan strongly suggests that the youth vote was concordant with the voting patterns of the older generation. It can be noted, again in the voting pattern of the 1972 presidential election, that there was a bimodal distribution of the vote for a mandate for change. The highest and lowest ends of the social scale (the elite and the disadvantaged) seemed to be the groups who preferred McGovern over Nixon. As judged by the 70 percent plurality in Washington, D.C., the size and solidarity of the black vote, both young and old, for McGovern was particularly striking. Some forecasters had anticipated that there would be a "youth bloc" of first-time, liberal voters. No such pattern materialized. Desire for social change did not break down along age lines.

Youth and Sex Roles

There is one area, however, in which contemporary youth does appear to be differentially responding along generational lines with respect to social change. This has to do with the roles of women. Up until fairly recently, at all ages, a conservative view about the role of women as homemaker and mother had been a dominant and deeply held American value. Opinion polls are now revealing that this traditional view, particularly among youth, is changing.

Over the past two decades there has been a gradual acceptance of women in work roles. In 1947, women made up 28 percent of the total labor force. By 1969, women were found to represent 37.8 percent of the working population.[91] Not only has the total number of women employed greatly increased but they now seek to occupy an ever-widening range of work roles. Their right to do so has been institutionalized by statute, Title VII of the Civil Rights Act prohibiting sex discrimination in hiring. By 1970, the Equal Employment Opportunity Commission had had some success in eliminating discriminatory wage differentials as well as in extending the hiring of women in new job categories. Coupled with this has been a shift in the acceptance of the working mother. In prior years there had been a deeply held belief that the young child needed his mother, specifically, and would be harmed if child-care arrangements were provided and the mother was employed out of the home. Youth has shown a far greater readiness to reevaluate this concept.

Particularly among the older generations there is still ambivalence about whether or not it is sound public policy to encourage mothers to work by establishing inexpensive, high quality and readily accessible child-care facilities. However, inasmuch as a legislative decision has been made that it is desirable to encourage welfare and disadvantaged mothers to work (and also to facilitate the hiring of women in industries with manpower shortages) public monies have been appropriated for the establishment of day care under federal auspices. This framework, coupled with accepting attitudes of young people, would seem to set the stage for a vast increase in day-care facilities in the near future and a consequent acceleration of the changing role of women as mothers.

In contemporary America, the attitudes of women in relation to mothering and childbearing have been greatly influenced by advances in biomedical technology for birth control, chiefly "the pill,"[19,20] and also by liberalized attitudes toward abortion. In the past, pregnancy was chiefly related to sexual motivation. Now, for a great many individuals it is increasingly a result of a desire to have and to rear children. Despite the lack of widespread support for Women's Lib per se, it would appear that all of these factors have caused contemporary young women to view their roles differently.

The current trend toward later first marriages[91] may be an indication of a lessened commitment to early marriage and children. Especially for women there is more emphasis on higher education, careers, and self-expression. These same attitudes may, in part, account for the unexpected, sharp drop in the birthrate, which is also being currently recorded.

There has been much interest among contemporary youth both in family arrangements that deemphasize a sex-role division of labor, and in the hierarchical, patriarchal family that was once traditional. On the one hand, there has been interest in a wide range of communal structures and, on the other hand, in new approaches to the more conventional nuclear family. The White House Conference on Children in 1970[95] identified five different communal-family types and seven variations on the traditional family in the section on "Changing Families in a Changing Society." It remains to be seen which of these experiments will be viable. One of the outcomes may very well be a general acceptance of the principle of a range of choices in life style. Acceptance of diversity is promoted by exposure to television. Individuals are vividly presented with direct exposure to perspectives and information in a way that was not possible prior to this TV generation. There is also a tendency by the media to focus on the most innovative developments of the time. The net result can be an apparent legitimatization of new freedoms and values.

Television and Youth

It would not be appropriate to conclude this discussion without commenting on the significance of television for contemporary youth. The influence of TV has been exerted throughout the entire course of their lives. It has played an important background role in shaping their attitudes, values, and behavior.

Unlike the printed word, TV is a direct experience. No decoding is necessary. Consequently, it is equally available to children, educated persons, illiterates, the rich and the poor. Studies have shown that TV has a preemptive quality and that when available, it tends to be preferred to other mass media.[41,75] The popularity of TV and its presence in 87 percent of all American homes, including poverty households, is truly phenomenal.[91] Gerbner[33] speaks of TV's ability "to from new bases for collective thought and action, quickly, continuously and pervasively across boundaries of time, space and class." With the advent of satellite communication, TV messages are now beamed all over the world.

As mentioned previously, TV has diluted the parental influence in shaping values by replacing their filtered information, which reflected a particular cultural perspective, with either "raw" information or, at other times, the opinions and judgments of nonfamily persons. In this way, TV opens up the possibility for the transmission of the culture among diverse groups.

An other effect of TV has been to enhance the cult of the personality. It elevates some persons to hero status. At the same time, with a relentless focus on the novel and the sensational there can be an emphasis on the unmasking of heroes, which can promote cynicism and loss of heroic figures with whom youth can identify. TV has also fostered a shrunken globe and "one-world" perspective. Through the evening news reports, world problems come to rest on the individual conscience.

The role of TV in promoting violence has been under scrutiny by the office of the Surgeon General,[92] and an extensive report has been issued. The findings would seem to implicate the viewing of television violence by children as a contributing factor to the violence of our society. The experimental evidence reviewed revealed that violence depicted on television can induce imitative behavior on the part of children. The effect was not uniform and it was noted that aggression-prone children were more likely to show an increase in aggressive behavior in response to television violence. It was also reported that there is very high television viewing among the three-to-twelve age span. The average home television is turned on six hours per day.

Many important issues are raised by the Surgeon General's inquiry. An important concern is the role of TV in the acquisition of aggressive tendencies in young children. The mutually reinforcing effects of environmental factors on aggressive behavior needs study.

There is little known, for example, about the shaping effects of TV in promoting a taste for violence in magazines, books, and movies or the translation of any of these into violent actions.

A more general issue can also be raised about the future of television programming. At present, the programs are geared for presentation to a mass audience. There are, however, alternatives of greater diversity and more specialized programming for pro-social goals, particularly with the advent of cable TV. Finally, there is need to review the underlying needs that have lead to such an extensive use of television. There may be important nontelevision avenues for use of leisure time that should be developed. It is possible that schools will need to place some emphasis, for example, on teaching children the uses and values of leisure-time pursuits and on giving them the skills and enthusiasm for seeking other activities.

❰ Conclusions

An effort was made to trace the impact of social change on American youth using the example of youth in the 1960s. This decade was chosen partly because of the turbulence of students in the universities during this period and partly because it may help us to better understand today's youth. The role of women in contemporary society is an issue that is of particular importance to youth.

It was proposed that response to social change is more closely related to membership in a particular cultural subgroup than to age or generational lines. Several major cohorts of youth were delineated. Within each group the continuity of values through the generations was discussed. Each group had a distinctive interpretation of basic American values that was transmitted to its children.

In order to understand the impact of social change on youth it is necessary to know something about the social context and the values of the parental generation who were responsible for the socialization of the individuals in question. The response to social change, in other words, is a function of a subculturally determined readiness to adapt. The parental generation under scrutiny is an interesting one because the families of that era were experiencing the stresses of urban, mobile, industrial society. The effects of television in further diluting the role of the family as a transmitter of values is discussed.

It was concluded that, despite difficulties, the family continues to provide its children with a basic-value structure. This set of values acts as a stable base for interpreting the environment and providing the individual with the range of possibilities of response to the changes that confront him. Even though the basic values are stable, each generation expresses its own version of these values and displays distinctive behavioral styles.

⟪ Bibliography

1. AMERICAN ALMANAC FOR 1971: STATISTICAL ABSTRACT OF THE UNITED STATES, 91st ed. New York: Grosset & Dunlap, 1971.
2. BELL, D. "Structural Changes in the United States," in F. Duchene, ed., *The Endless Crisis: America in the Seventies*, pp. 186–192. New York: Simon and Schuster, 1970.
3. BELL, R. and J. CHARLES, "Pre-Marital Sexual Experience Among Co-eds," *J. Marriage Fam.*, 32 (1970), 81–84.
4. BLOCK, J., N. HAAN, and B. SMITH. "Activism and Apathy in Contemporary Adolescents," in J. F. Adams, ed., *Understanding Adolescence: Current Developments in Adolescent Psychology*, pp. 198–231. Boston: Allyn & Bacon, 1968.
5. BLOOD, R. O., JR. "The Husband-Wife Relationship," in F. I. Nye and L. W. Hoffman, eds., *The Employed Mother in America*, pp. 282–305. Chicago: Rand McNally, 1963.
6. BOULDING, K. *The Meaning of the 20th Century*. New York: Harper-Colophon Books, 1964.
7. BRITTAIN, C. V. "Adolescent Choices and Parents-Peer Cross-Pressures," *Am. Sociol. Rev.* 28 (1963), 385–391.
8. BRONFENBRENNER, U. *The Two Worlds of Childhood: U.S. and U.S.S.R.* New York: Russell Sage Foundation, 1970.

9. BRZEZINSKI, Z. "America in the Technetronic Age: New Questions of Our Time," in F. Duchene, ed., *The Endless Crisis: America in the Seventies*, pp. 192–199. New York: Simon and Schuster, 1970.
10. BURCHINAL, L. "Trends and Prospects for Young Marriage in the United States," *J. Marriage Fam.*, 27 (1965), 243–254.
11. BURTON, R. V. and J. W. WHITING. "The Absent Father and Cross-identity," *Merrill-Palmer Q.*, 7 (1961), 85–95.
12. CALVERT, J. F. Commonwealth Club speech. San Francisco, March 24, 1972.
13. COHEN, A. S. and H. HODGES. "Lower Blue-Collar Class Characteristics," *Soc. Prob.*, 10 (1963), 3031–3033.
14. CONGER, J. J. "A World They Never Knew: The Family and Social Change," *Daedalus*, 100 (1971), 1105–1138.
15. COOPER, D. *Death of the Family*. New York: Pantheon, 1970.
16. D'ANDRADE, R. G. "Father Absence and Cross-sex Identification." Ph.D., Harvard University, 1962. Unpublished.
17. DAVIDSON, S. "Open Land: Getting Back to the Communal Garden," *Harper's*, June (1970), 91–102.
18. DAVIS, A. "Socialization and the Adolescent Personality," in *The 43rd Yearbook*, National Society for the Study of Education, Part 1, Chap. 11 (1944), 198.
19. DJERASSI, C. "Prognosis for the Development of New Chemical Birth-Control Agents," *Science*, 166 (1969), 468–473.
20. ———. "Birth Control After 1984," *Science*, 169 (1970), 941–951.
21. DOUGLAS, J. D. *Youth in Turmoil: America's Changing Youth Cultures and Student Protest Movements*. Public Health Service Publication No. 2058. Washington: U.S. Gov. Print. Off., 1970.
22. DOUVAN, E. and J. ADELSON. *The Adolescent Experience*. New York: Wiley, 1966.
23. DOUVAN, E. and M. GOLD. "Modal Patterns in American Adolescence," in L. W. Hoffman and M. L. Hoffman, eds., *Review of Child Development Research*, Vol. II, p. 485. New York: Russell Sage Foundation, 1966.
24. DUMPHY, D. C. "The Social Structure of Urban Adolescent Peer Groups," *Sociometry*, 26 (1963), 230–246.
25. EISENBERG, L. "Student Unrest: Sources and Consequences," *Science*, 167 (1970), 1688–1692.

26. EISENSTADT, S. N. *From Generation to Generation.* Glencoe: Free Press, 1956.

27. ELDER, G. H., JR. "Parental Power Legitimation and Effects on Adolescents," *Sociometry,* 26 (1963), 50–65.

28. EVELOFF, H. H. "Mass Media and Identity Formation," *Psychiatr. Op.,* 8 (1971), 6–9.

29. FLACKS, R. "The Liberated Generation: An Exploration of the Roots of Student Protest." *J. Soc. Iss.,* 23 (1967), 52–75.

30. GALDSTON, I. "The Rise and Decline of Fatherhood," *Psychiatr. Ann.,* 2 (1972), 10–17.

31. GALLUP, G. "Most Students Agree with the Aims of Campus Militants," *Los Angeles Times,* May 25, 1969.

32. GLAZER, N. "The Limits of Social Policy," *Commentary,* 52 (1971), 51–58.

33. GERBNER, G. "Communication and Social Environment," *Sci. Am.,* 227 (1972), 152–160.

34. GOSLIN, D. A. *The School in Contemporary Society.* Chicago: Scott, Foresman, 1965.

35. GRINKER, R. R., SR., R. R. GRINKER, JR., and J. A. TIMBERLAKE. "A Study of Mentally Healthy Young Males (Homoclites)," *Arch. Gen. Psychiatry,* 6 (1962), 27–74.

36. HAMBURG, B. "Coping in Early Adolescence: The Special Challenges of the Junior High School Period," in S. Arieti, ed., *American Handbook of Psychiatry,* Vol. 2, 2nd ed., pp. 385–397. New York: Basic Books, 1973.

37. HAMBURG, D. A. "Crowding, Stranger Contact and Aggressive Behavior," in L. Levi, ed., *Society, Stress and Disease,* Vol. 1, pp. 209–218. Oxford: Oxford University Press, 1971.

38. HARRIS, L. "Change, Yes—Upheaval, No," *Life,* 70 (1971), 22–27.

39. HERZOG, E. and H. LEWIS. "Children in Poor Families: Myths and Realities," *Am. J. Orthopsychiatry,* 3 (1970), 375–387.

40. HETHERINGTON, M. E. "Effects of Paternal Absence on Sex-Typed Behaviors in Negro and White Pre-adolescent Males," *J. Pers. Soc. Psychol.,* 4 (1966), 87–91.

41. HIMMELWEIT, H., A. OPPENHEIM, and P. VINCE. *Television and the Child.* London: Oxford University Press, 1958.

42. HOFFMAN, L. W. "Parental Power Relations and the Division of Household Tasks," *Marriage Fam. Liv.,* 22 (1960), 27–35.

43. ITANI, J. "On the Acquisition and Propagation of a New Food Habit in the Troop of Japanese Monkeys at Takasakigama," *Primates,* 1 (1958) 84–98.

44. KELLER, S. "Does the Family Have a Future?" *J. Comp. Fam. Stud.,* Spring (1971), 1–14.

45. KENISTON, K. *Young Radicals: Notes on Committed Youth.* New York: Harcourt, Brace and World, 1968.

46. KIELL, N., ed. "Rhetoric of Aristotle," in *The Universal Experience of Adolescence,* pp. 18–19. Boston: Beacon Press, 1964.

47. LASSITER, R. L. *The Association of Income and Educational Achievement.* Gainesville: University of Florida Press, 1966.

48. LEDERBERG, J. "Orthobiosis: The Perfection of Man," in A. Tiselius and S. Nilsson, eds., *The Place of Value in a World of Facts, Nobel Symposium* XIV, pp. 29–58. New York: Wiley Interscience, 1971.

49. ———. "Biological Innovation and Genetic Intervention," in J. A. Behnke, ed., *Challenging Biological Problems,* pp. 7–27. London: Oxford University Press, 1972.

50. LEWIS, L. "The Value of College to Different Sub-cultures," *School Rev.,* 77 (1969), 32–40.

51. LEWIS, O. "The Culture of Poverty," *Sci. Am.,* 215 (1966), 19–25.

52. LIPSET, S. M. "The Activist: A Profile," in D. Bell and I. Kristol, *Confrontation,* pp. 45–57. New York: Basic Books, 1969.

53. LIPSET, S. M. and P. G. ALTBACH. "Student Politics and Higher Education in the United States," *Comp. Ed. Rev.,* 10 (1968), 320–349.

54. LIPSET, S. and R. BENDIX. *Social Mobility in Industrial Society.* Berkeley: University of California Press, 1959.

55. LIPSET, S. M. and E. RAAB. "The Non-Generation Gap," *Commentary,* 50 (1970), 35–39.

56. MASON, W. "Determinants of Social Behavior in Young Chimpanzees," in A. Schrier, H. Harlow and F. Stollnitz, eds., *Behavior in Non-Human Primates,* Vol. II, pp. 335–364. New York: Academic, 1965.

57. McCORD, J., W. McCORD, and E. THURBER. "Some Effects of Paternal Absence on Male Children," *J. Abnorm. Psychol.,* 64 (1962), 361–369.

58. MENZEL, E. W., JR. "Spontaneous Invention of Ladders in a Group of Young Chimpanzees," *Folia Primatol.,* 17 (1972), 87–106.

59. MERTON, R. K. and A. ROSSI. "Contributions to the Theory of Reference Group Behavior," in R. K. Merton, ed., *Social Theory and Social Structure*, pp. 225–280. Glencoe: Free Press, 1957.

60. MILLER, D. R. and G. SWANSON. *The Changing American Parent*. New York: Wiley, 1958.

61. MILLER, W. B. "Lower Class Culture as a Generating Milieu of Gang Delinquency," *J. Soc. Iss.*, 14 (1958), 5–19.

62. NASH, J. "The Father in Contemporary Culture and Current Psychological Literature," *Child Dev.*, 36 (1965), 261–297.

63. NEWTON, D. "Mastery at Munich," *San Francisco Examiner and Chronicle*, August 27, 1972.

64. NYE, F. I. and L. W. HOFFMAN, eds. *The Employed Mother in America*. Chicago: Rand McNally, 1963.

65. OFFER, D. *The Psychological World of the Teenager: A Study of Normal Adolescent Boys*. New York: Basic Books, 1969.

66. OGBURN, W. F. *Social Change*. New York: B. W. Huebsch, 1922.

67. PARSONS, T. "The Impact of Technology on Culture and Emerging New Modes of Behaviour," *Int. Soc. Sci. J.*, 22 (1970), 607–627.

68. RAPOPORT, R. and R. N. RAPOPORT. "The Dual Career Family," *Hum. Rel.*, 22 (1969), 3–30.

69. REICH, C. *The Greening of America*. New York: Random House, 1970.

70. REMMERS, H. H. and D. H. RADLER. *The American Teenager*. Indianapolis: Bobbs, 1957.

71. ROBERTS, S. "Working Youth: The 17 Million 'Invisible' New Voters," *New York Times*, March 11, 1972, p. 1.

72. ROSENBERG, M. *Society and the Adolescent Self-Image*. Princeton: Princeton University Press, 1965.

73. ROSENTHAL, J. "Population Growth in U.S. Found Sharply Off," *New York Times*, November 5, 1971.

74. ROSZAK, T. *The Making of a Counter Culture*. Garden City, New York: Doubleday, 1969.

75. SCHRAMM, W., J. LYLE, and E. PARKER. *Television in the Lives of Our Children*. Stanford: Stanford University Press, 1962.

76. SHOSTAK, A. B. *Blue Collar Lives*. New York: Random House, 1969.

77. SIEGMAN, A. W. "Father Absence During Early Childhood and Anti-Social Behavior," *J. Abnorm. Psychiatry*, 71 (1966), 71–74.

78. SIMON, W., J. H. GAGNON, and S. A. BUFF. "Son of Joe: Continuity and Change Among White Working Class Adolescents," *J. Youth Adol.*, 1 (1972), 13–34.

79. SPOCK, B. *The Pocket Book of Baby and Child Care*. New York: Pocket Books, 1954.

80. STEINBECK, J. *Grapes of Wrath*. New York: Viking Press, 1939.

81. SUSSMAN, M. B. "Need Research on the Employed Mother," *Marriage Fam. Liv.*, 23 (1961), 368–373.

82. ———. "Family, Kinship and Bureaucracy," in A. Campbell and P. Converse, eds., *The Human Meaning of Social Change*, pp. 127–158. New York: Russell Sage Foundation, 1972.

83. TANNER, J. M. *Education and Physical Growth*. Indiana: Indiana University Press, 1970.

84. ———. "Sequence, Tempo, and Individual Variation in the Growth and Development of Boys and Girls Aged Twelve to Sixteen," *Daedalus*, Fall (1971), 907–930.

85. TOFFLER, A. "Value Impact Forecaster—A Profession of the Future," in K. Baier and N. Rescher, eds., *Values and the Future*, pp. 1–30. New York: Macmillan, Free Press Paperback, 1969.

86. ———. *Future Shock*. New York: Bantam, 1971.

87. TSUMORI, A. "Newly Acquired Behavior and Social Interactions of Japanese Monkeys," in S. A. Altman, ed., *Social Communication Among Primates*, pp. 207–219. Chicago: University of Chicago Press, 1967.

88. UNESCO. *Youth, 1969. The UNESCO Courier* (Special issue), 22 (1969), 5–34.

89. UNITED STATES BUREAU OF THE CENSUS. *U.S. Census of Population in 1960, Number of Inhabitants, U.S. Summary, Final Report*. Washington: U.S. Gov. Print. Office, 1960.

90. ———. *Historical Statistics of the United States, Colonial Times to 1957*. Washington: U.S. Gov. Print. Office, 1960.

91. ———. *Pocket Data Book, U.S.A., 1971*. Washington: U.S. Gov. Print. Office, 1971.

92. UNITED STATES PUBLIC HEALTH SERVICE. Report of the Surgeon General. *Television and Growing Up: The Impact of Televised Violence*, pp. 72–9090. Washington: Dept

of Health, Education and Welfare, 1972.

93. VINCENT, C. E. "Mental Health and the Family," *J. Marriage Fam.*, 29 (1967), 18–39.

94. WASHBURN, S. and F. C. HOWELL. "Human Evolution and Culture," in S. Tax, ed., *Evolution After Darwin*, Vol. 2, pp.33–58. Chicago: University of Chicago Press, 1960.

95. WHITE HOUSE CONFERENCE ON CHILDREN, 1970. Washington: U.S. Gov. Print. Office, 1970.

96. WILLIAMS, R. M., JR. *American Society: A Sociological Interpretation.* New York: Knopf, 1970.

97. WOLFENSTEIN, M. "Trends in Infant Care," *Am. J. Orthopsychiatry*, 23 (1953), 120–130.

98. WRIGHT, H. et al. "Children's Behavior in Communities Differing in Size," Department of Psychology, University of Kansas, 1969. Unpublished manuscript. Quoted by U. Bronfenbrenner in *The Two Worlds of Childhood: U.S. and U.S.S.R.*, pp. 96–97. New York: Russell Sage Foundation, 1970.

99. YARROW, M. R., P. SCOTT, L. DE LEEUW, et al. "Child Rearing in Families of Working and Non-working Mothers," *Sociometry*, 25 (1962), 122–140.

PART THREE

Frontiers in Psychopharmacology

CHAPTER 19

BASIC NEUROPHARMACOLOGY

George K. Aghajanian

I N THE PAST two decades, with the advent of the large scale use of drugs in psyiatric practice, the field of neuropharmacology has inevitably become closely linked to that of psychiatry. There has been an increasing involvement of psychiatrists as partners in basic as well as clinical neuropharmacological research. These developments are leading to a reversal of the previous trend toward an isolation of psychiatry from the biological sciences.

Basic neuropharmacology can be defined as the study of the actions and mechanisms of action of drugs on the nervous system. In a broad sense, efforts toward the elucidation of mechanisms of neurotropic drugs action depend for their success upon the growing sophistication of theory and methodology in neurobiology. At present, basic information about the action of drugs at multicellular, cellular, subcellular, microchemical, and molecular levels is approaching the point where we can soon expect a coherent and highly specific analysis of the mode of action of almost every

major drug of interest to psychiatry. These promising developments hopefully will lead to a transition from a "cookbook" use of drugs to a rational pharmacotherapy in the future.

A major emphasis of research in neuropharmacology has been upon presumptive transmitter substances and their vicissitudes. If the chemical transmission of impulses across synaptic junctions represents the common coin of communication in the central nervous system, then the alteration of such transmission is likely to represent a key site for the action of drugs that alter neural function. The specificity of drug action would then depend upon which synapse or transmitter is affected and the direction of the change (i.e., facilitation or inhibition). Although superficially such a formulation seems quite simple, on a practical level the study of transmitter substances and synaptic transmission in the mammalian central nervous system poses formidable technical problems for the neurobiologist and pharmacologist. The amounts of the transmitters may be very low (e.g., 10^{-6} to 10^{-7} g/kg of brain) the neurons under study exceedingly small (ten to twenty microns in diameter) and the synapses difficult to isolate. It will therefore be illuminating to examine first some basic neural mechanisms and the methods employed in their study. The economy of this approach is that a few fundamental principles apply to many drugs. The second portion of this review will deal with current concepts of the mode of action of specific classes of therapeutic and nontherapeutic psychotropic drugs.

(Mechanisms of Psychotropic Drug Action: Basic Approaches and Principles*

Biochemical

Presumably, since drugs are chemical agents, their primary site of action must be some kindred chemical site within the brain. Early on research on the central effects of neurotropic drugs was largely concerned with processes such as energy metabolism, which were not peculiar to the brain. It was natural to apply to studies on the brain knowledge about general biochemical processes previously gained from research on non-neural tissues. However, this approach has gradually been superceded by studies on substances that are specific for the essential functions of the nervous system. There is a great deal of experimental support for the assumption that in the mammalian brain neurotransmission is mediated by chemical substances, liberated at the nerve endings of one neuron (the *presynaptic cell*) that impinge upon the soma or dendrites of another neuron (the *postsynaptic cell*).[43] Thus, a great deal of attention is being given to the study of effects of psychoactive drugs upon putative transmitters in the brain. Substances in this category include acetylcholine, γ-aminobutyric acid, and the monoamines, serotonin (5-hydroxytryptamine), dopamine, and norepinephrine. In general, in order to

* For more extensive coverage of this area consult the recent excellent and succinct textbook by Cooper, Bloom, and Roth.[36]

qualify as a neurotransmitter a substance should be synthesized and stored in the presynaptic neuron, be released upon firing of that neuron, and produce the same physiological action (inhibition or excitation) upon the postsynaptic neurons as activation of the presynaptic nerve. Also, some mechanism for terminating the action of the transmitter must be available. As one might expect, each of these steps in the life cycle of the various candidate central transmitters is undergoing careful scrutiny as a possible site of drug action. While biochemical approaches to each of these processes are separately discussed, it is important not to lose sight of the fact that the ultimate importance of each step is in relation to its ability to modify synaptic transmission.

Synthesis is the initial stage at which a drug may effect the availability of a transmitter substance. It is generally assumed that when the synthesis of a transmitter is markedly inhibited, the transmission of impulses via this transmitter will be impaired. Similarly, if the synthesis of a transmitter substance is enhanced, then a facilitation of transmission may ensue. On this basis, a search has been underway in recent years for specific inhibitors or enhancers of neurotransmitter synthesis. Although none of the major drugs presently used therapeutically in psychiatry is believed to have as its primary action an alteration in synthesis (see below) there are a number of substances of this type whose actions are being explored in research studies in both animals and humans. One of these is para-chlorophenylalanine, a selective depletor of serotonin[77] that acts by inhibiting tryptophan hydroxylase,[70] the initial enzyme involved in the synthesis of serotonin from dietary tryptophan. The availability of this drug has prompted a multitude of research studies on the possible physiological function of serotonin.[106] These have included the interesting hypothesis that serotonin serves to mediate sleep mechanisms in the brain.[71] Another is alpha-methyl-p-tyrosine, a selective inhibitor of tyrosine hydroxylase,[99] the limiting enzyme in the synthesis of catecholamines.[103] This drug has been found to exacerbate some depressions in humans[24] and to produce a state resembling depression in monkeys.[91] Conversely, L-3,4-dihydroxyphenylalanine (L-Dopa) which increases brain catecholamine synthesis, has been found to induce manic episodes in bipolar depressive patients.[84] Such studies have implications for both the mechanism of action of psychotropic drugs and for theories about possible biological factors in these disease states. Moreover, this work underlines the potential influence of altering the rate of neurotransmitter synthesis. In the field of neurology, this strategy has led to the introduction of L-Dopa in the treatment of Parkinson's disease. Autopsy material from patients who died with this disease revealed a marked lowering of dopamine in portions of the extrapyramidal system.[67] On this basis it was reasoned that a deficiency in dopamine may account for the motor disturbance seen in this condition. Clinical trials with L-Dopa, the immediate precursor of dopamine, gave rise to dramatic therapeutic results that are now well known.[38] A parallel instance in psychiatry (i.e., of a drug producing a clear-cut therapeutic effect by altering the synthesis of a neurotransmitter) remains a possibility for the future.

The *storage* of neurotransmitters is believed to occur largely within synaptic vesicles. The latter are small membrane-bound structures that are clustered at the presynaptic terminals. Only a very small percentage (much less than 1 percent) of the total store is released with each nerve impulse. However, depletion of stores can interfere with the effective release of transmitter by nerve impulses. None of the therapeutic or even nontherapeutic drugs commonly used at this time acts primarily through this mechanism, but drugs that deplete stores of transmitter substances are nevertheless of considerable historical interest. In the mid 1950s, Brodie and his coworkers discovered that the drug reserpine, derived from the Indian plant *Rauwolfia serpentinia*, markedly reduced brain stores of serotonin.[21] Soon afterwards, it was found that catecholamines in the brain were also depleted.[15,65] Such a depletion of stores within the nerve terminals is sometimes referred to as "intraneuronal release," which is to be distinguished from "ex-

traneuronal release" (i.e., release from the nerve endings onto a postsynaptic cell). Reserpine was used as a tranquilizer to a limited extent during that period (i.e., 1950s) but it never achieved the great success and acceptance that was accorded the phenothiazines, which were also introduced during the same period. Nevertheless, the demonstration that dramatic changes in brain monoamine levels were caused by reserpine provided a great impetus to the belief that the action of psychotropic drugs could be explained in terms of alterations in neurohumoral or neurotransmitter functions.

The next stage in the life cycle of a neurotransmitter comes with its *release* from the presynaptic terminals onto the postsynaptic cell, where it presumably interacts with a "receptor" site. It is presumed that a transitory transmitter-receptor complex forms and then triggers an alteration in ionic conductance within the postsynaptic cell membrane. Such conductance changes (e.g., to the entry of Na^+ or Cl^-) are responsible for the altered functional state of the postsynaptic cell (either depolarization or hyperpolarization). A drug that releases a transmitter substance can therefore produce quite profound effects upon neural functioning. There is much evidence, for example, that amphetamine and other stimulant drugs produce their effects by releasing catecholamines from nerve terminals onto postsynaptic sites (see below). Conversely, drugs that block the action of neurotransmitters at receptor sites may have powerful antagonistic actions within these same systems. The phenothiazines appear to block the central effects of the catecholamines, and thereby act in opposition to the amphetamines. In general, the influence of psychotropic drugs on the release and subsequent action at postsynaptic receptors of neurotransmitters represents a key site in the consideration of their mechanism of action.

At the next stage, a drug may interfere with *termination of the action* of a neurotransmitter. The classical example of this is where a drug inhibits enzymes responsible for the transformation of the active transmitter into inactive products or metabolites. As a consequence, the transmitter will persist in the vicinity of the postsynaptic receptor site and continue to produce its effects. It has long been known that drugs that inhibit cholinesterases, the enzymes that hydrolyze acetylcholine into its inactive substituents, acetate and choline, potentiate the activity of this neurotransmitter. Ultimately, if sufficient acetylcholine accumulates the postsynaptic membrane may fail to recover from such excessive activation and a block in transmission can result. With the more commonly used psychotropic drugs, the monoamine oxidase inhibitors exemplify this paradigm of degradative enzyme inhibition. Monoamine oxidase is the principle route of destruction for serotonin and an important one for the catecholamines. Thus, monoamine oxidase inhibitors should promote the effects of these monoamines in the brain, and they have been used in the treatment of depressive illness. However, when monoamine oxidase is inhibited, "false" neurochemical transmitters may accumulate in nerve endings and, paradoxically, an impaired release of the normal transmitter can result.[78] Moreover, when an important degradative pathway in the body is blocked, serious side effects may ensue from the accumulation of toxic substances that require this pathway for their destruction. This proved to be the case for the monoamine oxidase inhibitors, since large amounts of sympathomimetic amines can accumulate, particularly after the ingestion of cheese and other foods high in these substances. In some cases, severe cardiovascular damage occurred in depressed patients who were being treated with monoamine oxidase inhibitors.[42] Therefore, a need for an alternate means of enhancing the activity of monoamines was created. An alternate mechanism came to light ex post facto when it was discovered that the tricyclic antidepressant drugs were powerful inhibitors of reuptake into presynaptic terminals.[29,57] The concept has emerged that reuptake of monoamines released from monoaminergic neurons represents the major mechanism for the termination of the action of these substances. By blocking uptake, the concentration of a transmitter at the synaptic junction should be elevated and

its action thereby enhanced. However, since degradative enzymes are still intact, an excessive accumulation of toxic substances is avoided. Thus, blockage of uptake represents an important mechanism to consider in assessing the action of psychotropic drugs.

Finally, drugs may alter the number or sensitivity of the postsynaptic receptor sites. The "receptors" per se are essentially theoretical constructions and are inferred to exist because of functional changes in postsynaptic cells. They are presumably macromolecules with proteolipid and glycoprotein constituents that interact with transmitter substances or drugs in a lock-and-key fashion. Drug-induced changes in receptor sites are no doubt of great importance, particularly for long-term, adaptive changes such as may occur in states of tolerance or addiction. A phenomenon resembling denervation supersensitivity, which is commonly seen at peripheral neuro-effector junctions, has been found to occur in the striatum following chronic disruption of the nigrostriatal dopamine pathway. The effects of L-Dopa and apomorphine (a dopamine agonist) are greatly enhanced under these circumstances.[104] Presumably, in response to postlesion reduction in dopamine, there is a compensatory increase in the number of receptor sites upon the striatal cells. It seems safe to predict that many other instances of long-term, receptor changes of relevance to the effects of narcotics and other drugs will be uncovered in the future.

Neurophysiological and Histochemical

To have physiological or behavioral meaning, the net effect of drugs interacting with neurotransmitters and receptors eventually must be expressed in terms of an altered rate of firing of neurons. On the simplest level, one can examine the effects of drugs on the firing of single neurons within homogenous populations. On a more complex level, the actions of drugs on systems of neurons within multisynaptic pathways can be investigated. Finally, an analysis of the read-out of such neuronal systems on a behavioral level is needed for a complete understanding of the "mechanism of action" of a psychotropic drug. Elsewhere in this volume the more complex indicators of neuronal function (e.g., EEG and behavior) will be discussed; this review will be limited primarily to drug actions at a cellular level.

During the past decade, techniques have been developed that permit not only the recording of action potentials (spikes or unit activity) from single neurons in the mammalian brain but also the application of minute amounts of drugs or transmitter substances through multibarreled micropipettes during such recording. The latter technique, which is termed "microiontophoresis" or "electrophoresis," was originally developed by Curtis and Eccles.[39] It provides a powerful tool for the analysis of drug action at a cellular level. Only by directly applying drugs or putative transmitters to individual neurons by such micromethods can it directly be established that a substance has a primary action upon a particular neuron under study. A second development during this same period has been the discovery of histochemical methods by which certain neurons within the brain can be identified according to their specific neurotransmitter content. Most prominently, this has been achieved for the monoamine-containing neurons in the brain. Heller and associates by means of selective brain lesions first provided evidence for the probable existence of monoamine neuronal pathways.[62,63] These investigators found that this pathway traversed the medial forebrain bundle in the lateral hypothalamus. Dahlstrom, Fuxe, and their associates, utilizing the formaldehyde-condensation, histochemical-fluorescence method of Falck and Hillarp,[47] directly determined and mapped the location of monoamine cell bodies and terminals in the brain.[10,40,53] Three principal monoamine pathways were discovered: (1) a nigrostriatal dopamine system whose cells of origin are situated in the zona compacta of the substantia nigra and projections in the caudate nucleus, accumbens nucleus, and olfactory tubercules; (2) a "noradrenergic" pathway with cell bodies in the locus coeruleus and brainstem, reticular formation, and projections to various parts of the forebrain, including the hypothalamus, hippocampus,

and molecular layer of the cerebral cortex; and (3) a "serotonergic" system with cell bodies in the raphe nuclei of the brainstem and projections to the hypothalamus, amygdala, and other portions of the limbic system. The far-reaching implications of this discovery are currently permeating all aspects of research in neuropharmacology. It should be apparent that the identification of chemically specific neuronal systems sets the stage for integrating biochemical and neurophysiological knowledge on the mechanism of drug action. Specific examples of drug effects on histochemically characterized brain neurons will be given in some of the sections that follow.

(Mechanism of Psychotropic Drug Action: Major Drug Classes

Antipsychotic Drugs

The principal drugs in this category are the phenothiazines and butyrophenones, as exemplified respectively by chlorpromazine and haloperidol. Chlorpromazine was first suggested for possible use in psychiatric patients in the early 1950s by Henri-Marie Laborit, a surgeon who had been testing a series of phenothiazine antihistamines as adjuncts to anesthesia.[26] It is interesting to note that the denotation applied to these drugs has changed since their introduction and early years of use. They were originally most commonly called "tranquilizers" or "neuroleptics," but partly as a result of the NIMH and VA hospital collaborative studies are now usually termed "antipsychotics."[25,34,58] This significant shift in terminology was based on the conclusion that although these drugs may initially have some sedative actions, in the long run they do more than merely quiet patients or reduce their anxieties. On the whole, schizophrenic patients seemed to become less withdrawn and more involved in affairs of reality, and in that sense "primary" symptoms of schizophrenia were ameliorated. The significance of these clinical findings for the pharmacologist is that studies on the mechanism of action of these drugs may give some insight into the nature of brain systems that may relate to the brain systems primarily disturbed in schizophrenia.

On a biochemical level, the search for sites of action of chlorpromazine and other antipsychotics has in the past included investigations upon tissue respiration (electron transport and oxidative phosphoylation), phospholipids, and a variety of enzyme systems.[83,88] In most such systems, some effect can be seen, but because rather high concentrations are usually necessary, the relevance of such changes to the behavioral actions of the drugs has been questioned. Of course, it is possible that the drugs may become concentrated at critical subcellular sites and thereby alter these basic biochemical systems. In any event, in recent years the main focus of work on the mechanism of action of these drugs has moved away from an examination of general metabolic systems. Instead, attention has focused upon putative neurotransmitters.

The occurrence of extrapyramidal side effects in patients who are being treated with phenothiazines and butyrophenones is well known to every clinician. It has been suggested that there is a high correlation between the potency (on a milligram basis) of the various antipsychotic compounds and their tendency to produce extrapyramidal side effects.[112] Thioridazine appears to be a partial exception to this pattern in that the incidence of extrapyramidal side effects is relatively low at clinically effective doses.[33] In any event, evidence has accumulated that the antipsychotic drugs may be powerful blockers of the putative transmitter dopamine.[11,30,41,85] The resulting reduction in dopamine activity is believed to be responsible for the extrapyramidal side effects seen with these drugs. Associated with this apparent receptor blockage is a marked acceleration in the synthesis of dopamine, which may represent a compensatory feedback mechanism. Consistent with this notion is the fact that when the synthesis of catecholamines is inhibited by alpha-methyl-p-tyrosine, the behavioral effects of antipsychotic drugs in animals is potentiated.[6,90] Horn and Snyder have recently determined, on the basis of calculations utilizing X-ray crystal-lography measurements, that the active phenothiazines are similar to dopamine in structural conformation.[66] Since there are several dopamine tracts outside the extrapyramidal system (e.g., to nucleus accumbens and olfactory tubercules[9]) Horn and Snyder have suggested that these may be involved in the antischizophrenic activity of the phenothiazines and butyrophenones. These investigators also point out that the "similarity of the phenothiazine conformation to that of dopamine would also apply to norepinephrine."

As in the periphery, certain actions of norepinephrine in the brain may be mediated by the "secondary transmitter," cyclic AMP ($3',5'$-adenosine monophosphate).[92] Norepinephrine stimulates the production of cyclic AMP in brain slices,[72] and the effects of norepinephrine on Purkinje cells appear to be mediated by cyclic AMP.[98] Phenothiazines have been found to block the norepinephrine-induced increase in cyclic AMP in a manner that correlates with relative antipsychotic potencies.[86,105] Phenothiazines may also block the release of norepinephrine from nerve terminals.[13] Single-unit recordings from norepinephrine-containing neurons of the locus coeruleus[59] and dopamine-containing cells of the substantia nigra[23] have shown that the antipsychotic drugs are potent antagonists of the effects of amphetamine upon the firing of these cells. Interestingly, amphetamine, a drug that enhances dopamine actions, regularly induces a paranoid psychosis in volunteer subjects.[60] Clinical effects of amphetamine can readily be reversed by the antipsychotic drugs.[46] However, this situation is complicated by the fact that under certain circumstances the phenothiazines, but not the butyrophenones, tend to retard the rate at which amphetamine is metabolized and therefore prolong its stay in the body.[17,80] In any case, on both a cellular and behavioral level the antipsychotic drugs and amphetamines appear to have opposing actions. It would appear that the blocking of dopamine and perhaps also norepinephrine by the antipsychotic drugs can account for both their extrapyramidal side effects and amphetamine antagonism.

In addition to their importance in the treatment of schizophrenia, the antipsychotic drugs in high doses have been of value in highly active stages of manic-depressive psychosis.[87,95] However, lithium carbonate appears to be more effective in long-term treatment of this condition.[95] There is little information on the basic mechanism of the action of lithium. Since lithium can displace sodium ions, it presumably may effect neuronal membrane potential, transport mechanisms and other sodium-dependent processes. In brain slices, lithium has been found to impair the release of putative transmitters such as serotonin and norepinephrine.[73] The relationship between these pharmacological findings and possible biochemical factors in naturally occurring psychoses such as mania and schizophrenia remains to be determined.[74] Nevertheless, the discovery that the antipsychotic drugs have pronounced interaction with the catecholamine systems in the brain represents an exciting new and fruitful development in our attempts to understand the mechanism of action of this important class of drugs.

Antidepressant Drugs

Of the many chemical agents that have been tested in the treatment of depressive illness, the so-called "tricyclic" compounds have emerged as the most useful clinically.[76] An inherent difficulty in the evaluation of the efficacy of antidepressant drugs is the self-limiting nature of most illnesses categorized as "depressive." Another difficulty is the fact that clinical response to these drugs tends to be delayed. Nevertheless, there is fairly wide agreement on the superiority of the tricyclic compounds as compared with placebo. The monoamine oxidase inhibitors are felt to be less effective than the tricyclic compounds, and their use has been limited by the occurrence of serious cardiovascular side effects.[42,75] In any case, interest in understanding the basic mechanisms of action of the various drugs in this category has been given its main impetus by the clinical finding of antidepressant efficacy.

Imipramine, a close structural analogue of chlorpromazine, was the first of the antidepressant tricyclics to be tested. It was presumed to be just another "tranquilizer" and its antidepressant properties were discovered serendipitously during a routine clinical trial of phenothiazine-related compounds.[79] Imipramine differs in chemical structure from chlorpromazine only in the substitution of an ethylene for a sulfide bridge in the middle ring and the absence of the 2-chloro substituent. Despite these similarities in chemical structure, the clinical and neuropharmacological actions of the tricyclic drugs are in most ways entirely distinguishable from that of antipsychotic phenothiazines. On a clinical level, although the tricyclic compounds have some sedative effects, they may aggravate rather than dampen psychotic symptomatology.[75] On a pharmacological level, effects upon the brain-dopamine system that are so characteristic of the phenothiazines and butyrophenones are lacking among the tricyclic drugs.

The first significant clue as to the mechanism of action of the tricyclic drugs was derived from the basic observations of Axelrod and his coworkers, that peripheral adrenergic nerves avidly accumulate radioactively-labeled catecholamines.[12] This work was extended into the central nervous system with the finding that tricyclic drugs, but not chlorpromazine, blocked the uptake of exogenous norepinephrine injected into the cerebral ventricles.[57] When the blood-brain barrier is circumvented by the latter route of administration, norepinephrine will enter the brain parenchyma and be taken up into catecholamine-containing neutrons.[1,54] Presumably, if imipramine or other tricyclic compounds block the uptake of exogenous norepinephrine, then endogenous norepinephrine, released by central noradrenergic nerves, would also be blocked. Since reuptake probably represents the primary mechanism for terminating the action of norepinephrine upon postsynaptic receptors, the tricyclic compounds may produce their behavioral effects by this means.

New data now require some modification and extension of what might be called the "catecholamine hypothesis" of the mechanism of action of the tricyclic drugs as presented above. It has been found that some of the tricyclic compounds are much more potent blockers of serotonin than of norepinephrine uptake.[28,94,96] The differential activity of the various tricyclic compounds on uptake seems to depend on the degree of methylation of the side-chain amine moiety. Those tricyclic drugs which have their side-chain nitrogen in the *tertiary* form (e.g., imipramine, amytriptyline, chlorimipramine) primarily block the uptake of serotonin. On the other hand, the demethylated analogues of these compounds, in which the side-chain nitrogen in *secondary* form (e.g., desmethylimipramine and protryptiline) are more active in blocking norepinephrine uptake. On this basis, Carlsson has suggested that these two subgroups within the general category of tricyclic drugs could have differing clinical actions.[28] For example, he suggests the tertiary amine forms may have their greatest effect on "mood," whereas the secondary amines might primarily influence "drive." The validity of this concept of differential uptake and clinical action remains to be tested. It is important to note that blockage of monoamine uptake may not be a necessary attribute of all tricyclic antidepressants. Iprindole, a tricyclic compound containing a ring indole moiety, has been reported to be an effective antidepressant, yet it appears to lack any effect on amine uptake.[48] Nevertheless, the studies on tricyclic antidepressants and amine biochemistry represent an excellent illustration of the mutuality among basic neuropharmacology and clinical psychopharmacology and therapeutics.

Stimulant Drugs

From the point of view of behavior, the principal drugs of interest in this category are the various isomers and analogues of amphetamine and methylphenidate. The therapeutic uses of these drugs are becoming progressively narrower as concern over their abuse potential increases. In psychiatry at the present time, their use is now almost entirely limited to the treatment of hyperkinetic children.[19] It has long been known from case histories and field observations that the ingestion of large amounts of amphetamines is associated with a paranoid psychosis that is often difficult to distinguish from paranoid schizophrenia. When unaccompanied by the use of barbiturates or other drugs, the person with the psychosis is free of the usual signs of confusion or disorientation classically associated with 'organic" mental states.[14,35,44,64] However, until the study of Griffiths and coworkers it was not established that amphetamine, if given in sufficient amounts, would induce a psychosis in volunteer subjects under controlled conditions.[60] In the latter study almost all subjects developed a paranoid psychosis within one to five days with cumulative doses of dextroamphetamine ranging from one hundred to seven hundred and fifty mg. Contrary to expectation, subjects appeared depressed rather than elated as the psychosis developed. Since it appears that a paranoid state can be induced in a regular fashion by amphetamine in most or all subjects at high-dose levels, this drug can be regarded as producing a true "model psychosis." These clinical observations have therefore stimulated much interest in the basic mechanisms of action of this class of drugs.

On an electrophysiological level it had been observed that d-amphetamine causes a decrease in the threshold required for producing EEG arousal by electrical stimulation of the reticular formation.[20] However, it is unclear by which neurochemical mechanism such effects are mediated. Of course, the amphetamines are structural analogues of the catecholamines and fall into the general category of sympathomimetic agents. However, it was not until the introduction of alpha-methyltyrosine, a selective inhibitor of catecholamine synthesis, that the means were available for testing the hypothesis that the amphetamines may produce their central effects through a catecholamine mechanism. It has been found that pretreatment with alpha-methyltyrosine blocked most of the behavioral effects of d-amphetamine. For example, the disruption of the conditioned avoidance response and excitatory responses produced by amphetamine in animals can all be blocked by alpha-methyltyrosine.[61,89,107] These studies appear to establish a direct requirement for the ongoing synthesis of brain catecholamines to sustain the actions of amphetamine, since the block by alpha-methyltyrosine occurs prior to any significant depletion of the amine stores.

The foregoing behavioral studies strongly suggest that the central actions of the amphetamines are mediated through the catecholamines. Biochemical and histochemical studies give support to this view. Indirect evidence suggests that the amphetamines can both release catecholamines from central catecholamine neurons and block their reuptake.[16,29][31,57] The fact that amphetamines have this dual action on catecholamines would seem to provide an explanation for the potent behavioral effects of these drugs, since extraneuronal release would result in enhanced catecholamine activity at postsynaptic receptor sites and the block in reuptake would prevent the removal of the catecholamines from such sites. The action of excessive amounts of catecholamines at postysnaptic sites may be expected to produce a compensatory feedback inhibition of the firing of the catecholamine neurons, and this has been demonstrated by direct, single unit recordings from catecholamine-containing neurons in the *locus coeruleus* and *substantia nigra*.[23,59]

Although much evidence now points to a direct mediation by brain catecholamines of the effects of amphetamine, the question still remains, which of the catecholamines—norepinephrine or dopamine—is primarily involved in the production of the paranoid psychosis in man? Since amphetamine produces several types of behavioral effects in animals, many studies have been carried out in an attempt to parcel out the relative contributions of the two catecholamines. The so-called stereotypic behaviors (e.g., compulsive gnawing) that may be most analogous to the amphetamine psychosis in man seem to be closely associated with dopamine and the dopamine tracts in the brain.[11,45,49] On the other hand, the increased locomotor activity induced by amphetamine may involve norepinephrine as well as dopamine in the brain,[27,100] Taylor and Snyder have studied this question by taking advantage of the fact that d-amphetamine is much more potent than l-amphetamine in blocking the neuronal uptake of norepinephrine, but that the two stereoisomers are essentially equipotent in blocking the uptake of dopamine by neuronal terminal in the corpus striatum.[101] They have found that d-amphetamine is ten times more effective than l-amphetamine in enhancing locomotor activity, but that the two have approximately the same potency with respect to compulsive gnawing behavior. If it is assumed that behavioral potency is a function of the degree to which uptake is blocked, then these results again suggest that norepinephrine is most important for mediating the activation and dopamine for the stereotyped behaviors induced by amphetamine. Taken together, these various results again underline the great importance dopamine and norepinephrine neuronal systems in the brain may have for abnormal behavioral patterns and their possible relevance to both amphetamine-induced and naturally occurring psychoses.

Psychotomimetic Drugs

A great many chemical substances, if ingested in large enough quantity, can alter fundamental metabolic processes and thereby produce a psychosis characterized by a generalized disturbance in perceptual, cognitive, affective, or vegetative functions. However, from a pharmacological standpoint the drugs of greatest interest are those which have selective actions and produce a well-defined "psychotic" state. The paranoid psychosis induced by amphetamine, discussed in the last section, is one example of this. Other well-defined drug psychoses include: (1) the delerium states produced by the anticholinergic drugs; and (2) the "psychedelic" state associated with D-lysergic acid diethylamide (LSD), mescaline, and related drugs. There has been much controversy over whether any of these drugs accurately mimic schizophrenia or other nondrug induced psychoses. Bowers and Freedman have reported that some acute psychoses begin with a psychedelic state, but that this may represent only a transient phase in the overall illness.[18] Thus, in some cases a psychotomimetic drug may be seen as mimicking phases or aspects of naturally occurring psychoses rather than the whole picture of an illness in a longitudinal sense. In any event, the significance of the psychotomimetic drugs for purposes of basic research is the fact that they can serve as tracers in the identification of chemical and neuronal systems in the brain that are of importance for the maintenance of normal mental or behavioral functions.

A specific hypothesis concerning chemical site of action was developed for LSD shortly after its introduction into pharmacological research in the early 1950s. Gaddum[55] and Woolley and Shaw[110] introduced the notion that LSD may produce its effects by interfering with the action of serotonin in the brain. It was found that LSD antagonized the effects of serotonin on certain smooth muscle preparations (e.g., isolated rat uterus).[55,56,110] Moreover, LSD resembles serotonin structurally (i.e., both contain an indole nucleus) and serotonin is present in the brain.[7,111] The hypothesis that LSD acts in the brain by antagonizing serotonin was soon questioned as a result of the finding that 2-brom LSD was as potent as LSD in antagonizing serotonin in peripheral systems, but had little behavioral effect.[32] Studies in man with a wide range of LSD congeners have confirmed this lack of relationship between peripheral antiserotonin potency and psychotomimetic effect.[69] However, it has also been found that LSD, particularly at low concentrations, could have a serotoninlike action in various smooth systems.[37][82,97,108] But it was apparent that studies with peripheral tissues could not settle the question of what, if any, interaction occurs between LSD and serotonin in the brain itself.

Freedman and Giarman, in a logical development from this earlier work dealing with LSD-serotonin interactions in the periphery, began to investigate the influence of LSD on the metabolism of serotonin in the brain.[50,51] They found that LSD produced a small (60–100 nanograms) but reproducible increase in the concentration of serotonin in the brain. The LSD-induced increase in serotonin could be interpreted as resulting from either increased synthesis or decreased breakdown.

However, the isolated measurement of serotonin concentration gave little clue as to which general mechanism may be involved. It has more recently been found that the concentration of 5-hydroxyindoleacetic acid (5-HIAA), the principal metabolite of serotonin in the brain, is decreased after the administration of LSD and other indoleamine type psychotomimetics.[52,93] Furthermore, the rate of synthesis of serotonin from labeled precursor (L-tryptophan) is also decreased.[81] These results point to the possibility that LSD acts to retard the turnover of brain serotonin.

Based on the dual observations that LSD reduced the turnover of brain serotonin and that electrical stimulation of the serotonin-containing neurons of the midbrain raphe nuclei increased turnover, it was suggested that LSD might depress the firing of raphe neurons.[4] A similar suggestion was based on the fact that LSD slowed the rate of depletion of serotonin that occurs after inhibition of synthesis.[9] By means of direct microelectrode recording from single raphe neurons in rats, it has been demonstrated that extremely small doses of LSD (10 μg/kg, i.v.) produced a total but reversible inhibition of firing.[2,3] This is an invariable finding and occurs both in anesthetized and unanesthetized animals.[22] This inhibitory effect of LSD was exceedingly selective and the firing of units outside the raphe nucleus was either unaffected or increased. The nonpsychotomimetic analogue of LSD, 2-brom-LSD, which is even more potent than LSD in blocking the actions of serotonin in smooth muscle preparations,[32] was found to have less than 1 percent of the activity of LSD in depressing raphe neurons. Taken together these results reinforce the original hypothesis that LSD might act in the brain by interacting somehow with serotonin. There are a number of possible mechanisms that might account for the observed inhibition by LSD of serotonin-containing (i.e., raphe) neurons. First, LSD might have a direct inhibitory action. In support of this possibility it has been found that raphe, but not other nearby neurons, were inhibited by direct, microiontophoretic administration of LSD.[5] However, the fact that raphe neurons may be inhibited directly by LSD does not exclude the interesting possibility that the drug also acts at postsynaptic sites.

The above studies represent only beginning efforts toward clarifying the interrelationship between the effects of LSD and the functional state of the serotonin-containing neurons of the raphe system. Although LSD has been the most thoroughly studied of the psychedlic drugs in this respect, other members of this class probably act through similar mechanisms. Indoleamines such as N,N-dimethyltryptamine and psylocybin, which are structurally related to LSD, as well as certain substituted phenethylamines (e.g., mescaline) and amphetamines (e.g., 2,5-methoxy-4-methylamphetamine) resemble LSD in many though not all behavioral effects and biochemical or neurophysiological actions.[3,52] In addition, mescaline and LSD show cross-tolerance toward one another in man.[109] On the other hand, marijuana or its active principle, Δ^9-tetrahydrocannabinol, although it may be classified as a psychedelic drug, does not exhibit cross-tolerance with LSD in man, suggesting that it acts through a different mechanism.[68] In any event, the elucidation of the mechanism of action of the psychedelic drugs will require more than simply isolated observations on their effects on serotonin-containing or other individual neurons. Ultimately, it will be necessary to integrate data from the unit level with knowledge about the interconnections and physiological role of the neuronal systems within which these units function.

❰ Conclusions

Neuropharmacology: Future Prospects

From the foregoing illustrations it can be seen that information about chemical and cellular sites of drug action is being elaborated on a wide front. Undoubtedly, trends that now seem promising will be discarded and other approaches that are not presently in vogue will supercede them. All drugs have multiple actions and it is possible that the currently known effects of certain drugs may not be the crucial ones in terms of behavior. However, there is every expectation that, in a relatively few years, given the current level of sophistication in methodology and approach, substantial progress will be made in the accurate characterization of the relevant mechanisms of action of most psychotropic drugs. We are closer to this goal in some areas than in others. The examples discussed in detail (i.e., antipsychotic, antidepressant, stimulant, and psychotomimetic drugs) seem to most clearly illustrate the current creative ferment in the field. In each case, a plausible and coherent basic mechanism of action has been proposed and is supported by a respectable amount of experimental work. On the other hand, in the case of the narcotics and antianxiety drugs, progress toward ascertaining the mechanisms of action has been less rapid. However, because of public concern over drug abuse, which is leading to increased support for research in this area, we can expect a marked expansion in our knowledge of the basic neuropharmacology of these drugs as well. A decade ago, these goals seemed much further from reach than they do at the present time.

Implications for Psychiatry

These developments in neuropharmacology will have a continued impact upon psychiatry in many spheres. First, in the area of training, as knowledge both about basic brain mechanisms as well as drug action increases, it will appear more relevant in the future than it has in the past to include a significant body of neuropharmacology and neurobiology in the training programs of departments of psychiatry. This will become more than simply an academic exercise if we reach a stage where an understanding of the mechanisms of drug action forms the basis for the intelligent clinical administration of drugs. In the area of psychiatric research, the concepts and methods of basic neuropharmacology are already having a major influence. One of the best examples of this is in biological research on the affective disorders. Neuropharmacological theories of the mechanism of action of antidepressant drugs (e.g., catecholamine or indoleamine) have led to investigations upon the status of such systems in patients with disturbances in affective states.* Finally, as our understanding of the mode of action of existing drugs increases, new drugs with improved efficacy or fewer unwanted effects can be developed. For example, if the antipsychotic drugs do, in fact, produce their therapeutic effects by blocking dopamine receptors, it would be useful to restrict this action to those dopamine pathways most directly concerned with the psychotic process. Since the dopamine pathway of the extrapyramidal motor system may not be directly involved in the therapeutic action of these drugs, it would be advantageous to have antipsychotic drugs that acted selectively upon dopamine receptors outside this system. Similar possibilities of increased specificity or efficacy exist for all of the presently used pharmacotherapeutic drugs. Through an understanding of their mode of action, rational procedures for improving known drugs or developing new drugs will thus be facilitated.

(Bibliography

1. AGHAJANIAN, G. K. and F. E. BLOOM. "Electronmicroscopic Autoradiography of Rat Hypothalamus after Intraventricular H³-norepinephrine," *Science*, 153 (1966), 308–310.

2. AGHAJANIAN, G. K., W. E. FOOTE, and M. H. SHEARD. "Lysergic Acid Diethylamide: Sensitive Neuronal Units in the Midbrain Raphe," *Science*, 161 (1968), 706–708.

3. ———. "Action of Psychotogenic Drugs on Single Midbrain Raphe Neurons," *J. Pharmacol. Exp. Ther.*, 171 (1970), 178–187. York: Academic, 1973.

4. AGHAJANIAN, G. K., and D. X. FREEDMAN. "Biochemical and Morphological Aspects of LSD Pharmacology," in D. H. Efron, ed.. *Psychopharmacology: A Review of Progress*, pp. 1185–1194. Washington: Government Printing Office, 1968.

5. AGHAJANIAN, G. K. and H. J. HAIGLER.

"Direct and Indirect Actions of LSD, Serotonin and Mescaline on Serotonin-Containing Neurons," in J. Barchas and E. Usdin, eds., *Serotonin and Behavior*. New York: Academic, 1973.

6. AHLENIUS, S. and J. ENGEL. "Behavioral Effects of Haloperidol after Tyrosine Hydroxylase Inhibition," *Eur. J. Pharmacol.*, 15 (1971), 187–192.

7. AMIN, A. H., T. B. B. CRAWFORD, and J. H. GADDUM. "The Distribution of Substance P and 5-Hydroxytryptamine in the Central Nervous System of the Dog," *J. Physiol.* 126 (1954), 596–618.

8. ANDÉN, N.-E., S. G. BUTCHER, H. CORRODI et al. "Receptor Activity and Turnover of Dopamine and Noradrenaline after Neuroleptics," *Eur. J. Pharmacol.*, 11 (1970), 303–314.

9. ANDÉN. N.-E., H. CORRODI, K. FUXE et al. "Evidence for a Central 5-Hydroxytryptamine Receptor Stimulation by Lysergic Acid Diethylamide," *Br. J. Pharmacol.*, 34 (1968), 1–7.

10. ANDÉN, N.-E., A. DAHLSTRÖM, K. FUXE et al. "Ascending Monoamine Neurons to the Telencephalon and Diencephalon," *Acta Physiol. Scand.*, 67 (1966), 313–326.

11. ANDÉN, N.-E., A. RUBENSON, T. HÖKFELT. "Evidence for Dopamine Receptor Stimulation by Apomorphine," *J. Pharm. Pharmacol.*, 19 (1967), 627–629.

12. AXELROD, J., H. WEIL-MALHERBE, and R. TOMCHICK. "The Physiological Deposition of H³-Epinephrine and its Metabolite Metanephrine," *J. Pharmacol. Exp. Ther.*, 127 (1959), 251–256.

13. BALDESSARINI, R. J. and I. J. KOPIN. "The Effect of Drugs on the Release of Norepinephrine-H³ from Central Nervous System Tissues by Electrical Stimulation *In Vitro*," *J. Pharmacol. Exp. Ther.*, 156 (1967), 31–38.

14. BELL, D. S. "Comparison of Amphetamine Psychosis and Schizophrenia," *Br. J. Psychiatry*, 111 (1965) 701–707.

15. BERTLER, A., A. CARLSSON, and E. ROSENGREN. "Release by Reserpine of Catecholamines from Rabbits' Hearts," *Naturwissenschaften*, 43 (1956), 521.

16. BESSON, M. J., A. CHERAMY, P. FELTZ et al. "Release of Newly Synthesized Dopamine from Dopamine-Containing Terminals in the Striata of the Rat," *Proc. Natl. Acad. Sci. USA*, 62 (1969), 741–745.

---

* Developments in this and similar areas are described in some other chapters of this volume.

17. BORELLA, L., F. HERR, and A. WOJDAN. "Prolongation of Certain Effects of Amphetamines by Chlorpromazine," *Can. J. Physiol. Pharmacol.*, 47 (1969), 7–13.

18. BOWERS, M. B. and D. X. FREEDMAN. "Psychedelic Experiences in Acute Psychoses," *Arch. Gen. Psychiatry*, 15 (1966), 240–248.

19. BRADLEY, C. "Benzedrine and Dexedrine in the Treatment of Children's Behavior Disorders," *Pediatrics*, 5 (1950), 24–36.

20. BRADLEY, P. B. and B. J. KEY. "The Effect of Drugs on the Arousal Responses Produced by Electrical Stimulation of the Reticular Formation of the Brain," *Electroencephalogr. Clin. Neurophysiol.*, 10 (1958), 97–110.

21. BRODIE, B. B., A. PLETSCHER, and P. A. SHORE. "Evidence that Serotonin has a Role in Brain Function," *Science*, 122 (1965), 968.

22. BUNNEY, B. S. and G. K. AGHAJANIAN. Unpublished data.

23. BUNNEY, B. S., J. R. WALTERS, R. H. ROTH et al. "Dopaminergic Neurons: Effect of Antipsychotic Drugs and Amphetamine on Single Cell Activity," *J. Pharmacol. Exp. Ther.*, 185 (1973), 560–571.

24. BUNNEY, W. E., JR., H. BRODIE, H. KEITH et al. "Studies of Alpha-methyl-para-tyrosine, L-Dopa, and L-Tryptophan in Depression and Mania," *Am. J. Psychiatry*, 127 (1971), 48–57.

25. CAFFEY, E. M., L. E. HOLLISTER, C. J. KLETT et al. "Veterans Administration (VA) Cooperative Studies in Psychiatry," in W. G. Clark and J. del Giudice, eds., *Principles of Psychopharmacology*, p. 429. New York: Academic, 1970.

26. CALDWELL, A. E. "History of Psychopharmacology," in W. G. Clark and J. del Giudice, eds., *Principles of Psychopharmacology*, p. 9. New York: Academic, 1970.

27. CARLSSON, A. "Amphetamine and Brain Catecholamines," in E. Costa and S. Garattini, eds., *International Symposium on Amphetamines and Related Compounds*, p. 289. New York: Raven Press, 1970.

28. CARLSSON, A., H. CORRODI, K. FUXE et al. "Effects of Some Antidepressant Drugs on the Depletion of Intraneuronal Brain Catecholamine Stores Caused by 4, Alpha-Dimethyl-meta-Tyramine", *Eur. J. Pharmacol.*, 5 (1969), 367–373.

29. CARLSSON, A., K. FUXE, B. HAMBERGER et al. "Biochemical and Histochemical Studies on the Effects of Imipramine-Like Drugs and (+)-Amphetamine on Central and Peripheral Catecholamine Neurons," *Acta. Physiol. Scand.*, 67 (1966), 481–497.

30. CARLSSON, A. and M. LINDQVIST. "Effect of Chlorpromazine on Haloperidol on Formation of 3-Methoxytyramine and Normetanephrine in Mouse Brain," *Acta Pharmacol. Toxicol. (Kbh)*, 20 (1963), 140–144.

31. CARR, L. A. and K. E. MOORE. "Norepinephrine: Release from Brain by d-Amphetamine *In Vivo*," *Science*, 164 (1969), 322–323.

32. CERLETTI, A. and E. ROTHLIN. "Role of 5-Hydroxytryptamine in Mental Diseases and Its Antagonism to Lysergic Acid Derivatives," *Nature*, 176 (1955), 785–786.

33. COLE, J. O. and D. CLYDE. "Extrapyramidal Side Effects and Clinical Response to the Phenothiazines," *Rev. Can. Biol.*, 20 (1961), 565–574.

34. COLE, J. O., S. C. GOLDBERG, and J. M. DAVIS. "Drugs in the Treatment of Psychosis: Controlled Studies," in P. Solomon, ed., *Psychiatric Drugs*, pp. 153–180. New York: Grune & Stratton, 1966.

35. CONNELL, P. H. "Amphetamine Psychosis," *Maudsley Monographs*, No. 5, p. 62. London: Chapman and Hall, 1958.

36. COOPER, J. R., F. E. BLOOM, and R. H. ROTH. *The Biochemical Basis of Neuropharmacology*. New York: Oxford University Press, 1970.

37. COSTA, E. "Effects of Hallucinogenic and Tranquilizing Drugs on Serotonin Evoked Uterine Contractions," *Proc. Soc. Exp. Biol. Med.*, 91 (1956), 39–41.

38. COTZIAS, G. C., P. S. PAPAVASILION, and R. GELLENE. "Modification of Parkinsonism—Chronic Treatment with L-Dopa," *N. Engl. J. Med.*, 280 (1969), 337–345.

39. CURTIS, D. R. and R. M. ECCLES. "The Excitation of Renshaw Cells by Pharmacological Agents Applied Electrophoretically," *J. Physiol.*, 141 (1958), 435–445.

40. DAHLSTRÖM, A. and K. FUXE. "Evidence for the Existence of Monoamine-Containing Neurons in the Central Nervous System. I. Demonstration of Monoamines in the Cell Bodies on Brain Stem Neurons," *Acta Physiol. Scand.*, 62 (1965), Suppl. 232, 1–55.

41. DAPRADA, M. and A. PLETSCHER. "Acceleration of the Cerebral Dopamine Turnover

by Chlorpromazine," *Experientia*, 22 (1966), 465–469.

42. DAVIES, B. E. "Tranylcypromine and Cheese," *Lancet*, 2 (1963), 691–692.

43. ECCLES, J. C. *The Physiology of Synapses.* New York: Springer-Verlag, 1964.

44. ELLINWOOD, E. H. "Amphetamine Psychoses: I. Description of the Individuals and Process," *J. Nerv. Ment. Dis.*, 144 (1967), 273–283.

45. ERNST, A. "Mode of Action of Apomorphine and Dexamphetamine on Gnawing Compulsion in Rats," *Psychopharmacologia*, 10 (1967), 316–323.

46. ESPELIN, D. E. and A. K. DONE. "Amphetamine Poisoning: Effectiveness of Chlorpromazine," *N. Engl. J. Med.*, 278 (1968), 1361–1365.

47. FALCK, B., N.-A. HILLARP, G. THIEME et al. "Fluorescence of Catecholamines and Related Compounds Condensed with Formaldehyde," *J. Histochem. Cytochem.*, 10 (1962), 348–354.

48. FANN, W. E., J. M. DAVIS, D. S. JANOWSKY et al. "Effect of Iprindole on Amine Uptake in Man," *Arch. Gen. Psychiatry*, 26 (1972), 158–162.

49. FOG, R. L., A. RANDRUP, and H. PAKKENBURG. "Aminergic Mechanisms in Corpus Striatum and Amphetamine-induced Stereotyped Behavior," *Psychopharmacologia*, 11 (1967), 179–183.

50. FREEDMAN, D. X. "Effects of LSD-25 on Brain Serotonin," *J. Pharmacol. Exp. Ther.*, 134. (1961), 160–166.

51. FREEDMAN, D. X. and N. J. GIARMAN. "LSD-25 and the Status and Level of Brain Serotonin," *Ann. N.Y. Acad. Sci.*, 96 (1962), 98–106.

52. FREEDMAN, D. X., R. GOTTLIEB, and R. A. LOVELL. "Psychotomimetic Drugs and Brain 5-Hydroxytryptamine Metabolism," *Biochem. Pharmacol.*, 19 (1970), 1181–1188.

53. FUXE, K. "Evidence for the Existence of Monoamine Neurons in the Central Nervous System. IV. Distribution of Monoamine Nerve Terminals in the Central Nervous System," *Acta Physiol. Scand.*, 64 (1965), Suppl. 247, 41–85.

54. FUXE, K. and U. UNGERSTEDT. "Localization of Catecholamine Uptake after Intraventricular Injection," *Life Sci.*, 5 (1966), 1817–1824.

55. GADDUM, J. H. "Antagonism between Lysergic Acid Diethylamide and 5-Hydroxytryptamine," *J. Physiol.*, 121 (1953), 15.

56. GADDUM, J. H. and K. A. HAMEED. "Drugs which Antagonize 5-Hydroxytryptamine," *Br. J. Pharmacol.*, 9 (1954), 240–248.

57. GLOWINSKI, J. and J. AXELROD. "Effects of Drugs on the Deposition of H^3-Norepinephrine in the Rat Brain," *Pharmacol. Rev.*, 18 (1966), 775–785.

58. GOLDBERG, S. C. "Brief Resume of the National Institute of Mental Health Study in Acute Schizophrenia," in W. G. Clark and J. del Giudice, eds., *Principles of Psychopharmacology*, p. 443. New York: Academic, 1970.

59. GRAHAM, A. W. and G. K. AGHAJANIAN. "Effects of Amphetamine on Single Cell Activity in a Catecholamine Nucleus, the Locus Coeruleus," *Nature*, 234 (1971), 100–102.

60. GRIFFITH, J. D., J. CAVENAUGH, J. HELD et al. "Dextroamphetamine: Evaluation of Psychotomimetic Properties in Man," *Arch. Gen. Psychiatry*, 26 (1972), 97–100.

61. HANSON, L. C. F. "Evidence that the Central Action of Amphetamine is Mediated Via Catecholamines," *Psychopharmacologia*, 10 (1967), 289–297.

62. HELLER, A., J. A. HARVEY, and R. Y. MOORE. "A Demonstration of a Fall in Brain Serotonin Following Central Nervous System Lesions in the Rat," *Biochem. Pharmacol.*, 11 (1962), 859–866.

63. HELLER, A. and R. Y. MOORE. "Effect of Central Nervous System Lesions on Brain Monoamines in the Rat," *J. Pharmacol. Exp. Ther.*, 150 (1965), 1–9.

64. HERMAN, M. and S. H. NAGLER. "Psychoses Due to Amphetamine," *J. Nerv. Ment. Dis.*, 120 (1954), 268–272.

65. HOLZBAUR, M. and M. VOGT. "Depression by Reserpine of the Noradrenaline Concentration in the Hypothalamus of the Cat," *J. Neurochem.*, 1 (1956), 8–11.

66. HORN, A. S. and S. H. SNYDER. "Chlorpromazine and Dopamine: Conformational Similarities that Correlate with the Antischizophrenic Activity of Phenothiazine Drugs," *Proc. Natl. Acad. Sci. USA*, 68 (1971). 2325–2328.

67. HORNYKIEWICZ, O. "Dopamine (3-Hydroxytryptamine) and Brain Function," *Pharmacol. Rev.*, 18 (1966), 925–964.

68. Isbell, H. and D. R. Janiski. "A Comparison of LSD-25 with $(-)$-Δ^9-Trans-Tetrahydrocannabinol (THC) and Attempted Cross Tolerance Between LSD and THC," *Psychopharmacolgia*, 14 (1969), 115–123.

69. Isbell, H., E. J. Miner, and C. R. Logan. "Relationships of Psychotomimetic to Anti-Serotonin Potencies of Congeners of Lysergic Acid Diethylamide (LSD-25)," *Psychopharmacologia*, 1 (1959), 20–28.

70. Jequier, E., W. Lovenberg, and A. Sjoerdsma. "Tryptophan Hydroxylase Inhibition: The Mechanism by which p-Chlorophenylalanine Depletes Rat Brain Serotonin," *Mol. Pharmacol.*, 3 (1967), 274–278.

71. Jouvet, M. "Biogenic Amines and the States of Sleep," *Science*, 163, (1969), 32–41.

72. Kakiuchi, S. and T. W. Rall. "The Influence of Chemical Agents on the Accumulation of Adenosine 3′,-5′-Phosphate in Slices of Rabbit Cerebellum," *Mol. Pharmacol.*, 4 (1968), 367–378.

73. Katz, R. I., T. N. Chase, and R. J. Kopin. "Evoked Release of Norepinephrine and Serotonin from Brain Slices: Inhibition by Lithium," *Science*, 162 (1968), 466–467.

74. Kety, S. S. "Current Biochemical Approaches to Schizophrenia," *N. Engl. J. Med.*, 276 (1967), 325–331.

75. Klein, D. G. and J. M. Davis. *Diagnosis and Drug-Treatment of Psychiatric Disorders*. Baltimore: Williams & Wilkins, 1969.

76. Klerman, G. L. and J. O. Cole. "Clinical Pharmacology of Imipramine and Related Antidepressant Compounds," *Pharmacol. Rev.*, 17 (1965), 101–141.

77. Koe, B. K. and A. Weissman. "p-Chlorophenylalanine: A Specific Depletor of Brain Serotonin," *J. Pharmacol. Exp. Ther.*, 154 (1966), 499–516.

78. Kopin, I. J., J. E. Fischer, J. Musacchio et al. "Evidence for a False Neurochemical Transmitter as a Mechanism for the Hypotensive Effect of Monoamine Oxidase Inhibitors." *Proc. Natl. Acad. Sci. USA*, 52 (1964), 716–721.

79. Kuhn, R. "The Treatment of Depressive States with G-22355 (Imipramine Hydrochloride)," *Am. J. Psychiatry*, 115 (1958), 459–464.

80. Lemberger, L., E. D. Witt, J. M. Davis et al. "The Effects of Haloperidol and Chlor-promazine on Amphetamine Metabolism and Amphetamine Stereotype Behavior in the Rat," *J. Pharmacol. Exp. Ther.*, 174 (1970), 428–433.

81. Lin, R. C., S. H. Ngai, and E. Costa. "Lysergic Acid Diethylamide: Role in Conversion of Plasma Tryptophan to Brain Serotonin (5-Hydroxytryptamine)," *Science*, 166 (1969), 237–239.

82. Mansour, T. E. "The Effect of Lysergic Acid Diethylamide, 5-Hydroxytryptamine, and Related Compounds on the Liver Fluke. Fasciola Hepatica," *Br. J. Pharmacol.*, 12 (1957), 406–409.

83. McIlwain, H. *Biochemistry of the Central Nervous System*. London: J. & A. Churchill, 1966.

84. Murphy, D. L., H. K. Brodie, F. K. Goodwin et al. "Regular Induction of Hypomania by L-Dopa in 'Bipolar' Manic-Depressive Patients," *Nature*, 229 (1971), 135–136.

85. Nyback, H. and G. Sedvall. "Effect of Chlorpromazine on Accumulation and Disappearance of Catecholamines Formed from Trysoine-C^{14} in Brain," *J. Pharmacol. Exp. Ther.*, 162 (1968), 294–301.

86. Palmer, G. C., G. A. Robeson, A. A. Manian et al. "Modification by Psychotropic Drugs of the Cyclic AMP Response to Norepinephrine in the Rat Brain *In Vitro*," *Eur. J. Pharmacol.*, (1972), in press.

87. Prien, R. F., E. M. Caffey, and C. V. Klett. "Comparison of Lithium Carbonate and Chlorpromazine on the Treatment of Mania," *Arch. Gen. Psychiatry*, 26 (1972), 146–153.

88. Quastel, J. J. "Metabolic Effects of Some Psychopharmacological Agents in Brain *In Vitro*," in W. G. Clark and J. del Giudice, eds., *Principles of Psychopharmacology*, p. 142. New York: Academic, 1970.

89. Randrup, A. and I. Munkrad. "Role of Catecholamines in the Amphetamine Excitatory Response," *Nature*, 211 (1966), 540.

90. Rech, R. H., L. A. Carr, and R. E. Moore. "Behavioral Effects of Alpha-Methyltyrosine after Prior Depletion of Brain Catecholamines," *J. Pharmacol. Exp. Ther.*, 160 (1968), 326–335.

91. Redmond, D. E., Jr., J. W. Maas, A. Kling et al. "Social Behavior of Monkeys Selec-

tively Depleted of Monoamines," *Science,*
174 (1971), 428–431.

92. ROBESON, G. A., R. W. BUTCHER, and E. W.
SUTHERLAND. "On the Relation of Hormone
Receptors to Adenyl Cyclase," in J. F.
Danielli, J. F. Moran, and D. J. Truggle,
eds., *Fundamental Concepts in Drug-
Receptor Interactions,* p. 59. London: Aca-
demic, 1969.

93. ROSECRANS, J. A., R. A. LOVELL, and D. X.
FREEDMAN. "Effects of Lysergic Acid
Diethylamide on the Metabolism of Brain
5-Hydroxytryptamine," *Biochem. Pharmacol.,* 16 (1967), 2011–2021.

94. ROSS, S. B. and A. L. RENYI. "Inhibition of
the Uptake of Tritiated 5-Hydroxytrypt-
amine on Brain Tissue," *Eur. J. Pharmacol.,*
7 (1969), 270–277.

95. SCHOU, M. "Special Review: Lithium in
Psychiatric Therapy and Prophylaxis,"
J. Psychiatr. Res., 6 (1969), 67–95.

96. SHASKIN, E. G. and S. H. SNYDER. "Kinetics
of Serotonin Accumulation into Slices from
Rat Brain: Relationship to Catecholamine
Uptake," *J. Pharmacol. Exp. Ther.,* 175
(1970), 404–418.

97. SHAW, E. and D. W. WOOLLEY. "Some Serotonin Activities of Lysergic Acid Diethylamide," *Science,* 124 (1956), 121–122.

98. SIGGINS, G. R., B. J. HOFFER, and F. E.
BLOOM. "Cyclic Adenosine Monosphos-
phate: Possible Mediator for Norepinephrine Effects on Cerebellar Purkinje
Cells," *Science,* 165 (1969), 1018–1020.

99. SPECTOR, S., A. SJOERDSMA, and S. UDEN-
FRIEND. "Blockade of Endogenous Norepinephrine Synthesis by Alpha-Methyl-
Tyrosine, an Inhibitor of Tyrosine Hydroxylase," *J. Pharmacol. Exp. Ther.,* 147
(1965), 86–95.

100. SULSER, F., M. OWENS, M. NORVICH et al.
"The Relative Role of Storage and Synthesis of Brain Norepinephrine in the
Psychomotor Stimulation Evoked by Amphetamine or by Desiprimine and Tetra-
benzine," *Psychopharmacologia,* 12 (1968),
322–331.

101. TAYLOR, K. M. and S. H. SNYDER. "Amphetamine: Differentiation by *d* and *l*
Isomers of Behavior Involving Brain Nore-
epinephrine or Dopamine," *Science,* 168
(1970), 1487–1489.

102. TWAROG, B. M. and I. H. PAGE. "Serotonin
Content of Some Mammalian Tissues and
Urine and a Method for Its Determinations," *Am. J. Physiol.,* 175 (1953), 157–
161.

103. UDENFRIEND, S., P. ZALTZMAN-NIRENBERG,
R. GORDON et al. "Evaluation of the Biochemical Effects Produced *In Vivo* by Inhibitors of the Three Enzymes Involved in
Norepinephrine Biosynthesis," *Mol. Pharmacol.,* 2 (1966), 95–105.

104. UNGERSTEDT, U. "Postsynaptic Supersensitivity after 6-Hydroxydopamine Induced
Degeneration of the Nigro-Striatal Dopamine System," *Acta Physiol. Scand.,*
Suppl. 367 (1971), 69–93.

105. UZUNOV, P. and B. WEISS. "Effects of
Phenothiazine Tranquilizers on the Cyclic
3′, 5′-Adenosine Monophosphate System
of Rat Brain," *Neuropharmacology,* 10
(1971), 697–708.

106. WEISSMAN, A. "Behavioral Pharmacology of
PCPA," in J. Barchas and E. Usdin, eds.,
Serotonin and Behavior, New York: Aca-
demic, 1973.

107. WEISSMAN, A., B. S. KOE, and S. S. TENEN.
"Amphetamine Effects Following Inhibition of Tyrosine Hydroxylase," *J. Pharmacol. Exp. Ther.,* 151 (1966), 339–352.

108. WELSH, J. H. "Serotonin as a Possible Neu-
rohumoral Agent: Evidence Obtained in
Lower Animals," *Ann. N.Y. Acad. Sci.*
USA, 66 (1957), 618–630.

109. WOLBACH, A. B., H. ISBELL, and E. J.
MINER. "Cross Tolerance Between Mescaline and LSD-25 with a Comparison of the
Mescaline and LSD Reactions," *Psychopharmacologia,* 3 (1962), 1–14.

110. WOOLLEY, D. W. and E. SHAW. "A Biochemical Pharmacological Suggestion
about Certain Mental Disorders," *Proc.*
Natl. Acad. Sci. USA, 40 (1954), 228–
231.

111. WOOLLEY, D. W. and E. N. SHAW. "Evi-
dence for the Participation of Serotonin in
Mental Processes," *Ann. N.Y. Acad. Sci.*
USA, 66 (1957), 649–665.

112. ZIRKLE, C. L., and C. KAISER. "Antipsychotic Agents," in A. Burger, ed., *Medi-
cinal Chemistry,* p. 1410. New York:
Wiley-Interscience, 1970.

CHAPTER 20

LINKAGE OF BASIC NEUROPHARMACOLOGY AND CLINICAL PSYCHOPHARMACOLOGY

James W. Maas and David L. Garver

(Introduction

THE INVESTIGATIVE EFFORTS and consequent production of new information
in basic neuropharmacology and clinical psychopharmacology in recent years has
been enormous. In the relatively short period
of the preceding twenty years specific pharmacological treatments for the major psychopathological states have become available.
Clinically effective psychopharmacological
agents have not only been helpful to patients,
but they have also turned out to be powerful
investigative tools for the elucidation of basic
neurobiological processes that in turn have led
to the development of specific hypotheses as

to the biological genesis of psychopathological
states. The literature dealing with linkages between basic neuropharmacology and clinical
psychopharmacology is huge in that almost any
paper dealing with a drug which affects the
psyche or a neurobiological process could be
rightfully included in this chapter, given its
title. Such a review would be not only beyond
the authors' abilities but also redundant in
that many excellent reviews of the relationship
of a variety of classes of psychopharmacological agents to neurobiological processes, and
vice versa, have been written. For these reasons the choice of a more focused review of a
particular area of relationship between basic
and clinical psychopharmacology was chosen.

Such a choice inevitably depends upon the judgment of the writers, but it is felt that a great many investigators would agree that the publication by Dahlström and Fuxe in 1965[34] indicating that the biogenic amines DA, NE, and 5-HT* are to be found in discrete and specifically identifiable groups of neurons was seminal. Subsequent work indicated that these amines, and probably their synthetic enzymes, are made in discrete groupings of cell bodies and then transported down the axons, which themselves are found in specific tracts, to nerve endings existing at a considerable distance from their cell bodies in some cases. It is now clear, although the specifics are only beginning to emerge, that the different aminergic systems regulate or modulate separable and to a certain extent discrete kinds of behavior. Further, it has been found that some clinically useful classes of psychopharmacological agents have specific actions on one of these aminergic systems but not others. Since studies of the relationships of specific brain amine systems, behavior, and psychopharmacological agents are relatively recent and because the implications of such studies for increasing our understanding of the biological genesis of psychopathological states is clear, it is this area of brain amine systems, drugs, and behavior that has been chosen for review.

Briefly, the general scheme of presentation is to first review our present knowledge as to the existence and localization of brain amine systems, to describe some kinds of behavior that may be modulated by them, to review the experimental evidence that indicates that some clinically useful psychopharmacological agents have specific actions upon these brain amine systems, to describe possible amine system interactions, and, finally, to conclude with suggestions as to the possibility that specific amine systems are centrally involved in the genesis of specific psychopathological states.

* Abbreviations used in this chapter are: DA, dopamine; NE, norepinephrine; 5-HT, serotonin; ACh, acetylcholine; NM, normetanephrine; HVA, homovanillic acid; Dopa, dihydroxyphenylalanine; 5-HIAA, 5-hydroxyindoleacetic acid.

([The Neuroanatomy of the Brain Amine Systems

History of Development of Techniques

The development of techniques for the localization of groups of cells responsible for DA, NE, 5-HT, and ACh production and release has added a new dimension to the study of neurotransmitters. For the first time amine-specific, cell-body areas can be defined, their axonal bundles can be demonstrated, and their terminal areas, at which there is release of specific neurotransmitter and activation of receptor site, can be localized and studied chemically, ultrastructurally, and electrophysiologically. Further, the behavioral effects that occur as a consequence of altering these systems by a variety of techniques may be studied.

Attempts at defining pathways of monoamine systems began with the work of Heller and Moore who, by making small lesions in various parts of the brain, could differentially effect whole brain levels of NE, DA, and 5-HT. Their work suggested that major tracts connecting with 5-HT and NE rich areas in the forebrain ran in the dorsomedial brainstem tegmentum and through the median forebrain bundle in the lateral hypothalamus. Ventrolateral tegmental lesions reduced only brain NE and central gray lesions lowered 5-HT only.[57] Their inability to trace degenerating fibers to the cortex and other structures that showed marked decreases in amine levels after lesions suggested to them that the monoamine systems might be multisynaptic with the reduction in amine content being secondary to a lesion of neurons which transsynaptically activated monoamine neurons.

A further development in technique for mapping out the catecholamine and indoleamine systems (NE, DA, 5-HT) began with the work of Falck and Hillarp[38] who devised a method of condensing these monoamines in tissue sections with formaldehyde vapor to produce an intense fluorphor, which could be visualized by fluroescence microscopy. Recent developments in microspectrophotofluorimetry have permitted excitation and emission differentials for the NE, DA, and 5-HT fluorophors,[17] permitting species identification for each of the catecholamines (NE and DA) and 5-HT.

Fluorescence histochemistry, together with lesioning techniques, provided the tools for clarifying some of the issues raised by the work of Heller and Moore, i.e., since monoamines accumulate proximal to axonal lesions, terminal and axonal regions can be destroyed selectively and specific pathways can be defined by following the development of increased fluorescence proximal to the lesioned stump. This approach, for example, has been used in studies in which the neostriatum was ablated with the subsequent accumulation of fluorescence in axons of the internal capsule and in the DA cells of the pars compacta of the substantia nigra, allowing definition of the now well-known nigro-striatal DA pathway.[9] Conversely, lesions in the DA cell-body area, the substantia nigra, caused a substantial loss of DA fluorescence in the neostriatum. Using the same apparoch it has also been found that many of the catecholamine containing nerve endings in the cerebral cortex are terminals of axons whose cell bodies are to be found in the brainstem. Alpha-m-NE also proved to be a useful tool in mapping amine systems as it is taken up and produces an intense fluorescence when injected into terminal areas and the fluorescence spreads retrograde toward the cells of origin.[119]

The fluorphors from 5-HT terminals and cell bodies are more difficult to visualize than those of catecholamines with the routine Falck-Hillarp method. In order to localize 5-HT more easily, pretreatment with a monoamine oxidase inhibitor is frequently used to increase tissue concentrations of 5-HT, which then makes recognition of the structures more possible. Even with such treatment many areas of the telencephalon and diencephalon, which are known from biochemical determinations to contain 5-HT, do not show fluorescence[64] and this is probably in part due to the fact that the 5-HT terminals are very fine and many are probably submicroscopic.[40] For these reasons negative findings in any given experiment, as to the 5-HT systems when the Falck-Hillarp method is used, must be interpreted with caution. While this problem is of particular concern with 5-HT systems, it may also occur with smaller terminals of the NE and DA systems. In terms of the limitations of this approach, it should also be noted that direct application of the histochemical-fluorescence method allows visualization only of those areas within the neuron that contain high concentration of monoamines. Highest concentrations of amines are found in terminal areas and adequate concentrations for visual recognition are also found in cell bodies, but axonal pathways contain too little monoamine to fluoresce, unless special manipulations are employed.[66]

Fluorescence histochemical mapping of several of the amine systems in rat brain, including the defining of cell bodies of origin, axonal pathways, and terminal areas, has been developed during the past several years by a group of investigators at the Karolinski Institute,[42,43] and these findings recently have been summarized and extended by Ungerstedt.[119] As of this writing this technique has permitted definition of six reasonably well-defined monoamine systems, i.e., two NE, one 5-HT, and three DA systems that supply primarily the diencephalon and telencephalon; and five of these have their cell bodies of origin in the medulla, pons, or mesencephalon. In this section, available data as to anatomical loci and possible interactions with other amine systems, including ACh systems, also defined herein and located in proximity, will be summarized. The following section will examine, when known, the behavioral effects of selective pharmacologic manipulations for each of these systems.

The assumption that identical monoamine systems as described in the rat are also present in higher species, including primates, must be approached with some caution. Preliminary evidence from work in progress suggests that although widespread similarities of cell-body and terminal areas exist, some interspecies dissimilarities in distribution of cell bodies and terminals in cat[112] and Rhesus brainstems (J. R. Sladek, Jr., personal communication) and squirrel and monkey brainstems (D. Felton, personal communication) are also present. Axonal pathways in species other than the rat have not as yet been systematically reported.

The Norepinephrine Systems (Figure 20–1.)

THE DORSAL NE SYSTEM[40,119]

The dorsal NE system arises from the cell bodies of the pontine nucleus locus coeruleus (A_6 according to the nomenclature of Dahlström and Fuxe[34]) and after giving off axons both to the cord and cerebellum, it ascends in the mid-reticular formation of the pons just ventral to the nucleus tractus solitarius. It passes in the dorsal part of the combined catecholamine bundle (dorsal and ventral bundle) between the pregenual fibers of the seventh cranial nerve. The dorsal NE fibers then separate from the ventral system, turning dorsomedially, ascending in a tight bundle just lateral to the oculomotor nucleus. Some axons leave the bundle to cross in the posterior commissure before it dives sharply ventrolaterally into the zona incerta at the junction

of the mesencephalon and diencephalon and rejoins the ventral NE system already in the median forebrain bundle. It gives off some branches dorsolaterally in the area of the nucleus subthalamus supplying NE terminals in the geniculate bodies and some branches dorsomedially to terminals in the nucleus anterior ventral thalamus and nucleus paraventricularis rotundocellularis. After contributing a small number of terminals (both crossed and uncrossed) to the hypothalamus, the bundle gives off, at a midhypothalamic level some axons which enter both the ansa lenticularis and the dorsal supraoptic commissure. There the axons spread both laterally toward the amygdala and basal cortical terminals, and medially, crossing the midline to end in the contralateral cortex. The bulk of the axons, however, ascend toward the septal region, where they give off terminals and then continue on in the cingulum on their way to terminals in the cortex and hippocampus. Terminal areas of the dorsal NE system are summarized in Table 20–1.

THE VENTRAL NE SYSTEM[40,119]

The ventral NE system arises from cell bodies at A_1, A_2, A_4, A_5, A_7 in the medulla and pons—there are very few cell bodies in the squirrel monkey A_3 A_4 and A_7,[121] (D. Felton, personal communication)—and it ascends in the mid-reticular formation. Its axons remain slightly ventral to the dorsal bundle in the pons and then they spread ventromedially along the medial lemniscus and continue rostrally, mainly in the median forebrain bundle in the mesencephalon. In the mesencephalon, it gives rise to NE terminal areas dorsally, in the ventrolateral part of the substantia griseum centralis (which are in intimate contact with 5-HT cells of group B_7 and to a lesser extent B_8) and to part of the mesencephalic reticular formation dorsal and dorsolateral to the medial lemniscus at the caudal level of the interpeduncular nucleus. The ventral NE system gives off terminals to the whole hypothalamus (especially the dorso-medialis hypothalami, nucleus periventricularis, area ventral to fornix, nucleus arcuatus, inner layer of median eminence, retrochiasmatic area, nucleus para-

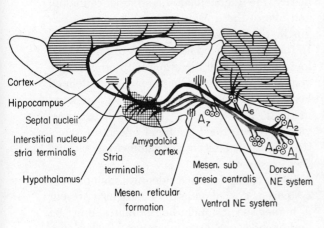

Figure 20–1. Saggital projection of the ascending norepinephrine (NE) pathway of the rat. Horizontal stripes indicate major terminal areas of the dorsal NE system. Vertical stripes indicate major terminal areas of the ventral NE system.

ventricularis, nucleus supraopticus, preoptic area) both ipsilaterally and contralaterally. Continuing in the median forebrain bundle, it ascends rostrally in the stria terminals, giving off NE terminals to the ventral part of the nucleus interstitialis stria terminalis before continuing on to supply terminal areas in the amygdaloid cortex. Terminal areas of the ventral NE system are summarized in Table 20–1.

The Dopamine Systems (Figure 20–2.)

NIGRO-STRIATAL SYSTEM[119]

The nigro-striatal system originates in the *substantia nigra* (A_9) especially the *zona compacta*, adjacent tegmental area, and an area just caudal to the substantia nigra and dorsal to the medial lemniscus (A_8) and it sends dopaminergic axons rostral in the lateral hypothalamus, entering the cerebral peduncle in the mid-hypothalamus, ascending in the internal capsule, fanning out in the globus pallidus, and finally entering and terminating in the caudate and putamen. DA terminals in the central amygdaloid nucleus are extensions of DA axons in the putamen and originate from axons running lateroventrally in the internal capsule. Terminal areas of the nigro-striatal DA system are summarized in Table 20–1.

MESO-LIMBIC DOPAMINE SYSTEM[119]

DA cell bodies that are located at A_{10} (around the interpeduncular nucleus and extending in the midline up to the level of the dorsal motor nucleus of the third cranial nerve) contribute axons that run just dorsal to

TABLE 20–1.   **Major Terminal Areas of Monoamine Systems**

	SYSTEMS						
TERMINAL AREAS	Dorsal NE	Ventral NE	Meso-Limbic DA	Nigro-Striatal DA	Tubo-Infundibular and Intrahypothalamic DA	5-HT	ACh
Cerebellar Cortex	X					X	X
Brainstem: Pons and Medulla	X	X				X	X
Limbic Midbrain Area and Tectum		X				X	X
Thalamus	X					X	X
Hypothalamus	X	X			X	X	X
Preoptic-Suprachiasmatic Area	X?*	X?*				X	X
Septum	X					X	(X)†
Interstitialis Nucleus Stria Terminalis		X	X				
Nucleus Accumbens	X?*	X?*	X				X
Tuberculum Olfactorium			X				X
Neostriatum				X		X	X
Amygdala and Amygdaloid Cortex	X	X		X		X	X
Hippocampus	X					X	X
Cerebral Cortex	X					X	X

* Cells of origin of innervation uncertain.
† Although cell bodies are present, terminals have not been described except more anteriorly in the diagonal band. However, intraseptal ACh produces rage that is antagonized by atropine. See discussion below.

Nigro-Striatal, Meso-Limbic and
Tubo-Infundibular Systems

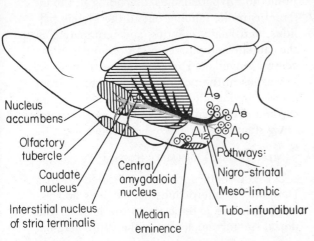

Figure 20–2. Saggital projection of DA pathways in the rat brain. Horizontal stripes indicate major terminal areas of the Nigro-striatal system. Vertical stripes indicate major terminal areas of the Meso-limbic system. Sloped stripes indicate major terminal areas of the Tubo-infundibular system.

the median forebrain bundle in the lateral hypothalamus and, at the level of the anterior commissure, give off a series of branches to supply terminals in the nucleus accumbens, the dorsal part of the interstitial nucleus of the stria terminalis, and in the olfactory tubercle. (DA fibers to the amygdala arise from the adjacent A_9—substantia nigra—and enter the internal capsule, diving through the putamen to central amygdaloid nucleus.) Terminal areas of the meso-limbic DA system are summarized in Table 20–1.

TUBO-INFUNDIBULAR SYSTEM[119]

The cell bodies of the dopaminergic tubo-infundibular system are located within the nucleus arcuatus (A_{12}) and along the lateral border of the periventricular nucleus. A_{12} innervates the external layer of the median eminence and is concerned with neuroendocrine control, discussion of which is beyond the scope of this chapter. The cells along the periventricular border give rise to intrahypothalamic DA terminals and are noted in Table 20–1.

Catecholamine Terminal Areas and Cell-body Areas With Unknown Pathways

Noradrenergic terminals have recently been described in the posterior medial part of the nucleus accumbens, bordering on the septal nuclei, and the interstitial nucleus of the stria terminalis.[89] The cells of origin and pathways to these terminals are not known, although the adjacent septal nuclei are innervated by the dorsal NE system and the adjacent ventral part of the interstitial nucleus of the stria terminalis is innervated by the ventral NE system. Their function in the accumbens has not been studied.

A dense group of DA cell bodies (A_{13}) has been reported just dorsolateral to the dorsomedial hypothalamic nucleus. This group has been reported to give rise to ascending axons in the median forebrain bundle.[119] Terminal areas have not been described and the function of this group of DA cells has not been studied.

Serotonin System(s) (Figure 20–3.)

Owing to the difficulties noted above concerning the insensitivity of the fluorescence-histochemical technique in demonstrating 5-

5-HT System(s)

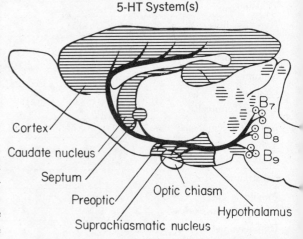

Figure 20–3. Saggital projection of ascending 5-HT pathway(s) of the rat. Horizontal stripes indicate terminal areas of the 5-HT system. Pathways to many of these areas are as yet undefined.

HT, such systems have been less clearly defined than those of catecholamines. The following description of known pathways is based on the work of Anden,[12] Dahlström and Fuxe,[34] Fuxe,[40] Fuxe et al.,[44] Heller and Moore,[57] and Ungerstedt.[119]

Although there exist a large number of bulbo-spinal 5-HT neurons that arise from 5-HT cells, many of which are innervated by NE terminals to the raphe nuclei and to the surrounding pyramidal tract of the medulla,[44] our interest here will be confined primarily to ascending 5-HT pathways.

An ascending system of 5-HT neurons arises from the 5-HT cell bodies in the raphe nuclei of the mesencephalon (nucleus of the dorsal raphe, B_7, and the nucleus of the median raphe, B_8). The axons run ventrally and then turn rostrally in the midbrain tegmentum as they approach the interpeduncular nucleus. Most of the axons lie close to the midline and become aggregated in a bundle lying medial to the fasciculus retroflexus on the border between the mesencephalon and diencephalon. The axons enter the median forebrain bundle by passing, laterally, close to the ventral outline of the fasciculus retroflexus, and most become aggregated close to the lateral surface of the fornix. At least one other smaller tract is seen running more laterally in the lateral hypothalamus ventral to the cerebral peduncle, and just dorsal to the lateral part of the optic tract. The cells of origin of the secondary tract have not been clearly defined, but it may be possible that this secondary tract amounts for the remaining 20 percent of tryptophan hydroxylase and 30 percent of the 5-HT that persists in the telencephalon and diencephalon after the complete electrolytic destruction of the raphe (B_7 and B_8) nuclei that leaves the more lateral 5-HT group (B_9) in the mesencephalic reticular formation intact.[75] The terminal area of the lateral secondary bundle has not been distinguished from that of the more medial primary bundle except as noted below. The primary bundle continues its route through the hypothalamus in the median forebrain bundle, running just ventral to the combined NE bundles, moving dorsally in front of the septal area, partly by the diagonal tract,

and into the cingulum and toward the superficial part of the white matter to supply the cortex. Lesions of both raphe nuclei produce electron microscopic signs of degeneration in the 5-HT rich suprachiasmatic nucleus[2] and reduce the overall 5-HT in whole brain by 70 percent, tyrosine hydroxylase by 80 percent.[75] Ventromedial tegmental lesions reduce tryptophan hydroxylase in at least caudate, anterior perforated substance, and septal area.[97] From these studies, the only clear localization of cell body to terminal area is that of the raphe (B_7 and B_8) supplying the suprachiasmatic nucleus. In addition to 5-HT terminals mentioned above (suprachiasmatic nucleus, cortex, septum, caudate, anterior perforated substance), the mesencephalon, telencephalon, and diencephalon show by fluorescent 5-HT terminals widespread areas of 5-HT innervation encompassing the dorsal tegmental nuclei, the zona reticulata of the substantia nigra, between the interpeduncular area and the median raphe nucleus, the interpeduncular nucleus, cranioventral to the interpeduncular nucleus, both colliculi, pretectal region, both geniculates, habenular nuclei, many of the thalamic and most of the hypothalamic nuclei, two of the preoptic nuclei, anterior amygdaloid nuclei, hippocampi and globi pallidus.[40] 5-HT cell bodies have not been reported anterior to the mesencephalon. It should be remembered, especially with 5-HT, that terminal areas may have relatively high amounts of monoamines and yet be invisible by fluorescent microscopy, i.e., that 5-HT terminals may be even more widespread than those noted. Demonstrated terminal areas of the 5-HT system(s) are noted in Table 20–1.

The Acetylcholine Systems[*]
(*Figures 20–4 and 20–5.*)

Unlike the catecholamines and indoleamines the neurotransmitter acetylcholine (ACh) does not form a fluorphor that can be visualized by fluorescent microscopy. The most successful attempts to define ACh path-

---

[*] ACh—a quaternary ammonium compound, not strictly classified as an amine, is commonly included among the monoamine neurotransmitters.

ways have depended not on the demonstration of ACh itself, but upon the presence of choline acetylase and especially acetyl cholinesterase in cell bodies, axons, and terminals of ACh neurons. Using the thiocholine method for esterase[71] and light microscopy, Shute and Lewis[78,111] mapped out ACh systems in the rat brain. They demonstrated three pathway systems of ACh with numerous interconnections, the terminal innervations of which are also summarized in Table 20–1.

THE DORSAL TEGMENTAL PATHWAY[111]

The dorsal tegmental pathway is a system of fibers that runs rostrally from the midbrain tegmentum and supplies the tectum, pretectal area, geniculate bodies, and thalamus. It arises primarily from the mesencephalic nucleus cuneiformis and supplies the inferior and superior colliculus (the latter transsynaptically), pretectal nuclei, medial and lateral geniculate bodies (especially the ventral nucleus of the lateral geniculate body), specific thalamic nuclei, including the centromedian and intralaminar thalamic nuclei, and especially the anteroventral thalamic nuclei of the anterior thalamic group. By long circuitous routes also supplied is the anterior colliculus and the pretectal nuclei, via the supraoptic decussation, and the lateral geniculate body via the medial strial bundle.

THE VENTRAL TEGMENTAL PATHWAY[111]

The ventral tegmental pathway arises from the ventral tegmental area and the pars compacta of the substantia nigra and supplies the oculomotor nucleus, mammillary bodies, subthalamus, anterior thalamic nuclei, especially the anteroventral thalamic nucleus, entopeduncular nucleus, and globus pallidus, the posterior and lateral hypothalamic areas, lateral preoptic area, paraventricular and supraoptic hypothalamic nuclei and olfactory tubercle, and, circuitously via the stria terminalis, the lateral amygdaloid nucleus. These fibers as they pass through the diencephalon enter the zona incerta, supramammillary region, and the lateral hypothalamic area, where there are many ACh-containing cells, before running rostrally to the basal areas of the forebrain.

The Cholinergic Dorsal and Ventral Tegmental Pathways

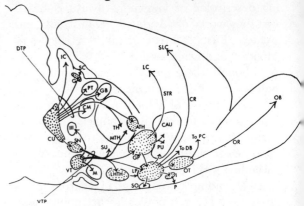

Figure 20–4. Diagram showing the constituent nuclei (stippled) of the ascending cholinergic reticular system in the mid-brain and fore-brain, with projections to the cerebellum, tectum, thalamus, hypothalamus, striatum, lateral cortex, and olfactory bulb. Abbreviations: ATH, antero-ventral and antero-dorsal thalamic nuclei; CAU, caudate; CM, centromedian (parafascicular) nucleus; CR, cingulate radiation; CU, nucleus cuneiformis; DB, diagonal band; DTP, dorsal tegmental pathway; G, stratum griseum intermediale of superior colliculus; GB, medial and lateral geniculate bodies; GP, globus pallidus and entopeduncular nucleus; I, islets of Calleja; IC, inferior colliculus; III, oculomotor nucleus; LC, lateral cortex; LHTH, lateral hypothalamic area; LP, lateral preoptic area; M, mammillary body; MTH, mammillo-thalamic tract; OB, olfactory bulb; OR, olfactory radiation; OT, olfactory tubercle; P, plexiform layer of olfactory tubercle; PC, precallosal cells; PT, pretectal nuclei; PU, patamen; SC, superior colliculus; SLC, supero-lateral cortex; SN, substantia nigra pars compacta; SO, supraoptic nucleus; STR, striatal radiation; SU, subthalamus; TH, thalamus; TP, nucleus reticularis tegmenti pontis (of Bechterew); VT, ventral tegmental area and nucleus of basal optic root; VTP, ventral tegmental pathway. Source: C. C. D. Shute and P. R. Lewis, *Brain*, 90 (1969), 529. By permission of the author.

The ventral tegmental system continues cholinergically from cell bodies located in nuclei already supplied by cholinergic terminals giving rise to centrifugal radiations to the neocortex, olfactory cortex and bulb, and to subcortical nuclei. The entopeduncular nucleus and globus pallidus give rise to cholinergic fibers that innervate the anteroventral nucleus of the thalamus, the caudate, and putamen and also give rise to striatal radiations to the lateral cortex above the rhinal fissure. The lateral preoptic (and anterior amygdaloid) areas give rise to cholinergic fibers supplying the amygdaloid nuclei—especially the pars ventralis of the lateral amygdaloid nucleus—give rise to fibers that run in the stria terminalis to the cortical and medial amygdaloid nuclei (olfactory part), and give rise to the amygdaloid radiation that pierces the amygdala, enters the ventral part of the external capsule and is distributed to the infernolateral cortex below the rhinal fissure. Arising also from the lateral preoptic area and augmented by contributions from the olfactory tubercle are innervations to the nucleus accumbens and fibers of the olfactory radiation that turn laterally from the preoptic area and travel rostrally in the lateral olfactory tract and in the olfactory peduncle and supply the nucleus of the lateral olfactory tract, the olfactory tubercle, and the olfactory bulb and the olfactory cortex (ventrolateral aspect of the hemisphere below the rhinal fissure). The lateral preoptic area also provides cholinergic innervation for the cortex on the superior aspect of the hemisphere through the cingulate radiation that ascends from the lateral preoptic area, anterior to the genu of the corpus callosum, and travels caudally in the cingulum and below the corpus, the latter piercing upward more caudally and reaching the cingulum on their way to the cortex.

THE CHOLINERGIC LIMBIC SYSTEM[78]

The cholinergic limbic system consists of an intermingling of cholinergic and noncholinergic neurons. It arises from cholinergic cell bodies, located in the medial septum, and the nucleus of the diagonal band, and it projects to the hippocampal formation via the septal radiation through the dorsal fornix, the alveus, and fimbria. Hippocampal efferents (noncholinergic) traveling via the fornix project directly or indirectly onto cholinergic neurons in the hippocampal commissure, anterior thalamus, habenular nuclei, dorsal and deep tegmental nuclei via the mammillo-tegmental

The Cholinergic Limbic System

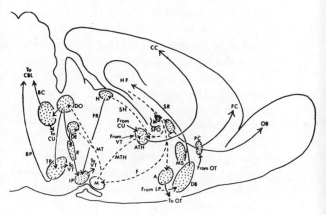

Figure 20–5. Diagram showing cholinesterase-containing nuclei of the mid-brain and fore-brain (indicated by stipple) connected with the hippocampus, their projections to the medial cortex, and their connexions with the ascending cholinergic reticular system. Abbreviations: A, nucleus accumbens; ATH, antero-ventral and antero-dorsal thalamic nuclei; BC, brachium conjunctivum; BP, brachium pontis; C, interstitial nucleus of the ventral hippocampal commissure; CBL, cerebellum; CC, cingulate cortex (cingular and retrosplenial areas); CU, nucleus cuneiformis; DB, diagonal band; DE, deep tegmental nucleus (ventral tegmental nucleus of Gudden); DO, dorsal tegmental nucleus; F, fornix; FC, frontal cortex (area infralimbica and anterior limbic area); FR, fasciculus retroflexus (habenulo-interpeduncular tract); H, habenular nuclei; HF, hippocampal formation; IP, interpeduncular nucleus; LD, laterodorsal tegmental nucleus; LP, lateral preoptic area; M, mammillary body; MS, medial septal nucleus; MT, mammillo-tegmental tract; MTH, mammillo-thalamic tract; OB, olfactory bulb; OT, olfactory tubercle; PC, precallosal cells; R, dorsal and median nuclei of raphe (nucleus centralis superior); SFO, subfornical organ; SH, stria habenularis; SR, septal radiation; TP, nucleus reticularis tegmenti pontis (of Bechterew); VT, ventral tegmental area. Source: P. R. Lewis and C. C. D. Shute, *Brain*, 90 (1969) 508. By permission of the author.

tract, and in the nucleus accumbens. These cholinergic cell-body areas then project cholinergic fibers: from hippocampal commissure to the precallosal cells and on to the frontal cortex and olfactory bulb; from anterior thalamus to the cingulate cortex; from habenular nuclei to the interpeduncular nucleus that connects with the ventral tegmentum area (ventral tegmental pathway); from dorsal tegmental nuclei to the cholinergic nucleus reticularis tegmenti poitis (that connects with the ventral tegmental pathway), to laterodorsal tegmental nuclei (cholinergic) that send fibers to the nucleus cuneiformis (dorsal tegmental pathway); and from both dorsal and deep tegmental nuclei to the dorsal and medial nuclei of the raphe that, through another cholinergic connection in the interpeduncular nucleus, also connect back to the ventral tegmental pathway; and from the accumbens nucleus to the olfactory tubercle.

❪ The Amine Brain Systems and Behavior

The demonstration of specific aminergic systems innervating specific loci within the brain opens the avenue to clarification of monoamine function in the regulation or modulation of behavior controlled at specific loci. Such clarification of function at specific loci can be expected to increase our understanding of the genesis of certain kinds of psychopathology. (See section on Specific Brain Aminergic Systems, p. 451.) Only a few experimental studies have been reported in which the relationship of these specific amine systems to behavior have been studied. There is, however, a great deal of activity in this area and it is expected that by the time of publication of this chapter much more experimental data will be available. To date, data as to the behavioral consequences of altering, by a variety of techniques, one or more portions of the aminergic systems are summarized below.

Dopaminergic Systems

The Nigro-striatal Pathway

The dopaminergic, nigro-striatal pathway, with the exception of its projection to the amygdala, has been studied more extensively than any other of the catecholamine pathways, probably because this system is reason-

ably discrete and because of its demonstrated involvement in a well-defined pathological condition, Parkinsonism.

Experimentally the nigro-striatal pathway can be lesioned so as to produce an ipsilateral deficiency in the terminals of the neostriatum of both DA and the synthetic enzymes, tyrosine hydroxylase and Dopa decarboxylase.[88] Unilateral lesions of the substantia nigra produce an ipsilateral hypokinesia and cause rats to rotate toward the lesioned, DA-depleted side, particularly after treatment with a monoamine oxidase inhibitor and reserpine or with amphetamine, both of which treatments presumably increase the quantities of DA at receptors on the nonlesioned side. Haloperidol, which blocks DA receptors (see below), very quickly interrupts such rotation as produced by amphetamine. The development of a postsynaptic receptor supersensitivity on the denervated side allows DA receptor agonists, such as apomorphine, to activate differentially the denervated side and produce a rotation away from the lesioned side when given systemically.[120] DA or apomorphine, injected directly into the neostriatum, produces rotation away from the side of injection.[122]

Stereotyped movements (interruption of normal grooming, feeding, and drinking, and the appearance of continuous sniffing, licking, gnawing, repetitive motor movements of the head extremities) are also seen after intraneostriatal administration of DA and amphetamine, and are antagonized by systemic administration of haloperidol.[28] Intraneostriatal administration of chlorpromazine antagonizes the stereotyped behavior induced by systemic administration of amphetamine.[39] That phenothiazines and butyrophenones exhibit DA blocking properties is suggested by the above and by their secondary effect of increasing DA turnover after presumed blockade of receptor sites. (See section on Actions of Clinically Useful Pharmacological Agents, p. 434.)

That the nigro-striatal DA systems control more than motor behavior is shown by Ungerstedt's recent work with the "lateral hypothalamic syndrome." He was able to produce adipsia and aphagia by total destruction of the nigro-striatal pathway bilaterally. Moreover, in animals so lesioned he noted severe hypokinesia, difficulty in initiating activity, and loss of exploratory behavior and curiosity. He concluded that it is probable that the nigro-striatal DA system may control the general arousal or drive level that is necessary for performing a number of vital activities such as eating and drinking.[121]

Of considerable interest is the possibility that the dopaminergic systems may have a role in mental function beyond that of regulating movement per se. The association of the antipsychotic actions of the phenothiazines, butyrophenones, etc., with extrapyramidal reactions in man and the antagonism of these same drugs to stereotyped behavior in animals (and perhaps stereotypy in schizophrenia) suggests that all of these kinds of behavior may be related to DA systems. In terms of this issue, it should be remembered that the antipsychotic or neuroleptic drugs probably block DA receptors related to the terminals of the meso-limbic DA system as well as the nigro-striatal.

The Mesolimbic Pathway

As noted above, one might speculate that it is the blockade of DA receptors in meso-limbic terminals that is responsible for the antipsychotic action of some neuroleptics. An attempt to separate the function of the dopaminergic meso-limbic terminals in the nucleus accumbens and olfactory tubercle from the dopaminergic nigro-striatal terminals has been made by removing the neostriatum of rats by bilateral electrocoagulation and then treating the animals with cataprezen, a NE receptor stimulating agent, both with and without apomorphine, which would be expected to activate the remaining DA receptors on the meso-limbic terminals (but not the destroyed DA terminals of the neostriatum). In such a preparation, apomorphine elicits a peculiar behavior consisting of jerky, very rapid movements with periods of complete rest.[7,44]

The Tubo-infundibular System

The dopaminergic tubo-infundibular system is believed to be concerned primarily with neuroendocrine function and is beyond the scope of this chapter. The reader is referred to recent reviews by Fuxe and Hokfelt,[41] and by Fuxe et al.[44]

The Norepinephrine Systems

The Dorsal NE System

The dorsal NE system can clearly be implicated in but one type of behavior: bar pressing for electrical self-stimulation. An electrode placed in the area of the locus coeruleus of the pons and just lateral to the central gray in the mesencephalon (the site of passage of the dorsal NE bundle) produces reinforcement, "reward," or "pleasure" when a small current is passed through it into the tissue; that is, a rat will bar press to receive electrical stimulation to his dorsal NE bundle at rates over 500/hr.[32,33]

It is clear, however, that fibers other than those of the dorsal NE bundle may also produce self-stimulation-reinforcing behavior since similar self-stimulation can be produced by stimulating the median forebrain bundle from its origin in the mesencephalon to the septal area.[32,95]

Ventral NE System

The specific functions of the ventral NE system have been sparsely studied. The intimate contact of its terminal area in the ventral substantia gresia centralis with 5-HT cell bodies of the (B_7) group[40] implies an interrelation between the ventral NE system and the 5-HT system, but the functional significance of such direct communication is obscure.

To date a single study has appeared involving a lesion of the ventral NE bundle. A behavioral response in rats to such a lesion was a hyperphagia, with increases in food consumption by 40 percent. Moreover, the animals so lesioned were refractory to the anorexogenic action of amphetamine.[3]

The Serotonin Systems

Electrical stimulation of the raphe nuclei (B_7 and B_8) of the mesencephalon produces behavioral signs of calmness and an EEG pattern similar to that found in sleep.[74] It also produces an increase in brain 5-HIAA and a decrease in 5-HT levels.[1,72] Destruction of mesencephalic raphe nuclei in cats caused a decrease in slow wave sleep, which significantly correlated with selective diminution of cerebral 5-HT (but not with NE content).[67,68] Behaviorally, these lesioned animals showed increases in spontaneous motor activity, aimless rotatory movements, and hypersensitivity to auditory stimuli.[73,75]

The Acetylcholine Systems

As mentioned previously (see nigro-striatal system) stereotyped behavior, felt by some to be the animal model of psychosis, occurs after a systemic administration of a number of psychostimulant drugs (especially amphetamines), and after microinjections of DA into the neostriatum, but this stereotypy can also be produced by injection of anticholinergics into the neostriatum.[98] Further, the stereotypy induced by psychostimulants is antagonized by the administration of anticholinesterases or by choline esters[14,61] as well as by injections of chlorpromazine and haloperidol into the neostriatum.[39]

Systemic administration of the anticholinesterase physostigmine depresses self-stimulation behavior and such effects are antagonized by atropine,[37,115] although the area of brain involved in stimulation may be a critical variable.[69] This suggests that ACh predominance results in decreased bar pressing for electrical stimulation (the operational paradigm for "reward") by increasing CNS cholinergic tone. Cholinergic agents (carbachol, muscarine, and physostigmine) injected into the medial hypothalamic area decreased the rate of punished behavior. Anticholinergic agents (scopolamine, atropine) similarly injected caused disinhibition of punished behavior.[81,82]

Margules[80] has demonstrated that the anticholinergic atropine *lessens* the effect of punishment in the passive-avoidance-deficit paradigm when injected into the entopeduncular nucleus. Introduction of cholinergic and cholinesterase inhibitors to certain sites may produce aggressiveness or even killing behavior in animals. Such aggressiveness and hyperactivity results from local application of amitone (an anticholinesterase agent) in the lateral septal nucleus of the rat and such behavior was inhibited by pretreatment with atropine.[60] Killing behavior in mice is induced by intra-hypothalamic injection of carbachol or neostigmine and is antagonized by prior intra-hypothalamic administration of methyl atropine.[113] Such demonstrations of the multiple effects of a single neurotransmitter (ACh) in various areas should not be surprising in view of the various functions of different discrete parts of the brain.

(Specificity of Actions of Clinically Useful Psychopharmacological Agents upon Brain Amine Systems

The Tricyclic Antidepressants (Thymoleptics)

In this section the terms tricyclic drugs or tricyclic amines are used to refer to a group of drugs that are chemically similar and that have been demonstrated to be of use in the treatment of depression in man. The structure of four of these tricyclic drugs, which are frequently referred to in this chapter, are shown in Figure 20–6. It is of interest that the secondary amines, desipramine and nortriptyline, are natural metabolic products of the tertiary amines and there is evidence that a part or all of the antidepressant actions of the tertiary amines are mediated via their desmethylated products.* Some of the published data as to structure-activity relationships will be briefly reviewed in this section and then considerable attention will be given to the differential effects of these drugs upon specific brain aminergic systems.

STRUCTURE-ACTIVITY RELATIONSHIPS FOR THE TRICYCLIC ANTIDEPRESSANTS

Bickel and Brodie noted that treatment of animals with a benzoquinolizine produced a reserpinelike syndrome and that desipramine

---

* See references 15, 37, 50, 58, and 86.

blocked all signs of this syndrome and, in higher doses, desipramine was even able to produce a hyperactive animal. Taking this as a model situation, these investigators tested a large number of drugs, as well as a number of structurally altered analogues of desipramine, in terms of their potency in reversing the benzoquinolizine syndrome. They noted the following. Activity was restricted to compounds having two or three carbons on the side chain whereas compounds with branch chains or chains containing more than four carbons tended to be inactive or toxic. In terms of N-substitution it was noted that activity was confined to methyl-substituted or unsubstituted amines, whereas ethyl or higher alkyl groups on the side chain nitrogen resulted in compounds that were either inactive or toxic. A number of ring-substituted compounds were active, i.e., the 3-chloro, 10-methyl, or the 10, 11-dimethyl. Changes in the bridge between

the two phenyl groups from CH_2–CH_2 to $CH=CH$ did not change activity. Removal of the ring nitrogen and substitution with a carbon made little difference in terms of activity. Given work that will be reviewed later as to the differential effects between tertiary and secondary tricyclic amines on uptake of 5-HT and NE, it is of interest that Bickel and Brodie noted that "almost all antidepressant compounds are primary and secondary amines . . ." and, "The possibility exists that the antidepressant action of the two active tertiary amines are mediated through the rapid formation of their secondary analogues in the body."[16]

Maxwell et al.[83,84,85,102] explored in some detail the molecular features of the tricyclic antidepressants as they may affect the inhibition of the uptake of NE. Although most of the work of this group has been done with rabbit aortic strips, there is one publication that suggests that the general conclusions reached by these workers can be applied to brain.[102] Their data agree with other work that has been or will be cited as to the greater potency of desipramine, as compared to imipramine, in blocking the uptake of NE, and they also found that at lower concentrations of NE the inhibition of NE uptake by desipramine departs markedly from linearity. For example, at a concentration of NE of 1×10^{-7} M there was a much more marked inhibition of uptake of NE than at a concentration of 4×10^{-7} M. This deviation from linearity was not observed for imipramine, nortriptyline, or a primary amine derivative. They note that at lower concentrations of NE the potency of desimpramine in blocking NE uptake relative to imipramine may be therefore much greater than the factor of ten, which is usually quoted (q.v.). This group has also made some interesting and important observations about mechanisms by which structural differences may alter the inhibition of uptake. They compared systems in which the bridge between the two phenyl groups was either absent or was formed by sulfur, a $-CH^2-CH^2-$, a $-CH=CH-$, an oxygen, or a bond between two carbons of the phenyl groups. They found that high potency (in blocking uptake of NE)

Tricyclic Antidepressants

Imipramine

Amitriptyline

Desipramine

Nortriptyline

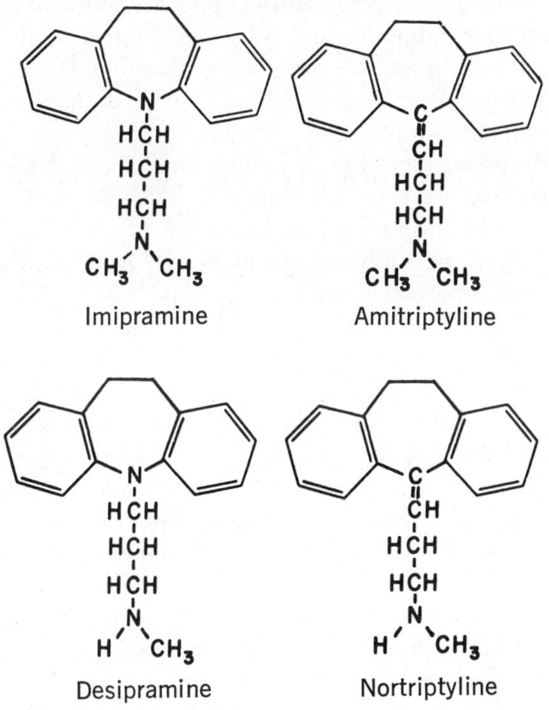

Figure 20–6. Structures of tricyclic antidepressant drugs frequently referred to in the text.

occurs with tricyclic compounds in which the phenyl groups are held at considerable angles to one another (examples of this would be, imipramine, amitriptyline, phenothiazines, or protriptyline); intermediate potency occurs with tricyclic drugs in which the two phenyl groups are held at slight angles or in which there is no bridge between the diphenyl systems. Tricyclics in which the phenyl rings are coplanar, such as carbazole, are only weakly active. They suggest that if the assumption is made that the receptor site is the best fit by the extended confirmation of phenylethylamine, then the presence of two phenyl rings that are not in the same plane will allow the side chain amine group of the drug to be inserted into the receptor site, and, further, that the phenyl ring that is above the plane can occupy a position somewhat analogous to that of the hydroxyl group on the β carbon of NE. Theoretical considerations led to the suggestion that the fit of the secondary amine into the receptor site is a tight one of the lock and key type. They calculated the difference in total free energy of binding for desipramine and its primary amine analogue and noted that the difference is of the order of -1.4 KC, which is quite close to the sum of -700 calories, occurring with the transfer of a methyl group from water to a nonaqueous phase, and -600 calories, the maximal increment for Van der Waals interactions of a methyl group with methylene groups in an enzyme. It is also apparent that since these drugs are not capable of blocking the uptake of DA (q.v.) which lacks a hydroxyl group on the β carbon, the interaction of the raised phenyl ring with another portion of the receptor must be of considerable importance.

STUDIES DEALING WITH THE UPTAKE OF DOPAMINE, NOREPINEPHRINE, AND SEROTONIN AS INFLUENCED BY TRICYCLIC ANTIDEPRESSANT DRUGS

Glowinski and Axelrod demonstrated that desipramine and imipramine, but not chlorpromazine, decreased the uptake of intraventricularly administered NE.[52,53] Subsequent studies, in which a variety of techniques have been used, have in general supported these original observations, but it has also been found that there are differences in the degree to which the various tricyclic antidepressants are able to block the uptake of NE within brain and further that there are differential effects upon specific amines and aminergic systems. Some of the published reports bearing upon this specificity of drug action are summarized in the following portion of this chapter.

Carlsson et al. pretreated rats with reserpine to deplete brain stores of biogenic amines and administered a monoamine oxidase inhibitor, nialamide, and then gave L-Dopa and studied the reappearance of catecholamine fluorescence. It was found that the reappearance of fluorescence was blocked in both brain and heart by desipramine and protriptyline and that these effects were restricted to NE fibers, in that the drugs did not alter the reappearance of fluorescence in DA fibers. Similar results as to differential drug effects on DA and NE neurons were obtained with the use of an in vitro, brain slice technique.[26] Glowinski et al. also found that while desipramine decreased the uptake of intraventricular administered $^3H - NE$ into several areas of brain, this drug was without effect on DA uptake.[53] Ross and Renyi, however, noted that the differential effects of the tricyclic drugs on blockade of uptake on DA and NE systems were not absolute. For example, desipramine in the incubating media produced a 50 percent inhibition of uptake of NE in brain slices at a concentration of 3×10^{-8} M and a 50 percent inhibition of uptake of DA into striatal slices at a concentration of 5×10^{-5} M, i.e., a blockade of DA uptake equal to that of NE required an approximate one thousand-fold increase in drug concentration. Similar differences in the concentration of imipramine required to produce a 50 percent inhibition of uptake in noradrenergic and dopaminergic systems were found. These workers also made the interesting discovery that there were marked differences in the concentrations of desipramine and imipramine that were needed to block uptake of NE into cerebral slices by 50 percent, whereas there was relatively little difference in the quantities of these two drugs required to give a 50 percent blockade of uptake of DA into striatal slices. They calculated, for example, that a 50 percent inhibition of uptake of NE by brain slices could be produced by incubating the slices with 3×10^{-7} M imipramine or 3×10^{-8} M desipramine (to produce the same degree of blockade of uptake by pretreatment of the animals it was necessary to give 6 mg/kg of imipramine but only 2 mg/kg of desipramine). These in vivo and in vitro biochemical findings were buttressed by physiological data, i.e., the amount of imipramine required to give significant inhibition of a reserpine produced ptosis was 7 mg/kg, and for hypothermia 5 mg/kg, whereas desipramine in doses of 0.8 mg/kg and 0.5 of mg/kg respectively produced the same antagonistic effects.[100] (These dose-blockade relationships suggest that the finding by Schanberg et al.[103] that desipramine and imipramine both significantly block the uptake of ^{3}H-NE into the cisterna magna was due to the dosage used, i.e., 25 mg/kg.) Häggendal and Hamberger also produced data that is in essential agreement with the preceding work. They pretreated rats with reserpine and nialamide, prepared slices from cerebral cortex and neostriatum, and examined the uptake of NE in both of these areas with and without desipramine. They demonstrated that the amine pump in the striatum was quite active for NE, i.e., NE was concentrated against a gradient, as it was in cerebral cortex, but that the blockade of the uptake in these two areas by desipramine and chlorpromazine was rather different, i.e., at a concentration of 1×10^{-5} M there was a significant blockade of uptake of NE by cortical slices, but that this effect was much reduced in slices of striatum.[56] That these actions of tricyclic drugs on the uptake of NE also occur in an in vivo situation was established by Sulser et al. This group pretreated rats with reserpine and desipramine and, with the use of a push-pull cannulae implanted in the hypothalamus, assayed labeled NE and NM in the perfusate. As expected desipramine produced an increase in both NE and NM in the perfusate.[117]

In general, the cited studies as a group are consistent in that they indicate that the tricyclic drugs, desipramine and imipramine, markedly block the uptake of NE by neural tissues and that these effects are either absent or much less marked in DA systems, viz., the concentration of desipramine or imipramine required to give a 50 percent inhibition of uptake in striatum is one hundred to one thousand times greater than that for the cerebral cortex. In addition to the differential effects on DA-versus-NE neurons, there is also agreement that desipramine is a more potent inhibitor of NE uptake than is imipramine, i.e., depending upon the experimental conditions, the amount of desipramine required to give the same effect is three to ten times less than that of imipramine.

Interestingly, in most of these studies the effects of these drugs upon the uptake of 5-HT was ignored. This omission, however, was soon rectified with some interesting results. Blackburn et al., using rat brain slices, found that at concentrations of 1×10^{-4} and 1×10^{-5} M, imipramine, desipramine, and chlorpromazine were all inhibitory of 5-HT uptake. However, at the 1×10^{-5} M concentration imipramine blocked uptake by 38 and 30 percent.[18] In partial contradiction to this work, Palaic et al. found that desipramine in doses of 10 mg/kg, when given intraperitoneally twenty minutes before sacrifice, did not affect the uptake of labeled 5-HT in an experimental situation in which the brain was perfused with labeled 5-HT and later assayed for both 5-HT and 5-HIAA. (They did find, however, that drug treatment produced a decrease in endogenous 5-HIAA, which is of interest in terms of work described in another section of this chapter regarding the effects of these drugs on amine turnover.)[96] Other published reports by different groups of investigators gave information relevant to the apparent discrepancy between the work of Blackburn et al. and Palaic et al. For example, Alpers and Himwich, using slices from rat brainstems, estimated the concentrations of imipramine, amitriptyline, and desipramine required to give a 50 percent inhibition of 5-HT uptake.[4] The concentrations required for imipramine and amitriptyline were essentially the same, i.e., 3 to 4.5×10^{-5} M, whereas for desipramine the concentration required was ten times greater, i.e., 3×10^{-4} M. Ross and Renyi[101] and Carlsson[24] also found that the tertiary tricyclic amines, imipramine and amitriptyline, were more potent in blocking 5-HT uptake than were their demethylated derivatives, desipramine and nortriptyline. For example, the latter authors found that a 50 percent inhibition of uptake of 5-HT by brain slices occurred at a concentration of imipramine of 6×10^{-7} M, whereas the concentration required for desipramine was 4×10^{-6} M. A similar difference, albeit not as marked, was found between amitriptyline and nortriptyline. Both Ross and Renyi[101] and Carlsson[24] noted that the difference in the inhibitory potency for the uptake of 5-HT by brain slices was exactly the opposite of that which had been found for NE. Carlsson further investigated the structural specificity for the inhibition of 5-HT uptake by cerebral slices obtained from mice that had been pretreated with reserpine and nialamide and found that chlorimipramine was somewhat more potent than imipramine.[23] Glowinski and coworkers have used a somewhat different but important technique to assess the differential effects of the secondary and tertiary tricyclic amines on serotonergic, noradrenergic, and dopaminergic systems. Their approach has been to dissect out specific structures such as the hypothalamus, medulla oblongata, or striatum, to make slice preparations from these areas and incubate the tissues for fifteen minutes with labeled tyrosine or tryptophan. Given the short period of incubation, they feel that they may be specifically focusing on the release and reuptake of newly synthesized amines that may be preferentially released during nerve stimulation. The data as obtained with this technique are essentially in agreement with the work that has been reviewed above, i.e., desipramine markedly increased the content of labeled NE in the media in which slices of medulla oblongata were incubated, whereas there were no effects on the quantities of labeled DA found under similar conditions with slices of striatum. Similarly, with slices of hypothalamus, imipramine resulted in marked increases in the quantities of labeled 5-HT found in the media. In general, these results were obtained whether the drugs were administered in vivo or were added to the incubating media.[51]

Given the agreement among the studies cited above as to the differential effects of the secondary and tertiary tricyclic amines on blockage of uptake of the three amines DA, NE, and 5-HT, a logical inference is that these different drugs might have specific effects on aminergic systems as morphologically defined. As expected this issue has been explored with the use of histochemical-fluorescent techniques. Fuxe and Ungerstedt pretreated experimental animals with reserpine and then gave intraventricular injections of DA, 5-HT, or NE. In some cases, prior to the injection of the amines, the animals were pretreated with desipramine or imipramine. They found that with the control animals, i.e., those which had been pretreated with reserpine but not with the tricyclic drug, there was a partial to marked increase in fluorescence following injection of DA, NE, or alpha-methyl-NE, in areas close to the ventricle. They further found that pretreatment with desipramine or protriptyline prevented the increase in fluorescence in NE terminals, but not in DA terminals. This effect was dose dependent. The blockage was greatest in those terminals just beneath the fourth ventricle and in the subarachnoid space of the medulla and pons, but little blockage was observed in NE nerve terminals of the hippocampal formation or septal area, where the concentration of injected amine would have been expected to be high. In contrast to the findings with desipramine or protriptyline, they found that pretreatment with imipramine only slightly decreased the return of fluorescence following the injection of the DA or NE. Further, pretreatment with desipramine did not block the accumulation of fluorescence following the injection of 5-HT in any of the areas examined, whereas there were partial effects following pretreatment with imipramine.[45] While these findings agree with and extend those obtained by biochemical or pharmacological approaches there remains the problem of the unphysiological route of administration of the amines. To avoid this potentially confounding problem Carlsson et al. injected rats and mice intraperitoneally with 4, alpha-dimethyl-meta-tyrosine (H77-77), which causes the depletion of NE and DA in both central and peripheral pools, and by the use of biochemical- and histochemical-fluorescent techniques examined the effects of imipramine, desipramine, or protriptyline on the drug-induced amine depletions. The H77-77 induced depletion of NE, but not DA, was prevented by pretreatment with desipramine and protriptyline, and this blocking effect appeared to be dose dependent. In contrast, pretreatment with imipramine or amitriptyline blocked NE nerve-terminal depletion by H77-77 only at the highest doses. Data obtained by biochemical analysis of brains for NE and DA content were, in general, in agreement with those obtained with the histochemical-fluorescence technique.[25] Carlsson[24] also found that an analogue of H77-77, 4-methyl-alpha-ethyl-meta-tyrosine (H75-12), was capable of causing depletion not only of catecholamines but also of 5-HT stores in the brain and, as before, he used this agent to examine the action of the tricyclic drugs on serotonergic systems in the brain. In these investigations the 5-HT nerve terminals examined were mainly in the mesencephalon and diencephalon, particularly the nucleus suprachiasmaticus. It was found that chlorimipramine and imipramine were the most potent drugs in blocking the H75/12 induced amine depletion in 5-HT nerve terminals, whereas drugs such as protriptyline, desipramine, and nortriptyline had little blocking activity in the doses studied. The biochemical data was supportive of and consistent with the histochemical-fluorescent data.

In summary, the available biochemical data indicate that the tricyclic antidepressant drugs do not block, or do so only weekly, the uptake of DA. Further, while the tricyclic drugs block the uptake of both 5-HT and NE by brain tissue there are differential effects in that the tertiary tricyclic amines, such as imipramine, are more potent inhibitors of 5-HT uptake than are the secondary amines, such as desipramine. In contrast, the secondary amines are more potent blockers of NE uptake than are the tertiary amines. As might be expected from this biochemical data, histochemical-fluorescent studies indicate that the tricyclic drugs are without effects upon dopaminergic systems per se, whereas the secondary and tertiary tricyclic drugs exert their principal effects respectively upon noradrenergic and serotonergic brain systems.

EFFECTS OF TRICYCLIC ANTIDEPRESSANTS ON TURNOVER OF DOPAMINE, NOREPINEPHRINE, AND SEROTONIN

In 1966, Neff and Costa published data that indicated that if rats were given protriptyline (20 mg/kg) or desipramine (10 mg/kg) × 5 over a three-day period, an increase of turnover of brain NE, but not DA, was produced.[90] In terms of issues to be discussed in other parts of this chapter, it should be noted that these investigators also found that in contrast to the lack of an effect of the tricyclic drugs on DA turnover, chlorpromazine in doses of 5 mg/kg did increase the turnover of DA. Corrodi and Fuxe pretreated experimental animals with imipramine and inhibitors of tyrosine hydroxylase or tryptophan hydroxylase and by biochemical- and histochemical-fluorescent techniques estimated the rates of disappearance of catecholamines and indoleamines. They found that, even with high doses of imipramine, there were no changes in the rates of depletion of NE or DA, whereas there was a significant slowing of the decrease in the disappearance of 5-HT.[30] This finding as to an effect of imipramine on the turnover of 5-HT and the lack of an effect on NE or DA systems, of course, "fits" with studies cited earlier in this chapter indicating that the tertiary tricyclic amines act primarily on serotonergic systems, whereas the secondary amines have a more specific action on noradrenergic systems. In later work Corrodi and Fuxe examined the effects of amitriptyline, chlorimipramine, and nortriptyline on brain 5-HT turnover by assessing the effects of these agents on the depletion of brain 5-HT and the rates of disappearance of fluorescence in serotonergic areas following the administration of a tryptophan hydroxylase inhibitor. They found that it was necessary to use extremely high doses to obtain significant slowing of turnover of 5-HT, and even then the results were very modest. (These findings are in contrast to the rather marked effects of some of these drugs in blocking 5-HT uptake, as noted in studies cited elsewhere in this chapter.) Using a somewhat different technique and approach, Meek and Werdinius[87] found that, following the administration of chlorimipramine and probenecid, there was a decrease in the accumulation of 5-HIAA in the brain, which is consistent with and supportive of the earlier suggestion that the imipraminelike drugs slow the turnover of 5-HT.

Schubert et al. approached the problem of turnover time, as influenced by the tricyclic drugs, by giving labeled tryptophan or tyrosine, either as a single pulse or as an infusion, and then measuring the amount of labeled 5-HT, DA, or NE that accumulated during the infusion or the amount of labelled amine that was found in brain at some point after the pulse was given. Drugs evaluated were imipramine, desipramine, amitriptyline, and nortriptyline. It was very clear from their data that none of these drugs affected DA accumulation or disappearance. For 5-HT the disappearance was decreased by imipramine and amitriptyline, but was unaltered by desipramine or nortriptyline. The accumulation of 5-HT was decreased by imipramine, but not by the other drugs. In general these findings may be considered to be consistent with the notion that imipramine slows the turnover of 5-HT, whereas desipramine or nortriptyline are without an effect. The accumulation of NE was not increased by any of the drugs, but the disappearance was increased by desipramine and nortriptyline, which would suggest that these two drugs may increase the turnover of this amine. Since only single time points are available, however, these conclusions as to effects of these four agents on turnover must be quite tentative, and it can only be firmly concluded that these drugs appear to be without effect on DA systems, but do have effects on the quantities of labeled 5-HT and NE found in brain.[110]

In an investigation of the effects of psychoactive drugs on 5-HT metabolism, Schildkraut et al. noted that when ^{14}C-5-HT was administered by intracisternal injection and imipramine was subsequently injected intraperitoneally (the animals were sacrificed two hours following the injection of the labeled amine) there was a significant increase in levels of ^{14}C-5-HT in those animals which had been treated with imipramine. This finding is consistent with the work noted above, which indicates that imipramine results in a slowing of the turnover of brain 5-HT.[107] Schildkraut has also presented data that indicates that the length of time of drug administration is a significant factor in determining potential effects on turnover time of the amine under study. For example, he noted that when rats were given imipramine (10 mg/kg) twice daily for three weeks, there appeared to be an increase in the rate of disappearance of ^{3}H-NE from the brain, following an intracisternal injection of the labeled amine. Again, this data is difficult to interpret with certainty, in that only two time points were presented and there were alterations in the endogenous NE content and, as such, specific activities were probably altered.[100,108,109]

Glowinski and coworkers, using a technique that was described earlier in this chapter, examined the effects of some tricyclic antidepressant on the synthesis of NE, DA, and 5-HT from labeled precursors. They found that the total labeled 5-HT found (media and tissue) was decreased if imipramine was present in the media or if tissue was obtained from animals that had been pretreated with this drug. Desipramine produced marked increases in NE synthesis in slices of medulla, but no effects on the synthesis of DA in striatum were noted.[51]

In summary, the available data indicate that the tricyclic drugs, whether of the tertiary or secondary amine type, do not alter the turnover or disposition of DA. Tricyclic drugs of the tertiary amine type produce effects that are consistent with a slowing of the turnover of 5-HT. In contrast, tricyclic drugs of the secondary amine type produce effects on NE that are consistent with an increase in turnover of this amine. These differential effects (or lack thereof) of the teritiary and secondary tricyclic amines on the turnover of DA,

NE, and 5-HT are also consistent with the demonstrated differential blockage of uptake of these three biogenic amines as produced by the tertiary and secondary tricyclic amines.

ACTIONS OTHER THAN THOSE ON UPTAKE AND TURNOVER

As is indicated by the foregoing there has been a great deal of attention paid to the effects of tricyclic drugs on the neuronal membrane pump for NE, DA, and 5-HT. It should be noted, however, that this may reflect the focus of the investigating spotlight rather than a total description of modes of action. For example, Mandell has presented data that indicates that imipramine in doses of 25 mg/kg (two times per day) for three days and at 10 mg/kg (two times per day) for eight days produces significant decreases in midbrain tyrosine hydroxylase activity.[79] It is also probable that the tricyclic drugs have some effects upon the uptake of amines into organelles within the neurons. The magnitude of this effect in determining the pharmacological actions of the drugs is uncertain, but it should not be overlooked. Brodie et al. found that desipramine blocks the uptake of small doses of tyramine by a rat heart, but if the tyramine is given in doses of 20 mg/kg, desipramine (20 mg/kg) does not alter the intracellular concentrations of tyramine, but it is able to prevent the depletion of NE by the tyramine.[20] Similarly, Leitz showed that while desipramine was able to prevent the efflux of NE from heart slices, following treatment with metaraminol, this effect was much greater than the blockage of the uptake of metaraminol per se. He interprets this data to indicate that while desipramine blocks the uptake of metaraminol at the neuronal membrane, it also blocks the entrance of metaraminol into the granules and thus has an intraneuronal action.[77] Steinberg and Smith, using rat-brain slices, found that low doses of desipramine did not prevent the uptake of ³H-tyramine at the neuronal membrane and subsequent synthesis of ³H-parahydroxyphenlyacetic acid, but that it did prevent the uptake of ³H-tyramine into intraneuronal sites, as indicated by the decreased formation of labeled octopamine.[116]

The Neuroleptic or Antipsychotic Drugs

These classes of drugs, for example, the butyrophenones and phenothiazines, are of particular interest in that although they differ chemically, they share the ability to decrease manifest psychotic behavior and ideation in schizophrenic subjects, whereas they are not particularly helpful in reversing depressive mood and psychomotor retardation in the depressive disorders.* Because of this specific clinical usefulness in the neuroleptics, a demonstrated action on specific aminergic systems would assume importance in that leads might be provided as to the possibility that one or more of the brain aminergic systems has a central role in the genesis of some, if not all, components of schizophrenia. This general line of pharmacological reasoning, of course, is similar to that which has been used to develop hypotheses as to the involvement of specific biogenic amines in the affective disorders.[104, 106] Investigation of the specificity of action of the neuroleptics has, however, posed methodological problems in that these drugs have a multiplicity of biological effects,[37] and the manipulation of a particularly important effect, receptor blockage, requires in vivo, function-type preparations, in contrast to other types of studies in which homogenates, brain slices, synaptosomes, ventricular-perfusion techniques etc., may be used. In general, studies of receptor blockage within specific amine systems have either utilized "functional-test" methods or a biochemical marker, i.e., amine turnover time, which changes as a consequence of drug administration.

STUDIES USING "FUNCTION" TYPE METHODS

Anden et al.[11] examined the effects of a variety of drugs on rats in which the DA pathway had been destroyed by either an electrolytic lesion in the crus cerebri at the level of the mammillary bodies or by unilateral re-

---

* They may, however, be quite helpful in decreasing the anxiety that is an integral part of some depressive states and, in fact, many clinicians prefer to give these drugs in combination with an antidepressant when anxiety is an important component of the clinical picture.

moval of the corpus striatum. Reserpine produced a turning of the tail and head to the side opposite from the lesion as did haloperidol and chlorpromazine, whereas promethazine was without effect. Pretreatment with a monoamine oxidase inhibitor accentuated the reserpine effect, but the turning was now toward the operated side and this was blocked by haloperiodol. Similarly, pretreatment with a monoamine oxidase inhibitor followed by L-Dopa, but not 5-hydroxytryptophan, resulted in a turning toward the operated side. These findings can be taken as supporting the possibility that chlorpromazine and haloperidol block dopaminergic receptors, but the question as to an effect on other types of central receptors is left unanswered.

Snyder et al.[114] noted that d-amphetamine is a more potent inhibitor of NE uptake than is l-amphetamine, whereas the two isomers are about equally active in inhibiting DA uptake, and, as such, suggested that this differential effect might be used to dissect out the noradrenergic versus dopaminergic-mediated behavior that is produced by amphetamine. It was found that d-amphetamine was about ten times more potent than the l-isomer in producing locomotor stimulation and only twice as potent in producing stereotypical gnawing and mouthing movements. It was concluded that the locomotor activity was predominantly mediated via noradrenergic systems, whereas the stereotypy was due primarily to dopaminergic systems with some contribution from the noradrenergic. These data can be used to reinterpret some earlier reports as to the effects of a variety of neuroleptic agents on the amphetamine-induced behavior. For example, Randrup et al. found that chlorpromazine, haloperidol, and ethoxybutamoxane were all effective antagonists of amphetamine-induced behavior that, as described by them, seems to be similar to gnawing and mouthing movements. In terms of later work to be reviewed, it is of particular interest that they found haloperidol was effective at lower doses than chlorpromazine.[99] Janssen et al. studied an amazingly large number of drugs of the neuroleptic type in terms of their ability to antagonize amphetamine- or apomorphine-induced

chewing and agitation. Given the correctness of Snyder's interpretation of his data as indicating that stereotyped gnawing behavior is due primarily to DA systems and the agitation to the noradrenergic, the data of Janssen can be used to categorize a large number of neuroleptics in terms of their potency for blockage of dopaminergic and/or noradrenergic receptors. For example, Janssen et al. noted that haloperidol is a more potent antagonist of amphetamine- or apomorphine-induced chewing than it is of agitation, which would imply a greater potency in blocking dopaminergic receptors.[65] Despite the great detail of the Janssen et al. report, however, it is clear that conclusions regarding the blockage of dopaminergic-versus-noradrenergic receptors rests upon inference, and it is for this reason that a relatively recent report by Anden et al.,[7] in which information was obtained as a specificity of receptor blockage by a more direct experimental approach is of particular interest. As noted, Anden et al. found that rats which had been unilaterally striatomized, when treated with apomorphine, turn toward the operated side. The dosages of a variety of neuroleptic agents required to block this behavior were noted, and this data was then taken as a measure of potency of dopaminergic-receptor blockage. For a test of central, noradrenergic-receptor blockage the ability of a series of neuroleptics, in varying dosages, to block the hind-limb flexor-reflex activity of a spinal animal after NE receptor stimulation, as produced by L-Dopa, was examined. It was found that two drugs of the diphenylbutylamine class, pimozide and fluspiriline, blocked only DA receptors, and even at very high dosage these drugs did not block NE receptors. A second group of drugs, among which were haloperidol, spiroperidol, and fluphenazine, had marked blocking activity for DA receptors, but only small to modest activity in blocking NE receptors. A third group of neuroleptics were reasonably good blockers of both dopaminergic and noradrenergic receptors and an example from this group is chlorpromazine.

The detailed report by Janssen et al. regarding the pharmacology and toxicology of pimozide contains data, which is consistent with the work of Anden et al., that indicates that this drug is a potent blocker of DA receptors.[64] Further, there is a report[19] that indicates that this drug is a potent antipsychotic, and that, in terms of regional distribution, the highest concentrations in the brain are to be found in the caudate nucleus and pituitary, which, given the anatomy of aminergic systems, supports the concept that this drug has its primary effects on dopaminergic systems.

In summary, the available data indicate that the neuroleptic drugs as a group block DA and/or NE receptors in the brain, but some of these drugs which have antipsychotic properties have been found to be selective blockers of dopamine receptors. This, of course, raises the possibility that brain DA systems, and not NE systems, are involved in the production of psychotic behavior.

Effects of Neuroleptic Drugs on the Disposition of Dopamine, Norepinephrine, and Serotonin

In 1963, Carlsson and Lindquist published data that indicated that chlorpromazine or haloperidol did not alter endogenous brain NE and DA levels, but that these agents did produce increases in NM and 3-methoxytyramine. Furthermore, these changes were not produced with either phenoxybenzamine or promethazine.[27] This report was seminal in that it suggested that chemically different drugs that have in common antipsychotic effects alter the turnover of two important brain amines, whereas a phenothiazine, promethazine, which does not have antipsychotic properties, was without effect. These findings led the authors to postulate that these drugs produce a receptor blockage that, via a neuronal feedback mechanism, results in increased transmitter release and, consequently, an increased turnover. Work compatible with and supportive of the increased turnover of DA, as induced by these neuroleptic drugs, was published by Anden et al. in 1964.[13] Laverty and Sharman also published data that were generally supportive of these earlier observations, but which raised questions as to problems of dosage and the capacity of neuro-

leptics to deplete amine stores. These investigations examined the effects of four different phenothiazines on brain levels of DA, NE, 5-HT, 5-HIAA and HVA. They noted that chlorpromazine when given acutely did not alter brain NE, 5-HT, or 5-HIAA, but that it did significantly decrease DA and increase HVA. Thioridazine, in contrast, did not affect 5-HIAA or DA, but it did increase NE and, in higher doses (50 mg/kg), treatment with this drug produced decreased brain 5-HT and increased HVA. In chronic experiments in which animals were treated with either chlorpromazine (20 mg/kg for fourteen days), trifluoperazine (8 mg/kg for twelve days) or thioproperazine (100 mg/mg for fourteen days) it was found that all drugs resulted in an increase in brain HVA, whereas there were no effects on brain NE, DA, 5-HT, or 5-HIAA (NE was measured in the hypothalamus, DA, and HVA in the caudate nucleus, and 5-HT and 5-HIAA in the thalamus). Atropine in doses of 25 mg/kg in cats had no effects on any of the assayed amines or metabolites.[76] Da Prada and Pletcher reported that chlorpromazine markedly increased, in a dose-dependent fashion, brain HVA but not 5-HIAA, and that this increase of HVA could be abolished by treatment with a monoamine oxidase inhibitor. They noted that the endogenous content of DA was not changed by chlorpromazine.[35]

Neff and Costa,[90] using a nonisotopic method, found that while treatment with chlorpromazine (5 mg/kg twice a day for three days) produced a significant increase in the turnover of brain DA, there was no change in the turnover of brain NE. This report represents the first direct demonstration that chlorpromazine does indeed alter the turnover of brain DA inasmuch as previous methods relied upon the analysis of changes in the metabolites of brain amines. Furthermore, the data in this paper, in terms of drug amine system specificity, set the stage for a controversy, which has not as yet been completely resolved, i.e., Neff and Costa found no change in the turnover of brain NE due to chlorpromazine, whereas the work of Carlsson suggested that this drug induced changes in the turnover of both DA and NE. Burkard et al. found that pretreatment of animals with chlorpromazine resulted in an increased conversion of peripherally administered tyrosine to ³H catechols in brain. The increase was major, being of the order of 80 to 100 percent, and lasted for one and a half to six hours.[22] In an extension of this work, Gey and Pletscher[47] found that the increase in labeled catechols that occurred as a function of treatment with chlorpromazine was due to an increase in the specific activity of DA, whereas there was no change in the specific activity of NE. Also, these investigators found that if they gave C[14]-Dopa and then gave chlorpromazine, the specific activity of DA at one hundred and twenty to one hundred and eighty minutes was significantly decreased, whereas that of NE was decreased less markedly and only at one hundred and twenty minutes as compared with controls. (The chlorpromazine treatment produced significant decrements in brain tyrosine levels, but this decrease was not of sufficient magnitude to negate the finding regarding turnover.) This data then supports the results of Neff and Costa as to an increase in DA turnover and a lack of change in NE turnover after chlorpromazine treatment.

Corrodi et al. presented both biochemical- and histochemical-fluorescence data that indicated that with rats acutely treated with haloperidol or chlorpromazine and sacrificed four hours after tyrosine-hydrosylase inhibition, there was a greater depletion of NE as a function of the neuroleptic drugs, whereas this was not found for DA. Treatment of rats for three days with chlorpromazine, followed by sacrifice six hours after enzyme inhibition, resulted in there being significantly less brain NE and DA in comparison to a control group. It should be noted that this latter "multiple" treatment schedule of Corrodi was similar to that of Neff and Costa; both groups used an inhibitor of tyrosine hydroxylase to assess the effects of neuroleptics on brain amine depletion, but Neff and Costa assayed for DA and NE at multiple time points, after tyrosine hydroxylase, and as such were able to calculate the actual slope of the rate of disappearance

of amines following enzyme inhibition, whereas the Corrodi group had only one or two time points.[31]

Nyback and coworkers published a series of articles[91,92,93,94] dealing with the problem of alterations in the turnover of brain amines as induced by neuroleptic drugs, using a technique in which rats or mice were pretreated with neuroleptic drugs and then either infused with labeled tyrosine or given a pulse of this catecholamine precursor. Immediately following infusion, or one and a half hours after the pulse, animals were sacrificed and the brains assayed for labeled tyrosine, DA or NE. Their data indicate that chlorpromazine resulted in an increased accumulation of ^{14}C-DA, no change in ^{14}C-tyrosine, and a small increase in the accumulation of ^{14}C-NE. Further, this result for DA was maximal if the chlorpromazine was given one hour before the infusion and absent if the chlorpromazine was given twelve hours previously. If they gave chlorpromazine one hour after the labeled tyrosine, there were no effects on labeled tyrosine or NE, but ^{14}C-DA was decreased. They also found that haloperidol increased the accumulation and disappearance of ^{14}C-DA. The disappearance, but not the accumulation of ^{14}C-NE, was increased by haloperidol, and promethazine did not alter the accumulation of labeled amines but did slightly increase the disappearance of ^{14}C-NE. It was also demonstrated that analogues of phenothiazines, possessing neuroleptic activity (chlorpromazine, levomepromazine, perphenazine, and chlorprothixene), in comparison to promethazine, altered the incorporation and loss of labeled DA from the brain, and that there was a tendency for the clinically most potent neuroleptics to have marked effects on DA formation and disappearance. At the highest dosages all drugs, except promethazine, increased the disappearance of NE and, at lower dosages, three of the four did.

Anden et al.,[5] as noted, classified drugs in terms of their ability to block DA and NE receptors within the central nervous system and then examined the effects of these same neuroleptic agents on the turnover of DA and

NE, as assessed by the rates of decrease of DA and NE in the rat brain following treatment with a tyrosine-hydroxylase inhibitor, as well as by following changes in histochemical fluorescence due to catecholamines. The authors found that the two drugs of the dipheny-buty-lamine type (pimozide and fluspiridene) which blocked only central DA receptors increased DA turnover and, in somewhat higher doses, NE turnover. In general, there was a relationship between the type and degree of receptor blockage and increased turnover of DA and/or NE.

Although the above reports clearly indicate that the neuroleptics alter brain DA turnover, the mechanism by which this change is induced is uncertain. As noted, in 1963 Carlsson and Lindquist originally speculated that this increase in turnover occurred as the consequence of receptor blockage that, via a direct or indirect neural feedback, initiated increased neural activity, increased transmitter (DA) release, and then increased synthesis. Anden et al.[6] investigated the problem as follows. It was noted that chlorpromazine, haloperidol, and an alpha receptor blocker, all prevented the Dopa-induced increase in the hind-limb flexor reflex in spinal animals. These drugs (but not a β blocker) also resulted in increased disappearance of NE after tyrosine-hydroxylase inhibition above the lesion, but not below, which led to the suggestion that the effect on NE turnover was due to an increase in nerve-impulse flow and not due to a direct action of the drugs themselves, i.e., the experimental data was consistent with Carlsson's original hypothesis. Tagliamonte et al., however, have suggested a somewhat different mechanism.[118] These authors found that chlorpromazine, in doses ranging from 5 to 20 mg/kg, was able to produce significant decreases in DA in the caudate nucleus with a corresponding increase in HVA. They further noted that with chlorpromazine there was a decrement in the 3-methoxy-tyramine content of brain. They concluded that it is probable that chlorpromazine may, like reserpine, produce an increased intraneuronal destruction of DA and that this then leads to the increase in

turnover. Himwich et al. found that haloperidol even in the lowest doses used (1mg/kg), produced significant decreases of dopamine in the caudate nucleus whereas with the same dosage no effect was noted in the rabbit.[59] Other authors have also noted that chlorpromazine or haloperidol at higher doses produces decreases in brain DA (see Laverty and Sharman), and these data give some support to Tagliamonte's suggestion. In contrast, much of the data reported by Swedish workers indicate that increases in turnover of brain DA can occur without decreases in endogenous DA content.[5,8,27] It is of interest that amphetamine is able to diminish the rate of DA synthesis from ^{3}H-tyrosine in brain slices in vitro, which raises the possibility that the effects observed are due to factors other than neural feedback mechanisms.

Relative to DA and NE, the biochemical effects of neuroleptics on brain 5-HT has not been intensively studied. Gey and Pletscher found that chlorpromazine and chlorprothixene did not alter the endogenous content of rat brain 5-HT, but it did counteract the increase of this amine after monoamine oxidase (MAO) inhibition or following 5-hydroxy-tryptophan as well as the decrement in 5-HT produced by reserpine. They conclude that the drug may affect the intracellular disposition of 5-HT.[46] Anden et al. found that 5-HT content in cell bodies and nerve endings were unchanged as assessed by the histochemical-fluorescent method, nor were there changes demonstrated with biochemical assays.[8] Giacalone and Kostowski found that for both forebrain and brainstem chlorpromazine (5 mg/kg) did not alter 5-HT content, but it did result in significant increases in 5-HIAA.[48] Guldberg and Yates found that chlorpromazine in dosages of 2.5 to 10 mg/kg resulted in increases of 5-HIAA in the ventricular-cerebrospinal fluid and caudate nuclei of dogs (but not of other brain areas) whereas higher doses (10 to 15 mg/kg) were without effect on 5-HIAA in either CSF or brain tissues.[54] Gumulka et al. found that chlorpromazine in doses of 1, 5, and 10 mg/kg did not alter brain 5-HT, but, in confirmation of Guldberg and

Yates, they found that the 5 mg/kg of chlorpromazine increased brain 5-HIAA, whereas this was not found with the lower or higher dose of the drug.[55] As noted elsewhere, Laverty and Sharman[76] found that acute chronic administration of chlorpromazine (at doses of 10 and 20 mg/kg respectively) did not alter brain 5-HT or 5-HIAA. It thus appears that the phenothiazine neuroleptics do not alter brain 5-HT, whereas, within a selected dose range, they do produce increases in 5-HIAA. However, because of the possibility that chlorpromazine will alter intraneuronal processes that are involved in the disposition of 5-HT and because of dose relationship, it cannot be assumed that this drug affects turnover. The relationship of neuroleptics to the 5-HT systems awaits more definitive investigation.

In summary, whether the brain DA systems have been examined in terms of alterations in brain metabolites, changes in DA content as produced by tyrosine-hydroxylase inhibition, or by the rates of formation of labeled DA, or disappearance of labeled DA following an intravenous pulse of labeled tyrosine, the results are consistent and in good agreement, i.e., treatment with neuroleptic drugs that may differ chemically but share antipsychotic effects, all produce increases in turnover of DA in brain. In contrast to DA, the data dealing with the effects of these antipsychotic or neuroleptic drugs on the turnover of brain NE is less consistent. Some authors have found no alterations in turnover of brain NE as a function of treatment with neuroleptics, whereas others have found small but statistically significant changes, depending upon the type and amount of drug administered. In comparison to DA, the effects on NE turnover produced by the neuroleptics would appear to be minimal. It has been postulated that the neuroleptic-induced increases in amine turnover occur as a consequence of receptor blockage, but definitive experimental data as to the exact mechanism by which the neuroleptics alter turnover is not available. Studies dealing with the effects of the neuroleptics on 5-HT systems are few, and this area needs further exploration.

(Lest We Forget

The function of specific aminergic systems has been approached artificially by the dissection, as much as methods allow, of each system from the influence of other amine systems. While the role of each system can be studied thereby, it is easy to lose the perspective that the brain is a complex organ or group of organs, all of whose component systems operating *together* yield the final measurable end product, behavior. Moreover, the aminergic systems described herein (NE, DA, 5-HT, ACh) make up only a small portion of brain neurons. While they may be the more critical neurotransmitter systems so far as psychopathologic states are concerned, it can be appreciated readily that other candidates also exist but as yet have not been either defined or investigated.

The relationships among the presently described systems are of considerable interest, especially the relationships of cholinergic to dopaminergic and noradrenergic systems. Recently, clinical studies in which brain ACh systems were altered by the anticholinesterase physostigmine have shown the induction of a short-lived depressive state with lethargy, withdrawal, and psychomotor retardation.[62] Physostigmine was also able to move manic patients toward the euthymic state.[63] For the moment these studies must remain a curiosity, since there is no evidence implicating a defect in ACh metabolism in the brain in depressive states, but the frequent coincidence of terminal areas of ACh and NE systems, noted in Table 20-1, raises the possibility that ACh and NE systems may be acting at specific sites, balancing one another's inhibitory or facilitory effect on a postsynaptic neuronal system that mediates affect, depression occurring when ACh receptor activation predominates over NE receptor activation.

The stereotypy induced by increasing DA in the neostriatum has been shown to be antagonized by ACh and by physostigmine[14,61] as well as by haloperidol. Here again the coincidence of DA and ACh terminals in the neostriatum suggest that the two monoamines, DA and ACh, may be balancing one another's inhibitory or facilitory effect on a postsynaptic neuronal system that mediates stereotypy, stereotypy appearing when DA receptor activation predominates over ACh receptor activation.

A specific neuronal system may also terminally innervate another neuronal system. The intimate contact of ventral NE terminals with 5-HT raphe cell bodies (B_7) as seen by fluorescent histochemistry[40] suggests such innervation. Such innervation of one system by another may not be unique to the raphe, but as yet it has not been described in other areas. The functional significance of such innervation is unknown at this time, but such findings open the possibility of further relationships among specific aminergic systems.

(Specific Brain Aminergic Systems and the Genesis of the Affective and Schizophrenic Disorders—Some Speculations

In this final section an attempt is made to integrate data, from previously cited reports, around the possibility that specific amine systems within the brain are crucially involved in the production of specific psychopathological states. Before proceeding, however, a couple of caveats about this approach are needed. First, the comments and paradigms herein give short shrift to the issue of interactions between amine systems that are, without question, of importance in the regulation of behavior. It is, for example, clear that there are cholinergic and dopaminergic nerve endings in the neostriatum and that these two transmitters produce antagonistic effects. It is also well-known that the tricyclic antidepressant drugs, in addition to their actions on other amines, possess anticholinergic properties. Secondly, given the complexity of the brain and of behavior, it is likely that a one-amine–one-psychiatric-disease* concept is too

* With apologies to George Beadle and E. L. Tatum.

simple, but it is felt that from the investigators' standpoint there is heuristic value in constructing reasonably simple paradigms that may contain at least partial truths.

Aminergic Brain Systems and Depression

If one tabulates the data reviewed above, there are some remarkably consistent findings that emerge from the studies with the tricyclic antidepressant drugs. These can be used to develop and buttress the idea that specific aminergic systems within the central nervous system are (or are not) involved in the production of severe depressive states in man† Some of this data has been tabulated in Table 20–2. Perhaps the most consistent finding is that the tertiary and secondary tricyclic amines, when administered in doses used clinically, are without effect on the uptake of DA into dopaminergic fibers. Further, these drugs do not have a significant effect on the turnover of DA. In contrast, drugs such as the phenothiazines and butyrophenones, which are without significant antidepressant activity, do have pronounced effects on the turnover of DA (q.v.). By inference then, it seems possible to exclude the dopaminergic systems as having a central role in the genesis of some depressive states, and, given the experimental data as reviewed, the question arises concerning the role that noradrenergic and/or serotonergic systems may play in depression. There also appears to be general agreement among different workers that tertiary amines are more potent inhibitors of the uptake of 5-HT than of NE, whereas the effectiveness of the blockage of uptake of 5-HT and NE is reversed with the secondary tricyclic amines. The data as to alterations in turnover of NE and 5-HT that occurs as a consequence of administration of the tertiary and secondary

† There are, of course, many other studies that indicate that the functional amounts of brain amines, particularly NE, are involved in the affective disorders, and these have been well summarized elsewhere.[104, 106] The focus in this chapter, however, is on the possibility that specific amine systems are involved in the genesis of depression. Hence cited references and speculations are directed toward this issue of specificity.

TABLE 20–2.   **The effect of secondary and tertiary tricyclic antidepressants on DA, NE and 5-HT uptake and turnover.**

Amine	Blockade of Uptake		Effects on Amine Turnover	
	Tertiary Tricyclic Amine (viz Imipramine)	Secondary Tricyclic Amine (viz Desipramine)	Tertiary Tricyclic Amine (viz Imipramine)	Secondary Tricyclic Amine (viz Desipramine)
DA	No Effect	No Effect	No Effect	No Effect
NE	+	+++	−	Increases
5-HT	+++	+	Slows	−

tricyclic amines is not quite as clear as that for blockage of uptake. But, on the balance, the available information indicates that the turnover of 5-HT is slowed by the tertiary tricyclic amines, whereas the turnover of NE is increased by the secondary tricyclic amines.

Given the above findings, one might reasonably conclude that both noradrenergic and serotonergic, but not dopaminergic brain systems, are involved in depressive disorders. This is essentially the position that Carlsson has taken, in that he posits a role for 5-HT in regulating mood and for NE in regulating drive energy and activity.[25] While such a view cannot, of course, be disproved and must be respected until definitive data is available, we feel that if one examines the situation a bit more closely, the evidence favors an involvement of noradrenergic rather than the serotonergic systems in the genesis of depression. The reasoning behind this position briefly is as follows. It is by now well-established that the tertiary tricyclic amine, imipramine, following administration to animals, undergoes rapid demethylation to form the secondary amine, desipramine. Direct experimental evidence has been obtained from a human subject who died as a result of an accidental overdose of imipramine, indicating that significant quantities of the demethylated product were formed. There are species differences, in that rat and man rapidly metabolize imipramine to desipramine, which is then itself metabolized less rapidly, with the net result being that there is a gradual accumulation of desipramine in tissues. In those animals in which rapid metabol-

ism of imipramine, and the less rapid metabolism of the demethylated product, do not occur, one finds that the ability of the tertiary amine to antagonize the effects of reserpine, or the experimental drug benzoquinolazine, is less marked.[*] Further, the available data on turnover would indicate that while the secondary tricyclic amines may increase NE synthesis, there is a decrease in turnover of 5-HT induced by the tertiary tricyclic amines. A slowing of turnover, accompanied by a blockage of reuptake, may produce a system in which quantities of amine available at receptors is the same as that found before drug treatment. An increase in synthesis, accompanied by blockage of reuptake as probably occurs with NE as a consequence of the tricyclic drug administration, should, on the other hand, make more amine available to the receptor. This data, particularly that dealing with the metabolism of the tricyclic drugs, suggests that the secondary tricyclic amine is the therapeutic agent. Given the data as summarized in Table 20–2, it is inferred that the noradrenergic rather than the serotonergic brain systems are primarily involved with depression. However, there are obvious problems with this reasoning, in that small amounts of the tertiary amine could still be available for changing the 5-HT systems. Against this argument is the fact that there is now a great wealth of clinical data available as to the effects of desipramine per se in the treatment of depressive states. The available

---

[*] See references 15, 37, 50, 58, and 86.

information indicates that desipramine is as effective as imipramine in the treatment of depressive disorders.[70] Since it is known that N-methylation of desipramine (to form imipramine) does not occur to any significant degree, it is suggested that the clinical effectiveness (in terms of mood and activity) of this secondary tricyclic amine, when coupled with its effects upon NE versus 5-HT systems (see Table 20–2) provides perhaps the most compelling argument that the principal systems involved in the depressive disorders are of the noradrenergic type.

Given the above reasoning, the next question is: Is it possible that a particular central, noradrenergic system is involved in the genesis of depression? The data relative to this point are very soft and nonspecific, but a few comments can be made. In general, the studies of changes in histochemical fluorescence of NE systems, as induced by pharmacological manipulations, do not indicate that the tricyclic amines of the secondary type are exerting their effects on any one of the specific NE systems. This, of course, may be a function of the investigative use of a drug that generally blocks the NE neuronal pump mechanism.

In summary, it is suggested that specific brain NE systems are intimately related to the genesis of depression. Studies of the regulation of behavior (including depressive mood and psychomotor activity) by specific NE systems can be expected to emerge in the next few years and this new information will undoubtedly be of major value, whatever the demonstrated relationship of NE systems to depression may ultimately be.

Aminergic Brain Systems and Schizophrenia

The data as to the specificity of action of neuroleptics on aminergic brain systems are somewhat less clear than are those for the tricyclic antidepressant drugs, but in some areas there has been remarkable agreement. We feel that there is heuristic value in suggesting that specific aminergic systems may be involved in the production of psychotic states, particularly schizophrenia. Neuroleptics that are clinically effective, whatever their chemical structure, block central DA receptors and increase the turnover of this amine in dopaminergic systems. This increase in DA turnover, as a consequence of neuroleptic drug treatment, has been demonstrated by studies that have measured metabolite accumulation, changes in amine level following enzyme inhibition, alterations in histochemical fluorescence in dopaminergic systems, formation of DA from labeled precursors, or the rate of the disappearance of labeled DA from the brain. The data from function-type studies are generally consistent and can be reasonably interpreted as indicating that many of the potent neuroleptics block central DA receptors. The mechanism by which DA receptor blockage is linked to increased DA turnover per se needs further investigation. In the aggregate the available data clearly indicate that neuroleptic drugs have marked effects upon brain DA systems.

The neuroleptic agents may also affect noradrenergic systems, but it would seem that this action is not crucial to the drugs' clinical effectiveness. There is disagreement as to the neuroleptic's ability to produce increased NE turnover. Some investigators find no effects, whereas others do. In those cases where changes in NE turnover have occurred as a consequence of treatment with the neuroleptics, the magnitude of the effect has been modest, inconsistent, and frequently occurred only at higher doses. The Swedish group of investigators, who in general have produced the affirmative data as to increased NE turnover after neuroleptics, have also produced data indicating that some potent neuroleptics are without effect on NE turnover.[5] Function-type studies indicate that while some neuroleptics block both DA and NE receptors, viz., chlorpromazine, others block principally or only DA receptors, viz., fluphenazine, spiroperidol, pimozide. Most importantly, those drugs which chiefly block DA receptors are among the more potent, at least in terms of dosage, of the neuroleptics. Phrased differently, the effectiveness of the neuroleptic drugs seems to be more related to their effects upon DA than to noradrenergic systems.

In the aggregate then, it is felt that a good case can be made for the hypothesis that dopaminergic systems, and not noradrenergic systems, are involved in the genesis of psychotic behavior that can be effectively treated with the neuroleptic drugs.

The neuroleptic drugs alter brain 5-HT systems, but this area has been less extensively studied; and the interpretation of the available data is made difficult by variations in results as a function of dose, and questions as to mechanisms by which the drugs produce their effects.

Finally, the question arises as to the possibility that a *specific* dopaminergic system may be involved in the production of psychotic states. As before, sufficient data to even modestly approach this question is unavailable. Histochemical-fluorescent techniques do not indicate a differential action of the neuroleptics on the meso-limbic or nigro-striatal brain DA systems. The future development of drugs that block DA receptors, but are without extrapyramidal side effects, may help with this issue, in that the retention or loss of the antipsychotic properties may allow one to differentiate between the neuroleptic activity being mediated via nigro-striatal versus meso-limbic DA systems. In this respect it is of interest that Bobon et al.[19] reported that pimozide produces a low incidence of Parkinsonismlike side effects, but caution is needed, in that in experimental animals this drug clearly blocks DA receptors in the striatum and is concentrated in the caudate nucleus.

❰ Bibliography

1. AGHAJANIAN, G. and F. BLOOM. "Electron Microscopic Localization of Tritiated NE in Rat Brain: Effect of Drugs," *J. Pharmacol. Exp. Ther.*, 156 (1967), 407–416.
2. AGHAJANIAN, G., F. BLOOM, and M. SHEARD. "Electron Microscopy of Degeneration Within the Serotonin Pathway of Rat Brain," *Brain Res.*, 13 (1969), 266–273.
3. AHLSKOG, J. and B. HOEBEL. "Hyperphagia Resulting From Selective Destruction of an Ascending Adrenergic Pathway in the Rat Brain," *Fed. Abstr.*, 1002 (1972), 397. Also personal communication.
4. ALPERS, H. S. and H. HIMWICH. "An In Vitro Study of the Effects of Tricyclic Antidepressant Drugs on the Accumulation of ¹⁴C-5HT by Rabbit Brain," *Biol. Psychiatry*, 1 (1969), 81–85.
5. ANDEN, N., S. BUTCHER, H. CORRODI et al. "Receptor Activity and Turnover of Dopamine and Noradrenaline after Neuroleptics," *Eur. J. Pharmacol.*, 11 (1970), 303–314.
6. ANDEN, N., H. CORRODI, K. FUXE et al. "Increased Impulse Flow in Bulbospinal NA Neurons Produced by CA Receptors Blocking Agents," *Eur. J. Pharmacol.*, 2 (1967), 59–64.
7. ANDEN, N., H. CORRODI, K. FUXE et al. "Evidence for a Central NE Receptor Stimulation by Clonidine," *Life Sci.*, 9 (1970), 513–523.
8. ANDEN, N., A. DAHLSTRÖM, K. FUXE et al. "The Effect of Haloperidol and Chlorpromazine on the Amine Levels of Central Monoamine Neurons," *Acta Physiol. Scand.*, 68 (1966), 419–420.
9. ANDEN, N., A. DAHLSTRÖM, K. FUXE et al. "Further Evidence for the Presence of Nigro-Neostriatal DA Neurons in the Rat," *Am. J. Anat.*, 116 (1965), 329–333.
10. ——. "Mapping Out CA and 5-HT Neurons Innervating the Telencephalon and Diencephalon," *Life Sci.*, 4 (1965), 1275–1291.
11. ——. "Functional Role of the Nigro-Neostriatal Dopamine Neurons," *Acta Pharmacol. Toxicol.*, 24 (1966), 263–274.
12. ANDEN, N., A. DAHLSTRÖM, K. FUXE et al. "Ascending Monoamine Neurons to the Telencephalon and Diencephalon," *Acta Physiol. Scand.*, 67 (1966), 313–326.
13. ANDEN, N. E., B. E. ROOS, and B. WERDINIUS. "Effects of Chlorpromazine, Haloperidol and Reserpine on the Levels of Phenolic Acids in Rabbit Corpus Striatum," *Life Sci.*, 3 (1964), 149.
14. ARNFRED, T. and A. RANDRUP. "Cholinergic Mechanisms in Brain Inhibiting Amphetamine Induced Stereotyped Behavior," *Acta Pharmacol. Toxicol.*, 26 (1968), 384–394.
15. BICKEL, M. H. "Metabolism and Structure-Activity Relationships of Thymoleptic Drugs," in S. Garattini and M. N. G.

Dukes, eds., *Antidepressant Drugs*, pp. 3–9. Milan: Excerp. Med. Found., 1966.

16. BICKEL, M. H. and B. B. BRODIE. "Structure and Antidepressant Activity of Imipramine Analogues," *Int. J. Neuropharmacol.*, 3 (1964), 611–621.

17. BJARKLUND, A., B. EHINGER, and B. FALCK. "A Method for Differentiating DA from NE in Tissue Sections by Microspectrofluorometry," *J. Histochem. Cytochem.*, 16 (1968), 263–270.

18. BLACKBURN, K. T., D. C. FUNCH, and R. J. MERRILLS. "5-HT Uptake by Rat Brain In Vitro," *Life Sci.*, 6 (1967), 1653–1663.

19. BOBON, J., J. COLLARD, A. PINCHARD et al. "Neuroleptiques a longue durée d'action II. Étude pilote du pimozide (R6238)," *Acta Neurol. Belg.*, 68 (1968), 137–153.

20. BRODIE, B. B., E. COSTA, A. GROPPETTI et al. "Interaction Between Desipramine, Tyramine, and Amphetamine at Adrenergic Neurones," *Br. J. Pharmacol.*, 34 (1968), 648–658.

21. BUNNEY, W. E., JR. and J. M. DAVIS. "Norepinephrine in Depressive Reactions," *Arch. Gen. Psychiatry*, 13 (1965), 483–494.

22. BURKARD, W. P., K. F. GEY, and A. PLETSCHER. "Activation of Tyrosine Hydroxylation in Rat Brain In Vivo by Chlorpromazine," *Nature*, 213 (1967), 732.

23. CARLSSON, A. "Structural Specificity for Inhibition of [14C]-5-hydroxytryptamine Uptake by Cerebral Slices," *J. Pharm. Pharmacol.*, 22 (1970), 729–732.

24. CARLSSON, A., H. CORRODI, K. FUXE et al. "Effect of Antidepressant Drugs on the Depletion of Intraneuronal Brain 5-hydroxytryptamine Stores Caused by 4-Methyl-*a*-Ethyl-Meta-Tyramine," *Euro J. Pharmacol.*, 5 (1969), 357–366.

25. ——. "Effects of Some Antidepressant Drugs on the Depletion of Intraneuronal Brain Catecholamine Stores Caused by 4,*a*-Dimethyl-Meta-Tyramine," *Eur. J. Pharmacol.*, 5 (1969), 367–373.

26. CARLSSON, A., K. FUXE, B. HAMBERGER et al. "Biochemical and Histochemical Studies on the Effects of Imipramine-Like Drugs and (+)−Amphetamine on Central and Peripheral Catecholamine Neurons," *Acta Physiol. Scand.*, 67 (1966), 481–497.

27. CARLSSON, A. and M. LINDQUIST. "Effect of CPZ on Haloperidol on Formation of 3-Methoxytyramine and Normetanephrine

28. COOLS, A. and J. VAN ROSSUM. "Caudal Dopamine and Stereotype Behavior of Cats," *Arch. Int. Pharmacodyn.*, 187 (1970), 163–173.

29. CORRODI, H. "Decreased Turnover in Central 5-HT Nerve Terminals Induced by Antidepressant Drugs of the Imipramine Type," *Eur. J. Pharmacol.*, 7 (1969), 56–59.

30. CORRODI, H. and K. FUXE. "The Effect of Imipramine on Central Monoamine Neurons, *J. Pharm. Pharmacol.*, 20 (1968), 230–231.

31. CORRODI, H., K. FUXE, and T. HOKFELT. "The Effect of Neuroleptics on the Activity of Central Catecholamine Neurons," *Life Sci.*, 6 (1972), 767–774.

32. CROW, T. "A Map of the Rat Mesericephalon for Electrical Self-Stimulation," *Brain Res.*, 36 (1972), 265–273.

33. CROW, T., P. SPEAR, and G. ARBUTHNOTL. "Intracranial Self-Stimulation With Electrodes in the Region of the Locus Coeruleus," *Brain Res.*, 36 (1972), 275–287.

34. DAHLSTRÖM, A. and K. FUXE. "Evidence for the Existence of Monoamine Containing Neurons in the CNS: I. Demonstration of Monoamines in the Cell Bodies of Brain Stem Neurons," *Acta Physiol. Scand.*, Suppl., 232 (1965), 1–55.

35. DA PRADA, M. and A. PLETSCHER. "Acceleration of the Cerebral Dopamine Turnover by Chlorpromazine," *Experientia*, 22 (1966), 465–466.

36. DINGELL, J. V., SULSER, F., and J. R. GILLETTE. "Species Differences in the Metabolism of Imipramine and Desmethylimipramine (DMI)," *J. Pharmacol. Exp. Ther.*, 143 (1964), 14–22.

37. DOMINO, E. and M. OLDS. "Cholinergic Inhibition of Self-Stimulation Behavior," *J. Pharmacol. Exp. Ther.*, 211 (1968), 164–202.

38. FALCK, B. "Observations on the Possibilities of the Cellular Localization of Monoamines by a Fluorescence Method," *Acta Physiol. Scand.*, Suppl. 197, (1962), 1–25.

39. FOG, R., A. RANDRUP, and H. PAKKENBURG. "Neuroleptic Action of Quarternary Chlorpromazine and Related Drugs Injected into Various Brain Areas in Rats," *Psychopharmacologia*, 12 (1968), 428–432.

40. FUXE, K. "The Distribution of Monoamine

Terminals in the CNS," *Acta Physiol. Scand.*, Suppl. 247, (1965), 38–86.

41. FUXE, K. and T. HOKFELT. "Catecholamines in the Hypothalamus and the Pituitary Gland," in W. Ganong and L. Martini, eds., *Frontiers in Neuroendocrinology*, pp. 47–96. New York: Oxford University Press, 1969.

42. FUXE, K., T. HOKFELT, and U. UNGERSTEDT. "Localization of Indolealkylamines in the CNS," *Adv. Pharmacol.*, 6 (1968), 235–251.

43. ———. "Central Monoaminergic Tracts," *Princ. Psychopharmacol.*, 6 (1970), 87–96.

44. ———. "Morphological and Functional Aspects of Central Monoamine Neurons," *Int. Rev. Neurobiol.*, 13 (1970), 93–126.

45. FUXE, K. and U. UNGERSTEDT. "Histochemical Studies of the Effect of (+)−Amphetamine, Drugs of the Imipramine Group, and Tryptamine on Central Catecholamine and 5-HT Neurons After Intraventricular Injection of Catecholamines and 5-HT," *Eur. J. Pharmacol.*, 4 (1968), 135–144.

46. GEY, K. F. and A. PLETSCHER. "Influence of Chlorpromazine and Chlorprothixene on the Cerebral Metabolism of 5-Hydroxytryptamine, Norepinephrine and Dopamine," *J. Pharmacol. Exp. Ther.*, 133 (1961), 18–24.

47. ———. "Alteration of Turnover of ^{14}C-Catecholamines in Rat Brain by Chlorpromazine," *Experientia*, 24 (1968), 335–336.

48. GIACALONE, E. and W. KOSTOWSKI. "5-Hydroxytryptamine and 5-Hydroxyindoleacetic Acid in Rat Brain: Effect of Some Psychotropic Drugs and Electrical Stimulation of Various Forebrain Areas," *Br. J. Pharmacol.*, 34 (1968), 662–663.

49. GILLETTE, J. R., J. V. DINGELL, and G. P. QUINN. "Physiological Distribution and Metabolism of Imipramine (Tofranil)," *Fed. Proc.*, Part I, 19 (1960), 137.

50. GILLETTE, J. R., J. V. DINGELL, F. SULSER et al. "Isolation from Rat Brain of a Metabolic Product, Desmethylimipramine, that Mediates the Antidepressant Activity of Imipramine (Tofranil)," *Experientia*, 17 (1961), 417–418.

51. GLOWINSKI, J. "Release of Monoamines In Central Nervous Systems," in H. J. Schumann and G. Kroneberg, eds., *New Aspects of Storage and Release Mechanisms of CA*, p. 301. Berlin: Springer-Verlag, 1970.

52. GLOWINSKI, J. and J. AXELROD. "Inhibition of Uptake of Tritiated-Noradrenaline in the Intact Rat Brain by Imipramine and Structurally Related Compounds," *Nature*, 204 (1964), 1318–1319.

53. GLOWINSKI, J., J. AXELROD, and L. L. IVERSON. "Regional Studies of Catecholamines in the Rat Brain. IV. Effects of Drugs on the Disposition and Metabolism of ^{3}H-NE and ^{3}H-Dopamine," *J. Pharmacol. Exp. Ther.*, 153 (1966), 30–41.

54. GULDBERG, H. C. and C. YATES. "Effects of Chlorpromazine on the Metabolism of Catecholamines in Dog Brain," *Br. J. Pharmacol.*, 36 (1969), 535–548.

55. GUMULKA, W., R. SAMANIN, and L. VALZELLI. "Effect of Chlorpromazine on 5-Hydroxytryptamine Metabolism in Hippocampal Stimulated Rats," *Eur. J. Pharmacol.*, 12 (1970), 276–279.

56. HÄGGENDAL, T. and B. HAMBERGER. "Quantitative In Vivo Studies on Noradrenaline Uptake and Its Inhibition by Amphetamines, Desimipramine and Chlorpromazine," *Acta Physiol. Scand.*, 70 (1967), 277–280.

57. HELLER, A. and R. MOORE. "Effect of CNS Lesions on Brain Monoamines in the Rat," *J. Pharmacol. Exp. Ther.*, 150 (1965), 1–9.

58. HERRMANN, B. and R. PULVER. "Der Stoffwechsel Des Psychopharmakons Tofranifl," *Arch. Int. Pharmacodyn*, 126 (1960), 454–468.

59. HIMWICH, W., J. DAVIS, K. LEINER et al. "Biochemical Effects of Haloperidol in Different Species," *Biol. Psychiatry*, 2 (1970), 315–319.

60. IGIC, R., P. STERN, and E. BASAGIC. "Changes in Emotional Behavior After Application of Cholinesterase Inhibitor in the Septal and Amygdala Region," *Neuropharmacology*, 9 (1970), 73–75.

61. JANOWSKY, D., J. DAVIS, M. EL-YOUSEF et al. "Physostigmine Reversal of Methyl Phenidate Induced Stereotyped Behavior." Submitted for publication, 1972.

62. JANOWSKY, D., M. EL-YOUSEF, and J. DAVIS. "Cholinergic Adrenergic Balance and Affective Disorders," Annu. Meet. Am. Psychiatr. Assoc., Dallas, Texas, 1972.

63. JANOWSKY, D., M. EL-YOUSEF, J. DAVIS et al. "Cholinergic Reversal of Manic Symptoms, *Lancet*, 1 (1972), 1236–1237.

64. JANSSEN, P. A. J., C. J. E. NIEMEGEERS, K. H. L. SCHELLEKENS et al. "Pimozide, a Chemically Novel Highly Potent and

Orally Long-Acting Neuroleptic Drug. Parts I, II, and III," *Arzneim. Forsch.*, 18, (1968), 261–287.

65. JANSSEN, P. A. J., C. J. E. NIEMEGEERS, K. H. L. SCHELLEKENS et al. "Is it Possible to Predict the Clinical Effects of Neuroleptic Drugs (Major Tranquillizers) From Animal Data?" *Arzneim. Forsch.*, 17 (1967), 841–854.

66. JONSSON, G. *The Formaldehyde Flourescence Method for the Histochemical Demonstration of Biogenic Monamines*, pp. 1–50. Stockholm: Ivar Haeggstroms Tryckeri AB, 1967.

67. JOUVET, M. "Neurophysiology of the States of Sleep," *Physiol. Rev.*, 47, (1967), 117–177.

68. ———. "Neuropharmacology of Sleep," in D. Efron, ed., *Psychopharmacology, a Review of Progress 1957–1967*, pp. 523–540. Washington: U.S. Govt. Print. Off., 1968.

69. JUNG, O. and E. BOYD. "Effects of Cholinergic Drugs on Self-Stimulation Response Rates in Rats." *Am. J. Physiol.*, 210, (1966), 432–434.

70. KLEIN, D. F. and J. M. DAVIS. *Diagnosis and Drug Treatment of Psychiatric Disorders*, p. 480. Baltimore: Williams & Wilkins, 1969.

71. KOELLE, G. and J. FRIEDENWALD. "A Histochemical Method for Localizing Cholinesterase Activity," *Proc. Soc. Exp. Biol. Med.*, 70 (1949), 617–622.

72. KOSTOWSKI, W. and E. GIACALONE. "Stimulation of Various Forebrain Structures and Brain 5HT, 5HIAA and Behavior in Rats," *Eur. J. Pharmacol.*, 7 (1969), 176–179.

73. KOSTOWSKI, W., E. GIACALONE, S. GARATTINI et al. "Studies on Behavioral and Biochemical Changes in Rats After Lesion of Midbrain Raphe," *Eur. J. Pharmacol.*, 4 (1968), 371–376.

74. ———. "Electrical Stimulation of Midbrain Raphe: Biochemical, Behavioral, and Bioelectric Effects," *Eur. J. Pharmacol.*, 7 (1969), 170–175.

75. KUHUR, M., R. ROTH, and G. AGHAJANIAN. "Selective Reduction of Tryptophan Hydroxylase Activity in Rat Forebrain After Midbrain Raphe Lesions," *Brain Res.*, 35 (1971), 167–176.

76. LAVERTY, R. and D. F. SHARMAN. "Modification by Drugs in the Metabolism of 3, 4-Dehydroxyphenylethylamine, Noradrenaline, and 5-Hydroxytryptamine in the

Brain," *Br. J. Pharmacol.*, 24 (1965), 759–772.

77. LEITZ, F. H. "Mechanisms by Which Amphetamine and Desipramine Inhibit the Metaraminol-Induced Release of Norepinephrine From Sympathetic Nerve Endings in Rat Heart," *J. Pharmacol. Exp. Ther.*, 173 (1970), 152–157.

78. LEWIS, P. and C. SHUTE. "The Cholinergic Limbic System," *Brain*, 90 (1967), 521–540.

79. MANDELL, A. J., D. S. SEGAL, T. KUCZENSKI et al. "Some Macromolecular Mechanisms in CNS Neurotransmitter Pharmacology and Their Psychobiological Organizations," in J. McGough ed., *Brain Mechanisms and Behavior*. New York: Plenum, forthcoming.

80. MARGULES, D. "Localization of the Anti-Punishment Actions of NE and Atropine in Amygdala and Entopeduncular Nucleus of Rats," *Brain Res.*, 35 (1971), 177–184.

81. MARGULES, D. and L. STEIN. "Cholinergic Synapses of a Periventricular Punishment System in the Medial Hypothalamus," *Am. J. Physiol.*, 17 (1969), 475–480.

82. ———. "Cholinergic Synapses in the Ventromedial Hypothalamus for the Suppression of Operant Behavior by Punishment and Satiety," *J. Comp. Physiol. Psychol.*, 67 (1969), 327–335.

83. MAXWELL, R. A., E. CHAPLIN, S. B. ECKHARDT et al. "Conformational Similarities Between Molecular Models of Phenethylamine and of Potent Inhibitors of the Uptake of Tritiated Norepinephrine by Adrenergic Nerves in Rabbit Aorta," *J. Pharmacol. Exp. Ther.*, 173 (1970), 158–165.

84. MAXWELL, R. A., S. B. ECKHARDT, and G. HITE. "Kinetic and Thermodynamic Considerations Regarding the Inhibition by Tricyclic Antidepressants of the Uptake of Tritiated Norepinephrine by the Adrenergic Nerves in Rabbit Aortic Strips," *J. Pharmacol. Exp. Ther.*, 171 (1970), 62–69.

85. MAXWELL, R. A., P. D. KEENAN, E. CHAPLIN et al. "Molecular Features Affecting the Potency of Tricyclic Antidepressants and Structurally Related Compounds as Inhibitors of the Uptake of Tritiated Norepinephrine by Rabbit Aortic Strips. *J. Pharmacol. Exp. Ther.*, 166 (1969), 320–329.

86. McMahon, R. E., F. J. Marshall, H. W. Culp. et al. "The Metabolism of Nortripty-line-N-Methyl-^{14}C in Rats," *Biochem. Pharmacol.*, 12, (1963), 1207–1217.

87. Meek, J. and B. Werdinius. "Hydroxy-tryptamine Turnover Decreased by the Antidepressant Drug Chlorimipramine," *J. Pharm. Pharmacol.*, 22, (1970), 141–143.

88. Moore, R., R. Bhatnagar, and A. Heller. "Anatomical and Chemical Studies of a Nigro-Neostriatal Projection in the Cat," *Brain Res.*, 30, (1971), 119–135.

89. Moore, R., A. Björklund, and U. Stenevi. "Plastic Changes in the Adrenergic Inner-vation of the Rat Septal Area in Response to Denervation," *Brain Res.*, 33, (1971), 13–35.

90. Neff, N. H. and E. Costa. "Effect of Tricyclic Antidepressants and Chlorpro-mazine on Brain Catecholamine Synthesis," in S. Garattini and M. N. G. Dukes, eds., *Antidepressant Drugs*. Milan: Excerp. Med. Found., 1966.

91. Nyback, H., Z. Borgecki, and G. Sedvall. "Accumulation and Disappearance of Catecholamines Formed From Tyrosine ^{14}C in Mouse Brain; Effect of Some Psy-chotrophic Drugs," *Eur. J. Pharmacol.*, 4, (1968), 395–403.

92. Nyback, H. and G. Sedvall. "Effect of Chlorpromazine on Accumulation and Disappearance of Catecholamines Formed From ^{14}C-Tyrosine in Brain," *J. Pharmacol. Exp. Ther.*, 162 (1968), 294–301.

93. ———. "Further Studies on the Accumula-tion and Disappearance of Catecholamines Formed From Tyrosine ^{14}C in Mouse Brain. Effect of Some Phenothiazine An-alogues," *Eur. J. Pharmacol.*, 10, (1970), 193–205.

94. Nyback, H., G. Sedvall, and I. J. Kopin. "Accelerated Synthesis of Dopamine-^{14}C From Tyrosine-^{14}C in Rat Brain After Chlorpromazine," *Life Sci.*, 6 (1967), 2307–2312.

95. Olds, M. and J. Olds. "Approach-Avoidance Analysis of Rat Diencephalon," *J. Comp. Neurol.*, 120 (1963), 259–295.

96. Palaic, D., I. Page, and P. Khairallah. "Uptake and Metabolism of [^{14}C] Sero-tonin in Rat Brain," *J. Neurochem.*, 14 (1967), 63–69.

97. Poirier, L., E. McGeer, L. Larochelle et al. "The Effect of Brain Stem Lesions on Tyrosine and Tryptophan Hydroxylases in Various Structures of the Telencephalon of the Cat," *Brain Res.*, 14 (1969), 147–155.

98. Pradham, S. and S. Dutta. "Central Cholinergic Mechanism and Behavior," *Int. Rev. Neurobiol.*, 14 (1971), 173–231.

99. Randrup, A., I. Munkvard, and P. Udsen. "Adrenergic Mechanisms and Amphet-amine Induced Abnormal Behaviors," *Acta Pharmacol. Toxicol.*, 20 (1963), 145–157.

100. Ross, S. B. and A. L. Renyi. "Inhibition of the Uptake of Tritiated Catecholamines by Antidepressant and Related Agent," *Eur. J. Pharmacol.*, 2 (1967), 181–186.

101. ———. "Inhibition of the Uptake of Tri-tiated 5-Hydroxytryptamine in Brain Tissue," *Eur. J. Pharmacol.*, 7 (1969), 270–277.

102. Salama, A. I., J. R. Insalaco, and R. A. Maxwell. "Concerning the Molecular Re-quirements for the Inhibition of the Up-take of Racemic ^{3}H-Norepinephrine into Rat Cerebral Cortex Slices by Tricyclic Antidepressants and Related Compounds," *J. Pharmacol. Exp. Ther.*, 173 (1971), 474–481.

103. Schanberg, S. M., J. J. Schildkraut, and I. J. Kopin. "The Effects of Psychoactive Drugs on Norepinephrine ^{3}H Metabolism in Brain," *Biochem. Pharmacol.*, 16 (1967), 393–399.

104. Schildkraut, J. J. "The Catecholamine Hypothesis of Affective Disorders: A Re-view of Supporting Evidence," *Am. J. Psychiatry*, 122 (1965), 509–522.

105. ———. "Changes in Norepinephrine-H^{3} (NE-H^{3}) Metabolism in Rat Brain After Acute and Chronic Administration of Tricyclic Antidepressants," *Fed. Proc.*, 28 (1969), 795.

106. Schildkraut, J. J. and S. S. Kety. "Biogenic Amines and Emotion, *Science*, 156 (1967), 21–30.

107. Schildkraut, J. S. Schanberg, G. Breese et al. "Effects of Psychoactive Drugs on the Metabolism of Intracisternally Adminis-tered Serotonin in Rat Brain," *Biochem. Pharmacol.*, 18 (1969), 1971–1978.

108. Schildkraut, J., A. Winokur, and C. Ap-plegate. "Norepinephrine Turnover and Metabolism in Rat Brain After Long-Term Administration of Imipramine," *Science*, 168 (1970), 867–869.

109. Schildkraut, J., A. Winokur, P. R. Dras-

KOCZY et al. "Changes in NE Turnover in Rat Brain During Chronic Administration of Imipramine and Protryptyline: A Possible Explanation for the Delay in Onset of Clinical Antidepressant Effects," *Am. J. Psychiat.*, 127 (1971), 1032–1039.

110. SCHUBERT, J., H. NYBACK, and G. SEDVALL. "Effect of Antidepressant Drugs on Accumulation and Disappearance of Monoamines Formed In Vivo From Labelled Precursors in Mouse Brain," *J. Pharm. Pharmacol.*, 22 (1970), 136–138.

111. SHUTE, C. and P. LEWIS. "The Ascending Cholinergic Reticular System," *Brain*, 90 (1967), 497–520.

112. SLADEK, J. R., JR. "Differences in the Distribution of Catecholamine Varicosities in Cat and Rat Reticular Formation," *Science*, 174 (1971), 410–412.

113. SMITH, D., M. KING, and B. HOEBEL. "Lateral Hypothalamic Control of Killing: Evidence for a Cholinoceptive Mechanism," *Science*, 167 (1970), 900–901.

114. SNYDER, S. H., K. M. TAYLOR, J. T. COYLE et al. "The Role of Brain Dopamine in Behavioral Regulation and the Actions of Psychotropic Drugs", *Am. J. Psychiat.*, 127 (1970), 199–207.

115. STARK, P. and E. BOYD. "Effects of Cholinergic Drugs on Hypothalamic Self-Stimulation Response Rates in Dogs", *Am J. Psychiat.*, 205, (1963), 745–748.

116. STEINBERG, M. I. and C. B. SMITH. "Effects of Desmethylimipramine and Cocaine on the Uptake, Retention and Metabolism of H^3-Tyramine in Rat Brain Slices," *J. Pharmacol. Exp. Ther.*, 173 (1970), 176–192.

117. SULSER, F., M. L. OWENS, S. J. STRADA et al. "Modification by Desipramine (DMI) of the Availability of Norepinephrine Released by Reserpine in the Hypothalamus of the Rat In Vivo," *J. Pharmacol. Exp. Ther.*, 168 (1969), 272–286.

118. TAGLIAMONTE, A., P. TAGLIAMONTE, and G. L. GESSA. "Reserpine-Like Action of Chlorpromazine on Rabbit Basal Ganglia," *J. Neurochem.*, 17 (1970), 733–738.

119. UNGERSTEDT, U. "Stereotaxic Mapping of the Monoamine Pathways in the Rat Brain," *Acta Physiol. Scand.*, Suppl. 367 (1971), 1–48.

120. ———. "Striated DA Release After Amphetamine or Nerve Degeneration Revealed by Rotational Behavior," *Acta Physiol. Scand.*, Suppl. 367, (1971), 49–68.

121. ———. "Adipsia and Aphagia After 6-OH-DA Induced Degeneration of the Nigro-Striatal DA System," *Acta Physiol. Scand.*, Suppl. 367 (1971), 95–122.

122. UNGERSTEDT, U., L. BUTCHER, S. BUTCHER et al. "Direct Chemical Stimulation of Dopaminergic Mechanisms in the Neostriatum of the Rat," *Brain Res.*, 14 (1969), 467–471.

123. WISE, C. and L. STEIN. "Facilitation of Brain Self-Stimulation by Central Administration of NE," *Science*, 163 (1969), 299–301.

CHAPTER 21

DEPRESSIONS AND BIOGENIC AMINES*

Joseph J. Schildkraut

Even in descriptive psychiatry the definition of melancholia is uncertain; it takes on various clinical forms (some of them suggesting somatic rather than psychogenic affections) that do not seem definitely to warrant reduction to a unity.

Sigmund Freud, *Mourning and Melancholia*

See also p. 478

❨ Introduction

THE STUDIES of biogenic amine metabolism in the depressive disorders were identified in the first edition of the *American Handbook of Psychiatry* as one of the most promising and rapidly evolving areas of biochemical research in psychiatry.[68] Examination of the present chapter, in relation to that earlier one, will serve to document the extensive development of this field during the past several years. Aspects of this expanding literature have been reviewed frequently.†

Advances in pharmacology have served to stimulate this area of neurochemical research in psychiatry through the introduction of drugs (e.g., monoamine oxidase inhibitor antidepressants, tricyclic antidepressants and lithium salts) which proved to be effective in the treatment of depressive and manic disorders, and through the elucidation of the effects of these drugs on biogenic amine metabolism.[189, 188,186] Various aspects of this area of neuropharmacology, as well as the basic biology of the biogenic amines, have been considered in a number of recent reviews.‡ Despite some discrepancies, most data seem compatible with the hypothesis that drugs which are effective in the treatment of depressions may increase one or another of the biogenic amines at receptor sites in brain, whereas drugs that

* I wish to thank Mrs. Gladys Rege and Miss Barbara Keeler for their assistance in the preparation of this chapter. This work was supported in part by USPHS Grant No. MH 15413 awarded by the National Institute of Mental Health.

† See references 28, 32, 44, 56, 57, 84, 102, 121, 158, 167, 186, 188, 199, and 227.

‡ See references 6, 13, 24, 58, 80, 103, 113, 155, 186, 188, 192, 199, 219.

cause depressions or are effective in the treatment of manias may decrease the activity of monoamines at receptors.

Studies of the metabolism and physiology of the biogenic amines in patients with affective disorders (depressions and manias) have focused on the catecholamines (norepinephrine, epinephrine, and dopamine) or the indoleamines (serotonin and tryptamine). Since direct biochemical assay of brain tissue in living man is not feasible, most research has involved the assay of monoamines or their metabolites in one or another body fluid under various clinical or pharmacological conditions. In accordance with the rationale described in the first edition of the *Handbook*, these studies have explored the biochemical differences between depressed, manic, and control subjects, utilizing cross-sectional research designs, and have also examined the biochemical changes that accompany alterations in affective state in depressed or manic patients studied longitudinally.[68]

The importance of differentiating among the different types of depressive disorders when prescribing treatment has been stressed by many investigators, and the differential responses of various types of depressions to one or another treatment modality have been documented in numerous studies.* Similarly, the heterogeneity of the depressive disorders has been emphasized in relation to the design and interpretation of biochemical studies.[188] Although many of the presently available systems for classifying the depressions on the basis of clinical signs, symptoms, and history are of some value in this regard, these classifications represent limited and temporary solutions to this very basic problem in psychiatry.

A common feature of several of these classifications is the separation, on the basis of clinical syndromes, of one particular group of depressions variously designated "endogenous," "vital," "major," or "retarded" depressions. These depressions, which may constitute only 10 to 20 percent of all depressive disorders, are generally unresponsive to interpersonal forms of treatment or the administration

of placebos, but they are relatively responsive to vigorous treatment with one or another of the antidepressant drugs or electroconvulsive therapy; and many neurochemical studies have focused on this group of depressions. A further subtype of the depressive disorders (of some biological importance) is based on the history of a prior manic or hypomanic episode, and is variably designated as the manic-depressive or bipolar disorders; these depressions are generally subsumed under the broader category of endogenous depressions. The manic-depressive depressions constitute what is probably the most homogeneous clinically defined subgroup of the depressive disorders, although the possibility of heterogeneity even within this subgroup cannot be excluded. The manic-depressive (i.e., bipolar) depressions are distinguished from the unipolar depressions, which are characterized by the absence of a prior episode of mania or hypomania. It is worth noting that this dichotomy of the depressive disorders (unless further subdivided) gives rise to a relatively homogeneous subtype, the manic-depressive depressions and the heterogeneous remainder, the unipolar depressions. Other dichotomous separations of the depressive disorders that have been employed in one or another study include: retarded versus nonretarded (or agitated or anxious); psychotic versus neurotic; endogenous versus nonendogenous, which embraces characterological, situational, or reactive depressions.

The problems inherent in these dichotomies, which in most instances separate a relatively homogenous subgroup from the heterogeneous remainder, as well as other issues related to more complex systems for classifying the depressive disorders on the basis of clinical signs, symptoms, and history are discussed in detail elsewhere.[188] While the need for systems of classification that are more meaningful biologically is widely recognized, it seems likely that further refinements in our capacity to differentiate among the depressive disorders and to prescribe treatment more rationally may be expected only when clinical distinctions can be augmented by biochemical or physiological criteria.[189]

* See references 1, 8, 94, 120, 122, 175, and 188.

note bearing of this on Fancher (letter) re testability of Freud's aetiology

For a number of years, investigators have recognized the possibility that different subgroups of patients with depressive disorders might exhibit different specific alterations in the metabolism of one or another of the monoamines; and it was suggested that studies of biogenic amine metabolism might ultimately contribute to the development of a more meaningful biochemical classification of the affective disorders and a more rational approach to the treatment of these disorders.[186,204] The present review, which is more representative than comprehensive, will examine the current status of research on biogenic amine metabolism in patients with depressive disorders, focusing on recent findings that indicate the possible emergence of biochemical criteria to predict differential responses to various modalites of treatment.

(Catecholamines and Related Substances

The alterations in catecholamine metabolism produced by drugs used in the treatment of the affective disorders have been studied extensively during the past decade.[188] On the basis of the initial findings of these studies, it was suggested that some, if not all, depressions may be associated with an absolute or relative deficiency of catecholamines, particularly norepinephrine at functionally important receptor sites in the brain, whereas manias may be associated with an excess of such monoamines. This formulation has come to be known as the catecholamine hypothesis of affective disorders.[186]

The functional deficiency of norepinephrine, suggested to occur in some (but not necessarily all) depressions may be seen as a final common pathway, since many environmental and constitutional factors could conceivably contribute to its development and several different biochemical mechanisms might be operative immediately in producing it.[204] These mechanisms could include decreased norepinephrine synthesis and output, impairment of norepinephrine binding and storage, increased enzymatic inactivation of norepinephrine by

deamination or O-methylation, increased inactivation by neuronal reuptake, and decreased receptor sensitivity to norepinephrine. The operation of these different mechanisms in one or another subtype of depressive disorder could possibly account for differences in clinical phenomenology and responses to pharmacological as well as psychotherapeutic interventions.[186]

Catecholamines, Normetanephrine and VMA in Urine and Blood

In a number of studies of manic-depressive patients, the urinary excretion of norepinephrine or dopamine (and, less consistently, epinephrine) has been found to be relatively lower during periods of depressions than during periods of manias or after recovery.* In one of these studies, a regular cycle of norepinephrine excretion was observed in cyclothymic manic-depressive patients, with increases starting during transition phases preceding manias and decreases starting in transition phases preceding depressions.[214] In another study that examined the transition from depression into mania in a small number of subjects, an increase in urinary norepinephrine was observed on the day prior to the onset of mania when patients exhibited a brief transition period of normal behavior and this increase of urinary norepinephrine continued during the manic period; although elevated dopamine levels were also observed during the manic phase, the increase in dopamine excretion, in contrast to norepinephrine, did not appear to precede the onset of mania.[34] Other investigators have also found increased dopamine excretion in manic patients.[138,216]

In a large series of manic patients, excretion of both norepinephrine and epinephrine was elevated above control values, but norepinephrine and epinephrine levels in a heterogeneous group of depressed patients were not different from control values; these depressed patients, however, did have a lowered catecholamine response to insulin stress.[10] Increased catecholamine excretion has been ob-

---

* See references 34, 96, 213, 214, 216, 217, and 220.

served in some depressed patients,[53] but mainly in those with agitated or anxious depressions.[95,216,227] In a recent study, elevated levels of plasma epinephrine and norepinephrine were observed in a group of patients with depression and anxiety most of whom were diagnosed as depressive or having anxiety neuroses; the correlation between the concentration of plasma catecholamines and the degree of anxiety was highly significant, whereas the correlation between plasma catecholamines and the degree of depression was not significant.[232] Depressed patients with delusions or hallucinations have been found to excrete higher levels of catecholamines (and metabolites) than patients who did not manifest these psychotic symptoms.[33,196] In one study, levels of norepinephrine in cerebrospinal fluid were reported to be higher in depressed and manic patients (as well as in schizophrenic patients) than in controls;[59] however, further studies will be needed to replicate these findings as well as to confirm the specificity of the method used to determine norepinephrine in cerebrospinal fluid.

A gradual rise in the excretion of normetanephrine, the O-methylated metabolite of norepinephrine that may reflect noradrenergic activity,[5,117,118] was observed during the period of definitive clinical improvement in a series of patients with endogenous depressions treated with the tricyclic antidepressant imipramine;[197] and this has recently been confirmed by other investigators.[*,126,169] Patients with retarded depressions had lower levels of normetanephrine excretion before treatment (when depressed) than after discontinuation of imipramine (when in clinical remission).[197] In some, but not all, patients with agitated depressions, normetanephrine as well as norepinephrine and epinephrine are higher during the depression than after improvement.[95]

---

* The tricyclic antidepressant imipramine as well as the monoamine oxidase inhibitor phenelzine was observed to decrease the urinary excretion of 3-methoxy-4-hydroxymandelic acid (VMA) in depressed patients, suggesting that the tricyclic antidepressants as well as the monoamine oxidase inhibitors might decrease the deamination of norepinephrine;[196,201] and this was subsequently demonstrated in studies in animals.[86,193,202]

In longitudinal studies, the excretion of normetanephrine has been observed to be relatively higher during manias or hypomanias than during depressions, with intermediate values observed in periods of remission; the magnitude of the normetanephrine elevations appears to be related to the clinical severity of the hypomanic symptoms.†

Although muscular activity may produce significant changes in catecholamine excretion,[109] the alterations in the excretion of the catecholamines or metabolites in association with changes in affective state did not appear to be a consequence of changes in motor activity in one study where this was specifically measured.[220] Moreover, the increases in urinary norepinephrine appeared to precede the onset of mania in two studies;[34,214] however, one cannot exclude the possibility that these increases in norepinephrine excretion might have been secondary to subtle behavioral or postural changes. Normetanephrine and metanephrine excretion have been reported to be elevated in association with agitated and unstable behavior in depressed patients and in other subjects.[144]

The urinary excretion of 3-methoxy-4-hydroxymandelic acid (VMA), a deaminated O-methylated metabolite of norepinephrine, has also been found to be relatively elevated during episodes of hypomania or mania when compared with normal or depressed phases.[36,183,220] The increase in VMA excretion appeared to be associated with the level of physical activity in one study,[183] but not in another.[220] In one longitudinal study, however, significant increases in urinary VMA were not observed during episodes of hypomania (relative to levels observed during retarded depressions or clinical remissions) despite significant increases in the levels of norepinephrine and normetanephrine as well as epinephrine during these hypomanic episodes;[96] this could conceivably reflect a relative decrease in the rate of deamination of norepinephrine and normetanephrine in some hypomanic patients, as suggested by the recent report of a decrease in platelet monoa-

† See references 96, 197, 198, and 220.

mine oxidase activity in some manic-depressive patients.[142]

After infusion with radioactive norepinephrine, patients with retarded depressions classified as manic-depressives were found to have an elevated ratio of radioactive amines to deaminated metabolites in the urine when compared with normal controls or patients with agitated unipolar depressions.[178,179] Many factors could account for this finding, including an alteration in the disposition of the infused radioactive norepinephrine as well as a decrease in the deamination of norepinephrine or normetanephrine in the manic-depressive depressed group.

Since all studies have not employed a uniform system for classifying the depressions, it is difficult to summarize the findings reviewed above. In general, however, norepinephrine and normetanephrine excretion appear to be relatively decreased in patients with retarded (endogenous) depressions and increased in patients with manias. The findings in patients with agitated or anxious depressions are less consistent and some of these patients seem to show increased excretion of norepinephrine and normetanephrine as well as epinephrine and metanephrine.

MHPG in Urine and Cerebrospinal Fluid

Because of the relatively effective brain-blood barrier to norepinephrine and normetanephrine,[87,127,185,228] it is probable that only a small fraction of urinary norepinephrine or normetanephrine derives from the brain. Thus, the urinary excretion of norepinephrine and normetanephrine may primarily reflect the activity of the peripheral sympathetic nervous system. It has been suggested recently that 3-methoxy-4-hydroxyphenylglycol (MHPG), a deaminated O-methylated metabolite of norepinephrine, may be the urinary metabolite of norepinephrine (and normetanephrine) that provides some index of the synthesis and metabolism of norepinephrine in the brain.[124,128] [184,185] All findings, however, do not support this,[41] and it is, moreover, generally recognized that the brain cannot be regarded as the

sole source of MHPG;[184] but recent studies in nonhuman primates suggest that approximately 50 percent of urinary MHPG may derive from norepinephrine originating in the brain.[124]

A number of studies have examined the excretion of MHPG in patients with affective disorders. In one of these studies, urinary MHPG was significantly lower in a diagnostically heterogeneous group of depressed patients than in a nondepressed control population.[126] Subsequent studies, however, indicate that all depressed patients do not excrete low levels of MHPG, but that this may be characteristic of a particular subgroup of depressive disorders and a criterion for predicting responses to specific forms of pharmacotherapy —as discussed below.[95,126,191,194]

In a longitudinal study of a small group of manic-depressive patients, levels of urinary MHPG were lower during depressions and higher during hypomanic episodes than after clinical remissions. The depressed patients in this study had agitated depressions, during which some showed relatively increased levels of norepinephrine and normetanephrine as well as epinephrine and metanephrine. Therefore, one cannot simply relate the reduced levels of MHPG in these depressed patients to a decrease in motor activity or a reduction in peripheral sympathetic or adrenomedullary activity.[95] Similar findings were observed in a longitudinal study of two manic-depressive patients in which urinary MHPG excretion was relatively elevated in the manic phases, decreased in the depressed phases, and intermediate during interval phases; these investigators felt that it was unlikely that the increased output of MHPG in the manic phase was simply a reflection of increased motor activity since the peaks of MHPG output occurred on different days and preceded the peaks of mania.[14]

The changes in MHPG excretion and affective state occurring in the context of amphetamine abuse and withdrawal were recently studied in a small group of patients.[205,226] During self-administration of amphetamines, the patients were clinically hypomanic and urinary MHPG excretion was elevated. Following the abrupt withdrawal of amphetamines, urinary MHPG excretion decreased and patients became depressed. Subsequently, there was a gradual increase in urinary MHPG excretion and a concurrent decrease in the depressive symptomatology. The changes in MHPG excretion occurred with or possibly preceded the clinical changes and were also associated with changes in REM sleep.[205,226] The changes in VMA excretion observed in this study were not similar to the changes in MHPG, suggesting that the latter were not simply a reflection of an increased output of norepinephrine or epinephrine from peripheral sympathetic nerves or adrenal glands during amphetamine administration, and a decreased output following withdrawal.[206]

However, the urinary excretion of MHPG has been shown to increase in response to various forms of stress[123,182] and may also vary in response to changes in motor activity or posture. Additional studies, therefore, will be needed to determine the extent to which these factors may have contributed to the changes in MHPG excretion observed to occur in association with changes in affective state.

Recent findings have suggested that the urinary excretion of MHPG may provide a biochemical basis for classifying depressed patients and for predicting the differential clinical responses to treatment with various tricyclic antidepressants. In one study it was found that patients who excreted relatively low levels of MHPG prior to treatment with imipramine or desmethylimipramine responded better to treatment with these agents than did patients who excreted relatively higher levels of MHPG. In this study, the patients who responded best to treatment excreted more normetanephrine and MHPG during drug treatment (relative to the predrug period), whereas those patients who responded least well had a decrease in the excretion of these two metabolites.[126] In another study of a small group of depressed patients, favorable responses to treatment with amitriptyline were observed in patients with relatively high levels of urinary MHPG but not in patients with lower levels of MHPG.[191,194]

While other possible interpretations cannot be excluded (as noted below) it has been suggested that the low levels of MHPG may reflect a reduced rate of synthesis of norepinephrine as well as a reduction in its net output from presynaptic neurons (i.e., a decrease in neuronal discharge or an increase in neuronal reuptake); whereas the higher levels of MHPG would be consistent with an increase in the enzymatic inactivation of norepinephrine or a deficiency in postsynaptic receptor sensitivity to norepinephrine, which is partially compensated by an increase in the output of norepinephrine from presynaptic neurons.[191] Findings compatible with these interpretations have been reported.[146,168,169] In these studies, patients with low MHPG excretion tended to have depressions that were often classified as manic-depressive, whereas patients with higher levels of MHPG tended to have depressions that were classified as chronic characterological (i.e., neurotic); but there were a number of exceptions to this association between MHPG excretion and clinical phenomenology or diagnostic subtype.

Another group of investigators was unable to confirm the finding that a favorable response to treatment with imipramine was associated with a low pretreatment level of MHPG; however, as the investigators noted, the patients in this study were drug free for as little as five days before the pretreatment MHPG levels were measured and residual drug effects may have influenced the initial MHPG values.[169] Further investigation will clearly be required to determine whether the level of MHPG excreted in the urine will provide a clinically useful criterion for classifying depressive disorders and predicting responses to pharmacotherapy.

Free and conjugated MHPG have been demonstrated in human cerebrospinal fluid,[93,184,229] and several studies have recently examined the levels of MHPG in the lumbar cerebrospinal fluid (CSF) of patients with affective disorders. In a small number of depressed patients (not classified with respect to diagnostic subtypes), MHPG levels were significantly lower than in control subjects.[93] Further studies from that laboratory have confirmed this decrease in CSF-MHPG levels in a larger series of depressed patients; CSF-MHPG levels were not different from control values in a small group of manic patients.[30] However, in another recent study, MHPG levels in CSF were not different from control values in a small heterogeneous group of depressed patients, but some manic patients showed markedly elevated levels of MHPG with a decrease to normal values during successful treatment with lithium carbonate.[230] In another small series of patients with recurrent (unipolar) depressions, manic-depressive depressions, and manias, there were no differences in the mean levels of MHPG between these various groups before treatment, nor did any significant changes occur after treatment; however, the investigators noted that there was a wide scatter in the concentrations of MHPG in the lumbar CSF of these patients (and this study differs from others in that a spectrophotofluorometric, rather than gas chromatographic, method was used to determine MHPG).[3]

While further studies of MHPG in the CSF of patients with affective disorders are clearly indicated, the available data suggest that levels of MHPG in the CSF may be decreased in some (but not all) depressed patients and increased in some patients with manias. However, some patients with affective disorders may have normal levels of MHPG in lumbar cerebrospinal fluid. As described above, similar findings have emerged from studies of urinary MHPG (as well as normetanephrine and norepinephrine) in patients with affective disorders. Differences in motor activity could conceivably contribute to these differences in levels of CSF MHPG, since the findings of a recent study demonstrated a statistically nonsignificant trend toward increases in CSF MHPG—as well as increases in homovanillic acid (HVA) and 5-hydroxy-indoleacetic acid (5HIAA)—after increased psychomotor activity was induced by simulating mania.[157] The differences in CSF levels of MHPG could also reflect differences in the rate of efflux of MHPG from the CSF rather than differences in its rate of production; simultaneous measurement of CSF MHPG and urinary MHPG

might help to clarify this—if the brain contributes as large a fraction (approximately 50 percent) of the urinary MHPG as recent findings suggest.[124]

HVA in Cerebrospinal Fluid

Homovanillic acid (HVA), a deaminated O-methylated metabolite of dopamine, can be determined in lumbar cerebrospinal fluid and may provide information about the cerebral metabolism of dopamine,[139] although some of the HVA in CSF may derive from brain capillaries.[7] Interpretation of such findings is further complicated by the fact that the concentration of HVA in lumbar CSF is considerably lower than in ventricular CSF, suggesting that there may be a transport system for the removal of HVA in the region of the fourth ventricle.[139]

Baseline levels of HVA in the CSF have been found to be lower in depressed patients than in control subjects in a number of recent studies.* In one study, decreased baseline HVA levels were observed in patients with retarded depressions but not in patients with nonretarded depressions,[163] but the decrease in CSF HVA did not appear to be related to motor activity in all studies.[149,157,230] In another study, patients with recurrent depressions (unipolar depressions) had lower HVA levels than patients with manic-depressive depressions (bipolar depressions)[3] but other investigators who found decreased levels of HVA in depressed patients (compared to controls) observed no differences in HVA levels between unipolar depressions and bipolar depressions.[137]

In one study the reduced levels of HVA observed in depressed patients did not increase after electroconvulsive therapy, although considerable clinical improvement was observed.[147] Another study indicated that the initial reduction of HVA in CSF in three depressed patients was followed by a relative increase after treatment; but one of these patients was noted to have shown little change in clinical condition and to have received large

* See references 22, 27, 137, 147, 149, 157, 177, and 230.

doses of L-Dopa for five weeks.[137] Other investigators observed no correlations between the changes in various clinical ratings and CSF-HVA values in a small group of depressed patients studied before and during treatment with amitriptyline; in this study HVA levels tended to decrease during treatment.[22]

Baseline levels of HVA in hypomanic and manic patients have been observed to be equal to or lower than control values in several studies.* In one of these studies, patients with severe mania, exhibiting a high degree of motor activity, had elevated levels of HVA, whereas levels of HVA in hypomanic patients were slightly lower than control values; the increased levels of HVA in patients with severe mania were attributed to increased motor activity and the fact that total bed rest often could not be maintained prior to the lumbar puncture.[157]

Because the rate of efflux of one or another metabolite from the CSF may vary over time and among subjects, measurements of the levels of these metabolites in lumbar CSF at an instant in time do not necessarily reflect the rates of production of the metabolites during a given time interval. Information of the latter sort may be obtained by blocking the efflux of acid metabolites from the cerebrospinal fluid with probenecid, a drug that inhibits the transport of the carboxylic acid metabolites of biogenic amines (e.g., HVA as well as 5-hydroxyindoleacetic acid (5HIAA), a deaminated metabolite of serotonin);[143] but in two clinical studies, probenecid did not appear to block the efflux of MHPG (a glycol) from the CSF.[93,119] Probenecid has been used more extensively in studies of 5HIAA, and the problems inherent in this technique are discussed in conjunction with these studies (see below).

Several studies have recently examined the accumulation of HVA in lumbar CSF following administration of probenecid in patients with affective disorders. (The difference between the level of HVA determined after probenecid administration and the baseline

level of HVA is referred to as the accumulation of HVA.) The accumulation of HVA following probenecid was decreased in a small group of depressed patients when compared with controls; the accumulation of HVA in manic patients was not different from control values.[177] In another study, the accumulation of HVA was significantly lower than control values in patients with retarded depressions, whereas the accumulation of HVA in patients with nonretarded depressions was slightly greater than control values.[163] The levels of HVA following probenecid administration (i.e., not accumulation since baseline levels were not subtracted) were higher in a diagnostically heterogeneous group of depressed patients than in a control population in one study.[20]

Tyrosine in Blood

The levels of tyrosine, an amino acid precursor of the catecholamines, in blood plasma of depressed patients have been examined by several investigators. In one study, manic-depressive patients showed no difference in the fasting levels of plasma tyrosine when compared with normal controls but both manic and depressed patients showed greater elevations of plasma tyrosine than did control subjects after an oral load of tyrosine.[221] In another study, plasma tyrosine levels of depressed patients were observed to be significantly lower at 8 A.M. when compared with normal controls, but this difference did not persist into the evening and it was suggested that depressed patients had an altered diurnal rhythm of plasma tyrosine.[12] In a third study, significantly lower levels of plasma tyrosine were observed at 11 A.M. in patients with endogenous depressions compared with neurotic depressives, schizophrenics, or healthy controls, but no significant differences were observed when tyrosine was measured at 8 A.M.; the response to an oral load of tyrosine was not significantly different in endogenous depressions when compared with controls.[9] Further investigations will be required to explore these apparent discrepancies.

* See references 22, 137, 157, 177, and 230.

Dopa Administration

Dihydroxyphenylalanine (Dopa), an amino-acid precursor of the catecholamines, can cross the blood-brain barrier, and under some conditions may elevate levels of dopamine or norepinephrine in the brain. Consequently, Dopa has been administered to patients with affective disorders, both to explore its clinical effects as well as to investigate the possible relationship of alterations in biogenic amine metabolism to changes in affective state. However, since the initial clinical trials of Dopa more than a decade ago, it has become apparent that in addition to increasing catecholamine levels, Dopa produces many other biochemical and neuropharmacological effects; consequently, the interpretation of the findings of such studies may not be as straightforward as was initially assumed.[110,187] One cannot be certain that the administration of Dopa will necessarily lead to an increased concentration of catecholamines at specific neuronal sites; nor can one be certain that any clinical effects observed are direct physiological effects of catecholamines derived from Dopa rather than the pharmacological effects of Dopa acting directly or indirectly upon other monoaminergic systems (i.e., by releasing monoamines, by displacing monoamines through the production of false transmitters, or by interfering with the metabolism of monoamines). Moreover, Dopa may affect many other diverse biochemical systems. The literature on the use of Dopa and other monoamine precursors in the treatment of depressions has been discussed recently in a detailed and extensive review.[37]

Early studies of the effects of Dopa in the treatment of depressions indicated that this substance was ineffective when relatively low doses of the d, l-isomer were used.[114,151] In other early studies, improvement in depressed patients was observed after intravenous administration of L-Dopa,[104,136] and elevation of mood was reported in a group of patients treated with a monoamine oxidase inhibitor and Dopa.[223] (This combination of drugs can produce severe hypertension and cardiac arrhythmias.)[200] More recent studies of relatively high doses of L-Dopa administered alone, or lower doses of L-Dopa administered in combination with a peripheral decarboxylase inhibitor, suggest that this drug may cause at least transient improvement in some depressed patients, particularly those with retarded depressions.[91,135,154] Transient hypomanic or manic episodes (characterized by increased motor and verbal activity with pressured speech, increased social involvement and intrusiveness, increased expression of anger, provocativeness, sleeplessness, euphoria, and feelings of grandiosity) occurred with regularity upon administration of L-Dopa in patients with manic-depressive depressions but not in patients with other types of depressions;[141] depressed mood often persisted during these episodes of hypomania and it has been suggested, on the basis of this observation,[141] that depression and hypomania may not represent opposite poles with respect to a catecholamine deficit (in depression) and an excess (in mania). However, this interpretation may be questioned since some investigators do not consider the symptom of depressed mood to be necessary for the diagnosis of endogenous depressions (which are characterized by psychic retardation, decreased interest and ambition, loss of initiative, impaired sense of vitality, inability to attain satisfactions or pleasures normally obtained from work or recreational activities); nor would they regard the persistence of depressed mood to be inconsistent with the remission of the core symptoms of endogenous depressions.[188] Further studies will be required to resolve this critical problem related to the clinical definition and diagnosis of the depressive disorders; and it is possible that these findings with L-Dopa, together with other pharmacological observations, may help us to better coordinate clinical concepts with underlying biological substrates.[187]

When L-Dopa has been used in the treatment of Parkinson's disease, improvement in depression and hypomaniclike states have been observed, but the precipitation of depressions has also been reported as a frequently occurring side effect of treatment with

L-Dopa. These and other behavioral effects of L-Dopa have been reviewed recently.[88] As noted above, the effects of Dopa on biogenic amine metabolism (i.e., indoleamines as well as catecholamines) are complex,* and it is not possible at the present time to definitively relate any of the clinical effects of Dopa to specific changes in catecholamine metabolism.

Alpha-methylparatyrosine

It was initially suggested that clinical studies with alpha-methylparatyrosine (a drug that inhibits catecholamine biosynthesis by blocking the conversion of tyrosine to Dopa) might provide crucial data to evaluate the catecholamine hypothesis of affective disorders.[186] Subsequent clinical studies have indicated that this drug regularly produces sedation when first administered and that some hypertensive patients may become depressed during treatment with alpha-methylparatyrosine, while transient hypomaniclike reactions frequently occur upon withdrawal of the drug.[70,72] In the course of these early clinical trials of alpha-methylparatyrosine, I had the opportunity to evaluate some of the patients treated with this drug. During the initial phase of treatment, some patients experienced a syndrome—characterized (in varying degrees) by psychic retardation, fatigue or loss of energy, decreased ambition or initiative, and an impaired sense of vitality—that could be descriptively classified as a mild endogenous depression, following the criteria that I have described elsewhere.[188] Upon withdrawal of alpha-methylparatyrosine, one could observe mild transient hypomaniclike states characterized by pressure of speech and an apparent decreased need for sleep. However, depressions were not observed in two studies of alpha-methylparatyrosine in schizophrenic patients.[40,83]

It has recently been reported that alpha-methylparatyrosine decreased mania in some manic patients, whereas it increased depression in a small number of depressed patients treated with this drug. During treatment with

alpha-methylparatyrosine, the levels of VMA, MHPG, and dopamine in urine decreased by more than 50 percent and cerebrospinal fluid levels of homovanillic acid decreased by more than 40 percent; thus catecholamine biosynthesis appeared to have been markedly but not completely inhibited. The authors concluded that under these conditions alpha-methylparatyrosine was therapeutically effective in some manic patients but that it was not as effective as lithium carbonate.[26]

In another recent study of subjects who abused amphetamine, the euphoric effects of large doses of intravenously administered d, l-amphetamine were reduced or abolished by alpha-methylparatyrosine. After one week of daily administration of alpha-methylparatyrosine, there was a reduction of this antiamphetamine effect (possibly the result of compensatory receptor supersensitivity). On the basis of these results and the findings from studies of the effects of drugs thought to block dopaminergic or noradrenergic receptors selectively, the investigators suggested that dopamine may be of importance for the euphoric effects of amphetamine.[107] However, as noted above, other investigators have found a relative increase in the urinary excretion of MHPG during amphetamine-induced hypomanias and a relative decrease in urinary MHPG during the depressions associated with amphetamine withdrawal; and these findings suggest that norepinephrine may also be of some importance in amphetamine-induced alterations in affective state.[205]

In nonhuman primates (*Macaca speciosa*), alpha-methylparatyrosine has been reported to produce changes in social behavior characterized by retarded motor activity, withdrawn posture, bowed head, as well as reduced initiated social interactions and facial expressions suggesting a lack of concern with the environment; the investigators regarded this behavioral state as similar, in some ways, to depressive states seen in man. The urinary excretion of MHPG and VMA was decreased during administration of alpha-methylparatyrosine and an attempt to reverse the behavioral syndrome in one animal using L-Dopa was unsuccessful.[171] In a further study, these

---

* See references 73, 89, 90, 145, 148, and 231.

investigators reported that parachloropheny-lalanine, the inhibitor of serotonin synthesis, did not produce a similar pattern of behavioral changes in *Macaca speciosa* in spite of a marked inhibition of serotonin synthesis as evidenced by a decrease in urinary 5HIAA excretion and the occurrence of weight loss, hair loss, ataxia, and debilitation in some of the animals.[170] After administration of parachlorophenylalanine to patients with carcinoid syndrome, nonspecific alterations in behavior including psychotic confusional states as well as nonpsychotic behavioral changes, sometimes with depressive components, have been observed in some patients.[31,71]

Beta-phenylethylamine

The urinary excretion of beta-phenylethylamine (both free and conjugated) has been found to be decreased in depressed patients by several groups of investigators;[15,78,105] and increased levels of phenylethylamine have been observed in manic as well as schizophrenic patients.[77] Treatment with imipramine or monoamine oxidase inhibitor antidepressants increases levels of phenylethylamine in animal brain as well as in the urine of depressed patients; whereas reserpine has been observed to decrease levels of phenylethylamine in animal brain.[77,105] Further studies will be required to confirm these interesting observations as well as to control for the possible effects of diet, concurrent drug administration, and other factors related to the clinical and psychiatric status of the patients.

Catechol O-Methyl Transferase Activity

The activity of catechol O-methyl transferase (COMT) in red blood cells of women with unipolar primary depressions was significantly lower than controls in a recent series of investigations,[43,66] whereas women with bipolar illnesses demonstrated COMT activities intermediate between unipolar women and the controls. (Red blood cell COMT, activity in schizophrenic women was not different from control values.) Within the group of women with primary affective disorders, red

blood cell COMT activity was independent of the phase of the illness (depression or mania) and did not change with recovery. In contrast to the differences observed in women with primary affective disorders, no differences in red blood cell COMT activity were found among comparable diagnostic groups of male patients.[43,66] It may be of interest to note in regard to these findings that another group of investigators hypothesized some years ago that malfunction of the catechol O-methyl transferase enzyme might cause some depressions by leading to the formation of noradnamine, a condensation derivation of norepinephrine;[172] however, direct evidence to support this speculative hypothesis is lacking.

(Indoleamines and Related Substances

Various aspects of indoleamine metabolism have been explored in patients with depressive disorders. These studies have provided further understanding of the biochemical pathophysiology underlying these clinical states.

5HIAA in Urine and Cerebrospinal Fluid

The urinary excretion of 5-hydroxyindoleacetic acid (5HIAA), a deaminated metabolite of serotonin, has been studied extensively in patients with affective disorders.* These findings have been considered in a recent comprehensive review[102] and will not be discussed in detail in this paper. Although there are many discrepancies, the findings reported in these various studies suggest that urinary 5HIAA levels may differ in different subtypes of depressive disorders and two studies indicate that the response to treatment with monoamine oxidase inhibitors may be more favorable in patients with relatively low levels of urinary 5HIAA than in patients with relatively higher levels,[151,166] but not all studies concur.[82] In longitudinal studies of manic-depressive patients, the levels of 5HIAA have been found to be relatively higher during epi-

* See references 82, 131, 151, 166, 176, 217, and 222.

sodes of mania than during episodes of depression. However, these findings must be interpreted cautiously since it is thought that a considerable fraction of urinary 5HIAA may derive from indoleamines in the gastrointestinal tract and that dietary factors may be of considerable importance.[52,176]

Various findings suggest that measurements of 5HIAA in lumbar cerebrospinal fluid (CSF) may yield information about the cerebral metabolism of serotonin,[139] although some of the 5HIAA in lumbar CSF may come from the spinal cord.[29] Concentrations of 5HIAA (like HVA) are considerably higher in ventricular CSF than in lumbar CSF, with intermediate values found in cisternal CSF, suggesting that there may be a transport system for the removal of 5HIAA from the CSF located in the region of the fourth ventricle.[139]

Since the initial report that 5-hydroxyindole compounds were decreased in the cerebrospinal fluid of depressed patients,[2] numerous investigators have confirmed the observation that CSF levels of 5-hydroxyindoleacetic acid are lower in depressed patients than in controls. In most studies statistically significant decreases,* or nonsignificant decreases,[22,149] in CSF 5HIAA levels have been observed in depressed patients. However, in several studies depressed patients were found to have essentially normal levels of 5HIAA in the cerebrospinal fluid.[92,147,177,230] Levels of 5HIAA in the CSF have been observed to be higher in subjects over the age of fifty-five than in middle-aged subjects;[21] and in one study, depressed patients over sixty years of age had significantly higher 5HIAA levels than did depressed patients under sixty years.[11] However, in several other studies no age correlation was observed.[92,147,149]

The variability observed in the many studies of CSF 5HIAA in depressions might be accounted for by a number of factors: the nature of the control group to which depressed patients were compared; differences in age or sex of the various groups; differences in the conditions under which the samples of cere-

* See references 3, 46, 60, 130, 137, 161, and 165.

brospinal fluid were obtained; and differences in techniques used for chemical determination, including the possibility that some of these methods may be relatively nonspecific. Possible differences in the diagnostic subgroups of depressive disorders, as well as in the clinical phenomenology of the patients examined in various studies, may also be of importance.

In two recent studies, patients with unipolar (recurrent) depressions had lower levels of 5HIAA in the CSF than did patients with bipolar (manic-depressive) depressions.[2,137] In one of these studies, normal levels of 5HIAA were observed in the patients with manic-depressive depressions.[2] Depressed patients classified as psychotic (on the basis of the presence of delusion) had lower CSF levels of 5HIAA than did nonpsychotic depressed patients in one study.[137] In another recent preliminary study of a small group of patients with endogenous depressions, patients with relatively low pretreatment levels of CSF 5HIAA did not improve clinically during treatment with nortriptyline, whereas patients with higher levels of 5HIAA responded favorably to treatment with this drug.[11]

In most studies the decrease in CSF 5HIAA levels in depressed patients persisted after recovery,[2,47,137] although a slow rise to normal values upon recovery from depression was noted in one study of a small number of patients.[60] During treatment with amitriptyline, imipramine, or nortriptyline, a further decrease in CSF 5HIAA has been observed in depressed patients.[11,22,149] No changes in CSF 5HIAA levels were observed in depressed patients after electroconvulsive therapy (ECT) in one study in which pretreatment levels of 5HIAA were not decreased.[147]

In some studies, low baseline levels of CSF 5HIAA have been observed in hypomanic or manic patients both before treatment and after recovery;[2,22,47,60] but the decreases in pretreatment levels were not statistically significant in all of the studies. Other investigators, however, have observed normal or increased CSF 5HIAA levels in manic patients.[3,92,177] CSF 5HIAA levels in lumbar cerebrospinal fluid have been shown to increase after exercise or periods of "simulated mania" with increased psychomotor activity;[79,157] since a concentration gradient of 5HIAA appears to exist within the cerebrospinal fluid system (with lowest levels observed in the lumbar CSF) this could conceivably result from an increased mixing of CSF from various levels during periods of increased physical activity.[3] In the light of these observations, the relatively low levels of CSF 5HIAA in manic or hypomanic patients, observed by a number of investigators, are of particular interest. However, in relation to these findings in patients with affective disorders, it should be pointed out that decreased levels of 5HIAA have been observed in other psychiatric conditions including schizophrenic disorders.[3,22]

The accumulation of 5HIAA in the CSF following administration of probenecid (i.e., the difference between levels of CSF 5HIAA after probenecid and before probenecid) was found to be decreased in a number of recent studies of depressed patients;[92,161,165,177] the differences were statistically significant in most but not all of these studies. The possibility has been suggested that decreased 5HIAA accumulation may be characteristic of only a subgroup of patients with endogenous (vital) depressions who are not otherwise distinguishable on the basis of psychopathological features or differences in motor activity.[161,165] (In one of these studies, the reduced accumulation of 5HIAA in the CSF following probenecid correlated significantly with reduced baseline levels of 5HIAA, but a similar correlation was not observed in the other study.) In another study, the levels (not the accumulation) of 5HIAA in CSF after probenecid administration were not different from control values in a group of patients with unipolar depressions; during treatment with amitriptyline, 5HIAA levels after probenecid administration markedly decreased.[20]

The accumulation of 5HIAA in CSF was compared before and after improvement in a small group of depressed patients; variable results were observed with 5HIAA accumulation increasing in some patients after improvement, but not in all.[162]

In one study, significantly lowered 5HIAA accumulation was observed in manic patients,[177] and CSF-5HIAA accumulation tended to be lower in manic patients in another study.[92]

The problems in interpreting data on the accumulation of acid monoamine metabolites in lumbar CSF following probenecid have been discussed elsewhere,[19,163] and will not be considered in detail here. Issues of relevance include: possible variations in the effects of probenecid from subject to subject, including differences in CSF probenecid levels or differences in the degree of blockade produced by a given concentration of probenecid; possible individual variations in transit time for 5HIAA (or HVA) to pass from brain to lumbar CSF; possible interindividual variations in the rate of transport of acid metabolites out of CSF; variations in the extent to which the transport of these metabolites is inhibited by the maximum dose of probenecid that may be administered to human subjects; possible variations in the volume of the cerebrospinal fluid; and possible effects of probenecid on monoamine metabolism apart from the inhibition of transport of acid metabolites. Since 5HIAA may not be the sole metabolite of cerebral serotonin, just as HVA is not the sole metabolite of dopamine, the possible contribution of the corresponding alcohol derivatives or other metabolites must also be considered when interpreting these findings.

In a pilot study of the effects of 5-hydroxytryptophan, a precursor of serotonin, in patients with vital (endogenous) depressions, three of five patients improved with 5-hydroxytryptophan, whereas none of five subjects improved with placebo; the three patients who improved during treatment with 5-hydroxytryptophan showed low pretreatment accumulations of 5HIAA in CSF after probenecid, whereas the two patients who did not improve had higher pretreatment accumulations of 5HIAA.[164] However, another group of investigators failed to demonstrate a therapeutic response to 5-hydroxytryptophan in six of seven depressed patients, although in this study 5-hydroxytryptophan administration was shown to produce increases in plasma 5-hydroxytryptophan, cerebrosplinal fluid 5HIAA and urinary 5HIAA; and the one patient who showed a moderate response to treatment with 5-hydroxytryptophan did not exhibit an exacerbation after withdrawal of the drug.[27] However, the results of this study need not necessarily contradict the preceding findings, since the accumulation of 5HIAA in the CSF after probenecid administration was not studied and baseline 5HIAA levels (although reduced) were not significantly lower in these depressed patients than in control subjects.

Other investigators have examined the changes in CSF 5HIAA following administration of tryptophan (an amino acid precursor of serotonin) in depressed patients. In one study,[17,18] L-tryptophan (in conjunction with vitamin B6) did not ameliorate either the depressive symptoms or the insomnia in a group of depressed patients. These depressed patients, however, showed less of an increase in CSF 5HIAA after tryptophan administration than did a group of schizophrenic patients.[18] On the basis of these and similar findings, it has been suggested that the synthesis of serotonin from tryptophan may be impaired in some depressed patients.[17,69] Another group of investigators, however, has observed that L-tryptophan produced an increase in platelet serotonin, urinary and CSF 5HIAA, as well as the accumulation of 5HIAA in the CSF after probenecid without an accompanying improvement in the depression in most of the patients.[35,67] In a recent study, levels of tryptophan in the cerebrospinal fluid of depressed and manic patients were found to be significantly reduced in comparison with control subjects; in a small number of patients following recovery from depression, normal CSF tryptophan levels were observed.[45]

Serotonin and 5HIAA in Brain after Suicide

Several studies have examined the levels of serotonin and 5HIAA in the brains of depressed patients after suicide. In one of these studies, levels of serotonin in the hindbrain were lower in depressed patients after suicide

than in a control group of subjects who had died from accidents or acute illnesses.[211] This difference in serotonin levels, however, was not replicated in a more recent study by some of the same investigators, but 5HIAA was reported to be lower in depressed patients after suicide than in control subjects after death from natural causes; statistically significant differences in the levels of norepinephrine were not observed.[16]

In another study,[152] serotonin levels were lower in the brain stem of patients after suicide than in control subjects; the major effect in this study was observed in patients with reactive depressions who committed suicide rather than in patients with endogenous depressions. Moreover, in this study a positive correlation was found between age and serotonin concentration and the authors note that the decrease observed in patients after suicide was offset to some extent by the difference in age between the suicide and control groups. There were no significant differences in the concentrations of 5HIAA in the brain stem, norepinephrine in hypothalamus or dopamine in caudate nucleus between suicides and controls in this study.[152]

Interpretation of these data is exceedingly difficult because of the many uncontrolled variables that may have influenced the results of these studies. These include: the ingestion of psychoactive drugs before suicide; differences in age between the suicide and control groups; and the fact that many of the low 5HIAA values, observed in patients after suicide in the study where this difference was significant, seemed to be associated with barbiturate ingestion. Another variable that has recently been commented upon is the length of time during which frozen specimens were stored between the necropsy and assay.[65]

Other Metabolites of Tryptophan in Urine

The urinary excretion of tryptamine was relatively reduced during depressions and increased after clinical improvement in several studies.[51,169,176] However, in another recent study, tryptamine levels were relatively elevated during depressions when compared with values obtained after recovery.[131] Most urinary tryptamine probably derives from the decarboxylation of tryptophan in the kidney and relatively little may be of central origin; dietary factors may also cause alterations in tryptamine excretion.[50,176] Depressed patients were reported to have relatively decreased rates of liberation of $C^{14}O_2$ from carboxy-labeled 5-hydroxytrytophan in one study,[50] but the group originally reporting this finding did not observe the phenomenon in a further study of depressed patients.[44]

A shift in the pathways of metabolism of tryptophan, possibly mediated by an increase in tryptophan pyrrolase leading to increased metabolism by the kynurenine pathway and decreased synthesis of indoleamines, has been suggested as a possible mechanism to account for some of the changes in indoleamine metabolism that have been reported to occur in depressive disorders,[54,121,133] and this has been explored by a number of investigators.

Excretion of xanthurenic acid, a product of the kynurenine pathway of tryptophan metabolism was found to be greater in depressed than in manic patients.[39] After a tryptophan load, female patients with endogenous depressions excreted more kynurenine and 3-hydroxykynurenine, but not the subsequent metabolite 3-hydroxyanthranilic acid, than did female control subjects in one recent study.[55]

In two manic-depressive patients studied longitudinally, the conversion of intravenously administered radioactive tryptophan to kynurenine was greater during episodes of depressions than during episodes of mania or during normal periods;[180] but the excretion of endogenous kynurenine was significantly lower during depression than during mania.[181] In another study, the excretion of kynurenine in depressive patients was significantly lower than in normal subjects.[12] However, these findings on alterations in levels in one or another of the urinary metabolites of tryptophan deriving from the kynurenine pathway are difficult to interpret in the absence of additional data on the other intermediary and final metabolites from this metabolic pathway.

Tryptophan and 5-Hydroxytryptophan Administration

A number of years ago, tryptophan, an amino acid precursor of the indoleamines, was found to be the only one of several amino acids that produced mood elevation in patients with chronic schizophrenia, when these amino acids were administered in conjunction with a monoamine oxidase inhibitor.[156] In depressed patients, the therapeutic effects of monoamine oxidase inhibitors have been reported to be potentiated by tryptophan,[48,85] [150] but not in all studies.[158] Some investigators have indicated that tryptophan administered alone (i.e., without the addition of a monoamine oxidase inhibitor) is effective in the treatment of depressions;[23,42,46,47] but all studies have not confirmed this.[18,35,38]

It has been suggested that these conflicting results may in part be explained by the finding that tryptophan does not increase levels of 5-hydroxyindoles in the CSF of all depressed patients,[17] but in one study, which failed to demonstrate a clinical antidepressant effect of L-tryptophan, increased levels of 5HIAA were observed in cerebrospinal fluid during L-tryptophan treatment.[35] It has also been suggested that these differences might be accounted for by the finding that all depressed patients do not show a decrease in serotonin turnover in the brain (as measured by 5HIAA accumulation in CSF after probenecid).[160] However, it must be remembered that tryptophan exerts many other biochemical effects besides increasing indoleamines; the complex biochemical pharmacology of tryptophan has been reviewed elsewhere.[37]

The antidepressant activity of monoamine oxidase inhibitors may also be potentiated by 5-hydroxytryptophan in some patients[115,116] but this effect has not been observed by all investigators.[84,151] One study reported a single case of a patient, refractory to both electroconvulsive treatments and amitriptyline, who responded to intravenous administration of 5-hydroxytryptophan administered in conjunction with barbiturates, diazepam, and a small dose of opium; this was accompanied by an increase in levels of 5HIAA in the cerebrospinal fluid.[153] Preliminary findings from another recent study suggest that patients with endogenous depressions who have decreased accumulation of 5HIAA in the cerebrospinal fluid following probenecid administration respond clinically to treatment with 5-hydroxytryptophan, but that those with higher accumulations of 5HIAA in the CSF do not.[164] In another recent study, 5-hydroxytryptophan was not effective in the treatment of a small number of depressed patients although it did produce a significant increase in levels of 5HIAA in the CSF; but the probenecid-induced accumulation of 5HIAA in CSF was not measured.[27] One cannot necessarily assume that alterations in mood which may be produced by 5-hydroxytryptophan result simply from an increase in indoleamines at specific receptors in brain; for example, 5-hydroxytryptophan may also release and displace catecholamines centrally.[25,81]

In the light of the complex biochemical pharmacology of tryptophan and 5-hydroxytryptophan, it would seem unwarranted to attempt to draw theoretical inferences concerning the possible roles of one or another of the monoamines in affective disorders on the basis of these data. Moreover, interpretations of the clinical results are complicated by the fact that different clinical diagnostic criteria may have been employed in the selection of patients in these various studies, and, as noted above, even depressed patients who appear similar clinically may be different in terms of underlying biochemical pathophysiology. Further investigations will be required to determine whether specific clinical or biochemical subgroups of depressed patients may be responsive to treatment with tryptophan or 5-hydroxytryptophan.

Methysergide and Related Substances

Methysergide, a serotonin (and tryptamine) antagonist, was initially reported to be effective in the treatment of manias by three groups of investigators employing various routes of administration including intrathecal.[61,99,100,225] Subsequent studies by a number of investigators failed to confirm these findings;* but some investigators have confirmed the therapeutic effects of methysergide in the treatment of a small number of manic patients, and the precipitation of depressions has been noted.[209,224] Cinanserin, another antiserotonin agent, has also been reported to be effective in the treatment of manias.[108] The clinical efficacy of methysergide (and cinanserin) in the treatment of manias, if substantiated, would suggest a disturbance of indoleamine metabolism in manic states; and one of the investigators reporting therapeutic effects with this drug has proposed that methysergide may exert its clinical effects in manias by antagonising tryptamine receptors in brain.[62,63] However, in the light of the several negative reports it would seem that methysergide is clearly not effective in the treatment of all manic disorders, and further studies will be required to determine whether methysergide when administered in adequate doses (or by specific routes of administration) may be effective in a particular subgroup of patients with manic disorders.[64,98]

⟨ Monoamine Oxidase Activity

In one study performed a number of years ago, the conversion of orally administered radioactive serotonin to radioactive 5HIAA recovered in the urine was examined in a group of depressed patients (clinical subtypes unspecified) and normal control subjects; no differences between these groups were observed and the investigators concluded that monoamine oxidase (and aldehyde dehydrogenase) functioned normally in the depressed patients.[75] In a more recent study,[112] plasma monoamine oxidase activity was significantly higher in a group of premenopausal depressed women (who did not require hospitalization) than in a group of control subjects. (The depressed patients in this study did not include "schizophrenic, psychotic, manic, reactive, and involutional depressives.") Orally administered conjugated estrogen produced a signifi-

* See references 46, 76, 97, 129, and 132.

cant decrease in plasma monoamine oxidase activity in the depressed patients and all of the depressed patients who received estrogen therapy reported an improvement in their mood; however, as the investigators noted, this study lacked the double-blind procedures adequate for a proper evaluation of the antidepressant effects of conjugated estrogens.[112]

Another group of investigators has recently reported that platelet monoamine oxidase activity was significantly higher in a large heterogeneous group of depressed patients than in a group of normal subjects matched for age.[146] In further studies, this group of investigators observed that there was a progressive increase in monoamine oxidase activities in the human hindbrain, platelets, and plasma with advancing age, starting at the age of thirty-five in platelets and brain and at the age of fifty-five in plasma, with maximal levels observed after the age of seventy. Women were found to have higher mean platelet monoamine oxidase activities than men at all age levels and higher mean plasma monoamine oxidase activities after the age of forty; the mean hindbrain monoamine oxidase activity in women was slightly, but not significantly, greater than in men. Levels of norepinephrine in the hindbrain (obtained at necropsy from patients who had died from a variety of causes) decreased significantly with advancing age, and the levels of norepinephrine in the hindbrain correlated negatively with hindbrain monoamine oxidase activity. Neither serotonin nor 5HIAA levels in the hindbrain correlated significantly with age, but levels of 5HIAA were positively correlated with hindbrain monoamine oxidase activity. It is tempting to speculate that these findings may help to explain the generally greater frequency of depressive illnesses in women than in men, and the increasing incidence of depressive illnesses during middle age in both sexes.[173,174]

In another recent study,[142] platelet monoamine oxidase activities were found to be significantly lower in bipolar depressed patients than in unipolar depressed patients or normal controls of similar age and sex distribution. The levels of platelet monoamine oxidase activity in the unipolar depressed patients were slightly higher than those of controls, but this difference was not statistically significant. There was a high negative correlation between platelet monoamine oxidase activity and tryptamine excretion with bipolar patients excreting significantly more tryptamine than unipolar patients. Preliminary results also indicate that the false transmitter octopamine (which accumulates in platelets after treatment with monoamine oxidase inhibitors) is present in platelets of individuals with endogenously reduced monoamine oxidase activity, particularly patients with bipolar depressions; and it has been suggested that endogenous false transmitters may play a role in the pathophysiology of some types of depressive disorders.[140] In a small number of bipolar patients studied longitudinally through both depressive and manic episodes, there was no consistent direction of change in platelet monoamine oxidase activities during either manic or depressed periods.[142]

Findings from one recent study indicate that at least some depressed patients have abnormal serum monoamine oxidase isoenzyme patterns. These preliminary data also suggest that serum monoamine oxidase isoenzyme patterns may differ in different subtypes of depressive disorders.[212]

It is difficult to compare the findings of these various studies, since different substrates were used in the assays of monoamine oxidase activities. Moreover, further investigation will be required to determine whether platelet (or plasma) monoamine oxidase activities provide an index of the monoamine oxidase activities in other tissues, particularly the brain, which may have different isoenzymes. However, in the aggregate, the findings of these studies do raise the possibility that the determination of monoamine oxidase activities or isoenzyme patterns may be of value in differentiating various subtypes of depressive disorders and possibly also in predicting differential responses to pharmacotherapy. In this regard, it should be noted that, in addition to the monoamine oxidase inhibitor antidepressants, many other drugs that alter affective state also appear to alter the deamination of monoamines.[188]

Tricyclic antidepressants (i.e., imipramine, desmethylimipramine, amitriptyline, nortriptyline, and protriptyline) produce a decrease in the deamination of norepinephrine in animal brain, which cannot be explained simply on the basis of an inhibition of neuronal uptake of norepinephrine;[193] and the findings from clinical studies of norepinephrine metabolism in patients treated with imipramine or amitriptyline are compatible with such a decrease in the deamination of norepinephrine.[194] [195,196] Stimulant and euphoriant drugs, such as amphetamine and cocaine, have similarly been observed to decrease the deamination of norepinephrine in animal brain; and it has previously been suggested that a decrease in deamination of norepinephrine or other monoamines may contribute to the clinical effects of many stimulants, euphoriants, and the tricyclic antidepressants as well as the monoamine oxidase inhibitors.[188] In contrast, lithium salts appear to increase the release and intraneuronal deamination of norepinephrine by monoamine oxidase in animal brain, and this has been suggested as a possible mechanism to account for the clinical effectiveness of lithium in the treatment of manias.[202,203] Moreover, this could conceivably also account for the reported antidepressant effects of lithium when used in combination with monoamine oxidase inhibitors,[101,233] and would lead to the prediction that lithium may exert antidepressant effects in those depressed patients with endogenously reduced monoamine oxidase activity.[190,192]

❲ Conclusion

It has long been recognized that hypotheses relating the affective disorders to alterations in biogenic amine metabolism were, at best, reductionistic oversimplifications of very complex biological states that undoubtedly involved many other biochemical, physiological, and psychological factors.[186,199] The body of research summarized in this review, however, attests to the heuristic value of these reductionistic hypotheses, initially formulated on the basis of the neuropharmacological effects of drugs used in the treatment of the affective disorders.

While it would be premature to attempt to integrate these diverse findings at the present time, it does appear that certain changes in biogenic amine metabolism (e.g., alterations in normetanephrine and MHPG excretion) may occur in association with changes in affective state, whereas other abnormalities in monoamine metabolism (e.g., as reflected by decreased 5HIAA in the CSF) may represent enduring constitutional factors in some patients with affective disorders.[111] Whether or not these or the other alterations in biogenic amine metabolism, reviewed here, ultimately prove to be of etiological importance, such findings will, nonetheless, increase our understanding of the pathophysiological changes that occur in patients with depressive disorders.[68]

In this connection, it is important to note that mere measurements of the levels of monoamines and their metabolites, in various tissues (including the brain) or body fluids (including the probenecid-induced accumulation of acid monoamine metabolites in CSF), do not enable one to distinguish among the varied physiological processes that may underlie alterations in these levels. For example, low levels of one or another monoamine or its metabolites might occur both with a primary deficiency in synthesis leading to a decrease of the monoamine at receptors, or with a feedback-induced decrease in synthesis secondary to an excess of the monoamine at receptors; similarly high levels of metabolites could occur both with an excess of the monoamine at receptors resulting from a primary increase in monoamine synthesis, or with a functional deficiency of the monoamine at receptors as a result of increased enzymatic inactivation of the monoamine, or a decreased receptor sensitivity to the monoamine, with a consequent feedback-induced increase in monoamine synthesis. However, our increasing understanding of the neurochemical effects of the drugs used in the treatment of affective disorders, including the effects of chronic administration since this is generally required for therapeutic effects,[207,208] may help us to clarify these underlying pathophysiological processes in patients with depressions and manias.[187,189]

While it has been strategic in individual studies, to focus on one or another of the monoamines, the physiological interactions of monoaminergic neuronal systems (noradrenergic, dopaminergic, and serotonergic) are generally recognized, and it appears that biochemical as well as physiological processes involving one monoamine may be modulated by another. Moreover, the balance between cholinergic as well as catecholaminergic and indolaminergic activity has been considered in relation to the effects of antidepressant drugs and reserpine,[8,24,218] and recent clinical findings suggest that physostigmine, an acetylcholinesterase inhibitor, can transiently decrease manic symptoms as well as precipitate depressions.[106]

The heterogeneity of the depressive disorders has been noted frequently in this chapter, and it appears that a major goal for future research will be to define the biochemical as well as other biological criteria that will enable us to classify patients with affective disorders more meaningfully, and to prescribe treatments more rationally, than is currently possible on the basis of clinical criteria alone. From the recent preliminary findings reviewed above, it seems not unreasonable to suggest that a number of variables related to biogenic amine metabolism (e.g., urinary and CSF MHPG; CSF 5HIAA, and HVA; platelet and plasma monoamine oxidase activity) may well be included among such biochemical criteria. In this context, additional attention should be directed toward possible differences in the biochemical as well as clinical effects of various antidepressant drugs, since a greater understanding of these differences will further increase our capacity to determine the specific antidepressant drug to be used in various clinically or biochemically defined subtypes of depressive disorders.

Many investigators expect this line of research to have a major clinical impact during the coming decade, and it is predicted that biochemical as well as physiological and provocative pharmacological tests will become as routine in the diagnostic workup of depressed patients as they are now in the evaluation of patients with endocrine or other medical disorders. Following the advances that have occurred in other areas of medical nosology, it seems quite conceivable that this approach will ultimately contribute to the development of a psychiatric nosology, based not only upon the clinical phenomenology of the depressive disorders but also upon a knowledge of the biological mechanisms underlying these phenomena.

❮ Bibliography

1. ANGST, J. "Vergleich der Antidepressiven Eigenschaften von Amitriptylin und Imipramin," *Psychopharmacologia*, 4 (1963), 389–401.
2. ASHCROFT, G. W., P. W. BROOKS, R. L. CUNDALL et al. "Changes in the Glycol Metabolites of Noradrenaline in Affective Illness." Presented 5th World Congr. Psychiatry, Mexico City, 1971.
3. ASHCROFT, G. W., T. B. B. CRAWFORD, D. ECCLESTON et al. "5-Hydroxyindole Compounds in the Cerebrospinal Fluid of Patients with Psychiatric or Neurological Diseases," *Lancet*, 2 (1966), 1049–1052.
4. ASHCROFT, G. W. and D. F. SHARMAN. "5-Hydroxyindoles in Human Cerebrospinal Fluids," *Nature*, 186 (1960), 1050–1051.
5. AXELROD, J. "Methylation Reactions in the Formation and Metabolism of Catecholamines and Other Biogenic Amines," *Pharmacol. Rev.*, 18 (1966), 95–113.
6. ———. "Noradrenaline: Fate and Control of Its Biosynthesis," *Science*, 173 (1971), 598–606.
7. BARTHOLINI, G., R. TISSOT, and A. PLETSCHER. "Brain Capillaries As a Source of Homovanillic Acid in Cerebrospinal Fluid," *Brain Res.*, 27 (1971), 163–168.
8. BENESOVA, O. and K. NAHUNEK. "Correlation Between the Experimental Data from Animal Studies and Therapeutical Effects of Antidepressant Drugs," *Psychopharmacologia*, 20 (1971), 337–347.
9. BENKERT, O., A. RENZ, C. MARANO et al. "Altered Tyrosine Daytime Plasma Levels in Endogenous Depressive Patients," *Arch. Gen. Psychiatry*, 25 (1971), 359–363.

10. BERGSMAN, A. "Urinary Excretion of Adrenaline and Noradrenaline in Some Mental Diseases: Clinical and Experimental Study," *Acta Psychiatr. Neurol. Scand.*, 54 Suppl. 133 (1959), 5–107.

11. BERTILSSON, L., M. ASBERG, B. CRONHOLM et al. "Indolealkylamine Metabolites in Cerebrospinal Fluid of Depressed Patients." Presented 5th Int. Congr. Pharmacol., San Francisco, 1972.

12. BIRKMAYER, W. and W. LINAUER. "Störung des Tyrosin-und Tryptophanmetabolismus bei Depression," *Arch. Psychiatr. Nervenkr.*, 213 (1970), 377–387.

13. BLOOM, F. E. and N. J. GIARMAN. "Physiologic and Pharmacologic Considerations of Biogenic Amines in Nervous System," *Annu. Rev. Pharmacol.*, 8 (1968), 229–258.

14. BOND, P. A., F. A. JENNER, and G. A. SAMPSON. "Daily Variations of the Urine Content of 3-Methoxy-4-Hydroxyphenylglycol in Two Manic-depressive Patients," *Psychol. Med.*, 2 (1972), 81–85.

15. BOULTON, A. A. and L. MILWARD. "Separation, Detection and Quantitative Analysis of Urinary β-Phenylethylamine," *J. Chromatogr.*, 57 (1971), 287–296.

16. BOURNE, H. R., W. E. BUNNEY, JR., R. W. COLBURN et al. "Noradrenaline 5-Hydroxytryptamine and 5-Hydroxyindoleacetic Acid in Hindbrain of Suicidal Patients," *Lancet*, 2 (1968), 805–808.

17. BOWERS, M. B., JR. "5-H.T. Metabolism in Psychiatric Syndromes," *Lancet*, 2 (1970), 1029.

18. ———. "Cerebrospinal Fluid 5-Hydroxyindoles and Behavior After L-tryptophan and Pyridoxine Administration to Psychiatric Patients," *Neuropharmacol.*, 9 (1970), 599–604.

19. ———. "Clinical Measurements of Central Dopamine and 5-Hydroxytryptamine Metabolism: Reliability and Interpretation of Cerebrospinal Fluid Acid Monoamine Metabolite Measures," *Neuropharmacol.*, 11 (1972), 101–111.

20. ———. "Cerebrospinal Fluid 5-Hydroxyindoleacetic Acid (5HIAA) and Homovanillic Acid (HVA) Following Probenecid in Unipolar Depressives Treated with Amitriptyline," *Psychopharmacologia*, 23 (1972), 26–33.

21. BOWERS, M. B. and F. A. GERBODE. "Relationship of Monoamine Metabolites in Human Cerebrospinal Fluid to Age," *Nature*, 219 (1968), 1256–1257.

22. BOWERS, M. B., JR., G. R. HENINGER, and F. GERBODE. "Cerebrospinal Fluid 5-Hydroxyindoleacetic Acid and Homovanillic Acid in Psychiatric Patients," *Int. J. Neuropharmacol.*, 8 (1969), 255–262.

23. BROADHURST, A. D. "L-tryptophan versus E.C.T.," *Lancet*, 1 (1970), 1392–1393.

24. BRODIE, B. B. "Some Ideas on the Mode of Action of Imipramine-Type Antidepressants," in *The Scientific Basis of Drug Therapy in Psychiatry*, pp. 127–146. Oxford: Pergamon, 1965.

25. BRODIE, B. B., M. S. COMER, E. COSTA et al. "Role of Brain Serotonin in Mechanism of Central Action of Reserpine," *J. Pharmacol. Exp. Ther.*, 152 (1966), 340–349.

26. BRODIE, H. K. H., D. L. MURPHY, F. K. GOODWIN et al. "Catecholamines and Mania: The Effect of Alpha-methyl-para-tyrosine on Manic Behavior and Catecholamine Metabolism," *Clin. Pharmacol. Ther.*, 12 (1971), 219–224.

27. BRODIE, H. K. H., R. SACK, and L. SIEVER. "Clinical Studies of 5-Hydroxytryptophan in Depression," in J. Barchas and E. Usdin, eds., *Serotonin and Behavior*. New York: Academic, forthcoming.

28. BUENO, J. R. and H. E. HIMWICH. "Dualistic Approach to Some Biochemical Problems in Endogenous Depressions," *Psychosomatics*, 8 (1967), 82–94.

29. BULAT, M. and B. ZIVKOVIC. "Origin of 5-Hydroxyindoleacetic Acid in the Spinal Fluid," *Science*, 173 (1971), 738–740.

30. BUNNEY, W. E., JR. Personal communication.

31. BUNNEY, W. E., JR., W. T. CARPENTER, JR., K. ENGELMAN et al. "Brain Serotonin and Depressive Illness," in T. A. Williams, M. M. Katz, and J. A. Shields, Jr., eds., *Recent Advances in the Psychobiology of Depressive Illnesses*, pp. 31–40. Washington: U.S. Gov. Print. Office, 1972.

32. BUNNEY, W. E., JR. and J. M. DAVIS. "Norepinephrine in Depressive Reactions: Review," *Arch. Gen. Psychiatry*, 13 (1965), 483–494.

33. BUNNEY, W. E., JR., J. M. DAVIS, H. WEIL-MALHERBE et al. "Biochemical Changes in Psychotic Depression: High Norepinephrine Levels in Psychotic vs. Neurotic Depression," *Arch. Gen. Psychiatry*, 16 (1967), 448–460.

34. BUNNEY, W. E., JR., D. L. MURPHY, and

F. K. GOODWIN. "The Switch Process from Depression to Mania: Relationship to Drugs Which Alter Brain Amines," *Lancet*, 1 (1970), 1022–1027.

35. BUNNEY, W. E., JR., D. L. MURPHY, F. K. GOODWIN et al. "Lack of Clinical Response to Large Doses of L-Tryptophan: Behavioral and Metabolic Studies," in J. Barchas and E. Usdin, eds., *Serotonin and Behavior*. New York: Academic, forthcoming.

36. CAMPANINI, T., A. CATALANO, C. DERISIO et al. "Vanilmandelic Aciduria in the Different Clinical Phases of Manic Depressive Psychoses," *Br. J. Psychiatry*, 116 (1970), 435–436.

37. CARROLL, B. J. "Monoamine Precursors in the Treatment of Depression," *Clin. Pharmacol. Ther.*, 12 (1971), 743–761.

38. CARROLL, B. J., R. M. MOWBRAY, and B. DAVIES. "Sequential Comparison of L-Tryptophan with E.C.T. in Severe Depression," *Lancet*, 1 (1970), 967–969.

39. CAZZULLO, C. L., A. MANGONI, and G. MASCHERPA. "Tryptophan Metabolism in Affective Psychoses," *Br. J. Psychiatry*, 1–12 (1966), 157–162.

40. CHARALAMPOUS, K. D. and S. BROWN. "A Clinical Trial of a-Methyl-para-tyrosine in Mentally Ill Patients," *Psychopharmacologia*, 11 (1967), 422–429.

41. CHASE, T. N., G. R. BREESE, E. K. GORDON et al. "Catecholamine Metabolism in the Dog: Comparison of Intravenously and Intraventricularly Administered (^{14}C)Dopamine and (^{3}H) Norepinephrine," *J. Neurochem.*, 18 (1971), 135–140.

42. COCHEME, M. A. X. "L-Trytophan versus E.C.T.," *Lancet*, 1 (1970), 1392.

43. COHN, C. K., D. L. DUNNER, and J. AXELROD. "Reduced Catechol-O-Methyltransferase Activity in Red Blood Cells of Women with Primary Affective Disorder," *Science*, 170 (1970), 1323–1324.

44. COPPEN, A. "Biochemistry of Affective Disorders," *Br. J. Psychiatry*, 113 (1967), 1237–1264.

45. COPPEN, A., B. W. L. BROOKSBANK, and M. PEET. "Tryptophan Concentration in the Cerebrospinal Fluid of Depressive Patients," *Lancet*, 1 (1972), 1393.

46. COPPEN, A., A. J. PRANGE, JR., P. C. WHYBROW et al. "Methysergide in Mania," *Lancet*, 2 (1969), 338–340.

47. COPPEN, A., A. J. PRANGE, JR., P. C. WHYBROW et al. "Abnormalities of Indoleamines in Affective Disorders," *Arch. Gen. Psychiatry*, 26 (1972), 474–478.

48. COPPEN, A., D. M. SHAW, and J. P. FARRELL. "Potentiation of Antidepressive Effect of Monoamine Oxidase Inhibitor by Tryptophan," *Lancet*, 1 (1963), 79–81.

49. COPPEN, A., D. M. SHAW, B. HERZBERG et al. "Tryptophan in Treatment of Depression," *Lancet*, 2 (1967), 1178–1180.

50. COPPEN, A., D. M. SHAW, and A. MALLESON. "Changes in 5-Hydroxytryptophan Metabolism in Depression," *Br. J. Psychiatry*, 111 (1965), 105–107.

51. COPPEN, A., D. M. SHAW, A. MALLESON et al. "Tryptamine Metabolism in Depression," *Br. J. Psychiatry*, 111 (1965), 996–998.

52. CROUT, J. R. and A. SJOERDSMA. "Clinical and Laboratory Significance of Serotonin and Catecholamines in Bananas," *N. Engl. J. Med.*, 261 (1959), 23–26.

53. CURTIS, G. C., R. A. CLEGHORN, and T. L. SOURKES. "Relationship Between Affect and Excretion of Adrenaline, Noradrenaline and 17-Hydroxycortico-steroids," *J. Psychosom. Res.*, 4 (1960), 176–184.

54. CURZON, G. "Tryptophan Pyrrolase—A Biochemical Factor in Depressive Illness?" *Br. J. Psychiatry*, 115 (1969), 1367–1374.

55. CURZON, G. and P. K. BRIDGES. "Tryptophan Metabolism in Depression," *J. Neurol. Neurosurg. Psychiatry*, 33 (1970), 648–704.

56. DAVIES, B. "Recent Studies of Severe Depressive Illnesses: Part 2," *Med. J. Aust.*, 1 (1969), 557–565.

57. DAVIS, J. M. "Theories of Biological Etiology of Affective Disorders," *Int. Rev. Neurobiol.*, 12 (1970), 145–175.

58. DAVIS, J. M. and W. E. FANN. "Lithium," *Annu. Rev. Pharmacol.*, 11 (1971), 285–303.

59. DENCKER, S. J., J. HAGGENDAL, and U. MALM. "Noradrenaline Content of Cerebrospinal Fluid in Mental Diseases," *Lancet*, 2 (1966), 754.

60. DENCKER, S. J., U. MALM, B.-E. ROOS et al. "Acid Monoamine Metabolites of Cerebrospinal Fluid in Mental Depression and Mania," *J. Neurochem.*, 13 (1966), 1545–1548.

61. DEWHURST, W. G. "Methysergide in Mania," *Nature*, 219 (1968), 506–507.

62. ———. "Cerebral Amine Functions in Health and Disease," in M. Shepherd and

D. L. Davies, eds., *Studies in Psychiatry*, pp. 289–317. London: Oxford University Press, 1968.

63. ———. "Cerebral Amines and Behavior," *Lancet*, 2 (1968), 514.

64. ———. "Methysergide in Mania." *Lancet*, 2 (1969), 490.

65. Dowson, J. H. "The Significance of Amine Concentrations," *Lancet*, 2 (1969), 596.

66. Dunner, D. L., C. K. Cohn, E. S. Gershon et al. "Differential Catechol-O-Methyltransferase Activity in Unipolar and Bipolar Affective Illness," *Arch. Gen. Psychiatry*, 25 (1971), 348–353.

67. Dunner, D. L. and F. K. Goodwin. "Effect of L-Tryptophan on Brain Serotonin Metabolism in Depressed Patients," *Arch. Gen. Psychiatry*, 26 (1972), 364–366.

68. Durell, J. and J. J. Schildkraut. "Biochemical Studies of the Schizophrenic and Affective Disorders," in S. Arieti, ed., *American Handbook of Psychiatry, Vol. 3*, 1st ed., pp. 423–457. New York: Basic Books, 1966.

69. Eccleston, D., G. W. Ashcroft, T. B. B. Crawford et al. "Effect of Tryptophan Administration on 5HIAA in Cerebrospinal Fluid in Man," *J. Neurol. Neurosurg. Psychiatry*, 33 (1970), 269–272.

70. Engelman, K., D. Horwitz, E. Jecquier et al. "Biochemical and Pharmacologic Effects of a-Methyltyrosine in Man," *J. Clin. Invest.*, 47 (1968), 577–594.

71. Engelman, K., W. Lovenberg, and A. Sjoerdsma. "Inhibition of Serotonin Synthesis by Para-chlorophenylalanine in Patients with Carcinoid Syndrome," *N. Engl. J. Med.*, 277 (1967), 1103–1108.

72. Engelman, K. and A. Sjoerdsma. "Inhibition of Catecholamines Biosynthesis in Man," *Circ. Res.*, 18 (1966), 104–109.

73. Everett, G. M. and J. W. Borchdering. "L-Dopa: Effect on Concentration of Dopamine, Norepinephrine and Serotonin in Brains of Mice," *Science*, 168 (1970), 849–850.

74. Fawcett, J. and V. Siomopoulos. "Dextroamphetamine Response as a Possible Predictor of Improvement With Tricyclic Therapy in Depression," *Arch. Gen. Psychiatry*, 25 (1971), 247–255.

75. Feldstein, A., H. Hoagland, K. K. Wong et al. "MAO Activity in Relation to Depression," *Am. J. Psychiatry*, 120 (1964), 1192–1194.

76. Fieve, R. R., S. R. Platman, and J. L. Fliess. "A Clinical Trial of Methysergide and Lithium in Mania," *Psychopharmacologia*, 15 (1969), 425–429.

77. Fischer, E. "Studies on Phenethylamine as a Brain Neurohumoral Agent." Presented Soc. Biolog. Psychiatry, Annu. Meet., May 1972.

78. Fischer, W., B. Heller, and A. H. Miro. "β-Phenylethylamine in Human Urine," *Arzneim. Fors.*, 18 (1968), 1486.

79. Fotherby, K., G. W. Ashcroft, J. W. Affleck et al. "Studies on Sodium Transfer and 5-Hydroxyindoles in Depressive Illness," *J. Neuro. Neurosurg. Psychiatry*, 26 (1963), 71–73.

80. Freedman, D. X. "Aspects of Biochemical Pharmacology of Psychotropic Drugs," in P. Solomon, ed., *Psychiatric Drugs*, pp. 32–57. New York: Grune & Stratton, 1966.

81. Fuxe, K., L. L. Blutcher, and J. Engel. "DL-5-Hydroxytryptophan-induced Changes in Central Monoamine Neurons After Peripheral Decarboxylase Inhibition," *J. Pharm. Pharmacol.*, 23 (1971), 420–424.

82. Gayral, L., R. Bierer, and A. Delhom. "L'excretion urinaire de l'acide 5-Hydroxyindolacetique dans les Depressions et les Melancolies sous l'influence du traitement par les inhibiteurs de la Monoamine-oxydase," in H. Brill, ed., *Neurospchopharmacology*, pp. 339–342. Amsterdam: Excerpta Medica, 1967.

83. Gershon, S., L. J. Hekimian, A. Floyd, Jr. et al. "a-Methyl-p-Tyrosine (AMT) in Schizophrenia," *Psychopharmacologia*, 11 (1967), 189–194.

84. Glassman, A. H. "Indoleamines and Affective Disorders," *Psychosom. Med.*, 31 (1969), 107–114.

85. Glassman, A. H. and S. R. Platman. "Potentiation of a Monoamine Oxidase Inhibitor by Tryptophan," *J. Psychiatric Res.*, 7 (1969), 83–88.

86. Glowinski, J., J. Axelrod, and L. L. Iversen. "Regional Studies of Catecholamines in Rat Brain IV. Effects of Drugs on Disposition and Metabolism of H^3-Norepinephrine and H^3-Dopamine," *J. Pharmacol. Exp. Ther.*, 153 (1966), 30–41.

87. Glowinski, J., I. J. Kopin, and J. Axelrod. "Metabolism of (H^3) Norepinephrine in Rat Brain," *J. Neurochem.*, 12 (1965), 25–30.

88. Goodwin, F. K. "Behavioral Effects of L-

Dopa in Man," *Semin. Psychiatry*, 3 (1971), 477–492.

89. GOODWIN, F. K., D. L. DUNNER, and E. S. GERSHON. "Effect of L-Dopa Treatment on Brain Serotonin Metabolism in Depressed Patients," *Life Sci.* [I], 10 (1971), 751–759.

90. GOODWIN, F. K., D. L. MURPHY, H. K. H. BRODIE et al. "L-Dopa, Catecholamines, and Behavior: A Clinical and Biochemical Study in Depressed Patients," *Biolog. Psychiatry*, 2 (1970), 341–366.

91. ———. "Levodopa: Alterations in Behavior," *Clin. Pharmacol. Ther.*, 12 (1971), 383–396.

92. GOODWIN, F. K. and R. M. POST. "The Use of Probenecid in High Doses for the Estimation of Central Serotonin Turnover in Patients: Differences in Diagnostic Groups and the Effects of Amine Precursors and Snythesis Inhibitors," in J. Barchas and E. Usdin, eds., *Serotonin and Behavior*. New York: Academic, forthcoming.

93. GORDON, E. K. and J. OLIVER. "3-Methoxy-4-Hydroxyphenylethylene Glycol in Human Cerebrospinal Fluid," *Clinica Chim. Acta*, 35 (1971), 145–150.

94. GREENBLATT, M., G. H. GROSSER, and H. WECHSLER. "Differential Response of Hospitalized Depressed Patients to Somatic Therapy," *Am. J. Psychiatry*, 120 (1964), 935–943.

95. GREENSPAN, K., J. J. SCHILDKRAUT, E. K. GORDON et al. "Catecholamine Metabolism In Affective Disorders III. MHPG and Other Catecholamine Metabolites in Patients Treated with Lithium Carbonate," *J. Psychiatric Res.*, 7 (1970), 171–183.

96. GREENSPAN, K., J. J. SCHILDKRAUT, E. K. GORDON et al. "Catecholamine Metabolism in Affective Disorders II. Norepinephrine, Normetanephrine, Epinephrine, Metanephrine and VMA Excretion in Hypomanic Patients," *Arch. Gen. Psychiatry*, 21 (1969), 710–716.

97. GROF, P. and P. FOLEY. "The Superiority of Lithium Over Methysergide in Treating Manic Patients," *Am. J. Psychiatry*, 127 (1971), 1573–1574.

98. HASKOVEC, L. "Methysergide in Mania," *Lancet*, 2 (1969), 902.

99. HASKOVEC, L. and K. SOUCEK. "Trial of Methysergide in Mania," *Nature*, 219 (1968), 507–508.

100. ———. "The Action of Methysergide in Manic States," *Psychopharmacologia*, 15 (1969), 415–424.

101. HIMMELHOCH, J. M., T. P. DETRE, D. J. KUPFER et al. Unpublished observations.

102. HIMWICH, H. E. "Indoleamines and Depressions," in H. E. Himwich, ed., *Biochemistry, Schizophrenia and Affective Illnesses*, pp. 230–282. Baltimore: Williams & Wilkins, 1970.

103. HIMWICH, H. E. and H. S. ALPERS. "Psychopharmacology," *Annu. Rev. Pharmacol.*, 10 (1970), 313–324.

104. INGVARSSON, C. G. "Orientierende Klinische Versuche Zur Wirkung Des Dioxyphenylalanins (l-Dopa) bei Endogener Depression," *Arzeim. Forsch.*, 15 (1965), 849–852.

105. INWANG, E. E., J. H. SUGARMAN, D. MOSNAIM et al. "Ultraviolet Spectrophotometric Determination of B-Phenyl-ethylamine-like Substances in Biological Samples and Its Possible Correlation with Depression." Presented Ann. Meet., Soc. Biolog. Psychiatry, May 1972.

106. JANOWSKY, D. S., M. K. EL-YOUSEF, J. M. DAVIS et al. "Cholinergic Reversal of Manic Symptoms," *Lancet*, 1 (1972), 1236–1237.

107. JONSSON, L.-E., E. ANGGARD, and L.-M. GUNNE. "Blockade of Intravenous Amphetamine Euphoria in Man," *Clin. Pharmacol. Ther.*, 12 (1971), 889–896.

108. KANE, F. J. "Treatment of Mania with Cinanserin, an Anti-serotonin Agent," *J. Psychiatry*, 126 (1970), 1020–1023.

109. KARKI, N. T. "Urinary Excretion of Noradrenaline and Adrenaline in Different Age Groups, Its Diurnal Variation and Effect of Muscular Work on It," *Acta Physiol. Scand.*, 39 Suppl. 132 (1956), 5–96.

110. KETY, S. S. "The Precursor-Load Strategy in Psychochemical Research," in A. J. Mandell and M. P. Mandell, eds., *Psychochemical Research in Man*, pp. 127–131. New York: Academic, 1969.

111. ———. "Brain Amines and Affective Disorders," in B. T. Ho and W. M. McIsaac, eds., *Brain Chemistry and Mental Disease*, pp. 237–244. New York: Plenum, 1971.

112. KLAIBER, E. L., D. M. BROVERMAN, W. VOGEL et al. "Effects of Estrogen Therapy on Plasma MAO Activity and EEG Driving Responses of Depressed Women," *Am. J. Psychiatry*, 128 (1972), 1492–1498.

113. KLERMAN, G. L. and J. O. COLE. "Clinical Pharmacology of Imipramine and Related

Antidepressant Compounds," *Pharmacol. Rev.*, 17 (1965), 101–141.

114. KLERMAN, G. L., J. J. SCHILDKRAUT, L. L. HASENBUSH et al. "Clinical Experience with Dihydroxyphenylalanine (Dopa) in Depression," *J. Psychiatric Res.*, 1 (1963), 289–297.

115. KLINE, N. S. and W. SACKS. "Relief of Depression Within One Day Using M.A.O. Inhibitor and Intravenous 5-HTP," *Am. J. Psychiatry*, 120 (1963), 274–275.

116. KLINE, N. S., W. SACKS and G. M. SIMPSON. "Further Studies on One Day Treatment of Depression with 5-HTP," *Am. J. Psychiatry*, 121 (1964), 379–381.

117. KOPIN, I. J. and E. K. GORDON. "Metabolism of Norepinephrine-H^3 Released by Tyramine and Reserpine," *J. Pharmacol. Exp. Ther.*, 138 (1962), 351–359.

118. ———. "Metabolism of Administered and Drug-Released Norepinephrine-7-H^3 in Rat," *J. Pharmacol. Exp. Ther.*, 140 (1963), 207–216.

119. KORF, J., H. M. VAN PRAAG, and J. B. SEBENS. "Effect of Intravenously Administered Probenecid in Humans on the Levels of 5-Hydroxyindoleacetic Acid, Homovanillic Acid and 3-Methoxy-4-Hydroxy-Phenylglycol in Cerebrospinal Fluid," *Biochem. Pharmacol.*, 20 (1971), 659–668.

120. KUHN, R. "Treatment of Depressive States with G22355 (Imipramine Hydrochloride)," *Am. J. Psychiatry*, 115 (1958), 459–464.

121. LAPIN, I. P. and G. F. OXENKRUG. "Intensification of the Central Serotoninergic Processes as a Possible Determinant of the Thymoleptic Effect," *Lancet*, 1 (1969), 132–136.

122. LAPOLLA, A. and H. JONES. "Placebo-Control Evaluation of Desipramine in Depression," *Am. J. Psychiatry*, 127 (1970), 111–114.

123. MAAS, J. W., H. DEKIRMENJIAN, and J. FAWCETT. "Catecholamine Metabolism, Depression and Stress," *Nature*, 230 (1971), 330–331.

124. MAAS, J. W., H. DEKIRMENJIAN, D. GARVER et al. "Excretion of MHPG After Intraventricular 6-OH-DA." Presented Ann. Meet., Am. Psychiatric Assoc., May 1972.

125. MAAS, J. W., J. A. FAWCETT, and H. DEKIRMENJIAN. "3-Methoxy-4-Hydroxyphenylglycol (MHPG) Excretion in Depressive States: Pilot Study," *Arch. Gen. Psychiatry*, 19 (1968), 129–134.

126. ———. "Catecholamine Metabolism, Depressive Illness and Drug Response," *Arch. Gen. Psychiatry*, 26 (1972), 252–262.

127. MAAS, J. W. and D. H. LANDIS. "Technique for Assaying Kinetics of Norepinephrine Metabolism in Central Nervous System *in vivo*," *Psychosom. Med.*, 28 (1966), 247–256.

128. ———. "*In vivo* Studies of Metabolism of Norepinephrine in Central Nervous System," *Pharmacol. Exp. Ther.*, 163 (1968), 147–162.

129. MCCABE, M. S., T. REICH, and G. WINOKUR. "Methysergide as a Treatment for Mania," *Am. J. Psychiatry*, 127 (1970), 354–356.

130. MCLEOD, W. R. and M. S. MCLEOD. "Serotonin and Severe Affective Disorders," *Aust. N.Z. J. Psychiatry*, 5 (1971), 289–295.

131. MCNAMEE, H. B., J. P. MOODY, and G. J. NAYLOR. "Indoleamine Metabolism in Affective Disorders: Excretion of Tryptamine Indoleacetic Acid and 5-Hydroxyindoleacetic Acid in Depressive States," *J. Psychosom. Res.*, 16 (1972), 63–70.

132. MCNAMEE, H. B., D. LE POIDEVIN, and G. J. NAYLOR. "Methysergide in Mania: A Double-blind Comparison with Thioridazine," *Psychol. Med.*, 2 (1972), 66–69.

133. MANDEL, A. J. "Some Determinants of Indole Excretion in Man," *Recent Ad. Biolog. Psychiatry*, 5 (1963), 237–256.

134. MANNARINO, E., N. KIRSHNER, and B. S. NASHOLD, JR. "Metabolism of (C^{14}) Noradrenaline by Cat Brain *in vivo*," *J. Neurochem.*, 10 (1963), 373–379.

135. MATUSSEK, N., O. BENKERT, K. SCHNEIDER et al. "Wirkung eines Decarboxylasehemmers (Ro 4-4602) in Kombination mit L-DOPA auf gehemmte Depressionen," *Arzneim. Forsch.*, 20 (1970), 934–937.

136. MATUSSEK, N., H. POHLMEIER, and E. RUTHER. "Die Wirkung von Dopa auf gehemmte Depressionen," *Klin. Wochenschr.*, 44 (1966), 727–728.

137. MENDELS, J., A. FRAZER, R. G. FITZERGERALD et al. "Biogenic Amine Metabolites in Cerebrospinal Fluid of Depressed and Manic Patients," *Science*, 175 (1972), 1380–1382.

138. MESSIHA, F. S., D. AGALLIANOS, and C. CLOWER. "Dopamine Excretion in Affective States and Following Li_2CO_3 Therapy," *Nature*, 225 (1970), 868–869.

139. MOIR, A. T. B., G. W. ASHCROFT, T. B. B.

CRAWFORD et al. "Cerebral Metabolites in Cerebrospinal Fluid as a Biochemical Approach to the Brain," *Brain*, 93 (1970), 357–368.

140. MURPHY, D. L. "Amine Precursors, Amines, and False Neurotransmitters in Depressed Patients," *Am. J. Psychiatry*, 129 (1972), 55–62.

141. MURPHY, D. L., H. K. H. BRODIE, F. K. GOODWIN et al. "Regular Induction of Hypomania by L-Dopa in 'Bipolar' Manic-Depressive Patients," *Nature*, 229 (1971), 135–136.

142. MURPHY, D. L. and R. WEISS. "Reduced Monoamine Oxidase Activity in Blood Platelets from Bipolar Depressed Patients," *Am. J. Psychiatry*, 128 (1972), 1351–1357.

143. NEFF, N. H., T. N. TOZER, and B. B. BRODIE. "Application of Steady-State Kinetics to Studies of the Transfer of 5-Hydroxyindoleacetic Acid From Brain to Plasma," *J. Pharmacol. Exp. Ther.*, 158 (1967), 214–218.

144. NELSON, G. N., M. MASUDA, and T. H. HOLMES. "Correlation of Behavior and Catecholamine Metabolite Excretion," *Psychosom. Med.*, 28 (1966), 216–226.

145. NG, K. Y., T. N. CHASE, R. W. COLBURN et al. "L-Dopa-Induced Release of Cerebral Monoamines," *Science*, 170 (1970), 76–77.

146. NIES, A., D. S. ROBINSON, C. L. RAVARIS et al. "Amines and Monoamine Oxidase in Relation to Aging and Depression in Man," *Psychosom. Med.*, 33 (1971), 470.

147. NORDIN, G., J.-O. OTTOSSON, and B.-E. ROOS. "Influence of Convulsive Therapy on 5-Hydroxyindoleacetic Acid and Homovanillic Acid in Cerebrospinal Fluid in Endogenous Depression," *Psychopharmacologia*, 20 (1971), 315–320.

148. O'GORMAN, L. P., O. BORUD, I. A. KHAN et al. "The Metabolism of L-3,4-Dihydroxyphenylalanine in Man," *Clin. Chim. Acta*, 29 (1970), 111–119.

149. PAPESCHI, R. and D. J. MCCLURE. "Homovanillic and 5-Hydroxy-indoleacetic Acid in Cerebrospinal Fluid of Depressed Patients," *Arch. Gen. Psychiatry*, 25 (1971), 354–358.

150. PARE, C. M. B. "Potentiation of Monoamine Oxidase Inhibitors by Tryptophan," *Lancet*, 2 (1963), 527.

151. PARE, C. M. B. and M. SANDLER. "Clinical and Biochemical Study of Trial of Iproniazid in Treatment of Depression," *J. Neurol. Neurosurg. Psychiatry*, 22 (1959), 247–251.

152. PARE, C. M. B., D. P. H. YEUNG, K. PRICE et al. "5-Hydroxytryptamine in Brainstem, Hypothalamus and Caudate Nucleus of Controls and of Patients Committing Suicide by Coal-gas Poisoning," *Lancet*, 2 (1969), 133–135.

153. PERSSON, T., B.-E. ROOS. "5-Hydroxytryptophan for Depression," *Lancet*, 2 (1968), 987–988.

154. PERSSON, T. and J. WÅLINDER. "L-Dopa in the Treatment of Depressive Symptoms," *Br. J. Psychiatry*, 119 (1971), 277–278.

155. PLETSCHER, A. "Monoamine Oxidase Inhibitors: Effects Related to Psychostimulation," in D. H. Efron, ed., *Psychopharmacology Review of Progress 1957–1967*, pp. 649–654. Washington: U.S. Govt. Print. Office, 1968.

156. POLLIN, W., P. V. CARDON, JR., and S. S. KETY. "Effects of Amine Acid Feedings in Schizophrenic Patients Treated with Iproniazid," *Science*, 133 (1961), 104.

157. POST, R. M., J. KOTIN, and F. K. GOODWIN. "Psychomotor Activity and Cerebrospinal Fluid Amine Metabolites in Affective Illness." Presented Ann. Meet., Am. Psychiatric Assoc., May 1972.

158. PRAAG, H. M. VAN. "Monoamines and Depression," *Phar. Psychiatrie Neur. Psychopharm.*, 2 (1969), 151–160.

159. ———. "Indoleamines and the Central Nervous System," *Psychiatr. Neurol. Neurochir.*, 73 (1970), 9–36.

160. PRAAG, H. M. VAN and J. KORF. "L-tryptophan in Depression," *Lancet*, 2 (1970), 612.

161. ———. "Endogenous Depressions with and without Disturbances in the 5-Hydroxytryptamine Metabolism: A Biochemical Classification?" *Psychopharmacologia*, 19 (1971), 148–152.

162. ———. "A Pilot Study of Some Kinetic Aspects of the Metabolism of 5-Hydroxytryptamine in Depressive Patients," *Biolog. Psychiatry*, 3 (1971), 105–112.

163. ———. "Monoamine Metabolism in Depression: Clinical Application of the Probenecid Test," in J. Barchas and E. Usdin, eds., *Serotonin and Behavior*. New York: Academic, forthcoming.

164. PRAAG, H. M. VAN, J. KORF, L. C. W. DOLS

et al. "A Pilot Study of the Predictive Value of the Probenecid Test in Application of 5-Hydroxytryptophan as Antidepressant," *Psychopharmacologia*, 25 (1972), 14–21.

165. PRAAG, H. M. VAN, J. KORF, and J. PUITE. "5-Hydroxyindoleacetic Acid Levels in the Cerebrospinal Fluid of Depressive Patients Treated with Probenecid," *Nature*, 225 (1970), 1259–1260.

166. PRAAG, H. M. VAN and B. LEIJNSE. Die Bedeutung der Monoaminoxydasehemmung als Antidepressives Prinzip. I.," *Psychopharmacologia*, 4 (1963), 1–14.

167. PRANGE, A. J., JR. "The Pharmacology and Biochemistry of Depression," *Dis. Ner. Syst.*, 25 (1964), 217–221.

168. PRANGE, A. J., JR., L. R. McCURDY, and C. M. COCHRANE. "The Systolic Blood Pressure Response of Depressed Patients to Infused Norepinephrine," *J. Psychiatr. Res.*, 5 (1967), 1–13.

169. PRANGE, A. J., JR., I. C. WILSON, A. E. KNOX et al. "Thyroid-Imipramine Clinical and Chemical Interaction: Evidence for A Receptor Deficit in Depression," *J. Psychiatr. Res.*, in press.

170. REDMOND, D. E., JR., J. W. MAAS, A. KLING et al. "Social Behavior of Monkeys Selectively Depleted of Monoamines," *Science*, 174 (1971), 428–430.

171. REDMOND, D. E., JR., J. W. MAAS, A. KLING et al. "Changes in Primate Social Behavior After Treatment with Alpha-Methyl-Para-Tyrosine," *Psychosom. Med.*, 33 (1971), 97–113.

172. ROBERTS, D. J. and K. J. BROADLEY. "Treatment of Depression," *Lancet*, 1 (1965), 1219–1220.

173. ROBINSON, D. S., J. M. DAVIS, A. NIES et al. "Aging, Monoamines, and Monoamine-Oxidase Levels," *Lancet*, 1 (1972), 290–291.

174. ROBINSON, D. S., J. M. DAVIS, A. NIES et al. "Relation of Sex and Aging to Monoamine Oxidase Activity of Human Brain, Plasma and Platelets," *Arch. Gen. Psychiatry*, 24 (1971), 536–539.

175. ROCKLIFF, B. W. "Measurement of Drug Effects in Newly Hospitalized Depressives," *Dis. Ner. Syst.*, 32 (1971), 532–537.

176. RODNIGHT, R. "Body Fluid Indoles in Mental Illness," *Int. Rev. Neurobiol.*, 3 (1961), 251–292.

177. ROOS, B.-E. and R. SJÖSTRÖM. "5-Hydroxy-indoleacetic Acid and Homovanillic Acid Levels in the Cerebrospinal Fluid After Probenecid Application in Patients with Manic-Depressive Psychosis," *Pharmacol. Clin.*, 1 (1969), 153–155.

178. ROSENBLATT, S. and J. D. CHANLEY. "Differences in Metabolism of Norepinephrine in Depressions: Effects of Various Therapies," *Arch. Gen. Psychiatry*, 13 (1965), 495–502.

179. ROSENBLATT, S., J. D. CHANLEY, and W. P. LEIGHTON. "The Investigation of Adrenergic Metabolism with 7H³-Norepinephrine in Psychiatric Disorders. II. Temporal Changes in the Distribution of Urinary Tritiated Metabolites in Affective Disorders," *J. Psychiatr. Res.*, 6 (1969), 321–333.

180. RUBIN, R. T. "Adrenal Cortical Activity Changes in Manic-Depressive Illness," *Arch. Gen. Psychiatry*, 17 (1967), 671–679.

181. ———. "Multiple Biochemical Correlates of Manic-Depressive Illness," *J. Psychosom. Res.*, 12 (1968), 171–180.

182. RUBIN, R. T., R. G. MILLER, B. R. CLARK et al. "The Stress of Aircraft Carrier Landings II. 3-Methoxy-4-Hydroxyphenylglycol Excretion in Naval Aviators," *Psychosom. Med.*, 32 (1970), 589–597.

183. RUBIN, R. T., W. M. YOUNG, and B. R. CLARK. "17-Hydroxycorticosteroid and Vanillylmandelic Acid Excretion in a Rapidly Cycling Manic-Depressive," *Psychosom. Med.*, 30 (1968), 162–171.

184. SCHANBERG, S. M., G. R. BREESE, J. J. SCHILDKRAUT et al. "3-Methoxy-4-Hydroxyphenylglycol Sulfate in Brain and Cerebrospinal Fluid," *Biochem. Pharmacol.*, 17 (1968), 2006–2008.

185. SCHANBERG, S. M., J. J. SCHILDKRAUT, G. R. BREESE et al. "Metabolism of Normetanephrine-H³ in Rat Brain—Identification of Conjugated 3-Methoxy-4-Hydroxyphenylglycol as Major Metabolite," *Biochem. Pharmacol.*, 17 (1968), 247–254.

186. SCHILDKRAUT, J. J. "The Catecholamine Hypothesis of Affective Disorders: A Review of Supporting Evidence," *Am. J. Psychiatry*, 122 (1965), 509–522.

187. ———. "Rationale of Some Approaches Used in Biochemical Studies of the Affective Disorders: The Pharmacological Bridge," in A. J. Mandell and M. P. Mandell, eds., *Psychochemical Research In*

Man, pp. 113–126. New York: Academic, 1969.

188. ———. *Neuropsychopharmacology and the Affective Disorders*. Boston: Little, Brown, 1970.

189. ———. "Neurochemical Studies of the Affective Disorders: The Pharmacological Bridge," *Am. J. Psychiatry*, 127 (1970), 358–360.

190. ———. "The Effects of Lithium on Norepinephrine Turnover and Metabolism: Basic and Clinical Studies," in S. Gershon, ed., *Amines and Affective Disease*. New York: Plenum, forthcoming.

191. ———. "Norepinephrine Metabolism in the Pathophysiology and Classification of Depressive Disorders," in J. O. Cole and A. Freedman, eds., *Psychopathology and Psychopharmacology*. Baltimore: Johns Hopkins Press, forthcoming.

192. ———. "The Effects of Lithium on Biogenic Amines," in S. Gershon and B. Shopsin, eds., *Lithium: Its Role in Psychiatric Research and Treatment*. New York: Plenum, forthcoming.

193. SCHILDKRAUT, J. J., G. A. DODGE, and M. A. LOGUE. "Effects of Tricyclic Antidepressants on Uptake and Metabolism of Intracisternally Administered Norepinephrine-H³ in Rat Brain," *J. Psychiatr. Res.*, 7 (1969), 29–34.

194. SCHILDKRAUT, J. J., P. R. DRASKOCZY, E. S. GERSHON et al. "Effects of Tricyclic Antidepressants on Norepinephrine Metabolism: Basic and Clinical Studies," in B. T. Ho and W. M. McIsaac, eds., *Brain Chemistry and Mental Disease*, pp. 215–236. New York: Plenum, 1971.

195. ———. "Catecholamine Metabolism in Affective Disorders. IV. Preliminary Studies of Norepinephrine Metabolism in Depressed Patients Treated with Amitriptyline," *J. Psychiatr. Res.*, in press.

196. SCHILDKRAUT, J. J., E. K. GORDON, and J. DURELL. "Catecholamine Metabolism in Affective Disorders. I. Normetanephrine and VMA Excretion in Depressed Patients Treated with Imipramine," *J. Psychiatr. Res.*, 3 (1965), 213–228.

197. SCHILDKRAUT, J. J., R. GREEN, E. K. GORDON et al. "Normetanephrine Excretion and Affective State in Depressed Patients Treated with Imipramine," *Am. J. Psychiatry*, 123 (1966), 690–700.

198. SCHILDKRAUT, J. J., B. A. KEELER, M. P.

ROGERS et al. "Catecholamine Metabolism in Affective Disorders: A Longitudinal Study of a Patient Treated with Amitriptyline and ECT." Presented Ann. Meet. Am. Psychosom. Soc., 1972.

199. SCHILDKRAUT, J. J. and S. S. KETY. "Biogenic Amines and Emotion," *Science*, 156 (1967), 21–30.

200. SCHILDKRAUT, J. J., G. L. KLERMAN, D. G. FRIEND et al. "Biochemical and Pressor Effects on Oral D, l-dihydroxyphenlyalanine in Patients Pretreated with Antidepressant Drugs," *Ann. N.Y. Acad. Sci.*, 107 (1963), 1005–1015.

201. SCHILDKRAUT, J. J., G. L. KLERMAN, R. HAMMOND et al. "Excretion of 3-Methoxy-4-Hydroxymandelic Acid (VMA) in Depressed Patients Treated With Antidepressant Drugs," *J. Psychiatr. Res.*, 2 (1964), 257–266.

202. SCHILDKRAUT, J. J., S. M. SCHANBERG, G. R. BREESE et al. "Norepinephrine Metabolism and Drugs Used in Affective Disorders: Possible Mechanism of Action," *Am. J. Psychiatry*, 124 (1967), 600–608.

203. SCHILDKRAUT, J. J., S. M. SCHANBERG, and I. J. KOPIN. "Effects of Lithium Ion on H³-Norepinephrine Metabolism in Brain," *Life Sci.*, 5 (1966), 1479–1483.

204. SCHILDKRAUT, J. J., S. M. SCHANBERG, I. J. KOPIN et al. "Affective Disorders and Norepinephrine Pharmacology," in E. Shneidman and M. J. Ortega, eds., *Aspects of Depression*, pp. 83–141. Boston: Little, Brown, 1969.

205. SCHILDKRAUT, J. J., R. WATSON, P. R. DRASKOCZY et al. "Amphetamine Withdrawal: Depression and MHPG Excretion," *Lancet*, 2 (1971), 485–486.

206. ———. Unpublished data.

207. SCHILDKRAUT, J. J., A. WINOKUR, and C. W. APPLEGATE. "Norepinephrine Turnover and Metabolism in Rat Brain After Chronic Administration of Imipramine," *Science*, 168 (1970), 867–869.

208. SCHILDKRAUT, J. J., A. WINOKUR, P. R. DRASKOCZY et al. "Changes in Norepinephrine Turnover in Rat Brain During Chronic Administration of Imipramine and Protriptyline: A Possible Explanation for the Delay in Onset of Clinical Antidepressant Effects," *Am. J. Psychiatry*, 127 (1971), 1032–1039.

209. SERRY, D. "Methysergide in Mania," *Lancet*, 1 (1969), 417.

210. SHARMAN, D. F. "Glycol Metabolites of Noradrenaline in Brain Tissue," *Br. J. Pharmacol.*, 36 (1969), 523–534.

211. SHAW, D. M., F. E. CAMPS, and E. G. ECCLESTON. "5-Hydroxytryptamine in Hindbrain of Depressive Suicides," *Br. J. Psychiatry*, 113 (1967), 1407–1411.

212. SHIH, J.-H., C. and S. EIDUSON. "Multiple forms of Monoamine Oxidase in Developing Tissues: The Implications for Mental Disorder," in B. T. Ho and W. M. McIsaac, eds., *Brain Chemistry and Mental Disease*, pp. 3–20. New York: Plenum, 1971.

213. SHINFUKU, N., M. OMURA, and M. KAYANO. "Catecholamine Excretion in Manic Depressive Psychosis," *Yonago Acta Med.*, 5 (1961), 109–114.

214. SHINFUKU, N. "Clinical and Biochemical Studies with Antidepressants," *Yonago Acta Med.*, 9 (1965), 100–102.

215. SJÖSTRÖM, R., "Steady-State Levels of Probenecid and Their Relation to Acid Monoamine Metabolites in Human Cerebrospinal Fluid," *Psychopharmacologia*, 25 (1972), 96–100.

216. SLOANE, R. B., W. HUGHES, and H. L. HAUST. "Catecholamine Excretion in Manic-Depressive and Schizophrenic Psychosis and Its Relationship to Symptomatology," *Can. Psychiatr. Assoc. J.*, 11 (1966), 6–19.

217. STROM-OLSEN, R. and H. WEIL-MALHERBE. "Humoral Changes in Manic-Depressive Psychosis with Particular Reference to Excretion of Catecholamines in Urine," *J. Ment. Sci.*, 104 (1958), 696–704.

218. SULSER, F., M. H. BICKEL, and B. B. BRODIE. "The Action of Desmethylimipramine in Counteracting Sedation and Cholinergic Effects of Reserpine-like Drugs," *J. Pharmacol. Exp. Ther.*, 144 (1964), 321–330.

219. SULSER, F. and E. SANDERS BUSH. "Effect of Drugs on Amines in the CNS," *Annu. Rev. Pharmacol.*, 11 (1971), 209–230.

220. TAKAHASHI, R., Y. NAGAO, K. TSUCHIYA et al. "Catecholamine Metabolism of Manic-depressive Illness," *J. Psychiatr. Res.*, 6 (1968), 185–199.

221. TAKAHASHI, R., H. UTENA, Y. MACHIYAMA et al. "Tyrosine Metabolism in Manic-Depressive Illness," *Life Sci.* [II], 7 (1968), 1219–1231.

222. TISSOT, R. "Connaissances Experimentales sur les Monoamines et Quelques Syndromes Psychiatriques," in J. De Ajuriaguerra, ed., *Monoamines et Systeme Nerveux Central*, pp. 169–207. Geneva: Georg, 1962.

223. TURNER, W. J. and S. MERLIS. "Clinical Trial of Pargyline and DOPA in Psychotic Subjects," *Dis. Ner. Syst.*, 25 (1964), 538–541.

224. VAN SCHEYEN, J. D. "Behandeling van Manie Met Methysergide," *Ned. Tijdschr. Geneeskd.*, 115 (1971), 1634–1637.

225. VERSTER, J. P. "Preliminary Report on the Treatment of Mentally Disordered Patients by Intrathecally Administered Phenothiazine Drugs and an Antiserotonin Substance," *S. Afr. Med. J.*, 37 (1963), 1086–1087.

226. WATSON, R., E. HARTMANN, and J. J. SCHILDKRAUT. "Amphetamine Withdrawal: Affective State, Sleep Patterns and MHPG Excretion," *Am. J. Psychiatry*, 129 (1972), 263–269.

227. WEIL-MALHERBE, H. "Biochemistry of Functional Psychoses," *Advances in Enzymology*, 29 (1967), 479–553.

228. WEIL-MALHERBE, H., J. AXELROD, and R. TOMCHICK. "Blood-brain Barrier for Adrenaline," *Science*, 129 (1959), 1226.

229. WILK, S., K. L. DAVIS, and S. B. THACKER. "Determination of 3-Methoxy-4-Hydroxyphenylethylene Glycol (MHPG) in Cerebrospinal Fluid," *Anal. Biochem.*, 39 (1971), 498–504.

230. WILK, S., B. SHOPSIN, S. GERSHON et al. "Cerebrospinal Fluid Levels of MHPG in Affective Disorders," *Nature*, 235 (1972), 440–441.

231. WURTMAN, R. J., C. M. ROSE, S. MATTHYSSE et al. "L-Dihydroxyphenylalanine: Effect on S-Adenosyl-Methionine in Brain," *Science*, 169 (1970), 395–397.

232. WYATT, R. J., B. PORTNOY, D. J. KUPFER et al. "Resting Plasma Catecholamine Concentrations in Patients with Depression and Anxiety," *Arch. Gen. Psychiatry*, 24 (1971), 65–70.

233. ZALL, H. "Lithium Carbonate and Isocarboxiad—An Effective Drug Approach in Severe Depression," *Am. J. Psychiatry*, 127 (1971), 1400–1403.

CHAPTER 22

FRONTIERS IN THE NEUROBIOLOGY OF EUPHORIA*

Arnold J. Mandell

❲ Introduction

THE RECOGNITION and then the evaluation of a particular human affect state by a culture at a time and place in history are indeed very complex. Those of us working in an area that is in the interface between sociocultural and psychobiological variables intuitively know that there are affect states which, due to our culture's lack of focus on them, go without a name. As an example, multivariate behavorial analyses frequently generate emotive factors that have no common name and researchers must assign them numbers or invent words to describe them. The role of cultural factors in the definition of affect states relates also to changes in the

values people assign to particular states. For example, we are aware of the interesting shift in features seen as highly valent in an excited young person of the Roaring Twenties compared to what was considered ideal in the cool, apparently relaxed, unresponsive young person of the Sixties. Yesterday's "flapper" is today's "up-tight;" yesterday's "schizo" is today's "cool" one. A dramatic example of this shift was clear to me when a recent freshman medical school class totally rejected a 1956 movie about a teenage borderline patient; in no way could they see his object relations and affect state as psychopathological.

A more common (and perhaps professionally exploited) shift relates to the current cultural view of anxiety. No longer is anxiety seen as a concomitant of living; in almost all forms it is seen as a treatable symptom. The recommended treatment for anxiety in the first

* This work is supported by USPHS Grants MH–14360–07; DA–00046–04; and DA–00265–03, as well as the Friends of Psychiatric Research of San Diego, Inc.

several decades of this century was psycho-therapy or psychoanalysis, and during the current era, it seems to be the use of an ever-burgeoning group of mild psychotropic drugs.

These cultural views of affect states have wide ramifications. For example, a person whose tendency is to be alert and to cope hyperactively in new, ambiguous circumstances may be made to feel abnormal. The hyperactivity may be seen as requiring some type of medical, pharmacological, or interpersonal intervention. In contrast, a person who withdraws emotionally may be seen as having a sense of mastery. This kind of issue has been of particular interest with respect to the drug treatment of some hyperactive children. In the case of a person manifesting features of the devalued affect state, the interpretation of this natural-for-him affect state as psychopathological may become in itself a stimulus for anxiety. Culturally determined positive and negative evaluations of various human affect states may be facilitated (at least within the diagnostic priesthood of medicine) by the advertising programs of pharmaceutical houses. It seems as though the effects of cultural consciousness, media management, and psychopharmacological discovery have and will lead to the birth and rationalization of many new dimensions of diagnosis and treatment in psychiatry.

This chapter focuses on an affect state that is emerging as important in the current era. Only very recently have even relatively sophisticated psychopharmacologists come to realize that euphoria can be chemically induced independent of the reduction of pain or anxiety or of hallucinatory propensity.[38,40] In addition to the increasing professional awareness of this potential for affecting human mood, there is a growing pressure from patients who insist that doctors help them with a new kind of depression, an existential crisis of meaning, an individually felt, but perhaps culturally determined, sense of anomie. Rather than serve as signals for change, renewal, reevaluation, or creative solutions, mild dysphoric states, catagorized under the rubric of depression, serve now as indications for treatment. Beyond the emergence of the chemical

tools and increased cultural awareness, the vast American folk pharmacology and a new era of self-medication by both patients and younger doctors are making euphoria an acceptable state, a desirable state. Our studies[9,10] have shown that young people are living through a period of polypsychotropic drug experimentation in which the drug family with the consistently unsaturated market is the euphorigen-hallucinogen class. Younger doctors and residents are sensitized to the dimensions of dysphoria and anhedonia and ask why these states are not treated specifically with the agents that they learned about through their folk pharmacology experiences.

The physician in his usual daily practice seldom sees euphoria apart from other drug actions like pain relief or antidepressant action. Some neurological syndromes that manifest aspects of euphoria have been described, however. The most dramatic would be the relaxed carefreeness of the middle and late stages of multiple sclerosis. Patients are described as being relatively happy while experiencing progressively crippling symptoms. In terms of clinical phenomena there isn't a more dramatic demonstration of the potential usefulness of this state in medicine. When discussing euphorigens, their method of action, and their potential uses in man, one encounters resistance to the topic even among scientists and medical men until the discussion is directed toward patients who have paid or soon will pay "their dues." It may be that the initial discussions of the development of drugs to produce primary euphoria (without attendant pain relief or antidepressant action) should be within the context of the clinical management of dying patients or their close relatives. Perhaps one should talk about these drugs as having the potential for the prevention or treatment of severe psychosomatic disorders attendant on the stressful experiences of life, such as the loss of a mate or child.

This paper will deal with four areas of the neurobiology of euphoria. The first section will be a brief discussion of some aspects of the physical chemistry of euphorigens in relation to naturally occurring neurotransmitters and their physiological and behavioral effects.

Second, there will be a description of some of the evidence that the brain may have the potential for the synthesis of euphorigens that could play some role in the normal regulation of subjective states in man. The third section will describe some of the barriers to developing euphorigens having long-term efficacy, i.e., the kinds of neurobiological adaptations that the brain can make to agents that alter normal synaptic function. The last section will suggest theoretical and experimental approaches for future research designed to deal with these adaptational processes.

(Euphorigens—Some Structures and Effects

In 1931, in a fascinatingly farsighted book, Lewin[20] created a useful typology of psychoactive drugs that focuses on five major affects: hypnotica, euphorica, phantastica, excitantia, and inebriantia. Increasing experience with human use of psychoactive agents suggests that, depending on the person and the dose, each drug can be euphorigenic, with the effect of higher doses depending upon drug class. Table 22–1 summarizes this concept with some examples. The euphorigenic properties of many drugs are not frequently acknowledged. For example, hypnotic drugs such as the barbiturates can produce a kind of "paradoxical" excitement early in the time course of their onset of action or at low doses. The "hit" that many barbiturate takers experience is described as euphoric. Mild to moderately depressed people especially frequently report euphoric relief from stimulants like the amphetamines.

An operational definition of euphoria for use in experimental work is most difficult. Using a wide variety of behavioral items and a relatively noneuphorigenic control drug that mimics such phenomena as central activation and autonomic effects (e.g. amphetamines) we can study the euphoric effect. The studies of Snyder, Faillace, and Weingartner on the methoxy-amphetamine derivatives,[40] and that of Szara on the N-methylated indoleamines[44] are good examples. We have summarized the clinical aspects of the effects of the euphorigen-hallucinogen family of drugs elsewhere.[30]

Two general categories of compounds are similar to naturally occurring neurotransmitters in the brain and relevant to the neurobiological issues addressed here. The first group consists of the indoleamines, exemplified in Figure 22–1. Note the indoleamine structure of serotonin and its obvious derivation from tryptophan via the 5-hydroxylation pathway. The dimethylation of the nitrogen group in serotonin produces a centrally active stimulant, N,N-dimethylserotonin (bufotenin). Because this compound will not cross the blood-brain barrier, it has not been demonstrated to have central action in man.[45] However, when the 5-hydroxy position is made less polar by methylation, 5-methoxy-N, N-dimethyltryptamine is formed, which is an extremely potent compound, active in doses of 3 to 5 μg/kg in man.[8] The other major group

TABLE 22–1   Typology of Psychoactive Drugs

| DRUG CLASS | EFFECT | | |
	LOW DOSE	INTERMEDIATE DOSE	HIGH DOSE
Stimulant	Euphoria	Excitement	Manic-paranoid state
Sedative	Euphoria	Sedation	Coma
Alcohol	Euphoria	Inebriation	Coma
Euphorigen, potent	Euphoria	Euphoria-hallucinosis	Psychosis
Euphorigen, mild	Euphoria	Euphoria	Euphoria

After L. Lewin.[20] Relative doses represent multiples of minimum psychoactive doses.

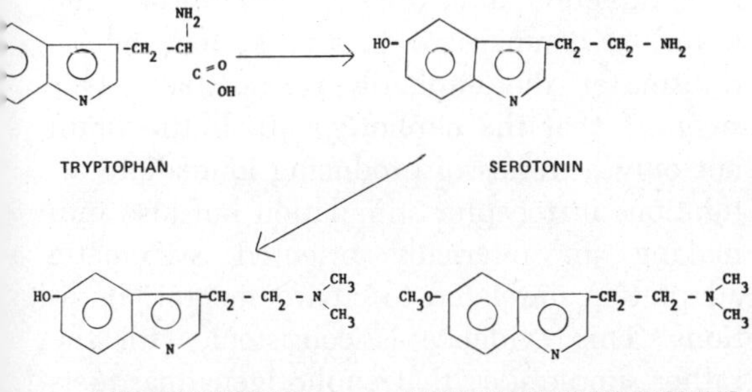

Figure 22–1. The metabolic derivation of indole(ethyl)amine euphorigens from the amino acid tryptophan.

of euphorigens that resemble neurotransmitters are noted in Figure 22–2, compounds structurally related to the brain catecholamines norepinephrine and dopamine. A well-known parent compound in this family is mescaline (3,4,5-trimethoxyphenylethylamine), and the relationship between this agent and dopamine is relatively clear. Another parent compound is one in which the aliphatic side chain is α-methylated, as in amphetamine. These two parent compounds can yield a wide variety of potentially euphorigenic derivatives, which have been reviewed by Shulgin and his associates.[39] The derivatives, such as 2,5-dimethoxy-4-methylamphetamine (STP) or 2,5-dimethoxy-4-ethylamphetamine (DOET), are euphorigenic at lower doses and have

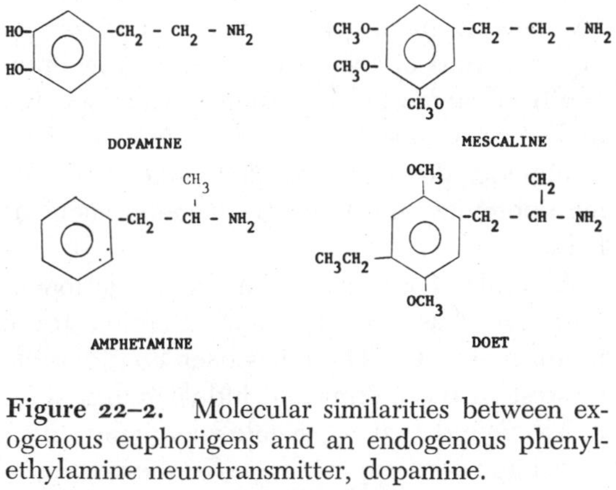

varying degrees of hallucinogenic activity at higher doses.

Structure-activity considerations involving these compounds have been theoretically elaborate,[39,41] but Shulgin has perhaps the most simple and straightforward formulation about the structure and electronic requirements for the euphorigen family. He suggests that at least three elements are necessary for central activity: (1) an aromatic system with potentially high molecular orbital energy, (2) an aliphatic carbon chain of optimal length separating the aromatic system from a (3) terminal nitrogen site. This scheme for euphorigenic activity is applicable to the indoleamines when we note that the five-membered pyrole part of the indole ring donates electrons to the substituted benzene ring. Electron donor groups on the nitrogen may increase basicity, thereby increasing the potency of the compound. If we view the pyrole ring as a methoxy group we can associate most psychoactive indoleamine compounds with the derivatives of mescaline or amphetamine. N-methylation apparently increases potency in the indoleamine series more effectively than in the phenylethylamine series. Alpha-methyl substitution may increase potency by hindering an enzymatic attack on the nitrogen of the amino group.

Various theories of action of these agents have been reviewed elsewhere, but the general assumption is that they interact with their analogous neurotransmitters and in so doing stimulate or inhibit receptor activity in an abnormal way or to an abnormal extent. Considerable evidence is accruing, from microelectrode studies in cell body and nerve ending regions of known biogenic amine pathways, that these agents result in abnormal activity associated with electrical evidence of various attempts at feedback compensation. Such evidence is available for the noradrenergic, dopaminergic, and serotonergic systems.[1]

The long-term effects of these agents present far more formidable challenges for mechanistic explanation. The post-hallucinatory glow that has been reported by a number of workers[44] can last several weeks. It could be viewed as either some sort of adaptation by

Figure 22–2. Molecular similarities between exogenous euphorigens and an endogenous phenylethylamine neurotransmitter, dopamine.

the brain to the action of the drug or the continuing action of the drug stored in nerve endings. In our laboratory we are considerably more impressed with the first concept, i.e. the potential importance of the behavioral expression of dramatically fast adaptation to these agents by the brain. Figure 22–3 summarizes data indicating very fast behavioral adaptation to a powerful hallucinogen when it was administered in such a way that hepatic mechanisms could not account for the tolerance. Note that within half an hour there was marked diminution in the behaviorally activating effects of both 5-methoxy-N,N-dimethyltryptamine and bufotenin. Work to be reviewed below demonstrates that these adaptations can last several hours, days, or weeks. Thus, in addition to the immediate neurophysiological compensation manifested by changes in action potentials and/or unit firing rates[1] there appear to be longer-term macromolecular changes that could change either the turnover of the neurotransmitter or the effectiveness of its receptor, or both.

Following the administration of an hallucinogen, a cell system's unit firing rate changes

in a direction indicating an attempt by the brain to compensate in the system whose transmitter the euphorigen resembles. This suggests that the euphorigen fools the brain not only in terms of producing immediate alterations in receptor stimulation but also into making an internally oriented systematic adaptation unrelated to environmental conditions. This evidence is consistent with the rather simple idea that euphorigens masquerade as transmitters and alter the function of synaptic systems both immediately *and* on long term bases.

❨ A Naturally Occurring Euphorigen

For a number of years evidence has been accruing that mammalian cells may be able to convert neurotransmitter biogenic amines into compounds in the euphorigen-hallucinogen category. The most common source of interest was the potential of such a transformation to cause various kinds of psychopathology, particularly the schizophrenias.[28] One of the best known speculations about conversion of a transmitter to a euphorigen was first reported by Friedhoff and Van Winkle.[6] They found a compound resembling dimethoxyphenylethylamine more frequently in the urine of schizophrenic patients than in that of a nonschizophrenic control group. This was confirmed as well as denied by other investigators.[3,17] The theory is that dopamine is converted from a normal neurotransmitter to a euphorigen-hallucinogen via an abnormal 4-o-methylation. The involvement of dopamine and/or its products and of the striate area in the brain has been suggested by others because of evidence concerning the site of action of psychotomimetic doses of amphetamine and the high-potency antipsychotic agents such as haloperidol.

A similar conversion, the dimethylation of serotonin, has occupied our attention for a number of years. There has been considerable interest in the methylated indoleamines since it was found that a psychic-energizing effect associated with euphoria and/or the precipita-

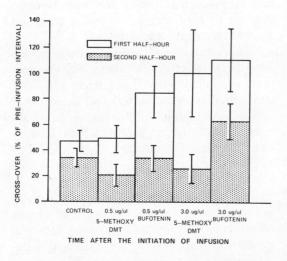

Figure 22–3. Effects of intraventricular infusion of 5-methoxy-dimethyltryptamine (DMT) and bufotenin on the gross motor activity of freely moving rats. The potency of these two compounds is comparable when they are administered directly to the brain. N = 6. Rate of infusion = 1 μl per 3 minutes.

tion of an acute attack of schizophrenia can result when an indoleamine source, such as tryptophan, is combined with a methyl source, such as betaine or methionine, and administered with a monoamine oxidase inhibitor.[4,18,33] In small doses exogenous tryptophan produces behavioral activation and an increased sense of well-being; in larger doses it activates latent psychotic symptoms.[11]

When we administered 5-hydroxytryptophan and a monoamine oxidase inhibitor to newborn white Leghorn chicks, the result was behavioral activation and abnormal posture that resembled patterns we had seen when we administered hallucinogens. The stereotypic response of these animals to psychotropic drugs made such comparisons possible.[29] The speculation followed that the monoamine oxidase inhibitor blocked the normal metabolic degradation of serotonin and shunted the transmitter to a methylation reaction. This scheme is diagrammed in Figure 22–4. A major reservation attendant on this theory was that there had been no demonstration of a specific indoleamine N-methyltransferase in brain that could make such a conversion.

Using isotopic loads of tryptophan, however, and S-adenosylmethionine as a methyl donor, we were able to demonstrate the presence of both monomethyl and dimethylserotonin in brain extracts.[42] Previous reports of a nonspecific lung enzyme that could methylate a variety of biogenic aromatic amines complicated the conclusion that the methylation of the indoleamines was occurring in the brain.[2] Because of the decreased blood-brain barrier in the newborn chick it was impossible to determine whether the radioactive bufotenin came from the lungs or the brain.

We then began to investigate whether the brain itself had an N-methylating enzyme for indoleamines. Our initial studies demonstrated that a chick brain homogenate could catalyze the production of radioactivity extractable in isoamyl alcohol when S-adenosylmethionine and either serotonin or tryptamine were used as substrates.[31] The enzymatic production of radioactivity was linear with time and protein concentration, and the protein fraction capable of catalyzing this reaction could be enriched over tenfold by ammonium sulfate precipitation and Sephadex G-200 column chromatography. The monomethyl and dimethyl products of this reaction were isographic with known standards on chromatograms in several solvent systems. This enzymatic activity was also demonstrated in the human brain.[26] We have since enhanced this indole(ethyl)amine N-methyltransferase (IENMT) activity twenty-five fold by progressive purification, including dialysis (Table 22–2). Table 22–3 summarizes experiments demonstrating the substrate specificity of the enzyme. Note that the imidazoleamine histamine and the catecholamines were not methylated by the enriched protein fraction. Saavedra and Axelrod[34] have confirmed our findings in temporal lobe material from the brains of nonpsychotic subjects. In addition, Frohman[7] has reported identification of dimethylated tryptamine from the human brain by the use of gas chromatography and mass spectroscopy.

The functional significance of brain indoleamine N-methyltransferase activity is far from settled. Its K_m for indoleamine substrates is about 50 μM. This suggests that under usual circumstances brain monoamine oxidase, which has higher specific activity and greater affinity for substrate, would probably degrade

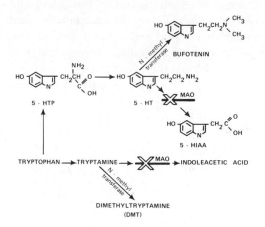

Figure 22–4. A hypothetical indole(ethyl)amine shunt that may be activated when the normal degradation of serotonin by oxidative deamination is blocked by a monoamine oxidase inhibitor (or a high dose of amphetamine).

TABLE 22–2.   Specific Activity of Indole(ethyl)amine N-Methyltransferase in Homogenate from Sheep Brain

FRACTION	ACTIVITY *pmoles tryptamine methylated per mg. protein per hour*
8,000 × g supernate	14.8
100,000 × g supernate	28.2
(NH₄)₂SO₄ precipitate 0–25%	8.9
25–35%	33.9
35–45%	71.5
45–55%	99.3
55–65%	24.4
65–80%	10.0
Sephadex G-200 fraction of 35–55% (NH₄)₂SO₄ precipitates	460.1

IENMT from sheep brain was progressively purified by centrifugation, ammonium sulfate precipitation and Sephadex column chromatography. The 35–55% ammonium sulfate precipitate was fractionated on a column equilibrated with potassium-phosphate buffer. Some portion of the 30-fold increase in activity probably reflects the removal of an inhibitor of the enzyme.

the indoleamines before methylation could occur unless compartmental variables prevented contact between the substrate and the oxidase. The other known inactivation mechanism for serotonin in the synapse is reuptake. The reuptake mechanism too has a higher affinity for the substrate than the methylation enzyme does. It thus appears that IENMT might function only under conditions of impaired presynaptic uptake or monoamine oxidase inhibition.

Table 22–4 demonstrates the relationship between IENMT and the nerve ending sero-tonin biosynthetic unit; note that the enzyme is present in nerve endings in more significant amounts. We have demonstrated adaptive changes in tryptophan hydroxylase, the rate-limiting enzyme in the biosynthesis of serotonin, after drug treatment or environmental manipulation.[27] Such changes could increase serotonin biosynthesis and, in turn, the probability that IENMT would function. So could exaggerated neural activity and the extraneuronal release of serotonin. Tryptophan loads increase the uptake of tryptophan into sero-tonergic nerve endings, and the combination

TABLE 22–3.   Substrate Specificity and Purification of Indole(ethyl)amine N-Methyltransferase from Sheep Brain

SUBSTRATE	SPECIFIC ACTIVITY *nmoles of substrate methylated/mg. of protein per /hour*		
	100,000 × g supernate	35–45% (NH₄)₂SO₄ precipitate	Sephadex G-200 fraction
Tryptamine	0.22	0.86	2.13
Histamine	7.13	1.23	0.17
Normetanephrine	0.04		
Norepinephrine			

Values below 0.02 were disregarded.

TABLE 22–4. **Regional Distribution of Indole (ethyl) amine N-Methyltransferase (IENMT) and Two Forms of Tryptophan Hydroxylase (TRYP-OH) in Rat Brain**

	ENZYME ACTIVITY		
	pmoles per mg. of protein per hour		
	synaptosomal		soluble
BRAIN REGION	TRYP-OH	IENMT	TRYP-OH
Caudate	100.6	83.5	0
Cortex	41.6	34.6	0
Medulla	29.8	36.4	3.7
Hypothalamus	29.3	36.1	29.8
Spinal cord	26.0	37.4	10.0
Midbrain	14.4	25.8	87.1
Whole brain	10.8	23.6	18.4

of tryptophan loads and monoamine oxidase inhibitors at lower doses elevates mood and promotes a sense of well-being, suggesting to us that serotonin may have become available to IENMT. The potency of bufotenin, once the blood-brain barrier has been overcome, is at least as great as that of 5-methoxy-N,N-dimethyltryptamine, which suggests that serotonin in the brain could be converted into a powerful euphorigen.[23]

Since "proof" of relationships between behavioral and neurobiological variables is so difficult, theorists talk about possibilities rather than probabilities. It can be said now only that the brain is capable of making an euphorigen that had been discussed previously only in pharmacological studies. Whether this capacity can be realized except under experimental circumstances has not been demonstrated.

The functional significance of a central euphorigen is obscured by myriad synaptic neurobiological compensatory mechanisms that would prevent prolongation of its action. This is particularly true of the drugs in the euphorigen class. It is clear that, in addition to agents that can induce euphoric feelings in man, the human brain may be able to produce such feelings with the biotransformation of a neurotransmitter. A major technical barrier to understanding how man can mobilize his own euphorigenic mechanisms and how we might be able to use drugs of this sort in the man-agement of long-term clinical problems appears to be the dramatic adaptation to the presence of such substances in the brain.

(Some Neurobiological Adaptive Mechanisms

The amount of neurotransmitter active at the synapse is thought to be determined by the release and reuptake of the transmitter, mediated by the activity of the neural system involved. Another component in the regulatory process seems to be the amount and/or the activity of the enzymes involved in transmitter degradation. In the case of the catecholamines, for example, the latter would involve O-methylation and/or oxidative deamination. The third factor in the regulation of the functional transmitter level in the brain is a sequence of biosynthetic enzymes.[21] An active neural system releases into the synapse newly synthesized transmitter in preference to stored transmitter.[14] Until very recently the only known regulatory mechanisms for tyrosine hydroxylase, the rate-limiting enzyme in the biosynthesis of catecholamines, appeared to be product-feedback inhibition.[19,32] Norepinephrine or its immediate precursor, the transmitter dopamine, as products of this pathway, can compete with tyrosine hydroxylase for its pteridine cofactor. Dopamine is ten times more effective as an inhibitor of the enzyme than norepinephrine is.[16] When more transmitter product is released, less product remains in the nerve ending to inhibit the enzyme activity, so more product is synthesized. When less product is released there is more remaining to inhibit the enzyme, and less transmitter is synthesized. This scheme is clearest for catecholamine biosynthesis in the adrenal where the amine is released into the general circulation and acts, as endocrine products do, on a distant target organ. The importance of product-feedback regulation compared to other regulatory mechanisms in nerve endings is less clear in both peripheral sympathetic systems and the brain. The cell's task is to convey information to the next cell in the system by affecting the receptor, and thus *effect* appears to be more critical than the amount of transmitter released. The regulatory significance of informational feedback from the receptor cell in activating mechanisms other than product-feedback inhibition is becoming prominent in experimental work on the brain.

Work from our laboratory has suggested that substrate supply, regulated by an energy-dependent, stereospecific uptake mechanisms, may account for some regulatory changes in transmitter synthesis.[12,13] For example, whereas morphine inhibits serotonin synthesis in the nerve ending by inhibiting tryptophan hydroxylase activity, cocaine accomplishes the same thing by the noncompetitive inhibition of the uptake of the substrate tryptophan. Too, changes in the physical state of an enzyme can alter synaptic transmission by allosteric activation or occlusion of the enzyme.[15,16,24] Tyrosine hydroxylase, when bound to nerve-ending membranes or altered from a tetramer to a monomer, gains affinity for its cofactor as well as its inhibiting products. This kind of change is represented schematically in Figure 22–5. A conformational alteration can be induced in the rate-limiting biosynthetic enzyme to "tune" it. We have shown that stimulants, like amphetamines, rapidly change the physical state of some of the enzyme tyrosine hydroxylase in the nerve ending from soluble to membrane-bound,[24] and so does the acute administration

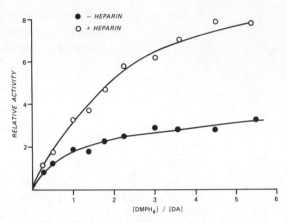

Figure 22–5. The sulfated mucopolysaccharide heparin activates native soluble tyrosine hydroxylase from the striatum of the rat. If the relative activity of the enzyme in the presence and in the absence of heparin is plotted as a function of various concentrations of artificial pteridine cofactor ($DMPH_4$) or catecholamine product (DA), it appears that activation by heparin sensitizes ("tunes") the enzyme to changes in the concentration of cofactor and/or end-product inhibitor.

of reserpine or the β-receptor blocker propranolol, with an apparent activation of the enzyme.[43]

Other adaptive mechanisms are associated with changes in the total amount of enzyme available in the nerve ending for synthesizing transmitter. Using various environmental, hormonal, and drug-induced changes in behavior as markers, we have demonstrated that some systems can be regulated by alterations in the amount of enzyme available,[5,35,37] which in turn are effected by changes in the rate of synthesis or degradation of the enzyme. A good example of such regulation comes from our studies of antidepressant drugs like the tricyclics, the monoamine oxidase inhibitors, or the amphetamines. Most of these drugs produce a systematic decrease in measurable tyrosine hydroxylase in the midbrain if they are administered over several days. Figure 22–6 summarizes the effects of the chronic administration of various drugs on midbrain tyrosine hydroxylase in the rat. Note that those that are generally antidepressant decrease the specific activity of the midbrain enzyme; those that are depressant increase it. The time course of these changes (which are, of course, dose-dependent) is several days. The time course of the functional or behavioral correlates of these enzymatic effects may reflect either the latency in enzyme turnover or the transport of the additional or reduced amounts of enzyme from the cell body to the nerve ending—a process called axoplasmic flow. The rate for this transport in our studies of tyrosine hydroxylase and tryptophan hydroxylase is on the order of 1 to 2 mm. per day.

The receptor, too, is sensitive to alterations in synaptic function, and it may play an important role in neurobiological adaptation. We have shown that thyroid hormone sensitizes central receptors to norepinephrine.[5] Preliminary experiments show a similar phenomenon in the brain after the intraventricular administration of 6-hydroxydopamine, a drug that selectively destroys catecholamine nerve endings.

So, neurochemical changes that apparently can regulate the amount or effect of neurotransmitter in a synapse in the brain include: (1) the amount of neurotransmitter released into the synapse; (2) the state of the neurotransmitter reuptake mechanism in the presynaptic nerve ending; (3) the amount, availability, and affinity of neurotransmitter-metabolizing enzymes; (4) the amount of product available in proximity to the rate-limiting enzyme to function as a feedback inhibitor; (5) the state of the supply and transport of precursors into the cell; (6) the physical state and/or conformation of the enzyme molecule as a regulator of activity or affinity for substrates; (7) increases or decreases in the amount of synthesizing enzyme in the nerve ending, regulated by its own synthesis, degradation, and the axoplasmic transport of enzyme protein; and (8) alterations in the sensitivity of the receptor.

The burgeoning vocabulary of central synaptic regulatory mechanisms that we have examined with the use of drugs and environmental manipulations has pointed toward one major principle of functional organization: the tendency of the adaptive mechanism to return the net function of the transmitter-receptor interaction to a baseline state. In addition, since even drugs with multiple actions do not impair all these mechanisms simultaneously, there appear to be some mechanisms always intact to carry through a serious attempt at compensation. Treatment with depressant drugs tends to lead to enzyme activation and/or increases in amount of enzyme, receptor sensitivity, or substrate supply. Stimulant or antidepressant drugs tend to decrease the excitability of the synapse though the opposite trend in the mechanisms. This rule of compensatory adaptation holds for the stimulant, narcotic, psychotropic, autonomic, and hallucinatory drugs that we have studied, and for environmental and genetic manipulations as well. For example, prolonged isolation appears to increase the activity of tyrosine hydroxylase, the rate-limiting enzyme in the synthesis of catecholamines, which activate behavior.[35] Genetic differentiation of six strains of rats on the basis of their levels of

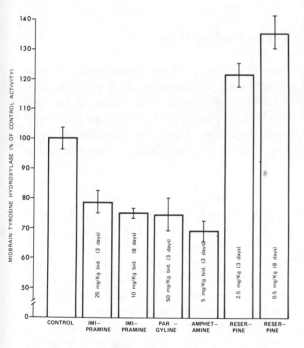

Figure 22–6. The effects of chronic drug treatment on the activity of tyrosine hydroxylase in the midbrain of the rat.

spontaneous motor activity shows a systematic inverse relationship between activity level and midbrain tyrosine hydroxylase activity.[36]

When we look for clinical evidence for adaptive changes to psychoactive drugs we do not have far to go. It is well known that tolerance develops very quickly to the potent euphorigen-hallucinogen lysergic acid diethylamide (LSD). A dose of 150 μg would be euphorigenic on Monday, mildly stimulating on Tuesday, and almost without effect on Wednesday, if the drug were taken daily. Furthermore, any one of a number of other euphorigens taken in an average dose on Thursday would have a markedly reduced effect because of cross-tolerance. The rapidity with which tolerance develops to amphetamines is another example of these adaptive mechanisms at work.

Thus, from both neurobiological and clinical points of view, it is clear that the extension of central euphorigen action over time has reached a technical barrier in the form of these acute and chronic mechanisms of adaptation. The acute responses may make a bad matter worse, or, the effects of the euphorigen may be modified or eliminated by the brain itself.

(New Frontiers

If the major impediment to the use of euphorigens for the long-term management of patients is the brain's capacity to adapt, there are still at least two useful ways to look ahead. The first and most straightforward is to consider the possibility that since most of the adaptations are macromolecular and subject to a prolonged time base, it may be possible to configure a management strategy to produce an end-state that *is* the adaptation, e.g. the tolerant state would be the treated state of the brain. Of course, further adaptations to induced tolerance could occur, but, at least superficially, this strategy is promising. We are speculating that some of the major psychotropic drugs, such as the tricyclic antidepres-

sants, may actually work by the creation of the tolerant state rather than by their primary effect. The delay of days to weeks for their behavioral effects to appear is similar to the time course of the macromolecular mechanisms described above. Mania, for example, has been thought to be a psychodynamic defense mechanism, but it is seductive to speculate that mania could represent an overdose of endogenous euphorigen in an effort to overcome a dysphoric state.

It might be useful to be able to modify the rate of development of these adaptive changes. Because new protein is probably involved with some presynaptic alterations of enzymatic activity and with postsynaptic alterations in receptor function, we are examining specific inhibitors of protein synthesis in an effort to find agents that may counteract adaptation. Parachlorophenylalanine is such an inhibitor for tryptophan hydroxylase.[12] It could also be useful to sensitize adrenergic receptors by means of the administration of thyroid hormone.[5]

(Concluding Remarks

Society currently adknowledges euphoria as a desired and sought-after affect state in man. Certain drugs that produce euphoria bear remarkable resemblance to two major, naturally occurring, neurotransmitter families. At least one of these compounds can be synthesized in the brain via N-methylation. A major obstacle to the use of euphorigens in the management of chronic diseases or dis-ease relates to the brain's metabolic adaptive processes. Adaptive mechanisms can be looked at in two ways. We might be able some day to induce these adaptations to achieve their ultimate behavioral and subjective consequences, or we might learn to alter or inhibit the rate of adaptation the brain makes to new treatments.

It appears that the age of euphorigens is upon us, and we are coming to it with far greater understanding of the biology of the brain than men have in earlier eras. Exciting times are ahead for those in the brain sciences. It wouldn't be surprising if over the next few years a wide variety of drugs that produce euphoria were available for use. The question of who will be in charge of them or how they will be used is, I think, beyond the legitimate purview of a brain scientist or a psychiatrist. Whether they can ever be used effectively, except on a periodic basis, awaits further research. It is perhaps philosophically important that drug-induced pleasure is habituated to quickly. It calls to mind a recent statement Heinz Lehmann made after hearing about some of this work: "It seems to me that puritanical attitudes toward pleasure must have as part of their bases these neurobiological mechanisms of adaptation." Perhaps pleasure can only be experienced against the background of its absence.

(Bibliography

1. AGHAJANIAN, G. K. "The Effects of LSD on Raphe Nuclei Neurons," in J. Smythies, ed., *The Modes of Action of Psychotomimetic Drugs, Neurosci. Res. Prog. Bull.*, 8 (1970), 40–54.

2. AXELROD, J. "Enzymatic Formation of Psychotomimetic Metabolites from Normally Occurring Compounds," *Science*, 134 (1961), 343.

3. BOURDILLON, R. E., C. A. CLARK, A. P. RIDGES et al. "Pink Spot in the Urine of Schizophrenics," *Nature*, 208 (1966), 453–455.

4. BRUNE, G. G. and H. E. HIMWICH. "Effects of Methionine Loading on the Behavior of Schizophrenic Patients," *J. Nerv. Ment. Dis.*, 134 (1962), 447–450.

5. EMLEN, J. W., D. S. SEGAL, and A. J. MANDELL. "Effects of Thyroid State on Pre- and Post-Synaptic Central Noradrenergic Mechanisms," *Science*, 175 (1972), 79–82.

6. FRIEDHOFF, A. J. and E. VAN WINKLE. "Isolation and Characterization of a Compound from the Urine of Schizophrenics," *Nature*, 194 (1962), 897–898.

7. FROHMAN, C. Personal communication, 1972.

8. GESSNER, P. K. "Pharmacological Studies of 5-methoxy-N,N-dimethyltryptamine, LSD and other Hallucinogens," in D. Efron, ed., *Psychotomimetic Drugs*, pp. 105–122. New York: Raven, 1970.

9. JUDD, L. L. and A. J. MANDELL. "A 'Free Clinic' Patient Population and Drug Use Patterns," *Am. J. Psychiatry*, 128 (1972), 1298–1302.

10. JUDD, L. L., E. GUNDERSON, G. R. ALEXANDER et al. "Youth Drug Use Survey of High School and College Students," in *Marijuana: A Signal of Misunderstanding*, Vol. 1, pp. 367–423. National Commission on Marijuana and Drug Abuse. Washington: U.S. Govt. Print. Off., 1972.

11. KLINE, N. Personal communication, 1971.

12. KNAPP, S. and A. J. MANDELL. "Parachlorophenylalanine—Its Three Phase Sequence of Interactions with the Two Forms of Brain Tryptophan Hydroxylase," *Life Sci.*, 2 (1972), 761–771.

13. ———. "Some Drug Effects on the Functions of the Two Physical Forms of Tryptophan-5-Hydroxylase: Influence on Hydroxylation and Uptake of Substrate," in, J. Barchas and E. Usdin, eds., *Serotonin and Behavior*, pp. 61–71, New York: Academic Press, 1973.

14. KOPIN, I. J., G. R. BREESE, K. R. KRAUSS et al. "Selective Release of Newly Synthesized Norepinephrine from the Cat Spleen During Sympathetic Nerve Stimulation," *J. Pharmacol. Exp. Ther.*, 161 (1968), 271–278.

15. KUCZENSKI, R. T. and A. J. MANDELL. "Allosteric Activation of Hypothalamic Tyrosine Hydroxylase by Ions and Sulfated Mucopolysaccharides," *J. Neurochem.*, 19 (1972), 131–139.

16. ———. "Regulatory Properties of Soluble and Particulate Rat Brain Tyrosine Hydroxylase," *J. Biol. Chem.*, 247 (1972), 3114–3122.

17. KUEHL, F. A., R. E. ORMOND, and W. J. A. VANDERHENVAL. "Occurrence of 3,4-dimethoxy-Phenylacetic acid in Urines of Normal and Schizophrenic Individuals," *Nature*, 211 (1966), 606–608.

18. LANER, J. W., W. M. INSKIP, J. BERNSOLM et al. "Observations on Schizophrenic Patients After Iproniazid and Tryptophan," *Arch. Neurol. Psychiatry*, 80 (1961), 122–130.

19. LEVITT, M., S. SPECTOR, A. SJOERDSMA et al. "Elucidation of the Rate Limiting Step

in Norepinephrine Biosynthesis in the Perfused Guinea Pig Brain." *J. Pharm. Exp. Ther.*, 148 (1965), 1–8.

20. LEWIN, L. *Phantastica; Narcotic and Stimulating Drugs, Their Use and Abuse.* London. Routledge and Kegan Paul, 1931.

21. MANDELL, A. J. "Drug Induced Alterations in Brain Biosynthetic Enzyme Activity—A Model for Adaptation to the Environment by the CNS," in, E. Datta, ed., *Biochemistry of Brain and Behavior*, pp. 97–121. New York: Plenum, 1970.

22. ———. "Discussion of A. T. Shulgin's paper in D. Efron, ed., *Psychotomimetic Drugs*, pp. 39–40. New York: Raven, 1970.

23. MANDELL, A. J., B. BUCKINGHAM, and D. S. SEGAL. "Behavioral, Metabolic and Enzymatic Studies of the Brain Indole(ethyl)-amine N-methylating System," in, B. T. Ho and W. McIsaac, eds., *Brain Chemistry and Mental Disease*, pp. 37–60. New York: Plenum. 1971.

24. MANDELL, A. J., S. KNAPP, and R. KUCZENSKI. "An Amphetamine Induced Shift in the Subcellular Distribution of Caudate Tyrosine Hydroxylase, *NAS-NRC Proc. Comm. on Prob. Drug Dependence*, pp. 742–766, 1971.

25. MANDELL, A. J., S. KNAPP, R. T. KUCZENSKI et al. "Methamphetamine-Induced Alteration in the Physical State of Rat Caudate Tyrosine Hydroxylase," *Biochem. Pharmacol.* 21 (1972), 2737–2750.

26. MANDELL, A. J. and M. MORGAN. "An indole-(ethyl)amine N-methyltransferase in Human Brain. *Nature*, 230 (1971), 85–87.

27. MANDELL, A. J., D. S. SEGAL, R. T. KUCZENSKI et al. "Some Macromolecular Mechanisms in CNS Neurotransmitter Pharmacology and Their Psychobiological Organization," in J. McGaugh, ed., *Chemistry of Mood, Motivation and Behavior*, pp. 105–148, New York: Plenum, 1972.

28. MANDELL, A. J. and C. E. SPOONER. "Psychochemical Research Studies in Man," *Science*, 162 (1968), 1442–1453.

29. MANDELL, A. J., C. E. SPOONER, and D. BRUNET. "Whither the Sleep Transmitter," *Biol. Psychiatry* 1 (1969), 13–30.

30. MANDELL, A. J. and L. J. WEST. "The Hallucinogens," in, A. M. Freedman and H. Kaplan, eds., *Comprehensive Textbook of Psychiatry*, pp. 247–253, Baltimore: Williams & Wilkins, 1966.

31. MORGAN, M. and A. J. MANDELL. "An Indole-(ethyl)amine N-methyltransferase in the Brain of the Chick," *Science*, 165 (1969), 492–493.

32. NAGATSU, T., M. LEVITT, and S. UDENFRIEND. "Tyrosine Hydroxylase: The Initial Step in Norepinephrine Biosynthesis," *J. Biol. Chem.*, 239 (1964), 2910–2911.

33. POLLIN, W., P. V. CARDON, and S. S. KETY. "Effect of Amino Acid Feedings in Schizophrenic Patients Treated with Iproniazid," *Science*, 133 (1961), 104–105.

34. SAAVEDRA, J. M. and J. AXELROD. "Psychotomimetic N-Methylated Tryptophan: Formation in Brain *in vivo* and *in vitro*," *Science*, 175 (1972), 1365–1366.

35. SEGAL, D. S., S. KNAPP, R. KUCZENSKI et al. "The Effects of Sensory Isolation on Tyrosine Hydroxylase and Tryptophan Hydroxylase Activity," *Behav. Biol.*, 8 (1973), 47–53.

36. SEGAL, D. S., R. T. KUCZENSKI, and A. J. MANDELL. "Strain Differences in Behavior and Brain Tyrosine Hydroxylase Activity," *Behav. Biol.*, 7 (1971), 75–81.

37. SEGAL, D. S., J. L. SULLIVAN, R. T. KUCZENSKI et al. "Effects of Long-term Reserpine Treatment on Brain Tyrosine Hydroxylase and Behavioral Activity," *Science*, 173 (1971), 847–849.

38. SHULGIN, A. T. "Psychotomimetic amphetamines: Methoxy-3-4-dialkoxyamphetamines," *Experientia*, 20 (1964), 366–369.

39. SHUGLIN, A. T., T. SARGENT, and C. NARANJO. "Structure-Activity Relationships of One-Ring Psychotomimetics," *Nature*, 221 (1969), 537–541.

40. SNYDER, S. H., L. FAILLACE, and H. WEINGARTNER. "DOM (STP), A New Hallucinogenic Drug and DOET: Effects in Normal Subjects," *Am. J. Psychiatry*, 125 (1968), 357–364.

41. SNYDER, S. H. and C. R. MERRIL. "A Relationship Between the Hallucinogenic Activity of Drugs and Their Electronic Configuration," *Proc. Natl. Acad. Sci.*, 54 (1965), 258–266.

42. SPOONER, C. E., A. J. MANDELL, D. BRUNET et al. "MAOI Reversal of 5-HTP Behavioral Depression: The Potential Role of Bufotenin," *Fed. Proc.*, 27 (1968), 540.

43. SULLIVAN, J. L., D. S. SEGAL, R. T. KUCZENSKI et al. "Propranolol Induced Rapid Activation of Rat Striatal Tyrosine Hy-

droxylase Concomitant with Behavioral Depression," *J. Biol. Psychiatry*, 4 (1972), 193–203.

44. Szara, S. "DMT (N,N-Dimethyltryptamine) and Homologues: Clinical and Pharmacological Considerations," in D. H. Efron, ed.,

Psychotomimetic Drugs, pp. 275–286. New York: Raven, 1970.

45. Turner, W. J. and S. Merlis. "Effect of Some Indolealkylamines on Man," *Arch. Neurol. Psychiatry*, 81 (1959), 121–129.

CHAPTER 23

THE PSYCHOBIOLOGY
OF MANIA

Dennis L. Murphy, Frederick K. Goodwin, and William E. Bunney, Jr.

MANIA is a complex behavioral syndrome that occurs episodically. It is characterized by a sustained increase in activity and speech, impaired judgment, provocative instrusiveness, manipulativeness, insomnia, and labile affect with prominent elation. Mania has been viewed as a psychological defensive effort to preserve self-esteem after a loss,[159] a triumphant fusion of ego and superego,[95] a disorder in biogenic amine metabolism,[235] a disorder in brain psychomotor activation regulation,[179] and an inherited mental illness.[138] Hippocrates originally used the word hypomania, which now designates mild manic symptoms, to describe the episodic development of a febrile delirium in some particular individuals.[88]

Almost all patients with manic episodes also manifest cyclic periods of depression, although only approximately 10 to 20 percent of all patients hospitalized for depression develop mania.[22,23,243] The occurrence of mania severe enough to require hospitalization or specific treatment has been used as the definitional characteristic in identifying the so-called bipolar patient group (individuals with both manic and depressive episodes) who manifest many familial, psychological, biological, and pharmacological features that differentiate them from the larger unipolar depressed patient group (those with depressive episodes only).

The manic phase in bipolar patients has been little studied, in good part because manic behavior is usually so disruptive of attempts at controlled investigation that reliable data beyond simple behavioral observation is uncommon. Nonetheless, in the last few years mania has come under increasing scientific scrutiny. This upsurge in interest in mania has resulted both from the discovery of an effective and specific antimanic drug, lithium carbonate, and from a spill over from widespread research interest in depression. In addition, the concept that mania represents an endogenous "high" is definitely of pertinence to the current interest in the motivation for drug-experience-seeking behavior.[35,216]

Not unexpectedly, these explorations have provoked interest in some old and new questions about mania. In having available a drug like lithium, with antimanic but not anti-schizophrenic properties, old questions of differential diagnosis have again become important, particularly in regard to the manic patient with delusions or paranoid behavior, and the schizoaffective patient group. Furthermore, the demonstrated therapeutic effects of lithium in acute depression, and in the prophylaxis of both depression and mania, have led to questions about how "opposite" these long-assumed "bipolar" states really are. Indeed, biologic and psychologic studies have delineated many similarities between these two "affective disorders," including quantitative documentation of the frequent co-occurrence of intense depressive affect during acute manic states. However, other studies have just as definitely identified nonaffective elements, such as some psychological and biological phenomena related to psychomotor activity, that closely fit the classical concept of depression and mania representing opposite manifestations of a single bipolar entity, "manic-depressive illness."

This chapter will review studies from the last decade of mania and of the bipolar patient group, concentrating in particular on investigations of biogenic amines, drug responses, sleep, other biologic changes, and some quantitatively assessed behavioral phenomena in manic individuals. This emphasis on biological and quantitative psychological studies reflects the dominant thrust of current research on this frontier of human behavior. It does not address the important but difficult-to-quantify and infrequently studied interpersonal aspects of mania that are responsible for much of the social morbidity of mania and occupy a large share of treatment program time for the manic individual. Some general clinical, intrapsychic and interpersonal aspects of manic-depressive individuals are considered in Volume 1 of the second edition of this

Handbook[6] and are the focus of several other recent reports and reviews.* The most comprehensive description of the clinical phenomena of mania is contained in Kraepelin's monograph.[151] Other monographs dealing with mania include those by Bellak,[15] Lewin,[159] and Winokur, Clayton, and Reich.[271]

(The Bipolar Patient and the Genetics of Mania

Although some early observers of patients with affective disorders noted that some individuals exhibited circular mood swings from elation to depression while others manifested only depression,[9,89] early studies of groups of patients with affective disorders did not clearly separate these patient groups. For instance, Kraepelin,[151] although allowing for the possibility that "later a series of subordinate forms (of 'manic-depressive insanity') may be described," felt in 1913 "more and more convinced that all of the above-mentioned states (periodic and circular insanity, simple mania, melancholia and delirious insanity) only represent manifestations of a single morbid process." He based this conclusion on the following characteristics: (a) the presence of common fundamental features in these disorders; (b) his observations indicating that "all the morbid forms brought together here as a clinical entity not only pass over the one into the other without recognizable boundaries, but . . . they may even replace each other in one and the same case"; (c) their uniform prognosis (they "never lead to profound dementia"), and (d) the lack of familial tendencies for a particular form of illness, since "in members of the same family we frequently enough find side by side pronounced periodic or circular cases, occasionally isolated states of ill temper or confusion, lastly very slight, regular fluctuations of mood or permanent conspicuous coloration of disposition."

In contrast, Perris,[203] Angst,[4] Winokur, et al.[271] and others[13,108,184,193] have presented

---

* See references 55, 133, 161, 198, and 265.

evidence supportive of Leonhard's[156] division of patients with primary-affective disorders into bipolar and unipolar subtypes. This information, taken together with many other studies of clinical features, physiologic and pharmacologic responses and genetic features, suggests that mania is the discriminating factor for a bipolar subgroup, representing approximately 10 to 20 percent of patients with severe affective disorders. This subgroup, generally identified on the basis of a history of manic symptoms of sufficient severity to require hospitalization or specific treatment, appears more homogeneous than the unipolar depressive group that includes the entire remaining clinical[57] and genetic[169,273] spectrum of depressive disorders (neurotic, involutional, psychotic, etc.). The position of another group of depressed patients who manifest periods of mildly increased activity or euphoria, frequently at the termination of a depressive episode or during treatment with antidepressant drugs or electroconvulsive therapy (ECT), remains uncertain. These "cyclothymic-depressive" or "bipolar II" individuals have biologic, pharmacologic, and genetic characteristics that, in some cases, more resemble the unipolar group and, in other instances, are closer to the bipolar group. Because their prevalence in the total depressive patient population equals or slightly exceeds that of the bipolar group, they need to be examined as a separate patient group for the present.

The Genetics of Mania

Evidence for a heritable factor in the occurrence of manic and depressive episodes in bipolar individuals is based on the higher incidence of bipolar-affective disorders in the relatives of bipolar patients compared to the general population, and on the higher concordance rate for the bipolar disorder in monozygotic compared to dizygotic twins. In addition, evidence from linkage studies has suggested that a specific mechanism of genetic transmission of affective disorders may be involved, namely a dominant factor localized to the short arm of the X chromosome. Alterna-

tively, an impairment in personality development or ego formation or the direct learning of some aspects of behavior and interpersonal relationships during early development might also account for a familial pattern of the bipolar disorder.[54] While the twin data more favor a major inherited contribution to the occurrence of the bipolar disorder, there are special problems in approaching psychiatric disorders from the twin-comparison approach.[131,142,143,225] The necessary and most informative twin study, that of separated monozygous twins, has not yet been accomplished for bipolar individuals.

Early, often-quoted studies by Kallmann,[138] Slater[245] and others presented evidence suggesting a heritable factor in the affective disorders, but did not consider bipolar patients separately from other patients with affective disorders. Leonhard, Korff, and Shulz[156] were the first to report a tendency for bipolar patients to have more relatives with bipolar illness compared to unipolar-depressed patients. More recently, several family-history studies have suggested that bipolar patients have a different and specific pattern of hereditability for their symptoms compared to patients with unipolar primary-affective disorders. Perris[203] reported a thirty-fold higher incidence of bipolar disorder among first-degree relatives of bipolar patients compared to unipolar patients. Angst[4] confirmed this finding, although a lower incidence of bipolar disorders among the bipolar relatives he studied (3.7 percent versus 10.8 percent in Perris' study) reduced the bipolar-unipolar incidence difference to thirteen-fold. Perris suggested that this discrepancy may be due to a shorter observation time in Angst's study, coupled with the fact that Angst did not include hypomanic phases requiring specific treatment at the termination of a depressive period as indicative of a separate bipolar episode.[5]

On the basis of comparisons of the family histories of 426 patients with affective disorders across two generations, Winokur[270] found evidence for a dominant type of direct familial transmission in bipolar compared to unipolar patients. Fifty percent of the bipolar patients had either parents or children with an affective disorder, in comparison to a similar history in 25 percent of the unipolar patients. In addition, only 6 percent of the bipolar patients had no family history for any kind of psychiatric disorder, while 32 percent of unipolar patients were without affected relatives. From a study of the relatives of a smaller number of bipolar patients, morbid risks for affective illness (either depression or mania) were calculated to be 34 to 41 percent for parents and 25 to 49 percent for siblings.[270] However, the incidence of bipolar disorder was lower, with mania occurring in only 25 percent of the parents and 41 percent of the siblings among those relatives with affective disorders.

Zerbin-Rüdin[278] reevaluated the twin studies in the literature, using those which provided sufficient data to identify individuals with bipolar symptoms. In thirty-four pairs of monozygotic twins, concordance was 82 percent for affective disorder (either mania or depression) and 62 percent for mania. In contrast, in nineteen pairs of dizygotic twins, concordance was 37 percent for affective disorder and 11 percent for mania.

Winokur, Clayton, and Reich[271] have suggested that a single, dominant gene located on the X chromosome represents the heritable factor in bipolar illness, basing their argument on the occurrence of bipolar disorders in successive generations, the presence of a higher female-male prevalence ratio, and the rarity of father-to-son transmission in their studies, although other reports are clearly not in agreement on the latter two points.[4,83,203] In addition, a significant linkage between bipolar illness and protan- and deutan-type color blindness in extended studies of two families,[220] and a suggestive association with the Xg blood group[272] provide direct evidence that a gene associated with bipolar illness may be located on the short arm of the X chromosome together with the sites of these other heritable traits. Recently reported data from a larger number of families have confirmed linkage of bipolar symptoms in some families with

color blindness (particularly the protan type) and also with the Xga blood group.[172]

On the basis of the frequency of affective disorders in the families of both parents of bipolar patients, and an unbalanced distribution of depression-only parents in these families, Winokur[270] suggested the possibility of a second genetic factor, possibly of an autosomal dominant type, that may be more explicitly related to the expression of mania than the X-linked factor and may more generally predispose the individual to either unipolar- or bipolar-affective disorder. Polygenic inheritance of bipolar symptoms was also suggested by the separate studies of Perris[203] and Slater, Maxwell, and Price,[247] using a computational model based upon maternal and paternal incidence figures.[98,246]

Characteristics of the Bipolar Individual

Mania is a dramatic existential state that provides the definitional characteristic of individuals with bipolar-affective disorders. However, because manic episodes represent a relatively small portion of the bipolar individual's life, and because some clues to the nature of the manic state may be better approached in individuals during nonmanic periods, a number of characteristics of the bipolar individual have been investigated during either normal or depressed periods.

Clinical and Psychological Characteristics. Age of onset of affective symptoms is lower in bipolar compared to unipolar individuals.[163,203,271] While there are more females in the unipolar patient group, there is no sex difference in the incidence of the bipolar disorder.[203] Bipolar individuals have a higher incidence of postpartum affective disorders,[10] and a higher frequency of celibacy (males only) and of divorce;[25,271] these latter two differences may well represent interpersonal side effects of manic episodes. Educational achievement and occupational level are higher in bipolar individuals as well as in their families compared to unipolar families and to the averages from national census data.[274] Early mortality from all causes is significantly higher in bipolar compared to unipolar individuals or to the general population; this difference is not explained by suicides, which are equally frequent in both patient groups.[203]

Bipolar patients in remission manifest differences from unipolar individuals on the Nyman-Marke temperament scale, including the presence of such traits as "sociability," "activity," and "syntony," while unipolar individuals are characterized by "insecurity," "obsessionalism," and "sensitivity."[208] Using the Maudsley personality inventory, Perris[202] found significantly lower neuroticism scores in bipolar compared to unipolar individuals. Beigel and Murphy[13] reported that bipolar-depressed patients had significantly lower ratings for overt expressions of anger, somatic complaints, physical activity, and anxiety compared to unipolar-depressed patients matched for behaviorally rated levels of depression. A comparison of Minnesota Multiphasic Personality Inventory (MMPI) self-ratings during depression revealed significantly lower D (depression) and Pt (psychasthenia) scale scores, and higher Ma (hypomania) scores in bipolar compared to unipolar patients.[79] As severity of depression had not been rated as being significantly different between these two groups on the basis of objective behavioral ratings on the Bunney-Hamburg scale, and as a high correlation between the MMPI and Bunney-Hamburg depression scores was found for the unipolar but not for the bipolar patients, it was suggested that the bipolar patients' subjective view of their depressed state as described by MMPI scores was inconsistent with or qualitatively different from that of the unipolar patients. However, bipolar individuals were considered, on the basis of clinical[54] and psychological examination of the evidence,[80,250] to be less psychodynamically minded and to excessively favor behavior and psychologic test responses that are conventional and socially desirable. These characteristics may contribute to the apparent "endogenous" presentation of symptoms in bipolar individuals, although whether these characteristics simply represent individual differences or are ego-defensive distortions is not clear.

While quantitative data are not available, bipolar patients have also been described as different from unipolar-depressed patients in several other characteristics. In keeping with the psychological test data, bipolar individuals have been more frequently described as "normal" between episodes, whereas neurotic or characterologic difficulties have been more frequently described in unipolar individuals.[4,156,202,228] During depressive episodes, bipolar patients have been described as most frequently manifesting psychomotor retardation, whereas agitation and anxiety appear to accompany depression in approximately one-half of the unipolar patients, with the other half manifesting some features of retardation.

Psychophysiologic and Biologic Characteristics. Bipolar patients have been described to have a lower sedation threshold for barbiturate drugs.[203] A lower flicker threshold and some EEG pattern differences have also been reported, although other psychophysiologic measures did not differentiate bipolar from unipolar patients.[203] Bipolar patients when depressed sleep longer at night but feel worse in the morning than do unipolar depressed patients.[75] In a study of visual average evoked responses (AER), bipolar patients showed relatively greater rates of increase of AER amplitude (augmentation) with increasing stimulus intensity than did unipolar patients.[31] This augmentation tendency appears to be a stable characteristic of the individuals that persists during depressed, manic and relatively normal states, but diminishes somewhat during treatment with lithium carbonate.[19,31]

Some biological differences have recently been reported between the two patient groups. Levels of catechol-O-methyltransferase, a major enzyme in the degradation of catecholamines, have been reported as reduced in erythrocytes when female depressed patients were compared to controls; the greatest reduction was found in unipolar patients, who had levels significantly lower than those in the bipolar patients.[82] Reduced levels of monoamine oxidase (MAO), another major enzymatic route of biogenic amine degradation, have been found in blood platelets from both male and female bipolar patients compared to unipolar patients and controls.[193] Urinary tryptamine excretion is greater in bipolar- compared to unipolar-depressed patients,[189] a difference compatible with the possibility of reduced monoamine oxidase activity in these patients, since tryptamine is almost exclusively degraded via MAO. Blood platelet levels of octopamine are also higher in bipolar patients compared to unipolar patients and controls.[186] Although potentially of interest because of the evidence that octopamine may function as a false neurotransmitter in man,[147,178] this finding is also compatible with the reported change in MAO activity, since octopamine accumulates in animals and man during the administration of MAO-inhibiting drugs.[147,186] Depressed bipolar patients also have reduced urinary 17-hydroxycorticosteroid levels compared to depressed unipolar patients and to normal controls.[84]

Pharmacologic Characteristics. Different responses to a number of psychoactive drugs have been described in comparative investigations of bipolar- and unipolar-depressed patients. In a study evaluating the antidepressant effects of lithium using double-blind methodology, thirty-two of forty bipolar patients (80 percent) improved significantly during treatment, while only four of eleven unipolar patients (30 percent) exhibited similarly reduced depression ratings.[108] Preliminary data from a study of tricyclic drugs in these two patient groups suggest that unipolar patients respond more frequently to these drugs, while bipolar patients either do not regularly respond or, as described below, may develop a manic episode during treatment.[33,38] The differential development of hypomania in bipolar compared to unipolar individuals treated with L-Dopa[184] is also described below in the discussion of the "switch" into mania. Bipolar patients have also been reported to have a modest antidepressant response to l-tryptophan administration, while unipolar patients were unchanged,[181,182,211] suggesting that one factor in the conflictual reports of the antidepressant efficacy of this drug may represent patient population selection factors.

(Clinical, Behavioral, and Cognitive Features of Mania

The clinical phenomena of the manic state have been described in detail in Kraepelin's monograph[151] and in other texts.* The typical acute manic state is generally clinically differentiable from other psychiatric syndromes on the basis of a marked increase in motor and verbal hyperactivity, interpersonal provocativeness and manipulation, distractibility, a clear sensorium, and, most often, elation and grandiosity. A state of labile affect, with a breakthrough of depressive or dysphoric affect with irritability and anger, is frequently observed. Sleeplessness, impaired judgment, and an increase in aggressive and sexual impulses are also common. In some instances, delusional thinking, hallucinations, and confusion may develop, particularly as the course of the manic state peaks or becomes prolonged, with minimal interruption for sleep or nutritional input.

Despite the apparent distinctiveness of the typical manic state, it has been suggested that frequent misdiagnosis, especially of individuals exhibiting labile affect or psychotic phenomena associated with mania, may account for the reported decreased incidence of manic-depressive illness in the United States in the last several decades.[152,226,264] A diminished interest in patient classification, and the efficacy of phenothiazine drugs in the treatment of most acute psychoses including both mania and schizophrenia, contributed to this problem. In contrast, the advent of lithium treatment has recently been accompanied by an apparent increase in the reported incidence of mania,[11] and reawakened interest in the phenomenology of manic behavior.

Behavioral Changes During Mania. The symptoms occurring during manic episodes in one hundred patients were cataloged by Winokur, Clayton, and Reich.[271] While euphoria was present in almost all patients, the affective state was generally highly labile, with over two-thirds of the patients exhibiting

* See references 55, 159, 195, 248, and 271.

depression. Reactive irritability and hostility were prominent, and the greatest degree of motor hyperactivity was associated with the most severe thought disorder and the presence of delusions.

It has recently been demonstrated that some manic symptoms are common to all patients, but that others are characteristic of only some manic individuals on the basis of data from a rating scale permitting continuous quantitative behavioral monitoring of manic patients.[12,14,183] The behavioral symptoms that correlated most clearly with severity of mania (as rated independently by psychiatrists), and that were found on a factor analysis of the scale to represent a single, dominant "core-mania factor" in all patients, included such symptoms as increased motor activity, increased speech, distractibility, poor judgment, diminished impulse control, anger, irritability, argumentativeness, and interpersonal demandingness.[12,183] Mania-scale items reflecting euphoria and grandiosity were less uniformly found elevated in all manic patients, and were found to be inversely correlated with items reflecting paranoid and destructive behavior, which were elevated in only some individuals. On the basis that similar ratings on the core-mania items were found in both the 70 percent of patients with high elation-grandiosity ratings but low paranoid-destructive ratings, and in the 30 percent of patients with low elation-grandiosity but high paranoid-destructive ratings, it was suggested that these differences might provide a quantitative definition of two subgroups of manic patients for evaluation in pharmacologic and other clinical studies.[12,14,183]

Psychotic Phenomena During Mania. Delusions occur in approximately one-half of all patients with mania, while hallucinations occur in one-third of manic episodes.[44,52,222,271] Ideas of reference, persecutory, and other paranoid thinking, passivity delusions, symbolism, and confusion may also occur during mania.[44,52,163,271] The presence of a thought disorder on Bannister's grid test for schizophrenic thought disorder did not differentiate manic from schizophrenic individuals.[23] Significant numbers of typically manic pa-

tients (15 to 30 percent) also exhibit Schneider's first-rank symptoms of schizophrenia.[47] These recent observations, emphasizing the difficulties in diagnostic evaluations based on Bleulerian and other symptom-related schema, have raised questions concerning the validity of earlier genetically oriented studies that suggested a clear separation between affective disorders and schizophrenia.

The occurrence of borderland conditions between mania and schizophrenic excitement was recognized by Meyer,[174] Bleuler[18] and Brill[24] and has sometimes been designated as "schizoid-manic" states. Separate "delusional" and "delirious" types of mania were differentiated by Kraepelin[151] from "acute" mania. Some of these patients exhibited clinical pictures as diverse as recurrent excited paranoid states and severely disorganized, generally undifferentiated psychotic states with some manic features. They were grouped together primarily on the basis of their tendency to remit and to not lead to chronic personality disorganization as in schizophrenia. Similar, more modern data on remission rates have been interpreted both to indicate a more favorable prognosis for schizophrenia (when these episodes have been included in the statistics of acute schizophrenic episodes) and an equally favorable prognosis for such "schizoaffective" patients or other manic patients with psychotic phenomena, compared to manic patients without delusions or hallucinations.*

Differentiating manic-psychotic individuals from schizophrenic individuals may be difficult and in some instances impossible in the midst of an acute episode.[44,144] Longitudinal analysis or reconstruction of the symptomatologic picture in the earliest stages of the psychotic episode may reveal typical manic behavior that was superseded by a less well differentiated psychosis. In addition, it has been suggested that factors other than symptoms may be of help, in that manic episodes are more likely to occur in individuals with a history of periodic recurrences who have symptom-free intervals associated with suc-

* See references 44, 53, 222, 261, and 266.

cessful interpersonal relationships. During the acute episode, and particularly at its onset, purposeful hyperactivity and interpersonal involvement in provocative, manipulative ways are far more characteristic of typical manic behavior than the more panicky, disorganized activity associated with the primarily autistic preoccupations of the schizophrenic individual. Fluctuating or fleeting delusional and hallucinatory phenomena are also more characteristic of mania than is a fixed, detailed delusional structure.

Nonetheless, criteria based on symptoms alone may be insufficient to reliably discriminate in all cases between patients with affective disorders, schizoaffective states, and schizophrenia. One discriminant function analysis of clinical phenomena in a large number of patients with affective psychoses and schizophrenia concluded that the distribution of patients was not different from a normal distribution,[141] a finding in agreement with other data from a variety of sources, including some genetic studies, and suggesting a continuum of clinical states from schizophrenia through schizoaffective disorders to the affective disorders.[*] It is not clear yet whether psychotic phenomena during mania represent a secondary form of response to an especially severe or prolonged manic state[44] or whether they only occur in certain individuals separately predisposed to a disorganization or disintegration of the personality.

Depressive Affect During Mania. Although depression and mania have often been considered "opposite" affective states, the existence of bursts of depressive affect and thought content during manic episodes has occasionally been described.[†] More recently, quantitative evidence of the coexistence of a depressive affect during manic episodes has been provided, verifying that most manic patients do exhibit some depressive affect during manic episodes and that depression is not negatively correlated with total mania ratings or even with rated elation in manic patients over an eight-hour assessment period.[12,183] This suggests that most manic patients manifest to

some degree a combined manic-depressive picture, although fewer manic individuals (20 to 35 percent) have the more marked "mixed" or labile state described in some patients by Kraepelin.[12,151,183,271]

In addition to frank depressive thought content and depressive affect, a more diffuse dysphoria together with irritability and expressed hostility has been observed in some manic patients exhibiting mood lability.[12,44,271] Manic episodes are immediately preceded by depressive periods in over 50 percent of patients,[39,44,271] and one study also documented the occurrence of depressive episodes within one month subsequent to a manic period in over half of the patients studied.[271]

Cognition During Mania

Reduced attention span, distractibility, impaired memory, and flight of ideas with clang associations, rhyming, and punning have all been described as clinical phenomena during mania. However, there have been only a few quantitative investigations of cognitive characteristics of the manic state. In a study of time sense, hypomanic individuals grossly overestimated a three-second time interval.[175] Reaction time to auditory and light stimuli was found to be reduced and to be inversely correlated with severity of mania in several studies.[66,67,162] Impaired self-judgment of symptomatologic behavior was observed in hypomanic and manic individuals compared to the results in the same individuals when nonmanic.[208]

Verbal learning was found to be impaired in individuals studied while manic compared both to nonmanic periods in the same patients and to normal controls.[121] Increased errors of commission and a substitution of intrusive responses for those presented were characteristics differentiating impaired learning during mania from the learning impairment seen in depressed and psychotomimetic drug-treated patients. In particular, it appeared that the co-occurrence of a deficit in word associations, representing a shift to less common and more idiosyncratic associative responses, which were also less stable, was an important con-

---

[*] See references 47, 53, 153, and 253.
[†] See references 107, 150, 151, 184, and 271.

tributory factor to the learning impairment. The number of idiosyncratic associations (defined according to the expected frequency of responses found in age- and sex-matched normals) was over 50 percent greater than the number in schizophrenic patients and several-fold greater when compared to patients with spontaneous, and drug-induced, psychotic symptoms.[121]

This thinking disorder in manic patients was fully reversible in that verbal associations reverted to normal patterns after manic behavior ceased. Of particular note was the occurrence of some identical idiosyncratic associations in subsequent manic periods, suggesting that some cognitive aspects of the individual are differentially available to him during this altered behavioral state.[122] While it has recently been demonstrated in studies with drugs that learning which occurs in a particular state (e.g., information acquired during alcohol administration) is less retrievable in a nondrug state, and vice versa,[197] evidence concerning the possibility that clinical-psychiatric states may represent the emergence of cognitive or behavioral patterns distinct from those usually available to the individual has not previously been presented.

Hypomania versus Mania. Hypomania has generally been considered as simply a milder form of mania, involving, in particular, less impairment of judgment and self-control and an absence of psychotic symptoms. While hypomanic symptoms are seen in patients who exhibit full-blown manic episodes, particularly toward the end of a treated episode, hypomanic behavior also occurs in other individuals who never develop mania, e.g., the cyclothymic or "bipolar II" patient group. Such individuals, who do not require specific treatment for spontaneously developing periods of increased activity or euphoria, or who develop such symptoms during treatment with antidepressant drugs, have been found to manifest some differences from both typical bipolar ("bipolar I") patients and also from unipolar-depressed patients. While their visual cortical evoked response patterns and their high incidence of antidepressant responses to lithium[31,108] suggested that these patients most

resembled the bipolar group, their responses to other drugs,[33,179] some biologic measures, including monoamine oxidase and 17-hydroxy-corticosteroid determinations,[84,193] and some clinical features, suggested either a closer resemblance to the unipolar group or the possibility that they represented a discrete subgroup of patients separate from other depressed individuals. A particularly high incidence of suicide was found in this group in one study.[83]

A prolonged, sometimes chronic or even fixed "characterologic" hypomanic state may be seen in some individuals who maintain a state of increased activity with diminished sleep, extraversion, often youthful appearance (frequently enhanced by acting and even dressing somewhat like a little boy or girl), and cheerful optimism.[3,157,158] While sometimes adaptive and successful as a life style, difficulties arise from overinvolvement and distractibility, labile affect, and replacement of ready conversation and wit by flamboyant argumentativeness; these personality characteristics often lead to marital and occupational instability. Many of these individuals may never experience a full-blown manic-psychotic episode.

(Biologic Phenomena Associated With the Steady-State of Mania

Mania is associated with profound alterations in many bodily functions that complicate the assessment of the specificity and significance of other biologic changes observed during the manic state.[191] In addition, the tolerance of the manic individual for the restrictions of a controlled study is limited, and greater than normal variance in experimental results related to impaired cooperation, if not outright sabotage, may occur. Some of the changes occurring as concomitants of mania that may contribute to some of the biologic (and possibly psychologic) alterations observed include: (a) markedly increased physical activity; (b) decreased sleep; (c) altered dietary intake, ranging from hyperbulimia to the more common reduced intake resulting from distractibility and excess activity; (d) similar extremes of fluid intake and urinary output, ranging from marked increases to states of dehydration; and (e) associated alterations in gastrointestinal function.[43,191]

Mania and Catecholamines. Evidence from pioneering studies in animals and in man, of drugs capable of altering behavior and mood, suggested that mania might be related to excess activity of central adrenergic neurons.[235,237] Early investigations of urinary catecholamines had generally indicated elevated norepinephrine and epinephrine excretion in hypomanic and manic patients, especially when manic and depressed phases were compared in cycling patients.* However, interpretation of these results is confounded by the preponderant contribution to urinary catecholamines and catecholamine metabolites from the peripheral autonomic nervous system and the adrenal gland rather than the brain, especially since marked alterations in physical activity regularly accompany manic behavior, and physical activity can elevate urinary and even cerebrospinal fluid amines and their metabolites. The relevance of these observations can by no means be dismissed, since catecholamine excretion in disproportionate excess to pedometer-measurement motor activity has been observed in some studies of mania,[255] and one catecholamine metabolite, 3-methoxy, 4-hydroxyphenylglycol (MHPG) has been suggested to yield an estimate of central nervous system catecholamine activity.[164]

More recently, increased urinary dopamine excretion has also been reported in manic patients.[173,249,254] While dopamine excretion in urine has been suggested to be little affected by muscular work,[116] no confirmatory evidence of increased brain dopamine release was obtained from studies of the principal metabolite of dopamine, homovanillic acid (HVA) in the cerebrospinal fluid, since HVA levels have not generally been found to be any higher in manic patients compared to depressed patients or controls.[224] However, one more recent study observed higher cerebrospinal fluid HVA levels during mania, al-

* See references 113, 114, 232, 236, 238, 242, 254, and 255.

though these levels were not as high as those found to be associated with increased physical and mental activity.[210]

Three-methoxy, 4-hydroxyphenylglycol (MHPG), a major metabolite of norepinephrine in the brain, was found not to be regularly elevated in the cerebrospinal fluid of manic patients, although a few patients had high levels.[210,268] It was also demonstrated that physical activity could produce elevations in MHPG, both in cerebrospinal fluid and in urine,[210] further indicating the difficulties in evaluating catecholamine changes in this disorder.

Mania and Indoleamines. Much of the pharmacologic evidence used to implicate catecholamines in affective disorders, such as that based on the effects of MAO inhibitors, tricyclic drugs, and reserpine, has been used to implicate the indoleamines as decreased in depression[154,262] and possibly, at least in the case of tryptamine,[77] as increased in mania. However, the application of this indirect pharmacological reasoning to mania does not hold well, probably because of the nonspecificity of action of the drugs studied.[51]

In direct studies of cerebrospinal fluid levels of 5-hydroxyindoleacetic acid (5-HIAA), this major metabolite of serotonin was found to be decreased during mania in two studies,[59,74] but slightly increased[210,224] or not different from control values in other studies.[7,20] These discrepant results may be related to differences in psychomotor activity in the different patient groups, since CSF 5-HIAA is increased after exercise and after increased physical and mental activity ("simulated mania").[93,210] However, in two studies manic patients (as well as depressed patients) were found to respond to the administration of probenecid with a smaller increase in 5-HIAA than in controls.[109,224]

Also against the theory that an excess of an indoleamine like serotonin might be contributory to manic symptoms is the evidence that methysergide, an indoleamine receptor blocker, was found to be ineffective in treating mania in a controlled, double-blind study by Coppen et al.[64] and in another study by Fieve et al.,[91] although several earlier studies had suggested a possible rapid therapeutic effect with this agent.[76,118] In fact, l-tryptophan, the amino acid precursor of serotonin, has been shown to have some antimanic action in a small number of patients.[181,182,212] The possible contribution of l-tryptophan's sedative effects[275,276] to this proposed antimanic action has not yet been evaluated. Thus, the current evidence would be more congruent with a decrease in serotonin or serotonin metabolism during mania than an increase in this or other indoleamines, although the evidence certainly is not conclusive.

Carbohydrate Metabolism in Mania. Glucose tolerance (as measured by the rate of glucose utilization following an intravenously administered glucose load) is higher in patients studied while manic compared to values obtained during remission induced by two weeks of lithium carbonate treatment.[120] The hypoglycemic response to injected insulin is also increased during mania compared to remission values. Since the patients who did not improve with lithium had negligible changes in glucose utilization and insulin sensitivity, these changes were thought to be produced by the change in behavior rather than to represent a pharmacologic effect of lithium. However, several studies in animals and man have indicated that lithium has some anti-insulin effects.[240]

The increased glucose tolerance observed in manic patients is an opposite finding from the decreased glucose tolerance observed in some[177,214,215,263] but not all[123] studies of depressed patients. Again, in contrast to manic patients, insulin sensitivity was decreased in psychotically depressed patients.[176]

Electrolyte and Water Metabolism in Mania. Patients when manic have generally been found to manifest increased urinary volume and increased sodium excretion during mania; elevations in total body water and calculated extracellular fluid space have also been described;* however, all studies are not in full agreement.† In investigations using isotope dilution techniques to measure sodium distribution among the different body compartments, Coppen et al.[63] found that calculated residual sodium was markedly increased in manic patients, and moderately increased in depressed patients, compared to control values from the literature. Residual sodium is thought to represent intracellular plus some bone sodium. Neither extracellular sodium nor the twenty-four-hour exchangeable sodium was significantly changed in their patients. Recovery from mania was associated with a return toward normal residual sodium values.[63] A more recent study did not replicate these findings.[8]

In studies of sodium transport, no difference was found in the rate of transfer of ^{24}Na and ^{42}K from plasma to cerebrospinal fluid in manic compared to depressed and normal patients.[50] However, sodium reabsorption from salivary ducts was reduced in both the manic and depressed patients studied by Glen.[103] Several studies have indicated that manic patients appear to excrete a smaller proportion of administered lithium during the initial phase of treatment.‡ Similar lithium retention has been shown experimentally to result from sodium depletion produced by low dietary intake or increased urinary sodium loss.[204,206] However, it is unlikely that the increased urinary sodium loss observed during mania represents the full explanation for lithium retention during mania. Contrary to the rapid rise in serum lithium levels and increased side effects that follow sodium restriction or diuretic-drug-induced sodium loss, manic patients generally have a remarkable tolerance for lithium and demonstrate lower lithium levels per dose administered and fewer side effects compared to other patients.§

Adrenal Corticosteroids in Mania. Plasma cortisol levels are normal[46,101,128,205] or slightly elevated[160] in manic patients, although diminished diurnal variation in plasma steroid levels has been observed,[46,205] a change reflecting primarily a diminished reduction in plasma levels in the latter part of the day. Cortisol production rates in hypo-

* See references 61, 63, 70, 127, 145, 146, 168, 214, and 230.
† See references 61, 63, 70, 73, 127, 145, 146, 168, and 230.

‡ See references 100, 111, 112, 129, and 257.
§ See references 100, 111, 112, 129, and 257.

manic patients are normal.[233] While one patient with regular forty-eight-hour cycles between mania and depression had markedly diminished urinary 17-hydroxycorticosteroids during mania,[37] other cycling patients have not exhibited similar patterns,[229,241] and it appears that individual patients may have either reduced, unchanged, or increased plasma cortisol levels and urinary 17-hydroxycorticosteroid levels during mania.* These results suggest that hypomania or mania per se do not result in any regular alteration in corticosteroids, although steroid changes may occur in manic just as in other psychiatric patients in relation to changes in circadian activity or to individually significant stresses resulting from interpersonal conflicts[241] or personality disintegration.[233]

Another adrenal corticosteroid, aldosterone, has been studied in manic patients because of its role in sodium and water metabolism. Although one manic-depressive patient with forty-eight-hour cycles was found to exhibit reduced aldosterone excretion during manic campared to depressed days,[134] two other studies have demonstrated increased urinary aldosterone excretion[2,190] and increased aldosterone production rates[2] in manic patients. While these aldosterone changes have been shown to correlate with sodium balance and extracellular fluid shifts, it is also likely that activity, diet, and weight differences in the manic patients may contribute to these results.[2,190,191]

Other Biologic Changes During Mania. Tyrosine administration leads to higher and more sustained elevations in plasma tyrosine levels ("impaired tyrosine tolerance") in manic patients compared to normals.[256] Increased urinary adenosine 3, 5′ cyclic monophosphate (cyclic AMP) excretion has been reported during mania in some studies[1,200] but not others.[28] Cyclic AMP excretion is reduced in association with a therapeutic response to lithium.[200] However, cerebrospinal fluid levels of cyclic AMP were not found to be elevated during mania.[223] Serum levels of the muscle enzyme, creatinine phosphokinase, are ele-

* See references 27, 37, 41, 46, 48, 101, 128, 160, 205, 229, 233, and 241.

vated in some manic individuals, as has also been reported in individuals with schizophrenia, other psychotic states, and certain central nervous system and muscle disorders.[171]

Sleep in Mania. Although sleeplessness is a cardinal feature of mania, manic patients report sleeping well and feeling rested after only a short sleep period.[207] EEG sleep studies have documented a marked reduction in total sleep time and in rapid eye movement sleep time during mania; slow wave sleep is less disturbed.[117,119] The "switch period" into mania is associated with an abrupt decline in REM sleep in both spontaneous and L-Dopa-induced hypomanic and manic episodes.[36,94] In general, drugs that increase functional brain catecholamines (e.g., L-Dopa) or reduce brain indoleamines (e.g., para-chlorophenylalanine) decrease rapid eye movement sleep, while drugs with reverse effects on catecholamines (e.g., alpha-methyl-para-tyrosine) or indoleamines (5-hydroxytryptophan) enhance rapid eye movement sleep.[275]

(Behavioral and Biological Changes During the "Switch Process" in Manic-Depressive Cycles

The process of the switch into and out of mania has recently been studied in some detail.[35,36,38,39] These transitional periods are of special theoretical interest because of their potential for revealing contributory behavioral and biochemical events prior to the development of nonspecific changes secondary to altered activity, diet, sleep deprivation, and other aspects of the steady-state of mania.

Spontaneous Switches into Mania

A review of the behavioral phenomena observed in ten spontaneous switches from depression into mania and seven switches from mania into depression revealed several characteristic features of each of these transition times.[35,36,39] Most switches into mania were preceded by a depressive period of moderate intensity characterized by withdrawn, self-seclusive behavior with reduced speech and motor activity accompanied by drowsiness. Immediately prior to the development of manic symptoms, all of the patients manifested a brief "normal" period with the sudden appearance of increased environmental and interpersonal interests and appropriate speech and activity.

The buildup of the manic phase following the normal period ranged from a few hours to a few days in duration. Three frequently observed phases were characteristic. Phase one was the first day of the onset of mania and was typified by a sudden marked increase in talking and physical activity. The second phase was characterized by incessant speech and shouting, constant movement, poor judgment, sexual preoccupations, the demanding of staff attention, anger, aggressiveness, and, at times, elation, and laughing. Phase three was characterized by grandiose and sometimes paranoid psychotic ideation, flight of ideas including rhyming and punning, and inability to accept limits.

A number of psychologically significant events occurred prior to the switches into mania. Discussion of discharge plans from the hospital appeared to be the environmental event that occurred most commonly prior to mania in this study.[39] It is a clinical impression that home visits from the hospital, along with impending discharge, are frequently occasions of considerable psychological stress to bipolar patients.[39] However, obtaining passes and discharge-planning status may also simply signifying increasing activity prior to the onset of a manic episode, rather than representing an active precipitant of mania.

In another study, the question of precipitating events prior to manic episodes was assessed by evaluating the number of premania stresses that were severe, unusual in the patient's life, and judged "likely to precipitate mania."[271] In one hundred manic episodes, thirty stressful events could be documented; however, eighteen of these events represented discontinuation of phenothiazine or lithium medication (six patients) or treatment with antidepressant drugs or ECT (twelve patients), conditions known to be associated with triggering the onset of mania. Thus, known significant psychological stresses were thought to be present in only 12 percent of the patients developing mania. This low incidence of psychological precipitants has been reported in other studies,[17] although serious methodological problems limit the meaningfulness of such statistics.[17,155]

The amount of total sleep and rapid eye movement sleep were both decreased immediately prior to and during the switch into mania.[36] Urinary norepinephrine excretion was significantly elevated on the day prior to and during the manic episodes, while smaller and nonstatistically significant changes were observed in the excretion of epinephrine, dopamine, 3-methoxy, 4-hydroxyphenylglycol (MHPG) and 5-hydroxyindoleacetic acid.[36] Urinary cyclic AMP excretion exhibited a brief peak on the day of the switch into mania and decreased subsequently.[199] Changes in urinary levels of cyclic AMP may well reflect the associated alterations in catecholamines or other hormones accompanying the behavioral changes, or may be directly involved in the switch process itself.[199]

The switch from mania to depression is characterized by a number of different features. Unlike the switch into mania, this transition period rarely occurred abruptly. Rather, the patients manifested the following gradual behavioral shifts, often extending over a period of weeks: mania, hypomania, a short, unstable transitional period with labile mood and activity, followed by the onset of depression, with prominent psychomotor retardation. A diagrammatic representation of typical switch sequences is presented in Figure 23–1.

Drug-Related Switches into Mania

The occurrence of some hypomanic and manic attacks in apparent relationship to the administration of psychoactive drugs that alter biogenic amines may be of some importance in understanding the "switch process."

Switches During Tricyclic Antidepressant Administration. In one study, three bipolar patients given tricyclic antidepressants devel-

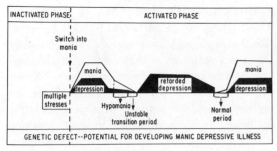

BIPOLAR MANIC DEPRESSIVE PROCESS WITH RAPID SWITCHES
(Theorized Schema)

Figure 23–1. Bipolar manic depressive process with rapid switches (theorized schema).

oped typical manic episodes that were characterized by sequential changes in mood and behavior very similar to those observed in spontaneous switches, including the presence of a brief "normal" period.[38] In two of these three cases, the switches occurred after four days of tricyclic drug treatment, i.e., much earlier than the antidepressant effects of these drugs usually occur. No manic episodes developed in the nonbipolar patients, although some of these patients exhibited increased activity and mild hypomanic symptoms after several weeks of treatment.

In papers from the literature dealing with the possible association between tricyclic medication and the onset of mania, data were available concerning previous psychiatric disorders in sixty-seven of one hundred and sixty patients who were reported as developing mania or hypomania during tricyclic drug treatment.[38] Of the fifteen patients who developed full-blown mania in this group, 66 percent had a past history of mania, 27 percent a past history of depression, 7 percent a past history of schizophrenia, and none of the patients lacked a history of mental illness.

Thus, bipolar patients appear to have the highest predilection for mania during tricyclic drug administration. An additional five patients with past histories of mania received equal or greater doses of tricyclic drugs in this study and did not develop mania. Thus, it appears likely that other variables in addition to

the medication may play a role in the onset of these manic episodes.

The mechanism by which the tricyclic drugs might act as a pharmacological trigger for mania is not yet clear. The antidepressant activity of these drugs has been most frequently assigned to a central potentiation of adrenergic neuroactivity resulting from inhibition of biogenic uptake. Recently, potentiation of norepinephrine effects[212] as well as inhibition of biogenic amine uptake[187] have been reported in patients receiving these drugs. It is possible that patients with manic histories are unusually sensitive to these effects of tricyclic drug treatment.[179]

Switches During L-Dopa Administration. In the course of a study designed to evaluate the possible antidepressant effects of L-Dopa (L-3,4-dihydroxyphenylalanine),[184] the amino acid precursor of the catecholamines dopamine and norepinephrine, eight of nine bipolar patients developed hypomanic episodes during the time of L-Dopa treatment. Only one of thirteen unipolar-depressed patients developed a similar episode, despite similar dosage and similar duration of L-Dopa administration in both groups. Antidepressant effects of L-Dopa were minimal in the patients as a whole, with only 25 percent of the patients exhibiting some improvement. However, it was noteworthy that all of the patients who improved had features of psychomotor retardation as part of their depressive symptomatology, and that among these patients who improved several relapsed following placebo substitution.[106]

The hypomanic episodes during L-Dopa treatment were generally similar to the patients' prior episodes in that they began abruptly and were characterized by increased speech, hyperactivity, increased social interaction, intrusiveness, sleeplessness, grandiosity, and some minimal euphoria. They were different from the spontaneous switches into mania and the switches associated with tricyclic drugs in their brevity (they usually were only two or three days in duration) and in their mildness. Only two of the patients developed full-blown manic episodes requiring specific treatment beyond the discontinuation of

L-Dopa. Only one of the patients who became hypomanic was considered to have become clearly less depressed while receiving L-Dopa.[184]

In the patients developing hypomania and mania during both L-Dopa and tricyclic antidepressant drug treatment, total sleep and rapid eye movement sleep were reduced, as in the patients developing mania spontaneously.[36,38,94] Urinary dopamine excretion was markedly increased, as expected, during L-Dopa administration. In a small subsample of patients studied during L-Dopa administration, some smaller elevations of urinary norepinephrine metabolites were also observed.[106]

The induction of hypomania by the catecholamine precursor L-Dopa supports the postulated importance of catecholamines in the manic phase of affective disorders.[34,235] However, these results do not provide conclusive evidence indicating a disorder in catecholamine metabolism in manic-depressive patients, since large doses of L-Dopa have stimulant properties in animals and may well have similar effects in man. These results do indicate a greater susceptibility to the excitant effects of L-Dopa in the manic-depressive patients who develop hypomanic episodes. Further study is needed to determine whether this susceptibility represents a specific abnormality in catecholamine metabolism, for example, a reduced metabolic capacity for an amine excess produced by an L-Dopa load. Alternatively, it may be that the patient prone to a manic or hypomanic episode is more sensitive to the stimulant effects of L-Dopa and other agents such as tricyclic antidepressants, monoamine oxidase inhibitors, electroshock treatment, or psychological stresses on some other genetic or developmental basis.[179] In any case, the regular occurrence of typical hypomanic symptoms in bipolar patients treated with L-Dopa, and the development of acute manic episodes in other bipolar patients in close association with tricyclic drug administration, serves to implicate a change in brain amines, specifically an increase in catecholamines, in the switch process. The fact that L-Dopa can produce hypomania in susceptible individuals without reversing depression sug-

gests that mania and depression are not simply opposite poles of the same continuum.

Monoamine Oxidase (MAO) Inhibitors. These drugs are of particular interest because, like L-Dopa and imipramine (and possibly the amphetamines), they act as behavioral activating agents via effects on the neurotransmitter amines.[179] In normal individuals, as well as in medical patients without psychiatric histories, their administration can produce mood lability and behavioral alterations,[71] [72,104] including the precipitation of manic episodes and the production of exacerbations in psychotic symptomatology in some schizophrenic patients.[29,110,218] They also appear to potentiate the psychotomimetic effects of some amino acids, including L-methionine and possibly L-Dopa.[16,209,259] The possibility of endogenously reduced MAO activity acting as a predisposing factor in the behavioral switch mechanism is a particularly intriguing question.[193]

Amphetamines. These agents can provoke behavioral, mood, and motor activity changes in animals and man and appear to act via effects on catecholamines.[65,136,217] Normal individuals as well as psychiatric patients generally develop transient hyperactivity and sometimes euphoria and with smaller doses hypomania and manic episodes have been precipitated in some individuals receiving amphetamines or other direct-acting sympathomimetic agents. Larger doses given over a longer duration often lead to behavioral depression and psychosis with paranoid symptoms predominating.[58,115] The postdrug period is typified by a "crash" period of severe, depressive-like symptoms.

Adrenal Corticosteroids. The administration of exogenous steroids in the treatment of various medical disorders, as well as the increased endogenous production of steroids in Cushing's syndrome, is associated with mood lability and other psychiatric symptoms.[102] Euphoria and full-blown manic episodes are apparently more common during exogenous steroid treatment, while depressive symptoms occur more often in Cushing's syndrome.[90] [139,167] The possible role that the adrenal corticosteroids may play in the triggering of psychopathology on the basis of their effects on electrolytes and biogenic amines at the neuronal membrane has been the subject of several reviews.[35,90,165,231]

Direct Brain Stimulation. Increased communication and mild euphoria have been reported to follow electrode stimulation of the median forebrain bundle,[252] as well as direct physical stimulation during surgery involving hypothalamic areas.[130] Stimulation of the amygdala in one instance yielded increased activity, rushing thoughts, and pressure of speech, and, in other instances, anger and a delayed-rage reaction.[86]

(Drugs in the Treatment of Mania

Lithium carbonate, the phenothiazines, and the butyrophenones are the drugs most used in the treatment of mania. Electroconvulsive therapy, although effective in some patients, has been mostly replaced by drug treatment. Most manic patients (more than 80 percent) respond to drugs, although large doses of the antipsychotic drugs and treatment with lithium carbonate for over a week may be required for full therapeutic benefit. Several recent reviews of the efficacy of lithium and other drugs in the treatment of mania are available,[99,105,240] and this section will focus only on the ways in which the effects of these drugs may contribute to the understanding of the pathogenesis of mania.

Lithium Carbonate. A large series of studies, reviewed elsewhere,[99,105,240] have demonstrated the efficacy of this drug in the treatment of mania. Used in doses of 1.2 to 2.4 grams per day which yield serum levels of 0.9 to 1.5 millequivalents per liter, an apparently specific antimanic effect can usually be seen after five to ten days of treatment. Negligible sedative or antipsychotic effects are produced by lithium carbonate, and some atypical schizoaffective patients appear more psychotic when hyperactivity diminishes.[107,135]

The ability of lithium carbonate to interact with sodium, potassium, magnesium, and calcium in a variety of biological systems[239,240] may be involved in its therapeutic effects.

Lithium treatment of manic patients has been shown to alter exchangeable and residual (cellular plus bone) sodium, total body potassium, and the urinary excretion of sodium and other electrolytes as well as the hormones (e.g., aldosterone) regulating electrolyte balance.* Whether these changes are important in relation to the alterations in water and electrolyte metabolism, reviewed above, or have some direct cellular relationship to the transport, storage, and release of biogenic amines, as reviewed elsewhere,[35] has not been conclusively demonstrated. Lithium has been demonstrated in animal brain and human platelet preparations to lead to actions antagonistic to biogenic amine effects, including an increase in amine reuptake, a decrease in amine release, an increase in intraneuronal amine destruction and an increase in amine turnover,[140,187,211,234] as well as to an antagonistic effect on cyclic AMP production.[92,188] This series of effects represent the most likely biochemical mechanism of action for the antimanic effect of lithium, based upon the theoretical support from human and animal studies that antagonistic effects on biogenic amine function would be consistent with antimanic efficacy; however, the relationship of these biochemical effects to the prophylactic[240] and partial antidepressant actions of lithium[107,108] remains problematic.

Phenothiazines and Butyrophenones. These antipsychotic drugs are effective in some manic patients, particularly in rapidly diminishing severely disruptive behavior.[213,219] While these drugs have multiple biochemical effects, they possess antagonistic actions on α-adrenergic and dopaminergic receptors in brain and in the periphery,[45,277] which have been suggested to be related to their antipsychotic and antimanic efficacy.[125]

Alpha-methyl-p-tyrosine. This drug is a blocker of dopamine and norepinephrine synthesis via direct inhibition of tyrosine hydroxylase, the rate-limiting enzyme in catecholamine synthesis, and was found to temporarily decrease manic symptomatology in most manic patients, some of whom showed a con-

---

* See references 8, 60, 62, 129, 185, 190, 191, 204, 240, 257 and 258.

sistent pattern of relapse with repeated pla-cebo substitution.[26] In these patients, de-creased urinary excretion of dopamine, 3-methoxy, 4-hydroxyphenolic acid (VMA), and 3-methoxy, 4-hydroxyphenylglycol (MHPG) was observed, as well as decreased levels of homovanillic acid (HVA) and MHPG in the cerebrospinal fluid. These clini-cal and biochemical data are consistent with the hypothesis that mania is associated with an increase in catecholamines. However, alpha-methyl-p-tyrosine is neither as practical a drug to use clinically (because of hypotension and other side effects) nor is it as effective as lith-ium or the antipsychotic phenothiazines in leading to a complete remission of manic symptoms.

❮ Affect, Catecholamines and Psychomotor Activation in Mania

Mania has been relegated to the category of the "affective disorders" and has been found to be the differentiating characteristic of "bi-polar" compared to unipolar patients among individuals with primary affective disorders. One implication of the studies reviewed in this chapter is that the use of these terms may be imprecise and perhaps misleading, in that the conception of mania and depression as repre-senting "opposite," pathologic extremes of af-fective expression appears overly simplistic and reductionistic.

While all depressive states share the com-mon affect of sadness, mania appears to be not as well characterized by elation but rather by a state of heightened affective expression overall together with lability of affect. The co-occurrence of marked depressive thought con-tent and behavior (like crying) with elation and heightened anger and other affects in sep-arately varying intensities in the same manic individual suggests that the equation of elated mood with mania represents an overemphasis and oversimplification of the phenomena of mania.

Various models attempting to relate mania, depression, and normality have been pro-posed: (a) the traditional bipolar model with

normality in the middle and mania and de-pression as pathologic extremes; (b) a con-tinuum model reflecting the suggested relative severity of these disorders, with normality at the bottom, depression intermediate, and mania at the top;[67,68] and (c) a triangular, tripolar model that, in its several variants,[35][180,192,267] essentially posits that mania and de-pression are separate and independent states. These different models all have some firm sup-port, but none fits all of the data, although the least constraining, the triangular model, comes closest to encompassing both the psychologi-cal and biological phenomena observed in these patients.

However, several crucial ingredients appear not to have been taken into account in the construction of conceptual models for manic-depressive illness: (a) the phenomena of de-pression observed in both unipolar and bi-polar patients have previously been grouped together for contrast with mania, although depression in bipolar patients is now known to have features different from that in other de-pressed patients,[13,79] while mania only occurs in bipolar patients; and (b) the dimension of psychomotor activity has been underempha-sized, while the affective state has been over-emphasized, particularly disproportionately in mania.

The Question of the Primacy of Psychomotor Activity in Mania

The data reviewed in this paper, as well as observations dating from the time of Kraepe-lin,[12,121,151] suggest that motor, speech, and cognitive hyperactivity may be more specifi-cally characteristic of mania than is elation. In fact, it seems more economic to consider mania and depression in the bipolar individual as more primarily representing extremes on the axis of psychomotor activity or arousal, rather than of mood. Depression in bipolar patients is more frequently characterized by psychomotor retardation, social withdrawal, anergia, and hypersomnia,[13,39,75,117] and ap-pears to be a distinctly different syndrome in other respects from depression in nonbipolar patients.[13,79] Manic hyperactivity, on the other hand, is accompanied by boundless energy, little need for sleep, and a high level of motor, verbal, and cognitive activity, and social interchange. It is of interest that some psychoanalytic interpretations of mania have emphasized its similarity to the elevated mood and omnipotence that attend the practicing period in early development associated with increased motor and exploratory activity.[198]

A case might even be made for considering the psychomotor hyperactivity with its cognitive components of distractibility and associated impairment of memory and judgment as capable of producing a near totally "present time only" pleasure-orientation as a basis for the elated mood. It is also possible that affective expression is regulated by the same mechanism as psychomotor activity, and, as suggested above, mania is associated with heightened expression or amplification of all affects, while phenomena like "not being able to cry" represent suppressed affective expression during depression. Similarly, other mechanisms regulating sleep, "reward" or pleasure, and other functions may be subject to independent activation, with the resulting combination of effects yielding each individual's manic syndrome.

However, direct evidence to prove the primacy of activity over mood, or vice versa, is lacking. Until more evidence is at hand, it would seem best to consider affect and psychomotor activity as separate dimensions or axes of behavior that can contribute independently to the final syndrome of mania. Some of the complexity in understanding depression may also be related to separate contributions of the affect-regulating mechanisms and activity-regulating mechanisms. For example, the severely agitated depressed patient with a marked motor component to his symptoms may not resemble other depressed patients when studied, but may rather be closer to manic patients in some phenomena.

Catecholamines, Brain Mechanisms, and Mania

On the basis of the impressive evidence linking brain dopamine and norepinephrine to the regulation of psychomotor activity,[40,87] sleep,[137] emotion,[142] reward mechanisms,[251] as well as to arousal mechanisms such as the reticular and limbic activating systems,[81,166,196,227] it seems especially pertinent to reemphasize the evidence linking brain catecholamines to mania. Methods capable of demonstrating increased catecholaminergic neuronal activity in man have not yet been devised. Perhaps the direct measure closest to providing a reflection of catecholamine metabolism in the brain, the measurement in the cerebrospinal fluid of levels of the norepinephrine metabolite, MHPG, has suggested an increase in norepinephrine turnover during mania.[268] However, it appears that physical activity alone may produce an equally large increase.[210]

Nonetheless, indirect evidence from drugs with the greatest relative specificity for affecting catecholamines indicate that the precursor of dopamine and norepinephrine, L-Dopa, can precipitate dose-related hypomanic episodes, while the catecholamine synthesis inhibitor, α-methyl-para-tyrosine, can dampen manic symptoms. Collaborative evidence from other psychoactive drugs including the tricyclic antidepressants, MAO inhibitors, antipsychotic drugs, reserpine, amphetamines, and lithium are also compatible with their mania-related effects being mediated via central catecholamines. While evidence for the primary involvement of serotonergic (see above), cholinergic,[132] and other biogenic amine mechanisms[77] in mania exists, as well as other metabolic interactions (see above), the most weighty current evidence implicates brain dopamine and/or norepinephrine as principal mediators of the symptomatology of mania. Cholinergic[132] and serotonergic[211,269] modulation or antagonistic "balancing" of some catecholamine effects may also be present.

In attempting to tie together the evidence pointing to the importance of psychomotor activity and arousal with the evidence implicating catecholamines in mania, it is necessary to consider the localization in the brain of dopamine and norepinephrine and of the brain sites involved in the regulation of activity and arousal. Recent histofluorescence studies[97,124,260] have verified and extended regional chemical analyses and indicate the existence of several different noradrenergic and dopaminergic neural pathways.

Most of the cell bodies of noradrenergic and dopaminergic neurons are present in the brainstem, i.e., the medulla, pons, and mesencephalon, but their terminals extend to almost all parts of the brain and spinal cord. The major dopaminergic pathways (the nigro-neostriatal tract) originates in the pars compacta of the substantia nigra and ascends through the mesencephalic tegmentum, crus cerebri, and internal capsule, terminating in the caudate nucleus and putamen; this system is important in the regulation of motor activation and posture. Another dopaminergic neuronal pathway ascends in the median forebrain bundle and terminates in the tuberculum olfactorum, the nucleus accumbens and the nucleus interstitialis striae terminalis. A small dopaminergic pathway extends into the hypophyseal capillary portal area.

A prominent noradrenergic neuronal group also ascends through the median forebrain bundle to terminate in widely distributed parts of the hypothalamus, most areas of the forebrain limbic system (the septal area), the preoptic area, the amygdaloid cortex, the cingulate gyrus, the nucleus interstitialis striae terminalis, and the neocortex. Their cell bodies are derived from the locus coeruleus in the pons and the reticular formation in the medulla. These noradrenergic neurons give off many collaterals, and it appears that a single neuron may send fibers to brain areas as distant as the cerebellum and the telencephalon. Monosynaptic connections have been described between both the limbic forebrain area and the neocortex and the reticular formation core of the lower brainstem.

Although normally catecholamines are localized in the above-described tracts, it should be noted that altered catecholamine formation, such as that which follows administration of L-Dopa, also affects serotonergic neurons[194] as well as other brain biochemical processes,[42] and since some of these mechanisms may operate in "balance" or permissive ways with catecholaminergic systems, it is possible that catecholamine-mediated behavioral and psychological changes may not be primarily effected through the catecholaminergic tracts themselves.

Nonetheless, there exists a close correlation between the catecholamine pathways and the sites that brain-lesion and electrode-stimulation studies indicate as important in the regulation of psychomotor activity, reward mechanisms, and arousal. These areas include: (a) dopaminergic corpus striatum areas, lesions of which produce slowed psychomotor activity, and Parkinsonian-type symptoms in animals and man;[126] (b) the various noradrenergic areas included in the limbic- and reticular-activating systems, which are well known for their role in arousal mechanisms;[196,227] and (c) some specific noradrenergic areas such as those in the septum which appear to function in the mediation of exploratory activity, rage responses, and reward mechanisms.[21,96,170,251]

Arousal, Psychomotor Activation, and Mania

There is very little direct information to relate the neurochemical state of these specific catecholaminergic brain areas to altered behavior in the manic state and to the hypothesized existence of altered arousal or activation regulation in the bipolar patient group. Indirect evidence based upon drug effects provides suggestive evidence to implicate catecholamine pathways, as discussed above, but cannot yield conclusive proof because of the multiplicity of effects of the drugs studied.[51] Lesion studies such as those which relate such manic-like phenomena as "rage," increased exploratory activity, and a lack of response inhibition to septal area destruction in animals[21,96,170] provide interesting models for abnormal behavioral syndromes, but are obviously severely limited by species differences and the nonspecificity of even small lesion production.[51,96] However, when several separate threads of evidence can be gathered together from different study approaches, a stronger line of argument is produced. For example, there already exists a body of data suggesting that hyperarousal may be present in some schizophrenic individuals. This theory is based in part on psychophysiologic evidence[85] and also on indirect data and models constructed from phenothiazine drug effects.[148,149] In some ways, an even stronger case can be made for hyperarousal in mania[179] as some similar psychophysiologic alterations occur in mania and as phenothiazines are effective antimanic drugs as well. In addition, the L-Dopa and antidepressant drug-related switches into mania described above also would be compatible with an inherent hypersensitivity of the bipolar individual to these drugs, all of which have activating effects.

From this viewpoint, manic and schizophrenic individuals may be postulated to share a common state of hyperarousal that predisposes them to maladaptive responses to further psychologically or pharmacologically based arousal. The specificity of the responses in these patients and in other individuals susceptible on different bases (e.g., brain damage) to impaired stimulus regulation is suggested to lie in other aspects of the personality structure.[179]

The information from the cortical evoked response studies of bipolar patients[31] provides direct evidence of altered stimulus-intensity modulation compatible with hyperarousal in these individuals, compared to normal people and especially to unipolar patients. The greater EEG augmentation responses in reaction to increasing intensities of light in bipolar patients is increased further during hypomanic and manic episodes and in response to L-Dopa administration.[30,31] In contrast, successful treatment of manic episodes with lithium carbonate and with the catecholamine synthesis inhibitor, a-methyl-para-tyrosine, is associated with decreased evoked response amplitudes in these patients.[19,30,31]

If the averaged EEG responses evoked by light can indeed be considered an index of stimulus intensity modulation as has been suggested,[19,32,244] an interesting model of maladaptive activation regulation is suggested. The bipolar manic-depressive patient in this model would appear to be operating in a state of positive feedback as evidenced by sensory input amplification. In control systems theory, positive feedback usually implies the liability of exaggerated overswings and a susceptibility to being driven by external stimuli. Such a state is clearly analogous to many features of the manic-depressive condition, including lability in mood and activity a swell as other characteristics of mania such as distractibility.[121] If, as has been suggested above, activation is alterable by catecholamine-mediated changes, an impaired control mechanism, regulating activation responsiveness to stimulate intensity in these patients, might well be found in the cellular events concerned with catecholamine synthesis, storage, release, reuptake, metabolism, and receptor function. Several examples of the most likely types of changes have been discussed elsewhere.[35,178,193]

For future exploration remains the more precise testing of this and other postulated mechanisms and models of the manic state. Of particular interest is the interaction between the apparently inherited susceptibility to mania and the precipitation, as well as different manifestations, of the bipolar disorder in individual instances. Indeed, the question of whether the inherited factor may lie directly in biogenic amine metabolic pathways,[82,193] or neural synaptic membranes,[35] or in other brain mechanisms only indirectly affected by psychologic or biochemical activating agents[179] is only beginning to be the subject of speculation. Pharmacologic and other animal models[49,78,221] for as complex a human behavioral phenomenon as mania are some distance from meaningful utility. It appears that continuing, clinically based research studies remain the proving ground for hypotheses concerning human behavior and its disorders, including mania.

(Conclusions

The review has focused on recent studies of mania and of the individuals who develop mania—the group with the so-called "bipolar-affective disorders." Some evidence indicating that mania and depression are "opposite" bipolar states in some ways only, and clearly not in others, was reviewed. Other evidence suggesting that mania represents more a disorder of activity than of affect was also considered.

Whether mania, schizoaffective states, and some or all forms of schizophrenia may be related in some way requires reinvestigation. Some of the evidence reviewed suggests that these disorders can be placed along a continuum, and other evidence indicates that they share some clinical and biologic phenomena, although the majority of family-history studies continue to suggest a low cross-incidence in the same family of schizophrenia and the affective disorders considered together.

Mania is the definitional characteristic of the bipolar subgroup of depressed patients. These individuals differ from other (unipolar) depressed patients in some clinical characteristics seen during depression and in remission. They also differ in familial incidence ("genetic") patterns; while an X-linked mode of genetic transmission has been suggested, current evidence is more compatible with a polygenic mode. Differences in psychophysiologic and biologic studies, ranging from EEG and cortical evoked response data to the activity of biogenic amine metabolizing enzymes, have also been observed. In addition, bipolar patients have been demonstrated to manifest a differential susceptibility to drugs such as lithium, L-Dopa and imipramine.

Information from animal studies concerning the mode of action of drugs that suppress and precipitate mania points toward the mediation of these effects in man via changes in central neurotransmitter amines, especially norepinephrine and dopamine. A contributory role of other neurotransmitters, especially the cholinergic and serotonergic systems, may also be integrated with the catecholamines in the regulation of psychomotor activity, arousal, and affective expression.

(Bibliography

1. ABDULLA, Y. H. and K. HAMADAH. "3'5' Cyclic Adenosine Monophosphate in Depression and Mania," *Lancet*, 1 (1970), 378–381.

2. ALLSOPP, M. N. E., M. J. LEVELL, S. R.

STITCH et al. "Aldosterone Production Rates in Manic-Depressive Psychosis," *Br. J. Psychiatry*, 120 (1972), 399–404.

3. ANGEL (KATAN), ANNY. "Einige Bemerkungen über den Optimismus," *Int. Z. Psychoanal.*, 20 (1934), 191–199.

4. ANGST, J. "Zur Ätiologie und Nosologie endogener depressiver Psychosen," *Monogr. Gesamtgeb. Psychiatr.*, 112 (1966), 1–118.

5. ANGST, J. and C. PERRIS. "Nosology of Endogenous Depression, a Comparison of the Findings of Two Studies," *Arch. Psychiatr. Nervenkr.*, 210 (1968), 373–386.

6. ARIETI, S., ed., *American Handbook of Psychiatry*, Volume 1, 2nd ed. New York: Basic Books, 1975.

7. ASHCROFT, G. W. and D. F. SHARMAN. "Drug-Induced Changes in the Concentration of 5-OR Indolyl Compounds in Cerebrospinal Fluid and Caudate Nucleus," *Br. J. Pharmacol.*, 19 (1962), 153–160.

8. BAER, L., J. DURELL, W. E. BUNNEY, JR. et al. "Sodium Balance and Distribution in Lithium Carbonate Therapy," *Arch. Gen. Psychiatry*, 22 (1970), 40–44.

9. BAILLARGER, J. G. "Note sur un Genre de Folie Dont les Accès Sont Caractérisés par Deux Periodes Régulières, l'une de Dépression et l'autre d'Excitation," *Bull. Acad. Natl. Méd. Paris*, 19 (1854), 340–352.

10. BAKER, M., J. DORZAB, G. WINOKUR et al. "Depressive Disease: The Effect of the Postpartum State," *Biol. Psychiatry*, 3 (1971), 357–365.

11. BALDESSARINI, R. J. "Frequency of Diagnoses of Schizophrenia Versus Affective Disorders from 1944 to 1968," *Am. J. Psychiatry*, 127 (1970), 759–763.

12. BEIGEL, A. and D. L. MURPHY. "Assessing Clinical Characteristics of the Manic State," *Am. J. Psychiatry*, 128 (1971), 688–699.

13. ———. "Unipolar and Bipolar Affective Illness. Differences in Clinical Characteristics Accompanying Depression," *Arch. Gen. Psychiatry*, 24 (1971), 215–220.

14. BEIGEL, A., D. L. MURPHY, and W. E. BUNNEY, JR. "The Manic-State Rating Scale: Scale Construction, Reliability and Validity," *Arch. Gen. Psychiatry*, 25 (1971), 256–262.

15. BELLAK, L. *Manic-Depressive Psychosis and Allied Conditions*. New York: Grune & Stratton, 1952.

16. BERLET, H. H., K. MATSUMOTO, G. R. PSCHEIDT et al. "Biochemical Correlates of Behavior in Schizophrenic Patients," *Arch. Gen. Psychiatry*, 13 (1965), 521–531.

17. BJARSCH, H. "Anankasmus und partielle Asthenie," *Psychiatr. Clin.*, 4 (1971), 19–39.

18. BLEULER, E. "Die Probleme der Schizoidie und der Syntonie," *Z. Gesamte Psychiatr.*, 78 (1922), 373–399.

19. BORGE, G., M. BUCHSBAUM, F. K. GOODWIN et al. "Neuropsychological Correlates of Affective Disorders," *Arch. Gen. Psychiatry*, 24 (1971), 501–504.

20. BOWERS, M. B., G. R. HENINGER, and F. A. GERBODE. "Cerebrospinal Fluid 5-Hydroxyindoleacetic Acid and Homovanillic Acid in Psychiatric Patients," *Int. J. Neuropharmacol.*, 8 (1969), 255–262.

21. BRADY, J. V. and W. J. H. NAUTA. "Subcortical Mechanisms in Emotional Behavior: Affective Changes Following Septal Forebrain Lesions in the Albino Rat," *J. Comp. Physiol. Psychol.*, 46 (1953), 339–346.

22. BRATFOS, O. and J. O. HAUG. "The Course of Manic-Depressive Psychosis," *Acta Psychiatr. Scand.*, 44 (1968), 89–112.

23. BREAKEY, W. R. and H. GOODELL. "Thought Disorder in Mania and Schizophrenia Evaluated by Bannister's Grid Test for Schizophrenic Thought Disorder," *Br. J. Psychiatry*, 120 (1972), 391–395.

24. BRILL, A. A. "The Schizoid Concept in the Neuroses and Psychoses," in *Schizophrenia*, pp. 31–43. New York: Hoeber, 1928.

25. BRODIE, H. K. H. and M. J. LEFF. "Bipolar Depression—A Comparative Study of Patient Characteristics," *Am. J. Psychiatry*, 127 (1971), 1086–1090.

26. BRODIE, H. K. H., D. L. MURPHY, F. K. GOODWIN et al. "Catecholamines and Mania: The Effect of Alpha-Methyl-Para-Tyrosine on Manic Behavior and Catecholamine Metabolism," *Clin. Pharmacol. Ther.*, 12 (1971), 218–224.

27. BROOKSBANK, B. W. L. and A. COPPEN. "Plasma 11-Hydroxycorticosteroids in Affective Disorders," *Br. J. Psychiatry*, 113 (1967), 395–404.

28. BROWN, B. L., J. G. SALWAY, J. D. M. ALBANO et al. "Urinary Excretion of Cyclic AMP and Manic-Depressive Psychosis," *Br. J. Psychiatry*, 120 (1972), 405–408.

29. BRUNE, G. G., G. R. PSCHEIDT, and H. E. HIMWICH. "Different Responses of Urinary Tryptamine and of Total Catecholamines During Treatment with Reserpine and Isocarboxazid in Schizophrenic Patients," *Int. J. Neuropharmacol.*, 2 (1963), 17–23.

30. BUCHSBAUM, M., F. K. GOODWIN, D. L. MURPHY et al. "Average Evoked Responses in Affective Disorders." Presented Am. Psychiatr. Assoc., San Francisco, May, 1970.

31. ———. "Average Evoked Responses in Affective Disorders," *Am. J. Psychiatry*, 128 (1971), 19–25.

32. BUCHSBAUM, M. and J. SILVERMAN. "Stimulus Intensity Control and the Cortical Evoked Response," *Psychosom. Med.*, 30 (1968), 12–22.

33. BUNNEY, W. E., JR., H. K. H. BRODIE, D. L. MURPHY et al. "Psychopharmacological Differentiation Between Two Subgroups of Depressed Patients," *Proc. Am. Psychol. Assoc.* Sept., 1970.

34. BUNNEY, W. E., JR. and J. M. DAVIS. "Norepinephrine in Depressive Reactions," *Arch. Gen. Psychiatry*, 13 (1965), 483–494.

35. BUNNEY, W. E., JR., F. K. GOODWIN, and D. L. MURPHY. "The 'Switch Process' in Manic-Depressive Illness. III. Theoretical Implications," *Arch. Gen. Psychiatry*, 27 (1972), 312–317.

36. BUNNEY, W. E., JR., F. K. GOODWIN, D. L. MURPHY et al. "The 'Switch Process' in Manic-Depressive Illness. II. Relationship to Catecholamines, REM Sleep and Drugs," *Arch. Gen. Psychiatry*, 27 (1972), 304–309.

37. BUNNEY, W. E., JR., E. L. HARTMANN, and J. W. MASON. "Study of a Patient with 48-Hour Manic-Depressive Cycles: II. Strong Positive Correlation Between Endocrine Factors and Manic Defense Patterns," *Arch. Gen. Psychiatry*, 12 (1965), 619–625.

38. BUNNEY, W. E., JR., D. L. MURPHY, F. K. GOODWIN et al. "The 'Switch Process' from Depression to Mania: Relationship to Drugs Which Alter Brain Amines," *Lancet*, 1 (1970), 1022–1027.

39. ———. "The 'Switch Process' in Manic-Depressive Illness. I. A Systematic Study of Sequential Behavioral Change," *Arch. Gen. Psychiatry*, 27 (1972), 295–302.

40. BUTCHER, L. L. and J. ENGEL. "Behavioral and Biochemical Effects of L-Dopa after

Peripheral Decarboxylase Inhibition," *Brain Res.*, 15 (1969), 233–242.

41. BUTLER, P. W. P. and G. M. BESSER. "Pituitary-Adrenal Function in Severe Depressive Illness," *Lancet*, 1 (1968), 1234–1236.

42. CALNE, D. B. and M. SANDLER. "'L-Dopa and Parkinsonism," *Nature*, 226 (1970), 21–24.

43. CAMERON, N. "The Place of Mania Among the Depressions from a Biological Standpoint," *J. Psychol.*, 14 (1942), 181–195.

44. CARLSON, G. and F. K. GOODWIN. "The Stages of Mania: A Longitudinal Analysis of the Manic Episode," *Arch. Gen. Psychiatry*, in press.

45. CARLSSON, A. and M. LINDQVIST. "Effect of Chlorpromazine or Haloperidol on Formation of 3-Methoxytyramine and Normetanephrine in Mouse Brain," *Acta Pharmacol. Toxicol.*, 20 (1963), 140–144.

46. CARPENTER, W. T., JR. and W. E. BUNNEY, JR. "Diurnal Rhythm of Cortisol in Behavior," *Arch. Gen. Psychiatry*, 25 (1971), 270–273.

47. CARPENTER, W. T., JR., J. S. STRAUSS, and S. MULEH. "Are There Pathognomic Symptoms in Schizophrenia? An Empiric Investigation of Kurt Schneider's First Rank Symptoms," *Arch. Gen. Psychiatry*, 28 (1973), 847–852.

48. CARROLL, B. J., F. I. R. MARTIN, and B. DAVIES. "Resistance to Suppression by Dexamethasone of Plasma 11-O.H.C.S. Levels in Severe Depressive Illness," *Br. Med. J.*, 3 (1968), 285–287.

49. CARROLL, B. J. and P. T. SHARP. "Rubidium and Lithium: Opposite Effects on Amine-Mediated Excitement," *Science*, 172 (1971), 1355–1357.

50. CARROLL, B. J., L. STEVEN, R. A. POPE et al. "Sodium Transfer from Plasma to CSF in Severe Depressive Illness," *Arch. Gen. Psychiatry*, 21 (1969), 77–81.

51. CHASE, T. N. and D. L. MURPHY. "Serotonin and Central Nervous System Function," *Annu. Rev. Pharmacol.*, 13 (1973), 181–197.

52. CLAYTON, P., F. N. PITTS, JR., and G. WINOKUR. "Affective Disorder: IV. Mania," *Compr. Psychiatry*, 6 (1965), 313–322.

53. CLAYTON, R. J., L. RODIN, and G. WINOKUR. "Family History Studies: III. Schizoaffective Disorder, Clinical and Genetic Factors," *Compr. Psychiatry*, 9 (1968), 31–49.

54. COHEN, M. B., G. BAKER, R. A. COHEN et al. "An Intensive Study of Twelve Cases of Manic-Depressive Psychosis," *Psychiatry*, 17 (1954), 103–138.

55. COHEN, R. A. "Manic-Depressive Reactions," in A. M. Freedman and H. I. Kaplan, eds., *Comprehensive Textbook of Psychiatry*, pp. 676–687. Baltimore: William & Wilkins, 1967.

56. COHEN, S. M., M. G. ALLEN, W. POLLIN et al. "Relationship of Schizoaffective Psychosis to Manic Depressive Psychosis and Schizophrenia," *Arch. Gen. Psychiatry*, 26 (1972), 539–545.

57. COMMITTEE ON NOMENCLATURE AND STATISTICS OF THE AMERICAN PSYCHIATRIC ASSOCIATION, *Diagnostic and Statistical Manual of Mental Disorders II.* Washington: Am. Psychiatr. Assoc., 1968.

58. CONNELL, P. H. "Review and Evaluation of Published Cases of Amphetamine Psychosis," in *Amphetamine Psychosis*, pp. 4–19. London: Chapman & Hall, 1958.

59. COPPEN, A., B. W. BROOKSBANK, and M. PEET. "Tryptophan Concentration in the Cerebrospinal Fluid of Depressive Patients," *Lancet*, 1 (1972), 1393.

60. COPPEN, A., A. MALLESON, and D. M. SHAW. "Effects of Lithium Carbonate on Electrolyte Distribution in Man," *Lancet*, 1 (1965), 682–683.

61. COPPEN, A. and D. M. SHAW. "Mineral Metabolism in Melancholia," *Br. Med. J.*, 2 (1963), 1439–1444.

62. ———. "The Distribution of Electrolytes and Water in Patients After Taking Lithium Carbonate," *Lancet*, 2 (1967), 805–806.

63. COPPEN, A., D. M. SHAW, A. MALLESON et al. "Mineral Metabolism in Mania," *Br. Med. J.*, 1 (1966), 71–75.

64. COPPEN, A., P. C. WHYBROW, R. NOGUERA et al. "The Comparative Antidepressant Value of L-Tryptophan and Imipramine With and Without Attempted Potentiation by Liothyronine," *Arch. Gen. Psychiatry*, 26 (1972), 234–241.

65. COSTA, E. and S. GARATTINI. *Amphetamines and Related Compounds.* New York: Raven Press, 1970.

66. COURT, J. H. "A Longitudinal Study of Psychomotor Functioning in Acute Psychiatric Patients," *Br. J. Med. Psychol.*, 37 (1964), 167–173.

67. ———. "Manic-Depressive Psychosis: An

Alternative Conceptual Model," *Br. J. Psychiatry*, 114 (1968), 1523–1530.

68. ———. "The Continuum Model as a Resolution of Paradoxes in Manic-Depressive Psychosis," *Br. J. Psychiatry*, 120 (1972), 133–141.

69. COURT, J. H. and F. M. M. MAI. "A Double-Blind Intensive Crossover Design Trial of Methysergide in Mania," *Med. J. Aust.*, 57 (1970), 526–529.

70. CRAMMER, J .L. "Water and Sodium in Two Psychotics," *Lancet*, 1 (1959), 1122–1126.

71. CRANE, G. E. "Further Studies on Iproniazid Phosphate, Isonicotinil-Isopropyl-Hydrazine-Phosphate Marsilid," *J. Nerv. Ment. Dis.*, 124 (1956), 322–331.

72. ———. "Iproniazid (Marsilid) Phosphate, a Therapeutic Agent for Mental Disorders and Debilitating Diseases," *Psychiatr. Res. Rep.*, 8 (1957), 142–152.

73. DAWSON, J., R. P. HULLIN, and B. M. CROCKET. "Metabolic Variations in Manic-Depressive Psychosis," *J. Ment. Sci.*, 102 (1956), 168–177.

74. DENCKER, S. J., V. MALM, B.-E. ROOS et al. "Acid Monoamine Metabolites of Cerebrospinal Fluid in Mental Depression and Mania," *J. Neurochem.*, 13 (1966), 1545–1548.

75. DETRE, T., J. HIMMELHOCH, M. SWARTZBURG et al. "Hypersomnia and Manic-Depressive Disease," *Am. J. Psychiatry*, 128 (1972), 1303–1305.

76. DEWHURST, W. G. "Methysergide in Mania," *Nature*, 219 (1968), 506–507.

77. ———. "New Theory of Cerebral Amine Function and Its Clinical Application," *Nature*, 218 (1968), 1130–1133.

78. DHASMANA, K. M., K. S. DIXIT, B. P. JAJU et al. "Role of Central Dopaminergic Receptors in Manic Response of Cats to Morphine," *Psychopharmacologia*, 24 (1972), 380–383.

79. DONNELLY, E. F. and D. L. MURPHY. "Primary Affective Disorder: MMPI Differences Between Unipolar and Bipolar Depressed Subjects," *J. Clin. Psychol.*, 29 (1973), 303–306.

80. DONNELLY, E. F. and D. L. MURPHY. "Social Desirability and Bipolar Affective Disorder," *J. Clin. Psychol.*, 41 (1973), 469.

81. DUFFY, E. "The Patterning of Activitation," in E. Duffy, *Activation Behavior*, pp. 82–91. New York: Wiley, 1962.

82. DUNNER, D. L., C. K. COHN, E. S. GERSHON et al. "Differential Catechol-O-Methyltransferase Activity in Unipolar and Bipolar Affective Illness," *Arch. Gen. Psychiatry*, 25 (1971), 348–353.

83. DUNNER, D. L., E. S. GERSHON, and F. K. GOODWIN. "Heritable Factors in the Severity of Affective Illness." Presented at the Annu. Meet. Am. Psychiatr. Assoc., San Francisco, May 1970.

84. ———. "Excretion of 17-Hydroxycorticosteroids in Unipolar and Bipolar Depressed Patients," *Arch. Gen. Psychiatry*, 26 (1972), 360–363.

85. EPSTEIN, S. and M. COLEMAN. "Drive Theories of Schizophrenia," *Psychosom. Med.*, 32 (1970), 113–140.

86. ERVIN, F. R., V. H. MARK, and J. STEVENS. "Behavioral and Affective Responses to Brain Stimulation in Man," *Proc. Am. Psychopathol. Assoc.*, 58 (1969), 54–65.

87. EVERETT, G. M. and R. G. WIEGAND. "Central Amines and Behavioral States: A Critique and New Data," *Proc. 1st Int. Pharmacol. Meet.*, 8 (1962), 85–92.

88. FALK, F. "Studien uber die Irrenheilkunde der Alten," *Allg. Z. Psychiatrie*, 23 (1866).

89. FALRET, J. P. "Mémoire sur la Folie Circulaire," *Bull. Acad. Natl. Méd. Paris*, 19 (1854), 382–400.

90. FAWCETT, J. and W. E. BUNNEY, JR. "Pituitary Adrenal Function and Depression: An Outline for Research," *Arch. Gen. Psychiatry*, 16 (1967), 517–535.

91. FIEVE, R. R., S. R. PLATMAN, and J. L. FLEISS. "A Clinical Trial of Methysergide and Lithium in Mania," *Psychopharmacologia*, 15 (1969), 425–429.

92. FORN, J. and F. G. VALDECASAS. "Effects of Lithium on Brain Adenyl Cyclase Activity," *Biochem. Pharmacol.*, 20 (1971), 2773–2779.

93. FOTHERBY, K., G. W. ASHCROFT, J. W. AFFLECK et al. "Studies on Sodium Transfer and 5-Hydroxyindoles in Depressive Illness," *J. Neurol., Neurosurg. Psychiatry*, 26 (1963), 71–73.

94. FRAM, D. H., D. L. MURPHY, F. K. GOODWIN et al. "L-Dopa and Sleep in Depressed Patients," *Psychophysiology*, 7 (1970), 316–317.

95. FREUD, S. (1921) "Group Psychology and the Analysis of the Ego," in J. Strachey, ed., *Standard Edition*, Vol. 18, pp. 69–143. London: Hogarth, 1955.

96. FRIED, P. A. "Septum and Behavior: A Re-

view," *Psychol. Bull.*, 78 (1972), 292–310.

97. FUXE, K., T. HOKFELT, and U. UNGERSTEDT. "Central Monoaminergic Traits," in W. G. Clark, and J. del Giudice, eds., *Principles of Psychopharmacology*, pp. 87–96. New York: Academic, 1970.

98. GERSHON, E. S., D. L. DUNNER, and F. K. GOODWIN. "Toward a Biology of Affective Disorders," *Arch. Gen. Psychiatry*, 25 (1971), 1–15.

99. GERSHON, S. "Lithium Salts in the Management of the Manic-Depressive Syndrome," *Annu. Rev. Med.*, 23 (1972), 439–452.

100. GERSHON, S. and A. YUWILER. "Lithium Ion: A Specific Psychopharmacological Approach to the Treatment of Mania," *J. Neuropsychiatry*, 1 (1960), 229–241.

101. GIBBONS, J. L. and P. R. McHUGH. "Plasma Cortisol in Depressive Illness," *J. Psychiatr. Res.*, 1 (1962), 162–171.

102. GLASER, G. H. "The Pituitary Gland in Relation to Cerebral Metabolism and Metabolic Disorders of the Nervous System," *Res. Pub. Assoc. Res. Nerv. Ment. Dis.*, 32 (1953), 21–39.

103. GLEN, A. I. M., G. C. ONGLEY, and K. ROBINSON. "Diminished Membrane Transport in Manic-Depressive Psychosis and Recurrent Depression," *Lancet*, 2 (1968), 241–243.

104. GOLDMAN, D. "Clinical Experience with Newer Antidepressant Drugs and Some Related Electroencephalographic Observations," *Ann. N.Y. Acad. Sci.*, 80 (1959), 687–704.

105. GOODWIN, F. K. and M. H. EBERT. "Lithium in Mania: Clinical Trials and Controlled Studies," in S. Gershon and B. Shopsin, eds., *Lithium: Its Role in Psychiatric Research and Treatment*, pp. 237–252. New York: Plenum, 1973.

106. GOODWIN, F. K., D. L. MURPHY, H. K. H. BRODIE et al. "L-DOPA: Alterations in Behavior," *Clin. Pharmacol. Ther.*, 12 (1971), 383–396.

107. GOODWIN, F. K., D. L. MURPHY, and W. E. BUNNEY, JR. "Lithium in Mania and Depression: A Longitudinal Double-Blind Study," *Arch. Gen. Psychiatry*, 21 (1969), 486–496.

108. GOODWIN, F. K., D. L. MURPHY, D. L. DUNNER et al. "Lithium Response in Unipolar Versus Bipolar Depression," *Am. J. Psychiatry*, 129 (1972), 44–47.

109. GOODWIN, F. K. and R. M. POST. "The Use of Probenecid in High Doses for the Estimation of Central Serotonin Turnover in Patients," in J. Barchas and E. Usdin, eds., *Serotonin and Behavior*, pp. 469–480. New York: Academic, 1972.

110. GREENBLATT, M., G. H. GROSSER, and H. A. WECHSLER. "A Comparative Study of Selected Antidepressant Medications and EST," *Am. J. Psychiatry*, 119 (1962), 144–153.

111. GREENSPAN, K., F. K. GOODWIN, W. E. BUNNEY, JR. et al. "Lithium Ion Retention and Distribution. Patterns During Acute Mania and Normothymia," *Arch. Gen. Psychiatry*, 19 (1968), 664–673.

112. GREENSPAN, K., R. GREEN, and J. DURELL. "Retention and Distribution Patterns of Lithium, a Pharmacological Tool in Studying the Pathophysiology of Manic-Depressive Psychosis," *Am. J. Psychiatry*, 125 (1968), 512–519.

113. GREENSPAN, K., J. J. SCHILDKRAUT, E. K. GORDON et al. "Catecholamine Metabolism in the Affective Disorders. III. MHPG and Other Catecholamine Metabolites in Patients Treated with Lithium Carbonate," *J. Psychiatr. Res.*, 7 (1970), 171–183.

114. GREENSPAN, K., J. J. SCHILDKRAUT, E. K. GORDON et al. "Catecholamine Metabolism in Affective Disorders. II. Norepinephrine, Normetanephrine, Epinephrine, Metanephrine and VMA Excretion in Hypomanic Patients," *Arch. Gen. Psychiatry*, 21 (1969), 710–716.

115. GRIFFITH, J. D., J. H. CAVANAUGH, J. HELD et al. "Experimental Psychosis Induced by the Administration of D-Amphetamine," in E. Costa and S. Garattini, eds., *Amphetamines and Related Compounds*, pp. 897–904. New York: Raven Press, 1970.

116. HAGGENDAL, J. and B. WERDINIUS. "Dopamine in Human Urine during Muscular Work," *Acta Physiol. Scand.*, 66 (1966), 223–225.

117. HARTMANN, E. "Longitudinal Studies of Sleep and Dream Patterns in Manic-Depressive Patients," *Arch. Gen. Psychiatry*, 19 (1968), 312–329.

118. HASKOVEC, L. and K. SOUCEK. "Trial of Methysergide in Mania," *Nature*, 219 (1968), 507–508.

119. HAWKINS, D. R., M. LIPTON, and J. MENDELS. "Sleep Studies in a Hypomanic Patient," *Psychophysiology*, 4 (1968), 394.

120. HENINGER, G. R. and P. S. MUELLER. "Car-

bohydrate Metabolism in Mania," *Archives of General Psychiatry*, 23 (1970), 310–319.

121. HENRY, G. M., D. L. MURPHY, and H. WEINGARTNER. "Idiosyncratic Patterns of Learning and Word Association During Mania," *Am. J. Psychiatry*, 128 (1971), 564–574.

122. HENRY, G. M., H. WEINGARTNER, and D. L. MURPHY. "Influence of Affective States and Psychoactive Drugs on Verbal Learning and Memory," *Am. J. Psychiatry*, 130 (1973), 966–971.

123. HERZBERG, B., A. J. COPPEN, and V. MARKS. "Glucose Tolerance in Depression," *Br. J. Psychiatry*, 114 (1968), 627–630.

124. HILLARP, N. A., K. FUXE, and A. DAHLSTROM. "Demonstration and Mapping of Central Neurons Containing Dopamine, Noradrenaline, and 5-Hydroxytryptamine and their Reactions to Psychopharmaca," *Pharmacol. Rev.*, 18 (1966), 727–741.

125. HORN, A. S. and S. H. SNYDER. "Chlorpromazine and Dopamine: Conformational Similarities that Correlate with the Antischizophrenic Activity of Phenothiazine Drugs," *Proc. Natl. Acad. Sci. U.S.A.*, 68 (1971), 2325–2328.

126. HORNYKIEWICZ, O. "Dopamine: Its Physiology, Pharmacology and Pathological Neurochemistry," in J. H. Biel and G. Abood, eds., *Biogenic Amines and Physiological Membranes in Drug Therapy*, Chap. 6. New York: Marcel Dekker, 1970.

127. HULLIN, R. P., A. D. BAILEY, R. McDONALD et al. "Body Water Variations in Manic-Depressive Psychosis," *Br. J. Psychiatry*, 113 (1967), 584–592.

128. ———. "Variations in 11-Hydroxycorticosteroids in Depression and Manic-Depressive Psychosis," *Br. J. Psychiatry*, 113 (1967), 593–600.

129. HULLIN, R. P., J. C. SWINSCOE, R. McDONALD et al. "Metabolic Balance Studies on the Effect of Lithium Salts in Manic-Depressive Psychosis," *Br. J. Psychiatry*, 114 (1968), 1561–1573.

130. IRONSIDE, R. "Disorders of Laughter Due to Brain Lesions," *Brain*, 79 (1956), 589–609.

131. JACKSON, D. D. "A Critique of the Literature on the Genetics of Schizophrenia," in D. D. Jackson, ed., *The Etiology of Schizophrenia*, pp. 37–91. New York: Basic Books, 1960.

132. JANOWSKY, D. S., M. K. EL-YOUSEF, J. M. DAVIS et al. A Cholinergic-Adrenergic Hypothesis of Mania and Depression," *Lancet*, 2 (1972), 632–635.

133. JANOWSKY, D. S., M. LEFF, and R. S. EPSTEIN. "Playing the Manic Game," *Arch. Gen. Psychiatry*, 22 (1970), 252–261.

134. JENNER, F., L. GJESSING, J. Cox et al. "A Manic-Depressive Psychotic with a Persistent Forty-Eight Hour Cycle," *Br. J. Psychiatry*, 113 (1967), 895–910.

135. JOHNSON, G., S. GERSHON, and L. J. HEKIMIAN. "Controlled Evaluation of Lithium and Chlorpromazine in the Treatment of Manic States: An Interim Report," *Comp. Psychiatry*, 9 (1968), 563–573.

136. JONAS, W. and J. SCHEEL-KRUGER. "Amphetamine Induced Stereotyped Behavior Correlated with the Accumulation of O-Methylated Dopamine," *Arch. Int. Pharmacodyn. Ther.*, 177 (1969), 379–389.

137. JOUVET, M. "The Role of Monoamines and Acetylcholine-Containing Neurons in the Regulation of the Sleep-Waking Cycle," *Ergeb. Physiol.*, 64 (1972), 166–308.

138. KALLMANN, F. "Genetic Principles in Manic-Depressive Psychosis," in J. Zubin and P. Hoch, eds., *Depression, Proceedings of the American Psychopathological Association*, pp. 1–24. New York: Grune & Stratton, 1952.

139. KANE, F. J., JR. and M. H. KELLER. "Mania Seen with Undiagnosed Cushing's Syndrome," *Am. J. Psychiatry*, 119 (1962), 267–268.

140. KATZ, R. I., T. N. CHASE, and I. J. KOPIN. "Evoked Release of Norepinephrine and Serotonin from Brain Slices: Inhibition by Lithium," *Science*, 1962 (1968), 466–467.

141. KENDELL, R. E. and J. GOURLAY. "The Clinical Distinction Between the Affective Psychoses and Schizophrenia," *Br. J. Psychiatry*, 117 (1971), 261–266.

142. KETY, S. S. "Biochemical Theories of Schizophrenia, Part I," *Science*, 129 (1959), 1528–1532.

143. ———. "Biochemical Theories of Schizophrenia, Part II," *Science*, 129 (1959), 1590–1596.

144. KLEIN, D. F. and J. M. DAVIS. *Diagnosis and Drug Treatment of Psychiatric Disorders*. Baltimore: Williams & Wilkins, 1969.

145. KLEIN, R. "Clinical and Biochemical Investigations in a Manic-Depressive with Short

Cycles," *J. Ment. Sci.*, 96 (1950), 293–297.

146. KLEIN, R. and R. F. NUNN. "Clinical and Biochemical Analysis of a Case of Manic-Depressive Psychosis Showing Regular Weekly Cycles," *J. Ment. Sci.*, 91 (1945), 79.

147. KOPIN, I. J. "False Adrenergic Transmitters," *Annu. Rev. Pharmacol.*, 10 (1968), 377–394.

148. KORNETSKY, C. and M. ELIASSON. "Reticular Stimulation and Chlorpromazine. An Animal Model for Schizophrenic Overarousal," *Science*, 165 (1969), 1273–1274.

149. ———. "Reticular Stimulation and Chlorpromazine," *Science*, 168 (1970), 1122–1123.

150. KOTIN, J. and F. K. GOODWIN. "Depression During Mania: Clinical Observations and Theoretical Implications," *Am. J. Psychiatry*, 129 (1972), 679–686.

151. KRAEPELIN, E. *Manic-Depressive Insanity and Paranoia*. Edinburgh: Livingstone, 1921.

152. LACHMAN, J. H. and A. L. ABRAMS. "The Decline and Fall of Manic-Depressive Psychosis, Manic Type." *Am. J. Psychiatry*, 120 (1963), 276–277.

153. LANGFELDT, G. "The Prognosis in Schizophrenia," *Acta Psychiatr. Scand., Suppl.* 110 (1956), 18.

154. LAPIN, I. P. and G. F. OXENKRUG. "Intensification of the Central Serotonergic Processes as a Possible Determinant of the Thymoleptic Effect," *Lancet*, 1 (1969), 132–136.

155. LEFF, M. J., J. F. ROATCH, and W. E. BUNNEY, JR. "Environmental Factors Preceding the Onset of Severe Depressions," *Psychiatry*, 33 (1970), 293–311.

156. LEONHARD, K., I. KORFF, and H. SHULZ. "Die Temperamente in den Familien der monopolaren und bipolaren phasischen Psychosen," *Psychiatr. Neurol.*, 143 (1962), 416–434.

157. LEWIN, B. D. "A Type of Neurotic Hypomanic Reaction," *Arch Neurol. Psychiatry*, 37 (1937), 868–873.

158. ———. "Comments on Hypomanic and Related States," *Psychoanal. Rev.*, 28 (1941), 86–91.

159. ———. *The Psychoanalysis of Elation.* New York: Norton, 1950.

160. LINGAERDE, P. S. "Plasma Hydrocortisone in Mental Disease," *Br. J. Psychiatry*, 110 (1964), 423–432.

161. LIPKIN, K. M., J. DYRUD, and G. G. MEYER. "The Many Faces of Mania," *Arch. Gen. Psychiatry*, 22 (1970), 262–267.

162. LUNDHOLM, H. "Reaction Time as an Indicator of Emotional Disturbances in Manic-Depressive Psychosis," *J. Abnorm. Psychol.*, 17 (1922–23), 293–318.

163. LUNDQUIST, G. "Prognosis and Course in Manic-Depressive Psychosis," *Acta Psychiatr. Neurol. Scand. Suppl.* 35 (1945), 1–96.

164. MAAS, J. W., J. A. FAWCETT, and H. DEKIRMENJIAN. "Catecholamine Metabolism, Depressive Illness and Drug Response," *Arch. Gen. Psychiatry*, 26 (1972), 252–262.

165. MAAS, J. W. and M. MEDNICKS. "Hydrocortisone-Mediated Increase of Norepinephrine Uptake by Brain Slices," *Science*, 171 (1971), 178–179.

166. MALMO, R. B. "Activation: A Neurophysiological Dimension," *Psychol. Rev.*, 66 (1959), 367–386.

167. MANDELL, A. J. and R. T. RUBIN. "ACTH Induced Changes in Tryptophan Turnover Along Induceable Pathways in Man," *Life Sci.*, 5 (1966), 1153–1161.

168. MANGONI, A., V. ANDREOLI, F. CABIBBE et al. "Body Fluids Distribution in Manic and Depressed Patients Treated with Lithium Carbonate," *Abstract, 2nd Int. Meet. Int. Soc. Neurochem.*, p. 279. Milan, 1969.

169. MARTEN, S. A., R. J. CADORET, G. WINOKUR et al. "Unipolar Depression: A Family History Study," *Biol. Psychiatry*, 4 (1972), 205–213.

170. McCLEARY, R. A. "Response-Modulating Functions of the Limbic System: Initiation and Suppression," in E. Stellar and J. M. Sprague, eds., *Progress in Physiological Psychology*, Vol. 1, pp. 210–266. New York: Academic, 1966.

171. MELTZER, H. "Creatine Kinase and Aldolase in Serum: Abnormality Common to Acute Psychoses," *Science*, 159 (1968), 1368–1370.

172. MENDLEWICZ, J. and R. R. FIEVE. "Linkage Studies in Affective Disorders. I. Color Blindneses and Manic-Depressive Illness," *Psychopharmacologia Suppl.* 26 (1972), 90–91.

173. MESSIHA, F. S., D. AGALLIANOS, and C. CLOWER. "Dopamine Excretion in Affective States and Following $Li_2 Co_3$

Therapy," *Nature*, 225 (1970), 868–869.

174. MEYER, A. *The Commonsense Psychiatry of Adolf Meyer.* A. Lief, ed. New York: McGraw-Hill, 1948.

175. MEZEY, A. G. and E. J. KNIGHT. "Time Sense in Hypomanic Illness," *Arch. Gen. Psychiatry*, 12 (1965), 184–186.

176. MUELLER, P. S., G. R. HENINGER, and R. K. MCDONALD. "Insulin Tolerance Test in Depression," *Arch. Gen. Psychiatry*, 21 (1969), 587–594.

177. ———. "Intravenous Glucose Tolerance Test in Depression," *Arch. Gen. Psychiatry*, 21 (1969), 470–477.

178. MURPHY, D. L. "Amine Precursors, Amines, and False Neurotransmitters in Depressed Patients," *Am. J. Psychiatry*, 129 (1972), 141–148.

179. ———. "L-Dopa, Behavioral Activation and Psychopathology," in I. J. Kopin, ed., *Neurotransmitters, Res. Publ. Assoc. Res. Nerv. Ment. Dis.*, 50 (1972), 472–493.

180. ———. In preparation.

181. MURPHY, D. L., M. BAKER, F. K. GOODWIN et al. "Behavioral and Metabolic Effects of L-Tryptophan in Unipolar Depressed Patients," in J. Barchas and E. Usdin, eds., *Serotonin and Behavior*, pp. 529–537. New York: Academic, 1973.

182. MURPHY, D. L., M. BAKER, F. K. GOODWIN et al. "L-Tryptophan: Antidepressant and Antimanic Effects in Bipolar and Unipolar Patients." In preparation.

183. MURPHY. D. L., A. BEIGEL, H. WEINGART-NER et al. "The Quantitation of Manic Behavior," in P. Pichot, ed., *Modern Problems in Pharmacopsychiatry*, pp. 203–220. Basel: S. Karger, 1974.

184. MURPHY, D. L., H. K. H. BRODIE, F. K. GOODWIN et al. "L-Dopa: Regular Induction of Hypomania in Bipolar Manic-Depressive Patients," *Nature*, 229 (1971), 135–136.

185. MURPHY, D. L. and W. E. BUNNEY, JR. "Total Body Potassium Changes During Lithium Administration," *J. Nerv. Ment. Dis.*, 152 (1971), 381–389.

186. MURPHY, D. L., D. CAHAN, and P. B. MOLINOFF. "Occurrence, Storage and Transport of Octopamine in the Human Platelet." *Clin. Pharmacol. Ther.*, in press.

187. MURPHY, D. L., R. W. COLBURN, J. M. DAVIS et al. "Imipramine and Lithium Effects on Biogenic Amine Transport in Depressed and Manic-Depressed Patients,"

Am. J. Psychiatry, 127 (1970), 339–345.

188. MURPHY, D. L., C. DONNELLY, and J. MOS-KOWITZ. "Inhibition by Lithium Treatment of Prostaglandin E_1 and Norepinephrine Effects on Cyclic AMP Production in Human Platelets." *Clin. Pharmacol. Ther.*, 14 (1973), 810–814.

189. MURPHY, D. L. and T. C. GOLDMAN. "Urinary Tryptamine Excretion as an Index of Endogenous Differences in MAO Activity and of Decarboxylase Inhibition." In preparation.

190. MURPHY, D. L., F. K. GOODWIN, and W. E. BUNNEY, JR. "Aldosterone and Sodium Response to Lithium Administration in Man," *Lancet*, 2 (1969), 458–461.

191. ———. "Electrolyte Changes in the Affective Disorders: Problems of Specificity and Significance," in T. A. Williams, M. M. Katz, and J. A. Shield, Jr., eds., *Recent Advances in the Psychobiology of the Depressive Illnesses*, pp. 59–70. Washington: Govt. Print. Off., 1972.

192. ———. "Clinical and Pharmacological Investigations of the Psychobiology of the Affective Disorders," *Int. Pharmacopsychiatry*, 6 (1973), 137–146.

193. MURPHY, D. L. and R. WEISS. "Reduced Monoamine Oxidase Activity in Blood Platelets from Bipolar Depressed Patients," *Am. J. of Psychiatry*, 128 (1972), 1351–1357.

194. NG, K. Y., T. N. CHASE, R. W. COLBURN et al. "L-Dopa-Induced Release of Cerebral Monoamines," *Science*, 170 (1971), 76–77.

195. NOYES, A. P. and L. C. KOLB. *Modern Clinical Psychiatry.* Philadelphia: Saunders, 1963.

196. OLDS, J. "Hypothalamic Substrates of Reward," *Psychol. Rev.*, 42 (1962), 554–604.

197. OVERTON, D. A. "Discriminative Control of Behavior by Drug States," in T. Thompson and R. Pickens, eds., *Stimulus Properties of Drugs*, pp. 87–109. New York: Appleton-Century-Crofts, 1971.

198. PAO, P.-N. "Elation, Hypomania, and Mania," *J. Am. Psychoanal. Assoc.*, 19 (1971), 787–798.

199. PAUL, M. I., H. CRAMER, and W. E. BUN-NEY, JR. "Urinary Adenosine 3'5'-Monophosphate in the Switch Process from Depression to Mania," *Science*, 171 (1971), 300–303.

200. PAUL, M. I., H. CRAMER, and F. K. GOOD-WIN. "Urinary Cyclic AMP Excretion in Depression and Mania," *Arch. Gen. Psychiatry,* 24 (1971), 327–333.

201. PERRIS, C. "Abnormality on Paternal and Maternal Sides: Observations in Bipolar (Manic-Depressive) and Unipolar Depressive Psychoses," *Br. J. Psychiatry,* 118 (1971), 207–210.

202. ———. "Personality Patterns in Patients with Affective Disorders," *Acta Psychiatr. Scand. Suppl.* (221), 47 (1971), 43–51.

203. ———. "A Study of Bipolar (Manic-Depressive) and Unipolar Recurrent Depressive Psychoses," *Acta Psychiatr. Scand. Suppl.* (194), 42 (1966), 1–188.

204. PLATMAN, S. R. and R. R. FIEVE. "Biochemical Aspects of Lithium in Affective Disorders," *Arch. Gen. Psychiatry,* 19 (1968), 659–663.

205. ———. "Lithium Carbonate and Plasma Cortisol Response in the Affective Disorders," *Arch. Gen. Psychiatry.* 18 (1968), 591–594.

206. ———. "Lithium Retention and Excretion," *Arch. Gen. Psychiatry,* 20 (1969), 285–289.

207. ———. "Sleep in Depression and Mania," *Br. J. Psychiatry,* 116 (1970), 219–220.

208. PLUTCHIK, R., S. R. PLATMAN, and R. R. FIEVE. "Self-Concepts Associated with Mania and Depression," *Psychol. Rep.,* 27 (1970), 399–405.

209. POLLIN, W., P. V. CARDON, and S. S. KETY. "Effects of Amino Acid Feedings in Schizophrenic Patients Treated with Iproniazid," *Science,* 133 (1961), 104–105.

210. POST, R. M., J. KOTIN, F. K. GOODWIN et al. "Psychomotor Activity and Cerebrospinal Fluid Amine Metabolites in Affective Illness," *Am. J. Psychiatry,* 130 (1973), 67–72.

211. PRANGE, A. J., JR., R. L. McCURDY, and C. M. COCHRANE. "The Systolic Blood Pressure Response of Depressed Patients to Infused Norepinephrine," *J. Psychiatr. Res.,* 5 (1967), 1–13.

212. PRANGE, A. J., JR., J. L. SISK, I. C. WILSON et al. "Balance, Permission, and Discrimination Among Amines: A Theoretical Consideration of the Actions of L-Tryptophan in Disorders of Movement and Affect," in J. Barchas and E. Usdin, eds., *Serotonin and Behavior,* pp. 539–548. New York: Academic, in press.

213. PRIEN, R. F., E. M. CAFFEY, and C. J. KLETT. "Comparison of Lithium Carbonate and Chlorpromazine in the Treatment of Mania," *Arch. Gen. Psychiatry,* 26 (1972), 146–153.

214. PRYCE, I. G. "Melancholia, Glucose Tolerance and Body Weight," *J. Ment. Sci.,* 104 (1958), 421–427.

215. ———. "The Relationship between Glucose Tolerance, Body Weight and Clinical State in Melancholia," *J. Ment. Sci.,* 104 (1958), 1079–1092.

216. RADO, S. "The Psychic Effect of Intoxicants," *Int. J. of Psychoanal.,* 7 (1926). 396–413.

217. RANDRUP, A. and I. MUNKVAD. "Pharmacological Studies on the Brain Mechanisms Underlying Two Forms of Behavioral Excitation: Stereotyped Hyperactivity and 'Rage,'" *Ann. N.Y. Acad. Sci.,* 139 (1969), 928–938.

218. REES, L. and S. BENAIM. "An Evaluation of Iproniazid (Marsilid) in the Treatment of Depression," *J. Ment. Sci.,* 106 (1960), 193–202.

219. REES, L. and B. DAVIES. "Study of the Value of Haloperidol in the Management and Treatment of Schizophrenic and Manic Patients," *Int. J. Neuropsychiatry,* 1 (1965), 263–266.

220. REICH, T., P. CLAYTON, and G. WINOKUR. "Family History Studies: V. The Genetics of Mania," *Am. J. Psychiatry,* 125 (1969), 1358–1369.

221. REIS, D. J., D. T. MOORHEAD, and N. MERLINO. "Dopa-Induced Excitement in the Cat," *Arch. Neurol.,* 22 (1970), 31–39.

222. RENNIE, T. A. C. "Prognosis in Manic-Depressive Psychosis," *Am. J. Psychiatry,* 98 (1942), 801–814.

223. ROBISON, G. A., A. J. COPPEN, P. C. WHYBROW et al. "Cyclic A.M.P. in Affective Disorders," *Lancet,* 2 (1970), 1028–1029.

224. ROOS, B.-E. and R. SJOSTROM. "5-Hydroxyindoleactic Acid (and Homovanillic Acid) Levels in the Cerebrospinal Fluid after Probenecid Application in Patients with Manic-Depressive Psychosis," *Pharmacol. Clin.,* 1 (1969), 153–155.

225. ROSENTHAL, D. *Genetic Theory and Abnormal Behavior.* New York: McGraw-Hill, 1970.

226. ROSENTHAL, S. H. "Changes in a Population of Hospitalized Patients with Affective Disorders, 1945–1965," *Am. J. Psychiatry,* 123 (1966), 671–681.

227. ROUTTENBERG, A. "The Two-Arousal Hypothesis: Reticular Formation and Limbic System," *Psychol. Rev.*, 75 (1968), 51–80.

228. ROWE, C. J. and D. R. DAGGETT. "Prepsychotic Personality Traits in Manic Depressive Disease," *J. Nerv. Ment. Dis.*, 119 (1954), 412–420.

229. RUBIN, R. T. "Adrenal Cortical Activity Changes in Manic Depressive Illness," *Arch. Gen. Psychiatry*, 17 (1967), 671–679.

230. ———. "Multiple Biochemical Correlates of Manic-Depressive Illness," *J. Psychosom. Res.*, 12 (1968), 171–180.

231. RUBIN, R. T. and A. J. MANDELL. "Adrenal Cortical Activity in Pathological Emotional States: A Review," *Am. J. Psychiatry*, 123 (1966), 387–400.

232. RUBIN, R. T., W. M. YOUNG, and B. R. CLARK. "17-Hydroxycorticosteroid and Vanillylmandelic Acid Excretion in a Rapidly Cycling Manic-Depressive," *Psychosom. Med.*, 30 (1968), 162–171.

233. SACHAR, E. J., L. HELLMAN, D. K. FUKUSHIMA et al. "Cortisol Production in Mania," *Arch. Gen. Psychiatry*, 26 (1972), 137–139.

234. SCHANBERG, S. M., J. J. SCHILDKRAUT, and I. J. KOPIN. "The Effects of Psychoactive Drugs on Norepinephrine-^{3}H Metabolism in Brain," *Biochem. Pharmacol.*, 16 (1967), 393–399.

235. SCHILDKRAUT, J. J. "The Catecholamine Hypothesis of Affective Disorders: A Review of Supporting Evidence," *Am. J. Psychiatry*, 122 (1965), 509–522.

236. SCHILDKRAUT, J. J. and J. DURELL. "Noradrenergic Activity During the Transition from Depression to Mania," *Lancet*, 1 (1971), 653.

237. SCHILDKRAUT, J. J. and S. S. KETY. "Biogenic Amines and Emotion," *Science*, 156 (1967), 21–30.

238. SCHILDKRAUT, J. J., E. K. GORDON, and J. DURELL. "Catecholamine Metabolism in Affective Disorders. I. Normetanephrine and VMA Excretion in Depressed Patients Treated with Imipramine," *J. Psychiatr. Res.*, 3 (1965), 213–228.

239. SCHOU, M. "Biology and Pharmacology of the Lithium Ion," *Pharmacol. Rev.*, 9 (1957), 17–58.

240. ———. "Lithium in Psychiatric Therapy and Prophylaxis," *J. Psychiatr. Res.*, 6 (1968), 67–95.

241. SCHWARTZ, M., A. MANDELL, R. GREEN et al. "Mood, Motility and 17-Hydroxycorticoid Excretion: A Polyvariable Case Study," *Br. J. Psychiatry*, 112 (1966), 149–156.

242. SHINFUKU, N., M. OMURA, and M. KAYANO. "Catecholamines Excretion in Manic Depressive Psychosis," *Yonago Acta Med.*, 5 (1961), 109–114.

243. SHOBE, F. O. and P. BRION. "Long-Term Prognosis in Manic-Depressive Illness," *Arch. Gen. Psychiatry*, 24 (1971), 334–337.

244. SILVERMAN, J. "A Paradigm for the Study of Altered States of Consciousness," *Br. J. Psychiatry*, 114 (1968), 1201–1218.

245. SLATER, E. "The Inheritance of Manic-Depressive Insanity," *Proc. R. Soc. Med.*, 29 (1936), 981–990.

246. ———. "Expectation of Abnormality on Paternal and Maternal Sides: A Computational Model," *J. Med. Genet.*, 3 (1966), 159–161.

247. SLATER, E., J. MAXWELL, and J. S. PRICE. "Distribution of Ancestral Secondary Cases in Bipolar Affective Disorders," *Br. J. Psychiatry*, 118 (1971), 215–218.

248. SLATER, E. and M. ROTH. *Clinical Psychiatry*. Baltimore: William & Wilkins, 1969.

249. SLOANE, R. B., W. HUGHES, and H. L. HAUST. "Catecholamine Excretion in Manic-Depressive and Schizophrenic Psychosis and its Relationship to Symptomatology," *Can. Psychiatr. Assoc.*, 11 (1966), 6–19.

250. SPIELBERGER, C. D., J. B. PARKER, and J. BECKER. "Conformity and Achievement in Remitted Manic-Depressive Patients," *J. Nerv. Ment. Dis.*, 137 (1963), 162–172.

251. STEIN, L. "Effects and Interactions of Imipramine, Chlorpromazine, Reserpine and Amphetamine on Self-Stimulation: Possible Neurophysiological Basis of Depression," *Recent Adv. Biol. Psychiatry*, 4 (1961), 288–309.

252. STEVENS, J. R., V. H. MARK, F. ERVIN et al. "Deep Temporal Stimulation in Man. Long Latency, Longlasting Psychological Changes," *Arch. Neurol.*, 21 (1969), 157–169.

253. STROMGREN, E. "Schizophreniform Psychoses," *Acta Psychiatr. Scand.*, 41 (1965), 483–489.

254. STROM-OLSEN, R. and H. WEIL-MALHERBE. "Humoral Changes in Manic Depressive

Psychosis with Particular Reference to the Excretion of Catecholamines in Urine," *J. Ment. Sci.*, 104 (1958), 696–704.

255. TAKAHASHI, R., Y. NAGAO, K. TSUCHIYA et al. "Catecholamine Metabolism of Manic Depressive Illness," *J. Psychiatr. Res.*, 6 (1968), 185–199.

256. TAKAHASHI, R., H. UTENA, Y. MACHIYAMA et al. "Tyrosine Metabolism in Manic Depressive Illness," *Life Sci.*, 7, Part II (1968), 1219–1231.

257. TRAUTNER, E. M., R. MORRIS, C. H. NOACK et al. "The Excretion and Retention of Ingested Lithium and its Effect on the Ionic Balance of Man," *Med. J. Aust.*, 2 (1955), 280–291.

258. TUPIN. J. P., G. K. SCHLAGENHAUF, and D. L. CRESON. "Lithium Effects on Electrolyte Excretion," *Am. J. Psychiatry*, 125 (1968), 536–543.

259. TURNER, W. and S. MERLIS. "A Clinical Trial of Pargyline and Dopa in Psychotic Subjects," *Dis. Nerv. Syst.*, 24 (1964), 538–541.

260. UNGERSTEDT, U. "Stereotaxic Mapping of the Monoamine Pathways in the Rat Brain," *Acta Physiol. Scand. Suppl.* 367, 1971, 1–48.

261. VAILLANT, G. E. "Manic-Depressive Heredity and Remission in Schizophrenia," *Br. J. Psychiatry*, 109 (1963), 746–749.

262. VAN PRAAG, H. M. "Indoleamines and the Central Nervous System," *Psychiatr. Neurol. Neurochir.*, 73 (1970), 9–36.

263. VAN PRAAG, H. M. and B. LEIJNSE. "Some Aspects of the Metabolism of Glucose and of the Non-Esterified Fatty Acids in Depressive Patients," *Psychopharmacologia*, 9 (1966), 220–233.

264. VINCENT, M. O. and C. F. STORY. "The Disappearing Manic-Depressive," *Can. Psychiatr. Assoc. J.*, 15 (1970), 475–483.

265. WADESON, H. S. and R. G. FITZGERALD. "Marital Relationship in Manic-Depressive Illness," *J. Nerv. Ment. Dis.*, 153 (1971), 180–196.

266. WELNER, J. and E. STROMGREN. "Clinical and Genetic Studies on Benign Schizophreniform Psychoses Based on a Follow-Up," *Acta Psychiatr. Scand.*, 33 (1958), 377–399.

267. WHYBROW, P. C. and J. MENDELS. "Toward a Biology of Depression: Some Suggestions from Neurophysiology," *Am. J. Psychiatry*, 125 (1969), 1491–5000.

268. WILK, S., B. SHOPSIN, S. GERSHON et al. "Catecholamines and Affective Disorders: Levels of MHPG in Cerebrospinal Fluid," *The Pharmacol.*, 13 (1971), 252.

269. WILSON, I. C. and A. J. PRANGE, JR. "Tryptophan in Mania: Theory of Affective Disorders," *Psychopharmacologia Suppl.*, 26 (1972), 76.

270. WINOKUR, G. "Genetic Findings and Methodological Considerations in Manic Depressive Disease," *Br. J. Psychiatry*, 117 (1970), 267–274.

271. WINOKUR, G., P. J. CLAYTON, and T. REICH, eds. *Manic Depressive Illness*. St. Louis: C. V. Mosby, 1969.

272. WINOKUR, G., and V. TANNA. "Possible Role of X-Linked Dominant Factor in Manic Depressive Disease," *Dis. Nerv. Syst.*, 30 (1969), 89–94.

273. WOODRUFF, R. A., JR., S. B. GUZE, and P. J. CLAYTON. "Unipolar and Bipolar Primary Affective Disorder," *Br. J. Psychiatry*, 119 (1971), 33–38.

274. WOODRUFF, R. A., JR., L. N. ROBINS, G. WINOKUR et al. "Manic Depressive Illness and Social Achievement," *Acta Psychiatr. Scand.*, 47 (1971), 237–249.

275. WYATT, R. J. "The Serotonin-Catecholamine-Dream Bicycle: A Clinical Study," *Biol. Psychiatry*, 5 (1972), 33–62.

276. WYATT, R. J., K. ENGELMAN, D. J. KUPFER et al. "Effects of L-Tryptophan (a Neutral Sedative) on Human Sleep," *Lancet*, 2 (1970), 842–846.

277. YEH, B. K., J. L. MCNAY, and L. I. GOLDBERG. "Attenuation of Dopamine Renal and Mesenteric Vasodilation by Haloperidol: Evidence for a Specific Dopamine Receptor," *J. Pharmacol. Exp. Ther.*, 168 (1969), 303–309.

278. ZERBIN-RUDIN, E. "Endogene Psychosen," in P. E. Becker, ed., *Humangenetic*. Stuttgart: Georg Thieme, 1967.

CHAPTER 24

PROMISING DIRECTIONS
IN PSYCHOPHARMACOLOGY

H. Keith H. Brodie and Robert L. Sack

T HE DISCOVERY and testing of most drugs used in clinical psychiatry today occurred between 1940 and 1960. Although the introduction of new drugs has slowed considerably since then, significant progress has been made in understanding the mechanisms by which the "old" drugs exert their effects. This has, in turn, generated a number of useful hypotheses concerning the pathophysiology of mental illness which have been tested with varying success (see Chapters 21 and 23 in this volume) by direct measurement of brain function. As a result, hope has been generated that new drugs can be developed rationally from hypotheses about the biochemical alterations associated with certain psychiatric illnesses.

In this chapter, we will present an overview of some of the newer directions in psychopharmacology with particular emphasis on the development of "rational" drug-mediated interventions—rational in the sense that drugs are used to alter specific metabolic processes based on hypotheses of mental illness. This approach is relatively recent; previously, drugs

have been developed by empirical or even serendipitous methods because knowledge of brain chemistry was simply too primitive to provide the basis for specifically planned interventions. This review focuses on current models of monoamine metabolism primarily because psychoactive drugs seem to have their most critical effects on neurotransmitter function.

The purpose of this chapter is to provide the practicing psychiatrist with an overview of developing trends in psychopharmacology by reviewing recent research in this field. Before presenting an outline for the rational development of new drugs, some of the more classical approaches will be reviewed.

(Classical Psychopharmacology

Animal Screening

One strategy for the development of new drugs is the random screening of compounds for biological activity in animals. The main ingredients of the animal-screening method have been patience, persistence, and luck. For example, in 1952, Leo Sternbach, a chemist working at Hoffman-La Roche, formed some forty derivatives of a compound he had been interested in twenty years earlier. All proved to be pharmacologically inert. So, discouraged, he put the forty-first on the shelf. A year and a half later, during a cleanup of the laboratory, his assistant suggested that they send the shelved compound to the screening section for routine testing. It not only proved to be active, but was later found to be a most useful antianxiety agent. It was named chlordiazepoxide (Librium).[5]

Currently animal screening for new psychoactive drugs is done for a number of reasons.[53] The most important is the necessary evaluation of drugs for toxicity, which can, in addition, produce information on probable pharmacological effects. For example, if animals die of intense sympathetic or parasympathetic stimulation, it is probable that the drugs will have autonomic effects at sublethal doses. Gross behavioral tests can sometimes give clues to the probable clinical effects of a drug; for example, spontaneous motor activity, ataxia, sedation, and blockade of tremors or convulsions induced by another drug such as metrazol or reversal of reserpine-induced hypothermia—all these effects are easily observed in animals and may relate to clinical efficacy in man.

Being able to predict psychopharmacological use in humans from animal-screening tests is difficult. Avoiding any preconceptions about the fundamental causes of anxiety, psychosis, or depression, experimenters have developed empirical-screening batteries of animal tests

that can reliably discriminate among drugs that have an antianxiety, antipsychotic, or antidepressant effect.[53] For example, the tests that best correlate with antipsychotic effects are shown in Table 24-1.[35] It is still uncertain which of the effects shown in the table may be most specifically related to antipsychotic activity. For several years the inhibition of apomorphine-induced vomiting in dogs was the test most highly correlated with antipsychotic activity, simply because most known antipsychotic drugs were also antiemetic.[35] The primary weakness of the empirical-screening methods is that they "find" drugs that are similar to the ones we already have and quite possibly miss drugs with different pharmacologic properties that might be useful in the treatment of patients.

In recent years, efforts have been directed to the evaluation of new drugs, employing parameters in animal testing that may have more meaning for predicting psychological effects in man.[53] Of importance has been the use of conditioning and learning techniques as formulated by the "behaviorist" psychologists. The behavioral paradigms are essentially derivatives of "classical" or "instrumental" conditioning. Utilizing these behavioral analyses, both antipsychotic and antianxiety agents have been shown to block avoidance conditioning. However, upon closer scrutiny, the avoidance behavior reduced by antipsychotic drugs is "active avoidance"; that is, the animal must actively make a response in order to avoid shock. In contrast, the antianxiety agents reduce "passive avoidance" in which animals are required to inhibit a usual response in order to avoid shock. Scheckel[53] has suggested that the distinction between "ac-

TABLE 24-1.   **Pharmacological Screening Tests for Phenothiazine-like Activity**

Reduce exploratory behavior without undue sedation.
Induce a cataleptic state.
Induce palpebral ptosis reversible through handling.
Inhibit conditioned avoidance behavior.
Inhibit intracranial self-stimulation in reward areas.
Inhibit amphetamine- or apormorphine-induced stereotypic behavior.
Protect against epinephrine- or norepinephrine-induced mortality.

tive" and "passive" avoidance characterizes to some degree the effects of these drugs in man: for example, he has speculated that phobias (in which antianxiety agents are useful) can be thought of as examples of passive avoidance, and the schizophrenias (in which antipsychotic medication is helpful) can be thought of as instances of active avoidance, particularly of social and interpersonal experience. Such speculations are preliminary, but they demonstrate how refined techniques of animal-behavioral analysis of conditioning and learning may produce some interesting theoretical insights into the mechanisms of action of pharmacological agents.

A promising direction, which may lead to more effective animal screening and which has more appeal to the dynamically oriented psychiatrist, is the production of psychiatric symptoms in animals, for example, depression produced in mother monkeys by isolating them from their young. Hopefully, this type of research will lead the way to "animal models" of psychiatric illness (see Chapter 15 in this volume) that can be used to test psychopharmacologic activity.

New Uses for Old Drugs

The gratuitous observation of psychotropic activity in a drug being used for other therapeutic purposes led to the discovery of both chlorpromazine and the MAO (monoamine oxide) inhibitors. In case of chlorpromazine, the path from synthesis to acceptance was most circuitous.[17] Although synthesized in 1944 by Paul Charpentier, chlorpromazine was initially rejected as having no therapeutic potential since it did not have very significant antihistaminic potency. Consequently, the clinical chapter of the chlorpromazine story began in 1949 when the surgeon Henri-Marie Laborit hypothesized that surgical shock was due to an overreaction of the autonomic nervous system. He began treating patients preoperatively with promethazine, a potent antihistaminic with sympatholytic and parasympatholytic properties. He noticed, to his surprise, that the patients treated with promethazine were calm and appeared to suffer less, even after major operations, than patients not treated with promethazine. His interests then changed course, and he began to consider the possibility of developing a technique of surgery without anesthesia by using drugs that had a calming effect but did not put patients to sleep. This hope was only partially realized with the combination of antihistamines called the "lytic cocktail."

Laborit began searching for a drug with more powerful central effects. In 1951, chlorpromazine was given a clinical trial and was found to produce a "disinterest" in the treated patients. Laborit became quite enthusiastic about his newly found drug and spread the word to many other specialties. Psychiatrists were at first quite reluctant to try it: so many drugs had been tested unsuccessfully on their patients that they were quite skeptical. When, in 1952, Laborit finally did persuade some of his psychiatric colleagues to try the drug, the results were dramatic. In the course of a single year, the treatment of psychosis was revolutionized in France and Italy. Acceptance in the United States came somewhat more slowly. Through numerous double-blind studies the effectiveness of chlorpromazine in the reduction of psychotic symptomatology was proven beyond reasonable doubt.[35]

Another example of serendipity in the development of a psychotropic drug was the discovery of the MAO class of antidepressants. Selikoff and Robitzek[55] reported that the antitubercular drug, iproniazid, had remarkable mood-elevating properties. The demonstration of this drug's main mechanism of action, that of monoamine oxidase inhibition, was made almost simultaneously.[66] Subsequently, the drug was recognized as a useful antidepressant.

Isolation of Active Plant Extracts

The rauwolfia alkaloids were first isolated from plant extracts. Reserpine, an alkaloid, is one of the most potent antihypertensive agents known to man. Possibly the folk remedies of primitive societies have not been mined thoroughly enough for psychoactive drugs. Perhaps some interesting new compounds, useful in the treatment of mental illness, will be developed from current research on the cannabis plant. Snyder[57] has noted euphorogenic effects of some tetrahydrocannabinol (THC) derivatives.

Modifying Existing Drugs

A more direct road to the development of psychopharmacologic agents has been the imitation of already existing, well-tested compounds. For example, the development of the thiozanthines was accomplished after recognition that the aromatic nitrogen atom of the phenothiazines could be replaced by a carbon. Imipramine was synthesized by replacing the phenothiazine sulfur atom with a dimethyl bridge. For amitriptyline, the central nitrogen atom of imipramine was replaced with a carbon atom. Thus, relatively minor structural changes can produce important differences in pharmacological activity. This approach is vigorously pursued by competing drug firms in their attempts to circumvent competing patent laws.

Serendipity

The use of lithium salts for the treatment of mania was discovered by a remarkable series of observations. In 1949, John Cade,[16] at the time an unknown psychiatric researcher working in a small hospital on limited funds in Western Australia, attempted to test the hypothesis that manic excitement was the result of intoxication from a normal body product analogous to thyrotoxicosis. His first step was the isolation of the toxic substance from the urine. After several experiments in which he injected urine from manic patients into guinea pigs, it was not too surprising that he found the most toxic substance in the urine to be urea. Cade became interested in the effect of urate salts on the toxicity of urea. Choosing the most soluble urate available, the lithium salt, he found that it produced a protective effect on the convulsive mode of death produced by urea and, as luck would have it, the

lithium ion, not the urate, was proven to be responsible for the effect. Furthermore, he noticed that animals injected with lithium salts became unusually placid. From these observations in animals, a trial of lithium in manic patients was initiated. As luck would again have it, the dose chosen was 600 mg. per day, close to the optimal range that has since been established. The only bad luck in this story was that during the year of the initial therapeutic success with lithium, a number of deaths were reported from lithium used in the treatment of congestive heart failure. Consequently, it required a large amount of research to validate the original observation sufficiently to allow the use of lithium in the treatment of mania.

Discoveries in psychopharmacology have been erratic and serendipitous. Little was known about the biochemistry of the brain when the afore-mentioned discoveries were made, so that a "rational basis" for the development of drugs was impossible. Although classical strategies continue to be practiced, many psychiatric researchers hope that an understanding of the pathophysiology of mental illness will bring even more significant discoveries than those made in relative darkness. However, this is a hope, and Jonathan Cole, one of the founders of the field of psychopharmacology offers this opinion on the development of antidepressants.

Of all the approaches, I believe that I have the most intellectual enthusiasm for the rational basic science approach to the development of new and better antidepressants. However, if I had to bet money, I would bet that the next new wonderful antidepressant would be developed by serendipity out of some strange irrelevant area of medicine rather than by design out of a series of rational procedures. I hope I am wrong. [p. 86][20]

❨ The Rational Approach

"Classical psychopharmacology" simplified the study of the effect of drugs on behavior largely by ignoring the intermediate levels.

The input was drug, the output was behavior, and what was between was dimly known and for many purposes considered a "black box."

Since the development of the first few psychopharmacological agents, a large amount of information on the biochemistry of neurohumoral synaptic transmission has become available. Furthermore, it has been discovered that most psychoactive agents have significant effects on some aspect of neurotransmitter metabolism. From the knowledge of the interactions of clinically useful drugs on the neurochemical events at the synapse, a number of hypotheses of the pathophysiology of mental illness have been developed. This approach to theorizing has been called the "pharmacological bridge." The "catecholamine hypothesis" of affective illness is the most coherent hypothesis of this type formulated thus far.[14,54] This hypothesis states that depression may be associated with a relative deficiency of catecholamines at functionally important receptor sites in the brain and, conversely, that mania may be associated with a relative excess. The catecholamine hypothesis of depression was largely derived from an analysis of the mechanisms of action of the effective drugs used in this illness. These compounds all seem to have the common characteristic of making catecholamines more available to the synaptic receptor, and thus intensifying or prolonging their effect. For example, the MAO inhibitors block degradation of monoamines and thus increase their concentration at the synapse. The tricyclic antidepressants block reuptake of monoamines, thus prolonging their effect at the synapse. Glassman[33] has reviewed the evidence that serotonin, an indoleamine, may be deficient in depression. His rationale is similar to the arguments used to support the catecholamine hypothesis.

Theories of schizophrenia have been derived both from an analysis of psychotomimetic agents as well as of antipsychotic drugs. A number of endogenously formed psychotogenic amine derivatives have been suggested as important in the etiology of schizophrenia, but, as yet, no unifying coherent theory comparable to the catecholamine hypothesis of depression has been formulated. Recently, effects of therapeutic agents used in schizophrenia on the dopamine receptor sites in brain have been noted and this may result in the development of a pharmacological bridge.

Synaptic Physiology and the Development of New Drugs

The brain is made up of ten[10] nerve cells that, although tightly packed together, are functionally quite isolated from each other, except for minute points along opposing membranes where information passes from one cell to another. These points, known as synapses, have been the focus of determined interest because they appear to be the anatomical locus of information transfer. Because synapses (in the periphery) and subsynaptic particles in the brain can be isolated for study, the knowledge of synaptic physiology has been greatly advanced since 1960.

In brief review, electrical impulses, the "markers" of neuronal information flow, are propagated along nerve cells in a stereotyped manner until they reach the area of the presynaptic membrane. Then, through a series of complex metabolic events, the electrical impulse is converted to a chemical message that effects the excitability of Neuron II by crossing the tiny gap between cells (see Figure 24–1). Depending on the type of neuroregulatory agent mediating this transmission, and the type of receptor on the postsynaptic membrane, the chemical message can be excitatory or inhibitory. If more than one nerve cell impinges on Neuron II, the net excitability produced by the impinging synapses will determine whether or not Neuron II will depolarize and propagate an electrical impulse down its axon to another neuron.

The metabolic events of transmission are pictured in Figure 24–1.

The elucidation of the biochemical events underlying synaptic transmission has been one of the important achievements of the past two decades, culminating in a Nobel Prize in 1970 for one of the most important contributors, Julius Axelrod.

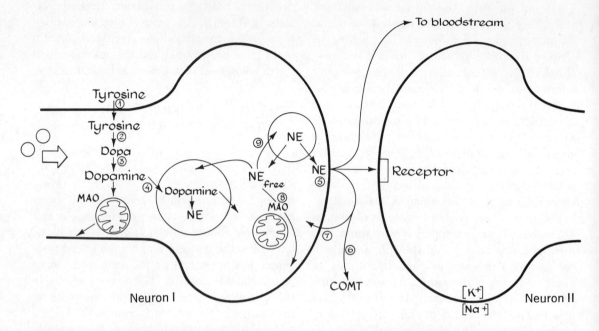

1. Uptake of tyrosine into cell
2. Conversion of tyrosine to dopa (rate limiting)
3. Conversion of dopa to dopamine
4. Uptake of dopamine into vessicle
5. Release of NE at synapse

6. Deactivation of NE by COMT
7. Reuptake of NE into cell
8. Deactivation of NE by MAO
9. Uptake of NE into storage granule

Figure 24–1.   The biochemistry of synaptic transmission.

Adrenergic Transmission

Norepinephrine (NE) is synthesized in the region of the presynaptic membrane. It is made primarily from the amino acid tyrosine, which must be actively transported into the cell from the blood stream. The formation of Dopa from tyrosine by the enzyme tyrosine hydroxylase seems to be the slowest in the series of enzymatic reactions, so that this enzyme regulates, under ordinary circumstances, the amount of norepinephrine ultimately formed. Decarboxylation occurs in the cytoplasm of the cell by way of the enzyme, L-amino acid decarboxylase. The product, dopamine (which may act as a transmitter itself) is taken up by the tiny vesicles and, therein hydroxylated, to form norepinephrine. Storage in the vesicle sequesters the synthesized norepinephrine and protects it from the intracellular

enzyme, monoamine oxidase (MAO) that inactivates norepinephrine by deamination. As the electrical impulse activates the presynaptic membrane, norepineprine is released into the synaptic cleft. Axelrod[4] has hypothesized that the NE is squeezed into the cleft by contractile fibers in the vesicle membrane, a process that requires the presence of Ca^{++} and is accompanied by the release of dopamine beta hydroxylase. Once the norepinephrine has activated the receptor site on Neuron II, it is conserved by a process of reuptake back into Neuron I, although a portion is deactivated by an enzyme, located outside the cell and known as catechol-O-methyl transferase (COMT).

Table 24–2 reviews these processes and shows some of the actions of specific drugs on neurotransmission. Table 24–3 shows similar processes for the serotonergic synapses. Theoretically, for each metabolic step there is a possible pharmacological intervention.

TABLE 24-2.   Synthesis and Metabolism of Norepinephrine

METABOLIC STEP	EFFECTED BY
1. Uptake of tyrosine into the cell.	1. Unknown.
2. Conversion of tyrosine to Dopa.	2. (Tyrosine hydroxylase) Blocked by alpha methyl tyrosine. May be effected by NE via negative feedback.
3. Conversion of dopa to dopamine.	3. (Dopa Decarboxylase) Rarely a critical step because of plentiful supply of decarboxylase enzyme.
4. Uptake of dopamine into storage vesicle.	4. Blocked by reserpine.
5. Conversion of dopamine to NE.	5. (Dopamine β-hydroxylase) Inhibited by disulfiram (chelating agent).
6. Release of NE into the synaptic cleft.	6. Stimulated by nerve impulses.
7. Deactivation of NE by COMT.	7. (Catechol-O-methyl-transferase) Inhibited by pyrogallol, N-butyl gallate.
8. Reuptake of NE into the cell.	8. Blocked by tricyclic antidepressants.
9. Intracellular deactivation of NE by MAO.	9. (Monoamine oxidase) Blocked by MAO inhibitors.
10. Uptake of NE into storage vesicle.	10. Blocked by reserpine.
11. Production of synaptic vesicles and transport down the axon.	11. Unknown.

Creveling and Daly[24] have published an excellent review of the drugs that have been shown to have an effect on each of the steps in neurotransmission. As the steps of biogenic amine synthesis have been described, it has been possible to set up screening methods that test the effect of a particular drug on a specific process of neurotransmission.

Tyrosine Hydroxylase

Recently, a rapid, sensitive radiometric assay for tyrosine hydroxylase has been developed, based on the stichiometric loss of tritium during hydroxylation of 3,5-ditritiotyrosine. This assay may be conveniently employed as a screen for potential inhibitors of tyrosine hydroxylase. Such screening procedures do not have any direct relationship to the effect of the drug clinically, but, in com-

bination with a theory about the disease process, a hypothesis about the therapeutic benefits of the drug may be formulated. For example, a drug that is a potent inhibitor of tyrosine hydroxylase would be expected to have a beneficial effect in mania, according to the catecholamine theory of affective disease, which relates mania to a functional excess of catecholamines.

As stated earlier, the hydroxylation of tyrosine is probably the rate-limiting step in catecholamine biosynthesis; consequently, any drug that affects the activity of this enzyme could be expected to have a prominent pharmacological effect on those moods or behavior related to neurotransmission involving catecholamines. A drug of this type which has received the most interest so far is a-methyl-p-tyrosine (AMPT). This drug is a potent inhibitor to the enzyme and is safe for clinical

TABLE 24-3.   Synthesis and Metabolism of Serotonin

METABOLIC STEP	EFFECTED BY
1. Uptake of tryptophane into the cell from the bloodstream.	1. Plasma tryptophane concentration, diet, diurnal variation in tryptophane?
2. Conversion of tryptophane to 5 HTP.	2. (Tryptophane hydroxylase) Blocked by parachlorophenylalanine. May be effected by serotonin via negative feedback.
3. Conversion of 5 HTP to 5 HT.	3. (L aromatic amino acid decarboxylase) Rarely a critical step.
4. Uptake of 5 HT into storage vesicle.	4. Blocked by reserpine.
5. Release of 5 HT.	5. Stimulated by nerve impulse.
6. Reuptake of 5 HT into the cell.	6. Blocked by tricyclic antidepressants.
7. Intracellular deactivation of 5 HT.	7. (Monoamine oxidase) Blocked by MAO inhibitors.
8. Production of synaptic vesicles.	8. Blocked by protein inhibitors.
9. Interaction with the receptor site.	9. Blocked by LSD? Blocked by methysergide?

use. Studies by Brodie[12] indicate that this drug may have some benefit in the treatment of mania.

It is likely that through the use of *in vitro* screening methods for drugs with tyrosine hydroxylase inhibiting activity other active compounds will be found that warrant a clinical trial in mania.

Jonsson has shown that the euphorogenic effects of amphetamine can be blocked by AMPT, thus providing evidence that the effects of amphetamine depend on intact catecholamine synthesis.[38] It is possible that AMPT, or some other tyrosine hydroxylase inhibitor, may find use in the treatment of amphetamine abuse.

Tryptophane Hydroxylase

The pathway for serotonin biosynthesis has many parallels to the pathway for norepinephrine synthesis. The synthesis of norepinephrine involves the hydroxylation of an amino acid as the first enzymatic step; for serotonin biosynthesis, the first step is the hydroxylation of tryptophane to form 5-hydroxytryptophane. There is evidence that this hydroxylation step is rate limiting, and thus the ultimate concentration of serotonin may be regulated by the activity of this enzyme. However, tryptophane hydroxylase is not ordinarily saturated by substrate; therefore, increases in available tryptophane may readily produce increases in brain concentrations of serotonin.

The most effective inhibitor of tryptophane hydroxylase is p-chlorophenylalanine (PCPA). The specific action of this drug is unknown, but it is probably related to a long-term process such as protein synthesis. One of the most striking findings has been the production of insomnia in cats treated with PCPA. The use of this drug in psychiatry has been limited. Clinical trials in mania and perhaps schizophrenia are warranted since in both of these syndromes there is some rationale for decreasing the production of serotonin. Other inhibitors of tryptophane hydroxylase, such as the 6-halo-tryptophanes and certain chelating agents, are available for animal studies. Interestingly, catechols, including norepinephrine, inhibit this enzyme. Such interactions between the serotonergic and adrenergic systems seem to be the rule, making specific interventions in and on the other system difficult.

L-Aromatic-Amino Acid Decarboxylase

This enzyme is plentiful in the brain and elsewhere in the body. The same enzyme is active in the decarboxylation of Dopa to form dopamine and of 5-hydroxytryptophane (5-HTP) to form serotonin. The main clinical usefulness of decarboxylase inhibitors has been in association with the administration of large doses of precursors of biogenic amines. For example, in the treatment of depression with L-Dopa, the concomitant administration of a hydrazine-type decarboxylase inhibitor, which does not itself cross the blood-brain barrier, results in less peripheral decarboxylation of Dopa and in increased amounts of Dopa passing into the brain, for conversion to dopamine.[11]

Dopamine Beta Hydroxylase (DBH)

This enzyme catalyzes the final step in the formation of NE from dopamine. Specific inhibitors of this step in norepinephrine formation may prove therapeutically useful.

Until recently, disulfiram (Antabuse) was the only inhibitor of DBH available for clinical use. However, recently a new nontoxic DBH inhibitor, fusaric acid, has been discovered and reported to be useful in the treatment of hypertension.[62] Both fusaric acid and disulfiram deserve clinical trials in mania on the basis that excessive concentrations of NE have been suggested as associated with the manic state.

Catechol-O-Methyl-Transferase

The metabolic inactivation of catecholamines proceeds by two major pathways: O-methylation produced by catechol-O-methyl transferase (COMT) and deamination carried out by monoamine oxidase (MAO). Various classes of compounds have been found to inhibit COMT. Perhaps the most potent are the pyrogallols. However these compounds are both quite toxic and short acting. The recent discovery of a nontoxic inhibitor of COMT available for use in man may prove of great importance in the study and treatment of psychoses.[28]

Monoamine Oxidase

Evidence from a number of investigators indicates that MAO is not a single enzyme but a family of isozymes with differing substrate specificities.[21] MAO is the enzyme responsible for intraneuronal metabolism of catecholamines and serotonin, as well as other indoleamines such as tyramine and tryptamine. Since the discovery of the therapeutic value of the MAO inhibitor iproniazid, a large number of compounds have been discovered that have MAO inhibiting activity. Much of the research in recent years on MAO inhibitors has focused on drugs that have fewer adverse side effects. This work has shown that the hydrazine-type MAO inhibitors are more often responsible for the liver damage and blood dyscrasias that occasionally occur with these drugs; consequently, efforts have been directed toward the discovery of nonhydrazine inhibitors. If safer and more effective MAO inhibitors can be found, use of these compounds in the treatment of depression may find renewed popularity. In addition, chemical testing of the spinal fluid from depressed patients may reveal which neurotransmitter is functionally deficient. The administration of a MAO inhibitor that blocks the isozyme specific for the deamination of that neurotransmitter may prove to be the treatment of choice.

Transport, Storage, and Release of Biogenic Amines

The processes of active membrane transport, intracellular storage, and release of amines upon stimulation, all affect the functional activity of amines. The tricyclic antidepressants are thought to be effective in depression because they inhibit reuptake of the amines into the nerve cell and thus prolong their action.

Cocaine, chlorpromazine, and imipramine are drugs that block the uptake of norepinephrine in sympathetic nerve tissue. Although they have similar effects on sympathetic nerves, they have very different behavioral effects. Less is known about the uptake of serotonin, since there is no convenient peripheral system available for study as there is for norepinephrine. However, serotonin uptake in brain slices is similar in many respects to the uptake of norepinephrine. Some of the tricyclic drugs are more potent in their action on norepinephrine uptake, whereas others affect serotonin uptake to a greater extent. The future will bring more understanding of the differential effect of drugs on these two systems, and on other less well studied transmitter agents.

Ordinarily, the transmitter substance is released as the electrical impulse depolarizes the presynaptic membrane. Calcium ions are essential for this release; lithium and bromide ions antagonize the release. The toxic effects of bromides and the effectiveness of lithium in manic stress may be explained by these actions. Reserpine releases norepinephrine by inhibiting the granule storage mechanism within the nerve, thus making norepinephrine susceptible to deamination. Other releasing compounds, such as tyramine and guanethidine, cause release by direct displacement of norepinephrine; this type of release is more physiological since the release transmitter interacts with the receptor and is metabolized by COMT. One of the recently discovered releasing drugs, 6-hydroxydopamine, causes irreversible damage to the adrenergic nerve cell, thus producing a selective neuronal lesion. Stein[58] has suggested that a small amount of this compound, formed endogenously, could be responsible for the production of schizophrenia; this suggestion remains highly speculative. However, the selective ablation of adrenergic nerves with 6-hydroxydopamine will be an important research tool in the future.

In summary, the ease with which amines cross certain membranes in the CNS (central nervous system) is a most important factor in their biological activity. The effect of drugs on these membrane-mediated functions is an area of intense research; in the future we may well expect that new drugs that affect these activities will be important tools for the psychopharmacologist. It may be that uptake, storage, and release are more important targets for intervention than synthesis and metabolism.

Receptor Site

Less is known about events at the postsynaptic membrane than at the presynaptic membrane. The study of receptor-site physiology is growing rapidly. Of importance is the finding that cyclic AMP (adenosine monophosphate) may play a role as a "second messenger" in the effects mediated by biogenic amines. Activation of adenyl cyclase by biogenic amines may catalyze the formation of cyclic AMP, which may activate further enzymatic activity within the neuron. The enzyme phosphodiesterase, which breaks down cyclic AMP, has been shown to be highly concentrated at the postsynaptic membrane.[32] Beer[9] has shown that there is a strong correlation between antianxiety effect and the inhibition of cyclic AMP phosphodiesterase. The use of drugs designed to affect adenyl cyclase or phosphodiesterase may be appropriate in the treatment of some mental illnesses.

There is some evidence that the propagation of the subsynaptic impulse may be the result of local release of cyclic AMP and that the neurotransmitters may act on the cyclic AMP system rather than on the subsynaptic membrane. Certain mild stimulants, e.g., caffeine and theophylline, inhibit phosphodiesterase, the enzyme that hydroxylyzes cyclic AMP. It is quite possible that in the future more potent stimulants (or antidepressants) will be developed as a result of understanding this system.

Prange[51] and his associates have administered thyroid extract (T-3) concomitantly with tricyclic antidepressants. They have shown a significantly briefer onset of action if this combination is employed as compared to tricyclics alone. The exact mechanism for this interaction remains unknown. It may involve an effect of T-3 on the receptor enzyme adrenyl cyclase. If this finding is substantiated, it may remove one of the serious disadvantages to the use of this group of tricyclic antidepressants. Kastin[40] has shown that the thyrotropic releasing hormone (TRH) may also have antidepressant properties.

Precursor Loading in Depression

The administration of the dopamine precursor L-Dopa has proven effective in the treatment of Parkinson's disease, an abnormality in which a deficiency of brain dopamine had been documented by autopsy studies. This has increased interest in this strategy as a possible means of treatment of various psychiatric illnesses. As Kety[41] has stated, the strategy of precursor loading involves three steps: first, the formulation of a hypothesis relating the concentration of some substance in the brain with a particular mental state; second, producing evidence, ordinarily derived from animal research, to show that administration of the precursor does in fact increase the concentration of the presumed deficient substance in the brain; third, testing the hypothesis clinically by administering the precursor and making carefully controlled observations of the patient's behavioral state.

In order to utilize a precursor, it must be able to cross the blood-brain barrier (BBB) (most of the transmitter substances themselves are not able to cross the BBB) and must be converted to the deficient substance without loss via alternate pathways. Using these criteria, there are but a handful of precursors that are practicable for altering monoamine concentration in the brain. For the catechol system, L-Dopa has been the most often used. It has the advantage of crossing the blood-brain barrier and of having a demonstrated pharmacological effect in Parkinson's syndrome.[18] It has the disadvantage that most exogenously administered Dopa is converted to dopamine, leaving norephinephrine concentrations relatively unaffected.[11] Efforts have been made to produce precursors of norepinephrine. For example, dihydroxyphenylserine

was at one time thought to be an effective precursor since it is converted directly to norepinephrine.[24] However, recent studies cast doubt on the ability of this metabolite to form NE intraneuronally.[48]

Clinical success with Dopa in the treatment of depression has been limited. There have been a few reported cases of Dopa sensitive depressions, but only a few.[11] As mentioned above, this failure may be due to the fact that Dopa primarily increases dopamine concentrations and not norepinephrine.

The clinical trials to date of the serotonin precursors, tryptophane and 5-hydroxytryptophane have been well-reviewed by Carroll.[18] In summary, tryptophane seems to have some effect when used in combination with MAO inhibitors, but not when employed by itself.[18] Claims for 5-HTP have been varied and this drug may still have clinical usefulness, although the more recent studies have not been encouraging.[13]

The major difficulties in using both Dopa and 5-HTP are related to the finding that the drugs have peripheral effects so that dosages must be increased slowly.[18] Furthermore, as additional knowledge becomes available about compartmentalization within the nerve cell, the more likely it becomes that monoamine concentrations may be increased by precursors without increasing the pool of amines that would be necessary to effect a change in physiological function.[43] Furthermore, it is possible that the neurotransmitter synthesized from the administered precursor will be stored and released in neurons not normally utilizing this neurotransmitter, e.g., dopamine storage and release in a serotonergic neuron. If this were to occur, the newly synthesized biogenic amine would act as a false transmitter, decreasing neurotransmission. Lastly, there has been the problem of selecting patients for precursor loading; even though most of the patients studied to date failed to respond to precursor administration, there might be a subgroup of patients with a specific biochemical abnormality that could make them amenable to precursor therapy. More will be said about predicting drug response in a later portion of this chapter.

Future Directions in the Use of Lithium and Rubidium

Lithium was first demonstrated to be effective in the manic phase of manic-depressive illness. Although the prophylactic use of lithium had been suggested earlier, Baastrup and Schou[6] were the first to report a systematic study that showed that lithium was effective in reducing the frequency and intensity of both manic and depressive episodes when used prophylactically. Recently Coppen[23] and Hullin[36] have shown that lithium may be an effective prophylactic agent in both bipolar and recurrent unipolar depressions. It is possible that in the future the spectrum of use for prophylactic lithium will widen considerably and perhaps exceed in importance the role of the drug in the treatment of acute mania.

Recently, Fieve[31] has reported preliminary pharmacological studies with rubidium. Rubidium belongs to the same series of alkali metals as lithium, sodium, and potassium. Interestingly, rubidium and lithium have contrasting behavioral, EEG, and biochemical properties. In contrast to lithium, which increases the uptake of norepinephrine into nerve cells, rubidium appears to augment the release of stored norepinephrine, thus increasing its turnover rate. Because preliminary studies in animals showed that the effects of rubidium were opposite to those of lithium, Fieve and his group have initiated clinical trials of rubidium in depressed patients. These experiments are proceeding cautiously since the toxicity of rubidium is unknown and since the metabolic half-life is long. Too few patients have been treated with the drug to allow clinical evaluations to be made as yet.

New Drugs for Mania

If manic illness is considered to be biochemically as well as behaviorally the converse of depression, then drugs that decrease the amounts of amine available at the synaptic cleft should have therapeutic potential. Both antiadrenergic and antiserotonergic drugs are currently being utilized in clinical trials. Administration of AMPT, a specific inhibitor of dopamine and norepinephrine synthesis, to manic patients has been reported to be of some benefit,[12] as has propanolol a beta adrenergic blocker.[56] Methysergiside and cinanersin, both antiserotonin agents have been claimed as effective for manic symptoms, but the results of trials to date remain controversial.[56]

Approaches to Schizophrenia

Osmond and Smythies[47] first formulated the "transmethylation hypothesis" of schizophrenia in 1952, when they made the observation that mescaline could be derived from norepinephrine by the addition of two methyl groups and suggested that a transmethylation enzyme could produce an endogenous psychotogen. The transmethylation hypothesis gained support when it was shown that other hallucinogens were methylated amines, for example, DMT (N, N-dimethyltryptamine) and bufotenin.[29,61] Kety and others showed that feeding patients compounds that would increase the supply of "methyl donors" in the brain could exacerbate the symptoms of schizophrenic patients.[49]

The transmethylation hypothesis suggested a possible treatment approach to schizophrenia, namely, the administration of a methyl "acceptor," nicotinic acid.[46] Although positive reports continue to appear, the utility of nicotinic acid, either by itself or in combination with phenothiazines, is now considered minimal.[8] Positive reports continue to appear.[2] From a theoretical point of view, there is no direct evidence that nicotinic acid significantly affects the methylation capacity of the body.[7,27] Furthermore, this drug does not improve those patients who have been made worse by administration of methyl donors such as methionine.[2] Since the transmethylation hypothesis remains a possible explanation for schizophrenia, a promising direction for future inquiry is the search for drugs that affect methylation processes more directly and efficiently.

Administration of Precursors in Schizophrenia

One of the older theories of schizophrenia, first suggested by Woolley[63] and now being reconsidered by others,[64] is that the concentration of brain serotonin might be abnormally low in schizophrenia. The recent evidence for this proposal comes from a number of places: (1) it is suggested that the sleep abnormalities characteristic of schizophrenics may be due to insufficient quantities of serotonin;[64] (2) potent serotonin depleting drugs such as PCPA produce a syndrome in animals that is suggestive of schizophrenia.[26] Wyatt[65] has recently been conducting a clinical trial in which 5-HTP, the precursor or serotonin, is being given to schizophrenics. He reports improvement in chronic schizophrenics given high doses (6 to 12 g.) of 5-HTP with a peripheral decarboxylase inhibitor over a long-time course.

Recent reviews by Kety and Matthysse[42] and Snyder[57] highlight the importance of the dopaminergic system in schizophrenia. They note that phenothiazines and the butyrophenones affect dopamine receptors, and they hypothesize that some nigro-striatal tracks may be the site of action for the antipsychotic activity of these compounds. In addition, Kety and Matthysse have noted that the amphetamine psychosis, presumed to represent an exaggerated activity of dopaminergic synapses in the brain, is clinically quite similar to certain schizophrenic states. Electrical stimulation of certain dopamine-containing nuclei of the limbic system, specifically the nucleus of the diagonol band, has resulted in altered mental states in which thought regresses from the secondary to the primary process, and in which thought images are converted to hallucinations.[42]

If, indeed, schizophrenia is a disease of dopaminergic activity, agents that affect the activity of dopa decarboxylase or dopamine beta hydroxylase may be effective in the treatment of this disorder. Other agents that affect the dopaminergic receptor site should prove clinically useful.

Other Transmitter Systems in the Brain

The adrenergic and serotonergic systems have been the most thoroughly studied, not entirely because of their suspected importance, but because of the easy and sensitive fluorometric procedures for determining the pathways and metabolism of these systems.[22] There are undoubtedly other transmitter substances in the brain that may be of equal importance but are more difficult to measure. Until recently, physiochemical methods for detecting acetylcholine were so insensitive that bioassay methods are required, resulting in rather desultory progress in the understanding of this system. Undoubtedly, in the next few years there will be increased knowledge of the relationship of cholinergic systems to the action of psychopharmacological agents, perhaps in a pattern similar to the evolution of knowledge about drugs and norepinephrine. Some phenothiazine drugs are potently anticholinergic. Furthermore, other types of anticholinergic drugs have been shown to be psychotomimetic.[22,39]

Janowsky[37] has proposed that the adrenergic-cholinergic balance in the CNS may be an important factor in affective disease, depression being related to cholinergic dominance and mania the converse. As evidence, he cites the fact that reserpine, a drug that may trigger depression, has cholinomimetic properties as well as its better known NE releasing effects. In addition, he points out that physostigmine, which increases central acetylcholine levels in the brain, counteracts mania and may cause depression in some individuals. Other examples of adrenergic-cholinergic antagonism from animal studies are presented in his review, which supports the thesis that the relative balance between the two systems may be of more importance than the level of activity of either system considered independently.

Some compounds with neurotransmitterlike activity are gamma aminobutyric acid, glycine, glutamic acid, and histamine.[22] The effects of drugs on these neurotransmitter systems may be extremely important in the design of new and better psychopharmacologic agents.

❰ Predicting Drug Response

One of the important tasks in psychopharmacology is the prediction of who will respond and who will not. Particularly in the case of the antidepressants there is a long latency between onset of treatment and response—usually from two to six weeks. Fawcett and Siomopoulos[30] have reported the use of a trial treatment period with dextroamphetamine as a means of discriminating patients amenable to treatment with tricyclic antidepressants from nonresponders. In their study of thirteen patients, they found a very good correlation between patients whose mood shifted upward during three days of amphetamine administration and eventual improvement subsequent to imipramine administration. This kind of screening procedure could prove valuable in allowing alternative drugs such as MAO inhibitors, or ECT, to be administered earlier in those cases where improvement on tricyclic medications, as judged by the amphetamine trial, would not be predicted to occur.

With the recent development of sensitive methods of assaying psychotropic drugs in the plasma, it has been demonstrated that concentrations of tricyclic antidepressants in patients on a standard dose can vary considerably.[3,10,15] Similar variability has been described for phenothiazines.[25] Furthermore, a reduction in plasma antidepressant level was found in patients treated concomitantly with other drugs such as phenobarbital. Several investigators have reported that there is a positive correlation between plasma levels of tricyclic antidepressants and clinical response.[3,10] Asberg found that most responders had levels in an optimal range between 50 and 139 nonograms per milliliter. Below that level, and interestingly, above that level, a clinical response was less likely to occur. It now appears promising that measurement of plasma levels of psychotropic drugs will be useful in predicting the treatment course of some patients who, because of some difference in metabolism or because of concomitant treatment with other drugs, require higher or lower doses.

Alexanderson[1] has shown that individual differences in plasma concentrations of nortriptyline are largely under genetic control. In a study of nineteen identical and twenty fraternal sets of twins given nortriptyline for eight days, the identical twins achieved similar plasma concentrations of the drug while the fraternal twins had concentrations that were uncorrelated. Thus, it appears that the science of "pharmacogenetics" may in the future advance our knowledge of differential response to psychotropic drugs, allowing more precise prediction of drug response.

A more distant goal for the psychopharmacologist is the use of laboratory methods to determine differences in patients that cannot be discriminated on purely clinical, psychometric, or pharmacological grounds. As a research tool, the measurement of biogenic amine metabolites in the CSF has been rewarding and in the future may lead to a more scientific choice treatment method.

An up-to-date review of the literature on amine metabolites measured in the CSF (cerebrospinal fluid) of patients with affective disorders has been provided by Post.[50] In summary, discrepancies are prevalent. Some investigators have found a decreased level of 5-HIAA (5-hydroxyindoleacetic acid), the end product of serotonin metabolism, in depressed patients, but this finding is not confirmed by other studies. A similar state of confusion exists for HVA (homovanillic acid), the end product of dopamine metabolism, and for MHPG (3-methoxy-4-hydroxyphenylglycol), the primary end product of norepinephrine metabolism. Methodological difficulties may account for some of these inconsistencies; for example, Post[50] has shown that physical activity can have profound effects on CSF amine metabolite levels.

A refinement in the measurement of CSF amine metabolites has been accomplished through the use of probenecid, administered prior to the collection of CSF samples. Probenecid blocks the transport of organic acids (including 5-HIAA and HVA) out of the CSF, resulting in an accumulation of these metabolites that is roughly proportional to the turnover of the parent amine compounds in the brain. Thus, it is possible, using probenecid, to obtain an indication of the dynamics of amine metabolism that is more relevant to the functional activity of these systems than is the measurement of the steady-state concentrations of amine metabolites. Using this technique, Goodwin[34] has demonstrated significant alterations in CSF amine metabolites, not evident from "baseline" (no probenecid pretreatment) samples alone. In summary, the study of CSF metabolites is in a phase of methodological refinement. It has the potential of providing a clearer window into the brain than previous methods.

It is possible that as methods are improved and correlations more firmly established, categories of depression may become modified by our knowledge of pathophysiological changes as reflected in CSF metabolites. Such knowledge might improve the specificity of drugs. For example, there is evidence that the tricyclic antidepressants and MAO inhibitors differ with respect to their activity on adrenergic and serotonergic systems.[60] If it could be shown that some depressed patients have a decrease of adrenergic metabolites in the CSF, they might be treated more effectively with drugs that augment adrenergic activity. If some depressions are associated with deficiencies of serotonin metabolites, they might be best treated with drugs specifically designed to affect serotonergic systems.

Another approach that may provide useful laboratory correlations of psychiatric illness is the study of peripheral blood elements. Murphy[45] has studied the amine metabolism of platelets from affectively disordered patients because of the similarities between the amine metabolism of platelets and the amine metabolism of brain. If one assumes that certain biochemical abnormalities associated with affective illness are systemic and not confined to particular areas of the brain, then the enzymes of the peripheral blood cells may reflect the important changes related to affective illness.[45] Murphy[44] has reported significant reductions in platelet MAO activity in drug-free bipolar patients (patients with a history of both mania and depression) as compared to unipolar patients and normal controls. Cohn[19] has found red blood cell COMT to be

reduced in depressed female patients. Unfortunately, in both these studies of blood-cell enzymes, the overlap between patient groups and controls has been large. However, the approach of studying the amine metabolism of the peripheral blood elements may in the future be a helpful adjunct to diagnosis and a guide to appropriate drug therapy.

Stokes[59] reported a clinical test in which lithium "responders" could be discriminated from "nonresponders" on the basis of the rate of excretion of lithium after a standard dose. More recent reports on this simple biochemical test have been disappointing.[59]

⟨ Delivery Systems

From the most primitive days of pharmacology, the modes of delivery of therapeutic compounds have not changed much. Oral, intramuscular, and intravenous administration continue to be the exclusive routes for getting drugs to target organs. The obvious drawbacks of oral administration are the unreliability of the patient, the variability of the absorption process, and differences in factors that affect blood concentrations.[15] Furthermore, the concentrations of drugs orally administered are variable rather than static.

The discovery of long-acting, slow-release compounds has increased the physician's ability to decrease the frequency of drug administration. The use of depot injections of prolixin has added somewhat to the usefulness of phenothiazines by allowing physicians to medicate the unreliable patient at biweekly intervals rather than three to four times a day.

The blood-brain barrier, which has been the nemesis of many psychopharmacologists, may turn out to be a useful ally in the future. An example of the utilization of the blood-brain barrier for more discriminating drug delivery is the combined use of L-Dopa and a peripheral inhibitor of Dopa decarboxylase (MK 486). L-Dopa has a number of peripheral side effects that limit the amount that can be administered and the rate at which dosage can be built up. MK 486 blocks the effects of L-

Dopa, but since it does not cross the blood-brain barrier, it has no effects on the central action of the drug. Thus, by using these drugs in combination, the peripheral effects can be partially blocked and higher concentrations of the drug achieved in the brain. The utilization of the blood-brain barrier for discriminative delivery of drugs to the brain has probably not been used to full advantage.

Delivery systems have recently received increasing attention. One new pharmaceutical company is devoting itself exclusively to the development of improved delivery technology and has already developed some ingenious ways of administering drugs for certain non-psychiatric illnesses. For example, a very small plastic membrane, which is worn comfortably in the conjunctival sac and releases miniscule amounts of pilocarpine at the rate of ten micrograms per hour, is now being used in the treatment of patients with glaucoma. Another system under development is a tiny capsule that is fitted in the uterus for the release of very small amounts of progesterone for the purposes of contraception. The great potential advantage of this system is that it bypasses the systemic circulation and thus avoids the many unpleasant side effects of oral birth control pills. In the future, delivery systems may be developed that can be modulated by an external source, such as a radio-transmitted message or an internal assessment of chemical concentrations within the body. For example, it may be possible to devise a system that would release insulin in a rate proportional to the blood level of glucose. A more radical development, which is not inconceivable, is the stereotaxic placement of tiny seeds of slow-release medication in precise areas of brain.

(Conclusion

Most of the psychopharmacologic agents in use today were shown to have a therapeutic effect in the treatment of mental illness by processes best explained as serendipitous and fortuitous. From these chancy, yet astute, observations have come compounds that have

effectively decreased the number of inpatients in our state hospitals. Biochemical studies concerning the mode of action of these compounds have provided us with several hypotheses relating to the neurochemical substrates of schizophrenia and the major affective disorders. Most of these hypotheses originated in the midsixties. During the last few years, these hypotheses have provided the psychopharmacologist with a rationale for the design of compounds tailored to overcome the presumed biochemical defect in these illnesses. From further clinical trials with these compounds, as well as from new research on neuronal transmission, there should emerge a new science of psychopharmacology in which serendipity will be replaced by the rational construction of a therapeutic molecule.

(Bibliography

1. Alexanderson, B., D. A. Price-Evans, and F. Sjoqvist. "Steady-State Plasma Levels of Nortriptyline in Twins: Influence of Genetic Factors in Drug Therapy," *Br. Med. J.*, 4 (1969), 764–768.

2. Ananth, J .V., T. A. Ban, H. E. Lehman et al. "Nicotinic Acid in the Prevention and Treatment of Artificially Induced Exacerbation of Psychopathology in Schizophrenics," *Can. Psychiatr. Assoc. J.*, 15 (1970), 15–20.

3. Asberg, M., B. Cronholm, F. Sjoqvist et al. "Relationship between Plasma Level and Therapeutic Effect of Nortriptyline," *Br. Med. J.*, 3 (1971), 331–334.

4. Axlerod, J., R. A. Mueller, and H. Thoenen. "New Aspects of Storage and Release Mechanisms of Catecholamines," *Bayer Symposium 1900* Vol 2, p. 212. Berlin: Springer, 1970.

5. Ayd, F. J., Jr. and B. Blackwell, eds. *Discoveries in Biological Psychiatry*. Philadelphia: Lippincott, 1970.

6. Baastrup, P. C. and M. Schou. "Lithium as a Prophylactic Agent. Its Effect Against Recurrent Depressions and Manic Depressive Psychosis," *Arch. Gen. Psychiatry*, 16 (1967), 162–172.

7. Baldessarini R. J. "Factors Influencing

Tissue Levels of the Major Methyl Donor in Mammalian Tissue," in H. E. Himwich, S. Kety, and J. R. Smythies, eds, *Amines and Schizophrenia*, p. 199–208. New York: Pergamon, 1966.

8. BAN, T. "Nicotinic Acid and Psychiatry," *Can. Psychiatr. Assess. J.*, 16 (1971), 413–431.

9. BEER, B., M. CHASIN, D. CLODY et al. "Cyclic Adenosine Monophosphate Phosphodiesterase in Brain; Effect on Anxiety," *Science*, 176 (1972), 428–430.

10. BRAITHWAITE, R. A., R. GOULDING, G. THEANO et al. "Plasma Concentration of Amitriptyline and Clinical Response," *Lancet*, 1 (1972), 1297–1300.

11. BRODIE, H. K. H. and F. K. GOODWIN. "A Peripheral Decarboxylase Inhibitor in Depression," *Sci. Prov. Sum. Form, 123rd Annu. Meet APA* (1970), 64.

12. BRODIE, H. K. H., D. L. MURPHY, F. K. GOODWIN et al. "Catecholamines and Mania: The Effect of Alpha-Methyl-Para-Tyrosine on Manic Behavior and Catecholamine Metabolism," *Clin. Pharmacol. Ther.*, 12 (1971), 218–224.

13. BRODIE, H. K. H., R. SACK, and L. SIEVER. "Clinical Studies of L-5-hydroxytryptophane in Depression," in J. D. Barchas and E. Usdin, eds., *Serotonin and Behavior*, pp. 549–560. New York: Academic, 1973.

14. BUNNEY, W. E., JR. and J. M. DAVIS. "Norepinephrine in Depressive Reactions," *Arch. Gen. Psychiatry*, 13 (1965), 483–494.

15. BURROWS, G., B. DAVIES and B. SCOGGINS. "Plasma Concentrations of Nortriptyline and Clinical Response in Depressive Illness," *Lancet*, 2 (1972), 619–623.

16. CADE, J. F. J. "Lithium Salts in the Treatment of Psychotic Excitement," *Aust. Med. J.*, 1 (1949), 349–352.

17. CALDWELL, A. E. "History of Psychopharmacology," in W. G. Clark and J. del Giudice, eds., *Principles of Psychopharmacology*, pp. 9–30. New York: Academic, 1970.

18. CARROLL, B. J. "Monoamine Precursors in the Treatment of Depression," *Clin. Pharmacol. Ther.*, 12 (1971), 743–761.

19. COHN, C. K., D. L. DUNNER, and J. AXELROD. "Reduced Catechol-O-Methyltransferase Activity in Red Blood Cells of Women with Primary Affective Disorder," *Science*, 170 (1970), 1323–1324.

20. COLE, J. O. "The Future of Psychopharmacology," in R. Fieve, ed., *Depression in the 1970's: Modern Theory and Research*, pp. 81–86. Amsterdam: Excerp. Med., 1970.

21. COLLINS, G. G. S., M. SANDLER, E. D. WILLIAMS et al. "Multiple Forms of Human Brain Mitochondrial Monoamine Oxidase," *Nature*, 225 (1970), 817–820.

22. COOPER, J. R., F. E. BLOOM, and R. H. ROTH. *The Biochemical Basis of Neuropharmacology*. New York: Oxford University Press, 1970.

23. COPPEN, A., R. NOGUERA, J. BAILEY et al. "Prophylactic Lithium in Affective Disorders," *Lancet*, 2 (1971), 275–279.

24. CREVELING, C. R. and J. W. DALY. "The Application of Biochemical Techniques in the Search for Drugs Affecting Biogenic Amines," in J. H. Biel and L. G. Abood, eds., *Biogenic Amines and Physiological Membranes in Drug Therapy*, pp. 355–412. New York: Dekker, 1971.

25. CURRY, S., J. DAVIS, D. JANOWSKY et al. "Factors Affecting Chlorpromazine Plasma Levels in Psychiatric Patients," *Arch. Gen. Psychiatry*, 22 (1970), 209–215.

26. DEMENT, W., V. ZARCONE, J. FERGUSON et al. "Some Parallel Findings in Schizophrenic Patients and Serotonin-Depleted Cats," in S. Sankar, ed., *Schizophrenia: Current Concepts and Research*, pp. 775–811. Hicksville, N.Y.: P. J. D. Publ., 1969.

27. ELLERBROOK, R. C. and M. B. PURDY. "Capacity of Stressed Humans under Mega Dosages of Nicotinic Acid to Synthesize Methylated Compounds," *Dis. Nerv. Syst.*, 31 (1970), 196–197.

28. ERICSSON, A. D. "Potentiation of the L-Dopa Effect in Man by the Use of Catechol-O-Methyltransferase Inhibitors," *J. Neurol. Sci.*, 14 (1971), 193–197.

29. FABING, H. D. "On Going Berserk: A Neurochemical Inquiry," *Am. J. Psychiatry*, 113 (1956), 409–415.

30. FAWCETT, J. and V. SIOMOPOULOS. "Dextroamphetamine Response as a Possible Predictor of Improvement with Tricyclic Therapy in Depression," *Arch. Gen. Psychiatry*, 25 (1971), 247–255.

31. FIEVE, R. R., H. MELTZER, D. L. DUNNER et al. "Rebidium, Biochemical, Behavioral, and Metabolic Studies in Humans," *Am. J. Psychiatry*, 130 (1973), 55–61.

32. FLORENDO, N., R. BARNETT, and P. GREENGARD. "Cyclic 3', 5'-Nucleotide Phosphodiesterase; Cytochemical Localization in

the Cerebral Cortex," *Science*, 173 (1971), 745–747.

33. GLASSMAN, A. "Indoleamines and Affective Disorders," *Psychosom. Med.*, 31 (1969), 107–114.

34. GOODWIN, F. K., R. M. POST, D. L. DUNNER et al. "Cerebrospinal Fluid Amine Metabolites in Affective Illness: The Probenecid Technique," *Am. J. Psychiatry*, 130 (1973), 73–78.

35. HOLLISTER, L. "Chemotherapy of Schizophrenia," in B. T. Ho and W. M. McIsaac, eds., *Brain Chemistry and Mental Disease*, pp. 303–317. New York: Plenum, 1971.

36. HULLIN, R. P., R. McDONALD, and M. N. ALLSOPP. "Prophylactic Lithium in Recurrent Affective Disorders," *Lancet*, 1 (1972), 1044–1046.

37. JANOWSKY, D. S., M. K. EL-YOUSEF, J. M. DAVIS et al. "A Cholinergic-Adrenergic Hypothesis of Mania and Depression," *Lancet*, 1 (1972), 632–635.

38. JONSSON, L. E., L. M. GUNNE, and E. ANGGARD. "Blockage of Intravenous Amphetamine Euphoria in Man," *Clin. Pharmacol. Ther.*, 12 (1971), 889–896.

39. KARCZMAR, A. G. "Central Cholinergic Pathways and Their Behavioral Implications," in W. G. Clark and J. del Giudice, eds., *Principles of Psychopharmacology*, pp. 57–86. New York: Academic, 1970.

40. KASTI, A. J., R. H. EHRENSING, D. S. SCHAKH et al. "Improvement in Mental Depression with Decreased Thyrotropin Response after Administration of Thyrotropin-Releasing Hormone," *Lancet*, 2 (1972), 740–742.

41. KETY, S. S. "The Precursor-Load Strategy in Psychochemical Research," in A. J. Mandell and M. Mandell, eds., *Psychochemical Research in Man.* pp. 127–134. New York: Academic, 1969.

42. KETY, S. S., and S. MATTHYSSE. *Neurosciences Research Program Bulletin*, Vol. 10. Brookline: Neurosci. Res. Prog., 1972.

43. MOIR, A. T. B., and D. ECCLESTON. "The Effects of Precursor Loading in the Cerebral Metabolism of 5-Hydroxyindoles," *J. Neurochem.*, 15 (1968), 1093–1108.

44. MURPHY, D. "Amine Precursors, Amines, and False Neurotransmitters in Depressed Patients," *Am. J. Psychiatry*, 129 (1972), 141–148.

45. MURPHY, D. L., and R. WEISS. "Reduced Monoamine Oxidase Activity in Blood Platelets from Bipolar Depressed Patients," *Am. J. Psychiatry*, 128 (1972), 1351–1357.

46. OSMOND, H., and A. HOFFER. "Massive Niacin Treatment in Schizophrenia: Review of a Nine-Year Study," *Lancet*, 1 (1962), 316–319.

47. OSMOND, H., and J. SMYTHIES. "Schizophrenia: A New Approach," *J. Ment. Sci.*, 98 (1952), 309–315.

48. PLETSCHER, A. "Amine Precursors in the Study of Affective Disorders," *7th Int. Congr., Collegium Int. Neuropsychopharm*, Prague, 1970.

49. POLLIN, W., P. V. CARDON, and S. S. KETY. "Effects of Amino Acid Feedings in Schizophrenic Patients Treated with Iproniazid," *Science*, 133 (1961), 104–105.

50. POST, R. M., J. KOTIN, F. K. GOODWIN et al. "Psychomotor Activity and Cerebrospinal Fluid Amine Metabolites in Affective Illness," *Am. J. Psychiatry*, 130 (1973), 67–72.

51. PRANGE, A. J., JR., I. C. WILSON, A. M. RABON et al. "Enchancement of Imipramine Antidepressant Activity by Thyroid Hormone," *Am. J. Psychiatry*, 126 (1969), 457–469.

52. REID, W. D. "Turnover Rate of Brain 5-Hydroxy Tryptamine Increased by D-Amphetamine," *Brit. J. Pharmacol.*, 40 (1970), 483–487.

53. SCHECKEL, C. L. "Preclinical Psychopharmacology," in W. G. Clark and J. del Giudice, eds., *Principles of Psychopharmacology*, pp. 235–254. New York: Academic, 1970.

54. SCHILDKRAUT, J. J. "The Catecholamine Hypothesis of Affective Disorders: A Review of Supporting Evidence," *Am. J. Psychiatry*, 122 (1965), 509–522.

55. SELIKOFF, I. J. and E. H. ROBITZEK. "Tuberculosis Chemotherapy with Hydrazine Derivatives of Isonicotinic Acid," *Dis. Chest*, 21 (1952), 385–438.

56. SHOPSIN, B. and S. GERSHON. "Chemotherapy of Manic-Depressive Disorder," in B. T. Ho and W. M. McIsaac, eds., *Brain Chemistry and Mental Disease*, pp. 319–377. New York: Plenum, 1971.

57. SNYDER, S. H. "Amphetamine Psychosis: A 'Model' Schizophrenia Mediated by Catecholamines," *Am. J. Psychiatry*, 130 (1973), 61–67.

58. STEIN, L. and C. D. WISE. "Possible Etiology

of Schizophrenia: Progressive Damage to the Noradrenergic Reward System by 6-Hydroxydopamine," *Science*, 171 (1971), 1032–1036.

59. STOKES, J. W., J. MENDELS, S. K. SECUNDA et al. "Lithium Excretion and Therapeutic Response," *J. Nerv. Ment. Dis.*, 154 (1972), 43–48.

60. SULSER, F. and E. SANDERS-BUSH. "Effect of Drugs on Amines in the CNS," *Ann. Rev. Pharmacol.*, 11 (1971), 209–230.

61. SZARA, S. "Dimethyltryptamine: Its Metabolism in Man: The Relation of Its Psychotic Effect to the Serotonin Metabolism," *Experientia*, 12 (1956), 441–442.

62. TERASAWA, F. and M. MASAKUNI. "The Clinical Trial of a New Hypotensive Agent, 'Fusaric Acid' (5-Butylpicolinic Acid); The Preliminary Report," *Jap. Circ. J.*, 35 (1971), 339–357.

63. WOOLLEY, D. W. *The Biochemical Bases of Psychoses or the Serotonin Hypothesis About Mental Illness*. New York: Wiley, 1962.

64. WYATT, R. J., B. A. TERMINI, and J. DAVIS. "Biochemical and Sleep Studies of Schizophrenia: A Review of the Literature 1960–1970. Part II. Sleep Studies," *Schizo. Bull.*, 4 (1971), 45–66.

65. WYATT, R. J., T. VAUGHAN, M. GALANTER et al. "Behavioral Changes of Chronic Schizophrenic Patients Given L-5-Hydroxytryptophan," *Science*, 177 (1972), 1124–1126.

66. ZELLER, E. A. and J. BARSKY. "*In Vivo* Inhibition of Liver and Brain Monoamine Oxidase by 1-Isonicotinyl-2-Isopropyl Hydrazine," *Soc. Exp. Biol. Med.*, 81 (1952), 459–461.

CHAPTER 25

RESEARCH IN NONNARCOTIC DRUG ABUSE

J. Fred E. Shick and Daniel X. Freedman

(Introduction

MEDICINE and the social sciences have been challenged to respond to "drug abuse," to assess the nature and extent of problems, causes, and outcomes, and to design and evaluate treatment and prevention. Well-designed, thoughtful, and empirical research has been the exception, but the field has rapidly expanded. The impetus has been a political and public demand for immediately applicable information. This is not intrinsically possible with research, and, in fact, deliberateness is not characteristic of public policy or research response in such emotionally explosive areas.

The topic presents a problem of focus. The abuse of drugs is not solely a medical issue. Entailed is an array of philosophical, social, behavioral, economic, and psychological issues implicit in the manufacture, discovery, distribution, and consumption of medicinals. Social, educational, legal, regulatory, medical, legislative, and research-supporting agencies are potentially involved. As a model for all of psychiatry (involving interactions of individual and social, as well as bodily factors) the topic is heuristically interesting, but psychiatric expertise alone is insufficient. This elusive and complex topic concerns the consumption of items, the use of which depends on cultural values, economic factors, small and large group phenomena, drug effects, and intrapsychic (and probably intercerebral) determinants, as well as recurrent dimensions of human behavior, such as the search for both novelty and constancy, and the tasks of self-regulation and mastery of various states of pleasure and pain.

The fact is that drug use impinges on the nonrational, and thus various belief systems and ideologies influence the research process as well as the user. First of all, from infancy forward, there is a fundamental ambivalence toward incorporated substances. Either a substance is taboo and related to danger, poison, and morbidity or it is welcomed as "chicken soup," enhancing growth and potencies, relieving aches and warding off uncontrollable morbidity. Tutored by the mother, the child learns these fundamental attitudes, which reflect the subculture's beliefs. Fads for, and phobias against, food and chemicals are a visible consequence of this inevitable heritage.

A second intrinsic source of nonrational attitudes about drugs stems from the issues of autonomy and of control over bodily and mental states. No society is comfortable either with man's capacity to overindulge in pleasure, to pursue private purposes and meanings, or the ease with which he can substitute dream and denial for confrontation and challenge. This social anxiety is expressed either as "rules" about the time and place for pleasure or as taboos against or social outlets for excessive absorption in the self. But a gradient of social anxiety about retreat and pleasure-seeking beyond prescribed limits is discernible.

The fact that drugs simultaneously affect private experience and public behavior also produces concern about the control and predictability of expected behavior and response —of just what a person is capable of when intoxicated or medicated. Most societies sense the power of drug consumption to magically obliterate pain, to ignore social consequences, to change the world in a single gulp, and to privately revise its meaning and demands. They equally fear the potential for "enslavement" and surrendered autonomy to a foreign (albeit, chemical) agent. Thus, whether drug-taking individuals will respond reliably and within reasonable limits to the social signals and cues by which individuals normally influence and regulate themselves and each other is an intrinsic source of social anxiety about the

problem. Similarly, denial of the power of drugs to regulate thoughts and tensions and failure to anticipate the future consequence of the moment's imperative are characteristic responses to the fear of enslavement and to the wish for the power of magical mastery.

Drug use can either express or threaten established beliefs. The recent illicit use of drugs in Western societies has occurred without a concomitant growth in social regulatory norms to shape and contain it. There has been a striking breakdown in the social definition of occasion, sponsorship, and ritual in drug use. Group processes generally help man to share his limits with others, to yield total autonomy, and to reduce the strain of internal struggles thereby. The group defines not only what substances are ingestible and why but the way events are to be interpreted and managed during the drugged state and after. During intoxication, the bridge to reality lies in the customs of the group as internalized by the individual and interpreted by the occasion. One is generally tutored in what to expect with drug consumption and how to interpret his feelings. When events cannot be explicitly monitored and tracked (as with stuffs that disappear "inside") attitudes and customs will generally interpret the invisible and regulate anxieties. Belief, ritual, and religion, then, are intrinsic means by which man attempts to regulate and contain powerful feelings of omnipotence, and drug consumption is integrally involved in this.

Around the epidemic of drug use of the 1960s, social practices that seemed foreign and threatening to a valued heritage emerged among the youth. In the climate of concern over the values and the uses of products of nature and technology, there has been, at the same time, confusion as to what is required for appropriate and reliable administration of drugs. Medicine, as the social system for reliable, rational governance of the giving and getting of drugs, is less valued than it was once, and in transition. The sanctioned giver of medicines is no longer trusted nor—as with public agencies—charged to perform infallibly. There is a stern demand that the "crutch" of medication be avoided and withheld; there is also a strident clamor that each individual has the right to experience whatever he wishes —and sometimes whenever, often with the codicil: as long as it is private and does not harm others, even though a "civil right" to drug-induced experiences more often than not affects others, is rarely private, and requires a purchase in a market.

Medicine and psychiatry are involved whether drug abuse is a "disease" or not. This is a pseudoargument which artificially splits mind and body. The medical model is sometimes viewed as a "medicine's model," rather than one recognizing the unity of man with disordered behavior. Obviously there are molecular, psychosocial, and conditioning mechanisms involved in drug use. Such arguments are generally relevant to the question of who has the power to intervene; of who is accountable. What the physician generally attempts to do is enhance the patient's ability to regulate himself and his bodily processes. The medical model in this service is a rational, predictable, and accountable approach to certain aspects of drug-related problems, intentionally utilizing (or utilized by) other social resources at all levels of research and treatment.

The drug problem is, then, many problems. The "drug culture" has threatened social custom, and been appropriated as a cause célèbre by many emerging groups. Musto shows that frequently in history an unpopular subpopulation is attacked on the basis of its habits of food or drug consumption.[244] Such consumption practices can be badges of identity. Confusion, then, exists as to what drug use symbolizes and how and with what movements it is identified, and how decisions about drugs will affect ideals as well as daily practices. A ready assumption of moralistic, pseudomoralistic, or proselytizing attitudes ("the world is hypocritical" and "you too," as a response to criticism of drug habits) is common: the debates preceding and during the American prohibition experiment in which rural virtues were pitted against perennial urban corruption document this.[244] Accordingly, groups overlook, isolate, avoid, or—to counter doubt —overenthusiastically embrace or excoriate

drug use. Research is thus faced with consequences of the nonrational, and with multiple definitions of a "drug problem."

The sixties presented an epidemic of drug "interest" far more distracting than the actual patterns of use and misuse. Drugs are now a fact of contemporary life and another option for risk taking about which to formulate attitudes and decisions. The psychiatric response has been a mixture of reassurance, attempts at understanding, and proselytizing for a youthful sector of the population with a new set of heroes, villains, and spokesmen—a sector with an unprecedented influence of technology, media, and fads, yet itself subject to an unparalleled, and exponential, expansion of information (and, occasionally, of knowledge). Suspended judgment and reflection within the psychiatric, medical, research, legislative, and legal sectors have been lacking. Sermons, called "The Literature on Drugs," and forced "drug education," have been one unhappy result. Thus, the problem in assessing research in drug abuse is one of focus and perspective, of explicit goals, and the level and quality of inquiry required for the specific and multiple questions.

Research into the pharmacology and neurochemistry of the various illicit drugs (hallucinogens, stimulants, sedatives, and derivatives of marijuana) has burgeoned. This extensive literature is beyond the scope of this chapter which, rather, focuses on the social-psychological research on the use and abuse of nonnarcotic drugs (excluding alcohol and tobacco) from a historical, social, and epidemiological perspective. Drug abuse, then, is a social and personal phenomenon that has a history in the culture. Drug use poses numerous problems for the psychiatrist in diagnosis, treatment, and education of the individual patient. He is expected to appreciate the causes and outcomes of such behavior. Research generally promises an extension of knowledge about the mind and body. What is known (and yet to be learned) about the motives and forces that initiate drug intake, sustain it, and lead to controlled or uncontrolled use, to stopping, and to relapse? This chapter will focus on such questions.

❨ Historical Research

Historical and ethnological study[81,36,48] indicate nothing novel in the use of chemicals to achieve social and ritual effects. Epidemics of drug interest and panic have occurred before, and societies have sought to regulate attitudes on the consumption of new or familiar substances, such as tobacco, or new forms of alcohol, such as gin. Historical and anthropological research, analyzing recurrent factors leading to the adoption, condemnation, acculturation, and regulation of particular substances within a specific segment of the population at a particular time, would be of value.[80,243,244] It is probable that cultural change and social stress are relevant prior variables or, at least, drug use taps such forces and factors, as well as generating consequences. Both transcultural and historical study, as well as the microhistory of recent contemporary events, contain data of general interest to the social and political sciences, to applied social research in communications (attempts at education, as well as studies of acculturation), and to the still crude arts of evaluation research in studies of designed or naturalistic social change.

T. G. Coffey's account of the gin epidemic of eighteenth-century Britain is a useful semi-analytic account.[62] A rural to urban migration, the politics of urban renewal following the great London fire of 1666, rural domination of Parliament, poverty and disorganization, the introduction of Dutch gin into England by soldiers returning from wars, led, between 1720 and 1750, to the despair evident in Hogarth's *Gin Street*, to high mortality from alcohol-related disease, to rampantly excessive infant mortality, and to general chaos in the streets. Prohibition of gin failed, and the eventual decline of consumption seemed directly related to: high gin taxes; new political powers gained by urban dwellers; legislation regulating the traffic of grain and the use of credit in sales to and from distillers; legislation forbidding alcohol consumption on the street and confining it to selected and dispersed taverns; the appearance of coffee shops for recreation; and—crucially—John Wesley's Methodism, directed to the poor and their customs, and evangelically enlisting them in alternatives to alcohol intoxication. While coffee and, later, tea ("witches' brew"), were also blamed for the moral deterioration of the poor, social reformers such as Henry Fielding and William Hogarth, who battled against both gin and beer, did not oppose these lighter beverages. Wesley even countenanced beer—the consumption of which markedly increased in the latter half of the seventeenth century. The marked decrease in gin consumption, achieved by the late eighteenth century, was thus related in part to legal, economic, and trafficking regulations, urban power, and alternatives, including a religious cause. There is no evidence that this occurred by special design, but rather by trial and error as other concerns, as well as those focused on alcohol, were dealt with. The recurrent questions requiring study are whether there are subtle factors in the excessive use of intoxicants that engender responses that lead to a self-limiting nature of epidemics over time: groups or generations, for example, reacting to the visible behavioral consequences of excess or exploiting talents (such as entrepreneurial and competitive competence) that may fill a vacuum and be visibly rewarding thereby.

Terry and Pellens's account of the opium problem in the United States up to 1928 is a landmark study.[338] The number of addicts per capita in the late nineteenth and early twentieth centuries was greater than at present. The post-Civil War "soldier sickness" and, later, the morphine sickness of women,[254] addicted through the prevalence of morphine in tonics and patent medicines, while alarming to a few vocal medical observers, did not provoke the community opprobrium reserved for contemporary narcotics users. The authors cite as causative the unrestricted use and popularity of opium for a variety of medical problems; educational laxness and ignorance about addictive processes among physicians and the laity; ". . . the influence of such writings as De Quincey and others of his day"; the hypodermic; the increased opium smoking spreading (through Chinese laborers) from the West

to the East Coast; the patent-medicine industry; introduction of heroin; ". . . all were natural factors leading to the increasingly widespread use of opium in all social groups."
Since patent-medicine remedies for morphine
sickness contained opium and alcohol, and
since such medicaments were used in the proliferating private sanatoriums, the phenomena
of substitute addictions was prevalent. Heroin
(the Bayer Company's trade name for diace-
tylmorphine) was apparently so used and
gradually adopted by the drug underground,
since its crystalline nature allowed it to be
more easily transported and adulterated. A
truly focused history of this drug and the dynamics of its flow from middle- to lower-class
use by the 1920s is still wanted.

Musto,[244] assembling and studying an impressive array of original documents, points
not only to the American focus on foreign
opiate traffic, as the U.S. consolidated its Far
Eastern influence in investments through
treaties, but also to the alliance of religious
and medical thought. Announcements by eminent authorities of cures (usually based on
theories about autointoxication and immune
mechanisms) mandated treatment by various
strong purges of the internal poisons. The
Harrison Act of 1914, aimed less at American
addicts than at trade and international concerns, nevertheless seemed to its authors not
only to contain moral virtue but to be humane, since "cure" was readily available. The
mushrooming morphine-maintenance clinics
after the First World War were surrounded by
growing controversy and doubt about such
confident medical theories. Sporadic scandals
concerning loosely monitored clinics generated, within a ten- or twelve-month period,
court interpretations and public opinion that
not only brought treatment to a halt but, by
1924, led physicians to abandon any attempts
to deal with addiction. Research on the problem of policy—indeed on the volatility of policy changes—are required. The feasibility of
goal setting and implementation by social
agencies to effect measures directed at economic, social, and consumption habits that
fundamentally are based on appetite, basic
drives for pleasure, and for physical and psy-

chic analgesia is the question. It presents political and social scientists with a still-challeng-
ing text for analysis.

Patrick Hughes' research on the heroin epidemic among Chicago Negro youths following
World War II (before which opium smoking
among Chinese was prevalent in the city)
shows that the epidemic reached its peak in
1949 and declined during the early 1950s.[150,157]
He documents the use of marijuana (for which
penalties were far higher than for heroin) in
the jazz scene by curious and vigorous young
experimenters. Later cocaine was introduced,
and the initial bold adventurers were replaced
by more delinquent groups whose later addiction to heroin finally emerged for treatment
in the methadone clinics of 1968. The careers
generated by the illegal manufacture and distribution of the drug are described along with
the social roles of the heroin "copping area."[154,156]
Strikingly, the legislative and judicial as
well as the short-lived therapeutic and mass-
media response to the epidemic occurred after
the peak incidence of new cases. While the
media distorted the "dope fiend"—borrowing
from the behavior of cocainized addicts—it
did precipitate police and legislative attention.
The enforcement effort appears to have prevented further spread (but with it the price of
heroin increased, the quality decreased) discouraging new cases but "taxing" the addicted,
whose criminalized status became entrenched.
Thus the contagious phase of this epidemic
went unnoticed, and the epidemic was already
in decline when the community, noting the
prevalence of heroin addiction, was finally
mobilized to respond. The drastic periodic
revisions of penalty structures seemed more
an affective than effective response. These
problems are part of the general legal and
penological questions involving the use of institutions and a variety of devices (from minimal mandatory sentencing to diversion of the
deviant into rehabilitation—however that is
defined) by which society attempts to deal
with deviance.

After World War II, the Japanese experi-
enced an epidemic of amphetamine abuse.[143,224,73] The war defeat led to widespread dis-
affection with traditional roles, customs, and

social controls centering on the family. Disillusionment and a raft of Japanese teen-agers discovering American ways contributed to the problem. Western style "coffee houses" and illicit entertainment centers became places for distribution of the drug, marketed as "Phikopon" ("Awake-Amine") or more familiarly "pone." The prewar family gangs were the first "collaborators" with the victorious Americans, purchasing large quantities of American and Japanese amphetamines (used by soldiers of both sides during the war and a standard part of survival kits) which were both plentiful and cheap. Postwar Japanese manufacturers probably diverted large supplies through these channels. Soldiers and students, followed shortly by night workers, prostitutes, and delinquents in the entertainment areas, used it orally and intravenously. Although there was drunkenness, opiates and marijuana were rarely used, but amphetamine was perhaps, as Heyman[143] explains, particularly suited to the Japanese—always an achievement-oriented society. At the height of the epidemic there was a popular saying: "Japan suffers from three evils—pone, pachenko [a gambling craze] and Premier Yoshita." Delinquency, particularly crimes of violence, increased sharply concurrently with the amphetamine epidemic, but subsequent studies and events "showed that although delinquency and drugs were linked, delinquency rates followed an independent course, even after the amphetamine epidemic was over."[143] Amphetamine psychosis became prevalent, and by 1954, when controls were placed on the drug, there were estimated to be more than 200,000 amphetamine addicts in Japan. Perhaps because Japan is a more authoritarian society, still emphasizing family reverence, "they were able to stem this epidemic (and an incipient heroin problem during the early 1960s) by mobilizing a broadly based social response centered on effective use of the criminal law and an education effort based in large measure on nation pride."[246] The broad discretionary powers of the Japanese police, prosecuting attorneys, and judges resulted in many compulsory hospitalizations. Legislation aimed at the sources of supply, the ability of police to work in the community, the expanding economy, increased employment, and social attitudes and cultural support inimical to drug abuse, all played a significant role in eliminating the problem. Sweden reported an epidemic of phenmetrazine that, though not so vast, attracted much attention,[14] and Griffith described the history of amphetamine use in this country.[125,127]

What so shocked the U.S. in the early 1960s was the noisy adoption of drugs other than alcohol for use and experimentation—specifically, and first, LSD—by the affluent white-college youth. Neither Havelock Ellis' description in 1889 of mescaline, nor the accounts of Baudelaire, Rimbaud, Moreau de Tours, Coleridge, De Quincey, and Poe in the nineteenth century, generated any truly widespread contagion of use, although *Lancet* warned editorially of problems that might occur if "this spreads to the streets." William James, K. Beringer and H. Kluver gave probing accounts of what Lewin called the "phantastica,"[201] but the imaginative attention of intellectuals in general was caught by Huxley in *The Doors of Perception and Heaven and Hell*,[162] published in the early 1950s. Psychiatric research into the effects of drugs—including LSD and the possible therapeutic use of it, of amytal, and methedrine—was of sporadic interest between 1930 and 1960. The midthirties had provoked a flurry of concern about marijuana, leading to several reports culminating in the comprehensive La Guardia Report of 1944 with its extensive psychopharmacological studies of the drug. Synthetics related to marijuana, e.g., Synhexyl,[3,364] were studied and dubiety concerning the unspecified social and psychiatric consequences of extensive use was amply expressed. In the late 1950s, several subcultures around the psychotherapeutic use of LSD sprang up on the East and West Coasts, and psychiatrists and various psychiatric camp followers reported a variety of attempts at cures, including simultaneous medication of patient and physician during sessions. There were serious studies as well.[50,281,198] These minor activities, coupled with some interest from the "beat underground,"[135] fueled a low-keyed but responsive interest among various subcommunities, and the attempt to try some of these remarkable drugs became stylish. With the vigorous and publicized activities in 1961 of T. Leary and R. Alpert at Harvard, a new and more socially consequential thrust was given to drug interest, and, coupled with the so-called psychedelic mystique and the cause of rebellion, the widespread epidemic of drug interest was launched.

Most veteran observers of the era are aware of the proselytizing, and the prescription for preferred behavior as the media led the imagination into a bold new future. Marijuana, endemic in bohemian subcultures and the ghetto, followed LSD and mescaline (in the form of peyote buttons). By 1965–66 there was sufficient concern about drug misuse for congressional investigations and action. Impressionistically, between 1966 and 1968, the rapid increase in the use of LSD on campuses began to level off, in part because of intrinsic boredom and in part with the discovery of "fractured chromosomes." The same mystiques and current of involvement in "turning off, in, up or down" on drugs spread to marijuana. This became a more likely and safe "cause" to expose the hypocrisy of laws and social institutions. There was a growth of hippie subcultures, of the drug and love movement heralded by the songs and styles of the 1960s, and the growing assertion that one's own experience was a sufficient guide for safety and sagacity. The purported "harmlessness" of marijuana generalized to "drugs." The era of pot and pills escalated after 1967, to be followed by (an as yet not well-analyzed) trial and use of heroin on campuses, in suburbs and ghettos, and among social classes hitherto immune. This pattern appeared transnationally. It moved from coastal campuses and large urban centers to inland campuses and smaller cities and towns, and from college age groups to the junior high schools, supported by the underground press and a variety of styles of dress and recreation that, at the least, did not provide "attitudinal barriers" against it.

In San Francisco, an actively proselytizing group of young people, sparked by the Leary influence and including a nucleus of the 1950s beat generation from the North Beach area, began to use LSD ritually as a "sacrament," proselytized for the hip life style, clustered in the Haight-Ashbury neighborhood in the early 1960s, and called themselves the New Community. Their attitudes and beliefs spread by word of mouth and by the underground press (primarily the Haight-Ashbury *Oracle*) to other areas of the nation, culminating in a pilgrimage of youth in the summer of 1967 ("Summer of Love") to the Haight. At its peak, the population—composed of runaway youth, college students, devout and weekend hippies, promoters, exploiters, and the curious —may have reached 20,000 persons within a twenty-square-block area.[300] Many stayed only days or weeks, but carried back with them experiences, attitudes, and myths of the hippie scene as well as the drugs in use. Pills (primarily LSD) were sold on the street under all sorts of names and disguises, and by May, 1967, rumors spread about "the superior properties of [a newly synthesized hallucinogen called] STP, said to be inexpensive and not yet illegal. . . . On June 21, 1967, at a celebration of the Summer Solstice held in Golden Gate Park, a familiar local figure distributed about 5000 STP tablets without charge [and] an additional smaller number were sold on the street," resulting in an estimated sixty cases of adverse reactions variously treated by the free clinic, local hospitals, and emergency centers.[235] A similar episode occurred four months later. By the end of that summer, small but significant fractions of the population had begun to use intravenous amphetamines,[300] the "death of hip" was celebrated by the community members, and large numbers of youth left the Haight-Ashbury for communes and other enclaves, in part because the more violent speed users and "acid heads" had begun to clash.[310] The most severely drug-dependent youth and those least productive stayed on. Microepidemics of barbiturate use occurred and later heroin appeared, and the Haight-Ashbury quickly declined in popularity.*

* See references 110, 247, 248, 312, 313, 318, and 320.

While observers are aware that LSD was "discovered" countless times by the media, that the mythologizing of youth and the coupling of their interest to psychedelic values was highly promoted in leading news journals, and while it was clear that leading philosophers, psychiatrists, and students of the romantic agony were quiet (if not diverted by the notion that perhaps drugs indeed were heralding a unique era) the microhistory of this spread of drug interest, trial, and misuse is still lacking, still challenging for sociopsychological study.

The initial research response was natural to the campus, where both investigators and users were clustered, including an expected concern of a panicked generation of parents and administrators. A number of studies of the scope, the extent, and the patterns of drug use began; psychiatric and other casualties were reported from those institutions in contact with these "fallouts" from the epidemic; and with the springing up of new "outreach" agencies, the motives, needs, and physical and psychological problems of various involved young users were reported.

Fear of arrest and hospitalization, a lack of effective medical treatment and knowledge about the new drugs and their adverse effects, and fear of the drastic treatments often employed encouraged subcultures to begin treating their own "bad trips," even where there were hippie-acceptable agencies.[313] This meant that drug victims were probably more prevalent than reported. Exactly how the communication of treatment norms, rationales, and mythology affected the avoidance of the medical agencies, the process of professional treatment of the users, and occasional adverse outcomes is unexplored.

The explosion of marijuana studies and technological developments for the production of tetrahydrocannabinol (THC); the description of scenes, myths, and subcultures leading to surveys of extent and scope and to studies determining the effects of the drugs on physiology, mentation, and behavior; the desperate, though to date futile, search for medical uses of the cannabinoids, as if to justify marijuana's recognition, all created pressures and fallouts.

The confidentiality of research and the fearless public reporting of findings when they were unpleasant to policy are some of the yet unreported struggles in research sectors during the 1960s.

A comprehensive cultural history of the drug movement would be a valuable contribution to the understanding of the epidemic propensity of fads. Whenever a piece of contemporary behavior is widely conveyed—or reacted to—it rapidly becomes significant, imitated, and consequential in terms of public style and habit. In a consumer-oriented economy, sharply responsive to novel fads (and with the distinct purchasing power of the young) there is an instantaneous communication network of TV, radio, books, and the underground press. Youth are highly mobile, obtaining drugs from one part of the country and demonstrating their use and distributing them in other parts. There is an increased reliance on psychoactive chemicals and an ambivalent mood about technology's ability to discover and market medicinals to influence the mind. But a social-psychological formulation of this epidemic—the output of information, the barriers and facilitators between the output and the receiver, and an analysis of how the receiver heard the message—is still lacking.

(Trend Studies and Epidemiological Models

Brief History of the Research

The voluminous research literature since 1960 on nonnarcotic drug abuse is primarily devoted to the assessment of the extent of use, defining patterns and subpopulations of users, attempts at understanding causes (including a few "process" studies—the social processes involved in the acquisition and consumption of drugs and the management of their effects) consequences and outcomes. Very few studies define treatment regimens or assess their efficacy.

Background knowledge about drugs and

drug use—psychopharmacologic profiles of primary drug effects and controlled studies on personality and performance related to drugs (the roots of psychopharmacology)—were largely done in the 1950s and before, culminating in Wikler's texts.[359,360] The vantage point of the social sciences was highly developed by Chein,[59] Lindesmith,[203,204] and Becker.[10,11,12] Physicians reported adverse effects (e.g., toxic psychoses) of psychotropic and other drugs, and the use of LSD in treatment was explored.[50,198,281] Finally, there were the reports of various commissions—Indian Hemp Drugs Commission,[163] La Guardia Report, and the landmark studies of the U.S. Public Health Service—reflecting the focus of biopsychosocial interest in drug use.

After the epidemic of the early 1960s, after the marijuana debates of 1967 and later, trend research into the "drug-abuse problem" began in earnest. The demand was to assess the scope of the "threat"—to quickly determine the extent of drug use and abuse and, hopefully, to cope with it as instantly. This community assessment research—almost entirely published after 1967—defined trends, described patterns, and communicated news of who had and was presently using illicit drugs. There was little inquiry into who had not used, who had stopped,[112,280] and who had relapsed and why. The ability to assess epidemic trends from this early data was disappointing, since most surveys focused on who had *ever* used drugs rather than assessing the more important epidemiological factors of incidence, prevalence, frequency, and rate and mechanisms of spread—statistics that best predict emerging trends and direction of current use. These early studies relied on self-report and utilized diverse samples (largely adventitious) and various methods and statistics that made comparison difficult.[23,245,246] Definitions of abuse were idiosyncratic; the reliability and validity of reports were, for the most part, unassessed, partly owing to the intrinsic difficulty of getting independent checks in this field. Factors that might serve as leads to prevention, regulation, therapeutic measures, and possible causes were only rarely investigated, and there was much repetition.

Definitional Problems and Patterns of Use

A predictable lack of precision in terminology has accompanied the proliferation of viewpoints on drug abuse. To remove illicit drug use from the moralistic arena, "abuse," replaced "addiction" in the early 1960s,[234] but this term also came to imply societal disapproval.[246] The public was found either to relate the term, drug abuse, to nonmedical use, to the medical consequences of such misuse, or simply to have no idea of what it meant.[246] A researcher's decision that a person is abusing a drug is somewhat arbitrary and depends upon the weight he gives to the consequences and outcomes of a subject's use (e.g., Bell's[19] use of amphetamine psychosis to indicate abuse), the frequency, duration, intensity, and amount of drug used on each occasion,[246,300] and the political and social orientation of the investigator or his subject (e.g., where social cost is considered). The precise distinction of the meanings of such terms as "addiction," "habit forming" or "narcotic hunger," is not necessarily explicit—nor always conscious to the investigator. At least, the connotations of each new term may bear the burden of cultural attitudes and overtones that are never quite explicit. For some investigators, addiction, dependence, or abuse, aside from its pejorative connotation, implies inability to cease drug use either because of withdrawal effects or out of a loss of control that the subject experiences.[359,360] The first marijuana commission[245] defined drug abuse as "the use of psychoactive drugs in a way likely to induce mental dysfunction and disordered behavior." By the second report, the term was discarded altogether: "The Commission believes that the term drug abuse must be deleted from official pronouncements and public policy dialogue. The term has no functional utility and has become no more than an arbitrary codeword for that drug use which is presently considered wrong. Continued use . . . with its emotional overtones, will serve only to perpetuate confused public attitudes about drug using behavior."[246] Another definition of abuse, i.e., the use of a drug to the extent that it interferes with one's health, social, personal, or economic functioning,[18,234,300] when applied to survey research rests upon decisions regarding the frequency and intensity of the drug used relative to anticipated consequences and outcomes of such use—decisions borne out of extensive personal experience with abusers. Such relationships vary from individual to individual, and an experience of an adverse effect implies nothing about an individual's patterns of use or dependency on the drug. Some studies have attempted to distinguish use from abuse on the basis of whether drugs are used under medical "supervision." The personal use of ethical or proprietary drugs, though hardly supervised, is generally time-limited and conservative.[256]

It is perhaps better to discuss drug use in terms of relative risks, and it is sometimes more enlightening, yet somewhat imprecise, to distinguish various *patterns*[246,300] of use such as experimentation, circumstantial-situational use, social, ritual, and recreational use, use for self-medication, intensified use, and compulsive or habitual or habitually episodic use, although at times, in any individual, the distinction between various patterns of use may be blurred. Drugs are used to counteract the effects of other drugs, and often, once a pattern of continued use is established, to ameliorate abstinence effects.

The abuse of drugs is easy to distinguish when a user is in trouble, but far more difficult when discussing large numbers of persons or the less incapacitating patterns. The pattern of use of a drug is determined by the interplay of a number of factors—political, legal, cultural, and economic influences, small and large group phenomena, personal goals, psychic structure and dynamics, family and interpersonal peer-group dynamics, primary and secondary reinforcement effects of the drug, ritual and social setting, as well as the effects of the drug on individual and group processes, and intrinsic factors such as abuse potential, tolerance, withdrawal effects, and adverse reactions. All these interact to determine when a person begins to use a drug, which drug he uses, and when he terminates use or evolves to

a different pattern. Various models, derived from epidemiologic data, personal experience with users, and, occasionally, free access to the drug in a clinical setting,[120,228] have appeared to describe patterns of use.*

Finally, the word drug was often equated with illicit drug, and researchers, as well as the public, had difficulty confronting the general category that would include alcohol and cigarettes. Upon studying the use of these drugs, important findings emerged.[116,246,300]

To be brief, we still do not know who is a "case," i.e., how—abstractly—to define an abuser (who need not be drug dependent) nor how to distinguish with one term the degree of harm of various dependencies. Practically, it is a matter of explicit operational definition: frequency, intensity, and duration of use, the dosage used or the need to increase it, age at introduction to use, number of drugs used, variety of drugs and their abuse liability, route of administration, the frequency of adverse reactions, the presence of an abstinence syndrome or tolerance, user's subjective or objective motivations for use, the occasion and sponsorship of use, social cost, or the effects and experience sought. Can criteria be developed that would predict with a fair degree of accuracy the outcome of a present level of use in terms of eventual morbidity and mortality? These questions, for the most part unanswered, nevertheless are employed in one way or another when a definition has been explicit.

Reliability, Validity, and Sampling Methods

The assessment of reliability and validity, and the sophistication of the sampling methods used, further complicate the design and evaluation of trend research. Problems of *response error* and the *reliability* and *validity* of the data gathered is an almost insurmountable problem when any research on deviant behavior is attempted. The fact that the use of drugs can be an illegal activity, decreases the validity and reliability of the self-report of drug use, particularly if the subject feels that the

* See references 15, 18, 97, 210, 234, 246, 168, 259, 270, 297, 300, and 374.

information that he supplies may eventually affect his ability to obtain more drugs.[240] The reliability and validity of the self-report of drug use and social history is largely unknown. Ball[8] discusses the reliability and validity of interview data obtained from narcotics addicts. Bell[19] reviews the literature on the reliability of the anamnestic interview in matters of the patient's history, and Haggard and associates [131] discuss the reliability of the interview in detail. Stimson and Ogborne[326] discuss the validity of interview data obtained from narcotics addicts. The problem of response error in survey studies raises two alternatives, i.e., anonymous versus identifiable questionnaires. Berg[23] discusses this dilemma in detail. The reliability of survey versus interview techniques for studying drug use is unresearched. Hawks[139] has suggested that the reliability of the self-report needs to be tested with respect to the amount, type, and frequency of drugs used, since it is unknown what effect the drugs themselves may have upon the data gathered. It is conceivable that if a subject is intoxicated with a particular drug, he might be more apt to honestly detail his past and present drug use, particularly if the researcher seems to him to be sympathetic to his drug use; he might also brag about and exaggerate his drug use; on the other hand, he might become suspicious and tend to minimize his use. Hughes and associates[159] cite evidence that the reports of drug use more than one year before the survey is conducted may be inadequate and unreliable. Hughes and associates,[160] Stimson and Ogborne,[326] de Alarcon,[74,75] Hawks,[139,140] and Blum and associates[37,38] have presented the clearest data with respect to the validity and reliability of their research.

Many studies give an inadequate description of their *sampling methods*. The majority have been of student, military, or hospitalized populations and have utilized "samples of opportunity," or word-of-mouth chains of referral.[117,133,300] Such research designs make extrapolations to the universe from which the sample is obtained unfounded. Random sampling, of course, avoids this difficulty, but it increases the numbers of subjects needed, since in many populations drug abuse is a rare phenomenon. Furthermore, some users sampled may simply be too "stoned" to fill out a questionnaire. Thus, it is important to assess the reasons for refusal. Most samples have been of student populations and only a few studies have assessed drug use among adults. Many studies in schools do not include absentees or school dropouts, which may lead to a serious underestimation of drug use.

A neglected and unexplored area is age-specific vulnerabilities to drug use. For example, those between sixteen and twenty-six who are no longer students—at that volatile time of life when roles are altering, identity becoming stabilized, peer relationships changing, where the youth has finished testing himself in the sheltered educational system and is embarking upon self-testing in the adult world, confronted by pressure, conflict and tension over how he is going to "make it," where there is still promise but much risk, and when, for some, it must be a relief to be a failure. These individuals are probably at a high risk to resort to drug use, as well as other "deviant activity."

The Trend Research

Epidemic drug use within a subpopulation changes considerably over time, and most trend studies have failed to specify when in the epidemic they have sampled. Regional and subcultural differences have rarely been stipulated and assessed. Many studies have attempted to find demographic, personal, and family variables that correlate with various patterns of use (see page 566, Research into the Causes). For the most part, demographic data in these trend studies indicate that drug use among youth as well as adults is influenced by age and education, occasionally by sex, and by regional and racial variation. Marijuana is most frequently the first *illicit* drug used and, next to alcohol, the most popular. Illicit drug experience among the general population tends to be greater among whites than nonwhites, among preteens than those over thirty; among those residing in metropolitan rather than in rural areas; among those in the Northeast and West than in the South and North Central areas. Experience with proprietary and ethical drugs is greater among women than men, whites than nonwhites, among persons reporting more formal education, among those in metropolitan areas, and among those residing in the West.[246] Some studies have found a decrease in alcohol consumption correlated with greater marijuana use and others have found no change. A few studies have been able to detect evidence for changing trends of use (see page 565).[134,246] Many studies find a positive relationship between frequency and intensity of drug use and polydrug use, but find that *most* marijuana users do not progress to polydrug use or more dangerous drugs. Many studies describe various patterns of use, and find certain drug combinations to be preferred, e.g., marijuana and hallucinogens among students. A few studies find that a lower age of introduction to illicit drug use correlates with increased chances for future extensive involvement with drugs.

Robins and Murphy[273] were the first to retrospectively study, by interview, drug use within a normal population (urban Negro males) unselected with respect to drug use. Among other issues, they attempted to discover the prevalence of drug use, which drugs were used and at what age their use began, what proportion of drug users became addicted, how age of first drug use related to the eventual extent of use, the rate of recovery from addiction, and what proportion received treatment. Although prevalence findings are dated, this study is a model of that design and answered many questions that later studies merely replicated, often less reliably. Blum and associates[37,38] randomly sampled a middle-class sector of students drawn from five universities in an attempt to determine prevalence and frequency of drug use and to characterize those who use drugs from those who do not. Walters[351] found that within a prestige college population the effects of illicit drug use on academic performance were minimal, and only alcohol use was consistently correlated with lower grades. Other college student populations have been studied by McGlothlin and Cohen,[219] Blum,[37,38] Schaps and Sanders,[284] Pearlman,[257,258] Robbins et al.,[271] Mizner et al.,[240] and Goldstein and Gleason.[116] The second NCMDA report has collected a bibliography of two hundred studies on students.[246] Rouse and Ewing[277] and Glass[111] studied coeds; high school populations were studied by Lombillo and Hain,[210] Kandel,[174] and Hughes et al.[160] Hospitalized patients were studied by Cohen,[65] Bowers,[41] Blumburg et al.,[40] Fischman,[96] and Shearn and Fitzgibbons.[297] Urban adults by Parry,[256] Gottschalk,[122] Mellinger,[226] and Manheimer;[223] high school dropouts by Berg;[23] hippies by Shick et al.[300] and Solomon;[324] political groups by Zaks;[371] medical students by Lipp et al.,[208] and soldiers by Greden and Morgan,[124] Black et al.,[31] and Callan;[53] a free-clinic population by Judd and Mandell;[173] a black ghetto population by Lipscomb;[209] samples of research subjects have been studied by McGlothlin,[219] Blum,[35] and Welpton;[355] and marijuana use among physicians has been studied by Lipp and Benson.[207] Zaks and associates indicated a tendency for the younger users to widen their drug use to many different drugs and for the older groups to constrict their use to one drug, usually marijuana, instead of many.[371]

Robbins and associates[271] have begun to study an especially large sample of students. Only Berg[23] and the second NCMDA report[246] have attempted a compilation of many trend studies, and both discussed the difficulty of comparing such diverse statistics. Drug use has been surveyed as part of a larger study not concerned with drug use in an attempt to get around the bias of researchers and the problem of reliability and validity of the self-report.[134,280] There have been no prospective studies published, although some are in preparation. McGlothlin[216] discussed national estimates of the marijuana market in terms of cost and expenditure, supply, and demand. Smart[305] has reviewed the trend studies on illicit drug use in Canada, and has discussed the log-normal distribution curve for drug use where there are many infrequent users, fewer moderate users, and even fewer heavy users.

Epidemiological Studies

The various trend-survey studies use many diverse measures to obtain data about the trends of drug use, which makes comparison difficult. Practically all studies report who has *ever used* a drug—i.e., the nonmedical use of the drug at least once. This measure includes both past and present use, and the use of drugs in all possible patterns, and it is the measure that is least useful to predict emerging trends. Hughes and associates,[153,159] Hawks,[140,142] de Alarcon,[72,73,74,75] Bejerot,[15] and Bewley[27,28] have all suggested an epidemiological method of standardization by employing incidence, prevalence, frequency, and exposure data derived from the contagious disease epidemiological model. These authors have compiled data about the trends of drug use among various population sectors over time, investigated the mode and rate of speed of heroin use within a community, and discussed the importance of the "initiator," "reinforcing agent," and "pathological prescribers" in communicability of drug use. They explain that *frequency* data (the number of times the person has used the drug illicitly) is helpful in defining patterns of use and ascertaining the numbers of persons who are dependent users—based upon an investigator's definition of dependence. *Prevalence* data indicates current regular use. One measures the active cases of drug use in a given year (or another time period) and this includes new cases as well as active cases. Few surveys include this data. Psychiatric hospital admissions or outpatient indices are of little value in estimating prevalence, since most users try to deal with the complications of drug abuse by themselves, avoiding admission. Psychiatrists may also underreport drug use or utilize other diagnostic labels.[116] Hughes explains that much of the drug use indicated by prevalence rates is due to a small group of multiple drug users. *Incidence* data measures the rate of new cases in a given year. Hughes explains that this measure may give the first clue to the spread of the disorder and also to the decline

of drug use. Very few studies report incidence data: they are difficult data to obtain, and interview effort and organization in case finding is required. The use of incidence data to justify the efficacy of treatment programs can be unwarranted when the decline in drug use is due to a saturation of the target area with the drug. Prevalence data avoids this difficulty.[153,159,160] Berg[23] discusses which studies employ each of these measures. Only Hughes[159,160] reports *remission rates* for polydrug users, although they are commonly employed in heroin research. He finds that remission rates are highest for amphetamines and lowest for marijuana. He cautions that investigators may attribute a favorable remission rate to program effectiveness, when, instead, it may be due to spontaneous remission because of the user's experience with various consequences of drug use, such as adverse reactions. *Relapse rates*, though valuable, have not been studied among polydrug using groups. *Exposure data* (how often a person uses a drug when it is immediately available) would include a concept of "host resistance" to drug use, which might be particularly valuable in understanding ways of preventing the spread of drug use, if the influencing factors could be defined.[159] Hughes finds that one-half of his sample exposed to marijuana in high school do not use the drug.[160] Such data indicate that exposure rates may not be as powerfully predictive of future prevalence and incidence as had been thought before. Exposure is more frequent among users than nonusers; Schaps and Sanders[284] have explained some of the factors involved and note that moderate users are least likely to be in treatment programs. Most studies have suggested that drug epidemics, as well as drug use by individuals, may be self-limiting. What drug and social factors and processes determine this limit within communities and among individuals are still largely unknown.

Current Trends in Drug Use

From currently available epidemiological and trend research, the marijuana commission has sought to describe trends of current illicit drug use among adult and student populations.[245,246] Newly marketed drugs do, at first, cause increased demand if only for experimentation with most drug users, and once demand in a target area is saturated and experimenters satisfy themselves about the effect and experience, incidence of use declines and demand decreases. The commission reports, "In sum [among adults and youth as a whole], the prospect of readily available marijuana elicits no substantial expectation of initiated or increased consumption among the general population."[246] Among secondary-school students the incidence of drug use has increased, and percentage increases in the number of students who have tried the illicit drugs have begun to approach, equal or surpass percentage increases in the incidence of alcohol use. At the college level, the proportion of students who reported ever using alcohol in 1972 declined somewhat, while the proportion who had ever used the other drug types, particularly the hallucinogens and marijuana, continues to increase. High-school students tend to have used hallucinogens more recently than college students, indicating the trend for the use of these drugs to be self-limiting. We are beginning to reach a saturation point in the incidence (ever use) of marijuana use among the college population, and the proportion of those experimenting with and continuing to use marijuana will stabilize and possibly decline within the foreseeable future. Experimentation with inhalants, such as glue and solvents, occurs primarily among junior high-school students. It has remained relatively stable since maximum popularity in 1969, and the use of these substances, once initiated, is quickly extinguished.

Occasional fads of stimulant and depressant use, alone or in combination, occurs sporadically. The use of heroin and other opiates among secondary-school and college students is comparatively low; the largest majority of these persons terminate use of opiates after experimenting with them once or a few times. Only a small proportion go on to become frequent users or reach dependent status.[265] The data on patterns of student drug use attests to the consistent occurrence of these patterns regardless of the location of the survey, the type of student body queried, their age, or the period of time since beginning drug use. Although the population at risk has increased, the relative proportions of frequent and regular drug users drawn from this pool have remained fairly constant.

Future drug use among those who have never used illicit drugs appears unlikely (except for the use of alcohol) and the future plans of those who have tried various drugs at least once are more uncertain and less predictable. The Marijuana Commission reports that most students had already made a decision either to continue using a drug or to discontinue using it; the question of the stability of such decisions is, of course, at issue. With the exception of alcohol, the majority of student drug users generally adopt and maintain patterns of low frequency, and low to moderate intensity, regardless of the duration of use. Furthermore, considerable attrition takes place as the students move from high school to college. Most of the high-intensity users represent the weekend-party marijuana, hallucinogen, hypnotic, or amphetamine user who generally confines taking these drugs to social occasions. Student drug use, though now beginning earlier than in the past, ordinarily remains a short-lived phenomenon, regardless of age or time since onset—except for marijuana and alcohol. Those who maintain relatively heavy and regular drug-usage patterns, particularly with the physical-dependence producing drugs, throughout high school and college stand a much greater chance of extending their drug use into adulthood. The use of any and all illicit or controlled drugs, particularly marijuana, is generally preceded by and highly correlated with the use of alcohol or tobacco. The majority of students generally confine the use of either controlled or illicit drugs to one drug type, although there is a relationship between greater frequency and intensity of drug use and the number of drugs used either concurrently or consecutively.

Conclusions

Epidemiological research, when properly designed and conducted, can yield much useful data about all of the various aspects of drug abuse. Hawks[138] explained that epidemiological research can be useful in describing the history of an epidemic, in providing a community diagnosis of the extent of a problem, patterns, and trends, in researching clues to causes, in ascertaining the individual's chances in terms of morbidity and mortality, in defining the efficacy of treatment programs, and in identifying various consequences and outcomes in terms of specific syndromes encountered. He naturally recommends that hypotheses should be constructed before the data is gathered, since the hypotheses determine the variables selected and "the data collected for wholly empirical ends will only be lent, post hoc, to theoretical rationale."[141]

Ideally, prospective studies of high-risk groups should be designed, and an agency rather than an individual should attempt such research, since long-term studies go beyond the time or ability of individual researchers.[141] Trend data when properly constructed can be useful in identifying new epidemics, new patterns of use, and newly emerging illicit drugs. It can also aid program planners to assess the extent of drug use within their community and, if so designed, the efficacy of intervention programs. The question is, generally, how timely and accurate such studies are. In general, trend studies do little more than illuminate some of the more important factors for further research.

❲ Research into the Causes

Introduction

Freud mentioned intoxication, together with ecstasy, neurosis, psychosis, humor, and self-absorption, as major ways of dealing with stress, danger, and suffering.[107,108] Intoxica-

tion served both the tasks of obtaining pleasure and avoiding pain. Lasting internal, autonomous regulation might provide some protection from suffering—but at the expense of omnipotence and the press for total or immediate satisfaction. Religion, rebellion, chronic intoxication, neurotic illness, and perversion are viewed as bringing some consolation for unsatisfied pleasure.

The bulk of analytic writing rests on a few cases of analytic or psychotherapeutic encounters describing the drug user's personality in a variety of terms. Research based on larger numbers and more extensive experiences has mainly been the trend study. A small though important body of epidemiological research has sought to define who is at risk in terms of demographic and personal variables, and has studied the communicability of patterns of drug consumption.* Both trend- and case-study approaches describe the user's rationale for starting or continuing use. Both attempt to define precipitating causes, and both point to what can broadly be said to be varying degrees of psychiatric difficulty among subpopulations of users. Intrapsychic and family determinants, social causes and reinforcement effects of the drug, the setting and the peer group have been cited to explain drug use. Many investigators touch upon the themes of risk taking and the search for recreation, or the need for both novelty and controls, as inherent in this behavior. Those factors which complicate definitions of the extent of "the problem" also apply to the research into causes.

The subtlety with which various factors can interrelate, and the minor changes in scrutiny and design that can bring one factor or another into focus, is demonstrated by Salzman and associates.[280] They studied hallucinogenic drug continuers and discontinuers. They found that the continuers were both more willing to make high-risk decisions that could impair health or life and also had a greater number of drug experiences than the discontinuers. On the other hand, if the number of drug experiences were held constant, the pre-

* See references 153, 154, 156, 140, 138, 141, 139, 75, 72, 73, and 74.

vious findings were altered and the risk-taking differences disappeared. Then, the continuers scored higher on measure of depression, anxiety, and psychiatric impairment. Thus, research must be flexible enough to notice unexpected findings.

The important fact is that most trend research is primarily of heuristic value in delineating the important variables and understanding which variables among specific groups are critical in the individual's "decision" to use drugs. Beyond asserting that minorities, the youth, and disturbed populations generally emerge in historical, transcultural, or current trend studies as relatively more vulnerable, it may not be a possible goal to specify by category who are members of the group at risk either to begin or to continue drug use, nor in whom the outcome will be constructive or hopelessly injurious. We do not yet fully understand the interrelationship of the broader human elements of the search for novelty, recreation, avoidance, and risk taking that underlie this behavior, as well as many others, nor the age-specific, developmental, neurochemical, or genetic predispositions that favor or oppose the exploitation of drug effects for a variety of purposes. That some persons' drug use seems to be self-limiting, and that for others the severity or intensity continues unchecked or recurrently interferes with organized social function remains unexplained.

Hawks[138] cites causative variables such as maternal deprivation, delinquency, parental separation and bereavement, truancy, social failure, work instability, character deficits, risk taking and precocity. He notes that many are effects as much as causes. Indeed, this is the crux of the problem. Few studies are (or can be) designed to clearly distinguish whether the characteristics found are antecedents, consequences, or independently developed concomitants of drug abuse. Without prospective studies, it is often impossible to decide which are the effects of the drug taking or the membership in a drug-taking clique, and which are the causes for the occasion of drug use itself. Crucially, the weighing of factors and the very delineation of sequences of causal and con-

tributory events mitigates against precision, even though various general constellations of social and psychological factors may be identified with fair confidence. Finally, as with all such discussions of behavior, one must be wary of ascribing motives and specify what is being explained and why. If curiosity is found as a motive, this does not rule out contributory pathological motives underlying it. If such individual pathology is not present, it is likely that continued drug-taking behavior can be more easily dealt with by both the individual and others—including the researcher!

Risk Taking, Recreation, the Search for Novelty and Control

In the present decade of heightened awareness and availability of drugs, many feel that not using LSD or marijuana is like having the electric light and not turning it on. An egalitarian and egocentric access to every available experience, rather than participation in socially prescribed mythical, heroic, or demonic presentations of the human potential, is part of contemporary style. If omnipotence or revealed truth is imprisoned within a pill, why not release it? Such thoughts readily become action, and, with the first act, it seems easier the next time, providing all goes well.

Novelty, risks, and recreation comprise a complicated, relatively unexplored psychology. The active or passive manipulation of a tension and of bodily sensation and action are involved. To control—or command—a change of state is a powerful human motive, tapping private, persevering, primitive, and peremptory wishes. The power of subjectively denying risks, consequences, and reality is not only essential in achieving many altered states and moments of pleasure but—in perspective—is awesome. The alcoholic's enthusiastic anticipation of the next intoxication is, for example, in marked contrast to the dysphoric affect experienced during the later stages of the drug state.[120] Observing drug abuse from the "outside," observer empathy is sometimes difficult, yet the drug-dependent patient gains something in achieving immediate and private change and in being able to act to reproduce it.

To specify both the anticipated and actual reinforcement in the drug state is difficult, and specific drugs may differentially enhance certain rewards (see page 581, Drug-specificity Hypotheses). It is clear that the consumer has some sort of hope for comfort or change that is somehow within his power to achieve; he cannot often correctly perceive what it is that he is gaining, nor regard the costs, even though they may be acknowledged. While speculation has been rife about the various motives enhanced by specific classes of drugs, there is little data on why some do become extensively involved in drug use and others do not, although the roles of magical thought, illusion, and denial are appreciated.

The power and potential of the self-administration of drugs to manage uncertainty is probably critical. The principle of familiarity and constancy is, particularly at the phase of dependency, impressive. The extent to which not only challenge but change can be warded off by ritual is at issue. In infancy, intrinsic barriers against the unwanted are achieved both by biological "screening," intrinsic adaptive features, and by empathic actions and intentions of the mother. The need, of course, both for barriers against stimuli and reassurances is enduring. In this vein psychoanalytic thought has implicated drugs as transitional objects[367] that perform such functions—ones the individual has not yet internalized. The drug state can become an integrating focus, subserving such parental ego functions. Many addicts simply do not feel like themselves without the familiar state produced by the drug. They learn, through the drug experience, ways to cope with stresses and to relate to others. They need only see, think, or encounter these conditioned signals to once again remember their power, their small assured mastery, while functioning in the drugged state. This self-provided "provider"— this deviation from sounder separation and individuation processes—represents the megalomanic and omnipotent power of narcissism,[188,189,190] and a symbiotic and egocentric view of relations that many therapists of alco-

holics, for example, have noted as an issue in treatment.

A person's capacity to interpose a screen and delay between himself and the world, or between himself and his impulses, and to have an assured experience, combine in any event to provide a powerful motive. Whatever our imaginative assumptions about the infant's expectation of omnipotent control of mind and body, observation of maturation indicates he gains control and finds pleasure through control. Similarly, states of feeling can to an extent be self-initiated and controlled.[1] Actions such as masturbation can be employed for mastery, relief, or increased self-esteem. There is a fine line, however, between control and manipulation resulting in mastery, increased self-esteem, decreased vulnerability, and a sense of self and the addiction to the act itself, where the internalization of the ability to regulate states of internal need and tension may be thwarted. This is why drug abuse is particularly disturbing in early adolescence, when bodily change occurs beyond will and control, and authentic mastery may be thwarted and dependency on drugs result. When does the use of drugs, masturbation, fantasy, and thought as trial action to make up for ego defects and to master feeling states serve to temporarily relieve stress and to promote growth, and when does it block growth and mastery? The use of masturbation and fantasy to transiently gain control of emerging sexuality, tenuously regulated self-esteem and aggressive drives until the youth can confidently delay gratification, tolerate aggression and sexual pressure, and develop adequate defenses is generally appreciated. The crucial question for research is when do the effects of drugs block development and when do they facilitate it, i.e., when is the drug for the occasional of testing oneself and recreational intoxication and when is it for dedicated escape?

Many authors have spoken of drug use as a search for novelty, and a correlation between drug use and increase in varied sexual activity may be an expression of this.[351] Some authors, e.g., Miller, have stated that "drugs turn banal thoughts into miraculous ones," and have spoken of the mythology that "boredom is beyond the possibility of being high."[238] The search for novelty is a universal aspect of mammalian behavior, and yet why some humans resort to drugs and others do not (indeed why animals do not—unless exposed) remains incompletely understood. Some users become bored with drug experiences, some turn to other drugs or other routes of administration, while others will decrease their use or stop altogether. Which persons and/or what reason they choose one or another alternative invites research. Why and for how long do some continue their drug use after boredom sets in? Do people repeat the drug experience to master it or merely to perfect it? That is, do certain states of partial discontrol present a challenge to increase the risks time and again with the hope of getting away with it at little or no cost? It would be constructive to learn how people perceive satiety and safety and how to train them (as culture-bound ceremonies somehow do) to do so. This is akin to a similar problem in obesity.[328,370] Drugs and their alternatives as recreational devices are imperfectly understood, and the uses of leisure and creative potential are issues long of concern and of increasing relevance in affluent Western societies.[167,229,296]

In summary, the extent to which man can control mind and body is limited in spite of an infinite capacity to dream to the contrary. Man's ability to recurrently substitute escapism, dream, and fantasy for confrontation with challenge is—banal as it may be to reiterate—astounding. Fantasy may serve a temporary purpose and the outcome may or may not be creative. By implication, research into self-regulatory behavior is important in the understanding of drug use and abuse.

Group Behavior as a Cause

The role of environment and interpersonal factors as contributory to the initiation and perpetuation of drug use has been emphasized; such factors are often a focus in the family or group therapy of alcoholics, for example. No studies have investigated the opposite: what cultural values, environmental variables, and interpersonal interactions serve to negatively reinforce or discourage drug use. What are the attitudinal "barriers" to interest in drug consumption? Such research might lead, if not to effective preventive measures, at least to an understanding of whether, and to what extent, they are important. Research into social causes, peer-group phenomena (including the role of the initiator and "reinforcing agents") the economics of supply and demand, and the group phenomenon of intoxication are relevant component questions. In general, drug use involves others, affecting expectations of performance and reliable response. This reciprocal expectancy means that personal motivations, patterns of use, drug of choice, the drug experience, and its management are, to varying degrees, altered by group processes.

Cultural norms and group ideals are obvious factors affecting both drug distributors and consumers, but they are also potent determinants of what emanates from research circles. The literature on drugs stems from various belief systems—from rationalistic to mystic—and implicit is a conflict of cultural priorities—material gratification, technical power, spiritual belief, or "inter-integration, harmony, and honesty."[369] Drug abuse is thus variously defined as a disease, a cultural menace, an illegal act, a personal freedom, a personal or cultural necessity, or an act of God-like enlightenment. Explicitness about such attitudes and review of them can lead to better designed and more precise research.

The value the individual attaches to the experience has its cognitive, behavioral, and symbolic aspects. The way he manages the effects of the drugs (controls the intoxication, for example) generates consequences. Both beliefs about and the behavior in the drug experience are related to the value placed upon the experience: those factors are also partly conditioned by cultural interpretation. If drugs were totally a private experience, there would not be any problem called drug abuse. But we have to acknowledge and give weight to the social context, as well as unconscious and personal determinants to account for drug abuse in an individual.

Social Causes

Attempts to understand the phenomenon of youthful drug use in the 1960s as part of a wider cultural change have been plentiful, and this is a continuing literature. There has been perhaps an excess of sociological mythologizing of youth, and announcements of new sources of consciousness and ahistorical and apsychological essays have appeared in abundance. Certainly the recent epidemic of drug interest and use has arisen along with other changes in our culture[137] that are elusive and sometimes difficult to describe: the impact of television; the Vietnam War; the very mass of youth flooding our unprepared institutions. A fine balance between empirical and ideological analysis is rare. The question, of course, is the independence or interdependence of cultural changes and the drug epidemic, and the values, ideologies, and behavior of a population variously construed as "youth."

The problems of sample and researcher bias are particularly applicable to this area. Lustman described such problems: "In this literature, students in general and radical students in particular are at one and the same time described as sick or sane; alienated or involved; arrogant or humble; immoral or religious; amoral or endowed with a super-morality which goes beyond the conventional morality; obscene or pure; selfish or generous; violent or gentle; cynical or idealistic."[213] In all such research, one fault stands out from many—the assumption that the participants in the sample actually *know* their motivations and are objective. As Lustman remarked, ". . . this seems a scientific regression to a purely conscious psychology. . . . It is an astonishingly idiosyncratic group of pseudoscientific papers which seems to have been markedly affected by the very political rhetoric and passion it seeks to describe and explain. . . . As a result, we have been left with a wide assortment of speculations: theories based on what students *say*; theories based on what students *feel*; theories based on what students *mean*,

regardless of what they say or feel; and on and on."[213]

Indeed, most of this "research" is little more than educated speculation and impassioned rhetoric by investigators who wittingly or unwittingly share the same convictions, and only rarely are the methods of investigation and the research samples presented and discussed, and rarely is it acknowledged that the apparently novel radical practices of youth have historical precedents.[276]

The youth particularly have attributed (rationalized?) their drug-taking behavior to their discontent with parental values as expressed in the culture. They assert that the old traditions are irrelevant to the modern age. Thus, the concept of a "counterculture"—a subculture of adolescents and young adults that does not emulate the dominant culture as (supposedly) did the youth in previous generations—has emerged. In the spirit of Paul Goodman's *Growing Up Absurd* and David Riesman's *The Lonely Crowd*, Theodore Roszak emerged after earlier prophets such as Timothy Leary as the leading interpreter and champion of the "psychedelic revolution" with his book *The Making of a Counter-Culture*.[276]

He depicts the counterculture as a youthful opposition to the technocratic society—i.e., "The social form in which an industrial society reaches the peak of its organizational integration," and he considers drug use an epiphenomenon of the youthful rebellion. Drugs, he says, are used for "temporary emotional liberation and perceptional diversion" and acknowledges the public's ambivalence—"a strange mixture of permissiveness and resistance." He feels youth have accurately emulated their parents' ideals and parents have blamed drugs for their own irresponsibility. He proposes that drug use will be accepted and integrated into society as a means of social control, if its use becomes divorced from its association with dissent.

Since the early 1960s there has been a continuing discussion of the cultural roots of the drug epidemic and the relationship of drugs to cultural change. Carey,[55] among many others, felt that the use of LSD and marijuana among the "new bohemians" was an expression of protest, grievance, and a "general vague dissatisfaction with the quality of our lives." The youthful population had no other channels through which to express their dissatisfaction, which stemmed from "a sense of powerlessness in the face of inflexible political structures." America's advanced industrialization, increase in urban population, and speed of internal migration, all contributed to the movement.[55] Messer[231] believed that youth perceived an end of an era—i.e., parents have lost their commitment to their own life style and have expressed their dissatisfaction with it. What the youth have done, he believes, is to create a different myth for their own generation, born out of historical and personal necessity in the face of their elders' disillusionment —a myth about which Gutmann[130] recently wrote: "*Somewhere within me, already formed, there is a domain of wholeness, of vital energy, of organic wisdom, of all possibilities and potential.* This perfection does not have to be created; it is there, already formed and waiting for the liberating action that will disperse the boundaries that a corrupt society has set between the mundane self and its reservoir of internal perfection." For him it is an outgrowth of the consumer society—"the consumption of life styles, rather than . . . material goods *per se.*"[130] Many have suggested that the new interest in religion and cosmology betrays such a search for a new ethos and new ideals.[231]

Zinberg[372] proposed that youth look at things with a different cognitive style, stemming from their exposure to McLuhanesque "soft" media, and he explained drug use as a natural outcome of their search for passive entertainment. Blum[36] described the demonology of drug use and how committed users advertise their escape from the fold. Bettelheim[26] described the campus unrest and drug use as the desperate search for meaning among "youth who consider themselves obsolete and are, at the least, peripheral to the economy." He, among others, considered their opposition to cultural norms as acting-out behavior of an oedipal conflict, a position which other authors, such as Keniston[180,181,183,184] and Lustman,[213] opposed as simplistic.

Keniston, in a discussion of drug use and student values, argued that, "In an age of debunking, conventional morality tends to suffice: individuals are pushed to higher levels of work development or to moral regression."[184] He felt that most youth adhered to the highest "post-conventional" morality, although acknowledging that some were morally regressed. But he felt that with most the difficulty lay in an imbalance in other sectors of development: "compassion, sympathy, capacity for love, and empathy."[184]

Adelson[2] faulted Keniston's *Young Radicals,*[182] explaining that in his "determination both to share and validate the radical world view" and his utilizing the "strategy of externalization" he shows "a persistent obtuseness to . . . negative qualities [of the youth]." The "joining of high moral purpose with violence" is common in history and "the moral passions are even more willful and imperious and impatient than the self-serving passions." He acknowledges that we like to think of our young "as possessing exemplary moral vision; it speaks so well of them and equally well of ourselves."

Gutmann[130] discussed the personal and social consequences of the new myth in Eriksonian stages of ego development (identity, intimacy, and generativity): a flight from identity, intimacy without loss, and only a fantasy of generativity. Youth, he says, have reached a premature senility: "they see metaphors and threats of death everywhere."

Many authors have speculated that the reception of the message about drug use and altered states of consciousness, the way it was interpreted, and its meaning to them was due to intrinsic aspects of youth—their confidence and gullibility, the tasks of adolescence, the burden and pain of autonomy, and the wish to escape adulthood or defer it.* Zinberg[372] hypothesized that drug use may be another way of working through a developmental task, and Wenkart[356] has explained drug use and

* See references 84, 85, 86, 87, 25, 278, 295, 293, 294, 322, and 323.

youthful rebellion in terms of E. Durkheim's concept of anomie. Yet other studies—and empirically quite impressive ones—on normal adolescence have noted that the presumptive upheaval of adolescence is far from universally expressed in behavior.[251,194,252,334] Goode[118,119] and Gusfield[129] among others have discussed the marijuana controversy as a political rather than a scientific debate. Just as Gutmann[130] noted that the "figure of the prophetic victim" tends to be politicized. It is, for Goode and Gusfield, an attempt to establish who is in control of power, ideology and morality. Gusfield has explained that public affirmation of a norm expressed the worth and power of a particular subculture vis-à-vis some other one, and that certain forms of deviance, e.g., drug abuse, threaten social norms more than others do. "Where consensus about the norm is lacking, movements for legal restrictions are most likely."[129]

Miller[237,238] described how, in the search for freedom and authenticity, youth turned to drugs, the encounter, romantic ethnicity, mystic philosophy, expressive politics, nomadism, and sexual freedom. He eloquently described one aspect of the problem of modern youth as the dilemma between conflicting ideals—between "hanging loose" and loving, between freedom and commitment.[238]

Freedman discussed the "new authoritarianism,"

. . . where authenticity derived from expertise is viewed with distrust, rejected without scrutiny, and verified data are labeled as a moralistic manipulation to serve the establishment. . . . Our youth appear to value leaders who *believe* in change; yet they simplistically believe that their own limited personal experience constitutes sufficient data not only to guide their personal behavior, but to reform society, if only by destruction of what prevails. . . . This gullibility leads not only to daringly useful "problem-posing," but to foolish risk-taking. . . . Perhaps the useful message is that there are many human complexities with which our technological age has not seriously bothered to grapple. This would require an intensive study of man and his behavioral potential in densely populated and technologically advanced societies for which man's adaptive techniques have never before been tested. [pp. 15–16][99]

The Role of the Peer Group

Knowledge about how drugs affect group interaction and how group interaction affects the drug experience, outcomes and drug-consuming behavior must not only be incorporated into the design, interpretation, and methodology of continuing drug research, but it is important in and of itself. That the effects of drugs can be contagious and that, in moderate dosage, drug effect is influenced by differences among specific individuals, specific situations, and specific tasks was predicted by Nowlis and Nowlis.[250]

Set and setting—terms popularized by Timothy Leary—become code words for how the user's expectations and the setting in which he takes the drug, as well as the cultural norms implicit in the group, affect the experience of being high, the interpretation of that experience, and the various outcomes that are possible.*

Jones,[172,169,170] in three papers, speaks particularly to the problems this raises for psychopharmacologic research methodologies. He speaks of the unreliability of the human assay, the differences of drug effects in the novice and experienced user, and the influence of expectation, setting, and previous drug experience. Some have explored the effects of LSD on group interaction,[304] and others have explored the group processes involved when alcoholics under controlled conditions become inebriated.[120,227,228,330]

Informal social systems can define the way events are to be interpreted and managed during the drug state. When one is intoxicated, the bridge to reality lies in the customs of the group as internalized by the individuals and interpreted by the occasion. Groups can also provide enormous relief from coping, tracking, and decision-making problems—if these problems can be shared. It is the sharing of painful autonomy, through the relaxation of the internal tension of decision making and a certain loss of self, that is characteristic of many shared group experiences.[97,104,105]

* See references 10, 12, 13, 32, 61, 172, 171, 170, and 283.

The social hierarchy within the groups—careers and roles—are also potent determinants of patterns of use, drug of choice, etc. A desire to belong to the group, and for status and power, makes users of some, dealers of others. Drugs can serve as symbols of solidarity as well as initiation, risk, and catastrophe. Youth seem to be more socialized by their peers than the former agencies of socialization—parents, teachers, families, government, and religion. Less willing to accept advice from elders and established agencies, youth continue to believe the shared myths of the "stoned group."

A sociological description of various drug-using groups emerged in studies by Carey,[54, 55,56] Finestone,[90] Sutter,[329] Goode,[117,118,119] Keniston,[180,182,183] Davis,[70,71] Becker,[10,11] Smith,[319,320] Schaps and Sanders,[284] Polsky,[264] and Preble.[266] Carey[54] described in detail the college drug scene, examined the organization of the drug-using colony in terms of involvement, attitudes, relationships, and living arrangements as well as the various roles of manufacturer, distributor, (middle- and top-level dealing) recreational user, and "head." Schaps and Sanders[284] studied various levels of involvement and found that within a college drug-using community, moderate users were the most secretive, and the light and heavy users the least so. They found that moderate users were wary of the "head" who might risk exposure and also wary of the novice who didn't understand the need for secrecy. Keniston[183] described the difference between campus "heads and seekers," and Davis[71] between the "heads and freaks." Becker[10,11] described the assumption of a career in deviance, the cultural context influencing such behavior, and the future of such deviance. Smith, documenting an episode of recent history, described how the wish for status influenced the patterns of use in the world of the Haight-Ashbury "speed freak,"[319] and the various roles involved in the illicit manufacture and distribution of amphetamine.[320] Blum[39] described the dealer in detail. Hughes and associates[154,156] described the social structure of the heroin-copping community; Carey[56] described the hierarchy of

social roles within the college drug scene and the Bay Area speed scene; and Zinberg,[373] the social context of drug use in Vietnam.

There has been some research into the determinants of joining and relinquishing membership within a group where drug use is one of the norms. For example, a person who stops using drugs may still maintain membership in the drug-using social group as long as he has signified in an initial affirmation "through public drug taking initiation and continues to espouse the group's point of view."[35]

Hughes and associates,[158,153] de Alarcon[75,72,73,74] and Hawks,[139] have discussed the various stages of the spread of heroin abuse within a community on the model of a contagious disease. They have discussed the role of an initiator and reinforcer as important to understanding the assumption of drug use by an individual.[72,73,259] Hartmann, Hawks, Blum, and Kandel, among others, discuss the role of siblings in initiating and reinforcing drug use. Drug users are first introduced to a drug by their friends, less often by siblings, and only rarely by persons not acquainted with the user.* Drugs are usually obtained from friends or acquaintances who deal in relatively small quantities, and the roles of dealer and purchaser may reverse themselves when another member of the peer group obtains a relatively larger supply of a drug than his peers.[72,73,54,56,117] McGloghlin discusses the marijuana marketplace on a national scale—annual consumption, source, importation, distribution, and retail expenditures. He discusses enforcement from the standpoint of arrests and seizures, and predicts current trends for the future use of marijuana.[216]

It has been widely asserted during this epidemic that all people, adults included, consume a wide variety of psychoactive medications and that their use has been ever increasing since the introduction of the major tranquilizers in the 1950s. Various authors have supported and refuted the thesis that there is as much abuse of proprietary and ethical drugs among adults as there is with illicit drugs among youth and that drug-using

---

* See references 37, 38, 39, 117, 136, 140, 139, 174, and 284.

youth come from (and are somehow caused by) drug-using parents.[37,38,305] "According to this view, drug use on the part of the young develops in response to parental [psychoactive] drug use."[174] Much of the presumed association between such adolescent and parental behavior, however, has so far been "based exclusively on the youth's perception of their parents' drug use." Kandel[174] has studied the problem with independent data from the adolescent, his parents, and the adolescent's best school friend that clearly indicate that peer influence on adolescent drug use is much stronger than parental influence. "There is a synergistic influence of parents and peers, so that the highest rates of [marijuana use] appear in situations in which both parents and peers use drugs."[174] Such studies, of course, do not answer whether drug use or drug-using friends come first. For such answers longitudinal data are necessary.

The effects of group norms, roles and status, the shared expectations and responsibility for the drug experience, as well as the effects of drug use on the mores and values of the group, combine with the economics of supply, distribution, and demand as well as cultural change to influence patterns of use, research viewpoints, and public response. It appears that a more complete understanding of these processes awaits further research of social-psychological and cultural anthropologists.

Adult Drug Use

The recent drug-abuse epidemic has arisen along with suggestions for changes in the role of government, advertising, and the medical community to protect the drug consumer from risk. There have been demands for free access to drugs and drug information, and the present system of controls and regulations has been called into question. The field of medicine is a reliable institution for researching and dispensing medicinals, but there is a need for social and anthropological research into the functioning of these systems. There has been a demand for evidence about prescribing practices and the consumption of proprietary and ethical drugs, and the results of various

studies are just beginning to emerge.* A number of recent studies have concentrated on the use of medication by adults, and prescribing practices by physicians.[197] Parry and associates[256] find that psychotherapeutic drugs are most often prescribed by general practitioners and internists. They believe that "there is no real evidence that the American people are 'over medicated' with respect to psychotherapeutic drugs, and, in fact, there is considerable evidence that they take them rather sparingly and under physician's orders . . . many of the users take them with . . . puritanical reservations. . . ." Women take such drugs almost twice as frequently as men; drug use is higher in the West; most users felt they were helped by these drugs; and adult drug use depends upon social class and age.

The findings suggest that the popular stereotype (of a pill-popping middle class housewife) has little foundation in fact. It is not among the typical middle class housewives that steady long term use of minor tranquilizers and sedatives is most common, but rather among the poor and least educated housewife.[256]

Mellinger and associates[226] explained that among young people marijuana seems to be an increasingly popular alternative to both alcohol and psychotherapeutic drugs obtained from a physician. Gottschalk and coworkers[122] found that youth tend to most frequently take stimulants, while adults seem to receive sedatives and analgesics from their physicians. Mellinger and associates[226] commented on the finding that young people tend to bypass the physician more often than adults to obtain drugs, and youth tend to downgrade the importance and relevance of medical judgments about the safety and specific indications of drugs.

There is public ambivalence about the role of the physician as a reliable dispenser of drugs. Although the role of the "pathologic prescriber" is well known, the prevalence of this phenomenon is unresearched.[72,74] How different sectors of the society treat the trend to trivialize drugs as a mere convenience or device is at issue. There have emerged cries to

* See references 122, 197, 223, 226, 242, and 256.

let people medicate themselves[13] to train paraprofessionals to dispense medication and become drug counselors[242] and on the other hand, to invoke limited licensure among physicians.[103] Muller[242] has described the forces in the marketplace of drugs and how the doctor, drug company, physician, pharmacist, and the hospital all make decisions based on factors and alternatives peculiar to their vested interests.

Certainly the individual's use of and access to trained professionals must be investigated, as well as approaches to a better reciprocal exchange of information between professional and laiety in the appropriate uses of medication. Yet the gap cannot be bridged completely. Professionals must make certain judgments borne out of experience, and they must count on the fact that both customs and social functions, including religion and recreational drugs, help people to solve, redefine, or contain some of their dilemmas and impulses. We could not, as a profession, adjudicate every anxiety to which people are prone. Individuals must learn to diagnose their own conditions, learn to tolerate and interpret pain and anxiety and define the reasons through extramedical resources. Intelligent or wise self-medication has a social role.[104] The extent to which psychotherapeutic drugs are abused is a question, and although such abuse appears in literature on occasion,[268] for the most part Americans tend to be conservative in their use of psychoactive drugs.

There is still little data about what social changes induce people to use drugs, cease their use, change drugs or prescribers, or move from legal to illicit sources, and the economics of this: the forces in the marketplace and the problems of supply, demand, and control invite research.

Rationales and Precipitants for Drug Use

Personal rationales for drug use have been investigated in an attempt to discover why people use illicit drugs. Most users have already begun drug use with alcohol or tobacco before trying illicit drugs, although this sequence may be changing.* No studies have inquired into the user's rationale for beginning alcohol or tobacco. Curiosity, experimentation, and challenge, the search for pleasure or meaning, self-discovery, heightened awareness, more meaningful communication with others and intimacy, violation of parental or societal standards, seeking answers to philosophical or personal problems, proof of maturity, intellectual depth and flexibility, enhancement of sexual pleasure and artistic creativity, and the production of mystical experiences, as well as the desire to go along with the peer group have all been listed by users as rationales to start or continue their illicit drug use.† Amphetamine use is generally associated with more specific rationales: to facilitate study, to control weight, or to ease tension.[240,271,371]

Mizner found that the rationales given for starting, as opposed to continuing drug use, are different.[240] Schaps and Sanders[284] explained that students had difficulty giving reasons for starting, but no difficulties giving rationales for continuing. As a subject's level of drug use increased, there was a greater use of rationales other than pleasure, since their sample of college students felt that these "more constructive rationales" were for them the more compelling reasons—given, the authors felt, out of a need to justify the violation of the larger group's reference standards. They also speculated that students may offer more compelling arguments, since they are more articulate and sophisticated, not necessarily more logical, than other groups. Curiosity as a rationale for beginning to use drugs is more often listed by older users than by younger ones.[371] For younger users, the desire to go along with the group and the use of drugs for pure pleasure are rationales most frequently found. Fads of a particular drug type or pattern of use within a community may also influence motivation. Mizner found that in trying to determine reasons for discontinuing the drug use, there is the greatest difficulty—62 percent of his sample checked

---

* See references 35, 66, 160, 271, 273, and 300.

† See references 51, 54, 206, 217, 240, 260, 271, and 371.

reasons other than those listed.[240] Motivations to discontinue drug use, although for the
most part unresearched, include experience of
adverse reactions,[176] hospitalization, the
user's awareness of his drug dependence, or
the fact that the drug experience did not live
up to expectations; include economic considerations, such as increase in cost or decrease in
supply, increase in the pressure from law-
enforcement agencies, or perhaps his guilt or
shame over drug use.[97,222] Motivations to relapse among polydrug users have not been
studied.

A much more important question, rarely
addressed, is whether the rationales given are
the same as objective motivations or precipitating causes, and will such questions asked of
users give us valid data as to why people start
or continue? Is not such trend research as we
have described investigating justification and
not motivations?

In an effort to objectively assess motivations
for use, various authors have investigated precipitants and environmental stress surrounding the onset of use or abuse. Stubbs has investigated environmental stress during the
formative years of young drug abusers.[327]
Whitlock has investigated precipitants in barbiturate dependence.[358] Glickman and Blumenfield have noted that their sample of fifteen patients, who were seen in a psychiatric
emergency area, had begun LSD ingestion at
a time of a sense of inadequacy in dealing
with a life crisis where "either greater pressure
was placed on the patient to assume a more
demanding and responsible adult role, or a
previously existing prop to the patient's self-
image as a mature and adequate adult was
lost."[114] Bell[19] explained that many users
commence the abuse of a drug after many
months or years of moderate use. He feels that
a precipitant—defined as a new circumstance,
associated in time with the onset of addiction,
that has some deeper psychological significance for the patient—is required to explain
the change in susceptibility of the individual
addict through time. He discovered precipitants in thirty-four of forty cases of amphetamine abuse, closely linked in time to the onset
of addiction, that, in twelve cases, resulted in

a "change in the patient's environment, allowing ready access to amphetamines for the first
time." He found the precipitants to be commonplace, yet stressful, life events of two
general types: rejection or separation from a
loved or admired object, and the transition to
a more demanding adult role. Both seemed to
resonate with important factors in the patient's psychological genetics and dynamics.

Although the determination of "precipitants" for investigating drug use or abuse are
useful in understanding and treating (see
page 590) this problem, such events are not
always traceable—group legitimatization of
drug-taking behavior can work and outweigh
many individual determinants and can make
determination of individual factors operationally sometimes impossible to define. This problem is not intrinsically different from sorting
out the necessary or sufficient precipitating life
events operative in any other psychiatric disorder. The user's verbalized rationales for
starting and continuing drug use have been
adequately researched; more objective interview studies are now needed to determine
possible precipitants surrounding the onset of
intensified use.

The question of who is at high risk to abuse
drugs has received scant attention. Who is at
risk to *begin* illicit drug use is unresearched
and might provide useful data about targeting
of preventive measures. Such data could provide a more efficient way of investigating the
more subtle psychological and social factors
involved in drug-abuse propensity.[141] There
are a number of retrospective studies of risk.
Robins and Murphy[273] studied a normal
population of urban Negro boys and found
that the earlier drug use begins, the greater
was the risk of going on to use heroin or amphetamines, the greater was the variety of
drugs eventually used, and the greater was the
risk of addiction or regular use; poor high-
school attendance and dropping out before
graduation were related to moving from marijuana to a more serious drug; delinquency
predicted a high risk of heroin use or heroin
addiction subsequently; socioeconomic status
and elementary-school performance did not
predict drug use, but the combination of an

absent father, delinquency, and dropping out of high school characterized a group of Negro boys who had a high risk of heroin addiction. More recent studies have often replicated these findings. Blum and associates[38] have concentrated on student responses on a "willingness" scale; earlier age of onset of illicit drug use (as well as alcohol and tobacco) correlates with high risk.[66,300,140] Many studies suggest that the occurrence of psychiatric difficulty, especially the diagnosis of antisocial personality disorder denotes a potential risk for drug abuse.[133] The question with such studies is whether the measures derived are reliable and valid over time and among different socioeconomic groups and subgroups of users.

Psychiatric Impairments

Implications of psychiatrically significant impairments associated with drug use are pertinent—whether from psychological measures, self-assessment, or observer data obtained from interviews—particularly in seriously dependent, individual drug users; from retrospective studies of populations at risk; or from unfiltered accounts of drug use in India and the Middle East. Yet whether the psychiatric difficulty, apart from toxic psychoses, predates the drug use or is subsequent is ultimately unanswerable except with prospective studies. Inquiry into neuropharmacological factors and organic damage is also relevant. Retrospective studies and post hoc case reports can do little more than provide shrewd speculation and leads about sequence, although certain findings such as truancy, sexual deviation, low grades in school, family difficulties, psychiatric help, school phobias, bed wetting, suicidal attempts, and the like among drug users prior to their first use of drugs tend to support a notion of preexisting pathology, at least in a fair number of dedicated users.[133]

The reliability and validity of the surveys, questionnaires, or interviews used are, of course, an issue. Drug users may have a need to deny psychiatric difficulties.[240,271] On the other hand, some people, especially contemporary students, are quick to admit confusion,

anger, anxieties, and problems, and "given a list of neurotic symptoms, may check them all."[183] Furthermore, students tend to define discomfort in sociological terms rather than by specific subjective symptoms.[351] As illicit drug use becomes more socially acceptable and the prevalence of drug use increases, the determination of "pathology" purely on the fact of illicit drug use becomes less valid.[134] Studies that contrast marijuana users to nonusers, especially in student populations, and attempt to assess differences in psychiatric difficulty, have rarely been able to detect significant differences for this very reason.[133,233,239]

High scores on measures of depression, anxiety, and neuroticism, self-descriptions of moodiness and unhappiness, visits to a psychiatrist, unusual sexual or aggressive activity, and problems with school or police authorities, have all been found among drug users and thought to indicate psychiatric difficulty.* A recent study by Halikas et al., interviewing a sample referred to them by word-of-mouth chains that consisted of one hundred regular marijuana users and fifty nonusing friends, found a strikingly high incidence of "definite" or "probable" psychopathology in *both* groups, and the incidence of psychiatric hospitalization and psychotherapy was about equal. They were able to determine that in most cases diagnosed psychiatric illness began before first marijuana use. Sociopathy did distinguish the two groups, appearing significantly more among the users.[133]

Particularly in the early phases of the recent epidemic, illicit drug use was "antisocial" in the sense that it was not normative behavior for the culture at large. But personality diagnosis based on behavior during an epidemic is not reliable. In some, drug use is clearly linked to a primary character problem of sociopathy, yet in others their antisocial acts seem to be confined to the realm of procuring and administering the drug, and this has been labeled "secondary deviance."[11,59,204] Others lose control during the drug intoxication, and as a result of the drug effects and/or group pressure,

* See references 66, 65, 134, 142, 183, 271, 351, and 274.

commit acts that are generally ego-alien and will display affects and impulses otherwise relatively controlled. The diagnosis of sociopathy is still highly debated; criteria for diagnosis must be accurately specified.[89,133]

Sociologists have consistently pointed out that labeling a person as deviant or criminal has important social and psychological ramifications for his own self-image and in the perpetuation of such behavior.[11,59,80,18] Even so, there is some evidence that among sociopathic individuals, and samples of incarcerated heroin addicts, the threat of further punishment, incarceration, and supervised parole seems to be a decisive factor in remission and improvement.[348,349,273] Among Robins' sample,[273] the first encounter with drugs was usually reported to have occurred in prison. Research into such phenomena as the hyperkinetic disorders among children show that some children may be quite disadvantaged in their ability to exercise self-control and are at risk of various "deviant" outcomes, including, perhaps, drug use.[229,230,354] Some have sought to define biobehavioral correlates of sociopathy as did Silverman, who suggests that ". . . cues which were ordinarily salient for other individuals are not sufficiently salient to capture the attention of psychopaths," and has suggested that drug use, particularly with stimulants and hallucinogens, serves to increase arousal.[303]

Closer scrutiny of the alcoholic[368,285] has enabled a separation between a primary disorder of alcoholism and alcoholism secondary to an underlying psychiatric illness that predated the onset of alcoholism. Many secondary alcoholic females show a primary affective disorder, developed independently or prior to the abuse of alcohol, and such studies indicate that alcoholism and antisocial behavior are highly correlated, more commonly in men than women.[368,285] Similar findings upon closer scrutiny of other forms of serious drug abuse would be anticipated.[133]

It seems clear that drugs may be used by some individuals as self-medication, where the regular or habitual user is treating himself: phobias, anxiety, depression, disorganization, and even schizophrenia. Some manage to be productive with such self-medication; for them, the only issue is the price.

Drug-abuse Personality

There is a continuing search for aspects of the drug abuser's personality that uniquely determine his preference for drugs as coping mechanisms. Why users have resorted to drugs and why nonusers with similar psychopathology have found other means to satisfy their needs is, at bottom, still unknown. It appears fruitless to expect to find a unique personality type who abuses drugs. On the other hand, in-depth elucidation of drug abusers' personalities may eventually highlight personality aspects and environmental variables that place a person in a high-risk category for drug use. Careful observation during the psychotherapy of suitable individuals may potentially prove useful for illuminating the most important treatment techniques, rationales, and decisions.

In his recent review of the pertinent psychoanalytic literature, Yorke has observed that particularly the early writers have concentrated on the impulse side of the problem; for example, ". . . not the toxic agent, but the impulse to use it, makes an addict of a given individual."[370] Wurmser,[369] Kohut,[189] Wikler and Rasor,[363] Welpton,[355] Calef and associates,[52] Gryler and Kempner,[128] Hartmann,[136] Bowers and associates,[44,45] Freedman,[97] Fischmann,[96] Weider and Kaplan,[352] Khantzian,[185] Chein,[59] Savitt,[282] and Pittel[262,261] have all recently written about the personality of one class or another of drug abusers. There is, in all, much agreement about the personality of those who abuse illicit drugs. Yet most samples are skewed toward hospitalized patients or patients seen in treatment, and few studies have investigated the personality of users not in treatment or who have appeared in crisis at some medical facility. A study such as Offer's on normal adolescents is a model for such future research.[251,252] Blacker and associates did study chronic users of LSD who were paid volunteers not in psychotherapy. "Although the . . . beliefs of chronic LSD users and schizophrenics are similar, . . . the clinical picture of . . . relatively intact interpersonal relationships and cognitive abilities suggests that these subjects are more similar to individuals usually termed eccentric than to individuals diagnosed as schizophrenic."[33]

E. Glover introduced the concept that drug abuse is a repair activity akin to that found in the psychoses, and has placed the syndrome in the diagnostic context of the transitional states between psychosis and psychoneuroses, as are the perversions.[370] Buckman,[51] Blos,[34] Vaillant,[348] Erikson,[84,85,86] Solnit,[323,322] and Settlage[293,294] specifically discuss drug use as part of adolescent development. Savitt,[282] on the other hand, recognizes that addiction as a symptom can occur in a variety of conditions such as schizophrenia, depressive states, psychoneuroses, character disorders, perversions, and borderline states. As Yorke says:

> . . . a somewhat abnormal ego must, at the very least, be involved, and that is, moreover, an ego with a rather curious kind of reality testing . . . the addict's disregard for reality is more generalized than the neurotic's, though it remains more adequate when it comes to obtaining supplies.[370]

Radford and associates focused on the diagnostic status of addicts, utilizing Anna Freud's diagnostic profile,[269] and indicated the promising directions of future research.

Drug abusers are commonly characterized as individuals who are often depressed, who have a low tolerance for frustration, are deficient in their capacity to delay gratification, and who have a dearth of meaningful and satisfying object relationships with others. They use drugs to maintain their sense of self-regard, to experience exalted states of fusion or merger, and to temporarily lessen intrapsychic conflict and feelings of depression or anxiety. Many writers agree that abusers have serious pathology in the narcissistic realm, i.e., in the maintenance of stable feelings of self-regard,[189] and recent theorists generally explain that drugs ameliorate ego defects in cognitive functions, affect, and impulse control, object relationships and superego functions.[52,128] Furthermore, drugs help satisfy a search for intimacy of the narcissistic type,

where there is a need to feel the same as others, and a wish for fusion or merger experiences with an idealized object.[189,136,370] Drug abusers are passive individuals who have difficulty in expressing neutralized aggression. Yorke comments that Glover most satisfactorily discussed the role of the superego, aggression, and sadism in the personalities of addicts.[370] For some, the drug seems to decrease uncontrolled outbursts of rage; others feel that they can express aggression more easily when using the drugs. Freedman and Blacker and associates speculate that among LSD users passivity and avoidance of aggression is a learned consequence of the use of psychedelics.[97,33]

Analysts reconstruct that in the narcissistic line of development, individuals who abuse drugs have experienced a sudden loss, severe frustrations, or traumatic disappointments in their relationships with their parents, who at an early age are experienced as idealized objects, not yet distinct from the person's own self-feelings. The parents have not been sufficiently empathic to the child's need for them as an adequate stimulus barrier or supplier of tension-relieving gratification at critical early periods. Taking (in) drugs symbolizes and partially gratifies a need to replace a disappointing unempathic parent or one who died or was lost through separation, divorce, or hospitalization; and it may be an unconscious motivation.[136] Hartmann found traumatic childhood histories involving deaths, severe illness, or operations among the genetic determinants.[136] The failure to phase—appropriately incorporate and internalize the idealized object, which in early childhood the parent represents—results in an ego structure that is defective in its ability to regulate a sense of well-being, to tolerate frustration, to delay gratification, and to live up to an ego ideal.[34,295]

Drug abusers appear to have impairments in their capacity for close, tender object relationships. They report a profound sense of psychological distance from others, which often predates their drug use. Many user's social contacts appear to be superficial, primarily with other individuals who take drugs. The drugs provide not only a sense of belonging to a group but also a consensual validation for the alienation that they feel from their parents, peers, themselves, and society as a whole.[25] Sexual relationships are usually infantile. Whether homosexual or heterosexual, they tend to be on an narcissistic, masturbatory level rather than intimate, emotional relationships with specific partners. Conflict in therapy seems to be in terms of "risking exposure of tender feelings and becoming vulnerable to some sort of rejection."[64]

The difficulty with drug experiences is that, although they temporarily provide gratifying affective experiences and often decrease the need for defensive operations, generally people are unable to assimilate such experiences in a way that would add to their psychological structure and modify ego defects. The drug experience is a prescribed time when reality testing and the inhibitions that reality imposes may be relinquished in favor of gratification through the expression of narcissistic grandiosity in fantasy, fusion, or omnipotent control over mind and body.

Some studies have concentrated on the self-destructive aspects of drug abuse and the suicidal ideation that accompanies massive doses. Often the anxiety users describe prior to ingesting a drug, or in the beginning of a drug experience—particularly with the psychedelics—is the result of threatened ego disruption, annihilation, and fragmentation,[189] which seems to be part of the psychedelic experience in particular. Drug abuse (and particularly self-destructive behavior) concerns important people in the user's environment. It tends to bring these need-satisfying objects closer to them.[64]

Drug use is found in better-organized individuals as well as extremely disorganized ones, and plenty of healthy individuals get drawn into the drug movement. Individuals who are at ease with intimacy and whose egos function more or less adequately generally use drugs in defiance of their parents or therapists to reassure themselves of their autonomy and personal definition, or out of peer-group pressure.[187]

Often associated with drug use in these individuals are feelings of guilt or shame over loss of control that tempts them to engage in acts that are ego-alien and do not measure up to their ego ideal. Such temptations may contribute to acute anxiety reactions during the intoxication or to depression after the intoxication has terminated. Borderline or psychotic individuals often use drugs in extreme amounts to reinstate feelings of closeness through merger and fusion experiences, to narcotize themselves against the psychic pain they feel, and sometimes in an attempt to feel something, even if that means to feel painfully, in order to break through the depths of despair and hollow, empty feelings. Lindeman and Clark stress the role of different drugs in providing a specific compensatory ego integration.[202,187]

In all drug-dependent individuals, the importance of magical wishes and demands is clear. They seem to be governed by a requirement for some kind of perfection, an uninterrupted and unchallenged serenity that also permeates their ideal demands for performance. This, of course, cannot be achieved in reality. Some of these individuals transfer their notions of power and perfection to the drug, the physician, or some other idol to whom they ascribe a sort of eternal presence, power, and perfection. They then become angry and crushed at the slightest disappointment either in themselves or in the idealized other. They engage in magical manipulations of supplies and needs. This is often socially evident as charm or blarney as the addict expresses his preoccupation with bringing others into the orbit of his control and inflated self-esteem. Narcissistic rage[190] and frustration over failure and the lack of assured protection along with the inability to perceive how others manage their imperfections, all are quite characteristic. All these factors refer to the same eternal problem: that man is indeed limited, his capacity to perceive perfection is not identical to prescription for real life, and, in all of this, the actual power to take the drug and its availability, no matter how this fact is masked, is crucial.

Drug-specificity Hypotheses

Drug users are a heterogeneous lot. Beyond certain general similarities in their personalities and behavior, the fact that they use illicit drugs—often multiple types of drugs—tempts investigators to group them together for purposes of diagnosis and treatment. Although multiple drug use is common, drug-specificity hypotheses have been proposed to explain that many individuals have a drug of choice.*

Most theories neglect the importance of changing patterns of drug use and the peer group and social determinants involved in the subject's choice of drugs. Nevertheless, such drug specificity implications seem operative at least in part. Griffith Edwards' personal communication notes that pharmacologic effects of specific drugs differ in terms of behavioral plasticity or variability. In terms of expected behavior sedatives, including alcohol and marijuana, have the most variable effects; heroin moderately so; and stimulants, the least variability. Freedman notes that the effect of LSD is to enhance variability, which nevertheless does not obliterate a basic sequence and patterning of drug effects.[97] Weider and Kaplan explained that withdrawal and the search for the relief-giving drug "induces artificial drive structures with their own rhythms and periodicity."[16,352] They discussed drug choice in terms of its psychodynamic meaning in a paper derived from intensive psychotherapeutic experiences with drug-using adolescents.[352] Alcohol and marijuana in low doses "lessen defenses against drive and impulse discharge," and increase internal and external perception while leading to increased propensity for sexual and aggressive discharge in action. LSD and related drugs induced regressive states of "union, reunion and fusion with the lost or yearned for object." Opiates seem to recover a "lost state of oneness with the drive-channeling, tension-reducing, idealized object where motor activity and perceptual input is diminished." Amphetamines and cocaine subserved

* See references 96, 99, 202, 214, 262, 300, 352, 363, and 369.

in their model a denial of passivity and a "real or illusory chemical increment in drive pressure," as well as reinforcing autonomous ego function, leading to increased self-assertiveness, self-esteem and frustration tolerance, while at the same time decreasing judgment and accuracy. Wurmser[369] explained:

[narcotics] appear to reduce the sensitivity and vulnerability to disappointment and to calm . . . anger. Amphetamines and cocaine . . . eliminate the sense of boredom and emptiness caused by the repression of feelings of rage and shame; and they give . . . a feeling of aggressive mastery, control, invincibility and grandeur. Psychedelic drugs have in common with the amphetamines their effect as antidotes to boredom, emptiness and meaninglessness. Also they reestablish an omnipotent, grandiose position but one centered less on aggressive mastery than on passive receptive merger through the senses. [pp. 17–18]

Fischmann found that among amphetamine addicts the preference for stimulants was determined "by the combined influence of cost, legal status of the drug, and their specific type of action . . . [and suggests] that the energizing effect was by far the most important motive for choice."[96] McCubbin disagrees with such generalizations. To him they suggest that internal psychodynamic needs can override pharmacogenic effects. He observes that most users show dramatic changes in drug preferences, not accompanied by dramatic changes in psychodynamics.[214]

A high dose of a drug generally produces the more typical drug effects, while a low dose increases the influence of situational and personality factors. Particularly among latency children and adolescents, "paradoxical" drug effects are often noted with low doses of amphetamines and barbituates.[229,230,354] McCubbin has evidence that they also occur with the psychedelic drugs.[214]

Although the meaning of the drug effects to the patient cannot be ignored and could lead to a deepened understanding of the dynamics of choice (and perhaps even quite useful treatment interventions) such differences are often obscured in the present, rapidly fluctuating, drug-abuse scene where social considerations, drug popularity and fad, and drug use to treat the side-effects and withdrawal syndromes of other drugs are often more important determinants of a person's drug choice at any one time.[300]

Family Characteristics

Characteristics of the drug user's family have been studied to find predictive factors that would place a child in a high-risk category. Trend studies of data obtained from users in the form of surveys or structured interviews, as well as a few case studies, have been the primary mode of research in this area. In such studies, one must ask to what extent the user's perception of his parent's drug use influences the data gathered and, therefore, how valid and reliable that data is. Adolescents who use illicit drugs *are* more likely to *report* that their parents use tranquilizers, amphetamines, or barbituates. But the validity of such reports is at issue.[174] It is a common supposition that the young who are reared in this culture and who see their parents using psychotropic drugs come to share the same behavior and start using mood-changing drugs themselves, albeit illicitly.[38,305] Kandel studied the relative importance of the parents, compared to peer-group and sibling influence, in introducing the subject to drugs and in perpetuating this behavior. She finds that among adolescent marijuana users, parental influence is relatively small compared to the influence of peers.[174] (see page 572, The Role of the Peer Group).

Family pathology is found among users, especially delinquent ones. Hawks investigated abusers of methylamphetamine. He found drinking problems, criminal behavior, and having consulted a psychiatrist were more prevalent among the subjects' fathers than mothers. A smaller percentage of the abusers' siblings had similar difficulties.[140] Robins and Murphy's investigation of drug use in a normal population of young Negro men found that among delinquents and dropouts the father had been absent at some time during elementary school—a factor that was rather acutely related to the risk of heroin addiction once any drug had been tried.[273] Data obtained from users often show a high incidence of parental loss or separation, particularly at an early age or during adolescence, that can often be associated in time with the onset of addiction.[19,37,38,138]

More extensive descriptions of such family pathology are available. Hartmann finds that in the twelve cases of drug-taking adolescents studied, there seemed to be more pathology among the mothers than the fathers. "Infantile libido and superego development prevailed among the mothers; with regard to aggression, the fathers seemed to show more controlled, the mothers more uncontrolled, aggression; seductive behavior was much more prevalent among the mothers; inconsistency and distance, more among the fathers."[136] Cohen and associates studied a group of adolescents referred for treatment of drug problems. They randomly selected a control group referred for other reasons. They found that although both groups had "disidentified" with their fathers and had lacked strong paternal ties, the group referred for drug problems "also disidentified with their mothers, whom they described as strong, narcissistic, and managerial." However, the authors felt that the homes would not be described as pathological, "since both parents were self-reliant, behaving adequately by societal standards, and living their lives in the pursuit of socially approved goals. Underlying this image, however, is often a family characterized by emotional, environmental deprivation and communication deficiencies."[64]

Blum and associates'[37,38] recent studies concentrate specifically on the family as a predictor of drug abuse among students. Contained therein is a review of the issues involved in such family studies and the pertinent literature. They randomly selected 101 white, middle-class families from the files of a university and interviewed the family and the student. On the basis of their offspring's drug history, families were classified as low-, moderate-, and high-drug-risk families. High-risk families used more prescribed medications and more alcohol and cigarettes than low-risk families. They were generally more permissive, less religiously involved, less cohesive.

They put less emphasis on child rearing, belief in God, and self-control than low-risk families. Traditional families of authoritarian fathers, emphasizing obedience and self-control, characterized low-risk families. The authors felt that such family factors "had a major predictive power for drug risk." The drug-using children of high-risk families had "more infant-health and feeding problems, more childhood-health problems, longer hospitalizations, and more psychosomatic disorders (bedwetting and headaches) . . . [they] receive more over-the-counter remedies of every sort and are given tranquilizers and, occasionally, alcohol, as infants and young children." They seem to "suffer from psychological problems during their youth and often cause their mothers to worry about their conduct. Mother–child relationships appear to be stressful for both," and occasionally mothers of high-risk youth applied food deprivation as punishment.[38]

The implication from Blum's study that family factors can prove predictive of drug risk among offspring needs adequate testing. It raises the question of how universal such "family factors" might be for other samples. The authors were able to construct a list of 176 items of family characteristics and narrow it down to thirteen items that they felt would be 75 percent accurate in predicting risk of drug use. These items were, however, bound to socioeconomic class; they were not reliable when applied to blue-collar or Mexican-American families.[38]

Blum attempted to show that the statistical surface measures, predictive of drug risk, reflected the family interior; he studied the family dynamics of thirteen families. In low-risk families, love, forgiveness for failure, physical expressions of affections, were emphasized, and criticisms of an offspring's mistakes centered on the mistake rather than on the child himself. Opposite findings were noted for high-risk families.[38] Vaillant, in a twelve-year follow-up of narcotics addicts, found that family pathology seemed unrelated to the outcome of eventual abstinence.[348,349]

The idea that drug-using youth come from families where parents use psychotropic drugs is a notion that has been both supported and refuted by various studies. It is certainly not a sufficient condition, nor is it, perhaps, even a necessary one for drug-using behavior to evolve. Family pathology and broken homes are prevalent findings in any study of deviant behavior, including mental illness, and there is little evidence that families of drug users are uniquely different from those of other psychiatric patients. Finally, the family constellation to be predictive must be predictive of some later condition that, in turn, will be related to current (and other) factors leading to some aspect of drug-taking behavior: the problem is to specify these sequences more sharply than with generalities about early experience and drug abuse.

Operant Conditioning Models of Drug Dependence

Experimental work on animals administered psychoactive drugs on various schedules of reinforcement—work pioneered by Wikler—has made an important contribution to the understanding of drug dependence, the development of tolerance, the effects of withdrawal, factors influencing relapse, and the assessment of abuse potential.* As Schuster and Thompson[287] have noted, such methods have "the obvious advantage of greater experimental control . . . and the investigator using infra-human organisms is less likely to invoke untestable mentalistic constructs as the factors generating the self-administration of drugs." These studies, based on behavioral conditioning models, "seek to determine the biological and environmental variables which modify a drug's reinforcing efficacy, that is, the extent to which a drug is self-administered."[287]

Primary reinforcement effects of various classes of psychoactive drugs have been intensively studied and compared, and Schuster and Thompson review this literature.[287] Deneau and coworkers compared the various classes of drugs usually abused by humans and found that those which appear to have the least abuse potential in humans, including chlorpromazine and mescaline, will not be self-

* See references 288, 287, 286, 359, 360, 361, 362, 115, and 78.

administered by monkeys. Cocaine and amphetamine will be self-administered by animals at very regular cyclical intervals, reminiscent of the high-dose cyclical pattern of intravenous amphetamine abuse in humans.[78,287]

Individual differences in the extent to which animals and humans become dependent on drugs, and display psychotoxicity or withdrawal, implicate various genetic (metabolic) sex and age variables with an unknown basis. These variables have been researched in animals.[287,288] Once physical dependence on opiates develops in animals, the reinforcement efficacy of the drug is amplified by the effect of withdrawal. However, the drive-reduction model of reinforcement, i.e., that abusers continue administering heroin in order to avoid the effects of withdrawal, is called into question, since physical dependence is not a necessary condition for opiates to act as reinforcers, and the drug can reinforce behavior independently of its ability to relieve abstinence.[362]

Various kinds of behavior and experience— particularly those in close temporal association with the drug taking—such as the rituals of "shooting up," procuring the drug, the neighborhood or room where the user takes the drug, or his associates, are associated with the primary reinforcement of the drug and become secondary reinforcers; when these are encountered again, even long after withdrawal, they may contribute to relapse. This is the basis for Wikler's "hustling theory."[360] Such observations have produced greater understanding about the determinants of the recurrent nature of drug-taking behavior and its intransigence. The acquired reinforcing effects of the ritual, setting, or acquaintances diminishes as extinction proceeds, but mere detoxification does not result in extinction of these conditioned responses. In treatment, active extinction, i.e., repeated elicitation of the conditioned response by the appropriate stimuli, is needed under conditions that preclude its reinforcing effects.[115,362] This is less difficult for opiates since the advent of methadone blockade and the development of narcotic antagonists, but it poses some research problems for nonnarcotic drugs. How, for in-

stance, could the reinforcement effect of a user's associates, home, or injection ritual, be actively extinguished? How effective would such procedures be in maintaining abstinence? No such studies of either opiate or nonnarcotic users have appeared.

Researchers have studied opiate abstinence and defined a primary as well as a secondary phase.[288,287] In humans the primary phase of opiate abstinence lasts for several months, followed by a secondary phase that lasts for at least an additional four months.[362] Whether the secondary abstinence stage is a major variable contributing to relapse, and what neurochemical mechanisms may be operating, must be determined, as well as similarly characterizing such phenomena from other drugs. With such reinforcement principles operating, "the sharp distinction between 'psychic dependence' and 'physical dependence' becomes untenable."[362]

C. Schuster explains that it is normal for animals to begin self-administration of reinforcing drugs; this drug abuse is not "abnormal" behavior, but rather "biologically normal." What *is* abnormal in drug abuse is the relative lack of competing behaviors. "Perhaps a mistake is made in studying human drug addiction in that the question to be asked may not be why one individual succumbs to drug abuse, but rather why most are capable of abstinence."*

Numerous studies assess the self-administration potential of the drugs of abuse. The question of how accurately an animal model[286,78] will predict abuse potential in human beings, for whom a variety of personality and social variables may be relatively more important, is at issue.[165]

Deneau and associates developed a method for assessing abuse liability of psychoactive drugs in animals, but explain, "While a drug must be self-administered before it is abused, a total assessment of its potential danger cannot be made from the fact that psychological dependence, as manifested by some degree of self-administration, occurs [in monkeys]. The major limitation [of this method] is that

* Personal communication.

drugs which are not water soluble cannot be tested."[78] The advantage of such a method is, of course, that abuse potential of new drugs could be estimated in advance of their widespread use. On the other hand, LSD, which will not be self-administered by animals, saw widespread—if only transient—abuse, which attests to the importance of social-psychological variables. Irwin has proposed that abuse liability or hazard indices take into account possibilities for mortality from chronic use, overdose and withdrawal, irreversible tissue damage, social and personal consequences, the production of violence or passivity, loss of control, psychomotor impairment, psychotic-like reactions, ease of overdose at use levels, and special hazards when taken intravenously or in combination with other drugs. He has proposed a classification of drugs along these lines.[165]

Policy research requires coming to grips with those issues. Often we have a vague or theoretical notion about the abuse potential of a drug from previous experience in clinical and experimental settings. While this should alert monitors, it is not useful to be drastic about regulating the availability of the drug until there is evidence of actual abuse. At that point what responses come about and which are legally sound, as well as the speed and effectiveness of these responses in deterrence, are all questions largely unresearched. The uses of drugs are culturally linked—and there is always the problem of predicting what will happen to cultural fads. It is important, of course, to monitor the climate of thinking about drug taking, as well as the actual prevalence of various patterns of use. Risks must be weighed against gains of availability of medically useful drugs. Toxic and lethal effects must be considered. Whether toxic effects can be readily diagnosed, treated and whether the drug signals toxicity to users or observers should be one consideration of relative availability of drugs of a similar class. It is important to consider how a drug lends itself to misuse—the dose and forms most likely to be misused, the assessment of physical dependence, withdrawal, and tolerance, as well as euphorigenic, sedative, or stimulant effects

—all factors that help predict drug-abuse potential.

Concluding Remarks on Research into Causes

The research into possible causes of drug use and abuse implicate not one determinant but many. Intrapsychic (personality) factors, family values, beliefs and dynamics, peer-group pressure and their norms, sibling's drug use and influence combine with cultural values and social change and economic aspects of availability and demand to influence the epidemic communicability of drug-taking behavior. The reinforcement effects of the drug, each experience and its setting add additional variables. All these factors can confound the researcher attempting to describe a single model in which to understand this multiple-determined behavior. Such factors are involved in any analysis of the critical factors in any deviant population, including mental illness.

Confusion still exists between what are causes and what are results of drug use, and which findings arise independently. Most studies of causes have been subsequent to the adoption of a particular drug, pattern, or peer-group identity. Assuming a factor predates drug abuse, can we be more precise as to what specifically has changed? If drugs are used to cope with stress, what coping mechanisms have been employed before that the drugs have now replaced?

How some persons succumb to drugs and why others utilize different means of dealing with their difficulties remains incompletely understood. There have been no set of reliable variables found that will predict drug-using behavior or outcome. Variables that place individuals in high-risk categories have been postulated, though not adequately validated. These variables often depend on the individual's socioeconomic background. The role of the initiator and reinforcing agents needs investigating to further understand the epidemic propensity of this behavior. How some persons refuse when invited to participate, and how others can maintain a pattern of oc-

casional recreational use, as well as what factors cause drug abuse in some to be self-limiting, invites research. The exchange of one
drug for another also requires scrutiny. While
the topic is no longer mysterious, and its dimensions are increasingly grasped, much remains to be learned about the causes of drug
abuse.

The pattern of an individual's drug use involves a beginning, peaks, remissions, relapses, and, at times, termination. Remission
may be drug specific or pattern specific. It
may reflect an experience with adverse reactions, treatment efficacy, epidemic outcomes,
changes in social groups, fads, and group
norms, or fluctuations in psychological variables and precipitating causes. Hawks suggests that any "universality" that exists to
explain the selectiveness of drug dependence
resides in a relationship *between* variables
studied, rather than in one variable itself. Due
to experimental design, usually only two variables can be correlated and multivariant
methods need to be utilized.[138] It is problematic whether we can identify high-risk
groups with precision; long-term prospective
studies should be designed to define them better and to ascertain more subtle factors in resistance as well as susceptibility to drug use at
all stages.

The last decade has witnessed an explosion
of interest in drugs that has widened into a
discussion of other altered states of consciousness,[332,333] accompanied by a public notion
that one drug will reliably produce a specific
effect, feeling, experience, altered state, or
behavior change. Instead, a wide variability of
effects is evident, dependent upon dose, reinforcement effects, social and personal expectations and personal psychology, as well as
metabolic, neurochemical, and tissue determinants as yet undefined.

❰ Treatment and Prevention

Since treatment and prevention of nonnarcotic drug abuse is not an advanced art,
but rather a tentative, fragmentary, and un-

certain array of ventures, research is relatively
undeveloped also. Probably—when the novelty dissipates—the same *principles* of diagnosis of situation, person, and his dysfunction,
the same *resources* that prevail in psychiatric
treatment generally, and the same *principles*
of group, individual, occupational, and pharmacotherapeutic treatment, will be applicable.
The phenomenon is recent and the natural history of multiple drug abusers, including mortality and morbidity statistics and the incidence of substitute addictions, is not yet well
recorded. Follow-up studies such as Vaillant's[347,348,349] represent a useful model.
Enough young adults and adolescents have
been heavily involved to warrant such study.
In general, trend studies indicate experimenters and most users—though not most
heavy users—shift their habits over time. The
long-term follow-up of narcotic addicts receiving one or another kind of treatment is only
beginning to be researched.[76,77,292] For multiple drug abuse, various modes of treatment
and prevention have been advocated, usually
without planning to evaluate the efficacy and
influence of such interventions on the individual and society at large.

Centers for drug analysis that disseminate
their findings to the individual users are a sort
of FDA for young consumers; the message
they convey and the way they are conducted
—a service to check out the pusher, to educate
toward caution, to give a general rather than
specific report of average sales—is rarely
thought through. That drugs are—more often
than not—falsely marketed is evident.[58]
Whether a service to the consumer for qualitative and/or quantitative analysis of samples
would be effectively used, before or after consumption, by whom (dealer or user), and most
importantly, whether the applicant would
alter his plans based on such information,
perhaps reducing the incidence of adverse
reactions, would need study. Drug-information education programs, the provision of alternatives to drug use, including meaningful
employment and meditation,[21,63,241] and efforts aimed at decreasing the availability of
drugs[164,74] have all been proposed to aid in

prevention. Self-help treatment programs, alternative activity programs, voluntary and compulsory hospitalization with or without supervised paroles, epidemiological field intervention, psychotherapy and drug maintenance have been proposed as treatment methods. The question of who will benefit from each type of treatment or preventive measure needs study; indeed, whether treatment—in the sense of skilled psychiatric intervention—is needed, and for whom, has been a crucial definitional question. Treatment for *what* remains the question, and drug use as often is a secondary issue in disturbed adolescents as it is a sustained problem; it may be that ticket of admission—and may require primary and initial attention—but life and adjustment problems, neuroses and character disorders become —sooner or later—a focus.

Goals

The implicit or explicit goals of therapeutic intervention must be known before efficacy is assessed. It is most evident that *process* research may be—at this juncture—more productive than *outcome* research. Practically all contemporary programs accept the elimination of psychological and physiological dependence as their ultimate, if not immediate goal. Some programs utilizing methadone maintenance seem to hold that—until the life situation and psychosocial problems are effectively managed—relief from drug dependence will fail; others are simply pill dispensing, and others utilize methadone as outreach and anticipate subsequent self-regulated withdrawal with or without the support of *residential* treatment; and still others seek to establish— through practices and personnel—sufficient trust and response to human needs to provide a range of services, of reentering stations for dropouts and job training, that comprise authentic rehabilitation. These programs may also have prevention aims emphasizing early detection, and community participation and interaction on the one hand, and special units for complicated problems—the addicted psychotic—on the other. The Public Health Service has advocated improved health prevention of disease among users, increased participation in conventional activities, decreased participation in criminal activities, and maximal social functioning and cessation of drug use other than in the treatment of illness as specific goals.[49] Meyer[232] discusses the three classic levels of prevention in a comprehensive public health approach: primary prevention of inappropriate drug use and drug abuse in vulnerable populations; secondary prevention that seeks to stop drug abuse in vulnerable populations; secondary prevention that seeks to stop drug abuse in an individual before he has become addicted, or before becoming solidly identified with a drug-abusing subculture; and tertiary prevention aimed at those individuals who are heavily involved with the abuse of drugs or in subcultures that support it. One can concentrate on treating the family or personality of the user, the symptom of addiction itself, or the social and medical consequences.[270] For what group complete abstinence or more moderate use of drugs is the more practical goal needs research.

Treatment and Prevention Aimed at Nonnarcotic Users

Aside from arguments about efficacy and goals, a widespread treatment response— aimed primarily at opiate abuse—has been mobilized in recent years toward those persons who are most severely drug dependent, and whose habitual drug use has precipitated the most serious adverse consequences. Although the present heroin epidemic seems to be waning, still a certain percentage of persons who try an illicit drug for the first time will eventually become drug dependent. One problem is how to minimize that number. The concern at this writing is the endemic problem of multiple drug use—generally in the underemployed, the sixteen-to-eighteen age group— that, with the unknown "right" circumstances, could become a heroin using population as well.[265]

Free Clinics and Crisis Centers

An outreach response was mobilized at a time when a "process factor"—trust in and access to institutions with skilled facilities, which were either not responsive or unprepared for the needs and attitudes of the clientele— surfaced. The young took care of each other with the help of a few professionals who were tested for trustworthiness. "Hot-line" telephone services and free medical clinics have emerged as a way of providing immediate, often anonymous, contact for a drug user in trouble or requesting information. Often privately endowed, organized under various guises by persons of varying skills, the effectiveness of these facilities is for the most part unresearched. Smith and Luce[313] document the establishment of the Haight-Ashbury Free Medical Clinic during the San Francisco drug epidemic of 1967 to 1969, and detail the history of the epidemic and the numerous problems involved in funding, accountability, conflicts with medical, social, and legal authorities, as well as with the population served. During the 1960s, conflicts between legal authorities and groups providing treatment, and conflicts in the minds of the doctors over the use of these illicit drugs and of accountability— whether to the patient, the community, or legal authorities—and how the youth interpreted these, tended to alienate patients in need of help. These conflicts also made it hard to gather data on the prevalence of use and adverse reactions. They generated a social structure within the drug-using community that advocated treatment of adverse reactions outside of medical settings, with the help of other users within the community. The myth was perpetuated that medical personnel were unwilling, incapable, or hostile to treating or advising on a drug problem. In short, community, legal, and medical policies toward the treatment of the drug user and his attitudes toward them served to further relegate drug use and treatment to an extramedical segment of the community.

Levy and Brown[200] report experience with a twenty-four-hour phone service called "Acid Rescue." Situated in the St. Louis metropolitan area, it received 1543 calls during 1970. This research assessed the types of calls received, the types of information given, times of maximal use, and the types of persons volunteering to work in such a program. In all, the authors felt that management of the crises, through supportive psychotherapy over the telephone in less than thirty minutes, was not difficult if the goal of the counseling was not to end the drug experience but to protect the individual from dangerous action and encourage a subjectively pleasant experience. Artificial separation of drug problems from other adolescent problems was impossible. Interestingly, the most common calls were for *drug information* from individuals contemplating using a drug or having recently used it, and only the second most common calls were about a *drug crisis*—usually from a youthful user. The action taken, information given, and counselor's accuracy and appropriateness of response, depended upon length of the counselor's experience. Only the correctness of the information given correlated significantly with the outcome. If the information given was appropriate, 65 percent of the callers altered their plans; if the information given was too detailed or unnecessarily frightening, no caller altered his plans. As the year wore on, as the counselors became more experienced, and as the correctness of the information given improved, the callers deciding not to take the drug increased from 9 to 21 percent. Two percent of the calls were unrelated to drugs and were mostly suicidal threats. The supervision of the employees of such a facility is discussed by Torop and Torop.[342]

The prolific increase in such facilities, and their utilization, may speak to a need for centers to disseminate accurate information, obtainable immediately, but only upon request, and for patient referral and treatment during an acute drug crisis.[344] The possibility that it is symptomatic of the loss and devaluation of institutional and parental functions is as likely. While ritualizing the use of dangerous drugs to diminish their fear and alienation, users also emphasize drug experimentation and use as the warrant for attention and response. As transitional institutions, these facilities offer the cultural anthropologist and social psychologist interested in age-specific social roles an interesting topic for study.

Information–Education

The drug-abuse, information–education explosion has been a visible societal response to concerns generated by the 1960s. Drug-abuse education classes in schools, churches, and community organizations, and the TV, film, radio, and news media recognize the topic. Federal agencies generate their own pamphlets and public-service broadcasts, diverting 67.6 million dollars in 1972 toward efforts called preventive and educational. "At the present time, no one can even accurately assess the scope of information–education efforts, much less measure its impact on behavior. There is no federal information exchange to which independent programs report; no description of all programs currently in operation; no assurance that the information disseminated is correct; no check to see that it is reaching its intended audience."[246] Youth generally obtain their drug information from peers, seeing drug messages on television, printed drug information, radio messages, the school lecture, and only rarely from parents.[246] Many materials about drug abuse are scientifically inaccurate; program sponsors add their own values to the facts; much of the information approaches drug use from the point of view that "any use is equally dangerous," which, from the recipient's point of view, tends to undermine the credibility of the information. Government has also utilized this information to rally support for its programs, and this confusion of objectives further undermines acceptance.[246] Experience with tobacco, alcohol, and venereal disease, demonstrates that knowledge about risks "in and of itself does not necessarily change behavior."[246] Certainly the various programs, even when objectively assessing risk versus gain, could arouse curiosity in an individual.[48] Blachly has discussed types of educational approaches which may minimize the possibilities for seduction.[30] The pressure on schools has often led to unprepared and unwise "shows of effort" by constructing artificial emergency "programs" to placate the press, legislators, or disturbed parents, rather than assessing parental attitudes and intraschool sentiment and practices as a start. The second marijuana commission recommends that "drug use prevention strategy, rather than concentrating resources and efforts in persuading or educating people not to use drugs, emphasize the alternative means of obtaining what users seek from drugs: means that are better for users and better for society. The aim of prevention policy should be to foster and instill the necessary skills for coping with the problems of living, particularly the life concerns of adolescents."[246] (A Chicago media program attempted to deglamorize drugs and was aimed at stimulating thought about nondrug issues relevant to the youths' dilemmas: how do you say no to a friend and still be a friend?) Information about drugs and the disadvantages of their use should be incorporated into more general programs, stressing benefits "with which drug consumption is largely inconsistent." The commission recommends that, from the standpoint of government, a single agency coordinate dissemination and screening of materials and recommend a moratorium on the production and dissemination of new drug-information materials and educational programs.[246]

In spite of the many efforts directed at education, the incidence of drug use for self-defined purposes has risen. It may be that the avalanche of drug information has been counterproductive "and that it may have stimulated rebellion, or simply raised interest in the forbidden."[246] For example, one as yet unreported study found that after "education" the youth were more comfortable using drugs. One aspect of such education that bears upon psychiatric interest in development and sociological and anthropological interest in societal change is the severe lack of interest in stimulating moral query: enlightened programs preach that the young should make up their own minds, but they rarely stimulate them to think beyond themselves or the moment. Making up their own minds is a challenge, not necessarily accepted out of enmity. Without more balanced, less "permissive" messages, the adolescent lacks even a feeble excuse for revolt against demand and is left without challenge to accountability by a seductively "free" counselor. Such subtle issues are factors little investigated. Without such research, programs are designed from relative ignorance about the specific needs (unrevealed by questionnaire) and about the developmental tasks of the audience.

Research into the media and its impact on the various population subsectors is only beginning.[255] The question of how the messages are presented and received, of how to advertize what you want the receiver *not* to do, and whether the target should be the behavior or the attitude, are all part of the larger issue of how people are influenced.

Psychotherapeutic Approaches

Psychotherapeutic encounters are most useful for persons least involved in a drug-using subculture, who evidence minimal intensity and duration of use, who are in various types of adolescent crises, and in whom a precipitant can be clearly identified. The efficacy, techniques, and especially the aims of such approaches, are largely unresearched. If precipitants (see page 590) can be identified, theoretically a focus upon the person's response to the precipitant, as well as explaining the link to him between the precipitant and his drug use, might be of benefit.[19] Similarly, if a person's illicit drug use is an attempt at self-medication for an underlying medical or psychiatric disorder (see page 577), the accurate diagnosis and treatment of the disorder should be a therapist's first order of business. Interpreting a person's drug use to him as beneficial in ameliorating fluctuations in self-esteem, stress, conflict, guilt, and shame, and providing a sense of personal and group identity, probably help him to understand, tolerate, and eventually relinquish his drug use.[52,189] Although the influence of families on drug use is still debated (see page 582), family counseling could relieve conflicts and stresses, as well as educate parents on how to modulate their often misconstrued fears.

The peer group (see page 572) is an important variable influencing drug use for social as well as developmental psychology of modern youth, and this fact requires scrutiny. The second marijuana commission report suggests that "peer influence toward drug use may be greater for junior and senior high school students than for college students." The novelty of drug use, the relative immaturity of the younger students, the desire to experience something new, a need to test the effects of a drug that the students have learned to expect or anticipate, as well as a drive to win peer approval and recognition, tends to generate among secondary-school students a focus upon the *act* of taking the drug and its attendant rituals and social activity. On the other hand, the greater maturity of the college students, their increased exposure to drug use among their peers, and their greater opportunity to observe the effects on friends in college, may serve to alter their own behavior and to "encourage greater discrimination as they seem to focus on the pleasure of the experience and its *outcome*, rather than the act itself."[246] It is unknown to what extent observations such as these—if valid—can be efficiently and effectively incorporated in a treatment approach. Participation in a group whose drug using is less serious, encouragement to form a relationship with a specific, highly valued partner, and changing residence to a community where drugs are not as available are important factors that help sustain abstinence. If drug abuse is viewed as a symptom of widespread social factors (see page 570), then attempts to understand, modify and alleviate social problems could be a long-range goal.[236,137] This is another way of indicating that community competence, responsive institutions, and rites of passage for the young can shift a variety of meanings and practices.

Wikler explains that verbal psychotherapy "might be utilized effectively to hasten extinction if it is directed toward 'cognitive' re-labeling of the conditioned responses."[362] He has outlined the use of "active extinction" models to prevent relapse with the help of methadone blockade and narcotic antagonists, and whether such models could be utilized in nonnarcotic abusers invites research.[115,362] The idea that drug abusers are unable to delay gratification led Wikler to conclude that "theoretically an 'ideal' vocation for such a person would be one that 'paid off' immediately on successful completion of a task," and perhaps that is one reason why illegal occupations are so often found among these people.[362]

Some socially useful kinds of behavior that are acquired during chronic drug intoxication may have to be relearned in the drug-free state, since they may be extinguished along with other conditioned behavior surrounding the drug abuse if active extinction is implemented.[362] Amphetamine users often report that they have developed useful and valued behavior while taking the drug. Such ideas are reminiscent of similar observations among alcoholics.[91,330] They deserve research. Much remains to be learned about "state-dependent" or "dissociative" learning and its application to the field of drug abuse.[91,92]

Theoretically, better ego strength, good object relationships, better tolerance for frustration and the ability to delay gratification, higher intelligence, and acute onset of drug use related to a precipitant are all factors that would predict a better result from intensive psychotherapy. Savitt,[282] Torda,[341] and Hartmann[136] report cases of successful psychoanalytically oriented psychotherapy with adolescents who abuse drugs. Hartmann found that drug use was resorted to surrounding the therapist's absence, misunderstanding or lapse in empathy, which is consistent with Kohut's formulations.[188,189,190] Savitt explicitly states that the nonpunitive management of the patient's acting out around drugs and sex is an important technique. Such advice may only apply to those with better ego strength, and other authors have indicated that setting limits is quite important when managing drug-using individuals.[185,270]

Premature dropping out of psychotherapy and failure to attend clinics regularly are major problems in attempting to provide treatment on an outpatient basis. Several explanations were proposed by Anderson and associates.[5,253] Patients may be "poorly motivated" or are coerced into seeking treatment;

patient's and therapist's expectations often are divergent since the patient wants to change immediately, cannot delay gratification, and does not return to the clinic after his expectations are not met. They feel that these two explanations only perpetuate the problem in that they blame the poor results on characteristics of the patients. Whether innovative techniques (as, for example, occurred with methadone maintenance) could be developed to immediately gratify such patients and surmount this ever-present difficulty is a question. The contention that the appropriate treatment was being used, but needed to be administered in higher doses by therapists of greater skill is another. The authors conclude that with the population these therapists could not compete with the immediate reinforcement inherent in drugs, since traditional psychotherapy offers no immediate solutions.

Cohen and associates[64] have written a most helpful article on the psychotherapeutic treatment of drug-abusing patients. They explain that drug abusers tend to alienate sources of help by assuming a help-rejecting stance and "by provoking feelings of competitiveness and resentment in the would-be helper. [They express] a wish to be passive and suspicious," engage in passive aggression and dependency, perhaps to ward off depression, and "can be described as angry, suspicious and self-doubting." They tend to be self-deceptive about their "assertive, . . . arrogant [and oppositional behavior, which are] almost the exact opposite of the passivity and dependence which they engage in. . . . Intervention which is explicitly defined as 'help' threatens [this] self-reliant facade and raises the spectre of being manipulated and exploited." Drug abusers "usually ask for help in an indirect way by requesting treatment for a 'bad trip' or in some other impersonal form which refers to the 'condition' rather than to themselves." The authors recommend that the therapist "be aware of the drug abuser's underlying despair about making an impact in a world perceived as critical, success-oriented, and unresponsive to needs which cannot be logically justified or even articulated directly . . . [and suggest] creating situations where he is in a position to offer something valued by the therapist, [and that the latter] present himself as a model who can risk exposing his tender feelings and the potential of experiencing rejection. [He must] empathize with the drug abuser's feeling of isolation and impotence [and focus away from details of drug abuse since] emphasizing [this] aspect of his behavior rigidifies his negative identity and restricts his possibilities for the future. Many resistances to involvement combined with acting out, [are] designed . . . to test the [therapist's] genuineness and stability of concern." [pp. 353, 355, 357][64]

Vaillant[347,348,349] recommends that the abuser be helped to find the best possible dependency objects, sustained employment with external support, and to discover a more mature way to deal with his instinctual needs. He contends that drug abusers can modify their defensive style to cope with traumatic events, which, in his patients, were handled by isolation, hypomanic suppression and denial, and a "deliberate search for the silver lining."

Psychotherapeutic approaches are useful for some drug-using persons and not for others. Difficulty enforcing drug abstinence and the failure to continue contact with a therapist are the most important reasons for disappointing results, and underlying factors are variously understood and communicated by both patient, therapist, and researcher. Continuing redefinition, description, and classification of patients and treatments is part of the meaningful categorization aimed toward prediction of who will benefit from psychotherapeutic approaches and exploration of the more subtle variables that lead to improvement or to relapse.[269] Outpatient facilities are not to be disparaged, for often adequate attention to the adverse effects of chronic drug use encourages rapport with a potentially beneficial treatment facility and is a step toward involvement in a more efficacious treatment modality.

Finally, inpatient psychiatric facilities are accumulating a vast experience with drug-using adolescents with relatively severe pathology—experience that should generate principles and variables for study. Whether the drugs add anything new to the research of delayed development, borderline states, severe character disorders, and schizophrenia prevalent in the 1950s is as yet unclear.

Self-Help Groups

Since the advent of Alcoholics Anonymous and, later, Synanon, the original model for self-help groups for drug abusers, a number of similar programs have emerged, such as Day Top, Marathon House, Phoenix House, and Crossroads. Khantzian[185] has discussed these programs which share in common several facts: they are residential programs staffed by ex-addicts; patients are expected to remain free of drugs; there is a heavy emphasis on work centered around responsibility for relatively mundane tasks within the program; residents gain status as they progress to the more sought-after job responsibilities dependent upon their improvement and length of stay; and encounter or confrontational methods are utilized in formal and informal situations around "the issues of addiction, problems in group living and analysis of each other's problems."[185] These confrontations often assume extremely aggressive proportions that may lead to "splitting" from the group (in some instances to psychiatric casualties) and the intense, affective experience may substitute for the drug "high."[185] There is, among these programs, a high dropout rate and much recidivism.[76,77,292] The common attitude that the person who leaves as a result of such encounters is "copping out" or avoiding confronting himself or others, generally underestimates "many addicts' limited capacity to deal with intense affect, particularly aggressive feelings and . . . seems to be incongruent, anti-therapeutic and destructive for many of the addicted patients. It leads to further . . . sense of failure in people who, too often in their life time, have suffered rejection and failure. For many borderline patients . . . failing to appreciate the dangers of prematurely forcing people to give up their defenses . . . is dangerous and most likely contraindicated."[185]

Residential treatment programs are helpful in removing the addict from his environment, and the emphasis on high expectation in the execution of their jobs serves to reinforce self-regulation and control. Khantzian explains:

. . . the forced work and humiliating tasks and activities to which the addict is subjected is effective because these exercises are in part successful manipulations of the addict's sado-masochistic tendencies. What is probably underestimated by the proponents of such an approach is how they may merely play into the addict's sado-masochism, and therefore offer little towards producing permanent change; to the extent that this is not appreciated, there exists the constant danger that the treatment becomes just a symptom of the illness.[185]

De Leon and associates have attempted follow-up studies comparing the persons who remain in the program with the persons who have left the program on measures of pathology and criminal activity.[76,77] No follow-up studies have appeared about the residential treatment of nonnarcotic and youthful drug abusers.

The advisability of using ex-addicts as role models and therapists is largely debated informally. Ex-addicts may indeed represent useful models for those who seek to become abstinent, and yet, because of their own psychopathology, sadistic impulses, and medical naiveté, ex-addicts may facilitate psychiatric casualties, be unempathic to a fault, and may not astutely observe when certain persons in the program are regressing toward decompensation.

Certainly the self-selection involved in clearly singling out those persons most "motivated" for treatment results in the high rates of improvement seen among those who complete the programs. The question of where the "failures" go for help is unresearched.

Fischmann[95] reviews the California Rehabilitation Center Program involving mostly minority males between seventeen and thirty-five years from a lower socioeconomic background, broken or incomplete homes, with a history of intravenous drug use and a history of juvenile or adult arrests, and describes their methods of therapeutic leverage. He remarks that "perhaps the most important single factor in the establishment of a therapeutic climate is the personality of the leader and that success in bridging the gap between patients and staff is paramount in establishing a therapeutic group culture." Wilmer[365,366] described his experience with an adolescent inpatient unit staffed by residents and utilizing videotape methods, group psychotherapy, and individual treatment. He has also discussed problems surrounding use of drugs smuggled into the ward. Hughes and associates[155,151] described the development of inpatient services in a general hospital for the treatment of narcotics addiction, and the tendency of hospitalized narcotics addicts to form an antitherapeutic patient subculture, which was reduced by giving ex-addicts equal responsibility with nurses for the operation of the unit. They discussed the important architectual considerations to insure control over outpatient traffic to and from the unit. They were successful in organizing the therapeutic potential of an addict-prisoner community by reducing the social distance between staff and prisoners, by replacing staff-disciplinary response to deviant behavior with a peer-group-helping response, by converting cliques into self-help interaction groups, by developing a rehabilitation-oriented, inmate-status and leadership hierarchy with important decision-making and rehabilitation functions, by structuring communication to and from inmate groups through rehabilitation-oriented representatives and by frequent community meetings to deal with rumors and distortions. They also described a model for precipitating identity crises in resistant sociopathic prisoners.[155]

Epidemiologic Models for Intervention During an Epidemic

Hughes and associates have shown how successfully an intervention method patterned after a contagious-disease model can rapidly and without coercion stem the tide of a heroin microepidemic in a community.* Their research concentrates on heroin epidemics, but it might be applied to epidemics of nonnarcotic nature as well. They have already de-

* See references 152, 153, 158, 161, and 106.

scribed a method for monitoring adolescent drug-abuse trends in a suburban high-school district that would be valuable in assessing the emergence of an epidemic.[159] Where in the epidemic to intervene and what methods of treatment should be offered and which would be effective are questions for research. Hughes and coworkers have found that newly involved cases of heroin addiction are much more "contagious" than chronic users. Whether the same applies to nonnarcotic users is at issue. Their work suggests that by organizing the therapeutic potential of a community, by organizing intervention around the drug-distribution system, and by enlisting adolescents in treatment as part of the rehabilitation staff, one form of drug abuse can be prevented in many who are at risk.[106]

De Alarcon[74] has researched the effectiveness of prompt governmental action restricting the availability of Methedrine on one urban area and three rural districts in Britain one-and-one-half years after abuse had begun there. He found a sharp drop in prevalence of injection three months after limitation of the supply; however, many tried injecting other forms of amphetamines and barbiturates and eventually switched to oral amphetamine and cannabis, LSD and barbiturates. Two years later the majority were still taking drugs, but only one-third were still injecting; only 10 percent on a regular basis.

The usefulness of epidemiologic models in detection and assessment of drug-using trends is well established. The particular type of intervention instituted has legal, ethical, and social implications, and the development and testing of a model for nonnarcotic epidemics awaits research.

Prognostic Factors in Abusers

There have been no systematic studies to date assessing the determinants of abstinence among treated or untreated persons who abuse nonnarcotic drugs. Several authors have speculated about prognostic factors in these persons on the basis of their experience.[57,185,300] Age of onset of drug use or abuse may perhaps prove to be a powerful predictive factor of future chronicity of addiction.[66,273] The question is how accurate such speculation of predictive factors may prove to be.

Studies of prognostic variables on institutionalized narcotic addicts have appeared.[199, 175,331] Vaillant[347,348,349] followed opiate addicts incarcerated at Lexington for twenty years and found that at the twenty-year follow-up "most of the variables that affected the addicts' prognosis twelve years after their Lexington hospitalization [the number of years of addiction; the amount of drugs used before Lexington; whether the addicts rapidly relapsed after the first hospitalization; whether they sought admission voluntarily; education, race and delinquency] appeared to be no longer important after twenty years." He found three variables that continued "to differentiate the best and worst outcomes": employment of four years or more prior to drug use; being raised in the same culture in which their parents had been raised; and having been married were associated with stable abstinence. The question of how closely his sample represents the nonnarcotic drug abuser is at issue. At the twelve-year follow-up, he found that his sample tolerated abstinence well. Incapacitating mental illness was not a major risk and when the symptom of drug addiction was given up, it was replaced by neither depressions nor psychosomatic illnesses, although many found substitute addiction with alcohol. Only 10 percent of his sample had, in twenty years, one or more brief psychiatric hospitalizations for reasons other than drug addiction. Only four men were diagnosed as psychotic.

Twenty-three percent of his sample were dead after twenty years, two from natural causes, four from murder or suicide, two from accidental death, two from secondary alcoholism, and ten from overdose or infection secondary to their heroin use. He discusses possible determinants of mortality differences. The five-year report from the Illinois Drug Abuse Program finds that the death rate is somewhat less for the nonnarcotic user than for the narcotics addicts.[292]

Never having been physiologically addicted, compulsory postinstitutional supervision, good premorbid adjustment (late onset of delinquency, high-school graduation, regular employment, and late onset of addiction) and ego strength ("the ability to live effectively, productively and happily over a period of time") were all associated with the favorable outcome of continued abstinence.[349] Similar prognostic factors among alcoholics, rather than psychiatric disorders, often predict remission more effectively than the severity of the manifest clinical symptoms. Employment, new meaningful nonparental relationships, and joining evangelical or mystical religious sects represent more constructive alternatives to addiction. Absence of a stable work history seemed, in Vaillant's sample, to be the best predictor of the chronicity of addiction. "Broken homes, per se, were not correlated with chronicity of addiction, but almost twice as many chronic addicts had broken homes before six."[349]

Vaillant[349] summarized his feeling that addicts improved "when they master their instincts and not when they burn out." He likens the abstinent addicts (as, indeed, many addicts do themselves) to the maturing adolescent in that both must achieve independence from their families:

. . . to which each finds himself bound and towards which he finds himself ambivalently angry and intolerant . . . each must find substitute objects to love and each must find appropriate channels for aggressive and sexual instincts that up to this point have either been focused toward family of origin, biologically latent, or, in the case of the addict, narcotized. If addiction is conceptualized as a form of immaturity, then it is not surprising to find that: (a) the disorder like adolescence gets better with time; (b) when symptoms are removed, they need not be replaced with others; and (c) ex-addicts can manifest new defenses.[349]

Tamerin and Neumann[331] studied several hundred cases of addicts from the upper-middle and upper-socioeconomic classes and found several factors that seemed predictive of successful outcome of short duration and could be classed under the rubric of motivation and a history of successful social and personal coping success.

When considering the wide range of degree and type of drug involvement in the nonnarcotic drug user, we are discussing factors such as the extent of his present involvement with drugs, the abuse potential of the drugs he presently uses, the total length of time he has used drugs—including alcohol—his present pattern of use and route of administration, the extent of his involvement in a drug-using subculture, and a consideration of possible precipitants for the addiction. Such factors may be more important among adolescents and early drug users than among heroin addicts of the type studied by Vaillant and others.

Conclusion

There are numerous problems involved with the diagnosis, prevention, and treatment of disorders associated with drug use as the primary influence disrupting psychosocial functioning. This is a self-reinforcing, risk-taking behavior, with immediate feedback that is often satisfying. What alternative kinds of behavior can be substituted for those where immediate sensate reinforcement accrues along with increased self-esteem, that have group-reinforcement potential, especially among peers, and that can satisfy a desire for novelty and recreation as well? The public may have become supersaturated with the notion of drug abuse, and further input may only serve to reinforce interest in a deviant activity that, in reality, only small numbers engage in with seriously incapacitating outcomes. The treatment response must be directed toward these few, but what sort of treatment is effective remains a research issue. The prevention response has been hurriedly implemented without planning to research the needs of the receiver or the effectiveness of the output. Knowledge is better than ignorance about drugs, but naive, sensationalized reporting has neither aided prevention nor supported dispassionate appraisal. New epidemics can be contained with a rapid and humane public-health approach. Intervention during the beginning years of illicit drug use requires cautious techniques at grade-school, high-school, and college-age levels. The question of how and who should intervene needs careful planning and study. Illicit drug use seems to beg for control, but whether schools should actively try to discover who is and who is not using drugs, and whether they should attempt to define who is at risk—assuming an accurate method could be developed—has numerous ethical, social, and legal implications. How parents can be educated toward effective response remains an avenue for exploration. To assess the needs of and resources available for those who ask for treatment is one issue; to assess the risk to public health of various sectors of other illicit users and their eventual outcome is another.

❰ Consequences and Outcomes

The discussion of treatment illustrates the definitional problems of just who represents a "case." A case is usually self-defined—a drug user in trouble requests help from a medical facility. Only rarely does research investigate such difficulties within the community, where a (so far) unknown number of users experience adverse consequences from their drug use, yet define their difficulties in terms obviating—in their minds anyway—medical intervention: they remain contained, tolerated or sheltered by their subculture. The user requesting help—diagnosis, treatment, or explanation—generally cannot be explicit as to precisely what has changed other than the simple notion that he took a drug and now is worried, confused, or helpless in the face of his difficulty. The researcher, too, has difficulty; usually, he must rely on the self-report and his clinical observation. Often patient and physician focus upon lurid drug details and accounts, which only further submerges the more important psychosocial variables. Adverse reactions, particularly, but attitude, value, and behavior changes as well, are linked to family and personal crises for which the drug serves, temporarily at least, as a focus of concern and a ticket of admission. The investigator's conscious and unconscious attitudes toward drugs and youth in general often underlie the characterization—or mischaracterization—of "the problem." Objective measures have been utilized, particularly in research about organicity and attitude, value and behavior change. Psychopharmacologic laboratory research has contributed more balanced accounts of the various consequences of drug intoxication. However, these drug-specific physical and behavioral changes (often with unknown bases) may only appear specific on the surface, since adolescent turmoil, latent schizophrenia, depression, and early sociopathy often underlie what presents itself as a drug complaint. Individual differences and response to drug effect are great, and the capacity to tolerate, assimilate, and integrate the drug experience varies widely.

Research into the consequences and outcomes attempts to define who is at risk, to identify a characteristic reaction, to understand a user's adaptation, and to assess the cost to the individual and society, as well as to delineate any neurochemical or tissue basis for a reaction and/or operative personal and social factors. Accordingly, this research comprises toxicological investigation, neurological assessment, morbidity and mortality studies, and descriptions of adverse behavioral reactions, as well as attitude, belief, and value changes. These depend upon adequate follow-up studies, which are rare. Whether drug use can selectively "catalyze" permanent or transient psychotic reactions and "amotivational states" in predisposed individuals, still presents a research challenge.

Toxicological Research

Clinical toxicological studies of drug users that attempt to relate the toxic syndromes encountered to a particular drug are intrinsically difficult since the purity, dose level, and schedule cannot be reliably assessed among users. Whatever the public-health interest of clinical studies, systematic animal-toxicity studies are needed to help define the mechanisms of toxic effects.

Research in toxicology of psychotropic

drugs describes various pathophysiological, and especially neuropathological (parenchymal) changes in animals and man. No such effects have been shown for LSD. The uterotonic effects of this ergot alkaloid conceivably could influence pregnancy, although clear and controlled data have not warranted any conclusion other than the general caution that unnecessary drugs in pregnancy should be avoided.[225] Jacobson and Berlin's report implies only that the milieu of the counterculture and multiple drug use are a hazard to birth.[166] Suspicions that the drug was a teratogen are not borne out to date.[221,225] Chromosomal changes in human lymphocytes have been neither verified as due to LSD nor linked to evidence of specific damage of genetic mechanism. While research might continue on the teratogenic effects of LSD, it cannot carry top priority from a public-health viewpoint.

Syndromes of "necrotizing angiitis" and abnormal cerebral angiographic findings associated with neurological complaints have been reported among intravenous users of multiple drugs.[60,279] The role of direct toxic effects of a certain drug, adulterants, sepsis, or other, unknown, factors is unsolved. How long such changes, when present, persist, whether they are reversible, and the extent to which thinking or behavior is contingently disturbed is unknown. Speculation that these findings are related directly to methylamphetamine abuse is not supported by studies of the chronic intravenous administration of methylamphetamine under aseptic conditions for as long as a year to monkeys who show no evidence of parenchymal damage at autopsy, although various behavioral effects, such as stereotyped behavior, are seen.[93,94]

Tennant and coworkers have reported, not surprisingly, various degrees of respiratory irritation associated with heavy use of hashish by soldiers in West Germany.[337] A more precise definition of such health risks with weak and potent preparations of marijuana awaits further study. Recent research with marijuana primarily concentrates on long-lasting and possibly cumulative effects of active metabolites of THC.[196]

Morbidity and Mortality

Understanding the relationship and measuring the effects of drug abuse on mortality is important in assessing the costs of the epidemic of multiple-drug use; however investigated, such statistics are often not specifically useful in determining the danger of various patterns of various drugs. The specific drug is often unknown, and the cause of death is not easily sorted out from the abuse pattern and life style with all its variability and adventitious factors.[141,48] For example, the headline-catching statistics on opiate deaths not only reflect the results of multiple-drug interaction (such as morphine, alcohol, and sedative hypnotics), infections, malnutrition, and other medical complications, but probably include other factors hitherto unexplained.

In any case, there has been a dearth of epidemiological research into the mortality and morbidity of various patterns of use of nonnarcotic, psychoactive substances. Mortality among intravenous users is especially high and septic conditions, violent death, and narcotic or sedative overdose, as well as conscious or unconscious suicide attempts, are generally implicated.* Morbidity figures that would assess the costs of different patterns of drug use to the individual are lacking, in part because there is little apparent problem with some commonly used agents. They would include the functional consequences of use, e.g., adverse reactions (which may or may not have a metabolic or tissue basis), accidents, hospitalizations, delinquency and imprisonment, progression to more dangerous drugs,[262] and medical complications such as hepatitis, malnutrition, abscesses, and the like.[211]

Neurological Consequences of Nonnarcotic Drug Use

Seizures associated with (but not shown to be necessarily contingent upon) LSD use have rarely been reported.[67] Seizures may be

---

* See references 27, 28, 75, 73, 140, 249, and 290.

the cause of death in overdosage of amphetamines, especially in accidental ingestions in children.[88] Perhaps because of tolerance, seizures occur rarely in chronic amphetamine abusers, except when barbiturates and amphetamines are used together. The diagnosis and treatment of the medical aspects of nonnarcotic dependence and withdrawal is discussed by Chambers,[57] Smith,[315,316] Wikler,[361] Tinklenberg,[339] and Shick et al.[301,299]

Studies of organicity among drug users that attempt to relate findings to a particular drug are complicated by the fact that many drugs have been used, of unknown purity and composition, by various routes of administration, generally predrug measures are unavailable and differences in test scores may be due to differences in motivation. The characterization of the nature of any "organicity" in LSD users have so far eluded strict definition. All such studies have been retrospective, and the time interval between the last dose of LSD and organicity assessment varies. The subjects of Blacker and associates[33] and S. Cohen and A. E. Edwards[218] had not used LSD for 48 hours prior to testing. Thus, the effects of metabolic changes or of long-lasting metabolites (unlikely with LSD) cannot be ruled out. Blacker and associates studied twenty-one paid, volunteer subjects living in the community who were chronic LSD users. They found only "scattered and inconclusive evidence" for minimal brain damage and no increased rate of abnormal EEGs among the users; a number of EEG records were judged abnormal by one or both readers at either the initial testing or six-month retest interval, but abnormal recordings did not correlate with the length of LSD ingestion; on auditory-evoked potentials (a measure found to be sensitive to intellectual disorganization in schizophrenia) the subjects showed no abnormality, yet visual-evoked potentials suggested that they were "uniquely sensitive to low intensity [visual] stimulation . . . [and] seemed to modulate and organize sensory input in a different fashion."[33] S. Cohen and A. E. Edwards, assessing organicity in thirty chronic LSD users, found significantly poorer performance on two tests of visual perception and spatial orientation.[218]

McGlothin and associates studied sixteen subjects drawn from a sample of 300 who had received LSD in a medical setting many years before the study, had no history of intravenous injections, and most of whom had not taken LSD for a period of about one year prior to testing, and matched them with a control group. The experimental design did not permit the implication of a causal relationship and could not exclude the possible influence of prior factors "associated with the decision to use LSD repeatedly."[218] Measures of organicity (including the Halstead-Reitan battery) did not replicate S. Cohen and A. E. Edwards' particular findings and confirmed previous studies "that there [was] no evidence of generalized brain damage [in the LSD group] related to the amounts of LSD ingested."[218] Evidence of moderate impairment of abstract ability suggestive of minimal brain dysfunction was provided by a significantly poorer performance on Halstead's category test—a nonverbal measure of ability to discern abstract principles, and involving memory for a sequence of presentations. No specificity of effects across users is shown, then, and slight and different changes observed cannot be clearly dissociated from motivational factors. No striking data of semipermanent effects of extended LSD usage is, then, available.

The prevalence of organic brain syndrome among illicit, intravenous drug users is unreported, although intravenous amphetamine abusers report subjective difficulties with memory, concentration, and fine motor coordination months after discontinuation.[301] Research involves the objective assessment of such complaints from intravenous users, the prevalence and outcome, as well as defining more precisely the tissue, metabolic, or neurochemical mechanisms involved. No studies have conclusively demonstrated central nervous system toxicity with amphetamine, and Freedman[101] has discussed the evidence usually cited. "In the light of parahydroxylated metabolites that leave the brain slowly, it is quite possible that a reversible biochemical effect is responsible for a change in behavior of this duration," in addition to drug-behavior interactions—learning under the drug state.

On the other hand, abnormal central nervous system signs in drug users either on EEG, brain scan or neurologic exam, suggest cardiovascular or infectious disease processes as a result of intravenous drug abuse.[211] Needle sharing is a phenomenon endemic to needle-using subcultures and Howard and Borges found that the sharing of needles is a social phenomenon dictated by pressures of group participation and inferred that "even if fits and points were legally available, sharing the needles would continue."[149] Intravenous drug users are exposed to a wide variety of other medical hazards relatively independent of the drug injected, including serum hepatitis, septic emboli, endocarditis, tetanus, syphilis, and malaria.[211,301]

Adverse Reactions to LSD

Various categorizations of *adverse* functional reactions for LSD have appeared.[*] These acknowledge psychotic and nonpsychotic varieties that can be acute (terminating as the intoxication dissipates) or chronic (lasting for various periods after the intoxication). Such adverse reactions include acute and prolonged anxiety states, depressive and paranoid states of psychotic or nonpsychotic proportions, schizophreniclike reactions, mild or severe confusional states dominated by magical thinking, and spontaneous recurrences ("flashbacks"). The use of LSD may also result in suicide, self-mutilation, homicide, assault, and other antisocial behavior, personality, attitude, and behavioral changes, and religious conversions (including irresponsibility and omniscience).[97,222,220,217] Schwarz[289] and Smart and Bateman[306] have reviewed the literature on adverse reactions with LSD prior to 1968.

Acute adverse reactions, ranging from mild anxiety to panic states of psychotic proportions, are known to occasionally occur with LSD and cogeners in social as well as research settings, and are related to a threatened loss of control over inner stability, variably experienced and symbolized. For some it is dread transcended ("death of the ego"), for others, unwelcome, denied, or projected fears ("fragmentation of the self").[189]

Some investigators have implied that acute panic states are fostered by fears generated by medical and research settings, and yet, perhaps just as often, the confidence engendered by the presence of competent and emphatic medical personnel leads to a diminution of such reactions.[169,170,171] McGlothlin[219] found no difference in harmful effects attributed to LSD between nonmedical as opposed to medically supervised exposure.

Clinical research into the acute effects of the intoxication cannot always be extrapolated to social drug use—reactions occur in the laboratory that may not occur in another setting and vice versa—and, furthermore, the results of such laboratory studies are influenced by the subjects' previous experience with drugs,[†] the research setting,[‡] and the variables investigated, as well as the techniques used and the investigator's bias.[172,169,170,171] Barr and Langs discuss the importance of control groups, the necessity for "active placebos," and the determinants of placebo responses with LSD in the laboratory;[9] the placebo for a drug of the potency and clarity of response characteristic of LSD has been found an abstract exercise by most competent investigators.

Research into the types of reactions that occur outside the laboratory, and their social management and interpretation, would be especially valuable since many such reactions are managed within the drug-using subculture[12] and only the most serious reactions or least involved users reach medical facilities.

Certain determinants of these reactions have been identified and include such drug-behavior interactions as dose,[§] social setting,[10,12,32,172,169,170,171] personality make-up,[178,177,299] expectations,[114,12] degree of drug experience and current life crises.[114] The role of a person's associates in precipitating and influencing such reactions is apparent.[97,12,104] Many of these determinants are

---

* See references 46, 68, 79, 114, 261, 97, 109, 142, 289, 306, 343, and 345.

† See references 12, 172, 169, 170, 171, and 233.
‡ See references 32, 9, 172, 169, 170, and 171.
§ See references 177, 178, 172, 169, 170, and 171.

not specific to drug use and can occur in other psychiatric patients as well. Glickman and Blumenfield[114] felt that reactions were more or less severe depending upon the patient's disappointment in the failure of LSD to avert threatened decompensation, his wish to attribute his symptoms to the drug, as well as the amount of pharmacologic effects, primarily dependent on dose. They characterized LSD users who later are hospitalized for an adverse reaction as having "pre-existing difficulties in adult social and sexual functioning, a tendency to use drugs to reduce tensions, a current life crisis [and] a fantasy . . . that LSD ingestion will enable them to overcome this crisis by introjecting strength. When this fantasy conflicts with reality, the patient may project upon LSD the cause of his decompensation."[114] Blacker and associates[33] found that the "bum trip" with LSD usually occurred in the context of anger and speculated that anger or hate was magnified into "nightmarish proportions and . . . experienced as demons or primitive, cannibalistic creatures who attack and destroy their creator." Silverman has hypothesized that fear of overstimulation accounts for the production of the bad trip and that various maneuvers observed in adverse reactions such as withdrawal, blocking, and constriction of movement and speech serve to reduce the amount of sensory stimulation experienced.[303] Intrusion of repressed material is no doubt also involved. Barr and Langs put it this way:

[Psychoactive drugs as potent as LSD are] . . . certain to stir up trouble, and sometimes seriously upsetting trouble, in persons who do not have flexible defenses and ready access to their primary processes without being threatened by their own unconscious fantasies. LSD does not work merely by lifting repression, anymore than alcohol really works by dissolving the superego, but many of the effects do seem to be attributable to alterations in important defenses. If this is the case, it is to be expected that most of the time what emerges into awareness will be frightening—since it has been held back precisely because it arouses anxiety. [p. 165][9]

Prolonged adverse reactions lasting beyond the usual duration of intoxication include psy-chotic decompensation, depressive reactions, acting out, and paranoid states. These have been described by many investigators.*

Characterization of prolonged reactions to LSD have so far eluded precise description. Even "good trips" occasionally produce a syndrome of rapid loss of will to exert competence—manifested by "dropping out," absorption in magical thinking, and generally retreating from complexity—a syndrome that is amotivational. Paranoid states and confusional states with an overreliance on magical thinking occur, as well as depression following the perception that the everyday world is not as stimulating as the drug state. Occasionally, impulsive acts based on misperception of reality occur.

In what respect prolonged drug psychoses (and the change that has occurred) are similar to and different from naturally occurring psychoses is incompletely understood. Historically, controversy centered around whether the LSD intoxication could be viewed as a "model psychosis."[97,45,46,9] "It was, at best, unwieldy to compare an acute drug response to a chronic behavior pattern."[42] The hallucinogens, particularly, are thought to occasionally precipitate psychosis in individuals so predisposed, although the nature of the vulnerability is undefined. The question of whether the acute or chronic use of such drugs can produce psychotic adaptations (e.g., Smith's "LSD and the Psychedelic Syndrome")[308] in individuals whose "premorbid personalities are not typical of pre-psychotic individuals" was broached by Glass and Bowers,[113] and more recent thinking asserts that "[hallucinogenic drugs] can by single or repeated administration lead to a syndrome which behaves much like nondrug induced psychosis in the long as well as the short run."[42] Whether an individual is "predisposed" is complicated, since "this judgment is always made retrospectively and involves some assumptions about schizophrenia which are unproven, including the idea that pre-schizophrenic states can be characterized and recognized. . . . The implication in these in-

* See references 113, 109, 186, 97, 206, 202, 179, 306, 114, 343, 289, 68, 79, and 142.

stances that the drugs play relatively unimportant roles in the emergence and perpetuation of psychotic symptoms may be unwarranted."[46] Vulnerability to a psychosis is something quite separate from prognosis, as Bowers explained, and the differentiating features between drug and nondrug psychoses "point in the direction of more favorable prognostic findings in the drug induced states." Although prognosis for the drug induced psychoses is generally better, they are not necessarily more benign since self-mutilation, suicide, and homicide sometimes, though rarely, occur.

Bower's retrospective measurements of spinal-fluid metabolites in drug psychosis are consistent either with the hypothesis that there is a persistence of an acute pharmacological effect of the drug or that a biochemical alteration present before the drug was taken "rendered the individual . . . more susceptible to the disruptive effect of these compounds."[43] Tucker and associates[343] found that those multiple-drug users with predominant LSD use who had "a longer history of use tended to show higher incidence of the disrupted thinking, boundary confusion, and to a degree a higher extent of over-specific, personalized, or idiosyncratic thinking, and also tended to show a lesser incidence of the appearance of affect in their responses." Neither "the age the drug use was started nor the variety of drug use was significantly related to thinking disturbance in the sample." Although selected aspects of drug-induced psychoses are similar to certain aspects found in schizophrenics,[343] Blacker and associates[33] found that in contrast to schizophrenics, chronic LSD users were "involved with people and skilled interpersonally." The clinical picture of unusual beliefs, relatively intact interpersonal relationships and cognitive abilities suggest that [their] subjects were more similar to individuals usually termed eccentric than to individuals diagnosed as schizophrenic.[33]

Drugs interact in a variety of nonspecific ways with personality and social setting, and nondrug situational and maturational stresses may predispose the subject to decompensation, influence both his coping ability and

original motivation to use the drug.[46] Whether such decompensation would have occurred without the drug cannot be definitely determined. McGlothlin[217,220] notes how often persons view even extreme adverse reactions as beneficial in the long run, and Kendall[179] believes that for some of his subjects drug use may have "halted the development of an organized disease syndrome" by reducing the intensity of drive conflict or redirecting the subject's attention away from conflictual material.[179] Yet, in most adverse reactions, the drug seems to have played a crucial role in enhancing conflict and loosening control.[9,44,46] The drug may "reactivate certain painful intrapsychic issues and heighten the experience of conflict at certain critical developmental periods."[46]

Various treatments for the acute adverse reactions from LSD have been recommended—generally sedative medication or supportive psychotherapy (often labeled the "talk-down approach") or a combination of these. Detailed discussions of the techniques and outcome of the talk-down approach are available,* and case descriptions are heuristically valuable. The viewpoints on the use of sedative medications and phenothiazines in treatment are discussed by Bowers,[42,43] Shick and Smith,[299] and Bowers and Freedman.[46] The studies on behavioral effects of the combination of phenothiazines and STP (DOM) that is, 2,5-dimethoxy-4-methylamphetamine, is reviewed by Shick and Smith.[299] Phenothiazines can simply complicate the "bad trip," but their use in prolonged drug-related psychotic reactions is often beneficial, and with amphetamines, phenothiazines seem speific.[46,88]

To predict who is at risk to develop an adverse reaction is at present difficult, although research into individual differences in response to LSD sheds some light on this problem, as well as addressing the difficulties in such research. G. D. Klee and W. Weintraub[9] found that "paranoidlike reactions under the drug were most frequent in persons who are usually mistrustful, suspicious and fearful, and

* See references 195, 299, 302, 315, and 335.

who often use projection as a defense." Tucker and associates[343] noted that hospitalized drug users, regardless of diagnosis (psychotic or nonpsychotic) tested during the first week of admission, have "more signs of increased intrusions of primitive-drive material, higher penetration scores, and higher responsivity" on standardized scoring of Rorschach evaluations than hospitalized nondrug users. Duration of drug use was more closely related to these thinking disturbances than the variety or intensity of the drug use. The old notion that schizophrenics are "tolerant" or "resistant" to LSD seems untenable now in light of more recent work.[9,46] Bercel and associates[22] reported that the Rorschach test could identify most psychotic reactors, but Rorschachs did not permit them to predict the form that these reactions would take. Hensala and coworkers,[142] Kleber,[186] and Frosh and associates[109] attempted to determine the correlates of adverse reactions resulting in hospitalization. Barr and Langs report the results of a two-year, double-blind study into the individual differences in response to 100µgs. of LSD—carried out before the LSD effects were well known—and have reviewed the prior research on LSD and individual differences.[9] They developed a typology of the LSD reaction at the level of *syndrome* (not symptom) and found that the reactions to the intoxication correlate well with personality. Regression did not occur uniformly across ego functions; drive-related and conflict-related contents attracted attention most readily in LSD states; and there was an impairment in active defensive functions and increased use of passive functions in the face of an LSD experience. They distinguished six groups of personalities that reacted differently and describe in detail those in whom the intoxication produced extreme anxiety and those who tolerated the experience well.

Our findings show a built-in danger in a drug such as LSD. It is likely to be tried first and written about by people of the kind to whom it is least dangerous, whose rhapsodic accounts of euphoria, increased insight, or experiences of great beauty make the drug irresistibly attractive to those who are most vulnerable to its harmful effects. For it

is the very people whose personalities make it likely that they will *not* have positive reactions who are likely to be allured by the promise of a quick and easy answer to their problem in living— boredom, anxiety, the feeling of being trapped in a conformist world, depression and the like. [p. 166][9]

Research by Becker[12] and discussions of peyote use by the Navajo[97,24,215] acknowledge that the culture's social ritual and tradition surrounding the use of psychoactive substances often serve to contain, explain and influence various aspects of the experience and outcome.

The *personal* ways individuals deal with the intoxication and how this affects outcome is crucial. Psychic defensive operations that correlate with personality have been described[9,187] and certainly assignment of meaning is important, and the search for synthesis and mastery universal.[97] There may be convictions of revelations, delusional mastery, and repeated attempts at mastery (flashbacks), and connotations often balloon into cosmic allusiveness and are experienced as religiosity, aesthetically, sensually, or in a variety of clear or confused frames of reference. Acting out, possibly out of a search for boundaries, is often seen, as well as aggressive and endless talking about experiences as if users were trying to explain and integrate them. Freedman[97] has said, "The *need* for synthesis not the *ability* to synthesize with due accounts to real limits, is what tends to be reinforced in the drug state." Severe rumination and depression may result from a realistic inability to recapture the lost illusory and brilliant drug world. Conflict and confusion about "what *is* reality" may ensue, as well as a variety of mild or severe symptomatic states of perplexity and disorganization.

In any event, variably determined needs or capacities to cope with the split or breach of normal experience can be expected. This may be a simple 'sealing over,' or even an enlightened and useful thought formation we call insight. Some react with a denial of inadequacy and anxiety about loss of control; borrowing the enhanced omnipotence of the drug state, they show a delusional autonomy. This may lead to various outcomes: that of the benevolent and foolish prophet, or the defensive, alienated therapist, angry at those who prevent his curing the rest of the world. Any threat to the values of the illusory experience of union and omnipotence—such as undrugged reality—could evoke defensive denial and strident proselytizing. [p. 338][97]

An individual can react to the acute experience of the drug intoxication with anxiety or panic, ecstasy or terror, awe or tempered judgment. "The *sense* of truth is experienced as compellingly vivid, but not the inclination to test the truth of the senses. Unlike the sleeping dreamer, the waking dreamer is confronted with the co-existence of two compelling and contradictory orders of reality—with the interface of belief and the orderly rules of evidence."[97]

The consideration of drug factors, the expectations of the user and the setting comprise a bewildering array of variables that, to different degrees, may precipitate and influence the adverse reaction as well as its outcome. Within the drug culture, many suggestions, rituals, and explanations born from experience, about how to manage the effects of the drug and minimize the possibilities for an adverse reaction—or how to cope with it if it occurs—have been concretized as shared myths. A systematic study of the content of these suggestions, as well as their effectiveness in averting adverse reactions or minimizing unfavorable outcomes, has not appeared.

Spontaneous Recurrences

The well-publicized, if not sensationalized, consequence of illicit drug use has been the occurrence of flashbacks among a small proportion of hallucinogen users.* Described as a "transient spontaneous recurrence of certain aspects of a drug experience occurring after a period of relative normalcy following the original intoxication," the flashback is not unique to LSD, but can occur with psychotomimetic amphetamines, such as methylenedioxyamphetamine (MDA), DOM, etc., and has been reported to occur with marijuana.[178] The

* See references 147, 275, 298, 325, and 219.

early accounts stressed the perceptual changes that sometimes occur and the anxiety over loss of control that is not universally found.[275] Flashbacks may occur in any sense modality and distort time sense, self-image, or reality.[147]

The prevalence of this phenomena is difficult to assess since, besides the fact that most adverse reactions are managed within the subculture, persons without anxiety rarely seek medical attention, and many confirmed drug users regard these recurrences as desirable.[298,219] Furthermore, these subjective experiences are difficult to characterize, for both the user and researcher and are usually related after they occur. Often they cannot be separated from other aspects of the user's personality, behavior, and life situation. The prevalence of reported flashbacks increased with the increased use of LSD in nonmedical settings and also as the phenomenon was labeled, advertised, and popularized. Therefore, estimates are probably unreliable.

Clinical impressions indicate that flashbacks often occur in association with a previous bad trip, and the flashback often contains elements of content, affects, and perceptions reminiscent of that experience.[147,298] Those persons with greater numbers of LSD experiences are more frequently reporters of LSD-like recurrences; serious psychiatric disorders are not overrepresented among them, and reporters of flashbacks score higher on tests of hypnotic susceptibility.[217] "In very few instances does there appear to be substantial evidence of a causal relationship between the LSD experiences and the incidents described. [In most] . . . nothing more than the association of two events bearing certain similarities."[217] Various degrees of dyscontrol, though usually quite short and mild, may occur during the flashback and can result in accidents, injury, or misperception.

Flashbacks occur frequently, but not exclusively with chronic use, and may occur after a single intoxication. The use of various licit and illicit psychoactive drugs can apparently "trigger" a flashback, and such associations indicate that the flashback may be explained in terms of "arousal—statebound recall" of experience or state-dependent learning.[91]

Various other explanations described by Horowitz[147]—a release theory, deconditioning theory, psychodynamic theory, and mystical theory—have been proposed to account for flashbacks. These recurrences may represent one type of repetitive symptom that is part of the larger search for synthesis of various aspects of the drug experience, and are similar to responses to overwhelming stressful stimuli seen in traumatic neuroses.[97] They have also been likened to preemptory ideation, obsessive rumination, and repetitive visual pseudohallucinations, as in hysterical psychoses.[147] Horowitz examined subjects' responses to stressful films and found that intrusive thought, repetition of film content in thought, and negative affect, all increased after the film.[148] A brief discussion after the film appeared to reduce, but not eliminate, this response.

The "barrier" against dereistic thinking in altered states of consciousness (and to what extent a person can control slipping into these states) merits investigation. Various treatments have been described by Shick and Smith,[298] and Horowitz explains that, with supportive psychotherapy, the elimination of the symptom may be "accomplished through establishing a positive relationship rather than resolution of a trauma or lifting repression per se."[147]

The behavior, social stress, and psychodynamics preceding these lapses from reality deserve close scrutiny. The effectiveness of various treatments, psychological coping mechanisms, and social myths and responses that aid reintegration, await study.

Attitude, Belief and Value Change with LSD

Those LSD users who feel they are never quite the same as before they took the drug, no matter what the outcome, are usually not able to specify to themselves or to the researcher what specifically has changed. Users may report a greater tolerance toward others; less defensiveness, materialism, anxiety, competitiveness, aggression, and rigidity; greater capacity for introspection; and increased creativity and appreciation of art and music since

their use of LSD. The question is, the extent to which such changes can be objectively verified.

McGlothlin and associates[220] studied outcomes of 200 μg. of LSD administered in a clinical setting to 24 naive subjects in the early 1960s before the effects of the drug were widely known. A matched control group received 20 mg. of amphetamine or a 25-μg. LSD dose. Tests of anxiety, including galvanic skin response, tests of personality, attitudes and values and aesthetic sensitivity and creativity tests, were administered before the LSD experience and again at two weeks and six months following the last session.

Although personality-test measures of anxiety were not significantly different between the experimental and control group, measures of galvanic skin response to traumatic words and neutral words, digit span, mental arithmetic and proper names, tended to support the hypothesis that the experimental group experienced less emotional response to laboratory stress in the postdrug period at the six-month but not the two-week interval. At the six-month follow-up, the experimental group reported a "greater feeling of detachment," and "more intense mood swings," yet no one reported a "tendency to feel depressed." They indicated they were "less easily disturbed by frustrating situations," as well as now having a "less materialistic viewpoint toward life." It is interesting that 15 percent to a quarter of the subjects who received amphetamine reported an "enhanced understanding of self and others, and a greater tolerance toward those with opposing viewpoints," and practically no one who had received 25 μg. of LSD reported similar positive responses. Approximately twice as many of the experimental group who had received 200 μg. of LSD in each session answered positively to those four items. Such findings attest to the influence of expectations and set and setting in reported changes, and the need for active placebos and dose response studies.

In contrast to the *reported* changes in personality, attitude, and values between the control and experimental groups, the psychological-test measures in these areas tend to agree in the predicted direction with the subjective reports, although the magnitude of the changes was generally small. Objective tests of increased creativity or aesthetic sensitivity did not support the subjective reports, although they were supported by increased behavioral activities such as number of phonograph records bought, spending more time in museums, and attending more musical events. Generally, the only evidence of lasting effect was the subjective report of personality, attitude, value, and behavior change. The authors felt that many of the self-perceived changes were related to the "capacity of the psychedelics to temporarily suspend firmly entrenched perceptions, beliefs and values, and the capacity for viewing any belief system as essentially arbitrary."[220]

McGlothlin and Arnold[217] explored the lasting effects of LSD on 247 randomly selected subjects from a population of 750 who had received LSD for psychotherapy or experimental purposes from three physicians in the 1950s; 25 percent of the sample had some nonmedical experience with LSD. These subjects were compared to matched-control patients who had received psychotherapy from the same physicians but who had never taken LSD. Subjective reports and testing of personality, beliefs and values, attitudes, alienation, and behavior revealed "very little evidence of LSD-related change" among those who had experienced LSD in medical settings when compared to a matched-control group. By contrast, those who had taken LSD prior or subsequent to their medical exposure "demonstrated relatively large and consistent differences in comparison to the control, both in terms of the proportion reporting changes and the scores on related measures." Such changes are probably explained by considering that nonmedical LSD use attracted a certain type of individual, or that LSD interacted with critical milieu variables to produce the change. The LSD experience itself seems insufficient in many people to produce the often reported changes.

Such studies generally indicate that the claims of those who proselytized for LSD use —states of religious ecstasy, union with God,

lasting personality change—were overenthusiastic. It appears that many of the alterations attributed to LSD use were subjective evaluations and were highly correlated with the expectations of the users reinforced by the group. Studies at NIMH on the army, before the psychedelic frenzy of the 1960s, did not produce cults of users. The only claims that appear to have some objective validation are a period of decreased anxiety in the postdrug period for some, and claims of increased passivity and decreased aggressiveness with chronic LSD use among some users.[33,222,219]

Adverse Amphetamine Consequences

Acute panic reactions can occur with amphetamine use, as well as with LSD, and some of the same determinants are involved. Kramer has described the syndrome of acute toxicity with an overdose that may result in "chest pain, immobilization and even brief comatose states."[192] Competitive "shoot outs" between users are described by Smith,[317] and the user may ingest or inject other drugs in an attempt to counteract the acute effect of overdose.[301] As with LSD, during acute panic the user may focus his attention on the physical symptomatology of the sympathomimetic effect, such as the profuse sweating, photophobia or tachycardia which accompanies high doses.

Chronic users often report apathy ("amphetamine blues"), psychomotor retardation and sleep disturbances after discontinuation. They commonly state that this syndrome is often the stimulus for resuming a new round of amphetamine use in an effort to counteract the dysphoria.[301,309] Such findings await more precise definition and explanation, since no such withdrawal is seen when the drug is abruptly discontinued in monkeys given chronic high doses.[93,94] Animals allowed to administer amphetamine intravenously ad lib show the same cyclical pattern of use which intravenous methamphetamine abusers demonstrate.[287]

Tolerance to a wide variety of the effects of amphetamines has been demonstrated in animals and in man.[191] Monkeys gradually made tolerant to increasing amounts of intravenously administered methamphetamine on a chronic schedule every three hours become tolerant to all the effects except the stereotypic behavior.[93,94] Stereotypic behavior in humans is visible in jaw grinding and formications ("crank bugs") which produce continued scratching of the body.

Connell, Ellinwood, Snyder, Griffith and associates, and Bell have described the amphetamine psychosis and proposed various neurochemical and neurobiological explanations.[*] The picture presented practically mimics paranoid schizophrenia and often goes unrecognized as a toxic psychosis in hospitalized psychiatric patients.[301] Bell and Snyder have sought symptoms by which the two can be distinguished.[17,321] Griffith and coworkers produced a paranoid state in all volunteer subjects by increasing oral administration of dextroamphetamine, although they found large individual differences in the dose needed to produce the psychosis.[126] These subjects were previous users of amphetamines with diagnoses of moderate personality disorder, and this "prior-state" factor has not been ruled out as a component of amphetamine psychosis. There is a close correlation between the hallucinatory experiences and paranoid thinking and the blood level of amphetamine, and the disappearance of these phenomena and the amphetamine excretion level in the urine.[6] The classic amphetamine psychosis is a transient affair, disappearing on abstinence, but it exhibits various characteristics of psychosis, and at times may be prolonged. The preexisting pathology that contributes to the paranoid state has not been characterized.[46]

"Many investigators consider this high dose amphetamine reaction the closest experimental analogue of the naturally occurring psychoses," supported by the specificity of clinically effective antipsychotic compounds to antagonize the effects of amphetamines.[46] However, Bowers and Freedman,[46] and Bell[20,17] describe psychedelic and visual perceptual changes in the very early onset of amphetamine psychosis, and Freedman[97]

emphasizes that the second "stage" (four hours) of an LSD trip shows ideas of reference in a clear sensorium so that the clinical specificity of the amphetamine psychosis is not at all established, nor is the occurrence and threshold of occurrence of amphetamine psychosis in normal people understood.

Adverse Reactions to Marijuana

Many of the various adverse reactions described for LSD use have occasionally been reported to occur with marijuana,[†] and similar psychosocial determinants operate.[‡] There have been case reports of memory loss, paranoid reactions, precipitated psychoses, various degrees of organic-brain dysfunction, perceptual distortion, and confusional states, depressive reactions, panic reactions, and "flashbacks." Weil and Bialos review this literature.[353,29] Jones[171] discusses the literature on the psychotomimetic potential of marijuana and the alleged schizophrenic's "sensitivity" to the drug. He discusses the precipitants of adverse reactions in his laboratory, and he asserts that reports of paranoid experiences on mild doses of the drug are best explained by the user's expectation of this effect, and the interaction with personality and social variables, rather than the effects of the drug per se. Bialos describes the criteria operating in the various conceptualizations of an adverse marijuana reaction.[29]

The dose of THC often correlates with these experiences, but there is great intersubject variability.[145,172,169,170,171] Although marijuana, as it is presently used in this country, seems to produce relatively few such reactions and constitutes a minor hazard from a public-health viewpoint, studies of the more potent preparations raise the possibility of the occurrence of acute toxic psychoses, panic reactions, and flashback phenomena (generally reported when hashish was used in combination with other drugs), transient or prolonged psychotic states, and long-term adverse effects

---

[*] See references 20, 17, 69, 82, 126, and 321.

[†] See references 29, 132, 145, 172, 169, 170, 171, 178, 177, and 353.
[‡] See references 176, 172, 169, 170, 171, 97, 133, 10, and 12.

—reminiscent of Smith's "amotivational syndrome"[314,311,336]—with chronic high doses. The further characterization of such effects and elucidation of the mechanisms involved await research.

Drugs and Antisocial Behavior

There has been much discussion and little data about the relationship of drugs to criminal activity. The British have assessed the extent of drug use among delinquents[249,291,290] and have found that drug use is associated with higher intelligence and unfulfilled educational aspirations in their delinquents.[249] Ellinwood has discussed cases of assault and homicide associated with amphetamine abuse.[83]

Tinklenberg[340] has most recently reviewed this literature in a study prepared for the National Commission on Marijuana and Drug Abuse. The research into associations between drugs and criminal behavior is complicated by the difficulty of replicating in the laboratory the critical nonpharmacological variables.

Naturalistic studies are appropriate but require careful design and large samples to assure appropriate control data.

A large number of studies indicate that alcohol, the most widely used drug in the world, is clearly linked with violent crime. In many assaultive and sexually assaultive situations, alcohol is present in both assailant and victim.

An increasing amount of data links barbiturate users and amphetamine users with criminal activity, especially assaultive crimes. In a recent large scale study, the users of either amphetamines or barbiturates were more likely to be arrested for criminal homicide, forcible rape, or aggravated assault than were the users of heroin, morphine, cocaine, marihuana, hashish, tranquilizers, psychedelics, methadone, and special substances. However, amphetamine and barbiturate users were no more likely to be charged with violent crimes than were individuals who were identified as nondrug users, a category that probably included alcohol users. [p. 266][340]

Tinklenberg recommends that future research in the relationship of crime and drug use should include assessment of the relative contributions of the pharmacologic properties and the nonpharmacological variables to the crime process. He explains that it is not correct to assume that the heavier drug use of the intravenous drugs is positively associated with violent behavior. He finds, to the contrary, that in his sample the *nonassaultives were much heavier users of all drugs,* especially marijuana, hashish, the psychedelics, and the opiates. Furthermore, the repeated association of violence with alcohol and barbiturates suggests that more extensive research with a large sample size may result in an important association between these drugs (used singly or together) and violent crimes.

Concluding Remarks on Consequences and Outcomes

Research into the consequences and outcomes of illicit drug use requires an even more precise understanding of the metabolic, molecular, and tissue bases for the adverse consequences. The prediction of who is at risk and how various outcomes are managed by the social group, the individual, and the clinical personnel is a major issue. Mortality and morbidity statistics are scant in this literature, and toxicological research, especially with chronic use of the higher potency THC compounds and the high doses of amphetamines, is just beginning. A more precise definition of the public-health risk of the various consequences described will require epidemiologic methods accurately defining prevalence of different patterns of use and sorting out the effects of the drug from the other social and psychological factors.

(Conclusion

Research in nonnarcotic drug abuse deals with a broad public-health issue that has involved many different segments of society. It spans the field of psychopharmacological and social-psychological studies, utilizing trend surveys, case studies, and epidemiologic, sociological, and psychiatric models (from psychoanalytic to operant conditioning) to describe and predict extent and trends of current use, to investigate causes, to define and implement treatment and prevention models (as well as to assess their efficacy), and to delineate and attempt to predict the consequences and outcomes. A thin cadre of knowledgeable research and treatment personnel in this area has been slowly growing.

Although knowledge and perspective have accrued, research is far from precisely and reliably defining who is at risk for a particular pattern of use or a particular outcome. What factors cause drug use and sustain it, as well as effects contingent on joining a subculture and factors arising independently, are still largely unspecified. Some observations of how subcultures grow are available but largely are unanalyzed. Why drug habits once entrenched are so hard to give up and are so rarely forgotten, how the search for novelty, recreation, risk taking and control influence drug use, how people medicate themselves and what they are treating, as well as how historical and cultural influences interact with drug-taking behavior, these are relevant dimensions and questions for further inquiry. In general, there is a grasp of the relevance of each issue to the entire range of issues. Placing each item in its context seems far more possible today than formerly. The definition of the problems to be solved and questions to be asked is beginning to be focused. The relationships of mental, bodily, behavioral, and social events can be studied through such psychopharmacological research, but psychopathological mechanisms have not been closely studied in drug-abusing individuals.

The research sector has been perhaps too involved in providing expertise to help mediate transitions in social customs centered about the giving, getting, and consumption of drugs, and the management of the outcomes. But while it is fair to warn the public about what is known—that there is always the unexpected that occurs with drugs, and that drugs are never given without weighing the risks—it is not appropriate for research to provide flimsy rationalizations for issues that require value judgments and public choice. All too frequently fragmentary findings have been lent to various social movements in attempts to influence public behavior with premature publicity. A crisis of trust, communication and understanding about the authenticity, validity, applicability (and intrinsic limitation) of research findings to the use and abuse—not only of illicit drugs but all medicines and their regulated traffic—has arisen. Scientific restraint is required to diminish the influence of those with vested interests in sensationalizing such issues.

Rapidly evolving social forms and redefinitions of personal purposes confront societies with truly severe crises. The uses of technology confuse and confound public decision. Adaptive man will probably confront and eventually construct answers to these complex problems—of which drug abuse is but a symptom. As with any symptom, it deserves and requires treatment in its own right as basic remedies are sought and researched. Precise definition of the kinds of harm of a particular drug or pattern of use is required. Initial diagnosis and goal setting, dispassionate assessment, selective fitting of means to ends, anticipation of consequences to the entire system of drug supply and use are essential principles in designing responses to concerns about drug use.

Perhaps the end of the epidemic of the 1960s is at hand; illicit drug abuse is again becoming a problem for *some* instead of a "problem for everybody." But drug misuse is an endemic problem and today's response may not be tomorrow's answer. Man's appetite for recreational drugs always has an epidemic or fadlike quality. Whether society will be better prepared for a future epidemic remains to be seen. The task will be to convert episodes of public panic into concern, and generally to encourage more selective and responsible patterns of drug taking.

Drug use, not just illicit drug use, is a complex legal, economic, social, and health issue. Essentially, a society regulates drug use by laws and by attitudes—establishing customs controlling both the manufacture of and access to drugs, and attempting to influence, interpret and control the drug-taking behavior of individuals. It is striking that the total drug and medicine network has never been looked at in a systematic way, nor has there been a responsible assembling of involved persons (manufacturers, educators, scientists, distributors, and consumers) to assess public needs and the consequences of randomly proposed solutions.

Policy formulation in support of research often fails because there is little public understanding of how research problems are approached and solved, how inquiry is, in fact, mounted (rather than engineered) how room must be left for the "surprising" finding, and how the scientific conclusions of the moment may be abandoned in the process of reaching the findings of the future. Neither the value, the limit, nor the intent of scientific method is widely comprehended even by some technically facile as well as administratively prominent scientists. The contingent status of a scientific finding, the "wasted activity" that bridges the gaps between occasional peaks of accomplishment, the unpredictability of the source of new knowledge, and respect for the complexity with which ultimately simple operations are organized as sequences of behavior are tasks for public education. So, too, is the existence of the system of inquirers ranging from the bench to the clinic, reciprocally posing problems and exchanging ideas—and adjudicating truth by critique and the logic of science.[105]

The defects in our total societal capacity to regulate medicines make us highly vulnerable to respond shortsightedly to the concerns about currently unpopular drugs and the persons using them. The piecemeal approach to drug abuse simply makes such fissures in the body politic more visible. Drugs *are* a vehicle for other issues, as the recent epidemic demonstrated. The research sector should recall that, while the rules of evidence belong to science, what is and is not legitimate research and medical practice is ultimately defined by society. The role of inquiry plays a part in all

of this, and its integrity and vitality rests on its freedom, its intrinsic limitations as well as its responsiveness to general social concerns.

(Bibliography

1. ADAM, K. S. and J. G. LOHRENZEO. "Drug Abuse, Self-abuse and the Abuse of Authority," *J. Can. Psychiatr. Assoc.*, 15 (1970), 79–81.
2. ADELSON, J. "The Invention of the Young Radical," *Commentary*, 51 (1971), 43–48 and 52 (1971), 26–31.
3. ALDRICH, C. K. "The Effects of a Synthetic Marijuana-like Compound on Musical Talent as Measured by the Reaction Test," *Publ. Health Repts.*, 59 (1944), 431–433.
4. ALLEN, J. R. and L. J. WEST. "Flight from Violence: Hippies and the Green Rebellion," *Am. J. Psychiatry*, 125 (1968), 364–369.
5. ANDERSON, W. H., J. E. O'MALLEY, and A. LAZARE. "Failure of Outpatient Treatment of Drug Abuse: II. Amphetamines, Barbiturates, Hallucinogens," *Am. J. Psychiatry*, 128 (1972), 122–126.
6. ANGRIST, B. N., J. SCHWEITZER, A. J. FRIEDHOFF et al. "The Clinical Symptomatology of Amphetamine Psychosis and Its Relationship to Amphetamine Levels in Urine," *Int. Pharmacopsychiatry*, 2 (1969), 125–139.
7. AUSBEL, D. P. *Drug Addiction: Physiological, Psychological and Sociological Aspects.* New York: Random House, 1958.
8. BALL, J. C. "Reliability and Validity of Interview Data Obtained from 59 Narcotic Addicts," *Am. J. Sociol.*, 72 (1967), 650–654.
9. BARR, H. L., R. J. LANGS, R. R. HOLT et al. *LSD: Personality and Experience.* New York: Wiley-Interscience, 1971.
10. BECKER, H. S. "Becoming a Marijuana User," *Am. J. Sociol.*, 59 (1953), 235–242.
11. ———. *Outsiders.* New York: Free Press, 1963.
12. ———. "History, Culture and Subjective Experience: An Exploration of the Social Bases of Drug-Induced Experiences," *J. Health Soc. Behav.*, 8 (1967), 163–176.

13. ———. "Knowledge, Power and Drug Effects," *Society*, 10 (1973), 26–31.

14. BEJEROT, N. "An Epidemic of Phenmetrazine Dependence—Epidemiological and Clinical Aspects," in C. W. M. Wilson, ed., *Adolescent Drug Dependence*, pp. 55–66. Oxford: Pergamon, 1968.

15. ———. "Social Medical Classification of Addictions," *Int. J. Addict.*, 4 (1969), 391–405.

16. ———. "A Theory of Addiction as an Artificially Induced Drive," *Am. J. Psychiatry*, 128 (1972), 842–846.

17. BELL, D. S. "Comparison of Amphetamine Psychosis and Schizophrenia," *Br. J. Psychiatry*, 111 (1965), 701–707.

18. ———. "Drug Addiction," *Bull. Narc.*, 22 (1970), 21–32.

19. ———. "The Precipitants of Amphetamine Addiction," *Br. J. Psychiatry*, 119 (1971), 171–177.

20. BELL, D. S. and W. H. TRETHOWAN. "Amphetamine Addiction," *J. Nerv. Ment. Dis.*, 133 (1961), 489–496.

21. BENSON, H. and R. K. WALLACE. "Decreased Drug Abuse after the Continued Practice of Transcendental Meditation." Unpublished manuscript.

22. BERCEL, N. A., L. E. TRAVIS, L. B. OLINGER et al. "Model Psychoses Induced by LSD in Normals, I and II," *AMA Arch. Neurol. Psychiatry*, 75 (1956), 588–611; 612–618.

23. BERG, D. "The Non-Medical Use of Dangerous Drugs in the U.S.: A Comprehensive View," *Int. J. Addict.*, 5 (1970), 777–834.

24. BERGMAN, R. L. "Navajo Peyote Use: Its Apparent Safety," *Am. J. Psychiatry*, 128 (1971), 695–699.

25. BERMAN, S. "Alienation: An Essential Process of the Psychology of Adolescence," *J. Child Psychiatry*, 9 (1970), 233–250.

26. BETTELHEIM, B. "Obsolete Youth," *Encounter*, 23 (1969), 29–42.

27. BEWLEY, T. H. "II: Recent Changes in the Pattern of Drug Abuse in London and the United Kingdom," in *The Pharmacological and Epidemiological Aspects of Adolescent Drug Dependence*, pp. 197–220. Proceedings of the Society of Addiction, London, September, 1966. Oxford: Pergamon, 1968.

28. BEWLEY, T. H., O. BEN-ARIE, and I. P. JAMES. "Morbidity and Mortality from Heroin Dependence," *J. Child Psychiatry*, 1 (1968), 725–732.

29. BIALOS, D. S. "Adverse Marijuana Reactions: A Critical Examination of the Literature with Selected Case Material," *Am. J. Psychiatry*, 127 (1970), 819–823.

30. BLACHLY, P. H. *Seduction: A Conceptual Model in the Drug Dependencies and Other Contagious Ills.* Springfield, Ill: Charles C. Thomas, 1970.

31. BLACK, S., K. L. OWENS, and R. P.WOLFF. "Patterns of Drug Use: A Study of 5,482 Subjects," *Am. J. Psychiatry*, 127 (1970), 420–423.

32. BLACKER, K. H. "Drugs and the Social Setting," *Clinical Toxicol.*, 2 (1969), 201–207.

33. BLACKER, K. H., R. T. JONES, G. C. STONE et al. "Chronic Users of LSD: The 'Acid Heads'," *Am. J. Psychiatry*, 125 (1968), 341–351.

34. BLOS, P. "The Function of the Ego Ideal in Adolescence," in *The Psychoanalytic Study of the Child*, Vol. 27, pp. 93–97. New York: International Universities Press, 1972.

35. BLUM, R. H. et al. *The Utopiates.* New York: Atherton Press, 1964.

36. ———. *Society and Drugs*, Vol. 1. San Francisco: Jossey-Bass, 1970.

37. ———. *Students and Drugs*, Vol. 2. San Francisco: Jossey-Bass, 1970.

38. ———. *Horatio Alger's Children.* San Francisco: Jossey-Bass, 1972.

39. ———. *The Dream Sellers.* San Francisco: Jossey-Bass, 1972.

40. BLUMBERG, A. G., M. COHEN, A. M. HEATON et al. "Covert Drug Abuse Among Voluntary Hospitalized Psychiatric Patients," *JAMA*, 217 (1971), 1659–1661.

41. BOWERS, M. B., JR. "Student Psychedelic Drug Use—An Evaluation by Student Drug Users," *Int. J. Addict.*, 4 (1969), 89–99.

42. ———. "Acute Psychosis Induced by Psychotomimetic Drug Abuse: I. Clinical Findings," *Arch. Gen. Psychiatry*, 27 (1972), 437–439.

43. ———. "Acute Psychosis Induced by Psychotomimetic Drug Abuse: II. Neurochemical Findings," *Arch. Gen. Psychiatry*, 27 (1972), 440–442.

44. BOWERS, M. B., JR., A. CHIPMAN, A. SCHWARTZ et al. "Dynamics of Psychedelic

Drug Abuse," *Arch. Gen. Psychiatry*, 16 (1967), 560–566.

45. BOWERS, M. B., JR. and D. X. FREEDMAN. "'Psychedelic' Experiences in Acute Psychosis," *Arch. Gen. Psychiatry*, 15 (1966), 240–248.

46. ———. "Psychosis Associated with Drug Use," in *American Handbook of Psychiatry*, S. Arieti, ed., Vol. 4, pp. 356–370. New York: Basic Books, 1975.

47. BRADEN, W. *Age of Aquarius*. Chicago: Quadrangle, 1970.

48. BRECHER, E. et al. *Licit and Illicit Drugs*. Boston: Little, Brown, 1972.

49. BROTMAN, R. and A. FREEDMAN. *A Community Mental Health Approach to Drug Addiction*. Washington: U.S. Govt. Print. Off., 1968.

50. BUCKMAN, J. "Theoretical Aspects of LSD Therapy," in H. A. Abramson, ed., *The Use of LSD in Psychotherapy and Alcoholism*, pp. 83–100. Indianapolis: Bobbs, 1967.

51. ———. "Psychology of Drug Abuse," *Med. Coll. Va.*, 7 (1971), 98–102.

52. CALEF, V., R. GRYLER, L. HILLES et al. "Impairment of Ego Functions in Psychedelic Drug Users." Presented at Conf. Drug Use and Drug Subcultures, Pacific Grove, Calif., 1970.

53. CALLAN, J. P. "Patterns of Drug Use among 19,948 Military Inductees." Presented at Am. Psychiatr. Assoc. Meet. Dallas, May 1972.

54. CAREY, J. T. *The College Drug Scene*. Englewood Cliffs, N.J.: Prentice-Hall, 1968.

55. ———. "Marijuana Use among the New Bohemians," in D. E. Smith, ed., *The New Social Drug*, pp. 94–104. Englewood Cliffs, N.J.: Prentice-Hall, 1970.

56. CAREY, J. T. and J. MANDEL. "A San Francisco Bay Area 'Speed' Scene," *J. Health Soc. Behav.*, 9 (1968), 164–174.

57. CHAMBERS, C. D. "The Treatment of Non-Narcotic Drug Abusers," in L. Brill and L. Liebermann, eds., *Major Modalities in the Treatment of Drug Abuse*, pp. 203–235. Boston: Little, Brown, 1972.

58. CHEEK, F. E., S. NEWELL, and M. JOFFE. "Deceptions in the Illicit Drug Market," *Am. Assoc. Advanc. Sci.*, 167 (1970), 1276.

59. CHEIN, I., D. L. LEE, and E. ROSENFELD.

The Road to H: Narcotics, Delinquency and Social Policy. New York: Basic Books, 1964.

60. CITRON, B. P., M. HALPERN, M. McCARRON et al. "Necrotizing Angiitis Associated with Drug Abuse," *N. Engl. J. Med.*, 283 (1970), 1003–1011.

61. CLAUSEN, J. A. "Social Pattern, Personality and Adolescent Drug Use," in A. H. Leighton, J. A. Clausen, and R. N. Wilson, eds., *Explorations in Social Psychiatry*, pp. 230–277. London: Tavistock, 1957.

62. COFFEY, T. G. "Beer Street: Gin Lane. Some Views of 18th-Century Drinking," *Q. J. Stud. Alcohol*, 27 (1966), 669–692.

63. COHEN, A. Y. "The Journey Beyond Trips: Alternatives to Drugs," *J. Psychedel. Drugs*, 3 (1971), 16–21.

64. COHEN, C. S., E. H. WHITE, and J. C. SCHOOAR. "Interpersonal Patterns of Personality for Drug Abusing Patients and Their Therapeutic Implications," *Arch. Gen. Psychiatry*, 24 (1971), 353–358.

65. COHEN, M. and D. F. KLEIN. "Drug Abuse in a Young Psychiatric Population," *Am. J. Orthopsychiatry*, 40 (1970), 448–455.

66. ———. "Age of Onset of Drug Abuse in Psychiatric In-patients," *Arch. Gen. Psychiatry*, 26 (1972), 266–269.

67. COHEN, S. "A Classification of LSD Complications," *Psychosomatics*, 7 (1966), 182–186.

68. COHEN, S. and K. S. DITMAN. "Prolonged Adverse Reactions to Lysergic Acid Diethylamide," *Arch. Gen. Psychiatry*, 8 (1963), 475–480.

69. CONNELL, P. H. *Amphetamine Psychosis*. Maudsley Monographs, 5. London: Chapman and Hall, 1958.

70. DAVIS, F. "Why All of Us May Be Hippies Some Day," in D. N. Michael, ed., *The Future Society*. Chicago: Aldine, 1970.

71. DAVIS, F. and L. MUNOZ. "Heads and Freaks: Patterns and Meanings of Drug Use among Hippies," *J. Health Soc. Behav.*, 9 (1968), 156–164.

72. DE ALARCON, R. "The Spread of Heroin Abuse in a Community," *Bull. Narc.*, 21 (1969), 17–22.

73. ———. "Drug Abuse as a Communicable Disease: The Public Health Value of Prevalence, Incidence and Mode of Spread Studies," Milroy Lectures, R. Coll. Phys., 1971.

74. ———. "An Epidemiological Evaluation of a Public Health Measure Aimed at Reducing the Availability of Methylamphetamine," *Psychol. Med.*, 2 (1972), 293–300.

75. DE ALARCON, R. and N. H. RATHOD. "Prevalence and Early Detection of Heroin Abuse," *Br. Med. J.*, 2 (1968), 549–553.

76. DE LEON, G., S. HOLLAND, and M. S. ROSENTHAL. "Phoenix House: Criminal Activity of Dropouts," *JAMA*, 222 (1972), 686–689.

77. DE LEON, G., A. SKODOL, and M. S. ROSENTHAL. "Phoenix House," *Arch. Gen. Psychiatry*, 28 (1973), 131–136.

78. DENEAU, G., T. YANAGITA, and M. H. SEEVERS. "Self-Administration of Psychoactive Substance by the Monkey," *Psychopharmacologia*, 16 (1969), 30–48.

79. DITMAN, K. S., W. TIETZ, B. S. PRINCE et al. "Harmful Aspects of the LSD Experience," *J. Nerv. Ment. Dis.*, 145 (1968), 464–474.

80. DUSTER, T. *The Legislation of Morality*. New York: Free Press, 1970.

81. EFRON, D. H., B. HOLMSTEDT, and N. S. KLINE, eds. *Ethnopharmacologic Search for Psychoactive Drugs*. Washington: PHS Pub., No. 1645, 1967.

82. ELLINWOOD, E. H. "Amphetamine Psychosis: I. Description of Individuals and Process," *J. Nerv. Ment. Dis.*, 144 (1967), 273–283.

83. ———. "Assault and Homicide Associated with Amphetamine Abuse," *Am. J. Psychiatry*, 127 (1971), 1170–1175.

84. ERIKSON, E. H. "Growth and Crises of the Healthy Personality," *Psychol. Issues*, 1 (1959), 50–100.

85. ———. "The Problem of Ego Identity," *Psychol. Issues*, 1 (1959), 101–171.

86. ———. *Identity: Youth and Crisis*. New York: Norton, 1968.

87. ———. "Reflections on the Dissent of Contemporary Youth," *Int. J. Psychoanal.*, 51 (1970), 11–21.

88. ESPELIN, D. E. and A. K. DONE. "Amphetamine Poisoning," *N. Engl. J. Med.*, 278 (1968), 1361–1366.

89. FEIGHNER, J. P., E. ROBBINS, S. B. GUZE et al. "Diagnostic Criteria for Use in Psychiatric Research," *Arch. Gen. Psychiatry*, 26 (1972), 57–63.

90. FINESTONE, H. "Cats, Kicks and Color," *Soc. Prob.*, 5 (1957), 3–13.

91. FISCHER, R. "The 'Flashback': Arousal—Statebound Recall of Experience," *J. Psychedel. Drugs*, 3 (1971), 31–39.

92. FISCHER, R. and G. M. LANDON. "On the Arousal State—Dependent Recall of 'Subconscious' Experience: Stateboundness," *Br. J. Psychiatry*, 120 (1972), 159–172.

93. FISCHMAN, M. W. "Behavioral Effects of Methamphetamines." Ph.D. thesis, University of Chicago, 1972.

94. FISCHMAN, M. W. and C. R. SCHUSTER. Behavioral Toxicity of Chronic Methamphetamine in the Rhesus Monkey," in B. Weiss and V. Laties, eds., *Behavioral Toxicology*. Appleton, forthcoming.

95. FISCHMANN, V. S. "Drug Addicts in a Therapeutic Community," *Int. J. Addict.*, 3 (1968), 351–359.

96. ———. "Stimulant Users in the California Rehabilitation Center," *Int. J. Addict.*, 3 (1968), 113–130.

97. FREEDMAN, D. X. "On the Use and Abuse of LSD," *Arch. Gen. Psychiatry*, 18 (1968), 330–347.

98. ———. "Implications for Research," *JAMA*, 206 (1968), 1280–1284.

99. ———. "Drug Abuse—Comments on the Current Scene," *Midway*, 9 (1969), 3–25.

100. ———. "What Is Drug Abuse?" in W. W. Stewart, ed., *Drug Abuse In Industry*, pp. 27–41. Miami: Halos, 1970.

101. ———. "Amphetamine and Cocaine Abuse," *Post. Grad. Med.*, 47 (1970), 57–59.

102. ———. "Drug Abuse and Medical Leadership," *Arch. Gen. Psychiatry*, 25 (1971), 289–290.

103. ———. "Symposium On Drug Abuse—Introduction," *Clin. Res.*, 19 (1971), 598–600.

104. ———. "Non-Pharmacologic Factors in Drug Dependence," in S. Btesh, ed., *Drug Abuse: Non-medical Use of Dependence-Producing Drugs*, pp. 25–34. New York: Plenum, 1972.

105. ———. "Psychosocial and Pharmacological Aspects of Opiate Addiction—Introduction," in S. Fischer and A. Freedman, eds., *Opiate Addiction: Origins and Treatment*, pp. 3–6. Washington: V. H. Winston, 1973.

106. FREEDMAN, D. X. and E. C. SENAY. "Heroin Epidemics," *JAMA*, 223 (1973), 1155–1156.

107. FREUD, S. (1930) "Civilization and Its Dis-

contents," in J. Strachey, ed., *Standard Edition*, Vol. 21, pp. 64–145. London: Hogarth, 1961.

108. ———. (1927) "Humour," in J. Strachey, ed., *Standard Edition*, Vol. 21, pp. 161–166. London: Hogarth, 1961.

109. FROSCH, W. A., E. S. ROBBINS, and M. STERN. "Untoward Reactions to Lysergic Acid Diethylamide (LSD) Resulting in Hospitalization," *N. Engl. J. Med.*, 273 (1965), 1235–1239.

110. GAY, G. R., J. J. WINKLER, and J. A. NEWMEYER. "Emerging Trends of Heroin Abuse in the San Francisco Bay Area," *J. Psychedel. Drugs*, 4 (1971), 53–64.

111. GLASS, G. S. "Marijuana and Other Drug Use by Coeds." Presented at Am. Psychiatric Assoc., Dallas, May, 1972.

112. ———. "The Psychology of Hallucinogenic Drug Discontinuers." Presented at Am. Psychiatr. Assoc., Dallas, May, 1972.

113. GLASS, G. S. and M. B. BOWERS. "Chronic Psychosis Associated with Long-Term Psychotomimetic Drug Abuse," *Arch. Gen. Psychiatry*, 23 (1970), 97–103.

114. GLICKMAN, L. and M. BLUMENFIELD. "Psychological Determinants of 'LSD Reactions'," *J. Nerv. Ment. Dis.*, 145 (1967), 79–83.

115. GOLDBERG, S. R. "Relapse to Opioid Dependence: The Role of Conditioning," in R. T. Harris, W. M. McIssac, and C. R. Schuster, eds., *Drug Dependence*, pp. 170–197. Austin: University of Texas Press, 1970.

116. GOLDSTEIN, J. W. and J. GLEASON. "On the Significance of Increasing Student Marijuana Use for Intended Use of Other Drugs." *Proc. 81st Annu. Conv. Am. Psychological Assoc.*, 1973.

117. GOODE, E. "Multiple Drug Use Among Marijuana Smokers," *Soc. Prob.*, 17 (1969), 48–64.

118. ———. "Marijuana and the Politics of Reality," in D. E. Smith, ed., *The New Social Drug*, pp. 168–186. Englewood Cliffs, N.J.: Prentice-Hall, 1970.

119. ———. *The Marijuana Smokers*. New York, Basic Books, 1970.

120. GOTTHEIL, E., A. I. ALTERMAN, T. E. SKOLODA et al. "Alcoholics' Pattern of Controlled Drinking." Presented at Am. Psychiatric Assoc. Meet., Dallas, May 5, 1972.

121. GOTTHEIL, E., L. O. CORBETT, J. C. GRAS-

BERGER et al. "Treating the Alcoholic in the Presence of Alcohol," *Am. J. Psychiatry*, 128 (1971), 475–479.

122. GOTTSCHALK, L. A., D. E. BATES, R. A. FOX et al. "Psychoactive Drug Use," *Arch Gen. Psychiatry*, 25 (1971), 395–397.

123. GOTTSCHALK, L. A., J. L. HAER, and D. E. BATES. "Effect of Sensory Overload on Psychological State," *Arch. Gen. Psychiatry*, 27 (1972), 451–456.

124. GREDEN, J. F. and D. W. MORGEN. "Patterns of Drug Use and Attitudes Towards Treatment in a Military Population," *Arch. Gen. Psychiatry*, 26 (1972), 113–117.

125. GRIFFITH, J. "A Study of Illicit Amphetamine Drug Traffic in Oklahoma City," *Am. J. Psychiatry*, 123 (1966), 560–569.

126. GRIFFITH, J., J. CAVANAUGH, J. HELD et al. "Dextroamphetamine," *Arch. Gen. Psychiatry*, 26 (1972), 97–100.

127. GRIFFITH, J., J. DAVIS, and J. OATES. "Amphetamines: Addiction to a Non-Addicting Drug," in O. Vinar, et al., eds., *Advances In Neuropharmacology*, pp. 251–260. Amsterdam: North Holland Pub. Co., 1971.

128. GRYLER, R. B. and P. A. KEMPNER. "Ego Impairments and Poly-Drug Abuse: A Case Study," *Bull. Menninger Clin.*, 36 (1972), 436–450.

129. GUSFIELD, J. R. "Moral Passage: The Symbolic Process in Public Designations of Deviance," *Soc. Prob.*, 15 (1967), 175–188.

130. GUTMANN, D. "The New Mythologies and Premature Aging in the Youth Culture," *J. Youth Adol.*, 2 (1973), 139–155.

131. HAGGARD, E. A., A. BREKSTAD, and A. G. SKARD. "On the Reliability of the Anamnestic Interview," *J. Abnorm. Soc. Psychol.*, 61 (1960), 311–318.

132. HALIKAS, J. A., D. W. GOODWIN, and S. B. GUZE. "Marijuana Effects: A Survey of Regular Users," *JAMA*, 217 (1971), 692–694.

133. ———. "Marijuana Use and Psychiatric Illness," *Arch. Gen. Psychiatry*, 27 (1972), 162–165.

134. HARMATZ, J. S., R. I. SHADER, and C. SALZMAN. "Marijuana Users and Non Users," *Arch. Gen. Psychiatry*, 26 (1972), 108–112.

135. HARRINGTON, M. "We Few, We Happy Few, We Bohemians," *Esquire*, 78 (1972), 99–103; 162–164.

136. HARTMANN, D. "A Study of Drug Taking Adolescents," in *The Psychoanalytic Study Of The Child*, Vol. 24, pp. 384–398. New York: International Universities Press, 1969.

137. HAUSER, P. M. "The Chaotic Society: Product of the Social Morphological Revolution," *Am. Sociol. Rev.*, 3 (1969), 1–19.

138. HAWKS, D. V. "The Epidemiology of Drug Dependence in the United Kingdom," *Bull. Narc.*, 22 (1970), 15–24.

139. ———. "The Dimensions of Drug Dependence in the United Kingdom," *Int. J. Addict.*, 6 (1971), 135–160.

140. HAWKS, D. V., M. MITCHESON, A. OGBORNE et al. "Abuse of Methylamphetamine," *Br. Med. J.*, 2 (1969), 715–721.

141. HAWKS, D. V., A. C. OGBORNE, and M. C. MITCHESON. "The Strategy of Epidemiological Research in Drug Dependence," *Br. J. Addict.*, 65 (1970), 363–368.

142. HENSALA, J. P., L. J. EPSTEIN, and K. H. BLACKER. "LSD and Psychiatric Inpatients," *Arch. Gen. Psychiatry*, 16 (1967), 554–559.

143. HEYMAN, F. "Amphetamine Abuse in Japan." Unpublished manuscript.

144. HOFER, R. and S. M. PITTEL. "Characteristics of Amphetamine Users in a Hippie Subculture." Presented at Am. Psychol. Assoc. Meet., Sept. 4, 1971.

145. HOLLISTER, L. E. "Marijuana in Man: Three Years Later," *Science*, 172 (1971), 21–29.

146. HOLMES, D. "Selected Characteristics of 'Hippies' in New York City: An Overview." Presented at Conf. on Drug Usage and Drug Subcultures, Asilomar, Calif., 1970.

147. HOROWITZ, M. J. "Flashbacks: Recurrent Intrusive Images after the Use of LSD," *Am. J. Psychiatry*, 126 (1969), 565–569.

148. HOROWITZ, M. J. and S. S. BECKER. "Cognitive Response to Stressful Stimuli," *Arch. Gen. Psychiatry*, 25 (1971), 419–428.

149. HOWARD, J. and P. BORGES. "Needle Sharing in the Haight: Some Social and Psychological Functions," *J. Psychedel. Drugs*, 4 (1971), 71–80.

150. HUGHES, P. H., N. W. BARKER, G. A. CRAWFORD et al. "The Natural History of a Heroin Epidemic," *Am. J. Pub. Health*, 62 (1972), 995–1001.

151. HUGHES, P. H., J. CHAPPEL, E. SENAY et al. "Developing Inpatient Services for Community-Based Treatment of Narcotic Addiction," *Arch. Gen. Psychiatry*, 25 (1971), 278–283.

152. HUGHES, P. H. and G. A. CRAWFORD. "Epidemiologic Field Projects to Reduce the Incidence and Prevalence of Heroin Addiction in Chicago," *J. Psychedel. Drugs*, 4 (1971), 95–98.

153. ———. "A Contagious Disease Model for Researching and Intervening in Heroin Epidemics," *Arch. Gen. Psychiatry*, 27 (1972), 149–155.

154. HUGHES, P. H., G. A. CRAWFORD, N. W. BARKER et al. "The Social Structure of a Heroin Copping Community," *Am. J. Psychiatry*, 128 (1971), 551–558.

155. HUGHES, P. H., C. M. FLOYD, G. NORRIS et al. "Organizing the Therapeutic Potential of an Addict Prisoner Community," *Int. J. Addict.*, 5 (1970), 205–223.

156. HUGHES, P. H. and J. H. JAFFE. "The Heroin Copping Area," *Arch. Gen. Psychiatry*, 24 (1971), 394–400.

157. ———. "Heroin Epidemics in Chicago." Proc. 5th World Congr. Psychiatry, Nov., Dec., 1971.

158. HUGHES, P. H., C. R. SANDERS, and E. SCHAPS. "The Impact of Medical Intervention in Three Heroin Copping Areas." *Proc. 4th Natl. Conf. Methadone Treat.*, pp. 81–83. San Francisco, Jan. 8–10, 1972. New York: Natl. Assoc. Prevtn. Addict. Narc., 1972.

159. HUGHES, P. H., E. SCHAPS, and C. R. SANDERS. "A Methodology for Monitoring Adolescent Drug Abuse Trends." Unpublished manuscript, 1972.

160. HUGHES, P. H., E. SCHAPS, C. R. SANDERS et al. "Drug Abuse Trends in Six Midwestern High Schools." Unpublished manuscript, 1972.

161. HUGHES, P. H., E. C. SENAY, and R. PARKER. "The Medical Management of a Heroin Epidemic," *Arch. Gen. Psychiatry*, 27 (1972), 585–593.

162. HUXLEY, A. *The Doors of Perception and Heaven and Hell.* New York: Harper & Row, 1954.

163. INDIAN HEMP DRUGS COMMISSION. *Marijuana, Report of the Indian Hemp Drugs Commission.* Simla: Govt. Cent. Print. Off., 1894.

164. IRWIN, S. "A Rational Approach to Drug

Abuse Prevention." Unpublished manuscript.

165. ———. "Drugs of Abuse: An Introduction to Their Actions and Potential Hazards," *J. Psychedel. Drugs*, 3 (1971), 5–15.

166. JACOBSON, C. B. and C. M. BERLIN. "Possible Reproductive Detriment in LSD Users," *JAMA*, 222 (1972), 1367–1373.

167. JAMES, W. *Varieties of Religious Experience.* New York: Collier, 1961.

168. JELLINEK, E. M. *The Disease Concept of Alcoholism.* New Haven: Hill House, 1960.

169. JONES, R. T. "Marijuana-Induced 'High': Influence of Expectation, Setting and Previous Drug Experience," *Pharmacol. Rev.*, 23 (1971), 359–369.

170. ———. "Tetrahydrocannabinol and Marijuana-Induced Social 'High', Or the Effects of the Mind on Marijuana," *Ann. N.Y. Acad. Sci.*, 191 (1971), 155–165.

171. ———. "Drug Models of Schizophrenia—Cannabis." Presented at Am. Psychopathol. Assoc. Meet., New York, 1973.

172. JONES, R. T. and G. C. STONE. "Psychological Studies of Marijuana and Alcohol in Man," *Psychopharmacologia*, 18 (1970), 108–117.

173. JUDD, L. L. and A. J. MANDELL. "A 'Free Clinic' Patient Population and Drug Use Patterns," *Am. J. Psychiatry*, 128 (1972), 1298–1302.

174. KANDEL, D. "Interpersonal Influences on Adolescent Illegal Drug Use," in E. Josephson and E. Carroll, eds., *Epidemiology of Drug Abuse.* Washington, D.C.: Winston, 1974.

175. KAPLAN, H. B. and J. H. MEYEROWITZ. "Psychosocial Predictors of Postinstitutional Adjustment among Male Drug Addicts," *Arch. Gen. Psychiatry*, 20 (1969), 278–284.

176. KEELER, M. H. "Motivation for Marijuana Use: A Correlate of Adverse Reaction," *Am. J. Psychiatry*, 125 (1968), 386–390.

177. KEELER, M. H., J. A. EWING, and B. A. ROUSE. "Hallucinogenic Effects of Marijuana as Currently Used," *Am. J. Psychiatry*, 128 (1971), 213–216.

178. KEELER, M. H., C. B. REIFLER, and M. B. LIPTZIN. "Spontaneous Recurrence of Marijuana Effect," *Am. J. Psychiatry*, 125 (1968), 384–386.

179. KENDALL, R. F. "Psychosis and Psychedelics." Presented at Calif. State Psychol.

Assoc. Meet., Coronado, Calif., Jan., 1971.

180. KENISTON, K. *The Uncommitted. Alienated Youth in American Society.* New York: Dell, 1965.

181. ———. "Why Students Become Radicals," *J. Am. Coll. Health Assoc.*, 17 (1968), 107–118.

182. ———. *Young Radicals.* New York: Harcourt, 1968.

183. ———. "Heads and Seekers," *Am. Scholar*, 38 (1968–1969), 97–112.

184. ———. "Student Activism, Moral Development, and Morality," *Am. J. Orthopsychiatry*, 40 (1970), 577–592.

185. KHANTZIAN, E. J. "Opiate Addiction: I. A Critical Assessment of Current Theory and Treatment Approaches." Unpublished manuscript.

186. KLEBER, H. D. "Prolonged Adverse Reactions from Unsupervised Use of Hallucinogenic Drugs," *J. Nerv. Ment. Dis.*, 144 (1967), 308–319.

187. KLEE, G. D. "Lysergic Acid Diethylamide (LSD-25) and Ego Functions," *Arch. Gen. Psychiatry*, 8 (1963), 461–474.

188. KOHUT, H. "Forms and Transformations of Narcissism," *J. Am. Psychoanal. Assoc.*, 14 (1966), 243–272.

189. ———. *The Analysis of the Self.* The Psychoanalytic Study of the Child Monogr. 4. New York: International Universities Press, 1971.

190. ———. "Thoughts on Narcissism and Narcissistic Rage," in *The Psychoanalytic Study of the Child*, Vol. 27, pp. 360–400. New York: International Universities Press, 1973.

191. KOSMAN, M. E. and K. R. UNNA. "The Effects of Chronic Administration of the Amphetamines and other Stimulants on Behavior," *Clin. Pharmacol. Ther.*, 9 (1968), 240–254.

192. KRAMER, J. C., V. S. FISCHMAN, and D. LITTLEFIELD. "Amphetamine Abuse," *JAMA*, 201 (1967), 305–309.

193. KRUS, D. M., S. WAPNER, H. FREEMAN et al. "Differential Behavioral Responsivity to LSD-25," *Arch. Gen. Psychiatry*, 8 (1963), 557–563.

194. KYSAR, J. E., M. S. ZAKS, H. P. SCHUCHMAN et al. "Range of Psychological Functioning in 'Normal' Late Adolescents," *Arch. Gen. Psychiatry*, 21 (1969), 515–528.

195. LAMPE, M. *Drugs: Information for Crisis*

Treatment. Beloit, Wisconsin: Stash Press, 1972.

196. LEMBERGER, L., J. L. WEISS, A. M. WATANABE et al. "Delta 9-Tetrahydrocannabinol," *N. Engl. J. Med.*, 286 (1972), 685–688.

197. LENNARD, H. L., L. J. EPSTEIN, A. BERNSTEIN et al. "Hazards Implicit in Prescribing Psychoactive Drugs," *Science*, 169 (1970), 438–441.

198. LEUNER, H. "Present State of Psycholytic Therapy and Its Possibilities," in H. A. Abramson, ed., *The Use of LSD in Psychotherapy and Alcoholism.* Indianapolis: Bobbs, 1967.

199. LEVY, B. S. "Five Years After: A Follow-up of 50 Narcotic Addicts," *Am. J. Psychiatry*, 128 (1972), 102–106.

200. LEVY, R. and A. BROWN. "An Analysis of Calls to a Drug Crisis Intervention Service," *J. Psychedel. Drugs*, 6 (1974), 143–152.

201. LEWIN, L. *Phantastica, Narcotic and Stimulating Drugs.* New York: Dutton, 1964.

202. LINDEMAN, E. and L. D. CLARK. "Modifications in Ego Structure and Personality Reactions under the Influence of the Effects of Drugs," *Am. J. Psychiatry*, 108 (1952), 561–567.

203. LINDESMITH, A. R. *Opiate Addiction.* Evanston: Principia Press, 1947.

204. ———. *The Addict and the Law.* Bloomington: Indiana University Press, 1965.

205. LINTON, H. B., R. J. LANGS, and I. H. PAUL. "Retrospective Alterations of the LSD-25 Experience," *J. Nerv. Ment. Dis.*, 138 (1964), 409–423.

206. LIPINSKI, E. and B. G. LIPINSKI. "Motivational Factors in Psychedelic Drug Use by Male College Students," *J. Am. Coll. Health Assoc.*, 16 (1967), 145–149.

207. LIPP, M. R. and S. G. BENSON. "Marijuana Use by Physicians." Presented at Am. Psychiatric Assoc. Meet., Dallas, 1972.

208. LIPP, M. R., S. G. BENSON, and Z. TAINTOR. "Marijuana Use by Medical Students," *Am. J. Psychiatry*, 128 (1971), 207–212.

209. LIPSCOMB, W. R. "Drug Use in a Black Ghetto," *Am. J. Psychiatry*, 127 (1971), 1166–1169.

210. LOMBILLO, J. R. and J. D. HAIN. "Patterns of Drug Use in a High School Population," *Am. J. Psychiatry*, 128 (1972), 836–841.

211. LOURIA, D. B., T. HENSLE, and J. ROSE. "The Major Medical Complications of Heroin Addiction," *Ann. Intern. Med.*, 67 (1967), 1–22.

212. LUDWIG, A. M. "Psychedelic Effects Produced by Sensory Overload," *Am. J. Psychiatry*, 128 (1972), 114–117.

213. LUSTMAN, S. L. "Yale's Year of Confrontation—A View from the Master's House," in *The Psychoanalytic Study of the Child*, Vol. 27, pp. 57–73. New York: International Universities Press, 1972.

214. McCUBBIN, R. J. "Drug Use: Predictions from Psychedelic Phenomenology." Presented at Calif. State Psychol. Assoc., Annu. Con., Coronado, Calif., Jan., 1971.

215. McGLOTHLIN, W. H. "Hallucinogenic Drugs: A Perspective with Special References to Peyote and Cannabis," *Psychedel. Rev.*, 6 (1965), 16–57.

216. ———. "Marijuana: An Analysis of Use, Distribution and Control," *Contemp. Drug Prob.*, 1 (1972), 467–500.

217. McGLOTHLIN, W. H. and D. O. ARNOLD. "LSD Revisited," *Arch. Gen. Psychiatry*, 24 (1971), 35–49.

218. McGLOTHLIN, W. H., D. O. ARNOLD, and D. X. FREEDMAN. "Organicity Measures following Repeated LSD Ingestion," *Arch. Gen. Psychiatry*, 21 (1969), 704–709.

219. McGLOTHLIN, W. H. and S. COHEN. "The Use of Hallucinogenic Drugs among College Students," *Am. J. Psychiatry*, 122 (1965), 572–574.

220. McGLOTHLIN, W. H., S. COHEN, and M. S. McGLOTHLIN. "Long Lasting Effects of LSD on Normals," *Arch. Gen. Psychiatry*, 17 (1967), 521–532.

221. McGLOTHLIN, W. H., R. S. SPARKES, and B. ARNOLD. "Effect of LSD on Human Pregnancy," *JAMA*, 212 (1970), 1483–1487.

222. McGLOTHLIN, W. H. and L. J. WEST. "The Marijuana Problem: An Overview," *Am. J. Psychiatry*, 125 (1968), 370–378.

223. MANHEIMER, D. I. and G. D. MELLINGER. "Marijuana Use among Urban Adults," *Science*, 166 (1969), 1544–1545.

224. MASAKI, T. "The Amphetamine Problem in Japan," *WHO Tech. Rep. Ser.*, 102 (1965), 14–21.

225. MAUGH, T. H. "LSD and the Drug Culture: New Evidence of Hazard," *Science*, 179 (1973), 1221–1222.

226. MELLINGER, G. D., M. B. BALTER, and D. I. MANHEIMER. "Patterns of Psychotherapeu-

tic Drug Use among Adults in San Francisco," *Arch. Gen. Psychiatry*, 25 (1971), 385–394.

227. MELLO, N. K. and J. H. MENDELSON. "Experimentally Induced Intoxication in Alcoholics: A Comparison between Programmed and Spontaneous Drinking," *J. Pharmacol. Exp. Ther.*, 173 (1970), 101–116.

228. ———. "A Quantitative Analysis of Drinking Patterns in Alcoholics," *Arch. Gen. Psychiatry*, 25 (1971), 527–539.

229. MENDELSON, W., N. JOHNSON, and M. A. STEWART. "Hyperactive Children as Teenagers: A Follow-up Study," *J. Nerv. Ment. Dis.*, 153 (1971), 273–279.

230. MENKES, M. M., J. S. ROWE, and J. H. MENKES. "A Twenty-five Year Follow-up Study of the Hyperkinetic Child with Minimal Brain Dysfunction," *Pediatrics*, 39 (1967), 393–399.

231. MESSER, M. "Running Out of Era: Some Non-pharmacologic Notes on the Psychedelic Revolution," in D. E. Smith, ed., *The New Social Drug*, pp. 157–167. Englewood Cliffs, N.J.: Prentice-Hall, 1970.

232. MEYER, R. E. *Guide to Drug Rehabilitation. A Public Health Approach.* Boston: Beacon Press, 1972.

233. MEYER, R. E., R. C. PILLARD, L. M. SHAPIRO et al. "Administration of Marijuana to Heavy and Casual Marijuana Users," *Am. J. Psychiatry*, 128 (1971), 198–203.

234. MEYERS, F. H., E. JAWETZ, and A. GOLDFEIN. *Review of Medical Pharmacology.* Los Altos, Calif.: Lange Medical Pub., 1972.

235. MEYERS, F. H., A. J. ROSE, and D. E. SMITH. "Incidents Involving the Haight-Ashbury Population and Some Uncommonly Used Drugs," *J. Psychedel. Drugs*, 1 (1967), 139–146.

236. MILGRAM, S. "The Experience of Living in Cities," *Science*, 167 (1970), 1461–1468.

237. MILLER, H. "A Youthful Celebration of Banality and Liability." Presented at Conf. Drug Use and Drug Subcultures, Pacific Grove, Calif. Feb., 1970.

238. ———. "On Hanging Loose and Loving: The Dilemma of Present Youth," *J. Soc. Issues*, 27 (1971), 35–46.

239. MIRIN, S. M., L. M. SHAPIRO, R. E. MEYER et al. "Casual Versus Heavy Use of Mari-

juana: A Redefinition of the Marijuana Problem," *Am. J. Psychiatry*, 127 (1971), 1134–1140.

240. MIZNER, G. L., J. T. BARTER, and P. H. WERME. "Patterns of Drug Use among College Students: A Preliminary Report," *Am. J. Psychiatry*, 127 (1970), 15–24.

241. MOLONEY, L. "Transcendental Meditation as an Alternative to Drugs." Unpublished manuscript.

242. MULLER, C. "The Overmedicated Society: Forces in the Marketplace for Medical Care," *Science*, 176 (1972), 488–492.

243. MUSTO, D. "The Marijuana Tax Act of 1937," *Arch. Gen. Psychiatry*, 26 (1972), 101–107.

244. ———. *The American Disease: Origins of Narcotic Control.* New Haven: Yale University Press, 1973.

245. NATIONAL COMMISSION ON MARIJUANA AND DRUG ABUSE. *Marijuana: A Signal of Misunderstanding.* First Report, Washington: U.S. Govt. Print. Off., 1972.

246. ———. *Drug Use in America: Problem in Perspective,* Second Report, Washington: U.S. Govt. Print. Off., 1973.

247. NEWMEYER, J. A. "Five Years After: Drug Use and Exposure to Heroin among the Haight-Ashbury Free Medical Clinic Clientele." Unpublished manuscript.

248. ———. "The End of the Heroin Epidemic of the San Francisco Bay Area." Unpublished manuscript.

249. NOBEL, P., T. HART, and R. NATION. "Correlates and Outcome of Illicit Drug Use by Adolescent Girls," *Br. J. Psychiatry*, 120 (1972), 497–504.

250. NOWLIS, V. and H. H. NOWLIS. "The Description and Analysis of Mood," *Ann. N.Y. Acad. Sci.*, 65 (1956), 345–355.

251. OFFER, D. *The Psychological World of the Teen-Ager.* New York: Basic Books, 1969.

252. OFFER, D., D. MARCUS, and J. OFFER. "Longitudinal Study of Normal Adolescent Boys," *Am. J. Psychiatry*, 126 (1970), 917–924.

253. O'MALLEY, J. E., W. H. ANDERSON, and A. LAZARE. "Failure of Outpatient Treatment of Drug Abuse: I. Heroin," *Am. J. Psychiatry*, 128 (1972), 99–101.

254. O'NEILL, E. *Long Day's Journey Into Night.* New Haven: Yale University Press, 1956.

255. PANEL ON THE IMPACT OF INFORMATION ON DRUG USE AND MISUSE. PHASE II REPORT.

"Evaluating Drug Information Programs,"
Washington: Assembly of Behav. Soc.
Scient. Natl. Res. Counc., Natl. Acad. Sci.,
July, 1973.

256. PARRY, H. J., M. B. BALTER, G. D. MELLIN-
GER et al. "National Patterns of Psychotherapeutic Drug Use," *Arch. Gen. Psychiatry*, 28 (1973), 769–783.

257. PEARLMAN, S. "Drug Use and Experience
in an Urban College Population," *Am. J.
Orthopsychiatry*, 37 (1967), 297–299.

258. PEARLMAN, S., A. PHILIP, L. C. ROBBINS
et al. "Religious Affiliations and Patterns
of Drug Usage in an Urban University
Population." *Proc. 1st Int. Conf. Student
Drug Surveys, Newark, Sept., 1972*, pp.
139–186. New York: Baywood, 1972.

259. PEARSON, M. M. and R. B. LITTLE. "The
Addictive Process in Unusual Addictions:
A Further Elaboration of Etiology," *Am.
J. Psychiatry*, 125 (1969), 1166–1171.

260. PHILIP, A. "The Campus Drug Problem,"
J. Am. Coll. Health Assoc., 16 (1967),
150–160.

261. PITTEL, S. M. "Psychological Effects of Psychedelic Drugs: Preliminary Observations
and Hypotheses." Presented at Meet. W.
Psychol. Assoc., June 21, 1969.

262. PITTEL, S. M. and R. HOFER. "The Transition to Amphetamine Abuse," *J. Psychedelic Drugs*, 5 (1972), 105–112.

263. PITTEL, S. M., A. WALLACH, and N. WIL-
NER. "Utopians, Mystics and Skeptics:
Ideologies of Young Drug Users—I." Un-
published manuscript.

264. POLSKY, N. *Hustlers, Beats and Others*. Chicago: Aldine, 1967.

265. POWELL, D. H. "A Pilot Study of Occasional
Heroin Users," *Arch. Gen. Psychiatry*, 28
(1973), 586–594.

266. PREBLE, E. and J. J. CASEY, JR. "Taking
Care of Business—The Heroin User's Life
on the Street," *Int. J. Addict.*, 4 (1969),
1–24.

267. PRESIDENT'S COMMISSION ON LAW ENFORCE-
MENT AND ADMINISTRATION OF JUSTICE.
"Task Force Report: Narcotics and Drug
Abuse." Washington: U.S. Govt. Print.
Off., 1967.

268. QUITKIN, F. M., A. RIFKIN, J. KAPLAN et al.
"Phobic Anxiety Syndrome Complicated
by Drug Dependence and Addiction,"
Arch. Gen. Psychiatry, 27 (1972), 159–
161.

269. RADFORD, P., S. WISEBERG, and C. YORKE.

"A Study of 'Main-Line' Heroin Addiction:
A Preliminary Report," in *The Psychoanalytic Study of the Child*, Vol. 27, pp.
156–180. New York: International Universities Press, 1972.

270. REDLICH, F. C. and D. X. FREEDMAN. *The
Theory and Practice of Psychiatry*. New
York: Basic Books, 1966.

271. ROBBINS, E. S., L. ROBBINS, W. A. FROSCH
et al. "College Student Drug Use," *Am. J.
Psychiatry*, 126 (1970), 1743–1751.

272. ROBINS, L. *Deviant Children Grown Up*.
Baltimore: Williams & Wilkins, 1966.

273. ROBINS, L. N. and G. E. MURPHY. "Drug
Use in a Normal Population of Young
Negro Men," *Am. J. Public Health*, 57
(1967), 1580–1596.

274. ROSENBERG, C. M. "Young Drug Addicts:
Background and Personality," *J. Nerv.
Ment. Dis.*, 148 (1969), 65–73.

275. ROSENTHAL, S. H. "Persistent Hallucinosis
following Repeated Administration of
Hallucinogenic Drugs," *Am. J. Psychiatry*,
121 (1964), 238–244.

276. ROSZAK, T. *The Making of a Counter-Culture*. Garden City, N.Y.: Doubleday, 1968.

277. ROUSE, B. A. and J. A. EWING. *Marijuana
and Other Drug Use by Coeds*. Unpublished.

278. RUBINS, J. L. "The Problem of the Acute
Identity Crisis in Adolescence," *Am. J.
Psychoanal.*, 28 (1968), 37–44.

279. RUMBAUGH, C. L., R. T. BERGERON, H. C. H.
FANG et al. "Cerebral Angiographic
Changes in the Drug Abuse Patient,"
Radiology, 101 (1971), 335–344.

280. SALZMAN, C., G. E. KOCHANSKY, and
R. SHADER. "The Psychology of Hallu-
cinogenic Drug Discontinuers," *Am. J.
Psychiatry*, 129 (1972), 131–137.

281. SAVAGE, C., J. FADIMAN, R. E. MOGAR et al.
"Process and Outcome Variables in Psychedelic (LSD) Therapy," in H. A. Abramson, ed., *The Use of LSD in Psychotherapy
and Alcoholism*, pp. 511-532. Indianapolis: Bobbs, 1967.

282. SAVITT, R. A. "Psychoanalytic Studies on
Addiction: Ego Structure in Narcotic
Addiction," *Psychoanal. Q.*, 32 (1963),
43–57.

283. SCHACTER, S. and J. E. SINGER. "Cognitive,
Social and Physiological Determinants of
Emotional State," *Psychol. Rev.*, 69 (1962),
379–399.

284. SCHAPS, E. and C. R. SANDERS. "Purposes,

Patterns and Protection in a Campus Drug Using Community," *J. Health Soc. Behav.*, 11 (1971), 135–145.

285. SCHUCKIT, M., F. N. PITTS, JR., T. REICH et al. "Alcoholism: I. Two Types of Alcoholism in Women," *Arch. Gen. Psychiatry*, 20 (1969), 301–306.

286. SCHUSTER, C. R. and C. E. JOHANSON. "The Use of Animal Models for the Study of Drug Abuse," in P. J. Gibbons, ed., *Research Advances in Alcohol and Drug Problems*, pp. 1–31. New York: Wiley, 1973.

287. SCHUSTER, C. R. and T. THOMPSON. "Self Administration of and Behavioral Dependence on Drugs," *Annu. Rev. Pharmacol.*, 9 (1969), 483–502.

288. SCHUSTER, C. R. and J. E. VILLARREAL. "The Experimental Analysis of Opioid Dependence," in D. H. Efron, ed., *Psychopharmacology: A Review of Progress 1957–1967*, pp. 811–828. Washington: PHS Pub., 1968.

289. SCHWARZ, C. J. "The Complications of LSD: A Review of the Literature," *J. Nerv. Ment. Dis.*, 146 (1968), 174–186.

290. SCOTT, P. D. and M. BUCHELL. "Delinquency and Amphetamines," *Br. J. Psychiatry*, 119 (1971), 179–182.

291. SCOTT, P. D. and D. R. C. WILCOX. "Delinquency and Amphetamines," *Br. J. Psychiatry*, 111 (1965), 865–875.

292. SENAY, E. C., J. H. JAFFE, J. N. CHAPPEL et al. "IDAP: Five Year Results." Proc. Natl. Conf. Methadone, Washington, April, 1973.

293. SETTLAGE, C. F., ed. "Anomie, Alienation and Adolescence: A Special Section," *J. Child Psychiatry*, 9 (1970), 202–281.

294. ———. "Adolescence and Social Change," *J. of Child Psychiatry*, 9 (1970), 203–216.

295. ———. "Cultural Values and the Superego in Late Adolescence," in *The Psychoanalytic Study of the Child*, Vol. 27, pp. 74–92. New York: International Universities Press, 1973.

296. SHAKOW, D. "The Education of the Mental Health Researcher: Encouraging Potential Development in Man," *Arch. Gen. Psychiatry*, 27 (1972), 15–28.

297. SHEARN, C. R. and D. J. FITZGIBBONS. "Patterns of Drug Use in a Population of Youthful Psychiatric Patients," *Am. J. Psychiatry*, 128 (1972), 1381–1387.

298. SHICK, J. F. E. and D. E. SMITH. "An Analy-sis of the LSD Flashback," *J. Psychedel. Drugs*, 3 (1970), 13–19.

299. ———. "The Illicit Use of the Psychotomimetic Amphetamines with Special Reference to STP (DOM) Toxicity," *J. Psychedel. Drugs*, 5 (1972), 131–138.

300. SHICK, J. F. E., D. E. SMITH, and F. H. MEYERS. "Patterns of Drug Abuse in the Haight-Ashbury Neighborhood," *Clin. Toxicol.*, 3 (1970), 19–56.

301. SHICK, J. F. E., D. E. SMITH, and D. R. WESSON. "An Analysis of Amphetamine Toxicity and Patterns of Use," *J. Psychedel. Drugs*, 5 (1972), 113–130.

302. SHOICHET, R. and L. SOLURSH. "Treatment of the Hallucinogenic Drug Crisis," *App. Ther.*, 11 (1969), 5–7.

303. SILVERMAN, J. "Research with Psychedelics," *Arch. Gen. Psychiatry*, 25 (1971), 498–510.

304. SLATER, P. E., K. MORIMOTO, and R. W. HYDE. "The Effects of LSD upon Group Interaction," *Arch. Gen. Psychiatry*, 8 (1963), 564–571.

305. SMART, R. G. "Illicit Drug Use in Canada: A Review of Current Epidemiology with Clues for Prevention," *Int. J. Addict.*, 6 (1971), 383–405.

306. SMART, R. G. and K. BATEMAN. "Unfavorable Reactions to LSD: A Review and Analysis of the Available Case Reports," *Can. Med. Assoc. J.*, 97 (1967), 1214–1221.

307. SMITH, D. E. "An Analysis of Variables in High Dose Methamphetamine Dependence," *J. Psychedel. Drugs*, 2 (1969), 60–62.

308. ———. "LSD and the Psychedelic Syndrome," *Clin. Toxicol.*, 2 (1969), 69–73.

309. ———. "Physical v. Psychological Dependence and Tolerance in High-Dose Methamphetamine Abuse," *Clin. Toxicol.*, 2 (1969), 99–103.

310. ———. "Speed Freaks v. Acid Heads," *Clin. Pediatr.*, 8 (1969), 185–192.

311. ———, ed. *The New Social Drug: Cultural, Medical, and Legal Perspectives on Marijuana*. Englewood Cliffs, N.J.: Prentice-Hall, 1970.

312. SMITH, D. E. and G. R. GAY. *Heroin in Perspective*. Englewood Cliffs, N.J.: Prentice-Hall, 1972.

313. SMITH, D. E. and J. LUCE. *Love Needs Care*. Boston: Little, Brown, 1971.

314. SMITH, D. E. and C. MEHL. "An Analysis

of Marijuana Toxicity," *Clin. Toxicol.*, 3 (1970), 101–116.

315. SMITH, D. E. and A. J. ROSE. "LSD: Its Use, Abuse, and Suggested Treatment," *J. Psychedel. Drugs*, 1 (1967), 117–124.

316. SMITH, D. E. and D. R. WESSON. "Phenobarbital Techniques for Treatment of Barbiturate Dependence," *Arch. Gen. Psychiatry*, 24 (1971), 56–60.

317. ———, eds. "The Politics of Uppers and Downers," *J. Psychedel. Drugs*, 5 #2 (1972), whole issue.

318. SMITH, D. E., D. R. WESSON, and R. A. LANNON. "New Developments in Barbiturate Abuse" in D. E. Smith, ed., *Drug Abuse Papers*. Berkeley: University of California Extension, 1969.

319. SMITH, R. C. "The World of the Haight-Ashbury Speed Freak," *J. Psychedel. Drugs*, 2 (1969), 77–83.

320. ———. "Traffic in Amphetamines: Patterns of Illegal Manufacture and Distribution," *J. Psychedel. Drugs*, 2 (1969), 20–24.

321. SNYDER, S. H. "Catecholamines in the Brain as Mediators of Amphetamine Psychosis," *Arch. Gen. Psychiatry*, 27 (1972), 169–179.

322. SOLNIT, A. J. "Youth and the Campus: The Search for Social Conscience," in *The Psychoanalytic Study of the Child*, Vol. 27, pp. 98–105. New York: International Universities Press, 1972.

323. SOLNIT, A. J., C. F. SETTLAGE, S. GOODMAN et al. "Youth Unrest: A Symposium," *Am. J. Psychiatry*, 125 (1969), 1145–1159.

324. SOLOMON, T. *A Pilot Study among East Village 'Hippies.'* Monogr. 35, New York: Associated YM-YWCA's, 1968.

325. STANTON, M. D. and A. BARDONI. "Drug Flashbacks: Reported Frequency in a Military Population," *Am. J. Psychiatry*, 129 (1972), 751–755.

326. STIMSON, G. U. and A. C. OGBORNE. "A Survey of a Representative Sample of Addicts Prescribed Heroin at London Clinics," *Bull. Narc.*, 22 (1970), 13–22.

327. STUBBS, V. M. "Environmental Stress in the Development of Young Drug Users." Presented at Calif. State Psychol. Assoc. Annu. Conv., Coronado, Jan., 1971.

328. STUNKARD, A. "New Therapies for the Eating Disorders: Behavior Modification of Anorexia Nervosa and Obesity," *Arch.*

Gen. Psychiatry, 26 (1972), 391–398.

329. SUTTER, A. G. "World of Drug Use on the Street Scene," in D. R. Cressey, and D. A. Ward, eds., *Delinquency, Crime and Social Process*, pp. 802–829. New York: Harper & Row, 1969.

330. TAMERIN, J. S. and J. H. MENDELSON. "The Psychodynamics of Chronic Inebriation: Observation of Alcoholics during the Process of Drinking in an Experimental Group Setting," *Am. J. Psychiatry*, 125 (1969), 886–899.

331. TAMERIN, J. S. and C. P. NEUMANN. "Prognostic Factors in the Evaluation of Addicted Individuals," *Int. Pharmacopsychiatry*, 6 (1971), 69–76.

332. TART, C. T., ed. *Altered States of Consciousness*. New York: Wiley, 1969.

333. ———. "States of Consciousness and State-Specific Sciences," *Science*, 176 (1972), 1203–1210.

334. TAUBE, I. and R. VREELAND. "The Prediction of Ego Functioning in College," *Arch. Gen. Psychiatry*, 27 (1972), 224–233.

335. TAYLOR, R. L., J. I. MAURER, and J. TINKLENBERG. "Management of Bad Trips in an Evolving Drug Scene," *JAMA*, 213 (1970), 422–425.

336. TENNANT, F. S., JR. and C. J. GROESBECK. "Psychiatric Effects of Hashish," *Arch. Gen. Psychiatry*, 27 (1972), 133–136.

337. TENNANT, F. S., JR., M. PREBEL, T. J. PRENDERGAST et al. "Medical Manifestations Associated with Hashish," *JAMA*, 216 (1971), 1965–1969.

338. TERRY, C. E. and M. PELLENS. *The Opium Problem*. New Jersey: Patterson Smith, 1970.

339. TINKLENBERG, J. "A Current View of the Amphetamines." Presented at the W. Inst. Drug Prob., Portland State University, Portland, Oregon, Aug. 17–21, 1970.

340. ———. "Drugs and Crime: A Consultant's Report," in Drug Use in America: Problem in Perspective, Vol. 1, *Patterns and Consequences of Drug Use*, pp. 242–299. Washington: U.S. Govt. Print. Off. (Stack #5266–00004), 1972.

341. TORDA, C. "An Effective Therapeutic Method for the LSD User," *Percept. Mot. Skills*, 30 (1970), 79–88.

342. TOROP, P. and K. TOROP. "Hotlines and Youth Culture Values," *Am. J. Psychiatry*, 129 (1972), 106–109.

343. TUCKER, G. J., D. QUINLAN, and M. HARROW. "Chronic Hallucinogenic Drug Use and Thought Disturbance," *Arch. Gen. Psychiatry*, 27 (1972), 443–450.

344. UNGERLEIDER, J. T. and H. L. BOWEN. "Drug Abuse in Schools," *Am. J. Psychiatry*, 125 (1969), 1691–1696.

345. UNGERLEIDER, J. T., D. D. FISHER, M. FULLER et al. "The 'Bad Trip'—The Etiology of the Adverse LSD Reaction," *Am. J. Psychiatry*, 124 (1968), 1483–1490.

346. UNGERLEIDER, J. T., D. D. FISHER, S. R. GOLDSMITH et al. "A Statistical Survey of Adverse Reactions to LSD in Los Angeles County," *Am. J. Psychiatry*, 125 (1968), 352–356.

347. VAILLANT, G. E. "A Twelve Year Follow-up of New York Narcotic Addicts: IV. Some Characteristics and Determinants of Abstinence," *Am. J. Psychiatry*, 123 (1966), 573–584.

348. ———. "A Twelve Year Follow-up of New York Narcotic Addicts: I. The Relation of Treatment to Outcome," *Am. J. Psychiatry*, 122 (1966), 727–737.

349. ———. "A Twenty Year Follow-up of New York Narcotic Addicts," *Arch. Gen. Psychiatry*, 29 (1973), 237–246.

350. WALLACH, A. "Varying Fates of Young Drug Users." Presented at Meet. Calif. State Psychol. Assoc. Annu. Conv., Coronado, Jan., 1971.

351. WALTERS, P. A., JR., G. W. GOETHALS, and H. G. POPE. "Drug Use and Life Style among 500 College Undergraduates," *Arch. Gen. Psychiatry*, 26 (1972), 92–96.

352. WEIDER, H. and E. H. KAPLAN. "Drug Use in Adolescents: Psychodynamic Meaning and Pharmacogenic Effect," in *The Psychoanalytic Study of the Child*, Vol. 24, 399–431. New York: International Universities Press, 1969.

353. WEIL, A. T. "Adverse Reactions to Marijuana," *N. Engl. J. Med.*, 282 (1970), 997–1000.

354. WEISS, G., K. MINDE, J. S. WERRY et al. "Studies of the Hyperactive Child: VIII. Five Year Follow-up," *Arch. Gen. Psychiatry*, 24 (1971), 409–414.

355. WELPTON, D. F. "Psychodynamics of Chronic Lysergic Acid Diethylamide Use," *J. Nerv. Ment. Dis.*, 147 (1968), 377–385.

356. WENKART, A. "Anomie or New Order," *Am. J. Psychoanal.*, 28 (1968), 196–200.

357. WHITE HOUSE CONFERENCE ON NARCOTICS AND DRUGS. *Proceedings*, Sept. 27–28, 1962. Final Report, President's Advisory Commission on Narcotics and Drug Abuse.

358. WHITLOCK, F. A. "The Syndrome of Barbiturate Dependence," *Med. J. Aust.*, 2 (1970), 391–396.

359. WIKLER, A. *Opiate Addiction; Psychological and Neurophysiological Aspects in Relation to Clinical Problems*. Springfield, Ill.: Charles C. Thomas, 1953.

360. ———. "On the Nature of Addiction and Habituation," *Br. J. Addic.*, 57 (1961), 73–79.

361. ———. "Diagnosis and Treatment of Drug Dependence of the Barbiturate Type," *Am. J. Psychiatry*, 125 (1968), 758–765.

362. ———. "Dynamics of Drug Dependence: Implications of a Conditioning Theory for Research and Treatment," *Arch. Gen. Psychiatry*, 28 (1973), 611–616.

363. WIKLER, A. and R. W. RASOR. "Psychiatric Aspects of Drug Addiction," *Am. J. Med.*, 14 (1953), 566–570.

364. WILLIAMS, E. G., C. K. HIMMELSBACH, A. WIKLER et al. "Studies on Marijuana and Pyrahexyl Compound," *Publ. Health Repts.*, 61 (1946), 1059–1083.

365. WILMER, H. A. "Drugs, Hippies and Doctors," *JAMA*, 206 (1968), 1272–1275.

366. ———. "Use of the Television Monologue with Adolescent Psychiatric Patients," *Am. J. Psychiatry*, 126 (1970), 102–108.

367. WINNICOTT, D. W. "Transitional Objects and Transitional Phenomena: A Study of the First Not-Me Possessions," *Int. J. Psychoanal.*, 34 (1953), 89.

368. WINOKUR, G., T. REICH, J. RIMMER et al. "Alcoholism: III. Diagnosis and Familial Psychiatric Illness in 259 Alcoholic Probands," *Arch. Gen. Psychiatry*, 23 (1970), 104–111.

369. WURMSER, L. "Psychology of Drug Abuse." Read at Adol. Med. Semin., Baltimore, March 13, 1972.

370. YORKE, C. "A Critical Review of Some Psychoanalytic Literature in Drug Addiction," *Br. J. Med. Psychol.*, 43 (1970), 141–159.

371. ZAKS, M. S., P. H. HUGHES, J. JAFFE et al.

"Young People in the Park." Presented at Am. Orthopsychiatr. Assoc. Annu. Meet., New York, 1969.

372. ZINBERG, N. E. "Drugs and Youth," in C. Brown and C. Savage, eds., *The Drug Abuse Controversy*. pp. 87–95. Baltimore: Natl. Ed. Consult., 1971.

373. ———. "Heroin Use in Viet Nam and the United States," *Arch. Gen. Psychiatry*, 26 (1972), 486–488.

374. ZINBERG, N. E. and D. C. LEWIS. "Narcotic Usage: I. A Spectrum of a Difficult Medical Problem," *N. Engl. J. Med.*, 270 (1964), 989–993.

CHAPTER 26

PHYSIOLOGICAL SOCIOLOGY: ENDOCRINE CORRELATES OF STATUS BEHAVIORS[*]

Patricia R. Barchas and Jack D. Barchas

(Introduction

INTERMITTENT CONCERN, variously expressed, with the relationship of individual physiology to social situations has been with social psychology at least since that field borrowed the concept of homeostasis from biology. The newer balance theories in the social sciences share with earlier views the central notion that disruption of the system produces effects on the social, psychological, and physiological levels and that the system will tend to

* We should particularly like to thank David Hamburg and Keith Brodie for their encouragement of this chapter. Our work has been graciously supported by the National Institute of Alcohol Abuse and Alcoholism (AA 00498), the National Institute of Mental Health (MH 23861), the Office of Naval Research, and the Grant Foundation. We would like to thank Lynn Hassler, Florence Parma, and Rosemary Schmele for their secretarial assistance.

attempt to reduce that tension by reestablishing balance (homeostasis). We would like to present some of the relationships and considerations in this chapter that have been made between a basic social process and endocrine measures that have been related to homeostasis and behavior.

Sociology is concerned in part with the ways in which group structure influences individual behavior. Status is viewed as one of the basic structural processes of social behavior in humans and other animals, although expressed differently in different species. The importance of status as a concept for social behavior would parallel the importance of the concept of the utilization of glucose for biochemistry. Although not generally recognized by persons with training in "psychological" areas, concepts such as status are the heart of investigation for social scientists involved in the study of interactional processes. We would like to examine some aspects of status as an example of a basic social behavior and present some of the correlations that have been made between status behavior and endocrine behavior.

We are presenting this system of organization for heuristic reasons: it permits a juxtaposition of two stances of inquiry, each of which seems relevant to psychiatry and can be made relevant to each other. However, utilizing such a system for some purposes does not preclude recognizing the value of other ways of inquiring into the relationships of physiology to behavior.

The physiological responses with which we will be concerned in relation to status behavior will emphasize hormonal patterns involving the adrenal-cortical steroids, adrenal-medullary and gonadal hormones, and brain neuroregulators. Each of these endocrine or neuroregulatory systems has, at some time, been considered as one of the body's systems of homeostatic mechanisms; each of the systems is activated or depressed under differing stimulus conditions; and each remains in effect for differing lengths of time, and influences other systems of response differentially. Individual variation is great, and, the data to date can in no way be applied as an explanation to any given single event. The knowledge that has been accumulated represents promise, but the needs for further information in the systems directly mentioned, and in systems which have not been studied, is very great.

We believe that investigation of these areas has great relevance for psychiatry. A variety of illnesses has been identified in which "psychological" factors may play a major role. These range from forms of allergy, hypertension and dermatoses to disorders of the gastrointestinal tract among others. For any processes that are so construed, social processes such as status, dominance, and role relationships and their complexities may be crucial parts of what has been considered "psychological." In the past, psychological processes in such illnesses have frequently been considered in terms of individual psychology rather than in terms of structural processes involving the individuals. In this paper we will deal exclusively with such structural explanations, although we are also convinced of the great importance of individual psychological processes.

We will present a general description of the concept of role and status. We will then proceed to a more detailed description of status behavior in a variety of human and nonhuman primate studies, studies that suggest powerful evolutionary aspects in this behavior. Some of the literature relating status behavior to endocrine function will be presented. Finally, we will consider aspects of the study of physiological sociology in terms of the relation of the physiological and behavioral events and the manner in which they may interact. We will take up some of the possible relations of these materials to psychiatric illness.

❲ Status as a Social Behavior

Some General Aspects of Role Therapy and Status in Human Groups

"Group dynamics" insofar as they are repeated group to group, independent of particular persons, may be considered as structural in nature. Groups themselves may be voluntary or involuntary, formal or informal, open or closed. But, without a structure (patterned relationships) no aggregate of people may be considered a group. One way of looking at group behavior, which permits us to relate it to physiology, is in terms of roles. Some of the basic ideas used by role theorists are: persons are the only actors in the social system and these persons occupy positions (statuses). To these positions are attached, to a greater or lesser degree, expectations about behavior. These expectations, of rights and obligations associated with the positions people take, constitute a role. There is room for individual style in carrying out rights and obligations. This is not part of the role. A position is delineated by shared expectations, and a role is delineated by behavior that reflects positional expectations. (It should be noted that the position—status—as well as the way in which a role is enacted, may be evaluated by self or others either positively or negatively. We will not be dealing with such evaluations, even though viewed as reward and punishment, we believe they bear upon status and physiological response to status.)

Relevant to role behavior are socialization into roles and maturational limitations on the abilities of actors to carry out roles. This area of development is of extraordinary importance and is essentially unexplored.

Any person carries about with him any number of role possibilities. Dependent upon the social situation, one or another may be activated. Each individual must be able to move from role to role, sometimes to juggle several simultaneously, and sometimes to find that role requirements are either ambiguous or in conflict with self-concept. Any and all of these can be termed role conflict; as such, for both literature and social psychology, as well as for psychiatry, they produce the stuff out of which the human drama is written.

Tension, its accompanying pains and consequent psychological or socially potential disruptions; inappropriate reduction mechanisms, again psychological or social in nature; and distortion of either self-concept or the social structure may result from role conflicts. It is not surprising that we may find physiological correlates of such powerful and ubiquitous human phenomena. Because of rapid social change, the roles for which children prepare, and the coping mechanisms they learn, may not meet the demands of their changing adult life situation.

Intrinsic to the idea of roles is the notion of reciprocity. For each status or position, there is a counterstatus; e.g., teacher–pupil; mother–child; friend–friend; employee–employer. Clearly, these may be hierarchically or horizontally arranged. Nevertheless, the rights and obligations that define the relationship are bidirectional, although not necessarily of equal intensity or frequency of emission. There are cases (probably most available to the therapist and difficult to document as to validity) in which the reciprocal roles for the individual in question are purely symbolic, as is the actor to whom the role is attached. Thus, we may have images of absent figures influencing our actions. These figures are sometimes constructed from childhood experiences, fantasy, literature, or mythology. For sociological studies, one would be concerned primarily with simultaneously present actors who simultaneously activate reciprocal roles.

One way to view notions of role is as a principle of organization that is meaningful, consciously or unconsciously, both to the individual actor and to the observer. We may view culturally held norms transmitted to the individual as general and specific attitudes. These attitudes are further organized around societal statuses or positions, and are emitted as kinds of behavior.

Remembering that the individual is more than the sum of his statuses and roles, we nevertheless may claim that much social behavior, if not all, is partially governed by role considerations. The specifications for behavior are more or less rigid and vary in degrees of clarity. Usually, individuals carry out their roles with a minimal amount of conflict and uncertainty. However, whenever a social situation activates two roles simultaneously, there is the possibility for conflict. In situations in which role requirements are highly specified, there is an increased possibility that required behavior will be at odds with the individual's conception of himself, or even with higher order role commitments as perceived by the individual. Plainly, situations in which role requirements are not clear can be stressful. Plainly, too, there is great individual variation in both the mode of dealing with, and the degree of, felt stress involved in these situations.

Areas of inquiry that may be organized in terms of role considerations—although they may equally well stand alone—include power relations, coalition formation, leadership phenomenon, and affiliative bonding.

Ubiquity of Status

We are working from the point of view that man is a biological organism, similar to other organisms, especially other primates, and that his biology is a determinant of the range of his behavior, social as well as physical. His particularly human characteristics we take to be derived from the cortex: these include plasticity, use of experience, use of symbols and language, and time sense.

Rejecting "social Darwinism," we nonetheless believe that social structures and social processes that are found to be most widely distributed in small human groups will be found in other primates as well. Should this be true, one could project to underlying mechanisms, perhaps biological, that partially determine such processes.[13] Casting our ideas in an evolutionary framework, we believe there is a substrate of social forms and processes, necessarily limited to small group interaction, that is common to the primates, including man.* We tentatively agree with Colter Rule who suggests that some kinds of social behavior, such as dominance "are as fundamental to human existence as such short rhythm phenomena as respiration and the heartbeat: intermediate (circadian) rhythms like sleeping, waking, eating, drinking; and longer rhythms like sexuality and seasonal changes."[89] We think it even more likely that some social processes involving structure are basic—such as some status processes, affiliative bonding of several types, and some depressive reactions.

The ubiquity of status orderings in small groups has been repeatedly confirmed by observers of mammalian behavior.† Whatever the nature of the population, status is generally thought to influence such social behavior as leadership, coalitions, aggression, priority of access to desired objects, intragroup conflict, conformity, and group structure.[25,36,41,66] Given these relationships and the current proclivity to compare human with nonhuman behavior—and to seek animal models for studying human social phenomena—it seems reasonable to explore the status phenomenon in a variety of mammals, so that methods and results can be compared with results from human studies. This is particularly true if there continues to be an increased tendency

among behavioral scientists to assume that basic social behavior is in part biologically determined, and that the similarity in the biology of nonhuman organisms and humans may dictate similar social processes at the most elementary level, although the specific social patterns and their meanings may rest on other foundations.

This view does not revive or take sides in the nature–nurture argument. It does, however, have evolution as its framework. It argues that the brain, like other organs, retains substrata, and that these substrata partially govern the most basic kinds of behavior, such as learning, emotional behaviors such as depressive reactions, and some social interactions. While the effect of both further evolution and the impact of language and culture is not denied, this view does present the possibility that some of man's social responses are more adapted to past patterns of small group interaction, given the lag between culture and man's biologic adaptation.[48] It also suggests that the most basic social responses may be studied in nonhuman populations with the same advantages and disadvantages as are found, for example, in the study of learning among nonhuman primates.

Approaches to Status and Findings in Humans

Status is, in general, an ordering of individuals by which rights, privileges, and responsibilities are distributed. The power and prestige order of a group is often considered synonymous with the status ordering.[19] Status is a ubiquitous phenomenon in human groups. Even gross knowledge of status positions explains and predicts many social behaviors.[17-19,40,41] A description of a group typically uses status to order observations.

There are three aspects to the phenomenon of status emergence: status orderings form, are maintained, and change. We will review the literature dealing with status formation, omitting the portion dealing with maintenance and change. Most studies of status formation focus on ad hoc, freely interacting task groups. (By task group, we mean any small group

* See references 7, 14, 15, 33, 76, and 86.
† See references 1, 2, 25, 31, 36, 58, 59, 63–66, 77, 78, 82, 90, 95–97, 104, 106, and 110.

brought together for the purpose of achieving a mutual goal through mutual efforts.)

In this context, it has been found that diffuse status characteristics, age, sex, race, which individuals bring to the group, are likely to determine the status ordering within the group.[18] Recently, Fisek and Berger presented material extending this approach to include any factor that discriminates among the actors, such as occupation, but not including personality and socialization variables.[19]

We note that in such groups, even when diffuse characteristics are held constant, a status ordering emerges.[17-19] The Balesian tradition has yielded most of the data on such groups. The status order in freely interacting task groups forms quickly, in as little as forty-five minutes and it is stable.[*] Working within this Balesian tradition, Fisek[40] found that the differentiation occurred rapidly.

Two routes to status formation have been studied, one in which the status order develops out of interaction, and one in which the status order precedes apparent interaction.[40] The work of Berger et al. may be taken as an exploration of the first route of formation, although it clearly deals with other matters as well.[19] In this approach, both formation and maintenance of the status or power and prestige order are systematically linked to the task through performance evaluations and consequent expectation states.

The Berger model does not account for those groups in which the differentiation has taken place prior to interaction, particularly those cases in which the observed initial order is stable over time. The simplest approach to explaining initially differentiated groups may be to look for variables that might operate in ways similar to diffuse status characteristics. Personality variables or socialization variables are often examples, both expressing themselves in "style," the cues for which could be extremely muted—carriage, posture, propensity for eye contact. If one were to predict which individual was to occupy a given position, one would probably need to take into account such variables systematically. The re-

sults may be culture bound, and, in addition, depend not only upon the background of the actor but upon the perceptions of other actors.

Status as a process is especially suited to comparative study. As a phenomenon, status has received attention from sociologists of human behavior for many years, and there is agreement that status is an important determinant of human behavior. A large body of descriptive, experimental, and theoretical literature has arisen concerning status. Those observations which have been made on established ongoing groups suggest that status differentiation occurs universally, and that status differentiations correlate highly with performance in a group.

Thus, status differentiation apparently occurs universally in human groups, and status can be observed in both ongoing and experimental groups. Further, when members of a group have a collective task, they evolve patterns of interaction that clearly reflect differences in power and prestige among the members of the group, even when they are strangers at the onset of observation and are matched for external status characteristics.

Findings on Status in Non-Human Primates

Similarly, observers of nonhuman mammals which live in groups have found some form of status differentiation to be generally present.[†] We restrict our comments in this section to nonhuman primates. Starting with Carpenter,[25] field observers have used the notion of status to order their observations. The term status has frequently meant dominance and has connoted priority of access.

Field workers and observers in seminatural habitats have described aspects of group structure for many species, cataloguing and describing behavior in context.[‡] These studies generally have been done either from a straight analogic approach or from an evolutionary approach to behavior. It has been assumed that there may be common forms of social behavior across related species, if not

---

[*] See references 4–6, 18, 22, 60, and 101.

[†] See references 58, 59, 63, 97, and 99.
[‡] See references 46, 47, 64–67, 69, 98, and 100.

common meaning for each form. From these studies comes the suggestion that there are intriguing similarities in the organization of social behavior across primate species, the similarities becoming greater as higher levels of abstraction are used in behavioral categories.

Observational categories have been developed that are apparently reliable across observers. There has developed a concurrence regarding the "meaning" of some kinds of behavior, relative to slightly higher order concepts, such as dominance and deference. There is seldom a report in the primate literature in which some reference is not made to a dominance order, if not a status order, among the group.

In general, the high-status animal has freedom of movement, other animals making way for the high-status animal who may take the desired objects, such as food, from the other animals.[36,66] Data have been interpreted to mean that disruption of the status ordering causes instability in the group and that such variables as extent of group territory correlate with the temperament of the highest status individual in the group.[25] It has been suggested[35] that the sleep of the high-status animal may be deeper and less disturbed than that of low-status animals. It has been found that the later status position of an infant is influenced by the present status of the mother. Further, it is suggested that types of mothering are affected by the status of the mother. In general, it has been found that adult males have higher status than adult females who, in turn, have higher status than young animals, although there may be considerable overlap in these orderings.[26,36,66]

Most observations of nonhuman primate groups have been made of single groups of mixed age and sex. There is consensus among observers that status relationships partially order behavior. It has generally been assumed that these relationships are the product of long term socialization in stable groups, and that the advent of status relations developing in new groups can be attributed to external differentiating characteristics in the animals, such as sex, size, and weight. Goodall and Hamburg suggest, on the basis of observations

of free-ranging chimpanzees, that motivation and "technical ingenuity" may be factors in an individual's rise in dominance.

Status differentiation has been found to be stable in naturally occurring groups, although there are clearly conditions under which status shifts occur, these being related to growth and development as well as to cyclical and other biological changes. Bernstein and Mason, reporting on a newly established, mixed group, state that status relationships formed within the first hour of interaction were stable for seventy-five subsequent days.[20]

Focusing upon the dominance aspect of status in groups of mixed status, Bernstein and Mason have demonstrated that dominance relations in mixed groups were quickly formed. Miller and Murphy[81] report that such relations are stable, and Warren and Maroney[108] and Kawai[67] have demonstrated them to be highly resistant to change. These features have been attributed to (1) external status differences, or (2) long-term socialization of the individuals with each other. However, in a study by Barchas[14] these two attributions were ruled out as both were controlled for. Thus, animals with fully developed social repertoires have the capacity to form status orderings out of interactions which are independent of broad differentiating cues and of interaction with known individuals.

In mixed groups, the fully adult male dominates females and younger animals, the larger animal the small, the animal in good condition the animal in poor condition. Most observations are upon groups of varying statuses.

Clearly, both human and nonhuman primates in field and laboratory settings have been observed to exhibit status orderings. As has been stated, in humans the basic finding about status orders comes from Bales and his associates, ". . . marked inequalities develop over time in the rate at which members are observed to initiate interaction [and] those who initiate action most frequently tend to be ranked highest on the criteria of 'best ideas' guidance and tend to receive actions from others at the highest rate." This occurrence has been further documented in a variety of contexts and its stability established with little question.* For specific information on contexts other than the original Bales study, see Berger et al.,[19] Investigation into the phenomenon as a process and on a theoretical and experimental level has been most vigorously pursued by a group of Stanford sociologists.[19,18]

(Some Endocrine Correlates of Status Related Behavior

Adrenal Cortical Functions

Until recently, the relationship between status and endocrine function has been investigated primarily in rodents.[32] Such studies have tended to focus on the relationship of adrenal cortical function to dominance (one dimension of status) and have yielded fairly consistent results. Thus, the studies of Barnett[16] regarding fighting behavior in wild rats suggested, in a dramatic fashion, that the adrenal cortical hormones may be markedly depleted following fighting in the subordinate animal, but not in the dominant animal, although both appeared to have had an equal overt stress. In a study of male mice derived from a wild strain, it was noted that there was an inverse correlation of the adrenal weight and social rank in animals having had social interaction over a ten-day period; high ranking animals have less adrenal weight than low ranking mice.[34] Such findings may be related to physiological changes occurring in crowded conditions, where it has been found that in rodents increased group density results in increased adrenal weight, but decreased body and testicular weights.[27,105] Isolated male mice display lower resting levels of plasma corticosterone and a decreased response to stress.[24] If mice are maintained in a paired situation for several weeks, the subordinate mice are characterized by higher adrenal weights and lower gonadal weights; however, if tested in a single trial against a new non-aggressive antagonist, the subordinate animals behave within the same range of behavior as

the dominant animals.[23] The author notes that it is not surprising that the later behavior is independent of the earlier behavior, since the behavior is part of an established hierarchical response and the response to an unfamiliar individual should be independent.

Direct measures of adrenal activity by measurement of plasma corticosterone as an indicator of adrenal-cortical activity have been obtained.[74] They confirmed the earlier impressions based upon adrenal weight: dominant mice had significantly lower levels of corticosterone than subordinate animals. The causal nature of the relationship has not been established.

Primate studies have provided a quite different view. Although such studies are difficult, the work of Leshner and Candland[72] is particularly interesting in the suggestion that higher status is associated with increased adrenal-cortical activity. Their work utilized assay of urinary 17-hydroxycorticosteroids with correlation to dominance ranking in an ongoing group of squirrel monkeys. Such a view is confirmed through adrenal weight measures, though without kinetic endocrine measures, in work with crab-eating monkeys.[57]

An interesting but difficult investigation to interpret in light of the preceding studies dealing with primates, comes from the work of Sassenrath[91] who studied the response in rhesus to adrenocorticotropic hormone (ACTH) on urinary steroids collected outside of the behavioral situation. In that study, the dominant animal has the lowest secretion of 17-hydroxycorticosteroids in response to ACTH. The interpretation would be that the response to ACTH is a test of the adrenal size, and that the lower the response, the less the activity of the adrenal. Although the interpretation is complicated, the results suggest powerful influences of social behavior on pituitary-adrenal function.

If one accepts the Leshner and Candland[72] and Hayama[57] data, there are profound differences between the rodent and primate in regard to pituitary-adrenal function. The differences are viewed by Leshner and Candland as due to the different styles of ongoing

* See references 6, 4, 5, 22, 41, 60, and 102.

interaction. Thus, in the rodent, dominance is established by direct physical attack, while in the primates that have been studied the dominance is settled by ritualized displays. These processes may relate to varying forms of aggressive interaction which have differing underlying endocrine and neurochemical mechanisms.[45]

Studies dealing with endocrine measures in primates are difficult because of the problems associated with obtaining adequate or appropriate samples of blood in relation to ongoing behavior. Thus, frequently the collection of the compound of interest is accomplished under conditions that are different from those involved in the status situation or social behavior situation per se. One could anticipate that for some kinds of behavior, there may be marked differences between the social situation and the collection situation in terms of endocrine response.

Gonadal Function in Males

Only very recently have procedures been developed that enable direct investigation of testosterone in relation to social behavior. Not only have the chemical assays required development, but the behavioral procedures for the collection of blood samples have also required development, so as to be able to obtain the samples very quickly in adapted animals. As a consequence of such development, important studies in which kinds of behavior could be determined with good reliability in relation to the endocrine measure have become possible.[88,87] From studies involving thirty-four animals in a one-third acre compound, it was established that dominance rank was positively correlated with testosterone concentration. The animals in the highest quartile had significantly lower levels of testosterone than those in the lower quartile, although there were no significant differences between animals in the second, third, or fourth quartiles. Aggression also correlated with testosterone, but the correlation of high submissiveness and low testosterone was not high. The complexity of the data is shown in the fact that the relationships are not always simply related. Thus, the most aggressive animals are not always the most dominant, and the most dominant animal need not have the highest testosterone. The studies led the investigators to a series of investigations of the relationship of behavior to endocrine changes, and an attempt to determine whether testosterone changes were preceded by changes in dominance. The data to investigate this possibility was obtained by using smaller groups and allowing animals to take a dominant position, in which case plasma testosterone increased; if the dominance position sharply decreased, the plasma testosterone decreased. These results are also of interest in light of the findings that plasma testosterone in humans is decreased by stress.[70]

Adrenal-Medullary Function

Relations of adrenal-medullary secretion to behavioral processes related to social behavior has proceeded upon two fronts. The first has been the area of measurement of adrenal-medullary hormones, epinephrine (adrenaline), and norepinephrine (noradrenaline), generally utilizing urinary samples. The second, in animals, has involved studies of the enzymes that form the catecholamines in the adrenal, as well as measurement of the catecholamines, with determination of changes associated with behavioral states. The rapid changes that can occur in the adrenal-medullary system and the powerful psychological effects of epinephrine[79,11] makes this system a particularly interesting one for investigation.

Several studies suggest that social behavior may alter the enzymatic processes involved in the formation of the catecholamines. Among those areas of investigation are studies dealing with social isolation and group housing, as exemplified by the studies of Welch and Welch.[109] They found decreased levels of catecholamines in the brain and adrenal of group-housed mice when contrasted with individually housed animals. Although the results of such studies may depend upon the species used,[103] it is clear that differential housing can markedly alter catecholamine mechanisms. More directly related to social interaction have been the investigations represented by the collaboration of Henry and Axelrod and their colleagues.[61,62] They have utilized a variety of mutual interaction situations including interconnected cages, a technique which leads to confrontations and severe social stimulation. In animals exposed to such severe social interaction, there were increases in the enzymes that form catecholamines in the adrenal, as well as increases in the levels of the hormones themselves. A decrease in the enzymes was noted in isolated animals. Preliminary studies have suggested that dominant animals may have lower levels of the enzymes that form catecholamines than the subordinate animals have. Many of the studies of the investigators utilized long-time bases (in some of the studies, periods as long as six months were used) and it will be of interest to see if changes associated with these and other social interaction paradigms can be demonstrated with short-time span interactions. Rapid changes in the enzymes that form catecholamines have been noted to occur within a few hours of certain forms of stress,[29] which suggests the possibility of investigations involving behavioral states with short-time parameters in the appropriate social situation.

Studies of adrenal-medullary function in humans have concentrated on determination of epinephrine and norepinephrine in urine. This has been necessary because of the difficulty in measuring the catecholamines in blood samples given the limitations of current assay procedures. Thus, samples that are assayed represent a pooling of many time-dependent processes, usually over a period of several hours, which is unfortunate, yet makes the fact that there are positive results even more tempting for future analysis with multiple time points. Ultimately, one would expect that assessment of adrenal-medullary function in humans would involve determinations at close time intervals by means of new techniques, which are now being developed, such as mass fragmentography.[37]

Several investigators have demonstrated powerful effects of psychosocial interaction variables on adrenal-medullary secretion. Many of the studies have demonstrated that a variety of behavioral situations that involve tense, anxious but passive emotional displays are associated with elevated epinephrine output.[38] This can be said of certain novel or distressing situations as well.[107] A variety of psychological states have been investigated in a pioneering series of studies conducted over many years by Levi[73] and brought together in a recent monograph. Urinary catecholamines were found to increase in a wide variety of arousing situations, such as viewing films with both "pleasant" and "unpleasant" aspects. Bland materials reduced the levels of excretion. Psychosocial stimuli were found to alter catecholamine secretion, depending upon the stimuli and on the starting point of the organism, without any simple relationships between anxiety and epinephrine secretion or aggression and norepinephrine secretion.

Frankenhaeuser[42] has conducted a series of careful investigations relating cognitive and emotional patterns with endocrine secretion. Among the most interesting studies has been a series of investigations in children.[43] These, while not specifically concerned with status, suggest powerful social interrelationships that may bear on status and power relationships. For example, there was a positive correlation between the norepinephrine secretion of mother and son, but not of father and son. There appeared to be a significant positive correlation between the mother's adrenaline output and the frequency with which the fathers punished their children. Such studies of interactional and developmental processes, particularly when combined with social processes, suggest outlines for the development of a new research area.

A means of studying the relationship of social processes to endocrine processes has emerged from investigations of free fatty acids and social behavioral states. Free fatty-acid levels are believed to correlate highly with sympathetic activation of which adrenal-medullary activity would be an important component. In a series of studies characterized by the use of rigorous behavioral parameters, as well as rigorous chemical measures, Back and Bogdonoff[3] have demonstrated correlations between chemical measures and behavioral measures of conformity and leadership in test situations in which these parameters could be directly controlled. Using changes in free fatty acids as an indicator, the authors of these pioneering studies note:

. . . if the social situation is perceived simply as a background to individual achievement, the dominant variable will be the potential for individual achievement and its meaning. In this situation, pressure to conform and pressure to assume leadership may be viewed as arousing stimuli, and the individual may seek to avoid these situations. If, however, the group relationship has the dominant meaning, the performance of the task may be seen in terms of the group interaction, and then deviation from the group norm becomes the arousing condition. Conforming behavior is then attended by decreased arousal. [p. 41][3]

A direct study of the relationship between social status processes and catecholamine secretion has just been completed by Barchas and Barchas. In this study, individuals of equal external status (education, age, race, sex) were brought together, and they interacted for a one-hour period. The status differential that was established between the individuals through interaction was assessed by observers and by questionnaires for the subjects. Urinary catecholamines (epinephrine, norepinephrine, and dopamine) were obtained before and after the session. There was no relationship between the urinary catechols taken before the interaction and the acquired status, but there was a pattern of association between acquired status and the urinary catechols sampled after interaction.

Brain Serotonin

Biogenic amines in the brain have been studied in terms of their relation to several kinds of behavior, including severe psychiatric disorders. Serotonin, an indoleamine, has been postulated to be a possible transmitter and to act as a regulator of neuronal function.[12] The compound has been linked to specific forms of behavior, but only limited studies related to social behavior have been conducted. A major procedure for investigating the effects of changes in brain serotonin involves use of parachlorophenylalanine (PCPA) which in-

hibits the formation of serotonin, although it may also act on other chemical systems. Studies in which PCPA has been administered to primates have been very few and suggest decreased activity. Boelkins[21] administered the drug to an ongoing group of three crab-eating macaques (*Macaca fascicularis*) and observed that the number of kinds of social behavior decreased, but that the time spent in social huddling increased, with no change in aggressive or other kinds of behavior.

Maas et al.[75] in studies with two groups of *Macaca speciosa* observed no changes in aggressive or submissive gestures, attacks, or hetero- and auto-grooming.

In each of these studies, the degree to which brain serotonin mechanisms have been interfered with is open to question, and larger doses of the inhibitor of serotonin formation caused the animals to appear ill, possibly due to peripheral effects. Thus, the role of serotonin in primate social behavior deserves further investigation.

Brain Catecholamines

Particular attention has focused on catecholamines as they relate to a variety of behavior.[10] By the use of specific inhibitors of the formation of catecholamines, studies have been performed suggesting important roles for catecholamines in social behavior. In a series of papers, the group associated with Maas[83,84,75] has investigated such processes in studies of macaque monkeys. In one set of investigations, the drug α-methyltyrosine, an inhibitor in the first step of catecholamine synthesis, was administered to some of the animals in a group-living situation, with monitoring of social behavior. It was found that the animals had a marked decrease in social initiation, including grooming, threats, and attack, although they responded to other animals. There also may be dominance shifts: an animal who was dominant did not have a change in social dominance, while two other animals had a decrease in dominance. In another study, a different drug, 6-hydroxydopamine, which destroys many of the neurons that contain norepinephrine in the central nervous system, was administered to free-ranging macaques. The treated animals were more peripheral to their social group, exhibited decreased social behavior, initiated fewer threats, less social grooming, and fewer social initiatives than the control animals.

The results of the Maas group demonstrate powerful effects of central catecholamines in social processes in nonhuman primates. Such studies would suggest that certain forms of social behavior may be mediated by catecholamine-containing neurons and be altered by drugs that alter catecholamine mechanisms. The processes that have been studied are related to basic social processes previously shown to be related in similar ways in nonhuman and human primates.[15] The findings that central catecholamine systems are profoundly involved in nonhuman primate social behavior raises questions as to the role of catechols in humans.

([Psychiatric Processes and Physiological Sociology

Some Aspects of Sociopathic Behavior

A number of psychiatric processes are observable in which there is clinical reason to believe that profound disturbances of sociological processes, including status, dominance relations, and affiliative bonding exist. One psychiatric illness that manifests itself in social structural relationships in a profound way is sociopathic behavior.

By the very nature of the sociopathic individual, persons with the disorder display altered social behavior.[85] The question as to whether in terms of their physiological responses such individuals respond differentially when compared to normal people has been raised by several investigators. Some evidence suggests that there are such differences.

Learning variables are among the factors that have been investigated. The studies of Hare and others have suggested that classical conditioning of autonomic responses and avoidance learning may be impaired.[54] For

example, it has been found that psychopathic criminals acquire conditioned electrodermal responses more slowly, that the formed responses are of lesser magnitude and are more quickly extinguished, and that, once acquired, the responses are generalized to a lesser degree than in nonpsychopathic criminals. These studies and others suggest that psychopaths may have normal attention to stimuli, but a decreased anticipatory fear.[56]

Particularly relevant from the standpoint of this review are a series of provocative studies dealing with the response to an injection of adrenaline by psychopaths when compared to other populations. The literature has been quite contradictory, but does strongly suggest that there are differences.[92,44,55] The experiments were performed under different conditions, including degree of ongoing activation. In the studies of Hare, which were able to take advantage of the earlier findings and to work with a carefully selected population, it was found that the change in skin conductance following the injection of adrenaline was smaller in a psychopathic group compared to a criminal nonpsychopathic group. In that study, differences in heart rate that had been noted in the earlier studies, with quite different subject-selection procedures and activities, were not found. Questions as to the hyper- or hyposensitivity of aspects of the autonomic nervous system have been raised by the various studies, although conclusions would require considerably more investigation.

Another side of the coin remains to be investigated—the effects of stresses on direct endocrine release. Such studies would involve, for example, in relation to the previous literature, determination of release of epinephrine and norepinephrine and the enzyme that converts dopamine to norepinephrine (dopamine-β-hydroxylase), which can be measured in the peripheral blood. Ideally, diurnal rhythms and the response to stress, and particularly the response to emotional conditioning, would be obtained. Studies of central brain mechanisms are clearly indicated.

The literature dealing with psychopathic behavior raises the question as to whether this form of social behavior, which involves a psychiatric diagnosis, may not have powerful biological aspects. One could imagine either biochemical differences based on genetic factors or on early experience. In either event, it is quite likely that psychopathic illness may reflect interactions between social behavior and biochemical processes.*

Frequently role enactment requires simultaneous action or interwoven action between two or more individuals. Discrepancies in perceptions of roles may lead to group stresses. Most frequently in this situation there is a mutual adjustment of expectations. When there is not, we may have such phenomenon as schism and skew in the family and scapegoating (here seen as a mode of releasing group tensions regarding roles to the detriment of the individuals involved). Similarly, the phenomenon of the double bind seen from the points of view of the sender and receiver of messages may be partially visualized as inadequate internalizations and expressions of role relations. Such social behavior could be expected to have profound effects on the types of parameters considered in this chapter. An additional example of the application of role theory and status processes to psychiatric illness could be made in the case of depressive illness.

Toward a Physiological Sociology

It is difficult at this early point in the development of physiological sociology to give an adequate general formulation of the potential relations between physiological events and sociological behavior. At this stage, it seems reasonable to assume that biochemical and sociological processes are intimately related. For example, biochemical processes may affect activity levels, emotional tones, and the susceptibility to stress. Sociological processes may set in motion processes that influence biochemical mechanisms; for example, changing the levels of particular compounds by producing shifts between pathways, altering utiliza-

tion of compounds, and inducing enzymatic changes. Biochemical events may profoundly alter the ability of the organism to respond to its environment.

If one visualizes a relationship between biochemical and social-structural events and assumes changes in response to a sociological event, then such changes become very important in relation to the length of time that they persist and the manner in which environmental and genetic factors interrelate. To account for long-term emotional behavior and alterability of behavior, one would have to assume alterability in underlying chemical events. In the simplest model, we would assume that sociological events affect the body chemistry and that the chemical change in turn affects the future sociological events. Thus, with particular genetic predispositions, chemical changes that are long-term in nature could, in effect, "lock in" certain psychological sets.

Different genetic strains have already been demonstrated to have a considerable variation in terms of the steroid hormones produced by the adrenal cortex and thyroid hormones.[49, 50,52,53] In a number of illnesses it has been demonstrated that there is a genetic difference in formation of adrenal-cortical hormones; several of these illnesses lead to marked behavior change.

Strong evidence now suggests that some of the other biochemical systems we have been concerned with in this chapter are also under genetic control. Thus, the levels of the enzymes that synthesize catecholamines (epinephrine, norepinephrine, and dopamine) vary in different inbred strains. The degree to which the level of the enzymes can be altered by stress and even the type of stresses to which there are responses varies in different inbred strains.†

An extensive listing could be made of how possible genetic differences in a system such as that involved in catecholamine production or utilization, both in the adrenal or in the brain, might affect social behavior. It has been shown that in response to stress differing amounts of adrenal-cortical steroids are re-

* The reader is referred to Leiderman and Shapiro[71] for a review of experiments that bear on the general subject.

† See references 8, 9, 28–30, 51, 68, and 80.

leased in different genetic strains. It is easy to imagine that in response to stress two individuals might send the same number of nerve impulses to the adrenal medulla, but, because of a genetic difference, one individual might form differential amounts of catechols, release differential amounts, metabolize the catechols at different rates, or have differential passage across the blood-brain barrier. If any of these possibilities were to occur, clearly there could be behavioral changes when the adrenaline reached various target organs, including the brain.

Other possibilities to be investigated include the presence of minor or abnormal pathways in adrenal-catechol metabolism, including the physiological controls on those pathways, and how they might be altered by social stress. Analogous factors could be relevant not only to adrenal catecholamines as hormones related to behavior but also to brain catecholamines and other putative transmitters between nerve cells, and to the various hormones we have considered in this chapter.

The hormonal systems have been related by physiologists to stress responses and it has been repeatedly suggested that feelings that accompany changes in levels of these hormones are interpreted by the individual according to past learning and present situational cues.[93,94] Using the conceptual framework of role theory, we may then direct our attention to those points at which stress may be expected and where pattern correlation between physiology and behavior is most likely to be seen within a culture. Conceptualization of these points should be at a level that cuts across specific roles. In addition to points of stress, there are expected to be physiological relationships to such aspects of roles as dominance or deference relations, and affiliative bonding.

For any individual, the relationship of physiological response to particular role-stress events may be posited as highly predictable. It would seem reasonable, however, when characterizing a population with regard to the relationships of physiology to role stress to think in terms of more general categories. Also, for some individuals, stress repeatedly

occurs with interaction in a nurturance system.

The idea of causality in the relations between endocrine and sociological events may be and has been helpful practically as experiments are set up and run. For some purposes the notion of causality is heuristically facilitative. However, if we are indeed dealing with a homeostatic system in terms of the individual's physiology as it adjusts to the psychological and social environment, then overemphasis on causality may, in the broad picture, obscure our vision. But it is not difficult to utilize those conditions on the one hand, while on the other we work toward a more intuitively satisfying understanding of how the individual makes his peace with his world, both physiologically and sociologically.

It is clear that more information, relative to the issue of the manner in which sociological events interact with physiological variables, will be needed. How do developmental patterns and behavioral states such as status orders or affiliation influence biochemistry? Can the response of endocrine agents or brain neurotransmitter agents to situations later in life be altered by early experience? What types of changes in the various mechanisms involving neuroregulatory agents can be found in different sociological states? What are the short- and long-term biochemical effects of different types of sociological situations? Does biochemical state influence social behavior? What is the possibility that behavior, such as repeated dominant or submissive behavior, may alter the propensity for long-term or repeated episodes of the behavior? Such studies involve animal investigation, but may lead to human studies. For example, to what extent does a sociological event, e.g., high status or low status, trigger biochemical changes that affect later events, thereby causing a cycle of actions that is neither wholly "sociological" or "psychological," nor wholly "biochemical?"

From the standpoint of psychiatry, one might well imagine psychiatric illnesses that meet the model of phenylketonuria in which a set of clear-cut, definable biochemical changes leads to severe behavioral changes. Understanding why *those* behavioral changes occur will be a crucial step. On the other hand, there may be other emotional illnesses that are more purely social structural or psychological than in the model just mentioned, and there may be still other illnesses in which a set of social-interaction events or psychological events in an individual with appropriate biochemical structures lead to an illness.

On the one hand, one encounters those who view mental illness and mind as apart from the brain, and, on the other, those who feel that a twisted thought, a twisted molecule. What is needed is a view that recognizes the subtle interplay of sociological, individual-psychological, biochemical, and physiological processes.

Recent research, including some presented in this paper, suggests the development of a new field of physiological sociology. Such a term is analogous to physiological psychology, and yet recognizes the new approaches and techniques that will be necessary for the field and its concern with behavior related to group structure and processes. The area is exciting in its conception, and yet poses many problems from technical to philosophical. Some of the problems include how to relate biochemical events to sociologically structured events, the effects of drugs on social structures, and developmental processes.

⟪ Concluding Remarks

We have chosen to examine some of the endocrine correlates associated with status behavior because status behavior can be viewed as one of the most basic building blocks of structural-social relations. Status structures are commonly found throughout mammalian species, status behavior has been sufficiently studied, and theories have been constructed, so that it is possible to begin to perform physiological investigations. Studies to date, although few in number with higher primates, suggest the potential of important correlations in a number of endocrine systems, with potential consideration of genetic and developmen-

tal processes. Such information can be of importance, theoretically, in terms of understanding aspects of the behavior, and, potentially, in altering some forms of behavior that may be deleterious to the individual. Further, such information may aid in understanding somatic processes in terms of aspects of social structure that profoundly alter somatic function. Such information may prove of value not only in theory, but also, potentially, in the treatment of psychiatric and psychosomatic conditions which would be a particularly important aspect of the new field of physiological sociology.

⟪ Bibliography

1. ALEXANDER, B. K. and M. J. BOWERS. "The Social Behavior of Japanese Macaques in the Corral," *Primate News*, 6 (1968), 3–10.
2. ALTMANN, S. A. "A Field Study of the Sociobiology of Rhesus Monkeys, *Macaca Mulatta*," *Ann. N.Y. Acad. Sci.*, 102 (1962), 338–435.
3. BACK, K. W. and M. D. BOGDONOFF. "Plasma Lipid Responses to Leadership, Conformity, and Deviation," in P. H. Leiderman and D. Shapiro, eds., *Psychobiological Approaches to Social Behavior*, pp. 24–42. 1964. Stanford: Stanford University Press.
4. BALES, R. F. "The Equilibrium Problem in Small Groups," in T. Parsons, R. F. Bales, and E. A. Shils, eds., *Working Papers in the Theory of Action*, pp. 111–161. Glencoe, Ill.: Free Press, 1953.
5. BALES, R. F. and P. E. SLATER. "Role Differentiation," in T. Parsons, R. F. Bales, and J. Olds, eds., *Family Socialization and Interaction Processes*, pp. 259–306. Glencoe, Ill.: Free Press, 1955.
6. BALES, R. F., F. L. STRODBECK, T. M. MILLS et al. "Channels of Communication in Small Groups," *Am. Soc. Rev.*, 16 (1951) 461–468.
7. BARCHAS, I. Personal communication, 1970.
8. BARCHAS, J. D., R. D. CIARANELLO, S. KESSLER et al. "Genetic Aspects of the Synthesis of Catecholamines in the Adrenal

Medulla," *Psychoneuroendrocrinology*. In press.

9. ———. "Genetic Aspects of Catecholamine Synthesis," *Psychoneuroendrocrinology*. In press.

10. BARCHAS, J. D., R. D. CIARANELLO, J. M. STOLK et al. "Biogenic Amines and Behavior," in S. Levine, ed., *Hormones and Behavior*, pp. 235–329. New York: Academic, 1972.

11. BARCHAS, J. D., J. M. STOLK, R. D. CIARANELLO et al. "Neuroregulatory Agents and Psychological Assessment," in P. McReynolds, ed., *Psychological Assessment*, Vol. 2, pp. 260–292. Palo Alto: Science and Behavior Books, 1971.

12. BARCHAS, J. D. and E. USDIN. *Serotonin and Behavior*. New York: Academic, 1973.

13. BARCHAS, P. R. "Approaches to Aggression as a Social Behavior," in R. Ofshe, ed., *Readings in Social Psychology*, pp. 388–401. Englewood Cliffs, N.J.: Prentice-Hall, 1971.

14. ———. "Differentiation and Stability of Dominance and Deference Orders in Rhesus Monkeys." Ph.D. thesis, Stanford University, 1971. Unpublished.

15. BARCHAS, P. R. and M. H. FISEK. "Status Formation in Ad Hoc Groups of Rhesus and Humans," submitted for publication.

16. BARNETT, S. A. "Competition among Wild Rats," *Nature*, 175 (1955), 126–127.

17. BERGER, J. and T. L. CONNER. "Performance Expectations and Behavior in Small Groups," *Acta Sociol.*, 12 (1969), 186–197.

18. BERGER, J., B. COHEN, JR., and M. ZELDITCH. "Status Characteristics and Expectation States," in J. Berger, M. Zelditch, and B. Anderson, eds., *Sociological Theories in Progress*, Vol. 1, pp. 47–73. Boston: Houghton-Mifflin, 1966.

19. BERGER, J. and M. H. FISEK. "A Generalization of the Theory of Status Characteristics and Expectation States," in J. Berger, T. L. Connor, and M. H. Fisek, eds., *Expectation States Theory: A Theoretical Research Program*, pp. 163–205. Cambridge, Mass.: Winthrop, 1974.

20. BERNSTEIN, I. and W. A. MASON. "Group Formation by Rhesus Monkeys," *Anim. Behav.*, 11 (1963), 28–31.

21. BOELKINS, R. C. "Effects of *Parachlorophenylalanine* on the Behavior of Monkeys," in J. D. Barchas and E. Usdin, eds., *Serotonin and Behavior*, pp. 357–364. New York: Academic, 1973.

22. BORGATTA, E. F. and R. F. BALES. "Interaction of Individuals in Reconstituted Groups," *Sociometry*, 15 (1953), 302–320.

23. BRAIN, P. F. "Endocrine and Behavioral Differences between Dominant and Subordinate Male House Mice Housed in Pairs," *Psychonom. Sci.*, 28 (1972), 260–262.

24. BRAIN, P. F. and N. W. NOWELL. "Isolation versus Grouping Effects on Adrenal and Gonadal Function in Albino Mice," *Gen. Comp. Endocrinol.*, 16 (1971), 149–154.

25. CARPENTER, C. R. *Naturalistic Behavior of Nonhuman Primates*, pp. 342–357; 365–385; 392–397. University Park, Pa.: Pennsylvania State University Press, 1964.

26. CHAMPNESS, B. Quoted in *Time Magazine*, Oct. 17, 1969, p. 74.

27. CHRISTIAN, J. J. "Effect of Population Size on the Weights of the Reproductive Organs of White Mice," *Am. J. Physiol.*, 181 (1955), 477–480.

28. CIARANELLO, R. D., P. R. BARCHAS, S. KESSLER et al. "Catecholamines: Strain Differences in Biosynthetic Enzyme Activity in Mice," *Life Sci.*, 11 (1972), 565–572.

29. CIARANELLO, R. D., J. N. DORNBUSCH, and J. D. BARCHAS. "Regulation of Adrenal Phenylethanolamine N-Methyltransferase Activity in Three Inbred Mouse Strains," *Mol. Pharmacol.*, 8 (1972), 511–520.

30. ———. "Rapid Increase of Phenylethanolamine N-Methyltransferase by Environmental Stress in an Inbred Mouse Strain," *Science*, 175 (1972), 789–790.

31. COLLIAS, N. C. "Social Behavior in Animals," *Ecology*, 34 (1953), 810–811.

32. CONNER, R. L. "Hormones, Biogenic Amines and Aggression," in S. Levine, ed., *Hormones and Behavior*, pp. 209–233. New York: Academic, 1972.

33. DARWIN, C. *The Expression of the Emotion in Man and Animals*. New York: Appleton, 1896.

34. DAVIS, D. E. and J. J. CHRISTIAN. "Relation of Adrenal Weight to Social Rank of Mice," *Proc. Soc. Exp. Biol. Med.*, 94 (1957), 728–731.

35. DEMENT, W. C. Personal communication, 1971.

36. DeVore, I., ed. *Primate Behavior: Field Studies of Monkeys and Apes.* New York: Holt, Rinehart & Winston, 1965.

37. DoAmaral, J. R. Personal communication, 1972.

38. Elmadjian, F., J. M. Hope, and E. T. Lamson. "Excretion of Epinephrine in Various Emotional States," *J. Clin. Endocrinol.*, 17 (1957), 608–620.

39. Etkin, W. "Theories of Animal Socialization and Communication," in W. Etkin, ed., *Social Behavior and Organization among Vertebrates*, pp. 167–205. Chicago: University of Chicago Press, 1964.

40. Fisek, M. H. "The Evolution of Status Structures and Interaction on Task Oriented Discussion Groups." Unpublished Ph.D. dissertation Standford University, 1968.

41. Fisek, M. H. and R. Ofshe. *The Process of Status Evolution.* Technical Report No. 33. Stanford, Calif.: Laboratory for Social Research, Stanford University, 1970.

42. Frankenhaeuser, M. "Behavior and Circulating Catecholamines," *Brain Res.*, 31 (1971), 241–262.

43. Frankenhaeuser, M. and G. Johansson. "Behavior and Catecholamines in Children," in L. Levi, ed., Society, Stress and Disease, Vol. 1: *The Psychosocial Environment and Psychosomatic Diseases.* London: Oxford University Press, forthcoming.

44. Goldman, H., L. Lindner, S. Dinitz et al. "The Simple Sociopath: Physiologic and Sociologic Characteristics," *Biol. Psychiatry*, 3 (1971), 77–83.

45. Goldstein, M. "Neuroscience Bases of Abnormal Behavior," *Arch. Neurol.*, 30 (1974), 1–35.

46. Hall, K. R. L. "Aggression in Monkey and Ape Societies," in P. Jay, ed., *Primates: Studies in Adaptation Variability*, pp. 149–161. New York: Holt, Rinehart & Winston, 1968.

47. ———. "Social Training in Monkeys," in P. Jay, ed., *Primates*, pp. 383–397. New York: Holt, Rinehart & Winston, 1968.

48. Hamburg, D. A. "Emotions in Perspective of Human Evolution," in P. Knapp, ed., *Expressions of the Emotions in Man*, pp. 300–317. New York: International Universities Press, 1963.

49. ———. "Genetics of Adrenocortical Hormone Metabolism in Relation to Psychological Stress," in J. Hirsch, ed., *Behavior —Genetic Analysis*, pp. 154–175. New York: McGraw-Hill, 1967.

50. ———, ed. *Psychiatry as a Behavioral Science.* Behavioral Social Sciences Survey Monograph Series. Englewood Cliffs, N.J.: Prentice-Hall, 1970.

51. Hamburg, D. A., B. Hamburg, and J. Barchas. "Anger and Depression: Current Psychobiological Approaches," in L. Levi, ed., *Parameters of Emotion.* London: Oxford University Press, Forthcoming.

52. Hamburg, D. A. and S. Kessler. "A Behavioral-endocrine-genetic Approach to Stress Problems," in S. Pickett, ed., Memoirs of the Society for Endocrinology No. 15: *Endocrine Genetics*, pp. 249–270. London: Cambridge University Press, 1967.

53. Hamburg, D. A. and D. Lunde. "Relation of Behavioral, Genetic, and Neuroendocrine Factors to Thyroid Function," in J. Spuhler, ed., *Genetic Diversity and Human Behavior*, pp. 135–170. Chicago: Aldine, 1967.

54. Hare, R. D. *Psychopathy: Theory and Research.* New York: Wiley-Interscience, 1970.

55. ———. "Psychopathy and Physiological Responses to Adrenalin," *J. Abnorm. Psychol.*, 79 (1972), 138–147.

56. Hare, R. D. and M. J. Quinn. "Psychopathy and Autonomic Conditioning," *J. Abnorm. Psychol.*, 77 (1971), 223–235.

57. Hayama, S. "Correlation between Adrenal Gland Weight and Dominance Rank in Caged Crab-eating Monkeys (*Macaca irus*)," *Primates*, 7 (1966), 21–26.

58. Hebb, P. O. and W. R. Thompson. "The Social Significance of Animal Studies," in G. Lindzy, ed., *Handbook of Social Psychology*, Vol. 1, pp. 532–561, New York: Addison-Wesley, 1954.

59. Hediger, H. *Wild Animals in Captivity: An Outline of the Biology of Zoological Gardens.* New York: Dover, 1964.

60. Heinicke, C. and R. F. Bales. "Developmental Trends on the Structure of Small Groups," *Sociometry*, 16 (1953), 7–38.

61. Henry, J. P., D. L. Ely, and P. M. Stephens. "Changes in Catecholamine-controlling Enzymes in Response to Psychosocial Activation of the Defense and Alarm Reactions," in *Physiology, Emotions, and Psychosomatic Illness*, pp. 225–251. London: CIBA Foundation, 1972.

62. HENRY, J. P., P. M. STEPHENS, J. AXELROD et al. "Effect of Psychosocial Stimulation on the Enzymes Involved in the Biosynthesis and Metabolism of Noradrenaline and Adrenaline," *Psychosom. Med.*, 33 (1971), 227–237.

63. HINDE, R. G. and L. E. REWELL. "Communication by Postures and Facial Expressions in the Rhesus Monkeys (*Macaca mulatta*)," *Proc. Zool. Soc. Inst.*, 138 (1962), 1–21.

64. IMANISHI, K. "Social Behaviors in Japanese Monkeys, *Macaca fuscata*," *Psychologiozea*, 1 (1957), 47–54.

65. ——— "Social Organization of Subhuman Primates in Their Natural Habitat," *Curr. Anthropol.*, 1 (1960), 393–407.

66. JAY, P., ed. *Primates: Studies in Adaptation and Variability.* New York: Holt, Rinehart & Winston, 1968.

67. KAWAI, M. "On the Rank System in a Natural Group of Japanese Monkeys," *Primates*, 1 (1958), 84–98.

68. KESSLER, S., R. D. CIARANELLO, J. G. M. SHIRE et al. "Genetic Variation in Catecholamine-synthesizing Enzyme Activity," *Proc. Natl. Acad. Sci.*, 69 (1972), 2448–2450.

69. KOFORD, C. B. "Population Dynamics of Rhesus Monkeys on Cayo Santiago," in I. DeVore, ed., *Primate Behavior*, pp. 160–174. New York: Holt, Rinehart & Winston, 1965.

70. KREUZ, L. E., R. M. ROSE, and J. R. JENNINGS. "Suppression of Plasma Testosterone Levels and Psychological Stress," *Arch. Gen. Psychiatry*, 26 (1972), 479–482.

71. LEIDERMAN, P. H. and D. SHAPIRO. *Psychobiological Approaches to Social Behavior.* Stanford, Calif.: Stanford University Press, 1964.

72. LESHNER, A. I. and D. K. CANDLAND. "Endocrine Effects of Grouping and Dominance Rank in Squirrel Monkeys," *Physiol. Behav.*, 8 (1972), 441–445.

73. LEVI, I., ed. "Stress and Distress in Response to Psychosocial Stimuli. Laboratory and Real Life Studies on Sympathoadrenomedullary and Related Reactions," *Acta Med. Scand.* (Suppl.), 528 (1972), p. 166.

74. LOUCH, C. D. and M. HIGGINBOTHAM. "The Relation between Social Rank and Plasma Corticosterone Levels in Mice," *Gen. Comp. Endocrinol.*, 8 (1967), 441–444.

75. MAAS, J. W., D. E. REDMOND, and R. GAUEN. "Effects of Serotonin Depletion on Behavior in Monkeys," in J. D. Barchas and E. Usdin, eds., *Serotonin and Behavior*, pp. 351–356. New York: Academic Press, 1973.

76. MCKINNEY, W. T., JR., S. J. SUOMI, and H. F. HARLOW. "Depression in Primates," *Am. J. Psychiatry*, 127 (1971), 1313–1320.

77. MARONEY, R. J., J. M. WARREN, and M. M. SINHA. "Stability of Social Dominance Hierarchies in Monkeys (*Macaca mulatta*)," *J. Soc. Psychol.*, 50 (1957), 285–293.

78. MASLOW, A. H. "The Role of Dominance in the Social Behavior of Infrahuman Primates: IV. The Determination of Hierarchy in Pairs and in a Group," *J. Genet. Psychol.*, 49 (1936), 161–198.

79. MASON, J. W. "A Review of Psychoendocrine Research on the Sympathetic-adrenal Medullary System," *Psychosom. Med.*, 30 (1968), 631–653.

80. MILKOVIC, K., C. WINGET, T. DEGUCHI et al. "The Effect of Maternal Manipulation on the Phenylethanolamine N-methyltransferase Activity and Corticosterone Content of the Fetal Adrenal Gland," *Am. J. Physiol.*, 226 (1974), 864–866.

81. MILLER, R. E. and M. V. MURPHY. "Social Interactions of Rhesus Monkeys: Food-getting Dominance as a Dependent Variable," *J. Soc. Psychol.*, 44 (1956), 249–255.

82. PORTMANN, A. *Animals as Social Beings.* New York: Harper & Row, 1961.

83. REDMOND, D. E., J. W. MAAS, A. KLING et al. "Changes in Primate Social Behavior after Treatment with Alpha-Methyl-*Para*-tyrosine," *Psychosom. Med.*, 33 (1971), 97–113.

84. REDMOND, D. E., J. W. MAAS, A. KLING et al. "Social Behavior of Monkeys Selectively Depleted of Monoamines," *Science*, 174 (1971), 428–431.

85. ROBINS, L. N. *Deviant Children Grown Up: A Sociological and Psychiatric Study of Sociopathic Personality.* Baltimore: Williams & Wilkins, 1966.

86. ROE, A. and G. G. SIMPSON, eds. *Behavior and Evolution.* New Haven: Yale University Press, 1958.

87. ROSE, R. M., T. P. GORDON, and I. S. BERNSTEIN. "Plasma Testosterone Levels in the Male Rhesus: Influences of Sexual and

Social Stimuli," *Science*, 178 (1972), 643–645.

88. ROSE, R. M., J. W. HOLADAY, and I. S. BERNSTEIN. "Plasma Testosterone, Dominance Rank and Agressive Behavior in Male Rhesus Monkeys," *Nature*, 231 (1971), 366–368.

89. RULE, C. "A Theory of Human Behavior Based on Studies of Nonhuman Primates," *Perspect. Biol. Med.*, 10 (1967), 153–176.

90. SADLEIR, R. M. F. S. "The Establishment of a Dominance Rank Order in Male *Peromyscus maniculatus* and Its Stability with Time," *Anim. Behav.*, 18 (1970), 55–59.

91. SASSENRATH, E. N. "Increased Adrenal Responsiveness Related to Social Stress in Rhesus Monkeys," *Horm. Behav.*, 1 (1969), 283–298.

92. SCHACHTER, S. and B. LATANÉ. "Crime, Cognition and the Autonomic Nervous System," in M. R. Jones, ed., *Nebraska Symposium on Motivation, 1964*, pp. 222–272. Lincoln: University of Nebraska Press, 1964.

93. SCHACHTER, S. and J. E. SINGER. "Cognitive, Social, and Physiological Determinants of Emotional State," *Psychol. Rev.*, 69 (1962), 379–399.

94. SCHACHTER, S. and L. WHEELER. "Epinephrine, Chlorpromazine, and Amusement," *J. Abnorm. Soc. Psychol.*, 65 (1962), 121–128.

95. SCHREIER, A. M., H. F. HARLOW, and F. STOLLMITZ, eds. *Behavior of Non-Human Primates*, Vols. 1 and 2. New York: Academic, 1965.

96. SCOTT, J. P. "Group Formation Determined by Social Behavior: A Comparative Study of Two Mammalian Societies," *Sociometry*, 8 (1945), 42–52.

97. ———. *Animal Behavior*. Chicago: University of Chicago Press, 1958.

98. ———. "The Effects of Early Experience on Social Behavior and Organization," in W. Etkin, ed., *Social Behavior and Organization among Vertebrates*, pp. 231–255.

Chicago: University of Chicago Press, 1964.

99. SIMMEL, G. In K. Wolfe, ed., *The Sociology of Georg Simmel*, pp. 181–303. New York: Free Press, 1950.

100. SOUTHWICK, C. H., ed. *Primate Social Behavior*. Princeton: Van Nostrand, 1963.

101. SOUTHWICK, C. H., M. A. BEG, and M. R. SIDDIGI. "A Population Survey of Rhesus Monkeys in Northern India: II. Transportation Routes and First Areas," *Ecology*, 42 (1961), 698–710.

102. STEPHAN, F. and E. G. MISHLER. "The Distributions of Participation in Small Groups and Exponential Approximation," *Am. Soc. Rev.*, 17 (1952), 598–608.

103. STOLK, J. M., R. CONNER, and J. D. BARCHAS. "Social Environment and Brain Biogenic Amine Metabolism," *J. Comp. Physiol. Psychol.*, in press.

104. TERRY, R. T. "Primate Grooming as a Tension Reduction Mechanism," *J. Psychol.*, 76 (1970), 129–136.

105. THIESSEN, D. D. and D. A. RODGERS. "Population Density and Endocrine Function," *Psychol. Bull.*, 58 (1961), 441–451.

106. TINBERGEN, N. *Social Behavior in Animals, with Special Reference to Vertebrates*. London: Methuen, 1955.

107. TOLSON, W. W., J. W. MASON, E. J. SACHAR et al. "Urinary Catecholamine Responses Associated with Hospital Admission in Normal Human Subjects," *J. Psychosom. Res.*, 8 (1965), 365–372.

108. WARREN, J. M. and R. J. MARONEY. "Competitive Social Interaction between Monkeys," *J. Soc. Psychol.*, 48 (1958), 223–233.

109. WELCH, B. L. and A. S. WELCH. "Greater Lowering of Brain and Adrenal Catecholamines in Group-housed than in Individually-housed Mice Administered DL-α-Methyltyrosine," *J. Pharm. Pharmacol.*, 20 (1968), 244–246.

110. ZUCHERMAN, S. *The Social Life of Monkeys and Apes*. London: Kegan, Paul, Trench, Trubner, 1932.

PART FOUR

New Directions in Treatment and Care

CHAPTER 27

INTRAUTERINE DIAGNOSIS AND GENETIC COUNSELING: IMPLICATIONS FOR PSYCHIATRY IN THE FUTURE*

Gilbert S. Omenn and Arno G. Motulsky

MANY PSYCHOLOGICAL BURDENS are associated with pregnancy, one of the most distressing being the fear of a deformed or defective baby. The fear has some basis in the fact that approximately 3 percent of all live births are severely retarded in mental development or have serious defects. For the family in which a child or another relative is already defective, the risks may be greatly magnified. In the past two decades, genetic

* This review was supported by grant GM15253 from the U.S. Public Health Service.

counseling clinics have been established to deal with the medical, genetic, and emotional aspects of such disorders.

The first requirement for genetic counseling is precise diagnosis in order to predict the course of the illness. Determination of the risk of a recurrent defect in subsequent children requires clear differentiation of heterogeneous causes of similar syndromes, often relying upon the detailed family history and upon various laboratory analyses such as radiologic studies, chromosome karyotypes, or enzyme assays. Nevertheless, even with the most detailed evaluation, families usually can be provided with only a statistical statement. For example, the risk of recurrence in subsequent children is about 1 percent for most cases of Down's syndrome (mongolism), about 5 percent for many other birth abnormalities, 25 percent for inborn errors of metabolism inherited as autosomal recessive disorders, and 50 percent for autosomal dominant conditions. Often, however, family counseling is complicated by variable severity of the illness, uncertainty of diagnosis, or the possibility that the affected child had a fresh mutation. For many common disorders, including schizophrenia and depression, for which there is good evidence of genetic factors of unknown mechanism, an "empiric risk figure" based upon reports of the frequency of recurrence in large series of families can often be given. It must be stressed that these risks for specific disorders are in addition to the approximately 3 percent risk of mental retardation or birth defects that every couple takes when having a child.

In the past few years, a dramatic development in counseling for some genetic disorders has occurred. For a small, but rapidly increasing number of diseases, it is possible to diagnose the condition *in utero* early enough in pregnancy to permit selective abortion of affected fetuses.* Unfortunately, treatment is unsatisfactory for so many conditions, especially those affecting mental development, that prevention of the birth of an affected child appears highly desirable to many parents and to their physicians. Diagnosis depends on the specific determination of chromosome karyotype or enzyme assays in cells of fetal origin obtained from the amniotic fluid around the fetus and grown in tissue culture medium in the laboratory. Though much speculation exists about the potential feasibility of "genetic engineering" by manipulation of the DNA in cells, many specific disorders can be prevented by what might be called "reproductive engineering."

* See references 8, 23, 44, 54, 57.

Amniocentesis

Amniocentesis is a procedure for obtaining amniotic fluid that contains fetal cells desquamated from respiratory and urinary tract endothelia and from skin and amnion. A transabdominal approach under local anesthesia has replaced the transcervical and transvaginal approaches, which carry a higher risk of bleeding, infection, and induced miscarriage. A small-gauge "spinal" needle is inserted under sterile conditions through the abdominal and uterine wall into the amniotic cavity. The procedure is done "blind"; success depends upon the skill and experience of the obstetrician. More accurate localization of the placental and fetal position using ultrasound techniques is being evaluated for reliability and safety.[1,33] The time at which amniocentesis is carried out must be a compromise. The more advanced the pregnancy, the more fluid and the greater the likelihood of obtaining an adequate sample for study. On the other hand, amniocentesis must be carried out early enough so that laboratory studies can be completed and abortion be done safely (and legally) if termination of the pregnancy is indicated. The volume of the amniotic fluid has been measured directly with the removal of the products of conception *in toto* in pregnancies interrupted by abdominal hysterectomy between ten and twenty weeks of gestation.[2,71,86] There is an average of 50 ml. of amniotic fluid at twelve weeks, 100 ml. at fourteen weeks, 150 ml. at fifteen weeks, and 450 ml. at twenty weeks (see Figure 27–1). Usually 10–20 ml. are removed for studies. The length of pregnancy or gestational age is calculated by obstetricians from the first day of the last menstrual period. Thus, the actual fetal age is approximately two weeks less than the "duration of pregnancy."

The hazards of amniocentesis are not yet fully evaluated. Early reports of several hundred procedures are remarkably free of serious immediate complications.[8,24,57] There are no known cases of severe maternal bleeding, infection, or uterine rupture; no induced miscar-

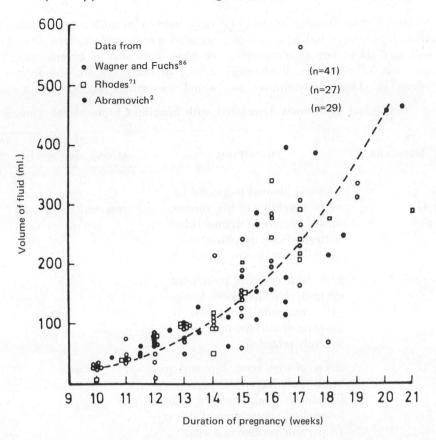

Figure 27–1. Volume of amniotic fluid as a function of gestational age. Note variation among individual specimens. Data from a total of ninety-seven cases.[2,71,86] (From Emery[23] with permission.)

riage; and no increase in the number of congenital malformations in the offspring. The fetus seems to "float away" from the amniocentesis needle, which presumably accounts for a lack of direct puncture wounds. The potential long-term hazards of amniocentesis are much more difficult to evaluate. Careful follow-up with appropriately matched control births must be carried out to assess mental and physical development in "normal" babies subjected to amniocentesis during pregnancy. The effect, if any, of disturbing the volume and possibly the dynamics of the amniotic fluid is simply unknown. It would be a tragedy if normal babies suffered mild depression of their later IQ levels or some other subtle damage because of a diagnostic procedure aimed at detecting an abnormal fetus. For this reason, parents in the early 1970s were being counseled in pregnancies with less than 1 per-

cent recurrence risk for a given disease that the risk of the procedure may be greater than the risk of a fetus affected with the avoidable condition. Depending on how abhorrent the disorder is to the parents, they may agree to forgo amniocentesis, or they may insist on accepting the risk of the procedure or else elect to have no more pregnancies.

【 Methods of Analysis of Amniotic Cells

Determination of Sex and Chromosome Karyotype of the Fetus

Not until 1956 were suitable techniques for spreading and staining the human chromosomes developed, so that the correct number of chromosomes could be established as 46 (not 48).[85] These chromosomes occur in pairs, 23 from each parent, including 22 sets of autosomes and one set of sex chromosomes, XX for females and XY for males. Beginning with mongolism or Down's syndrome in 1959, many clinical syndromes have been associated with specific abnormalities in number or gross structure of chromosomes[81] (Table 27–1). In the aggregate, these gross chromosomal aberrations occur in about one of 200

Table 27–1.   Clinical Syndromes Associated with Specific Chromosomal Abnormalities*

KARYOTYPE AUTOSOMAL DISORDERS	PHENOTYPE	FREQUENCY AMONG LIVE BIRTHS	DIAGNOSED IN UTERO
Trisomy 21 D/G, G/G translocation	Hypotonia, slanted palpebral fissures, speckling of iris, simian crease, abnormal dermal ridge patterns, bony dysplasia, congenital heart disease, leukemia	1/660 (marked maternal age effect)	yes
Trisomy 18	Feeble fetal activity, prominent occiput, clenched hand, low-set ears, congenital heart defects, 10 percent survive one year, severely retarded	1/3000	yes
Trisomy 13	Defects of eye, nose, hip and forebrain, polydactyly, hyperconvex fingernails, scalp defects, cardiac anomalies, severe mental defect; 18 percent survive one year	1/5000	
Partial deletion of short arm of chromosome 5	Catlike cry in infancy, microcephaly, antimongoloid slant, mental deficiency, simian crease	case reports (> 30 cases)	
Sex chromosome disorders XO	Gonadal dysgenesis, short stature, broad chest, lymphedema, webbed neck, aortic and renal anomalies; normal intelligence, defect in space-form perception. (95 percent of XO fetuses are lost as spontaneous abortions)	1/3000	yes
XXY	Hyalinized seminiferous tubules, small testes, gynecomastia, eunuchoid appearance, infertility. Mental retardation and psychopathology more common	1/450 males	
XYY	Variable phenotype with increased height, gonadal anomalies, increased risk of psychopathology	1/800 males	yes

* For additional chromosomal syndromes, consult Smith.[81]

births and are usually detectable at birth; thus they are congenital. However, except for unusual instances due to chromosomal translocations or mosaicism in a parent, these disorders are not "inherited"; other family members are not usually affected.

The four chromosomal disorders of greatest interest to neuropsychiatry are mongolism, trisomy 21; Turner's syndrome or gonadal dysgenesis, 45XO; Klinefelter's syndrome, 47XXY; and 47XYY (see below).

Sex of the fetus can be determined, of course, from the full karyotype. However, it is also possible to stain fetal cells directly to detect a Barr body,[7] which is a condensed inactive X chromosome, or a highly fluorescent Y chromosome,[14] the "flashing Y" sign of male cells. The Barr body is found in normal XX female cells and in various sex chromosome aberrations having at least two X chromosomes, such as XXY males or XXX females. Determination of sex is useful for detection both of these sex chromosome disorders and of males at risk for such X-linked recessive conditions as hemophilia and Duchenne-type muscular dystrophy. Technical artifacts of the two types of staining procedures can lead to errors, with obvious serious consequences in the genetic counseling. A full karyotype of cultured amniotic cells is therefore considered essential. The most important reason is that maternal cells may contaminate the amniotic fluid sample and give spurious results of a normal female. Fortunately, since adult cells have a shorter lifespan in culture than do fetal cells, the cells which grow out after two to three weeks in tissue culture appear to be exclusively of fetal origin.

Biochemical Studies

Inborn errors of metabolism may be recognized by abnormal accumulation of metabolites or by deficiency of specific enzyme activity. Amniocentesis late in pregnancy has been performed for many years to monitor bilirubin levels as a sign of hemolysis in Rh-incompatible pregnancies in sensitized mothers. Elevated concentrations of pregnanetriol and 17-ketosteroids can be detected at term in amniotic fluid of fetuses affected with adrenogenital syndrome,[43] but not at earlier times when abortion of affected fetuses might be desired. At least two conditions have been diagnosed on the basis of deficiency of enzymes normally detectable in the cell-free fluid; these are alpha-1, 4-glucosidase for Pompe's type of glycogen storage disease[58,77] and N-acetylhexosaminidase A for Tay-Sachs disease.[78] In both cases, the diagnosis was confirmed with uncultured and cultured amniotic fluid cells. Tests of the uncultured fluid are hazardous, because most enzymes are intracellular and not present normally in cell-free fluid, because the cell population of amniotic fluid may be highly variable, and because maternal contamination may give a falsely normal assay.

The rule of thumb applied to enzymatic analysis of amniotic fluid cells is the following: If the enzymes can be detected in cultured fibroblasts from skin biopsies, then the enzyme should be present in cultured amniotic fluid cells. This generalization is the basis for an extensive tabulation[44] of rare, inherited metabolic disorders for which prenatal diagnosis has not yet been demonstrated, but for which prenatal diagnosis is feasible. On the other hand, it is known that some enzymes first appear only at certain stages of development and that many others have different levels of quantitative activity at different times in fetal and postnatal life. Furthermore, the activity of certain enzymes may vary with the stage of the cell cycle in cultures in vitro.[76] Thus, it is essential for each enzyme that rigorous controls be established with normal amniotic cells in identical culture conditions. Inasmuch as each of the inborn errors of metabolism is rare (often occurring at a frequency of one case per 40,000 births), no laboratory should be expected to assay for each enzyme deficiency. In fact, major genetic centers are actively collaborating in providing amniotic fluid samples of various ages as controls and in carrying out different, specific assays.

CONSENT FOR AMNIOCENTESIS

Because amniocentesis is still considered an investigative procedure, current knowledge about the procedure and the tests required for prenatal diagnosis should be discussed as fully as possible with the parents. They should be asked to read and sign a consent form[24,41] containing the following major points:

1. There is an unknown, but low, risk to mother and fetus.

2. More than one amniocentesis may be required to obtain sufficient fluid.

3. Cell cultures may fail to grow.

4. Chromosomal or biochemical analyses may be unsuccessful.

5. In vitro results rarely may not reflect the status of the fetus, especially if a twin pregnancy is sampled.

6. Normal chromosomal or biochemical results on the tests that are performed do not eliminate the possibility of birth defects or mental retardation from other causes or both. Any condition not ruled out by a specific test can be expected to occur with a frequency similar to that in the general population.

❨ Types of Behavioral Syndromes Suitable for Prenatal Diagnosis

By far the greatest progress in prenatal diagnosis has come in the area of those chromosomal and metabolic disorders that grossly disrupt the normal processes of neurological and mental development in the central nervous system. The reason is simple: The "phenotype" of mental retardation has been sorted on clinical and laboratory grounds into numerous specific etiologic mechanisms, for which specific diagnostic tests can be applied.

Chromosomal Disorders Causing Mental Retardation

The most important single disorder suitable for prenatal diagnosis is Down's syndrome (mongolism).[17,65] One of every 660 births is a child with Down's syndrome, recognizable at birth by the clinical features of hypotonia, slanted palpebral fissures, flat facial profile, speckling of the iris, simian crease in the palms, and congenital heart defects. The risk of mongolism increases strikingly with age of the mother, from about 1/2000 at age twenty, to 1/1000 at age thirty, 1/500 at age thirty-five, 1/100 at age forty, and 1/40 at age forty-five. More than 95 percent of cases are due to trisomy 21, meaning that 47 chromosomes are present, with the No. 21 set occurring in triplicate rather than as a pair. The mechanism of trisomy 21 is nondisjunction, that is, the pair of No. 21 chromosomes in the mother's egg failed to separate normally. The added single No. 21 chromosome from the father's sperm produces a fertilized egg with three No. 21 chromosomes. Penrose[64] calculated that one-half of all the babies with mongolism are born to mothers over thirty-five years old. The number of children born with Down's syndrome can be decreased simply by social practices that reduce the average age of mothers or that discourage women from having children after age thirty-five. Alternatively, it is feasible, for those couples who accept selective abortion, to prevent the birth of such children by monitoring the pregnancies of older women for trisomy 21. The age for monitoring pregnancies is now arbitrarily set at age thirty-eight to forty, but is expected to fall to age thirty-five as genetics centers develop the capacity to handle more cases and if evaluation of the potential hazards of amniocentesis indicates that the risks of the procedure are sufficiently small.

There are other circumstances in which amniocentesis should be carried out for Down's syndrome. If the family has already had one child with Down's syndrome due to trisomy 21 and the parents appear normal, the recurrence risk is estimated to be about 1 percent. The level of risk combined with the emotional, social, and financial impact of one child already affected with Down's syndrome usually leads the parents and physicians to seek prenatal diagnosis of subsequent pregnancies. About 2 to 5 percent of children with Down's syndrome have a karyotype with a "translocation pattern," 46 chromosomes that include a structurally abnormal chromosome. The "extra" No. 21 (G group) chromosome is attached to one of the "normal" G or D group chromosomes, making the equivalent of a triplicate of the No. 21 chromosome. The likelihood of the translocation pattern is relatively greater with younger mothers, so chromosome studies are particularly important in children with young mothers. When a translocation pattern is found in the child, it is imperative to study the chromosomes of the parents. About half of the translocation cases occur *de novo* (in the formation of the egg or sperm) and have a recurrence risk similar to that for trisomy 21. The other half of translocation cases have a parent who is a healthy, balanced translocation carrier, having only 45 chromosomes, including the translocated G/D or G/G chromosome. Empirical studies have shown that the recurrence risk is 15 to 20 percent if the carrier parent is the mother and only 5 percent if the father is the carrier. One very rare form of translocation carrier (21/21) gives rise only to triplicated 21 or monosomic 21 (lethal) fertilized eggs, producing a 100 percent risk of recurrence in live-born children. These abnormalities can be recognized reliably in the karyotypes of cultured amniotic cells. If either parent is a translocation carrier, the aunts and uncles and other relatives should have chromosomal studies, since a significant proportion of relatives will also be translocation carriers with similar risk of transmitting Down's syndrome to their children.

The mean IQ for older patients with Down's syndrome is 24, with an upper limit of about 50.[81] Many children and most adults require institutionalization; in most states, Down's syndrome accounts for half of all the patients in institutions for the mentally retarded. The annual cost to society for custodial care is so high that extensive prenatal diagnostic screening and abortion for trisomy 21 can be justified on a cost-benefit basis alone.

Other autosomal chromosomal disorders (Table 27–1) occur much less frequently or are lethal early in life and will not be discussed further here. With new and fairly simple techniques that demonstrate specific banding patterns of human chromosomes,[18] the list of neuropsychiatric disorders associated with less severe chromosomal alterations may be extended in the near future to include milder abnormalities than gross mental retardation.

A variety of seemingly harmless chromosomal translocations is found among "normal" individuals. Sometimes the abnormality is found first in a mentally retarded child, and then the same abnormality is identified in cells of his unaffected siblings or parents. Several such variants of uncertain significance have been discovered while testing amniotic fluid specimens for trisomy 21 or for inborn errors of metabolism. Even when there is time to test the parents and find a similar variant, it is often impossible to be sure that the fetal chromosomal findings are harmless. Moreover, one cannot offer the parents the assurance that subsequent pregnancies could be monitored with any greater certainty. Another complication arises from mosaicism, the occurrence of more than one type of cell line. For example, a pregnancy at risk for Tay-Sachs disease was monitored, and normal enzyme levels were found; however, because of the mother's advanced age, chromosomes were analyzed as well. Cultured amniotic cells were 45 XO, but studies of the aborted fetus later showed only a normal 46 XY karyotype.[38] Presumably the fetus had the XY/XO karyotype. Also, the possibility that twins are present and only one is sampled must be noted. In the early series of cases reported by Nadler and Gerbie,[57] two instances of twin pregnancies were not recognized, but no untoward consequences resulted.

Inborn Errors of Metabolism

At least ten autosomal recessive and three X-linked recessive enzyme deficiencies have been demonstrated in amniotic fluid cell specimens, permitting abortion of affected fetuses (Table 27–2). Many but not all of these disorders are associated with mental retardation. As noted above, enzyme assays are feasible for many other conditions.[44] For several of these disorders with a recurrence risk of 25 percent, pregnancies at risk (previous child affected) have been monitored, and parents were correctly informed, on the basis of normal enzyme assays, that the fetus would be unaffected. (One cannot guarantee that the child

TABLE 27–2.   **Inborn Errors of Metabolism Already Diagnosed *in utero***

DISORDER	PHENOTYPE	DEFICIENT ENZYME	REFERENCE
Lipid Metabolism			
Gm$_2$ Gangliosidosis (Tay-Sachs)	Onset age five months, apathy, psychomotor deterioration, cherry red spot in macula, blindness	Hexosaminidase A	78
Metachromatic Leukodystrophy	Ataxia, hypotonia, paralysis; "schizophrenic" onset in adult form	Arylsulfatase A (Cerebroside-sulfatase)	57
Gaucher's disease	Hepatosplenomegaly, bone involvement, anemia, low platelets, retardation	Glucocerebrosidase	24
Niemann-Pick disease	Hepatosplenomegaly, cherry red spot in macula, retardation	Sphingomyelinase	24
Globoid Leuko-dystrophy (Krabbe)	Absence of myelin, presence of "globoid bodies," severe retardation	Galactocerebrosidase	24
Fabry's disease*	Distinctive rash, renal impairment, corneal opacities, peripheral neuralgias; not mentally retarded	Ceramide Trihexosidase	10
Carbohydrate Metabolism			
Galactosemia	Hepatosplenomegaly, cataracts; severe retardation prevented by excluding galactose (milk) from diet	Galactose-1-phosphate uridyl transferase	53
Pompe's disease	Hepatomegaly, cardiomegaly, failure to thrive, glycogen storage type II	a-1,4-glucosidase	58
Miscellaneous			
Lesch-Nyhan* syndrome	Hyperuricemia, choreoathetosis, self-destructive behavior, retardation	Hypoxanthine-guanine phosphoribosyl transferase	16
Lysosomal acid phosphatase deficiency	Vomiting, hypotonia, opisthotonus, infantile death	Acid phosphatase	56
Methylmalonic acidemia	Ketoacidosis, developmental retardation	Propionyl CoA Carboxylase Methylmalonyl CoA mutase	48
Hurler's syndrome Hunter's* syndrome	Mucopolysaccharidoses: hepatosplenomegaly, gargoylish skull and faces, retardation	"Correcting factors": a-L-iduronidase; Sulfa-iduronate sulfatase	26

* X-linked; all others autosomal recessive.

will be "normal" because of all the other un-
tested disorders that may occur.) Each of
these conditions is rare, so monitoring of
pregnancies is ordinarily restricted to families
in which a case has already been diagnosed.
Without the option of prenatal diagnosis, most
families faced with a 25 percent risk of a serious genetic disorder have elected in the past
to forgo further pregnancies.[12] Prenatal diagnosis and abortion make it possible for such
parents to have a normal child without fear of
recurrence of that disease.

Certain autosomal recessive conditions,
however, are not rare, especially when one
considers particular ethnic or racial groups.
Three examples are cystic fibrosis, which occurs in 1/2000 Caucasians; Tay-Sachs disease,
which occurs in 1/5000 Ashkenazi Jews; and
sickle-cell anemia, which occurs in 1/400
blacks in the United States. There is no reliable test on cultured cells for cystic fibrosis, so
prenatal diagnosis is not yet feasible. Tay-
Sachs disease causes severe mental and neurological disintegration and death by the age of
four years and is due to deficiency of the enzyme N-acetyl-hexosaminidase A, which is
demonstrable in amniotic cells in culture. This
enzyme can be measured accurately in human
serum samples, allowing detection of the heterozygous carriers. As a result, extensive
screening of the Jewish population in the Bal-
timore-Washington area is currently under
way. The high frequency of the gene in this
population has been confirmed, and young
couples in which both spouses are carriers
have been identified and have been offered
the option of prenatal monitoring for Tay-
Sachs during pregnancy. Heterozygote detection for many other autosomal recessive storage disorders is now feasible.[9] Finally,
extensive screening is in progress in many cities for carriers of the sickle hemoglobin trait.
The carriers are healthy, but if two carriers
marry, their children have a 25 percent risk of
sickle-cell anemia. In this case, carrier detection is technically very reliable, but no method
is available to obtain fetal blood cells for prenatal diagnosis. Since production of sickle
hemoglobin can be detected in eighty-day
fetuses,[35,63] direct visualization of the fetus

(amnioscopy) and sampling of even 10 μl. of
blood would allow diagnosis *in utero*.

One rare X-linked recessive disorder that
merits special discussion is the Lesch-Nyhan
syndrome, consisting of hyperuricemia, choreoathetosis, and a compulsive self-mutilating
behavior.[39] These boys bite their lips and fin-
gertips until the structures are destroyed. The
metabolic defect is a deficiency of the enzyme
hypoxanthine-guanine phosphoribosyl transferase (HGPRT), leading to overproduction
of uric acid and very high concentrations of
uric acid in blood and urine. This enzyme lies
in what was previously thought to be a minor
pathway of purine metabolism, but the devastating effects of its deficiency reveal the pathway to be physiologically important. The
highest activity of the enzyme in normal individuals is found in the basal ganglia of the
brain, providing an excellent correlation with
the major neurologic abnormality of this syndrome—the involuntary movements. But the
basis for the compulsive behavior is beyond
understanding at present. There is no very
effective therapy, even though the uric acid
production can be controlled to prevent damage to the kidney from uric acid stones. For
families in which this disorder has occurred,
the risk of recurrence is 50 percent for boys;
there is essentially no risk for girls, although
half of the girls will be carriers. Specific enzymatic assay allows detection of affected
male fetuses *in utero*.[16] In the common
X-linked disorders hemophilia and Du-
chenne's muscular dystrophy, specific tests to
distinguish affected from unaffected male fetuses are not yet available. These conditions
can be prevented by abortion of all male fetuses, when the mother is a carrier for the
disease. Such mothers could have unaffected
daughters, though half of these girls will also
be gene carriers for the disease.

Psychopathic
and Sociopathic Personality

There is no doubt that familial and social
milieu contribute importantly to personality
disorders and criminality. Nevertheless, in
similar environments remarkable individual

variation is found in personality and in the likelihood of getting into trouble with the law. Studies of twins indicate that even for indices of personality and temperament, genetic factors can be inferred,[79] though the genetic component seems much smaller than for IQ measures. Among men imprisoned for criminal behavior, cytogenetic screening has identified individuals with sex chromosomal abnormalities at frequencies much higher than in the general population.[13,36] Considerable controversy about the medical and legal interpretation of such findings has been generated with the XYY syndrome, even though little attention has been paid to the more frequently found XXY or Klinefelter syndrome.

The Klinefelter syndrome consists of testicular atrophy and infertility, occasional gynecomastia, tall eunuchoid appearance, and variable behavior, ranging from altogether normal men through individuals with mild to moderate mental deficiency or psychopathic and criminal problems. Screening for the XXY karyotype can be carried out simply with smears of the buccal mucosa and staining for the Barr body. For example, among 942 mentally abnormal inmates with a tendency to criminal behavior, 12 (1.3 percent) were found to have the XXY karyotype and 7 (0.7 percent) had the XXYY karyotype, compared with 0.2 percent and 0.02 percent, respectively, in the general population.[36] It has been suggested that the psychopathology is secondary to mental deficiency or hypogonadism, rather than an independent result of the chromosomal abnormality. XXYY males are more likely than XXY individuals to have mental deficiency, as are persons with even greater sex chromosome imbalance, such as XXXY. Rather than sampling a prison or psychiatrically abnormal population, Nielsen evaluated hypogonadal male patients of 46 XY (N=16) and 47 XXY (N=34) karyotypes at a sterility clinic in Denmark. The XXY patients had significantly more psychiatric symptoms and were particularly differentiated from the XY patients by signs of immaturity, insecurity, boastful and self-assertive behavior, and a record of legal offenses.[60,84] Differences in testis size, gynecomastia, and IQ were not related to the indices of psychopathology. With testosterone therapy, secondary sexual development like a normal male can be stimulated. However, the hyalinization of the tests cannot be reversed, and fertility is not possible. The overall frequency of XXY births is one in 450 males, with slightly increased risk with advancing maternal age. It is likely that a family in which amniocentesis is done and an XXY karyotype is found would opt for an abortion, given the likelihood of mild mental retardation and the approximately fivefold increased risk of psychopathology. Whether the frequency of this disorder or its medical and psychiatric findings warrant population screening by amniocentesis is an unresolved question that raises many social and ethical problems (see below).

The story of the XYY syndrome is one of the most curious in behavior genetics. XYY karyotypes were first reported in association with a variety of gonadal abnormalities. In 1965, an excessive incidence of XYY males was described after screening very tall men in maximum-security prisons in Scotland.[36] Presumably because males are considered more aggressive than females and because an extra Y seemed to be an intuitively reasonable basis for greater height and greater aggressiveness, stories from Australia and France about accused murderers having XYY karyotypes made front-page news in the United States.[46] A mass murderer of eight Chicago nurses was publicized, wrongly, as a (possible) XYY. Behavior geneticists have taken increased interest in the XYY syndrome for another reason. A psychosocial evaluation with family data on nine XYY and eighteen XY prisoners at the maximum-security prison at Carstairs in Scotland indicated that XYY criminals could be distinguished from XY counterparts by a lack of broken families, a lack of criminal records among their siblings, a tendency to get into trouble with the law earlier in their teens with crimes against property rather than people, and a greater lack of concern about their criminal behavior.[66,67] In other words, such individuals seemed to represent chromosomal accidents that made them "black sheep" of otherwise upstanding families. The analogy to mental retardation syndromes was obvious: a severely mentally retarded child in a family of normal parents and siblings is often the result of a particular chromosome or metabolic abnormality, while a mild or moderately retarded child in a family with parents and siblings of similar IQ reflects the interplay of multiple genetic and environmental influences.[64,73] Unfortunately, subsequent studies[6,31,46,59] have failed to confirm this striking differentiation between XYY and XY criminals. Furthermore, population screening by the laborious preparation of full chromosomal karyotypes demonstrated that 1/800 male births is XYY, many times the frequency of tall criminals in Western society. At present it appears that the XYY karyotype is associated with a severalfold increased risk of psychopathology and criminality. No parent populations are known to have an increased risk of producing XYY children. While screening women of age forty or older for Down's syndrome, Nadler[55] encountered one case of the XYY syndrome as well as three cases of Down's syndrome, among 104 pregnancies. Should the family desperately want a baby or disapprove of abortion, the knowledge that the child is born with an XYY karyotype may interfere with normal attitudes toward childrearing. It is obvious that moral, ethical, and legal problems arise from such situations, especially when knowledge of the natural history of the chromosomal syndrome is incomplete or biased. Screening of all pregnancies for XYY fetuses appears inappropriate at the present state of knowledge, but the fortuitous finding of an XYY fetus seems a reasonable indication for abortion.

Disorders of Sexual Differentiation of Behavioral Interest

Genetic and chromosomal disorders affecting every stage of differentiation and function of the gonads and the sex hormone-responsive tissues have been described. Several excellent reviews are available.[25,72] Federman, for example, has divided the syndromes into three categories: ambiguity of genital development without infertility; infertility without ambiguity; and both ambiguity and infertility.[25] Patients range from true hermaphrodites (containing functioning ovarian and testicular tissue) to those with gonadal dysgenesis (having no functioning germ tissue). Evidence in rats, guinea pigs, monkeys, and man demonstrates that sex hormones have important influences in the development of attitudes and many specific behaviors in addition to those directly involved in reproductive behavior.[30] Money and his colleagues have investigated in detail a variety of chromosomal disorders and inborn errors affecting sexual development, as well as other behavioral patterns for which no biological basis is yet known (homosexuals; transsexuals). The most intriguing findings are those from studies of patients with gonadal dysgenesis (Turner's syndrome).[3,4] These girls have short stature and lack functioning ovarian tissue, hence lack menstruation or breast development. Nevertheless, they have essentially normal intelligence and normal female gender identity. IQ testing revealed that scores for verbal performance regularly exceeded those for nonverbal subtests, but the difference lay in the tests of space-form perception, in which at least 80 percent of these girls are remarkably deficient. Similarly, the draw-a-person or figure-copying tests elicit bizarre and poorly formed outlines. It is not at all clear how a chromosomal abnormality present in all cells could so strikingly affect one particular cognitive function. There is some analogy[4] to the constellation of signs known as Gerstmann's syndrome (right-left disorientation, dyscalculia, finger agnosia, and dysgraphia) that can occur with tumors or strokes affecting the left (dominant) parietal region of the brain. The 45 XO karyotype can, of course, be recognized in amniotic cells; however, nearly half of the cases of gonadal dysgenesis are mosaics, leading to problems in diagnosis. Furthermore, the proportion of mosaic lines may be quite different in vitro than in vivo and may be variable between tissues, making a decision about the prognosis very difficult. A couple's decision about abortion of a 45 XO fetus will be influenced by their attitudes about abortion and their willingness to accept a "less than perfect" child.

Another interesting category of disorders is congenital adrenal hyperplasia, due to enzyme deficiencies at one of the several steps in the biosynthesis of cortisol and stimulation of the adrenal by pituitary ACTH to make more cortisol precursors. The resulting high levels of androgens cause the external genitalia of a female fetus to become masculinized, leading to mistaken identification of the baby as a boy. When the metabolic abnormality is recognized, sex is reassigned to female. Fifteen girls with the adrenogenital syndrome treated early with cortisone, compared with a control group matched for age, sex, IQ, and father's occupational level, had a much higher incidence of interest in masculine-associated clothing and toy preference and very little interest in infant care and feminine-associated clothing and toys.[20] They considered themselves and were considered by others to be tomboys. It was postulated that the tomboyish traits are a product of androgenization of the hypothalamus or related areas of the brain *in utero*. There was considerable individual variation, suggesting an interplay of social conditioning and fetal androgenic effects. Surprisingly, IQ testing of 70 patients with adrenogenital syndrome[47] gave a mean IQ of 110 ± 19, with 60 percent of the patients above IQ 110, instead of the expected 25 percent of a control population. Better control data, using unaffected sibs as controls, are needed to evaluate the significance of these findings. Because the enzymes responsible for steroid biosynthesis are not normally expressed in fibroblasts or amniotic fluid cells, direct assay in early pregnancy for these enzymes is not feasible. The accumulation of steroid precursors can be demonstrated late in pregnancy,[43] but not in time to intervene with abortion. In these disorders, treatment is quite effective and reasonably simple, so many families would be willing to accept the birth of an affected child, especially if diagnostic and therapeutic measures were instituted promptly. Other families, in our experience, have decided against further pregnancies, because they would not consign 25 percent of their children to lifelong treatment with cortisone.

Other evidence that androgens during pregnancy can affect the psychologic development of girls comes from cases in which synthetic progestational agents have been administered to pregnant mothers to prevent threatened miscarriages.[21] (Note that a high percentage —at least 25—of such threatened miscarriages reflect chromosomal aberrations and represent nature's way of avoiding some defective babies.) Of ten girls with progestin-induced hermaphroditism studied at ages three to fourteen years, six had IQ scores above 130, with a mean of 125 ± 12 and no significant difference between verbal and performance IQ, and nine of the ten were considered tomboys.[21]

Yet another instructive syndrome, determined by abnormality at a single gene locus, is testicular feminization.[72] These genetic males have a 46 XY karyotype, two intraabdominal testes, and produce testosterone, but their target tissues are "insensitive" to the action of testosterone. Phenotypically, these males appear at birth and through puberty to be females, then seek medical attention in their teens for amenorrhea or infertility. The external genitalia are those of a normal female. The vagina ends blindly. Breast size varies as in normal women. Psychologically, a series of ten such patients showed unmistakably feminine behavior and outlook with regard to marriage and maternalism.[46] For four married patients, interviews of the husbands confirmed these conclusions. The treatment of choice is to inform the "woman" that she is infertile, that the "gonads" in the inguinal hernia should be removed because they are not functioning normally and may become malignant, and that any difficulty with intercourse may be improved by plastic surgery procedures. It is unwise to advise such a person that "she" is cytogenetically a male, since physiologically, psychologically, socially, and legally she is a female. If the syndrome is recognized in a family, it is possible for a couple to avoid having affected children. Since the trait is inherited as an X-linked or sex-limited disorder, amniocentesis and determination of fetal sex would permit the parents to abort male fetuses, which have a 50 percent risk of being affected.

The indications and results of monitoring pregnancies, based upon published experiences, are summarized in Table 27–3.

(Psychiatric Disorders Not Now Feasible for Prenatal Diagnosis

Depression (Affective Disorders)

There is considerable evidence from twin and family studies that depression and especially manic-depressive psychosis is conditioned by genetic factors.[28,87] Among the relatives of a patient with manic-depressive psychosis, approximately 10 percent of parents, 10 percent of children, and 12 percent of sibs will have affective disorders.[75] When more knowledge is gained about the biochemistry of depression, it may be possible to assay specific enzymes or use pharmacologic challenges[62] in in vitro systems to identify healthy individuals or even fetuses at higher-than-normal risk of developing depression later in life.

Schizophrenia

Statisical analyses of family and twin data and comparisons of the incidence of schizophrenia in biological and adoptive relatives of probands who were adopted early in life suggest a major role for genetic factors in schizo-

phrenia,[22,34,74,75] though the exact mechanism or mechanisms of inheritance are unknown. No specific metabolic abnormalities have been discovered as the basis or bases of such a predisposition in the vast majority of cases. Genetic counseling for relatives of a schizophrenic patient, therefore, rests on empirical risk figures.[75]

One sure sign of heterogeneity is the mimicking of schizophrenia by specific inborn errors of metabolism, such as the adult form of metachromatic leukodystrophy.[5] The onset of metachromatic leukodystrophy has been recognized in at least nineteen patients over twenty-one years; their mental and emotional changes were so severe that they were institutionalized, usually with a diagnosis of schizophrenic illness. Only years later did neurological deterioration become manifest and lead to the pathological demonstration of sulfatide storage in the brain. Probably these patients have a less severe deficiency of the same enzyme that is deficient in the infantile presentation of metachromatic leukodystrophy, cerebroside sulfatase.

It would not be surprising if many other enzymes whose complete deficiency grossly disrupts the development of the central nervous system function were found to be causes of late-onset dysfunction manifested as psychoses, either as a result of a different mutation causing less severe deficiency or as the half-deficient heterozygous carrier of the gene causing infantile onset. Very few studies have been made of the parents (obligate carriers) or siblings (two-thirds are carriers) of chil-

TABLE 27–3.   **Summary of Data on 387 Monitored Pregnancies**[24,55]

INDICATION FOR AMNIOCENTESIS	NUMBER OF CASES	NUMBER AFFECTED
For Down's syndrome		
Maternal age $\geq$ 38 years	138	5
Previous Trisomy 21	91	2
Translocation carrier	42	11
Other chromsomal abnormalities	29	5
Sex determination for X-linked disorders	35	18 (males)
Autosomal recessive metabolic disorders	52	11
	387	52

dren affected with autosomal recessive inborn errors of metabolism. A disease like phenylketonuria, in which the abnormality lies in a liver enzyme with only secondary toxic effects on the brain from accumulated metabolites, would not be a good choice for such studies. Instead, a disorder in which the affected enzyme normally has high activity in the brain should be selected for study. Such a disorder is homocystinuria, in which there is a deficiency of cystathionine synthetase.[52] Cystathionine is normally present in remarkably high concentrations in brain, though its function is unknown. It is one of many amino acids now considered possible neurotransmitters. Individuals affected with homocystinuria have skeletal abnormalities, ectopic lens, marked tendency to venous and arterial thromboses, and about half are retarded. Why only half are retarded is not at all clear. Those who are considered of normal intelligence might have had higher IQs if not for the homocystinuria. Among the unaffected relatives in certain families, a seeming excess of schizophrenia has been noted,[11,19] but no systematic studies have been carried out with carriers of the homocystinuria gene. Homocysteine and methionine are involved in methylation reactions in the brain, offering another possible connection to schizophrenia, if methylated neurotransmitter metabolites are involved in the pathogenesis of schizophrenia.[82] Cystathionine synthetase deficiency can be demonstrated in amniotic fluid cells, and recent studies[29] of stimulated peripheral lymphocytes indicate that detection of heterozygotes may become feasible. Even for this rare recessive condition (disease frequency about 1/40,000) the frequency of heterozygous gene carriers is 1 percent in the general population.

Another rare autosomal recessive condition that can be present with schizophrenic-like symptoms in the early stages is progressive myoclonic epilepsy, or the Unverricht-Lundborg syndrome.[80] Centrencephalic epilepsy with petit- and grand-mal seizures is accompanied by deposition of amyloidlike Lafora bodies in the brain, retina, nerves, muscle, heart, liver, and fibroblasts. With elucidation of the biochemical abnormality, this condition should become diagnosable *in utero*.

Autosomal Dominant Disorders

Unfortunately, the biochemical basis for dominantly inherited disorders is still unknown. Often, the manifestations of the disease are not present at birth, and their appearance may be delayed even for decades into middle life. Also, it is characteristic of dominant conditions that the clinical manifestations vary considerably from patient to patient. The more severe the disorder, the less likely that the affected person will reproduce; thus, the more severe the disorder, the higher the probability that individual cases are due to fresh mutations (often associated with advanced paternal age), rather than transmitted from parents. Autosomal dominant disorders that may cause mental retardation include neurofibromatosis, tuberous sclerosis, and myotonic dystrophy.[64] Genetic counseling depends on making the diagnosis, then informing an affected parent that his children have a 50 percent risk of getting the abnormal gene and a variable risk (about 10 percent) of being retarded as a result of the genetic disease. Prenatal diagnosis for these conditions must wait for the development of specific biochemical tests or for the discovery of linkage of the gene for the disease to another marker gene, whose product can be detected *in utero*.

Two dominant disorders can present with depressive psychoses, indicating genetic heterogeneity for affective disorders. The porphyrias are metabolic disorders of hepatic heme biosynthesis, vertically transmitted through families as autosomal dominant traits. Episodes of colicky abdominal pain with constipation (due to autonomic neuropathy) occur together with variable central nervous system involvement, including flaccid paralysis, agitated and paranoid depression, or schizophrenic behavior.[42] In the Swedish type, or intermittent acute porphyria, biochemical diagnosis during the acute attack is highly reliable. However, the increased urinary excretion of porphyrin precursors may not be present before puberty or between attacks. Increased production of delta-amino-levulinic acid (ALA) and porphobilinogen is caused by higher than normal activity of the rate-limiting enzyme, ALA-synthetase, in the liver. The mechanism of the increased activity is not yet clear.[37,83] Several common drugs induce higher activity of the ALA-synthetase and may precipitate attacks in predisposed individuals. These drugs include barbiturates, certain sulfonamides, and the antifungal agent griseofulvin. Hepatic cells are required to demonstrate ALA-synthetase activity; either liver biopsy or some as yet unknown means of "turning on" the gene for ALA-synthetase in amniotic cells would be needed to attempt prenatal diagnosis.

Huntington's chorea is a degenerative neurologic and psychiatric disorder that is one of the major problems in counseling in medical genetics. Over a period of ten to twenty years, the affected person undergoes progressive deterioration of personality and of mental function, eventually requiring institutional care because of psychotic behavior or dementia or both. Irresponsible social behavior may lead to psychiatric evaluation and diagnosis of affective or schizophrenic processes before the neurologic signs become manifest or before the importance of the family history is appreciated. The age of onset of involuntary movements is usually in the thirties or forties, but may be delayed even longer. Thus, individuals at risk (50 percent if a parent is affected) have the dual misery of not knowing whether they will be transmitting the disease to their children and of worrying that any "normal" twitches or behavioral problems may be the early signs of the disease. The pathophysiology of the disease is unknown, and no specific diagnostic test is yet available. Since L-Dopa administration to patients with Parkinsonism may induce involuntary, choreiform movements, it has been speculated that carriers of the gene for Huntington's chorea might manifest such movements at a lower dose of L-Dopa than do normal people or Parkinson patients.[15] However, individuals at risk for this untreatable disease certainly will differ in their desire to know or to not know whether they will become affected later.

Possible Diagnosis by Genetic Linkage for Dominant Disorders

The gene for Huntington's chorea might be closely linked to some other gene whose product is easily tested, like a blood group. It is now feasible in suitable pedigrees to use linkage to the secretor locus to make an early, even a prenatal, diagnosis of myotonic dystrophy, another autosomal dominant disorder of late age of onset.[32] Although myotonia and other complications of this disease may not appear until middle life, it has been possible to identify gene carriers before age twenty by slit-lamp demonstration of a particular type of cataract. Thus, two- and three-generation data suitable for linkage analysis could be obtained. The locus that controls secretion of blood group substances into saliva and other body fluids, including the amniotic fluid,[32] happens to be closely linked on one of the chromosomes to the gene for myotonic dystrophy. Although linkage is sometimes mentioned as a powerful indirect diagnostic approach, even for this seemingly ideal example of close linkage (recombination only 8 percent), very few pedigrees are suitable. The carrier of the gene for myotonic dystrophy must also be heterozygous for secretor status (probability 0.5) and the spouse must be homozygous negative for secretor function (probability 0.25); in addition, the "phase" of the myotonic dystrophy and secretor genes on the two homologous chromosomes must be inferred from study of other relatives. Even then, incorrect conclusions will result 8 percent of the time due to crossing-over (recombination) between the two linked loci.

Computer-assisted programs to seek evidence for linkage of a postulated dominant gene for schizophrenia to some genetic marker have been proposed.[22] Because of the likely heterogeneity of mechanisms underlying so complex a phenotype as schizophrenia, individual large kindreds should be used for such studies.

Anticipated Technical Developments

As enzymatic assays are adapted to micromethods, the delay between the time of amniocentesis and the report of results should be shortened, relieving some of the tension of the wait and making abortion, if necessary, safer. As biochemical mechanisms of more diseases are elucidated, the list of conditions for which prenatal diagnosis will be feasible should continue to grow. Detailed evaluation of the potential hazards of amniocentesis will make more exact the patients' and physicians' balancing of benefit and risk in undertaking amniocentesis for disorders of low frequency. Hopefully, better methods of terminating pregnancies in mid-gestation may be developed.

For the common psychiatric phenotypes, it is expected because of heterogeneity that the mass of cases will be attacked only gradually, as in the case of mental retardation syndromes. Promising approaches include the application of new staining methods for abnormal chromosomal banding patterns, the evaluation of heterozygous carriers of genes that cause mental retardation in the homozygous state, the possibility of demonstrating linkage to easily tested genetic markers, and the development of *in vitro* methods for pharmacogenetic differentiation of cellular responses. Many biochemical functions or responses that are characteristic of the nervous system may not be expressed in amniotic fluid cells. Progress must then depend upon "turning on" the unexpressed genes in the amniotic cells[27] and upon harmless methods for biopsy of superficial tissues or organs of the fetus. Certain neurological conditions may be associated with congenital anomalies visible through a fiberoptic amnioscope. Other sensitive instruments may be able to detect fetal physiological and neurophysiological parameters. Monitoring of pregnancies will become more widespread and applicable to more diseases. Population screening for heterozygous carriers

will be initiated, requiring computerized data evaluation and regional or national networks for counseling family members.

([Special Issues Involving the Psychiatrist in Genetic Counseling

Stresses of Monitoring a Pregnancy

With the popularization of amniocentesis and prenatal diagnosis in magazines, many families have initiated contact with their physicians or counseling centers with the unfortunate expectation that tests can assure them of a normal baby or that many specific conditions can be tested, for which no tests are available. Sometimes a couple has tried for years to have a child or has waited many years after an affected child for the possibility of such prenatal monitoring. The many weeks of waiting before amniocentesis can be performed and before test results are available can be exceedingly stressful, especially when the hazards of a late abortion loom as a distinct possibility and the couple realizes that mistakes can be made in the testing procedures.[40] Occasionally a couple will seek amniocentesis in the hope that something will be found to be wrong with the baby, so that they can justify to themselves terminating the pregnancy. For example, Epstein et al.[24] described a couple who previously had a child with translocation Down's syndrome; when karyotypes of the amniotic cells indicated a 46 XY fetus, they requested an abortion anyway, for reasons of mental health. Husband and wife may have basic disagreement about abortion or child-rearing, of course, and in most states they still must contend with archaic laws restricting abortion. In states like California, Oregon, New York, Hawaii, and Washington, where liberalized abortion statutes are in effect, the genetic counselor and the family can deal more directly with the medical and psychological problems of the individual family. It is highly desirable that counseling be provided before the woman is pregnant. Sometimes extensive arrangements for specific enzymatic assays must be made or complicated testing of the woman for possible carrier status with regard to an X-linked disorder must be carried out. In any case, the stress is bound to be less if the couple can consider the genetic information and plan the pregnancy.

Severity of Disease and the Indications for Abortion

If the risk of recurrence is high and the disorder severe, such as the autosomal recessive conditions listed in Table 27–2, most couples will desire amniocentesis, unless they seek no more children. But when the risks are low, as in the cases of advanced maternal age and previous trisomy 21, the couple must decide whether to take the high probability (about 99 percent) that the fetus will not have trisomy 21 or whether to take the unknown risks associated with the procedure. Couples differ in their responses to this predicament. Therefore, it is important that detailed genetic counseling be offered before the obstetrician performs the amniocentesis. In one series,[24] twenty-seven of eighty-three couples decided against amniocentesis after receiving counseling. Many were reassured by the low recurrence risks; in three cases the condition could not be detected by available tests; one woman had no desire to have her pregnancy terminated whatever the outcome; and in another there was not time to do all the necessary tests because of the advanced stage of pregnancy. With the behavioral disorders of adult onset, the definition of "genetic disease" and of tolerable severity is complicated.[50] The available information from population, family, twin and adoption studies suggests that genetic factors predispose to affective disorders or schizophrenia, but do not indicate the probability of such a predisposed person developing severe disease. Similarly, in the cases of sex chromosomal abnormalities, for which prenatal detection is already feasible, most men with XYY karyotype are not psychopathic criminals and most individuals with XYY or XXY or XO karyotypes do not suffer serious mental impairment. Is the infertility associated with XXY or XO karyotypes a basis for the parents to insist upon abortion? Or the possibility of behavioral problems associated with XXY? The problem is vexing, because firm data on the absolute risks of such behavioral problems are not available and there is no basis for predicting which offspring will be affected later in life.[49] The physician is then faced with the dilemma of giving or withholding information that the parents cannot evaluate either. By analogy, the discovery of Huntington's chorea in a patient brings a pall over the family, because there is no treatment for the disease and no advantage of early diagnosis except the prevention of further offspring and the establishment of a diagnosis that saves the family fruitless medical inquiry. On the other hand, vigorous investigation of the family with polyposis of the colon is considered essential, since prophylactic removal of the affected colon will prevent fatal colonic carcinoma.[49] Although genetic counselors seek to provide detailed information and meaningful advice, the responsibility for deciding the course of action rests with the individual couple. It is our impression that families fear behavioral disorders even more than somatic anomalies and that the majority of families would request abortion of a XYY or XXY or XO fetus if informed of the results of the chromosomal tests.

Abortion nowadays is discussed as a simple and innocuous matter. Psychologically, of course, it is not: each couple must be evaluated and assisted. Surgically, abortion for conditions diagnosed in mid-pregnancy requires special techniques and carries substantially higher risks of maternal mortality or morbidity than does abortion before eight weeks of gestation. At present, abortion between twelve and twenty weeks is being done primarily by saline infusion or by hysterotomy, though newer agents, such as prostaglandins, may prove helpful. If the couple lives in a state that does not allow legal abortion for such indications, they face the ignominy of "fleeing" to another, more liberal state for the abortion, seeking a physician who will twist or violate the law, or taking no action. If no abortion can be obtained, amniocentesis can be justified only in exceptional circumstances. For instance, after the birth of one child with Down's syndrome an occasional couple who would not allow abortion may still seek amniocentesis for reassurance that the fetus is unaffected.

An alternative to selective abortion of affected fetuses is detection and counseling of unmarried teenagers and young adults who are heterozygous carriers for such diseases as Tay-Sachs and sickle-cell anemia. These young people could avoid the birth of affected children by avoiding marriage with carriers for the same disease. Most authorities agree that a massive educational effort would be required to affect mating patterns. It is not known whether the knowledge that one is a carrier for such a disease would influence a person to avoid marrying someone who is also a carrier, and it is not known how such an educational effort should be mobilized to properly inform, and yet not frighten, these healthy carriers. Several screening and educational programs have been started for sickle-cell anemia, since intrauterine diagnosis is not feasible for this disease. When feasible, the identification of couples who are both carriers and who wish to avoid the birth of affected children by selective abortion seems more practical. However, affected children would continue to be born of out-of-wedlock matings in such a program.

With abortion on demand in certain states and with increasing family planning, some families have sought to use the technology of intrauterine chromosome karyotyping to learn the sex of the fetus and assure themselves the birth of either a boy or girl. Obviously, the "risk" of the "wrong" sex is 50 percent, but a couple must have an overwhelming desire to select the sex of the child in order to accept the unknown risks of amniocentesis and a late abortion. A request for amniocentesis and chromosome karyotyping of cultured amniotic fluid cells for sex may be dismissed as a frivolous attitude or may be considered a cold-blooded approach to an "ideal" family of one son and one daughter, according to the attitudes of those involved. To many physicians in genetic counseling, the prevention of dev-astating disease provides moral justification for abortions, while the selection of the sex of one's children raises moral, social, and political issues far beyond the medical clinic.[68]

Society's Position with Regard to Genetic Diseases

With the decrease in deaths from acute infections and the recognition of so many specific inherited conditions, the medical profession and lay people are becoming increasingly aware of the nature and variety of genetic diseases that require hospitalization, cause deaths, and influence the lives of people in contact with those affected. Until recently, society has disapproved of abortion as a means of preventing unwanted children. Now most people approve of abortion to prevent the birth of defective children, if not simply "abortion on demand." Will amniocentesis be required for women above a certain age, just as testing for phenylketonuria is required by law in most states? How will society look upon the couple who refuse abortion and deliver a child with severe mental retardation who is dependent upon the society for his existence? Many of these questions transcend the realm of medicine.

One may ask, also, what effect intrauterine diagnosis and selective abortion will have on the frequency of inherited diseases. The impact of several types of public-health programs has been projected by Motulsky et al.[51] The total number of cases will be reduced slightly if intrauterine diagnosis is initiated only after the birth of an affected child, as for the rare autosomal recessive conditions listed in Table 27-2. Maximal case reduction requires detection of high-risk mothers or high-risk matings before marriage, as is feasible for Tay-Sachs and other lipid storage disorders and for sickle-cell heterozygous carriers. There is a slight "dysgenic" effect of selective abortion, in that an individual who would not have survived to pass on the deleterious gene is likely to be replaced in the sibship by another child with a substantial risk (two-thirds for autosomal recessive traits) of being a carrier. However, since changes in gene frequencies are significant only over many generations, medical and social efforts should be directed to the intrauterine diagnosis and prevention of affected cases, especially of the common genetic diseases.

(Concluding Remarks

Intrauterine diagnosis is possible for chromosomal disorders and many rare inborn errors of metabolism. Most common birth defects and genetic diseases, however, cannot yet be diagnosed *in utero*. Diagnosable disorders of particular interest to psychiatrists and the directions of anticipated future developments are stressed. Since intrauterine therapy of genetic disorders is not feasible in most cases, abortion of affected fetuses is usually practiced. Psychiatric and social problems surrounding abortion for genetic and chromosomal diseases affecting behavior merit further attention.

(Bibliography

1. ABDULLA, U., S. CAMPBELL, C. J. DEWHURST et al. "Effect of Diagnostic Ultrasound on Maternal and Fetal Chromosomes," *Lancet*, 2 (1971), 829–831.

2. ABRAMOVICH, D. R. "The Volume of Amniotic Fluid in Early Pregnancy," *J. Obstet. Gynaecol. Br. Commonw.*, 75 (1968), 728–731.

3. ALEXANDER, D., A. A. EHRHARDT, and J. MONEY. "Defective Figure Drawing, Geometric and Human, in Turner's Syndrome," *J. Nerv. Ment. Dis.*, 142 (1966), 161–167.

4. ALEXANDER, D. and J. MONEY. "Turner's Syndrome and Gerstmann's Syndrome: Neuropsychologic Comparisons," *Neuropsychologia*, 4 (1966), 265–273.

5. AUSTIN, J., D. ARMSTRONG, S. FOUCH et al. "Metachromatic Leukodystrophy (MLD) VIII. MLD in Adults; Diagnosis and Pathogenesis," *Arch. Neurol.*, 18 (1968), 225–241.

6. BAKER, D., M. A. TELFER, C. E. RICHARDSON et al. "Chromosome Errors in Men with Antisocial Behavior. Comparison of Selected Men with Klinefelter's Syndrome and XYY Chromosome Pattern," *JAMA*, 214 (1970), 869–878.

7. BARR, M., L. BERTRAM, and E. G. BERTRAM. "A Morphological Distinction between Neurones of the Male and Female, and the Behavior of the Nucleolar Satellite During Accelerated Nucleoprotein Synthesis," *Nature*, 163 (1949), 676–677.

8. BERGSMA, D. and A. G. MOTULSKY, eds. "Symposium on Intrauterine Diagnosis," *Birth Defects*, 7 (1971), 1–36.

9. BRADY, R. O., W. G. JOHNSON, and B. W. UHLENDORF. "Identification of Heterozygous Carriers of Lipid Storage Diseases," *Am. J. Med.*, 51 (1971), 423–431.

10. BRADY, R. O., B. W. UHLENDORF, and C. B. JACOBSON. "Fabry's Disease: Antenatal Detection," *Science*, 172 (1971), 174–175.

11. CARSON, N. A. J., D. C. CUSWORTH, C. E. DENT et al. "Homocystinuria: A New Inborn Error of Metabolism Associated with Mental Deficiency," *Arch. Dis. Child.*, 38 (1963), 425–436.

12. CARTER, C. O., J. A. F. ROBERTS, K. A. EVANS et al. "Genetic Clinic: A Followup," *Lancet*, 1 (1971), 281–285.

13. CASEY, M. D., L. J. SEGALL, D. R. K. STREET et al. "Sex Chromosome Abnormalities in Two State Hospitals for Patients Requiring Special Security," *Nature*, 209 (1966), 641–642.

14. CASPERSSON, T., G. LOMAKHA, and L. ZECH. "The 24 Fluorescence Patterns of the Human Metaphase Chromosomes, Distinguishing Characteristics and Variability," *Hereditas*, 67 (1971), 89–102.

15. CLAWANS, H. C., G. W. PAULSEN, and A. BARBEAU. "A Predictive Test for Huntington's Chorea," *Lancet*, 2 (1970), 1185–1186.

16. DEMARS, R., G. SARTO, J. S. FELIX et al. "Lesch-Nyhan Mutation: Prenatal Detection with Amniotic Fluid Cells," *Science*, 164 (1969), 1303–1305.

17. DOWN, J. L. H. "Observations on an Ethnic Classification of Idiots," *Clin. Lect. Rep., London Hosp.*, 3 (1866), 259.

18. DRETS, M. E. and M. W. SHAW. "Specific Binding Patterns of Human Chromosomes," *Proc. Natl. Acad. Sci. USA*, 68 (1971), 2073–2077.

19. DUNN, H. G., T. L. PERRY, and C. L. DOLMAN. "Homocystinuria: A Recently Dis-

covered Cause of Mental Defect and Cere-
brovascular Thrombosis," *Neurology*, 16
(1966), 407–416.

20. EHRHARDT, A. A., R. EPSTEIN, and J. MONEY.
"Fetal Androgens and Female Gender
Identity in the Early-treated Adrenogenital Syndrome," *Johns Hopkins Med. J.*,
122 (1968), 160–167.

21. EHRHARDT, A. A. and J. MONEY. "Progestin-
induced Hermaphroditism: IQ and Psychosexual Identity in a Study of Ten Girls,"
J. Sex Res., 3 (1967), 83–100.

22. ELSTON, R. C. and M. A. CAMPBELL.
"Schizophrenia: Evidence for the Major
Gene Hypothesis," *Behav. Genet.*, 1
(1970), 3–10.

23. EMERY, A. E. H. "Antenatal Diagnosis of
Genetic Disease," *Mod. Trends Hum.
Genet.*, 1 (1970), 267–296.

24. EPSTEIN, C. J., E. L. SCHNEIDER, F. A.
CONTE et al. "Prenatal Detection of Genetic
Disorders," *Am. J. Hum. Genet.*, 24 (1972),
214–226.

25. FEDERMAN, D. D. *Abnormal Sexual Development: A Genetic and Endocrine Approach
to Differential Diagnosis.* Philadelphia:
Saunders, 1967.

26. FRATANTONI, J. C., E. F. NEUFELD, B. W.
UHLENDORF et al. "Intrauterine Diagnosis
of the Hurler and Hunter Syndromes,"
N. Engl. J. Med., 280 (1969), 686–688.

27. FRIEDMAN, T., and R. ROBLIN. "Gene Therapy for Human Genetic Disease?" *Science*,
175 (1972), 949–955.

28. GERSHON, E. S., D. L. DUNNER, and F. K.
GOODWIN. "Toward a Biology of Affective
Disorders," *Arch. Gen. Psychiatry*, 25
(1971), 1–15.

29. GOLDSTEIN, J. L., B. K. CAMPBELL, and S. M.
GARTLER. "Homocystinuria: Heterozygote
Detection Using Phytohemagglutinin-
Stimulated Lymphocytes," *J. Clin. Invest.*,
52 (1973), 218–221.

30. GOY, R. W. "Early Hormonal Influences on
the Development of Sexual and Sex-Re-
lated Behavior," in F. O. Schmitt, ed., *The
Neurosciences, 2nd Study Program*, pp.
196–206. New York: Rockefeller University Press, 1970.

31. GRIFFITHS, A. W., B. W. RICHARDS, J. ZAR-
EMBA et al. "Psychological and Sociological Investigation of XYY Prisoners," *Nature*,
227 (1970), 290–292.

32. HARPER, P., W. B. BIAS, J. R. HUTCHINSON

et al. "ABH Secretor Status of the Fetus:
A Genetic Marker Identifiable by Amniocentesis," *J. Med. Genet.*, 8 (1971), 438–
440.

33. HELLMAN, L. M., G. M. DUFFUS, I. DONALD
et al. "Safety of Diagnostic Ultrasound in
Obstetrics," *Lancet*, 1 (1970), 1133–
1135.

34. HESTON, L. L. "The Genetics of Schizophrenia and Schizoid Disease," *Science*,
167 (1970), 249–256.

35. HOLLENBERG, M. D., M. M. KABACK, and
H. H. KAZAZIAN, JR. "Adult Hemoglobin
Synthesis by Reticulocytes from the Human Fetus at Midtrimester," *Science*, 174
(1971), 698–702.

36. JACOBS, P. A., M. BRUNTON, M. M. MEL-
VILLE et al. "Aggressive Behavior, Mental
Subnormality, and the XYY Male," *Nature*,
208 (1965), 1351–1352.

37. KAPPAS, A., H. L. BRADLOW, P. N. GILLETTE
et al. "Abnormal Steroid Hormone Metabolism in the Genetic Liver Disease Acute
Intermittent Porphyria," *Ann. N.Y. Acad.
Sci.*, 179 (1971), 611–624.

38. KARDON, N. B., P. R. CHERNAY, L. Y. HSU
et al. "Pitfalls in Prenatal Diagnosis Resulting from Chromosomal Mosaicism,"
J. Pediatr., 80 (1972), 297–299.

39. KELLEY, W. N., and J. B. WYNGAARDEN.
"The Lesch-Nyhan Syndrome," in J. Stan-
bury, J. B. Wyngaarden, and D. Fredrick-
son, eds., *The Metabolic Basis of Inherited
Disease*, 3rd ed., pp. 969–991. New York:
McGraw-Hill, 1972.

40. LIEBERMAN, E. J. "Psychosocial Aspects of
Selective Abortion," in D. Bergsma and
A. G. Motulsky, eds., *Birth Defects*, 7
(1971), 20–21.

41. MACINTYRE, M. N. "Chromosomal Problems
of Intrauterine Diagnosis," in D. Bergsma
and A. G. Motulsky, eds., "Symposium on
Intrauterine Diagnosis," *Birth Defects*, 7
(1971), 10–14.

42. MARVER, H. S. and R. SCHMID. "The Porphyrias," in J. Stanbury, J. Wyngaarden,
and D. Fredrickson, eds., *The Metabolic
Basis of Inherited Disease*, 3rd ed., pp.
1087–1140. New York: McGraw-Hill,
1972.

43. MERKATZ, I. R., M. I. NEW, R. E. PETERSON
et al. "Prenatal Diagnosis of Adrenogenital
Syndrome by Amniocentesis," *J. Pediatr.*,
75 (1969), 977–982.

44. MILUNSKY, A., J. W. LITTLEFIELD, J. N. KAUFER et al. "Prenatal Genetic Diagnosis," *N. Engl. J. Med.*, 283 (1970), 1370–1381, 1441–1447, 1498–1504.

45. MONEY, J., A. A. EHRHARDT, and D. N. MASICA. "Fetal Feminization Induced by Androgen Insensitivity in the Testicular Feminizing Syndrome: Effect on Marriage and Maternalism," *Johns Hopkins Med. J.*, 123 (1968), 105–114.

46. MONEY, J., R. J. GASKIN, and H. HULL. "Impulse, Aggression and Sexuality in the XYY Syndrome," *St. John's Law Review*, 44 (1970), 220–235.

47. MONEY, J. and V. LEWIS. "IQ, Genetics, and Accelerated Growth: Adrenogenital Syndrome," *Bull. Johns Hopkins Hosp.*, 118 (1966), 365–373.

48. MORROW, G., III, R. H. SCHWARZ, J. A. HALLOCK et al. "Prenatal Detection of Methylmalonic Acidemia," *J. Pediatr.*, 77 (1970), 120–123.

49. MOTULSKY, A. G. "Genetic Therapy: A Clinical Geneticist's Response," in M. Hamilton, ed., *The New Genetics and the Future of Man*, pp. 125–132. Grand Rapids, Mich.: Eerdmans, 1972.

50. ———. "Significance of Genetic Disease," in B. Hilton, D. Callahan, M. Harris et al., eds., *Ethical Issues in Human Genetics*, pp. 59–71. New York: Plenum, 1973.

51. MOTULSKY, A. G., G. R. FRASER, and J. FELSENSTEIN. "Public Health and Long-Term Genetic Implications of Intrauterine Diagnosis and Selective Abortion," in D. Bergsma and A. G. Motulsky, eds., Symposium on Intrauterine Diagnosis, *Birth Defects*, 7 (1971), 22–32.

52. MUDD, S. H., W. EDWARDS, P. M. LOEB et al. "Homocystinuria due to Cystathionine Synthase Deficiency: The Effect of Pyridoxine," *J. Clin. Invest.*, 49 (1970), 1762–1773.

53. NADLER, H. L. "Antenatal Detection of Hereditary Disorders," *Pediatrics*, 42 (1968), 912–918.

54. ———. "Prenatal Detection of Genetic Defects," *J. Pediatr.*, 74 (1969), 132–143.

55. ———. "Indications for Amniocentesis in the Early Prenatal Detection of Genetic Disorders," in D. Bergsma and A. G. Motulsky, eds., "Symposium on Intrauterine Diagnosis," *Birth Defects*, 7 (1971), 5–9.

56. NADLER, H. L., and T. J. EGAN. "Deficiency of Lysosomal Acid Phosphatase," *N. Engl. J. Med.*, 282 (1970), 302–307.

57. NADLER, H. L. and A. GERBIE. "Role of Amniocentesis in the Intrauterine Detection of Genetic Disorders," *N. Engl. J. Med.*, 282 (1970), 596–599.

58. NADLER, H. L. and A. M. MESSINA. "In-utero Detection of Type-II Glycogenosis (Pompe's Disease)," *Lancet*, 2 (1969), 1277–1278.

59. NIELSEN, J. "Klinefelter's Syndrome and the XYY Syndrome. A Genetical, Endocrinological, and Psychiatric-Psychological Study of Thirty-three Severely Hypogonadal Male Patients and Two Patients with Karyotype 47, XXY," *Acta Psychiatr. Scand.* (Suppl.), 209 (1969), 1–353.

60. NIELSEN, J., A. SØRENSEN, A. THEILGAARD et al. "A Psychiatric-Psychological Study of 50 Severely Hypogonadal Male Patients, Including 34 with Klinefelter's Syndrome, 47, XXY," *Acta Jutl.*, 41 (1969), 1–183.

61. O'BRIEN, J. S., S. OKADA, A. CHEN et al. "Tay-Sachs Disease. Detection of Heterozygotes and Homozygotes by Serum Hexosaminidase Assay," *N. Engl. J. Med.*, 283 (1970), 15–20.

62. OMENN, G. S. and A. G. MOTULSKY. "Psycho-Pharmacogenetics," in D. G. Fried, ed., *Yearbook of Drugtherapy*, pp. 5–26. Chicago: Yearbook Medical Publ., 1973.

63. PATARYAS, H. A. and G. STAMATOYANNOPOULOS. "Hemoglobins in Human Fetuses; Evidence for Adult Hemoglobin Production after the Eleventh Gestational Week," *Blood*, 39 (1972), 688–696.

64. PENROSE, L. S. *The Biology of Mental Defect*, 3rd ed. New York: Grune & Stratton, 1963.

65. PENROSE, L. S. and G. F. SMITH. *Down's Anomaly*. Boston: Little, Brown, 1966.

66. PRICE, W. H. and P. B. WHATMORE. "Behavioral Disorders and Pattern of Crime among XYY Males Identified at a Maximum Security Hospital," *Br. Med. J.*, 1 (1967), 533–536.

67. ———. "Criminal Behavior and the XYY Male," *Nature*, 213 (1967), 815.

68. RAMSEY, P. "The Ethics of a Cottage Industry in an Age of Community and Research Medicine," *N. Engl. J. Med.*, 284 (1971), 700–706.

69. RATCLIFFE, S. G., M. M. MELVILLE, A. C. STEWART et al. "Chromosome Studies on 3500 Newborn Male Infants," *Lancet*, 1 (1970), 121–122.

70. RENWICK, J. H., S. E. BUNDEY, M. A. FERGUSON-SMITH et al. "Confirmation of Linkage of the Loci for Myotonic Dystrophy and ABH Secretion," *J. Med. Genet.*, 8 (1971), 407–416.

71. RHODES, P. "The Volume of Liquor Amnii in Early Pregnancy," *J. Obstet. Gynaecol Br. Commonw.*, 73 (1966), 23–26.

72. RIMOIN, D. and R. N. SCHIMKE. *Genetic Disorders of the Endocrine Glands*. St. Louis: Mosby, 1971.

73. ROBERTS, J. A. F. "The Genetics of Mental Deficiency," *Eugen. Rev.*, 44 (1952), 71–83.

74. ROSENTHAL, D. *Genetic Theory and Abnormal Behavior*. New York: McGraw-Hill, 1970.

75. ROSENTHAL, D. and S. S. KETY, eds. *The Transmission of Schizophrenia*. Oxford: Pergamon, 1968.

76. RUSSELL, S. B., J. D. RUSSELL, and J. W. LITTLEFIELD. "β-glucuronidase Activity in Fibroblasts Cultured from Persons with and without Cystic Fibrosis," *J. Med. Genet.*, 8 (1971), 441–443.

77. SALAFSKY, I. and H. L. NADLER. "Prenatal Diagnosis of Pompe's Disease," *N. Engl. J. Med.*, 284 (1971), 732.

78. SCHNECK, L., C. VALENTI, D. AMSTERDAM et al. "Prenatal Diagnosis of Tay-Sachs Disease," *Lancet*, 1 (1970), 582–583.

79. SHIELDS, J. *Monozygotic Twins Brought Up Apart and Brought Up Together*. London: Oxford University Press, 1962.

80. SLATER, E. and V. COWIE. *The Genetics of Mental Disorders*. London: Oxford University Press, 1971.

81. SMITH, D. W. *Recognizable Patterns of Human Malformation*. Philadelphia: Saunders, 1970.

82. SMYTHIES, J. R. "Biochemistry of Schizophrenia," *Postgrad. Med. J.*, 39 (1963), 26–33.

83. STRAND, L. J., B. F. FELSHER, A. G. RADEKER et al. "Heme Biosynthesis in Intermittent Acute Porphyria: Decreased Hepatic Conversion of Porphobilinogen to Porphyrin and Increased Delta Aminolevulinic Acid Synthetase Activity," *Proc. Natl. Acad. Sci. USA*, 67 (1970), 1315–1320.

84. THEILGAARD, A., J. NIELSEN, A. SØRENSEN et al. "A Psychological-Psychiatric Study of Patients with Klinefelter's Syndrome, 47, XXY," *Acta Jutl.*, 53 (1971), 1–148.

85. TJIO, J. H. and A. LEVAN. "The Chromosome Number of Man," *Hereditas*, 42 (1956), 1–6.

86. WAGNER, G. and F. FUCHS. "The Volume of Amniotic Fluid in the First Half of Human Pregnancy," *J. Obstet. Gynaecol. Br. Commonw.*, 69 (1962), 131–136.

87. WINOKUR, G., P. J. CLAYTON, and T. REICH. *Manic-Depressive Illness*. St. Louis: Mosby, 1969.

CHAPTER 28

HUMAN SEXUALITY: RESEARCH AND TREATMENT FRONTIERS

Richard Green

(Introduction

THE MULTIFACETED NATURE of human sexuality imparts a wide array of research and treatment frontiers. During the past decade changes have been brought about by social experimentation and social evolution, developments in laboratory hardware, and the application of sophisticated research methods to sexual behavior. Human sexuality, in attitude and action, has undergone extensive change and has dated much previous psychiatric knowledge. Change continues. This chapter will attempt to capture the dawn on the research and treatment horizon.

(Developmental Strategies

Gonadal Hormones: Prenatal Influences on Behavior

Is behavior influenced by sex steroids *in utero*? As the fetus is exposed to gonadal hor-
mones derived from its own and maternal organs and as its central nervous system undergoes rapid growth and development, it is reasonable to ask whether levels of these steroids influence later behavior. As sexually dimorphic kinds of behavior have been clearly documented in many species, inquiry has been directed toward the possible relation between prenatal levels of androgens and estrogens and those kinds of postnatal behavior.

Young male and female rhesus monkeys behave differently, with males showing more chasing, aggressive, and rough-and-tumble play. Prenatal androgen levels have been shown to influence these activities.[135] Female rhesus monkeys exposed to large amounts of testosterone *in utero* behave more like young male monkeys than do untreated young females (they become "tomboy" monkeys). *Post*-natal androgen exposure does not have a comparable effect.

A human analogy exists. Females with the adrenogenital syndrome, in which excessive prenatal adrenal androgen is produced, have also been reported to differ from typical girls, behaviorally as well as anatomically.[30,31] When compared to their nonadrenogenital-syndrome sisters, these androgen-exposed girls are less often described as interested in doll play, playing with infants, and wearing dresses, and more often described as tomboys. A third study also showed a trend (not statistically significant) for adrenogenital girls to be described as tomboys, compared with a non-sibling control group.[88]

What of human males prenatally exposed to unusually large amounts of estrogen? For about two decades diabetic pregnant women have been administered estrogen and progesterone at Boston's Joslin Clinic. Sixteen-year-old and six-year-old males who were products of these pregnancies have been compared with same-aged males of nontreated, nondiabetic mothers.[134] The male offspring of female hormone treated mothers were reported as less rough-and-tumble, aggressive, and athletic. However, one important uncontrolled factor in the study was the influence of the experimental group mothers' chronic illness on their son's behavior (rather than hormone exposure per se).

These studies suggest that just as anatomic dimorphism is influenced by androgenic hormone (androgen induces maleness; no gonadal hormone is needed for femaleness),[67] so too may dimorphic behavior be influenced. Here, rough-and-tumble, physically aggressive play may be affected. In cultures that label such behavior masculine or feminine (as does our own) this influence could significantly affect psychosexual development. Peer-group socialization may be modified with a low level of aggressivity resulting in a boy's accommodating more easily to the activities and companionship of girls. "Boys play too rough!" is the typical cry of the behaviorally feminine boy, described later. Similarly, mother–son and father–son interaction may be modified, with a low level aggressive boy relating more easily to the domestic activities of his mother and avoiding the sports activities of his father.

A significant obstacle in studying the effects of steroid hormones on the developing behavioral system is assessment of the prenatal hormonal milieu. While some preliminary techniques are available, validity and feasibility are problematic. Strategies include repeated samplings of maternal plasma and urine during gestation, plus amniocenteses. Questions that remain are the degree to which any of these indirect approaches to the fetal milieu in fact reflect the fetal milieu, identification of critical gestational periods and whether the tissues of some individuals are more or less responsive to the same level of hormone. Should valid measures become attainable, then a series of longitudinal studies is possible, assessing high and low androgen- and estrogen-exposed children, of *both* sexes, on dimensions of neonatal and subsequent sex-typed behavior.

Neonatal Sex Differences

Studies of the human neonate hold promise of isolating the early roots of "innate," male–female dimorphism. Several sex differences have been reported, some replicated, others not, and most are difficult to interpret. They group into displays of greater muscle strength, sensory differences, and the degree of affiliative behavior to adults.

Newborn males are more able to lift their head from a prone position.[9] Mothers have been observed to stretch the limbs of their three-week-old boys more readily than those of their same-aged girls, but more often to imitate sounds made by the girls.[102] Mothers have been observed to hold their five-month-old daughters more than their sons, and, at thirteen months, these same daughters are more reluctant to move away from their mothers. The same thirteen-month-old children also show a different play style with toys and react differently to a barrier placed between themselves and the toys: boys tend to hurl toys about, girls tend to gather them together; boys more often crawl to the barrier's end (in an attempt to get around it) girls more often sit where placed and cry.[47]

In an elegant research design, differential mother-attachment behavior by *opposite-*

sexed co-twins was demonstrated. Female co-twins looked at, vocalized to, and maintained proximity to their mothers more than did their brothers.[17]

Other differences during the newborn period have been reported, sometimes of an obscure nature. Neonatal females increase their formula intake when a sweetener is added; boys do not.[103] At three months, females can be conditioned to an auditory reward while boys respond to a visual one.[132] At six months, girls show cardiac deceleration (a measure of attention) while listening to modern jazz, whereas boys decelerate to an interrupted tone.[69]

While sex differences on these several parameters are reported, intrasex differences exist, as well as considerable intersex overlap. Many measures have a bell-shaped distribution. Males and females who fall at the ends of the distribution could be longitudinally studied to determine correlations between neonatal behavior and developmental attributes. Of interest would be those infants whose physiologic patterns fall within the zone typically found for the other sex. For example, will males with a female pattern of taste preference or within the female range for elevating the prone head show later childhood behavior that is culturally feminine, e.g., preferring doll play to rough-and-tumble play?

Studying neonatal activity levels and responsivity to holding (cuddliness) also offers research promise. During the first year, children differ considerably regarding physical activity and their response to holding. These "temperamental" features influence parental perception of the child, parental attitudes toward the child, and affect the degree to which the child is held (notably by the mother). Mothers of the feminine boys described later typically describe their sons as having been the cuddliest of their children and Stoller[122] theorizes that excessive maternal holding promotes feminine identity in a young male. Objective measures of these variables can be developed. For example, children could be placed in the nucleus of a series of concentric circles and their movement measured, during a standard time period, from the

starting place across these lines. Nonparent males and females ("unbiased" raters) could pick up infants (prior to the development of stranger anxiety) and the degree of clinginess or withdrawal noted.

Again, it is expected that measures of activity level and response to holding would scatter across a bell-shaped curve. Males and females at both ends of the curve could then be longitudinally followed, and correlations made between these variables and later behavior, including rough-and-tumble play, and activity and toy preferences. The degree to which these variables could be correlated with prenatal hormone levels would depend on the extent to which the latter become measurable.

Intersexed (pseudohermaphroditic) infants could provide an intriguing research model here. If one or another of the above sex differences is replicated in normal infants (e.g., taste preference), would anatomically intersexed babies (e.g., adrenogenital females, or XXY males) be behaviorally intersexed?

Anatomically Intersexed Children

Studies with pseudohermaphrodites have demonstrated the extensive influence of early experiential factors on psychosexual development and bear significant treatment implications. Consider two gonadal and chromosomal females with ambiguous (masculinized) genitalia, appearing similarly intersexed at birth (the virilizing adrenogenital syndrome). One is neonatally designated female by the attending physician; the other is designated male. Each will typically develop a sexual identity consistent with the sex assigned at birth and consequent rearing experiences.[99,100] In the latter case, the person, though possessing ovaries and the 44 + XX female-chromosomal configuration, will have a male identity. This will manifest as typical masculinity and erotic attraction toward females. Environmental influences appear to have overruled whatever innate biological influences existed.

These "experiments of nature" have told us more. Sexual identity is set early in childhood. The evidence is from cases in which subsequent sex reassignment has been attempted when an "error" in the original sex designation is discovered. For example, if the person described above, assigned to male status, had been unambiguously raised as a male, an attempt at reassignment after about the fourth birthday would typically be unsuccessful.[100,122]

Some of these data, now nearly two decades old, have been the subject of criticism. Exceptions to the early critical-period concept of sexual identity have been collated[136] and alternative interpretations of the clinical data presented.[25] These latter writers either point to a few cases in which sex reassignment was apparently effected without significant psychological hardship after life's first years, or they reinterpret the establishment of sexual identity as due to prenatal neuroendocrine input, rather than postnatal socialization.

Problems have existed in evaluating many of the case reports of the anatomically intersexed. One has been the degree to which they are representative of the intersexed population, or represent a bias in the direction of "successful" or "unsuccessful" adjustment to either initial sex assignment or later reassignment. Also missing from many case studies is a detailed documentation of early socialization experiences. The full range of parental attitudes toward the intersexed status of the infant, the message(s) transmitted by physicians to parents during the earliest years, and the peer-group experiences of the child are rarely described.

Most recently, Lev-Ran,[80] a Soviet investigator now emigrated to Israel, has reported a series of intersexed patients supporting the classic thesis of Money, the Hampsons, and Stoller. Money et al. had stressed the importance of genital appearance as a contributing factor to the socialization experience of the intersexed child. This feature, if in conflict with assigned sex, might cause some intersexed children to question their sex of assignment. The recent Lev-Ran report is unique in that cases are described in which sexual identity is consonant with sex of assignment in spite of dramatic genital incongruity. One example is an adult female with the adrenogenital syndrome, feminine and heterosexual, whose clitoris measuring 9 cm. stands as the only significant obstacle to her participation in heterosexual intercourse, and another is a masculine boy with a 1.5 cm. penis.

Management of anatomically intersexed infants remains somewhat controversial. Although there are some "chromosomal fatalists" who assert that genetic sex determines male or female identity and that the roots of biological sex will invade contrary postnatal rearing, the consensus is that sex assignment should be dictated by genital appearance and potential genital functioning. Construction of a cosmetically and physiologically acceptable penis has not been perfected; development of a cosmetically and physiologically acceptable vagina has. Thus, a chromosomal, gonadal male, born with a micro- or absent penis, or who has lost his penis at age one or two years via trauma, should be raised as a female. This will avoid the lifelong distress of being a penisless male, and will permit functioning as a sexual person with an acceptable body image. The chromosomal, gonadal female with a markedly enlarged clitoris or an atretic vagina should be raised as a female, with appropriate repair of the genitals. Decisions regarding other states, e.g., a chromosomal, gonadal male, with third-degree hypospadias and bilateral cryptorchidism, would depend on the degree to which surgical constructive repair of the genitalia is possible. Sexual identity will typically follow the sex of assignment if parents are convinced of the wisdom of that assignment and raise their child accordingly.

It is important and helpful for parents of the anatomically intersexed to know the evidence behind the assertion that postnatal socialization is the chief determinant of human sexual identity. Additionally, a helpful analogy is that of language acquisition. Humans are born with the capacity to learn a language—which one is learned depends on the early environment. Humans are also born with the capacity for psychosexual differentiation (learning a male or female identity). As with language, which one is learned depends on the early environment. (Details of patient management have been fully described by Money.)[98]

One argument against using the anatomically intersexed as a model for *normal* psychosexual differentiation is that by virtue of their anomaly the gonadal hormonal milieu bathing their prenatal central nervous system has been atypical. Therefore, they may be more behaviorally "plastic" than normal children. However, an intriguing "experiment" is under way to test this criticism. A set of male monozygotic twins is currently being raised by their parents in opposite sex roles. Circumcision accident caused the penis of one genetic male co-twin to slough, and the child has been reassigned, female, to be raised as a girl. In this case, the prenatal hormonal milieu plus genetic factors are held relatively constant, with postnatal socialization being the significant variable.[99] Additionally, our own research[54] has uncovered two sets of monozygotic twins, one male set and one female, discordant for sexual identity. One twin pair consists of ten-year-old males, one of whom is very feminine and wants to become a girl. His brother is unremarkably masculine. The second twin pair consists of a twenty-five-year-old female graduate student who desperately wants sex-change surgery and her feminine college graduate sister. Different early life socialization experiences are reported for both twin pairs.

An increased incidence of cross-sexed behavior (typically transvestism and transsexualism) in males with sex chromosome anomalies has been suggested.[2,3,101] Most typically, these are males with an extra X chromosome. However, there is difficulty in evaluating a causal relation between anomalies of sex chromosomes and sexual identity due to the possibility of sample bias. Those patients with both anomalies are more likely to be reported. Whether the concordance between the two variables is higher than would be expected by chance is unclear, since while the incidence of sex chromosome aneuploidy is known, that of transvestism and transsexualism is not.

The incidence of the XXY chromosomal anomaly is 1 in every 700 males. Thus, a large number of such infants can be detected at birth with buccal smear or karyotyping procedures. These children could then be longitudinally assessed, hormonally and behavior-

ally. Coupled with detailed analyses of parental attitudes toward varieties of childhood play and other early socialization experiences, a complex developmental study becomes possible that could weigh the several variables of psychosexual development. At least one such study is currently underway.[131] However, future court decisions may block large-scale karyotyping procedures as a violation of the subject's rights (recently a screening for XYY boys was blocked). Secondly, dissecting the influence of the microscopic, longitudinal study process from the child's "natural" sexual identity development is problematic.

Atypical Sex-Role Behavior in Anatomically Normal Children

Studies of transsexuals, persons who want to change sex, reveal that there are anatomically normal adults with an intense, irreversible, inner conviction of belonging to the other sex who trace the onset of this cross-sex identity to childhood.[11,122,53] Invariably, these persons, recalling their childhood, report having role played as persons of the other sex, having dressed as children of the other sex, having preferred opposite-sexed children as playmates, and having avoided the toys and games typical of their sex.

Studies of transvestites, males who cross-dress with accompanying sexual arousal, also demonstrate the early life onset of atypical sexuality. Approximately half of five hundred transvestites in one series[107] reported commencing cross-dressing prior to adolescence.

Studies of homosexuals, persons whose primary sexual commitments are to partners of the same sex, again point to the enduring significance of childhood gender-role behavior. One study reported that about a third of one hundred homosexual adult male patients recalled playing predominantly with girls during boyhood (compared to 10 percent of the heterosexual control group) and 83 percent displayed an aversion to competitive group games (compared to 37 percent of the heterosexuals.[14]). Another study of a nonpatient homosexual sample reported that two-thirds of eighty-nine males recalled "girl-like" behavior during childhood (compared to only 3 percent of the heterosexual controls). For female homosexuals, over two-thirds of a group of fifty-seven were tomboyish during childhood (compared to 16 percent of the heterosexuals) with half of them persisting with tomboyism into adolescence (compared to none of the heterosexuals).[114]

What emerges from these retrospective studies is the fact that atypical sex-role behavior during childhood may persist as atypical sex-role behavior during adulthood. However, retrospective studies pose significant research obstacles. Objective indices of the child's behavior are not obtained and recollections of interpersonal experiences, notably those with parental figures, are distorted by the passage of time. Objective measures of parent–parent and parent–child behavior at the time when atypical behavior is emerging are not possible.

My own research design, initiated with John Money and continued with Robert Stoller, has been to generate a sample of young children behaving in a manner similar to that reported by adults with an atypical sexual identity. We have studied sixty-five anatomically normal boys, aged four to ten, who prefer the dress, toys, activities, and companionship of girls, role play typically as females, display feminine mannerisms, and may state their wish to be girls. These boys have undergone extensive psychological testing, behavioral observation, and interviewing. Their parents have been interviewed with structured formats, alone and together, and have also undergone psychological testing.

An attempt is being made to match each feminine boy with a same-aged child who is masculine, has the same configuration of younger and older siblings, and is from a family with a similar socioeconomic, ethnic, and marital background. To date fifty-five of the feminine-boy families have been matched. Detailed, behavioral descriptions of the feminine boys and their parents, plus preliminary testing data, are reported in *Sexual Identity Conflict in Children and Adults*.[51]

The boys test similarly to girls of the same age on a variety of psychological procedures and are significantly different from most same-aged boys. When they construct fantasies, they generally utilize female family figures and an infant (as do girls, whereas boys utilize male figures and pay less attention to an infant). When they are requested to draw a person, the figure drawn is usually female (girls do the same, most boys draw a male). Alone in a playroom, they play mostly with a "Barbie" doll (as do girls, while other boys play with a truck). On the It Scale for Children (in which a neuter figure "It" selects a variety of sex-typed preferences illustrated on cards[18]), their selection of toys, playmates, and articles are the same as girls and differ from most boys. When they complete card sequences in which a child of their own sex joins a parent engaged in a sex-typed activity, they join the female parent in a feminine activity (as do girls, but not most boys). A preliminary series of possible variables associated with this atypical development has been formulated:

1. An innate low level of aggressivity.
2. Parental indifference to or encouragement of culturally feminine behavior in a boy during his first years.
3. Maternal inhibition of boyish or rough-and-tumble play during the first years.
4. Cross-dressing of a young boy by a female.
5. Extraordinary maternal attention to and physical contact with a young male resulting in a lack of psychological separation between the two.
6. Absence of an older male identity model during a boy's first years, or paternal rejection during this period.
7. Physical beauty in a boy of sufficient degree that adults treat him in a culturally feminine manner.
8. Absence of male playmates during a boy's initial years of socialization.
9. Strong maternal dominance of a family.

A preliminary synthesis of how these variables may operate in a composite child is sequentially conceptualized as follows: A mother considers her male infant unusually attractive. She finds him to be extremely cuddly. She devotes considerable attention to this boy. Her other children are adequately separated in age so they do not infringe on this child's early mothering experience. Her other commitments are few for channeling feelings of caring and love. The child, beginning to explore the environment for playthings, finds the many colorful accessories belonging to his mother and initiates play with these objects (shoes, jewelry, and cosmetics). He imitates mother, the person with whom he is in primary contact. These kinds of behavior are considered cute, and the child receives additional attention and supportive laughter. The father is a much less significant person in the boy's life, and interacts minimally with him. His possessions and accessories are less attractive as early play objects. The father, too, may view his son's early play with feminine objects as funny or cute, or else ignores it. As peer relationships begin for the boy, girls are mostly available. Boys, if available, are more aggressive than he is, frighten him, and perhaps meet with parental disapproval. The child says boys are "too rough" and prefers girls. The father having anticipated a period when the boy would be amenable to father–son, roughhouse play, instead finds his son to have minimal interest in such activity. The boy is in tune with the domestic activities of his mother, and the father, experiencing this as rejection, dubs his son a "mamma's boy." The boy, aware of his father's demands and disapproval, moves further toward the accepting reactions of his mother. During the early school years his prior socialization in feminine skills poses an additional obstacle to same-sex peer integration. Accustomed to female playmates, he does not relate easily to males. In consequence of his culturally feminine interests and greater comfort with a female peer group, he is teased by boys, driving him further from the male group. The mother continues to respond positively to his interest in cross-dressing or improvising feminine costumes. She interprets boyish and girlish behavior during this life period as having no relation to later masculinity or femininity. The boy continues to show little interest in his father's activities. Emotional distance between the father and son escalates. The boy's increasing identification with females is revealed by a feminine affectation. This increases social stigmatization and the child is labeled "sissy."

Treatment of the Atypical Child

Intervention into the behavior of very feminine boys engages both research and ethical issues. First, some research questions. What do we know about the natural course of untreated boyhood femininity? What might intervention, of various types at various ages, do?

Follow-up studies tell us something of the "natural course" of boyhood femininity. Twenty-seven adult males previously seen clinically for boyhood femininity have been reevaluated. Fifteen are currently transsexual, transvestic, or homosexual.[79,137,50] The degree of treatment intervention with most of these patients is not clear. By contrast, the adult transsexuals, transvestites, and homosexuals in the series noted earlier were rarely evaluated during childhood.

Consider next "sexual identity." While complex, for the purpose of this discussion it can be viewed as including three components: (1) earliest: a person's self-awareness of being male or female—core-morphologic identity; (2) later: manifestations of culturally defined masculine and feminine behavior; and (3) still later: partner preferences for genital sexuality.

All three components of sexual identity are atypical for transsexuals (they consider themselves female, behave like women, and are attracted to anatomically same-sexed partners). Transsexuals report that their parents felt their atypical behavior was insignificant and would pass, and so they were not treated; sexual identity remained completely atypical. Although the feminine boys seen by Money and myself initially behaved in a way similar to that reported by many transsexuals, they did undergo evaluation and are not now transsexual. For example, at five, one boy prayed nightly to be changed into a girl and was repeatedly cross-dressing. His parents brought him for evaluation at seven. Today he does not want to be a woman, does not cross-dress, but is homosexual. Why did the first two components of sexual identity (core-morphologic identity and gender-role behavior) undergo change, and the third component, genital sexuality, remain atypical?

We can speculate. Core-morphologic identity appears to be crystallized during the first three years of life. While it continues to be significantly overlaid during the ensuing three years (and, to a degree, throughout life) a considerable portion of sexual identity has been set by the time the atypical child is initially evaluated. Gender-role behavior, a later identity component, may be more modifiable during childhood. Thus, one outcome of early intervention may be that a young male who feels he is or wants to be a female may be convinced that the change is not possible. Additionally, a sufficient number of nonrough-and-tumble activities may be found, along with nonrough-and-tumble male playmates, to promote comfort in anatomic maleness. If so, sufficient behavioral change will ensue so that the tortuous search for later sex change is averted. However, attention is not specifically addressed to the third component, genital sexuality, because such behavior is not manifested during these years.

The critical factor with respect to whether behavior of an atypical boy changes may be whether the parents seek evaluation. Those parents who request evaluation are initiating a new milieu for their son, one that discourages and rejects feminine gender-role behavior. By so doing, the second component of sexual identity, and perhaps indirectly the first component, may undergo change. If such is the case, the pretranssexual male may mature into a homosexual male. The degree to which the first two components influence the third component is not clear.

The effect of same-aged, peer group relations during grade school years is coming under more study. While it apparently has great import, the relationship between early peer group interaction and later genital sexuality is enigmatic. One possibility is that the feminine boy's lack of positive affective responses from males during earlier years (peer group and father) results in "male affect starvation," which is compensated for in adulthood in male–male romantic relationships. Another possibility is that the young male with a female peer group is socialized in that group to the point of evolving similar, later romantic interests (attachments to males). The manner in which preadolescent, *homosocial* peer group relationships typically evolve into adolescent and adult *heterosexual* relationships and *heterosocial* peer group relationships into *homosexual* ones is an intriguing, little understood facet of psychosexual development. Obviously, this active period, the "latency years," deserves closer scrutiny.

Ethics of Treatment

Should clinicians attempt to modify the behavior of the child whose sexual identity is dramatically atypical? The very feminine male child experiences considerable social conflict in consequence of his behavior. He is teased, ostracized, and bullied. The masculine girl is not stigmatized. Parents who bring their very feminine boy for professional consultation are concerned about his behavior and want something done. Parents do not bring their masculine girls for consultation unless the behavior is dramatically atypical. What, then, is the professional's responsibility toward the parents of the very feminine boy and their child?

It can be argued that the conflict experienced by the feminine boy is derived mainly from the culture in which he lives, a culture that dictates, for irrational reasons, that boys and girls behave in specified dimorphic ways. Many parents are attempting to raise their children in a less traditionally stereotyped manner, giving boys and girls a wider range of behavioral options. However, to a major degree this ethic has yet to engage the general population and great differences still exist for boys and girls in dress, toy, and game preferences. Other children continue to label feminine boys "sissy." Unless the entire society undergoes dramatic change during the next few years, the psychic distress and alienation experienced by the very feminine boy will augment during his teens. While the clinician may prefer that the whole society immediately change, there is more basis for optimism in helping a single individual to change.

But what kind of change? Treatment need not forge the feminine boy into an unduly aggressive, insensitive male. However, treatment can impart greater balance to a child's interests and behavior where previously skewed patterns have precluded comfortable social integration. For example, consider the exclusively female peer group of the feminine boy. Opponents of intervention argue that there is nothing wrong with a boy playing with girls. Advocates of limited intervention argue that there is nothing wrong with playing with boys. They observe that the very feminine boy is eliminated from interaction with one-half of the potential peer group (as is the traditionally masculine boy, but without consequent teasing). Intervention may help the feminine boy find unstigmatized boys, who prefer "sex-role-neutral" activities so as to widen his range of social interactions.

Do therapists reinforce societal sexism by treating the feminine boy? To a degree, yes. What are the alternatives? An attempt could be made to modify the attitudes of the peer group, so that teasing stops and the feminine boy is effectively integrated into the group. However, to rapidly change the pediatric society is clearly a formidible task. On the other hand, helping the boy cope with teasing can constitute part of the intervention program.

Clearly, the issue is not simple. The standard of many clinicians is to be nonjudgmental, with goals to be dictated by the patient. If (1) parents want their child to be happier, (2) the child is in serious conflict, and (3) the likelihood of reducing that conflict is greatest by some behavioral change, is it ethical to refuse intervention? More extended discussion of this dilemma is found in Green.[51]

Children of the Sexually Atypical

HOMOSEXUAL PARENTS

Contemporary social experiments may provide new information on psychosexual de-velopment. These involve children whose parents live an atypical sexual life style.

While the majority of divorcing mothers seek and find a new husband (and the majority of fathers seek and find a new wife) some enter into homosexual relationships. "Lesbian mothers" have received increasing attention in the press and in courts of law. Some female homosexual mothers are being challenged for child custody by former husbands with the contention that lesbianism signifies an unfit mothering status. At least one homosexual male father has been judged as not providing a suitable environment for overnight visits by his children.

What is the effect on children of being raised by one or two homosexual adults? Issues engaged include the significance for psychosexual development of having both sex-role models for parents during childhood and teens, the availability of both sex-role models in families in which parents of only one sex are represented, the effect on a child of recognizing that a parent is homosexual, the effect on a child of peer group reactions to a child's atypical household, and the influence of the attitude of the other (nonhomosexual) biological parent.

Role models of the other sex are not excluded from the lives of children who live in homosexual-parent households. Children are repeatedly exposed to heterosexual adults of both sexes in the persons of relatives, parents of the peer group, and at school. Additionally, the conventional nuclear-family model of mother, father, and children depicted on television, in books, and in moving pictures repeatedly bombards a child.

The effect on a child's later sexual preferences of knowing that at least one parent is homosexual is not fully determined. This will depend, in part, on the extent to which partner preference is a result of role modeling. Role modeling cannot account for the entire process of psychosexual development however, in that the vast majority of homosexuals were raised by heterosexual parents.

The view held by the homosexual parent, or couple, of persons of the other sex may be significant. The image painted of these absentee figures can be influential in shaping later affectional elements.

Yet another issue is a possible biological predisposition to homosexuality, perhaps inherited, such as atypical gonadal hormone levels. Should such a basis be firmly demonstrated (see below) it is questionable whether raising a child so predisposed in either a homosexual or a heterosexual household would significantly affect future sexuality.

TRANSSEXUAL PARENTS

Boys and girls may be raised by a parent (in either the mother or father role) who has undergone sex-change surgery. In some families, females married to men who were formerly women have become pregnant via donor insemination, and the couple then raises the child. In other instances, transsexual couples are raising a child who is a product of the wife's former marriage. And, in a recent court case, a chromosomal female who had previously borne a child and was currently living as a man, was granted authority to raise the child in the role of father.

These "social experiments" permit the testing of various assumptions regarding parental role modeling and identification. The long-term evaluation of such children is a study in which several standard components of the typical child-raising experience are altered.

The Homosexual's Parents

The parents of homosexuals have typically been "studied" by indirect means. Adults have been asked to recall traits of mother and father during the respondent's childhood. These methods are compromised by the inaccuracy of recalled experiences with conscious or unconscious distortions diluting their validity. A major study utilizing this approach was that of Bieber and his psychoanalytic colleagues[14] who were treating 100 homosexual males. Their conclusion was that the close-binding, intimate mother and the passive, distant, hostile, perhaps absent father contributed to the homosexual partner preference.

Several efforts at replicating the Bieber find-

ing have been attempted. Evans[33] confirmed this pattern using a nonclinical sample, but Greenblatt[56] found that the fathers of male homosexuals were described as generous, pleasant, and dominant and the mothers as neither overprotective nor dominant. A third study[119] with a large number of subjects, 307 male homosexuals and 138 male heterosexuals, utilized several psychometric instruments to retrospectively assess parental characteristics. For the entire subject sample the finding that homosexuals more often recall their fathers as rejecting and distant was confirmed. However, mothers were not more often described as protective, demanding, close, or dominant. Furthermore, reports of relative father-versus-mother dominance did not discriminate the two groups. Of considerable significance is the finding that when only those homosexuals and heterosexuals scoring low on neuroticism measures are compared, the differences in parental backgrounds between the groups *disappears*. Thus, it may be that the tendency for individuals, especially homosexuals in therapy, to report more rejecting fathers may be related more to the reporter's level of neuroticism than to sexual orientation per se.

Homosexuality and Gonadal Hormones

Following an era in which a hormonal basis of atypical sexual behavior in the human fell into disrepute, a revival of interest now exists. The introduction of exquisitely sensitive hormonal assays has opened a new era of investigation. Where previous studies utilizing gross, nonspecific measures failed to show differences between homosexuals and heterosexuals, several recent studies have found differences.

In 1970, the ratio of two stereoisomeric urinary metabolites of testosterone, androsterone, and etiocholanolone were found to discriminate twenty adult male heterosexuals from twenty male homosexuals.[89] However, three severely depressed heterosexuals and one diabetic heterosexual also had ratios like that of the homosexuals. During the same year Loraine and co-workers[84] reported four homosexual females with higher urinary androgen and lower estrogen levels than four heterosexual females, and two homosexual males with lower androgen levels than controls. Then, in 1971, Kolodny and co-workers[72] reported that thirty male homosexuals had significantly lower plasma testosterone levels than fifty male heterosexuals.

Questions of specificity abound. Rigorous attention has not been paid to possibly confounding variables, especially stress, drug intake, and recency of sexual activity. Heterosexual males under military stress also have testosterone levels lowered to the same degree as those reported for homosexuals.[113,74] Homosexuals, because of their stigmatized life style, may be under greater stress than heterosexuals. In the Kolodny et al. study, data on marijuana ingestion are given for the homosexual subjects, but not for the heterosexuals. This drug appears to reduce plasma testosterone (also Kolodny et al.).[73] Beyond this, three subsequent studies have failed to find differences in testosterone levels,[6,105,125] and a fourth found homosexuals to have higher levels.[16] Data are not given in the last study for sexual activity prior to plasma sampling. Sexual activity can influence plasma testosterone.[38,106] Finally, another study, while not noting a testosterone difference, did find an elevation of estradiol in homosexual males.[26] The only finding so far to survive replication is the androsterone-etiocholanolone study, which has been repeated by the original investigator[90] and also by an independent researcher.[34] The relevancy of this finding remains obscure.

Two investigations have indirectly looked at the hypothalamic-pituitary axis of males with a same-sexed partner preference to see whether it follows a female-type gonadotropin release pattern. Two male–female differences have been studied. The first is the well documented tonic release pattern in the male and the cyclic pattern in the female. The second is the less extensively studied gonadotropin feedback response resulting from an intravenous estrogen load (decrease followed by rebound above baseline in the female, decrease followed by return to normal in the male).

Male-to-female transsexuals (who have a male partner preference) were studied to determine whether their gonadotropin release pattern was tonic (male) or cyclic (female). It was tonic.[46] Male homosexuals and heterosexuals were given intravenous estrogen. The homosexuals' gonadotropin response showed a reduction, followed by a rise above baseline (female pattern). The heterosexuals' response showed no positive rebound after the initial reduction (male pattern—Dorner et al).[27] This provocative finding has yet to be replicated.

Bisexuality

Bisexuality (also called ambisexuality) is a term with many usages. It may imply an isolated or occasional sexual experience with one sex and most relations with the other sex. It has been used to imply innate sexual features of all persons or a "latent" impulse seething to find outlet. Usage here is narrowly restricted to those persons who would rate "3" on the 7-point Kinsey scale,[70,71] with 0 designating exclusive heterosexuality and 6 exclusive homosexuality. Individuals who are equally disposed in fantasy and overt behavior to males and females are not common.

True bisexuality raises a number of theoretical and research questions. Explaining homosexuality as an anxiety or phobic reaction to one genital configuration (typically the male reacting to the "castrated" female) meets with difficulty in understanding the individual capable of sexual satisfaction with both males and females. If future research documents that specific developmental routes, be they social or biological, promote either an exclusive male or female sexual partner preference, would bisexuals fall in the middle range on these attributes? Finally, will the changes in early childhood socialization that less clearly demarcate children's sex roles promote more bisexuality during adult years?

The bisexual population has been largely ignored until recently (Blumstein and Schwartz.[15]) It offers considerable promise in understanding the full potential of human sexual response in males and females.

(Clinical Management Strategies: Adulthood

Treatment of Sexual Dysfunction

A new era in sexual health has been opened by the pioneering research and treatment of Masters and Johnson.[92,93] "Sexual dysfunction" has been introduced into the medical vocabulary. This term is shorthand for a variety of sexual difficulties, most commonly erectile failure and premature ejaculation in the male and painful intercourse or nonorgasmia in the female. The great success of the Masters and Johnson treatment program has resulted in a rash of centers conducting "Masters and Johnson" therapy. Conspicuously absent from these economically successful enterprises, however, has been sophisticated evaluation of their efficacy.

Treating sexual dysfunction is more complex than training a male for greater ejaculatory control or a female for orgastic response. The complexity is underscored by Fordney-Settlage[36,37] who characterizes factors behind the problems of the individual or sexual couple. Problems may engage: (1) deficient sexual information; (2) restrictive sexual attitudes; (3) deficient or negative sexual experience; (4) inadequate sexual communication; (5) regressive sexual communication or behavior; (6) deficient or damaged individual self-concept; (7) individual intrapsychic factors; (8) nonsexual interpersonal distress; and (9) destructive reaction patterns. It is unlikely that any simple, inflexible intervention can address itself to this multiplicity of problems.

Research designs are needed in which groups begin therapy on an equal basis, all input to the patient(s) during the treatment period, except for the specific intervention modality are held constant, objective indices are given for pre- and postintervention behavior, and finally, long-term follow-up results are reported. Nontreatment control groups are also needed (waiting list) to accommodate the high degree of motivation brought by these patients to the treatment situation.

Which components of these programs are associated with symptom reversal in the several styles of sexual dysfunction must be ascertained.

Evaluating outcome as "successful" or "unsuccessful" is not simple. A couple may find the dysfunctional symptom removed but additional interpersonal problems to be of such magnitude that they separate or divorce. Or, symptom reversal may manifest itself only in sexual interactions with other partners. Treatment-outcome measures need to consider several dimensions, not merely presence or absence of specific symptoms. Whether a couple graduates from a dysfunction program "*magna cum* loudly" may not be the most important variable.

In the absence of specific dysfunctions, but "merely" general *sexual malaise*, valid behavioral criteria are needed. A step in this direction is the inventory developed by LoPiccolo and Steger.[83] This self-report cites seventeen kinds of sexual behavior, and for each kind both partners rate the activity as it applies to their relationship. Indices are obtained of satisfaction with the frequency and range of the couple's sexual behavior, as well as knowledge of the partner's sexual preferences. The inventory has been shown, in a preliminary study, to have good reliability, to be capable of separating sexually dysfunctional and functional couples, and to record changes associated with treatment.

Quality control and licensing of "sex clinics" is necessary to avoid exploitation and insure that responsible, effective intervention is being provided. Additionally, treatment programs are typically expensive and may not be covered by health insurance, thus rendering them unresponsive to the health needs of many people. Perhaps inexpensive, self-help materials can be developed on audio- and video-tape cassettes, providing effective home education and treatment.

The use of erotic materials and surrogate partners are controversial elements in some sexual dysfunction programs. Does viewing explicit sexual materials benefit an individual's sexual competence? Preliminary data were published in 1970 by the Commission on Obscenity and Pornography.[111] Questionnaires were given to patrons of "adult" film theaters. Based on responses of the one third who returned the forms (questionably representative, but real people nevertheless) 54 percent experienced sex as "more enjoyable since viewing sex films" and only 1 percent reported a negative effect. Seventy-nine percent reported that the films motivated them to introduce new variety into their sexual behavior, variety within the range of typical sexuality. While many people treat themselves with erotica, from adolescence through later years, learning and role rehearsing various sorts of sexual behavior and generally enriching their erotic fantasy,[41] this sexual-health view of erotica is not shared by law-enforcement officials who typically see erotica as sowing the seeds of moral decay. Surrogate sexual partners are discussed below in a section on the treatment of homosexuality but that discussion has parallel applicability here.

Two additional subjects merit note: pheromones and biofeedback. Pheromones are odoriferous substances that act as chemical messengers between individuals. The possibility exists that sex pheromones may operate in the human primate.[126] Unquestionably, they operate in the nonhuman primate. In the rhesus monkey, a vaginally secreted short-chain aliphatic acid dramatically activates male sexual interest.[95,96] Should such a human pheromone be isolated, it may be harnessed by enterprising therapists in the treatment of sexual dysfunction. A biofeedback design is briefly mentioned in the following section.

Male–Female Differences in Patterns of Erotic Arousal

The Kinsey et al.[70,71] data suggested that males and females respond differently to potentially erotic stimuli. Females were described as not responding to visual sexual materials while males clearly did. Now, two decades later, other studies have revealed no sex difference in responsiveness to visual materials, with both males and females reporting sexual arousal.[116] Another previously reported sex difference concerned the degree of

romantic content in the materials: females were reported to be more responsive to romantic narrative imagery and males to stories with an emphasis on "impersonal, mechanical" sex.[70,71] Again, more recent research has found no sex difference.[117] These studies have relied on verbally reported sexual arousal as experienced by genital sensation and coital activity before and after exposure to erotica. No physiologic measures of arousal were obtained.

In an effort to explain the differences in response patterns noted by the Institute for Sex Research in the U.S. in the 1940s (Kinsey) and the Institute for Sex Research in West Germany in the 1970s (Schmidt, Sigusch), Gebhard[42] has suggested that the wording of the Kinsey interview may have yielded an artifactual sex difference. To elicit a positive reply re erotica in the earlier studies, a strong genital response was necessary, or else the respondent was likely to reply negatively to the particular stimulus modality. Gebhard also reasons that females respond more gradually to erotic stimuli so that questions such as, "Do you become aroused if shown a photograph of coital activity?" would elicit a negative reply from women.

Until recently, research on the responsivity of females to potentially erotic stimuli relied on verbal reports. While male responsivity had been measured via penile plethysmography, in which penile volume change is recorded by a strain-gauge mercury loop,[5] no reliable device had been developed to provide an objective measure of female response. In 1970, Cohen and Shapiro[19] described a device for measuring changes in vaginal blood flow via two thermistors that recorded temperature changes, and in 1971 Jovanovic[68] noted a device designed to measure vaginal contractions via an intravaginal balloon, with another designed to record clitoral erections via a thermistor.

In 1974, Sintchak and Geer[120] described an easily inserted, intravaginal photoplethysmograph that measured vaginal blood volume and vaginal pressure pulse. These measures have been demonstrated to change in response to viewing erotic materials or listening to erotic recordings, but not to change in response to nonerotic stimuli.[44] Thus, the possibility exists of more sophisticated studies of the effects of various types of stimuli on both males and females. Also open to study are attempts to correlate arousal patterns with personality features and prior sexual experiences.[61]

Penile and vaginal plethysmography may find applicability in the treatment of sexual dysfunction. Objective indices of arousal to specific stimuli can be recorded and feedback provided to the subject. Biofeedback designs in which subjects are rewarded for increments in sexual arousal may enable a subject to enhance sexual responsivity—of obvious value in the treatment of male impotence and female nonorgasmia.

Nonpatient Homosexuals

Clinicians have largely ignored the questionable validity of generalizing from a psychiatric patient sample of homosexuals to the entire homosexual population. Early researchers to focus on this fallacy were Hooker[65] and Marmor.[91]

The homosexual life style has been traditionally viewed within a psychodevelopmental framework as *sine qua non* of mental disorder, or *prima facie* evidence of unresolved oedipal conflict, residual castration fear, and psychologic immaturity. Forearmed with this rationale, the life dilemmas bringing forth the homosexual patient have been construed as supportive of this mental-illness position. An alternative interpretation is that those homosexuals consulting psychiatrists have difficulties represented by only a minority of the homosexual population, that the difficulties experienced (maintaining stable object relations, anxiety, depression) are also found in the heterosexual-patient population, and that those homosexuals in conflict, or desirous of heterosexual reorientation, are responding to societal discrimination.

The 1970s brought a radical rethinking of the homosexuality-equals-mental-illness dictum. Forces operant were the increasingly strident voices of homosexual activists, criticism and questioning by psychiatrists (e.g., Marmor,[91] Hoffman,[64] Green[50]) and an increasing body of data from studies of nonpatient homosexuals challenging the illness theory.

Two important large-scale studies conducted of nonpatient homosexuals were those of Siegelman[118] and Saghir and Robins.[114] Three hundred and seven homosexual and 137 heterosexual males were studied by Siegelman, utilizing several psychometric tests. On the Scheir-Cattell Scale, homosexuals scored higher on tender-mindedness, submissiveness, anxiety, and neuroticism, and lower on depression. The two groups did not differ on measures of alienation, trust, self-acceptance, sense of self, and dependency, or for neuroticism on the McGuire Neuroticism Scale. Homosexuals were also found to be more "goal directed." When homosexuals and heterosexuals scoring low on femininity were compared, the difference in anxiety level disappeared.

Male and female homosexuals (about 150) and unmarried heterosexual contrast groups were compared in the comprehensive study by Saghir and Robins.[114] Twenty-six percent of the male homosexuals and 6 percent of the heterosexuals had had psychotherapy, usually of a brief nature. Treatment was typically for depression, with either the breakup of a relationship or guilt feelings instigating therapy. Only 9 percent of the homosexuals who sought psychiatric help did so to change to heterosexuality. There was no history of definable psychiatric disorder in 34 percent of the homosexuals and 40 percent of the heterosexuals. There were no significant differences with respect to any of the major psychiatric disorders, including affective states, drug abuse, alcoholism, and anxiety. At the time of study, 72 percent of each group was free of psychiatric disorder. Those homosexuals who had been feminine as boys (about two-thirds) had an adult history of anxiety phobia and psychophysiologic reactions; those not previously feminine did not.

For the homosexual females, a third had had some psychotherapy, compared to a quarter of the heterosexual female group. One-third of the homosexual patients had sought help for depression (typically secondary to the breakup of a love relationship) and nearly half for insight or alleviation of guilt. One-quarter of the heterosexual patients sought help for depression and three-fourths for insight and emotional growth. Problem drinking was significantly higher among the homosexual subjects.

The authors concluded: "Homosexuals are not necessarily sick within the limits of the definition of sickness or manifest pathology interfering with health or with function. . . . Homosexual men are psychologically very similar to single heterosexual men while homosexual women tend to show a greater degree of psychopathology (drinking problems) than heterosexual women. However, manifest neurotic disorders do not seem to be more prevalent among homosexual men or women."

Criticism may be leveled against the Siegelman study[118] on the grounds that the subjects were never interviewed, that psychometric tests do not fully tap mental functioning, and that the samples may not be representative of the homosexual population but reflect volunteer bias (just as psychiatrist patient samples are biased). The Saghir and Robins study may be criticized on the grounds that an unmarried heterosexual contrast group, while controlling for marital status and permitting better comparison of life-style experiences, is an atypical heterosexual sample, and one more prone to conflict and poor social adjustment.

Results from a large study conducted by the Institute for Sex Research (A. Bell and M. Weinberg) are promised within a year. It has assessed a large number of heterosexual and homosexual black and white males and females. The volume of data dealing with social and psychological adjustment as well as early life recalled events holds considerable potential.

Treatment of Homosexuality

Treatment of homosexuality has become simultaneously a better therapeutic prospect and an ethical dilemma. Psychiatry had historically found little for rejoicing in its attempts to reorient homosexuals (typically males). Freud[39] was less than optimistic when he noted that it was about as easy to reorient a homosexual as a heterosexual. But Bieber and colleagues[14] reported in 1962 that about a third of their highly motivated, masculine-appearing predominantly homosexual males reoriented after at least 300 hours of psychoanalysis. Hadden[58] reported reorientation in group therapy, and Bergler,[13] Socarides[121] and Hatterer[60] reported success (typically labeled "cures") with psychoanalytic or dynamically-oriented therapy.

Concurrently, behavior therapists instituted their strategies (following a largely unnoticed report in the 1930s)[94] and additional evidence demonstrated that some highly motivated homosexual males could reorient toward heterosexuality. A variety of behaviorist techniques were introduced, but generally there was pairing of a noxious stimulus (electric shock to the wrist) with a visual image of an erotic male and absence of the noxious stimulus with an image of a female.[40,85–87] Behavior therapy reorientation rates were comparable to insight-oriented therapies (about 20 to 40 percent) but the treatment time (two to four weeks) was considerably shorter. Follow-up evaluations in both types of studies indicated that the majority of those who reoriented remained so (for an extensive review, see Bancroft[4]).

It has occurred to some clinicians that heterosexuality is more than achieving an erection while viewing a slide of a female nude; consequently, additional other forms of retraining have been introduced. Social skills involved in meeting females, holding conversations, and requesting dates have been taught as well as techniques of advanced seduction. Social-skills training may include modeling, role playing, and behavior rehearsal.[78] Subjects are trained in appropriate verbal fluency and body and facial expression. Social-skill therapists insist that the appropriate interpersonal responses are not part of the subject's prior repertoire and must be taught in order for laboratory-conditioned erotic responses to generalize to the "real world." (Interestingly, the one male "transsexual" reported as aban-

doning his goal of sex-change surgery to female status did so after sequential programs of
social-skills training for heterosocial competence and aversion conditioning to male erotic
partners.[7])

Comparative study of these interventions is
difficult. Those patients who consult a psychoanalyst, a behavior therapist, or a social-skills
facilitator are not the same. The duration of
time involved in the intervention experience is
not the same, and it is difficult to control for
other variables entering the patient's life during a prolonged treatment period such as psychoanalysis.

Sex-partner availability and the feasibility
of putting into practice newly learned behavior is another practical treatment consideration and brings into question another frontier
—the sexual surrogate. The report by Masters
and Johnson[93] that they successfully utilized
female surrogates for sexual and emotional
support in their treatment program of heterosexual dysfunction has sparked new and more
open impetus for the use of professional partners. While a few therapists had formerly dis-
patched patients to prostitutes (programs for
"penises without partners") the past few years
have seen the surfacing of surrogate training
programs and surrogate associations.

The future role of surrogate partners is a
provocative topic. On the one hand, they may
experience difficulty in consequence of prose-
cutions for prostitution; on the other hand,
there is the possibility of more formalized
training and licensing, in the manner of other
physical therapists. The issue of quality control in training and practice would then need
be addressed, as in other areas of health-care
delivery.

Professional homosexual organizations have
strongly protested any treatment designed to
reorient a male or female to heterosexuality.
Their view is that homsexuality should be
treated as a human variant, in the manner of
left-handedness, and that any intervention
reinforces the societal second-class status of a
same-sexed partner preference. Supporters of
therapeutic intervention insist they treat only
volunteer patients, that the patient sets the
goals of therapy, and that to deny treatment

would be unethical. Homosexual activists assert that those who request heterosexual reorientation do so out of societal oppression and
not out of free will. For a more detailed discussion of this dilemma see Green[50] and
Money.[97]

Sex-reassignment Surgery

Since 1966 "sex-change" operations have
been openly performed at American medical
centers. While the controversy prior to the late
1960s was whether sex-change surgery was a
legitimate treatment for anyone,[55] the major
thrust of that dispute has been blunted and
the principal current question is *which* patients are the best candidates.

Several subgroups of male patients requesting sex change are being granted surgery. The
past history of one subgroup better fits the life
style of the feminine homosexual, another that
of the transvestite, and the third that of the
more classic transsexual. Those in the first
group have had extensive homosexual experience, have been markedly effeminate, and
have not experienced sexual arousal from
cross-dressing. Misfitted into the larger homosexual subculture, they experience a sense of
legitimization for their atypical behavior with
the designation "transsexual," and find new
hope in the destigmatized medical product—
the postoperative transsexual woman. The second group has been conventionally masculine
in most behavior except for periodically dressing in women's clothes, with accompanying
sexual arousal. Sexual behavior has been both
heterosexual and homosexual. Over time, the
frequency of cross-dressing has increased and
the degree of concordant genital arousal decreased. The person evolves a greater sense of
femininity and an increasing desire to become
a woman. The last group consists of those
males who were very feminine from earliest
years, have not experienced genital arousal
from cross-dressing, and whose sexual interests
have always been directed toward males.

It has been suggested by Stoller[122] that the
first two groups are probably poor candidates
for sex-change surgery in that their identity is

too heavily comprised of male components. Other clinicians neglect past history and require the surgical candidate to convincingly demonstrate the capacity to function adequately in the aspired-for gender role.[35] The degree to which the merits of these positions will be borne out by long-term follow-up evaluations is anxiously awaited.

As normal penises and breasts become surgical specimens in increasing numbers, the time is here for sophisticated follow-up studies. However, formidable difficulties are being encountered. Many patients wish to leave behind all painful memories of their siege and disappear into the "straight" community. They are uniquely reluctant to maintain any contact with their physician. Additionally, some physicians are disinterested in what becomes of the patient five years after leaving the operating room and paying all bills. I suggest that the $5000 charged these patients, rather than generating additional professional income, be placed in an interest-bearing, escrow "follow-up" account. With each return visit by the postoperative transsexual, biannually for ten years, a portion of that account would be returned to the patient. In this way, the patients would receive the treatment they request and science would learn more about how to best serve the transsexual.

Physical Disability

There are many categories of physical disability; only recently has much attention been paid to the ways they can impinge on sexuality. Disabilities can be grouped into (1) those which are *pre*pubertal and *stable*, such as brain injury, spinal-cord injury, skeletal deformity, altered body growth, heart disease, and blindness; (2) those which are *pre*pubertal and *progressive*, such as muscular dystrophy, cystic fibrosis, diabetes, and heart disease; (3) those which are *post*pubertal and *stable*, such as spinal cord injury, genital amputation, disfiguring injuries, enterostomies, and blindness; and (4) those which are *post*pubertal and *progressive*, such as heart disease, stroke, diabetes, muscular dystrophy,

multiple sclerosis, and end-stage renal disease. The number of patients affected is obviously enormous. Research, education, and counseling at the interface of human sexuality and these disabilities is a long overdue development, but still in its infancy.[20]

Two disabilities will be highlighted here, spinal-cord injury and heart disease. Spinal-cord injury and sexual behavior have traditionally been considered incompatible. This myth has been popularized by the D. H. Lawrence classic, *Lady Chatterly's Lover*. The number of spinal-cord-injured patients has grown at a tragic rate, in consequence of the successes of national foreign policy, and the sales campaigns of the automotive and motorcycle industries.

New optimism exists for sexual rehabilitation of the paraplegic or quadriplegic. Rates at which the spinal-cord injured engage in sexual activity appear to be largely dependent on therapists' early institution of discussions and education regarding 'the patient's sexual potential.[45] Spinal-cord-injured patients can be provided information regarding reflex erection from manual or oral penile manipulation, "stuffing" techniques for intravaginal penile containment, techniques of oral-genital pleasuring, and prospects for fertility.[20] Seventy percent of 150 male patients reported by Comarr[21] were capable of erection from mechanical stimulation, and the use of surgically implanted penile splints[76] may prove to be useful in the remaining cases (as with other patients with irreversible impotency). Fertility in spinal-cord-injured males has been reported with the administration of intrathecal prostigmin to induce ejaculation.[57]

Myocardial infarction and sexuality is significant for many older couples. Heart attack need not signal termination of one's sexual practices. Cardiovascular research indicates that the individual capable of ascending one or two flights of stairs should be able to tolerate the blood pressure and pulse changes accompanying coital activity with one's regular partner.[62] Intercourse with new partners is generally accompanied by · considerably greater cardiac output and may be contraindicated for *medical* reasons.[129]

Sexuality and Old Age

Sexual functioning during old age is an area of increasing social significance, as the aged population grows and sexuality becomes a more acceptable topic of discussion among all age groups.

Traditionally, old age and sexuality have been considered mutually exclusive. To a degree this mythology was debunked by the Kinsey data[70,71] of twenty-five years ago revealing that 75 percent of their males were sexually potent at the age of seventy and that couples in their sixties were engaging in weekly sexual intercourse. Physiological studies of the sex-response cycle by Masters and Johnson[92] also reveal that males and females remain sexually responsive into advanced age. Changes that accompany advanced years in the male are a higher threshhold to erotic stimulation for an erectile response, lessened ejaculatory force, and a longer postorgasmic refractory period. For the aged female on adequate sex-steroid maintenance, multiorgasmic response can be continued from earlier years.

Questions remain regarding gonadal hormone maintenance for sexual functioning. Some preliminary data on younger females suggest that rates of sexual intercourse are, in part, related to the stage of the menstrual cycle, with a rate decrease during the luteal phase.[126] This raises the possibility that varying combinations of exogenous estrogen and/or progestrone may affect sexual interest during postmenopausal years. Other evidence strongly links adrenal androgen to female drive,[132,63] and females given testicular androgens typically report enhanced sexuality.[115] Thus, low doses of androgen might be an effective hormonal stimulant. More compelling evidence from the aged female shows that atrophy of the vaginal mucosa, resulting in painful intercourse, plus the painful uterine contractions sometimes accompanying orgasm in this age group can be alleviated with gonadal hormone maintenance.[92]

Whether older males who experience significant reduction in sexual functioning may benefit from hormone administration is less clear. While such "therapy" with testosterone has been practiced in the past with enthusiastic reports,[10] controlled studies utilizing placebo administration are called for.

Sexual-partner availability for senior citizens is also problematic. Many older people lose their regular partner through death. Frequently, the surviving partner spends the final years of life in a home for the aged. In the past, the sexual health of residents of "nursing homes" has not been a primary concern. A decade ago Ullerstrom[127] suggested that "sexual services" be made available to the aged and infirm. Certainly, educational programs for the elderly are needed, providing input that sexuality is part of the entire life cycle. Additionally, the image of sexuality as the domain of the young and beautiful might be modified somewhat if the media specialists currently engaged in producing sexually explicit educational films would also feature geriatric "stars."

⟨ Other Social Issues

Erotica and Antisocial Behavior

Several studies have attempted to test the popular assumption that exposure to sexually explicit materials is causally related to the commission of antisocial sexual behavior. The United States Commission on Obscenity and Pornography funded several projects. In one, 3000 American psychiatrists and clinical psychologists were surveyed as to whether they had ever encountered a case in which pornography was a factor in producing antisocial sexual behavior. Seven percent indicated they had, and another 9 percent suspected so.[111]

Another approach has been obtaining the pornography histories of convicted male sex offenders. The Institute for Sex Research reported on 1350 offenders, 900 males incarcerated for nonsexual crimes, and 500 nonprisoners. There were no significant differences in exposure between the two offender groups and the nonoffender group. Nor were substantial differences reported in the degree of arousal to erotica.[43]

Exposure of sex offenders and nonoffenders to erotica during adolescence has also been studied. Exposure rates for sex offenders are reported as lower. In one study, 80 percent of the nonoffender control group reported seeing photographic depictions of coitus during their teens, compared to 54 percent of pedophiles and 62 percent of rapists.[49]

The age at first exposure to erotica has been another focus. Half the persons in one sample incarcerated for a nonsexual crime had seen erotica between the ages of six and ten, whereas only 28 percent of the sex offenders reported such an experience.[22] Similarly, a group of rapists was found to have had its initial experience with depictions of sexual intercourse more than three years later than nonsex offenders.[130]

Regarding *recent* exposure to photographic depictions of coitus, again rapists reported less during the year preceding incarceration than did the controls for the year preceding interview,[49] although no differences were found for other sexual depictions.[130] Though the study by Gebhard et al.[43] found no differences in reported response to erotica, other studies found one: sex offenders reported more often that they masturbated to the materials whereas nonsex offenders more often reported engaging in intercourse.[22,49]

Do convicted sex offenders implicate erotica as having been responsible for their antisocial acts? Three studies asked this of sex offenders. In the first, only one of forty-seven offenders blamed erotica. In the second, no difference in blaming erotica was found between sex offenders and other criminals. In the third, sex offenders were more likely to blame sexual materials.[111]

Reports of convicted offenders are difficult to interpret. Experiences may be consciously or unconsciously rendered invalid. Some sex offenders may deny experience with erotic materials in an attempt to put themselves in a more favorable moral light. On the other hand, reports of sex offenders who blame erotica for their crimes must be regarded with even greater suspicion. The "scapegoat" phe-

nomenon may be operant here, with an offender blaming some external agent rather than assuming responsibility himself.

The legal experience in Denmark has been of considerable interest to those concerned with the social significance of erotica. With the relaxation of laws controlling the availability of such materials to persons sixteen or older, reports of exhibitionism, voyeurism, and pedophilia were significantly reduced.[12] While it is difficult to demonstrate a cause-and-effect relationship between legal availability of erotica and diminution of certain sex crimes, the Danish experience does not appear to be the result of changes in the reportability of various crimes, or changes in laws which decriminalize some offenses.[12,75]

The studies of the Commission on Obscenity and Pornography[111] are not without flaws and a critical brief on their scientific merit has been assembled by V. Cline. However, the greatest importance of the commission may be that more research was conducted on the subject of erotica during a two-year period than ever before. That the legal recommendation of the commission to eliminate laws controlling the availability of materials to consenting adults was declared "morally bankrupt" by President Nixon may not have been a death blow to new legislation, as many public moral pronouncements of the abdicated president have become the object of unprecedented skepticism.

Clearly, better research is needed in this area in which heavy emotionalism is typically "balanced" against light facts. It is the responsibility of behavioral scientists and criminologists to conduct more careful investigations into the effects of erotic materials of various types, at various ages, and on various kinds of behavior. Behavior must include both antisocial sex acts, and an individual's sexual competence in socially appropriate circumstances.

Social Rehabilitation of Sex Offenders

A variety of interventions have been utilized in attempts to control sex offenders. Historically, the approach to "treating" sex offenders (habitual pedophiliacs, rapists) has been indefinite incarceration and surgical castration.[124]

Lately, somewhat more humane approaches have been introduced. Behavior therapists have attempted to recondition sexual responsivity away from inappropriate partners by pairing noxious stimuli (usually faradic stimulation) with pictures of children, or with fantasy and depictions of sexual assaults against adults.[112,23] Outpatient group therapy of probationed sex offenders has also been implemented and lower recidivism rates demonstrated.[104] Social-skills training for relating comfortably to appropriate sexual partners (discussed earlier) also holds promise here.

As an alternative to irreversible, surgical castration of sex offenders, newer research has been directed to reversible pharmacological intervention. An antiandrogenic agent has been utilized to treat offenders in Europe. The drug, cyproterone acetate, a progestational agent, may act through blocking the metabolic (and hence behavioral) actions of androgen at tissue receptors, or by inhibiting gonadotropin secretion, or perhaps through direct action on the testes.

The great majority of male patients treated with cyproterone acetate report profound reduction of sex drive. This antilibido effect has been achieved in 120 of 150 males in one series treated for a minimum of six months.[77] The antiandrogen effect reportedly proceeds in the following order: libido, erection, orgasm. Maximum effect is described between the twentieth and twenty-fifth day. Reversibility of erectile capacity may take up to six weeks, depending on dosage and duration of treatment. Reversibility of spermatogenesis inhibition occurs within five months of discontinuing the drug. Absent from these studies, however, has been a double-blind design in which the placebo effects of cyproterone acetate, as well as motivational impetus for incarcerated offenders to report low sex drive to obtain freedom, are ruled out.

If cyproterone acetate is pharmacologically effective, the possibility exists for a treatment program coupling diminished sex drive, in an outpatient setting, with social-skills training in appropriate sexual conduct, or other forms of psychotherapy. The drug could then be withdrawn when the patient is considered a good risk for continued control of socially inappropriate behavior.

In the United States the Food and Drug Administration has yet to approve the use of cyproterone acetate for the treatment of sex offenders, though approval has been given for its use in controlling androgen-responsive carcinoma of the prostate. Public reaction against the use of cyproterone has been considerable. The label "chemical castrator," has contributed much emotionalism to the issue, and cries have been heard that the drug would be used against political dissenters. At the other end of the political spectrum, opposition has been mobilized against the use of drugs that might release rapists and pedophiliacs from prison by those who feel these inmates should remain permanently incarcerated.

Research and ethical issues remain. Whether cyproterone acetate and other "antiandrogenic" drugs indeed reduce sex drive has yet to be adequately documented, and which subgroups of sex offenders might respond best to a true antiandrogen is also not known. In individuals for whom the significance of violence toward women is paramount, rather than a strong sex drive, the drug might have only minimal effect. Similarly, for those males lacking the social skills required to engage adult partners, the drug might also have only minimal effect.

Beyond this, the capacity of an incarcerated person to give a truly informed consent remains a dilemma. A prisoner confronted with the option of taking a drug or participating in a behavior-modification program that may shorten prison stay, and told the possible risks, may sign an "informed" consent, but still act under coercion. A variety of alternatives have been suggested, including uncoupling the duration of incarceration from participation in experimental treatment programs, or initiating the program *after* the individual is released. The different approaches are extraordinarily complex and have been debated at length. One example is found in the proposed policy regarding protection of human subjects published by the Department of Health, Education and Welfare.[24]

Common Illegal Sexual Behavior

In a trial in California in 1972, a defendant was charged with (and convicted of) conspiracy to commit oral copulation. The maximum sentence for this crime is fourteen years. The U.S. Supreme Court refused to consider the case. As of this writing, oral copulation is a crime in forty-two states, including when practiced by a married couple in the privacy of their bedroom. Oral copulation is a sexual act engaged in by about 80 percent of the adult population.[66]

In a trial in New Jersey in 1974, a defendant was charged with (and convicted of) fornication (sexual intercourse involving an unmarried, consenting adult female). As of this writing, the conviction is being appealed on constitutional grounds. Fornication and/or cohabitation is a crime in twenty-two states. Fornication is practiced by at least 50 percent of the population.[66,108–110]

In a trial in Texas in 1974, a man was convicted of publicly wearing women's clothes. There was no intent on the individual's part to perfect a disguise to elude police detection or attempt fraud. The U.S. Supreme Court refused to consider the case. Cross-dressing is practiced by thousands of transsexuals and transvestites to promote emotional well-being.

Anal intercourse, also called in the statutes "the crime against nature" (nineteen states) or "the act not to be mentioned among Christians" is a crime in forty-five states. The maximum penalty in California is ten years. Anal intercourse is reportedly practiced by some 20 percent of young (under age thirty-five) *het-erosexual* couples[66] and by a majority of homosexual males.[8]

What effect do these laws have on mental health? Many patients experience difficulties in sexual relationships due to guilt feelings when considering or practicing these common sexual behaviors (e.g., oral copulation). Legal pronouncement of such behaviors as criminal positively reinforces these feelings. Additionally, therapists treating varieties of sexual dys-

function and counseling couples or individuals with inhibitions about such behaviors are advocating criminal acts.

Persons with a strong need to wear clothes more typically worn by the other sex experience frustration when denied access to these garments. Additionally, many medical centers engaged in sex-reassignment surgery for transsexuals require that the patient live in the social role aspired to for one year prior to surgery. This trial period is critical in helping safeguard against disappointment after irreversible intervention.

The removal of homosexuality per se as a category of mental disorder by the American Psychiatric Association in 1974 reflected, in part, a growing awareness of the psychiatric consequences of labeling certain kinds of behavior as mentally disordered.[123] Similar psychiatric arguments exist for labeling certain kinds of behavior as criminal. Vulnerability to blackmail and police harassment are additional hazards.

Sex Education

Sex education, whether in medical school or kindergarten, remains controversial. Instruction on human sexuality in medical school came into vogue in the 1970s, with 95 percent of schools participating.[81] However, effective delivery of sexual knowledge and its clinical impact remain to be adequately evaluated.

The most widely used assessment instrument has been the Sexual Knowledge and Attitude Test (SKAT) developed by Lief, and modified by Lief and Ebert. In one of the few efforts at determining whether a course changed either knowledge or attitudes the test was given in a before-and-after design by Golden and Liston.[48] No student change was reported. However, Ebert (personal communication) points out that if the authors had statistically analyzed their data, significant student improvement would have been found. Irrespective of whether change in knowledge or attitude can be accurately measured, it is another matter whether change, if present, carries over into interpersonal relations at either the private or professional level. Most students bring to their medical experience sexual misinformation, conflicts, and blocks. These interfere with sexual history taking[52] and sexual counseling. Thus, the goal of providing information and facilitating a comfortable, objective patient–doctor exchange. How to effect this is controversial.

An explosive use of explicit sex films in educational settings occurred in the 1970s. Advocates of the use of erotica point to a wide range of benefits: "desensitization" to various aspects of sexual interaction, augmented student dialogue on sexuality stimulated by the material, greater comfort in interviewing in the area of sexuality, and general education regarding the range of sexual experiences. Detractors see the use of erotica as an unnecessary gimmick that depersonalizes sexuality and contributes to the voyeurism of student and teacher.

The major source of erotic films used in medical schools has been Multi-Media Resource Center in San Francisco, under the direction of Reverend Ted McIlvenna.[128] Twenty-minute films depicting a variety of sexual behaviors, including male–female typical, male–female atypical (male paraplegic–female able-bodied), male–male, female–female, and solo male or female have been produced. More recently commercial enterprises (e.g., Edcoa, Englewood, New Jersey) and psychiatrists (Paul Miller, University of Nevada, Reno) have been producing and selling erotic films for educational purposes. Multi-Media has also produced a film designed to treat premature ejaculation, and Edcoa released a film of a physician's "sexological" examination of a couple (both partners present and the genitalia demonstrated, examined, and explained).

Additional educational strategies include presentations by persons with various sexual life styles, and small group student interactions, which are seen as catalyzing comfortable communication and private attitude reassessment. The degree to which each or any of these strategies is successful is not well documented.

Evaluating the clinical effect of general information giving (and obtaining) is complex.

Assessments need to be made of knowledge imparted, attitude change, and capacity to conduct sexual interviews and counseling. Ratings of competence must utilize objective criteria by trained raters, and the subjective experience of the patient. Correlations could also be made between course information input and attitude change (if any) and ratings by self and partner(s) of sexual competence and satisfaction. Valid assessment instruments need to be constructed for such evaluations.

Sex education for children remains politically volatile. Most people believe that "sex education" is a good thing. What is not agreed upon is at *what age* education should begin, *who* should do the educating, and just *what* should be taught. Advocates of sex education in the earliest school years stress that sex can be removed from the arena of mystery and misinformation and that lack of education is associated with adult sexual dysfunctions[93] and the commission of sexual offenses.[49]

The primary source of sex information has been the peer group (true for 91 percent of 477 lower-class males, 89 percent of 888 incarcerated criminals, and 89 percent of 1395 sex offenders as recently as the mid ninteen-sixties).[43] The peer group has rarely been a source of accurate sexual counseling.

The public school system has not fared much better. Sex education courses have typically vacillated between lessons in "reproductive biology," depicting the heroic canine sperm swimming upstream to find its helplessly awaiting mate, and lectures on maintaining a hygienic body, powered by the energies of an aseptic soul.

The Sex Information and Education Council of the United States (SIECUS) in New York, founded by Mary Calderone, has been a catalytic force during the past decade in providing educational material and counsel for teachers and students. SIECUS also maintains an active index and reviewing system of available educational books and films.

Sex educators of the young optimistically believe that effective delivery of information at appropriate developmental periods will promote a positive attitude toward one's body (genitalia included) and will reduce the rates of venereal disease, unwanted pregnancy, sexual dysfunction, and sexual offenses. Firm data to support this prediction are awaited.

❮ Conclusion

These research-treatment frontiers are broadly based, reflecting the wide scope of human sexuality. The topics are not exhaustive, but encompass some areas of therapeutic, research, political, and social significance. Sexual attitudes and conduct are problematic. They are subject to what may appear as capricious change, dictated by an evolving social structure. Here is an area of science in which *a priori* knowledge has traditionally compromised dedication to fact and the search for greater wisdom. Here is an area of treatment in which personalized value systems can compromise the goal of implementing patient-activated guidelines. My hope is that this chapter will quickly become "dated," and that by the time the editors formulate the third edition of the *Handbook*, its research questions will be considered "quaint." If so, we will know much more about the bases of human sexuality and how to promote sexual health.

❮ Bibliography

1. ABEL, G., D. LEVIS, and J. CLANCY. "Aversion Therapy Applied to Taped Sequences of Deviant Behavior in Exhibitionism and Other Sexual Deviations," *J. Behav. Ther. Exper. Psychiatry*, 1 (1970), 59–66.
2. BAKER, H. and R. STOLLER. "Can a Biological Force Contribute to Gender Identity?" *Am. J. Psychiatry*, 124 (1968), 1653–1658.
3. ———. "Sexual Psychopathology in the Hypogonadal Male," *Arch. Gen. Psychiatry*, 18 (1968), 361–434.
4. BANCROFT, J. *Deviant Sexual Behaviour.* London: Oxford University Press, 1974.
5. BANCROFT, J., H. G. JONES, and B. R. PULLAN. "Simple Transducer for Measuring Penile Erection," *Behav. Res. Ther.*, 4 (1966), 239–241.
6. BARLOW, D., G. G. ABEL, E. BLANCHARD et al. "Plasma Testosterone Levels and Male Homosexuality: A Failure to Replicate," *Arch. Sex. Behav.*, 3 (1974), 571–575.
7. BARLOW, D., E. REYNOLDS, and S. AGRAS. "Gender Identity Change in a Transsexual," *Arch. Gen. Psychiatry*, 28 (1973), 569–576.
8. BELL, A. "The Homosexual as Patient," in R. Green, ed., *Human Sexuality: A Health Practitioner's Text*, pp. 54–72. Baltimore: Willams & Wilkins, 1975.
9. BELL, R. and J. DARLING. "The Prone Head Reaction in the Human Newborn. Relationship with Sex and Tactile Sensitivity," *Child Dev.*, 36 (1965), 943–949.
10. BENJAMIN, H. Personal communication.
11. ———. *The Transsexual Phenomenon.* New York: Julian Press, 1966.
12. BEN-VENISTE, R. "Pornography and Sex Crime: The Danish Experience," in *Technical Reports of the Commission on Obscenity and Pornography*, Vol. 7, pp. 245–261. Washington: U.S. Govt. Print. Off., 1970.
13. BERGLER, E. *1000 Homosexuals. Conspiracy of Silence on Curing and Deglamorizing Homosexuality.* Paterson, N.J.: Pageant, 1959.
14. BIEBER, I., H. J. DAIN, P. R. PRINCE et al. *Homosexuality: A Psychoanalytic Study.* New York: Basic Books, 1962.
15. BLUMSTEIN, P. and P. SCHWARTZ. "Lesbianism and Bisexuality," *Arch. Sex. Behav.*, in press.
16. BRODIE, H. K., N. GARTRELL, C. DOERING et al. "Plasma Testosterone Levels in Heterosexual and Homosexual Men," *Am. J. Psychiatry*, 131 (1974), 82–83.
17. BROOKS, J. and M. LEWIS. "Attachment in 13-Month-Old Opposite-Sexed Twins," *Child Psychol.*, 45 (1974), 243–247.
18. BROWN, D. "Sex Role Preference in Young Children," *Psychol. Monogr.*, 70 (1956), no. 421.
19. COHEN, H. and A. SHAPIRO. "A Method for Measuring Sexual Arousal in the Female," *Psychophysiology*, 8 (1971), 251–252.
20. COLE, T. "Sexuality and the Spinal Cord Injured," in R. Green, ed., *Human Sexuality: A Health Practitioner's Text*, pp. 142–170. Baltimore: Williams & Wilkins, 1975.
21. COMARR, A. "Sexual Function among Pa-

tients with Spinal Cord Injury," *Urol. Int.*, 25 (1970), 134–168.

22. COOK, R. and R. FOSEN. "Pornography and the Sex Offender," in *Technical Reports of the Commission on Obscenity and Pornography*, Vol. 7., pp. 149–162. Washington: U.S. Govt. Print. Off., 1970.

23. DAVISON, G. "Elimination of a Sadistic Fantasy by a Client-Controlled Counter-Conditioning Technique," *J. Abnorm. Psychol.*, 73 (1968), 84–90.

24. DEPARTMENT OF HEALTH, EDUCATION AND WELFARE. "Protection of Human Subjects. Proposed Policy," *Fed. Reg.*, 38 (194) (1974), 27881–27885.

25. DIAMOND, M. "A Critical Evaluation of the Ontogeny of Human Sexual Behavior," *Q. Rev. Biol.*, 40 (1965), 147–175.

26. DOERR, P. G. KOCKETT, H. G. VOGT et al. "Plasma Testosterone, Estradiol, and Semen Analysis in Male Homosexuals," *Arch. Gen. Psychiatry*, 29 (1973), 829–833.

27. DORNER, G., W. ROHDE, F. STAHL et al. "A Neuroendocrine Conditioned Predisposition for Homosexuality in Men," *Arch. Sex. Behav.*, 4 (1975), 1–8.

28. EBERT, R. K. Personal communication.

29. EBERT, R. K. and H. LIEF. "Why Sex Education for Medical Students?" in R. Green, ed., *Human Sexuality: A Health Practitioner's Text*, pp. 2–6. Baltimore: Williams & Wilkins, 1975.

30. EHRHARDT, A. "Maternalism in Fetal Hormonal and Related Syndromes," in J. Zubin and J. Money, eds., *Contemporary Sexual Behavior*, pp. 99–115. Baltimore: The Johns Hopkins University Press, 1973.

31. EHRHARDT, A., R. EPSTEIN, and J. MONEY. "Fetal Androgens and Female Gender Identity in the Early-Treated Adrenogenital Syndrome," *Johns Hopkins Med. J.*, 122 (1968), 160–167.

32. EHRHARDT, A., K. EVERS, and J. MONEY. "Influence of Androgen on some Aspects of Sexually Dimorphic Behavior in Women with the Late-Treated Adrenogenital Syndrome," *Johns Hopkins Med. J.*, 123 (1968), 115–122.

33. EVANS, R. "Childhood Parental Relationships of Homosexual Men," *J. Consult. Clin. Psychol.*, 33 (1969), 129–135.

34. ———. "Physical and Biochemical Characteristics of Homosexual Men," *J. Consult. Clin. Psychol.*, 39 (1972), 140–147.

35. FISK, N. Stanford University. Personal communication.

36. FORDNEY-SETTLAGE, D. Paper presented at NIMH Stony Brook Sex Conference, June 1974. Summary, *Arch. Sex. Behav.* 4 (1975).

37. ———. "Treating Sexual Dysfunction as a Solo Female Physician," in R. Green, ed., *Human Sexuality: A Health Practitioner's Text*, pp. 213–221. Baltimore: Williams & Wilkins, 1975.

38. FOX, C., A. ISMAIL, D. LOVE et al. "Studies on the Relationship between Plasma Testosterone Levels and Human Sexual Activity," *J. Endocrinol.*, 52 (1972), 51–58.

39. FREUD, S. (1920) "The Psychogenesis of a Case of Homosexuality in a Woman," in J. Strachey, ed., *Standard Edition*, Vol. 18, pp. 147–172. London: Hogarth, 1955.

40. FREUND, K. "Diagnosing Homo- or Hetero-Sexuality and Erotic Age Preference by Means of a Psychophysiological Test," *Behav. Res. Ther.*, 5 (1967), 209–228.

41. GAGNON, J. and W. SIMON. *Sexual Conduct*. Chicago: Aldine, 1973.

42. GEBHARD, P. "Sex Differences in Sexual Response," *Arch. Sex. Behav.*, 2 (1973), 201–203.

43. GEBHARD, P., J. GAGNON, W. POMEROY et al. *Sexual Offenders: An Analysis of Types.* New York: Harper & Row, 1965.

44. GEER, J., P. MOROKOFF, and P. GREENWOOD. "Sexual Arousal in Women: The Development of a Measurement Device for Vaginal Blood Volume," *Arch. Sex. Behav.*, 3 (1974), 559–564.

45. GEIGER, R. Personal communication, University of California Medical Center, 1973.

46. GILLESPIE, A. Paper read at the 2nd Int. Cong. Gender Identity, Elsinore, Denmark, 1971.

47. GOLDBERG, S. and M. LEWIS. "Play Behavior in the Year Old Infant: Early Sex Differences," *Child Dev.*, 40 (1969), 21–31.

48. GOLDEN, J. and E. LISTON. "Medical Sex Education: The World of Illusion and a Practical Reality," *J. Med. Educ.*, 7 (1972), 761–771.

49. GOLDSTEIN, M., H. KANT, L. JUDD et al. "Exposure to Pornography and Sexual Behavior in Deviant and Normal Groups," in *Technical Reports of the Commission on Obscenity and Pornography*, Vol. 7, pp.

1–89. Washington: U.S. Govt. Print. Off., 1970.

50. GREEN, R. "Homosexuality as a Mental Illness," *Int. J. Psychiatry*, 10 (1972), 77–98.

51. ———. *Sexual Identity Conflict in Children and Adults.* New York: Basic Books, 1974.

52. ———. "Taking a Sexual History," in R. Green, ed., *Human Sexuality: A Health Practitioner's Text*, pp. 9–19. Baltimore: Williams & Wilkins, 1975.

53. GREEN, R. and J. MONEY, eds. *Transsexualism and Sex Reassignment.* Baltimore: The Johns Hopkins Press, 1969.

54. GREEN, R. and R. STOLLER. "Two Monozygotic (Identical) Twin Pairs Discordant for Gender Identity," *Arch. Sex. Behav.*, 1 (1971), 321–327.

55. GREEN, R., R. STOLLER, and C. MacANDREW. "Attitudes Toward Sex Transformation Procedures," *Arch. Gen. Psychiatry*, 15 (1966), 178–182.

56. GREENBLATT, D. R. Semantic Differential Analysis of the 'Triangular System' Hypothesis in 'Adjusted' Overt Male Homosexuals. Ph.D. thesis, University of California, 1966.

57. GUTTMAN, L. and J. WALSH. "Prostigmin Assessment of Fertility in Spinal Man," *Paraplegia*, 9 (1971), 39–51.

58. HADDEN, S. "Treatment of Male Homosexuals in Groups," *Int. J. Group Psychother.*, 16 (1966), 13–22.

59. HAMPSON, J. L. and J. G. HAMPSON. "The Ontogenesis of Sexual Behavior in Man," in W. C. Young, ed., *Sex and Internal Secretions*, 3rd ed., pp. 1401–1432. Baltimore: Williams & Wilkins, 1961.

60. HATTERER, L. *Changing Homosexuality in the Male.* New York: McGraw-Hill, 1970.

61. HEIMAN, J. Personal communication, Ph.D. research, State University of New York at Stony Brook.

62. HELLERSTEIN, H. and E. FRIEDMAN. "Sexual Activity and the Post-Coronary Patient," *Arch. Intern. Med.*, 125 (1970), 987–999.

63. HERBERT, J. "Hormones and Reproductive Behavior in Rhesus and Talapoin Monkeys," *J. Reprod. Fertil.*, (Suppl.) 11 (1970), 119–140.

64. HOFFMAN, M. *The Gay World: Male Homosexuality and the Social Creation of Evil.* New York: Basic Books, 1968.

65. HOOKER, E. "The Adjustment of the Male Overt Homosexual," *J. Proj. Tech. Pers. Assess.*, 21 (1957), 18–31.

66. HUNT, M. *Sexual Behavior in the 1970's.* Chicago: Playboy Press, 1974.

67. JOST, A. "Recherches sur la différentiation sexuelle de l'embryon de lapin," *Arch. Anat. Microsc. Exp.*, 36 (1947), 151–200.

68. JOVANOVIC, V. "The Recording of Physiological Evidence of Genital Arousal in Human Males and Females," *Arch. Sex. Behav.*, 1 (1971), 309–320.

69. KAGAN, J. and M. LEWIS. "Studies of Attention in the Human Infant," *Merrill-Palmer Q.*, 11 (1965), 95–127.

70. KINSEY, A., W. POMEROY, and C. MARTIN. *Sexual Behavior in the Human Male.* Philadelphia: Saunders, 1948.

71. KINSEY, A., W. POMEROY, C. MARTIN et al. *Sexual Behavior in the Human Female.* Philadelphia: Saunders, 1953.

72. KOLODNY, R., W. MASTERS, J. HENDRYX et al. "Plasma Testosterone and Semen Analysis in Male Homosexuals," *N. Engl. J. Med.*, 285 (1971), 1170–1174.

73. KOLODNY, R., W. MASTERS, R. KOLODNER et al. "Depression of Plasma Testosterone Levels after Chronic Intensive Marijuana Use," *N. Engl. J. Med.*, 290 (1974), 872–874.

74. KREUZ, L., R. ROSE, and J. JENNINGS. "Suppression of Plasma Testosterone Levels and Psychological Stress," *Arch. Gen. Psychiatry*, 26 (1972), 479–482.

75. KUTCHINSKY, B. "Sex Crimes and Pornography in Copenhagen," in *Technical Reports of the Commission on Obscenity and Pornography*, Vol. 7, pp. 263–310. Washington: U.S. Govt. Print. Off., 1970.

76. LASH, H. "Silicone Implant for Impotence," *J. Urol.*, 100 (1968), 709–710.

77. LASHETT, V. "Antiandrogen in the Treatment of Sex Offenders," in J. Zubin and J. Money, eds., *Contemporary Sexual Behavior*, pp. 311–320. Baltimore: The Johns Hopkins University Press, 1973.

78. LAWS, R. and M. SERBER. "Measurement and Evaluation of Assertive Training," in R. Hosford and S. Moss, eds., The Crumbling Walls: Treatment and Counseling of the Youthful Offender. Urbana: University of Illinois Press, 1974.

79. LEBOVITZ, P. "Feminine Behavior in Boys—Aspects of Its Outcome," *Am. J. Psychiatry*, 128 (1972), 1283–1289.

80. LEV-RAN, A. "Gender Role Differentiation in Hermaphrodites," *Arch. Sex. Behav.*, 3 (1974), 339–424.

81. LIEF, H. and R. EBERT. "A Survey of Sex Education Courses in United States Medical Schools," Paper presented at WHO, Geneva, Feb. 1974.

82. LoPICCOLO, J. and W. G. LOBITZ. "The Role of Masturbation in the Treatment of Sexual Dysfunction," *Arch. Sex. Behav.*, 2 (1972), 163–171.

83. LoPICCOLO, J. and J. STEGER. "The Sexual Interaction Inventory: A New Instrument for Assessment of Sexual Dysfunction," *Arch. Sex. Behav.*, 3 (1974), 585–595.

84. LORAINE, J., D. ADAMOPOULOS, K. KIRKHAM et al. "Patterns of Hormone Excretion in Male and Female Homosexuals," *Nature*, 234 (1971), 552–555.

85. McCONAGHY, N. "Subjective and Penile Plethysmograph Responses following Aversion Relief and Apomorphine Aversion Therapy for Homosexual Impulses," *Br. J. Psychiatry*, 115 (1969), 723–730.

86. ———. "Subjective and Penile Plethysmograph Responses to Aversion Therapy for Homosexuality: A Follow-Up Study," *Br. J. Psychiatry*, 117 (1970), 555–560.

87. MacCULLOCH, H. and M. FELDMAN. "Aversion Therapy in Management of 43 Homosexuals," *Br. Med. J.*, 1 (1967), 594–597.

88. McGUIRE, L. and G. OMENN. "Congenital Adrenal Hyperplasia: Cognitive and Behavioral Studies," *Behav. Genet.*, in press.

89. MARGOLESE, S. "Homosexuality: A New Endocrine Correlate," *Horm. Behav.*, 1 (1970), 151–155.

90. MARGOLESE, S. and O. JANIGER. "Androgen-Etiocholanolone Ratios in Male Homosexuals," *Br. Med. J.*, 2 (1973), 207–210.

91. MARMOR, J. *Sexual Inversion.* New York: Basic Books, 1965.

92. MASTERS, W. and V. JOHNSON. *Human Sexual Response.* Boston: Little, Brown, 1966.

93. ———. *Human Sexual Inadequacy.* Boston: Little, Brown, 1970.

94. MAX, L. "Breaking Up a Homosexual Fixation by the Conditioned Reaction Technique: A Case Study," *Psychol. Bull.*, 32 (1935), 734–738.

95. MICHAEL, R. P. and E. B. KEVERNE. "Primate Sex Pheromones of Vaginal Origin," *Nature*, 225 (1970), 84–85.

96. MICHAEL, R. P., E. B. KEVERNE, and R. W. BONSALL. "Pheromones: Isolation of a Male Sex Attractant from a Female Primate," *Science*, 172 (1971), 964–966.

97. MONEY, J. "Strategy, Ethics, Behavior Modification, and Homosexuality," *Arch. Sex. Behav.*, 2 (1972), 79–81.

98. ———. "Sex Assignment in Anatomically Intersexed Infants", in R. Green, ed., *Human Sexuality: A Health Practitioner's Text*, pp. 109–123. Baltimore: Williams & Wilkins, 1975. Adapted from *Clin. in Plastic Surg.*, 1 (1974), 215–22, 271–74.

99. MONEY, J. and A. EHRHARDT. *Man and Woman; Boy and Girl.* Baltimore: The Johns Hopkins University Press, 1973.

100. MONEY, J., J. HAMPSON and J. HAMPSON. "An Examination of Some Basic Sexual Concepts: The Evidence of Human Hermaphroditism," *Bull. Johns Hopkins Hosp.*, 97 (1955), 301–319.

101. MONEY, J. and E. POLLITT. "Cytogenetic and Psychosexual Ambiguity: Klinefelter's Syndrome and Transvestism Compared," *Arch. Gen. Psychiatry*, 11 (1964), 589–595.

102. MOSS, H. "Sex, Age and State as Determinants of Mother–Infant Interaction," *Merrill-Palmer Q.*, 13 (1967), 19–36.

103. NISBETT, R. and S. GURWITZ. "Weight, Sex, and the Eating Behavior of Human Newborns," *J. Comp. Physiol. Psychol.*, 73 (1970), 245–253.

104. PETERS, J. and H. ROETHER. "Group Therapy for Probationed Sex Offenders," in H. L. Resnik and M. Wolfgang, eds., *Sexual Behaviors*, pp. 255–266. Boston: Little, Brown, 1972.

105. PILLARD, R., R. ROSE, and M. SHERWOOD. "Plasma Testosterone Levels in Homosexual Men," *Arch. Sex. Behav.*, 3 (1974), 453–458.

106. PIRKE, K., G. KOCKETT, and F. DITTMAR. "Psychosexual Stimulation and Plasma Testosterone in Man," *Arch. Sex. Behav.*, 3 (1974), 577–584.

107. PRINCE, V. and P. BENTLER. "Survey of 504 Cases of Transvestism," *Psychol. Rep.*, 31 (1972), 903–917.

108. REISS, I. "How and Why America's Sex Standards Are Changing," *Trans-Action*, 5 (1968), 26–32.

109. ———. *Heterosexual Relationships: Inside and Outside of Marriage.* Morristown: General Learning, 1973.

110. ———. "Heterosexual Relationships of Patients: Premarital, Marital, and Extramarital," in R. Green, ed. *Human Sexuality: A*

Health Practitioner's Text, pp. 37–52. Baltimore: Williams & Wilkins, 1975.

111. REPORT OF THE COMMISSION ON OBSCENITY AND PORNOGRAPHY. Washington: U.S. Govt. Print. Off., 1970.

112. RESNIK, H. and M. WOLFGANG, eds. "Treatment of the Sex Offender," *Int. Psychiatry Clin.*, 8 (1972).

113. ROSE, R., P. BOWNE, and R. POE. "Androgen Response to Stress," *Psychosom. Med.*, 31 (1969), 418–436.

114. SAGHIR, M. and E. ROBINS. *Male and Female Homosexuality.* Baltimore: Williams & Wilkins, 1973.

115. SALMON, U. and S. GEIST. "Effect of Androgens upon Libido in Women," *J. Clin. Endocrinol.*, 3 (1943), 235–238.

116. SCHMIDT, G. and V. SIGUSCH. "Sex Differences in Response to Psychosexual Stimulation by Films and Slides," *J. Sex Res.*, 6 (1970), 268–283.

117. SCHMIDT, G., V. SIGUSCH, and S. SCHAFER. "Responses to Reading Erotic Stories," *Arch. Sex. Behav.*, 2 (1973), 181–199.

118. SIEGELMAN, M. "Adjustment of Male Homosexuals and Heterosexuals," *Arch. Sex. Behav.*, 2 (1972), 9–26.

119. ———. "Parental Background of Male Homosexuals and Heterosexuals," *Arch. Sex. Behav.*, 3 (1974), 3–18.

120. SINTCHAK, G. and J. GEER. "A Vaginal Plethysmograph System," *Psychophysiology*, in press.

121. SOCARIDES, C. *The Overt Homosexual.* New York: Grune & Stratton, 1968.

122. STOLLER, R. *Sex and Gender: On the Development of Masculinity and Femininity.* New York: Science House, 1968.

123. STOLLER, R., J. MARMOR, I. BIEBER et al. "A Symposium: Should Homosexuality be in the APA Nomenclature?" *Am. J. Psychiatry*, 130 (1973), 1207–1216.

124. STURUP, G. "Castration: The Total Treatment," in H. L. Resnik and M. Wolfgang, eds., *Sexual Behavior.* Boston: Little, Brown, 1972.

125. TOURNEY, G. and L. HATFIELD. "Androgen Metabolism in Schizophrenics, Homo-sexuals and Controls," *Biol. Psychiatry*, 6 (1973), 23–36.

126. UDRY, J. R. and N. MORRIS. "Distribution of Coitus in the Menstrual Cycle," *Nature*, 220 (1968), 593–596.

127. ULLERSTROM, L. *The Erotic Minorities.* New York: Grove, 1966.

128. VANDERVOORT, H. and T. MCILVENNA. "Sexually Explicit Media in Medical School Curricula," in R. Green, ed., *Human Sexuality: A Health Practitioner's Text*, pp. 235–244. Baltimore: Williams & Wilkins, 1975.

129. WAGNER, N. "Sexual Activity and the Cardiac Patient," in R. Green, ed., *Human Sexuality: A Health Practitioner's Text*, pp. 173–179. Baltimore: Williams & Wilkins, 1975.

130. WALKER, C. "Erotic Stimuli and the Aggressive Sexual Offender," in *Technical Reports of the Commission on Obscenity and Pornography*, Vol. 7, pp. 91–147. Washington: U.S. Govt. Print. Off., 1970.

131. WALZER, S. Boston University. Personal communication.

132. WATSON, J. "Operant Conditioning of Visual Fixation in 14-Week-Old Infants," *Dev. Psychobiol.*, 1 (1969), 508–516.

133. WAXENBERG, S., M. DRELLICH, and A. SUTHERLAND. "The Role of Hormones in Human Behavior, Changes in Female Sexuality after Adrenalectomy," *J. Clin. Endocrinol.*, 19 (1959), 193–202.

134. YALOM, I., R. GREEN, and N. FISK. "Prenatal Exposure to Female Hormones—Effect on Psychosexual Development in Boys," *Arch. Gen. Psychiatry*, 28 (1973), 554–561.

135. YOUNG, W., R. GOY, and C. PHOENIX. "Hormones and Sexual Behavior," *Science*, 143 (1964), 212–218.

136. ZUGER, B. "Effeminate Behavior Present in Boys from Early Childhood," *J. Pediatr.*, 69 (1966), 1098–1107.

137. ———. "Gender Role Differentiation: A Critical Review of the Evidence from Hermaphroditism," *Psychosom. Med.*, 32 (1970), 449–463.

CHAPTER 29

PROMISING DIRECTIONS IN PSYCHOANALYSIS

Albert J. Solnit and Melvin Lewis

OUT OF the interplay between classical psychoanalytic theory and treatment, the experiences with direct observation, and the applications of psychoanalytic theory, several promising trends have emerged. Much of the data for these new directions are derived from more systematic studies and descriptions of the developing child.[5,17,21] Experimental studies of sucking[31] and direct observations of infants, for example, have refined questions and suggested modifications in psychoanalytic theory. Studies of the capacities of maternally deprived children to achieve partial or nearly complete recovery, as well as data from the psychoanalytic treatment of children and adults, have led to a synthesis of our understanding about normative growth. The socializing interactions between parents and children, beginning during the period of helplessness of the newborn child, have provided a basis for understanding not only the development of the child, but also for the changes that take place in the adult. These psychoanalytic studies portray young adulthood, parenthood, middle and old age as a dynamic unfolding of human experience.

In his earliest development the infant's psychology is his physiology. Yet, with the care of a responsive, competent adult—who herself, in an active role, is re-experiencing the helplessness of the young child—the infant is enabled to become progressively competent. He will give first evidence of social receptiveness in his responsive smile at the age of four to eight weeks. Though the earlier studies of Ribble[22,23] Spitz,[27,28] and Spitz and Wolf[29] furnished the basis for understanding the marasmic state, which in the preantibiotic era led to death in severe cases, more recent studies by Provence and Lipton,[21] Leonard, Rhymes, and Solnit,[15] Elmer and Gregg,[4] and others have enabled us to understand the failure-to-thrive syndrome. Certain children are more vulnerable to partial maternal deprivation, but recent studies have suggested that the mother's vulnerability must also be taken into account in the failure-to-thrive situation. This concept has been further elaborated by viewing both the abused child and the child who fails to thrive on a continuum of maternal deprivation in which the parents are also failing to thrive.

If the parents were deprived in childhood or had their stores of energy, love, and patience depleted by adverse conditions in their adult lives, then the conditions that predispose transmission of this vulnerability and depletion to their children are increased with the advent of each successive child. The marital relationship is a crucial index of the adult's resources. Whether it will culminate for the child in understimulation and in the lack of a loving bond between child and parents, or whether it will culminate in physical abuse and violence is more a function of the parents' psychopathology and deprivational state than of the child's vulnerability or socializing characteristics.

Psychoanalytic theory has increasingly demonstrated that the newborn does not have the ego capacities for adaptation, regulation, and synthesizing multiple demands and stimuli. The infant's immaturity in organizational capacities is temporarily provided for by the mother, the auxiliary ego without whom the child would not survive. It is this psychoanalytic conceptualization and the observations of infants by psychoanalysts that have still further advanced our knowledge of how children and their parents fail to thrive and develop.

(The Children—Failure to Develop

In many studies of children and their parents, socialization is often taken for granted as an implicit dimension of the investigation. When socialization is untroubled, it is silent; it becomes audible only when the process is disturbed or when conflicts exist. Studies of children who fail to thrive despite the absence of detectable organic abnormalities indicate that a major factor in the failure of growth is the mother's inability to socialize her relationships with the young child. Viewed on a continuum in which child and maternal development are assumed to parallel each other, the failure of the mother's development can be the essential cause of the child's failure to grow and mature according to expected norms.

Clinical observations suggest that the child's failure to thrive stems from two extremely opposite conditions. Under the first, the child is used by the mother or maternal figure as the basis for her own sexual and aggressive gratification. The child's normative characteristics and behavior are perceived as evocative stimuli that invite the adult's regressive reactions of unmodified impulsive behavior. It is the child of this mother who is most often physically abused. He becomes the object through whom the parent derives direct gratification of poorly modified sadistic impulses. These impulses become unbridled in response to the young child's stimulating behavior and helplessness, both of which set in motion the adult's regressive behavior. In many of these situations, the psychotic parents had been released from the psychiatric hospital under the influence of tranquilizers. Though medication permits them to be sustained outside of the hospital, they are not able to cope with their children's demands and needs; their behavior toward their children becomes damaging and depriving.

Under the second failure-to-thrive condition, the child is neglected or understimulated and undergratified. Here the mother's inability to activate the child's development reflects her own depressive or depleted state. These mothers are in need of being nurtured, of being mothered before they can respond appropriately to their children. When the mother's libidinal supplies are adequate, she can provide the maternal presence and responsiveness that are sources of the crucial stimulation and organizing influences—essential conditions for vigorous development in childhood. When the mother's psychic (and often physical) energies are depleted, the investment of interest in the child and his behavior is deficient.

Both of these extreme conditions or their combination require sustained interventions if the children are to be protected from the permanently corrosive effects of such experiences.

These sustained interventions are necessary for the mother's development. They should, therefore, be directed toward assisting parents in caring for their children and in advancing their own development.

Early socialization is viewed as a complex developmental phenomenon based on a relationship of the child to the mother that promotes his capacity to postpone impulsive behavior and to accept substitutes for the original gratifications. In studies of interventions for children who failed to thrive because of understimulation and neglect, socialization often appears as a restitutive phenomenon presenting a paradox of bewildering proportions. These phenomena were observed in children recovering from relative maternal deprivation in the home, and in those who were placed in a foster home after living in an institution. As the individual child recovered from the disadvantage of understimulation, his pathway to recovery, especially with respect to the reactions of increased social responsiveness, was often misinterpreted as undesirable wildness. The "coming alive" of the child, as his drives were awakened by affection and a responsive environment, was often found by parents and foster parents to be unacceptable and undesirable.

We have assumed that this "coming alive" or activation of dormant and often stunted drive capacities produces a disharmony or dysynchronization of impulsive energies and regulative capacities in the individual child. Viewed by the parents in this way, the deprived child's drives and his capacities to transform, channel, or ward off the pressures and demands of the drive energies are out of phase. Ironically, just as these children begin to respond, to "come alive," the (foster) parents often feel overwhelmed by their behavior, which they misperceive not only as rejection but as a lack of grace and gratitude as well. The foster parents, feeling let down, often bitterly invoke the "bad seed" syndrome, referring to the child's background which to them represents unacceptable social values.

In their follow-up study of institutionalized children placed in foster homes, Provence and Lipton[21] state:

As time passed the beneficial influence of maternal care, family life, and the enrichment of experience in many areas was increasingly manifest in all aspects of development. The children became more lively, more active, began to learn to play, and to solve everyday problems. They increasingly made relationships with others. In addition, there were other signs of improvement that were not always universally recognized by the parents as signs of growth: they began now to show some provocative, negativistic, and aggressive behavior. This was a time of crisis for some of the parents and children. If the parents saw this behavior as bad or as indicating that they were failing as parents or if they felt rejected by the child, some either gave up in actuality and asked that the child be removed from the home, or withdrew some of the emotional investment and interest that were so important to his improvement. Others realized that such behavior was a necessary step in the child's progress and were able to react to it in a helpful way. [p. 148][21]

Socializing is a broad concept. It pertains to people living together, forming a unit in which the whole is greater than the sum of the parts. It embraces considerations as widely separated as social values and biological adaptation. If, for example, the mother does not feed, stimulate, and protect the infant in the context of affectionate expectations, he will die or suffer severe developmental impairments. Emotional deficiency, as in institutionalization, can and often does lead to nutritional deficiency and failure to grow, with permanent residual impairments to physical, social, mental, and emotional capacities. All studies of the failure-to-thrive child have clearly indicated that the impact of institutionalization is not an all-or-nothing condition. Furthermore, children raised in disadvantaged families and those raised by depressed or severely constricted parents can also suffer from maternal deprivation.

(Parents—Failure to Develop

Studies of young children who failed to thrive despite the absence of organic disease or deficits have traced the condition to the vulnerability of the child, the failure of the depleted mother to have ample supplies of affection for her child, and the failure of the family and community to provide the personal interest, assistance, and protection for the mother and her child. The failure of adults to agree effectively on the kind of social world for which they are preparing their children to enter as adolescents and adult citizens has also to be considered. Studies of infants suggest that one of the most critical factors in a child's failure to thrive, can be described in terms of the mother's failure to thrive. These investigations indicate the following formulation:

Maternal or motherly feeling does not always immediately accompany biological motherhood. Motherhood is an unfolding developmental phase that is activated by pregnancy and the birth of a child. The adequacy of this developmental response is multiply determined by the mother's previous social experiences as well as by the physical, psychological, and emotional resources available to her during the successive phases of motherhood. The number of children the mother has borne and cared for, as well as the support she received from her husband, parents, and other relatives and friends, can nurture or deplete the mother's supplies of affectionate energies and her tolerances of frustration and conflict.

Maternal development is influenced by and dependent on a host of cultural, physical, and psychological considerations. Included among these factors are the quality and quantity of nurturing experiences the mother received in her own infancy and childhood, and the continuation of maturing and satisfying relationships with her husband and others on whom she depends for closeness and emotional support. With the birth of each child, maternal feelings surface as the mother is able to supply the needs of her dependent infant in a satisfying way and in turn is able to be gratified by his increasing responsiveness to her. Adequate development in motherhood is experienced by a woman as a sense of self-fulfillment in her activities as a mother. In mothering her child competently and with satisfaction, she can sublimate her instinctual drives in a uniquely creative way by adapting to the child as he responds to her affectionate demands and as he expresses his developmental needs and capacities. The experiences of mothering successive children are critical influences in shaping the mother's personality. When mothering experiences are altered by stressful or traumatic life situations, she needs considerable inner strength and environmental support to maintain an adaptive equilibrium.

Following our earlier studies of mothers of children who accidentally swallowed poison,[16] we found that the mothers of infants who fail to thrive were also depleted, overwhelmed, and deprived. In some instances these deficits were discernible in women who had retained infantile personality characteristics and for them the first child's needs and behavior expended the scanty resources available to them before they became pregnant. Many of the mothers whom we evaluated and assisted in this clinical action-research had such cumulative handicaps as inadequate or insufficient mothering themselves; minimal or no support from husbands; several children born in rapid succession, with the last one representing a magnified expression of the cumulative depletion of their physical, emotional, and mental resources.

Many of these mothers represented the second or third generation of a family who was poor, disadvantaged, disorganized, and living in a slum community. These women were failing to thrive in their own milieu. They found it a painful or impossible demand to respond to their baby's manifest needs and behavior. They described their despair, frustration, and anger at having to care for a child whose failure to grow and develop further undermined their own sense of worthlessness and inadequacies. In this context each infant and mother reciprocally contributed to the other's failure to thrive, an instance of mutual maladaptation. Often these families lived under crowded housing conditions that also contributed to the inadequate or deviant relationships in these social units.

Thus, the mother and infant influence each other's actions and attitudes reciprocally in a progressive manner. Physiological and behavioral characteristics and deficits of the infant often initiate difficulties in the mother–child socialization patterns. These difficulties are not readily understood as different from the interactional dissonance in mother–child conflicts. However, each of these patterns can be internalized, i.e., become an internal conflict for the child that is expressed in the infantile neurosis. Depending on the origin of the infantile neurosis there may be a modification of technique in child analysis. In the case of the child's ego deficit precipitating mother–child difficulties it may be desirable to adapt the treatment to assist the child with his or her ego deficits, often providing temporary and partial need satisfaction for the so-called "borderline" child. This facilitates development and enables the therapist to use the more classical analytic treatment with the child.

We noted at the outset that contemporary psychoanalysis is moving in several promising directions. In addition to new techniques in the treatment of children who fail to develop, there are also these new trends: First, a new approach to treatment and new developmental insights have resulted from the treatment of blind children. Second, psychoanalytic treatment of adolescents has undergone significant revision. A third trend can be discerned in the treatment of the so-called narcissistic personality in adults. Finally, there has been a rediscovery of psychoanalytic principles in the treatment of people who are underprivileged and indigent.

❨ The Blind Child

In the deviant congenitally blind child, the process of ego formation is impeded during the critical period of nine to eighteen months. Fraiberg and Freedman[6] note, for example, that the mouth remains the primary organ of perception, and the personality remains mouth-centered to an extent that is almost never encountered among sighted children, except perhaps for certain children who have suffered extreme deprivation in infancy. Language is rarely employed for communication or expression of need. The mother often fails to offer stimulation or make emotional contact with the sensorially deprived infant. Walking is markedly delayed. "The deviant blind children present a picture that begins to lag at the end of the first year and fall off progressively during the second year," say Fraiberg and Freedman, "In the third year we have the impression that development has come to a standstill."

On the basis of her understanding of the development of these blind children, Fraiberg applied analytic insights in their treatment. In a report of a treatment during two-and-one-half years of Peter, a blind boy eight-years and ten-months-old, Fraiberg describes a number of observations that offer great promise for helping children with similar problems. For example, when the mother was led to understand how need satisfaction and constancy were the indispensable first steps in establishing human ties, Peter's attachment to her became evident and his ability to speak expanded rapidly. As opportunities for free movement and exploration of his environment opened up to him, and as the range of his experiences expanded, his exploration and manipulation of objects became more and more absorbing. During Peter's treatment it also became clear that the hand behaved like a mouth, the fingernails like teeth, and the pinching activity like biting. Oral-incorporative aspects of mouthing and biting, mobilized during moments of fear of abandonment, had thus been transferred to the hand. Once this was understood, a useful interpretation could be made to Peter, and his clutching and clawing behavior were brought under control. Most important, the mother, too, was able to understand that the behavior she previously regarded as aggressive was in fact a kind of inarticulate terror. Gradually the hand, which had largely functioned as an auxiliary mouth, appeared to free itself of the oral mode, with corresponding neutralization of drive qualities.

Fraiberg points out that where vision mediates the evolution of hand autonomy in the sighted child, the absence of vision obstructs this crucial process in the otherwise healthy blind infant. Blindness, too, is an impediment to the achievement of locomotion. Without locomotion the development of the concept of objects independent of the blind child's perceptions is arrested. Fraiberg describes how the mother has to "teach" the blind infant about the permanence of objects.

What is promising about this work, and similar work done by others,[2,12,19,25] is the application of psychoanalytic insights to the successful treatment of handicapped children. In addition, a bridge between cognitive theory and psychoanalytic theory in the clinical field has been established here. Piaget's concept[20] of object permanence combined with the psychoanalytic theory of ego development can contribute to an understanding of the special care of the blind child, resulting in a useful therapeutic outcome.

(The Adolescent and Development

Another trend in psychoanalysis reflects the increasing recognition that many adolescents are able to benefit from psychoanalytic treatment.[1] In the past, analysts have been cautioned that applying the classical psychoanalytic method during this period of rapid developmental change and narcissistic preoccupation ran the risk of evoking undesirable regressive behavior and unanalyzable transference reactions.[7,8] During the past decade, however, the cumulative experience in adapting psychoanalytic technique to the developmental characteristics of adolescents has shown the usefulness of the psychoanalytic method in treating neurotic adolescents. Often the treatment has begun before puberty and has been completed during early adolescence, or the treatment has begun during mid or late adolescence and has been completed during early adulthood. There are still grounds for conservatism about beginning a psychoanalytic treatment during early adolescence, although it has been carried out effectively when the technique is adapted to the developmental tolerances of the adolescent. These adaptations are mainly centered on how and what to interpret and the activity of the analyst. Often in early adolescence the patient has

a low tolerance for silence and becomes too anxious about or rejects interpretations that are not ego syntonic or which encourage regressive attitudes and behavior. As the analysis proceeds, his tolerance for reflective thought and the capacity to utilize interpretations of his defenses will gradually increase if the analysis is progressing.

Another trend in psychoanalytic research and understanding of adolescents concerns the question: has the adolescent experience changed? There is a consensus that it has,[3,9,26] but the quality and rate of the alteration are currently in need of investigation. The psychoanalytic view of this change has encouraged analysts to combine direct observation with pooled psychoanalytic treatment observations and to move toward a greater emphasis on reconstructing the adolescent experience of adults who are undergoing psychoanalytic treatment.

The question is given added validity by the knowledge that puberty occurs earlier now than it did in the past.[30] This change in the biological timetable in the direction of a more rapid and elaborate maturation has been associated with improved nutrition and health care. At the same time, there has been a demand for more schooling over a longer period of time. These opposing pressures resulted in what has been perceived as the necessity for a longer and more complicated developmental stage in order to acquire what has been viewed as desirable education and training. The increasing discrepancy between biological timetables and social expectations appear to have intensified the conflicts and dilemmas of the adolescent in the 1970s.

Meanwhile, the psychoanalyst who works with an adolescent is sharply aware that internal psychological changes and conflicts continue as the youth copes with the developmental conflicts and the need to (1) relinquish childhood ties to parents and siblings, painfully opposed by the regressive attraction exerted by the revival of oedipal longings; (2) become aware of himself while striving to become an increasingly independent person, a process complicated by dependence on the persons against whom he feels compelled to rebel; (3) establish ties with new long-term friends while drifting apart from the "old" crowd of friends who provided much support during the earlier phases of adolescence; and (4) seek values and ideals that are his own, but which are often in conflict with powerful sexual and aggressive appetitive impulses.

These developmental conflicts and tasks of adolescence are responsive to a changing external and internal environment. Future psychoanalytic research will undoubtedly contribute to the efforts to better understand and appreciate our adolescents.

(The Narcissistic Personality

The treatment of character problems has become increasingly prominent in psychoanalysis. Among these is narcissism. People with a narcissistic personality seem to need and seek repetitive reinforcement of narcissistic supplies in order to maintain an inflated self-regard. They tend to use others for their own aggrandizement, with little if any feeling of guilt when they drop a person who no longer is expected to offer them any gains. They rarely truly depend on others. In spite of immense drive and productivity, their work is often empty and superficial. They appear to function well in society, and do not manifest any obvious neurotic symptoms or difficulties in controlling their impulses.

What is of interest here is the increasing success of analytic treatment for such people.[10,11,13,24] For example, Kernberg[11] describes the treatment of a twenty-year-old female who was initially diagnosed as having a "psychoneurotic reaction, mixed type," but who subsequently was found to have a narcissistic personality structure. The quality of her object relations, past and present, was crucial in the diagnosis. The intensity and chronicity of the patient's aloofness and estrangement was a result of a narcissistic withdrawal and denial of her pathological dependence. In this particular patient, Kernberg describes a characteristic transference paradigm: on the one hand the patient depreciated herself and felt worthless and guilty for all her extreme greediness and destructive fantasies; on the other hand, she denied and identified with her omnipotent ego ideal. Her narcissistic defenses were fully expressed and the intense negative transference was successfully analyzed. By the end of her treatment she had selected a man who permitted her to think of herself as attractive and wanted, and she began to think of herself as acceptable. Her professional activities had expanded, and she developed a more satisfactory social life.

The increased interest in persons with narcissistic characters, and the successful treatment of them, can be attributed to our broader and deeper knowledge in psychoanalysis of the complexity of ego development. Previous focus on the so-called transference neuroses was largely an outcome of earlier interest in the libido theory. The attention currently being paid to the treatment of the narcissistic character is a manifestation of the more recent developments in psychoanalysis, particularly in ego psychology and in studies of the vicissitudes in developing aggressive drives. Interestingly, the current importance given to the psychoanalytic treatment of character disorders coincides with the recent epidemiological shift in prevalence from neurotic disorders to character disturbances.

(The Underprivileged and Indigent Person

The rediscovery of psychoanalytic principles in the treatment of people who are underprivileged and indigent is particularly timely in the context of the burgeoning development of community psychiatry and community mental-health centers and programs. One example of this rediscovery is the work currently being done at the Tremont Crisis Center in New York under the direction of E. Hornick. Although called a "crisis" center, the treatment it offers to disturbed, underprivileged people is based on classical psychoanalytic principles and is highly effective.[14] Another example is the work being done with a lower income population in the so-called Blue Collar Project in New York under the direction of M.

Zaphiropoulos. Here, again, analytic principles guide the treatment of people in this restricted income group. The notion that psychoanalytically oriented treatment is the privilege of the well-to-do is thus outdated and unfounded.

These promising directions in psychoanalysis are particularly fortuitous in the face of current mental-health problems and trends. The need to provide service to large populations has sometimes prompted the innovation of treatment methods that remain to be tested. Hence the rediscovery of the value of psychoanalytic principles in treating the indigent and the underprivileged, who for so long have been denied adequate service, is particularly important.

❰ Bibliography

1. BLOS, P. *On Adolescence: A Psychoanalytic Interpretation.* New York: Free Press, 1962.
2. BURLINGHAM, D. "Some Notes on the Development of the Blind," in *The Psychoanalytic Study of the Child*, Vol. 16, pp. 121–145. New York: International Universities Press, 1961.
3. DEUTSCH, H. *Selected Problems of Adolescence.* New York: International Universities Press, 1967.
4. ELMER, E. and G. S. GREGG. "Developmental Characteristics of Abused Children," *Pediatrics*, 40 (1967), 596–602.
5. ESCALONA, S. K. *The Roots of Individuality: Normal Patterns of Development.* Chicago: Aldine-Atherton, 1969.
6. FRAIBERG, S. and D. A. FREEDMAN. "Studies in the Ego Development of the Congenitally Blind Child," in *The Psychoanalytic Study of the Child*, Vol. 19, pp. 113–169. New York: International Universities Press, 1964.
7. FREUD, A. *The Ego and the Mechanism of Defense.* New York: International Universities Press, 1946.
8. ———. "Adolescence," in *The Psychoanalytic Study of the Child*, Vol. 13, pp. 255–278. New York: International Universities Press, 1958.
9. ———. "Adolescence as a Developmental Disturbance," in G. Caplan and S. Lebovici, eds., *Adolescence*, pp. 5–10. New York: Basic Books, 1969.
10. KERNBERG, O. "Factors in the Psychoanalytic Treatment of Narcissistic Personalities," *J. Am. Psychoanal. Assoc.*, 18 (1970), 51–85.
11. KERNBERG, P. F. "The Course of the Analysis of a Narcissistic Personality with Hysterical and Compulsive Features," *J. Am. Psychoanal. Assoc.*, 19 (1971), 451–571.
12. KLEIN, G. S. "Blindness and Isolation," in *The Psychoanalytic Study of the Child*, Vol. 17, pp. 82–93. New York: International Universities Press, 1962.
13. KOHUT, H. "The Psychoanalytic Treatment of Narcissistic Personality Disorders. Outline of a Systematic Approach," in *The Psychoanalytic Study of the Child*, Vol. 23, pp. 87–113. New York: International Universities Press, 1968.
14. LEFER, J. Personal communications, 1971.
15. LEONARD, M. F., J. P. RHYMES, and A. J. SOLNIT. "Failure to Thrive in Infants," *Am. J. Dis. Child.*, 3 (1966), 600–612.
16. LEWIS, M., A. J. SOLNIT, M. H. STARK et al. "An Exploratory Study of Accidental Ingestion of Poison in Young Children," *J. Am. Acad. Child. Psychiatry*, 5 (1966), 255–271.
17. MAHLER, M. S. "Thoughts about Development and Individuation," in *The Psychoanalytic Study of the Child*, Vol. 18, pp. 307–324. New York: International Universities Press, 1963.
18. ———. "A Study of the Separation-Individuation Process: And Its Possible Application to Borderline Phenomena in the Psychoanalytic Situation," in *The Psychoanalytic Study of the Child*, Vol. 26, pp. 403–424. New York: International Universities Press, 1971.
19. OMWAKE, E. G. and A. J. SOLNIT. " 'It isn't fair.' The Treatment of a Blind Child," in *The Psychoanalytic Study of the Child*, Vol. 16, pp. 352–404. New York: International Universities Press, 1961.
20. PIAGET, J. *The Construction of Reality in the Child*, p. 12. New York: Basic Books, 1954.
21. PROVENCE, S. and R. LIPTON. *Infants in Institutions.* New York: International Universities Press, 1962.
22. RIBBLE, M. A. *The Rights of Infants.* New York: Columbia University Press, 1943.
23. ———. "Infantile Experience in Relation to Personality Experience," in J. McV. Hunt, ed., *Personality and the Behavior Dis-*

orders, pp. 621–651. New York: Ronald, 1944.

24. ROSENFELD, H. A. "On the Psychopathology of Narcissism: A Clinical Approach," in H. A. Rosenfeld, ed., *Psychotic States*, pp. 169–170. New York: International Universities Press, 1964.

25. SANDLER, A. M. "Aspects of Passivity and Ego Development in the Blind Infant," in *The Psychoanalytic Study of the Child*, Vol. 18, pp. 343–361. New York: International Universities Press, 1963.

26. SOLNIT, A. J. "Adolescence and the Changing Reality," in Irwin M. Marcus, ed., *Currents in Psychoanalysis*, pp. 98–110. New York: International Universities Press, 1972.

27. SPITZ, R. A. "Hospitalism: An Inquiry into the Genesis of Psychiatric Conditions in Early Childhood," in *The Psychoanalytic Study of the Child*, Vol. 1, pp. 53–74. New York: International Universities Press, 1945.

28. ———. "Hospitalism: A Follow-up Report," in *The Psychoanalytic Study of the Child*, Vol. 2, pp. 113–117. New York: International Universities Press, 1946.

29. SPITZ, R. A. and K. M. WOLF. "Anaclitic Depression: An Inquiry into the Genesis of Psychiatric Conditions in Early Childhood," in *The Psychoanalytic Study of the Child*, Vol. 2, pp. 313–342. New York: International Universities Press, 1946.

30. TANNER, J. M. *Growth at Adolescence*. Springfield, Ill.: Charles C. Thomas, 1962.

31. WOLFF, P. H. and M. A. SIMMONS. "Nonnutritive Sucking and Response Thresholds in Young Infants," *Child Dev.*, 38 (1967), 631–638.

32. ZAPHIROPOULOS, M. L. and L. CALIGOR. "Providing Organized Limited Income Groups with Mental Health Resources—Problems and Possibilities," *Conference Proceedings*, pp. 21–29. Oil City, Pa.: Psychiatric Outpatient Centers of America, 1966.

CHAPTER 30

NEW DIRECTIONS IN
GROUP THERAPY

Irvin D. Yalom

WHAT OF the future of group therapy? Group psychotherapists at the meetings of national professional associations may choose from an arresting display of training opportunities. A sprinkling of workshop titles[1] will provide us with the flavor of current directions: Marathon Group Therapy, Integrating Encounter and Gestalt Techniques into Analytic Group Therapy, Body-movement in Group Therapy, Multifamily Group Therapy, Marital Group Therapy, Video-tape Playback Group Therapy, Transactional Analysis and Contract Psychotherapy in Groups, Nude Marathon Group Therapy, Psychodrama in Groups, Non-verbal, Gestalt, and Encounter Games in Group Therapy.

If each of these approaches represents a substantial new trend, then there is scarcely any keeping abreast of the group-therapy field, much less in foreseeing future directions. It is my opinion, however, that these new developments do not constitute a coherent intellectual thrust; rather than prefigure the future they resemble more the aimless whirlings of a broken mechanical toy, more a flamboyant proliferation than a Renaissance. If this is true, then an interesting question arises: why has the youthful and robust group-therapy movement passed so quickly into a high-baroque phase? This chapter will address itself to this question and will then attempt to describe those foundations of group therapy which are likely to survive and shape the substance, if not the form, of the field of the future.

(The Baroque Period
in Group Therapy:
Evolution and Explanation

We gain better perspective of the field by examining the rather brief history of the evolution of group psychotherapy. Although for centuries the group has intuitively been used for support and succor of troubled individuals, the first explicit systematic attempts to harness the potential power of the small group for psychotherapeutic purposes occurred in the 1920s and 1930s. The technique was wrenched untimely from its adolescence by the advent of World War II. Group therapy's growth spurt was driven by an economic piston: the large number of military psychiatric patients and the small number of trained psychotherapists urged an immediate and widespread use of groups as a psychotherapeutic method. In the following years there was considerable attention paid to the application of small groups for different types of patients and in different clinical settings: groups were used in inpatient and outpatient clinics, in day hospitals, in prisons, in schools, in family service agencies, in psychoanalysts' private offices as well as on the back wards of state hospitals. Theoreticians—Freudian, Sullivanean, Horneyan, Rogerian—explored the application of their conceptual framework to the theory and practice of group therapy. The differences between the different approaches to group therapy thus paralleled the differences between the theoretical schools from which they sprang.

A major shift in the practice of group therapy occurred in the mid-1960s when the group-therapy tradition collided with a related but parallel and separate stream—the encounter-group movement.

"Encounter group" is a rough generic term under which may be classified a large number of group approaches. Examples may be gleaned from university bulletin boards, growth centers such as Esalen, free university catalogues, and mountains of second-class mail pamphlets. We know them by such names as t-groups, NTL groups, human-relations groups, human-potential groups, and personal-growth groups. Despite the colorful and varied nomenclature, these groups share several features. They are generally small enough (six to twenty members) to permit considerable face-to-face interaction; they focus on the here-and-now (e.g., the behavior of the members as it unfolds in the group); they encourage openness, honesty, interpersonal confrontation, and self-disclosure; they

encourage strong emotional expression; the participants are not usually labeled "patients," the experience is not ordinarily labeled "therapy"; the groups do strive, however, to increase awareness and to change behavior. The explicit goals of the groups may vary, and although occasionally they seek only to entertain, to "turn on," to provide joy, they generally strive toward some type of personal change—change of behavior, of attitudes, of values, or of life style.

The current term for these groups is encounter group. The older, superannuated term is "human-relations-training group (t-group)." The transition from one label to the other represents symbolically the evolution of the trend which some have referred to as the encounter group social movement.

The prototype of the present-day encounter group took place in 1946 when a group of social psychologists and educators first realized that an experimental group experience was a powerful way of teaching human relations. Members of the groups were helped to acquire interpersonal skills in the basic human-relations training group (which was later shortened to t-group, the "t" for training) or sensitivity group (for training in interpersonal sensitivity). A large organization—the National Training Laboratories—evolved, which sponsored large numbers of training groups for individuals to undergo a personal learning experience. T-group leaders described concepts such as "feedback" (the giving and receiving of interpersonal perceptions), the observer–participant role (studying that process of which one is a member) and designed some highly imaginative group techniques or exercises to accelerate development or explicate the dynamics of the group. Industrial organizations soon learned that it was good to have individuals in key personnel positions who had highly developed interpersonal abilities. Indeed, industry also discovered that large-scale organizational problems could be reduced through a group approach. For example, a unit with low morale, low productivity, high absenteeism, and personal turnover could be helped by holding a laboratory in which the entire unit could meet together in a group in order to work through the interpersonal friction so often underlying organizational conflict. A number of other institutions, for example, departments of education, organized religion, as well as agencies of local and federal government, began to utilize the experimental small group as a basic mode of lubricating organizational development.

The modern, swinging, let-it-all-hang-out encounter group appeared as a speck on the horizon early in the 1960s and derived from many sources. One important development occurred when several West Coast group leaders boldly questioned the concept of "education." Till then the goal of human-relations education had been the acquisition of interpersonal and leadership skills. Some leaders proposed a broader and humanistically based redefinition of education. Education, they argued, was synonomous with personal growth; the true educator helps each student discover and mine his hidden untapped resources. The emphasis thus shifted from technical education—from learning about group dynamics —to self-discovery and to the development of one's full potential. The groups were renamed personal-growth groups and later by Carl Rogers, the "basic encounter group."

I do not mean to imply that the encounter group has a single source, for the evolution from the human-relations training group to the personal growth or encounter group is as much manifestation as cause. California in the 1960s provided fertile soil for the cultivation of any experience that promised intimacy and a sense of community. For nowhere else had there been a more inexorable deconstitution of traditional, stabilizing, intimacy-sponsoring institutions. The extended as well as the nuclear family, the stable neighborhood or work group, the local merchants, the home-visiting general practioner, the neighborhood church —all had fallen prey to the demands of progress and a runaway technocracy. The small group thus masqueraded as a well of intimacy: one small oasis where people could drop the facades demanded by a fast-moving, competitive society and confront themselves and others with all the fears and doubts of the basic human condition.

The "third force" in psychology that emphasized a holistic humanistic concept of the person provided impetus for the personal-growth group from yet another direction. Psychologists such as Abraham Maslow eloquently argued for the need of a "liberating model" in addition to or instead of a teaching or a therapy model. Other derivative streams arose simultaneously but independently from the same soil: Synanon, gestalt therapy, the marathon, alternative life-style systems. They suggested that we are all patients. The disease is an uncontrolled, dehumanizing, technocratic culture, the remedy is a return to grappling with basic problems of the human condition, the vehicle of the treatment is ideally the small group that becomes "group therapy for normals." The differentiation between mental illness and health grew as vague as the distinction between treatment and education. Personal-growth group leaders claimed at the same time that patienthood is ubiquitous and that one need not be sick to get better.

The inevitable confluence or, as some would have it, collision between the two fields is by now readily apparent to the reader. With personal-growth group techniques purporting to offer group therapy for normals and with the "patienthood" label becoming ever increasingly relativistic, considerable confusion ensued.

Although in its first decade the t-group was generally led by an educator or social psychologist, recent years have seen the influx of an increasing number of clinicians into the field. Many psychotherapists were participants in t-groups and subsequently became t-group leaders, using these techniques in groups in their consultation work and in their teaching. Many have been impressed with the apparent potency of a number of t-group techniques and have applied these in their psychotherapeutic work. (We shall discuss some of these techniques in detail later in this chapter.)

A reciprocal development has occurred amongst encounter-group leaders who have had no specific clinical training, but whose experience has suggested to them that members of their group had therapeutic experiences and that, in fact, there was no difference between the psychotherapy group and the encounter group. Accordingly, many growth centers either intentionally or unwittingly advertised their groups in such a manner as to attract individuals with rather significant emotional problems, whose hopes for immediate, near-miraculous relief were augmented by an encounter-group mystique suggesting that it could condense months, even years, of psychotherapeutic work into a single, prolonged, intensive group experience. Many psychotherapists reacted vigorously to this development, not only because of such substantive issues as the incumbent risk and the ethical breech in offering more than could be delivered but also in fear of an invasion of their professional territorial rights. Indeed, in some sections of the country, the encounter-group network has served as an auxiliary mental-health system. One suspects that a very significant number of troubled individuals enter some type of small personal-growth group who, only a few years ago, would have applied for help from a traditional mental-health resource.

Of course, scurrying in between these tumbling pillars was the confused would-be patient, who was faced, on the one hand, with the mass-media promulgation of the effectiveness of encounter groups, and, on the other hand, with the medical professions warnings of high risks, but, nevertheless, themselves offering a profusion of varying group formats, many of which were indistinguishable from encounter-group approaches.

Some relevant research may rescue us from this quagmire of claims and counterclaims. My colleagues and I reported in 1972[3] the results of a large-scale research project that studied the process and outcome of encounter groups. The overall study is reported in detail elsewhere, but I shall describe some of the findings that are relevant to this discussion. We studied the leader behavior, the group process, and the short and long-term outcome of eighteen encounter groups representing ten different ideological schools: gestalt therapy, transactional analysis, t-groups (traditional human-relations or sensitivity groups), personal-growth groups (West Coast version of human-relations groups with the emphasis on

intrapersonal growth rather than on primarily interpersonal and group-dynamic learning), Synanon, psychoanalytically oriented encounter groups, marathon groups led basically in a Rogerian style, psychodrama groups, sensory awareness (Esalen groups) and encounter tape groups (these groups had no formal leader except for a tape recorder that each meeting provided the members with procedural instructions).

The leaders were all highly seasoned professionals, all had many years experience in the field, and many had national reputations. The subjects were Stanford University undergraduate students between the ages of eighteen and twenty-two. Each group lasted a total of thirty hours, some in a massed format with two or three time-extended (marathon) meetings. Others had shorter meetings, spaced approximately one week apart. Leader behavior was studied by trained observers who coded all their behavior during the groups, by questionnaires filled out by participants, and by transcripts of the meetings in which leader-verbatim comments were recorded. Outcome of the groups was measured by a massive battery of outcome instruments, including self-administered questionnaires, evaluations by friends and members of their social network, ratings by other group members, ratings by the leader, and from a number of other perspectives such as school performance, life decisions, etc.

Let us turn to several aspects of the results that are relevant. The research indicated that the encounter groups studied were all in all (comparing all the encounter-group participants with a large control population) ineffective change agents. When compared, for example, with well-designed outcome psychotherapy studies, the encounter groups produced far less positive change and more negative change ("casualties") than traditional therapy. We recognize that comparisons of this sort are risky—the participants of these groups did not enter as patients. The outcome measures were similar but not entirely comparable to psychotherapy outcome measures. The psychotherapy studies used as comparisons are individual psychotherapy studies, not group psychotherapy studies (there are no rigorous outcome studies on group psychotherapy). Nevertheless, despite these qualifications, there was convincing evidence to prove that, regardless of the criterion used, the encounter groups were nonproductive agents of change.

We do not suggest that, by other criteria, the groups were not "successful." The overwhelming majority of the participants liked the groups. They found the experience exciting, interesting, and often compelling. The groups were potent in that they aroused strong emotions and, for a small minority of individuals, they were successful in contributing to a very pronounced and very positive shift on a number of important outcome dimensions.

Another finding was that the ideological school to which leaders belonged told us little about the actual behavior of the leader in the group. We found that the behavior of the leader from one school—for example, transactional analysis—resembled that of another leader from the same school no more than it resembled the behavior of any of the other seventeen leaders. This finding was a general one. It leads to the rather obvious conclusion that one can know what a group leader does only by observing his behavior, which is not predictable from what he says, he does, or from his membership in a particular ideological school.

Although, in general, the members of the encounter groups did not experience significant positive change, there were, nonetheless, some very striking differences in outcome among the eighteen groups. Some groups were so ineffective that none of the participants experienced positive change and several experienced some type of negative result; other groups were so effective that the great majority of individuals experienced positive results and no members underwent any negative change. From the foregoing it is clear that the effectiveness of the leader is not a function of his ideological school but is very much a function of his behavior in the group. We constructed a new leader typology based on actual leader behavior and were able to demon-

strate that certain leader "types" were highly correlated with certain outcome patterns. The "provider" (the leader who provides both high-positive support and a considerable cognitive framework) for example, is likely to lead a high-yield, low-risk group, while the "energizer" (the leader who is highly charismatic, both highly supportive and attacking, very active, and very personally revealing) is likely to lead a high-risk and a moderate-to-low-yield group.

A study of the actual process of change in the participants was singularly illuminating. In brief, the research revealed that change does not revolve around the solitary sun of the leader; the data provided strong evidence that psychosocial relations in the group played an exceedingly important role in the process of change. For example, individuals in a role that included high influence, activity, and high-value congruence tended to have high-positive outcome, whereas members with low scores on this role tended to have low or casualty outcome. Members with little attraction to the group rarely finished with a positive outcome. Members who misperceived group norms or who were considered deviant by other members were quite likely to have had a negative-learning experience. In short, there were many factors, powerfully influencing the change process, that occurred in the substratum of the group outside of the leader's level of awareness.

The vast majority of the encounter-group leaders attributed far too much importance to their direct contribution, to their immediate effect on each of the members of the group. They placed paramount importance on their personal ability to offer members insight, to confront, to stimulate, to challenge, to help members become aware of their feelings, to help members reveal themselves, to help them become "in touch with" their body. We found, however, that the effective leader intuitively augments the psychosocial forces at work. He helps to create a group that is a potent agent of change and an atmosphere within that group which encourages the type of support, trust, and acceptance so necessary to the change process. We say that the leader "intuitively" performs these tasks. By and large, he is unaware of the importance of these indirect functions. Most leaders fashion their style and their theory of change on their own personal observations of their groups. Given the invisibility (without some type of systematic inquiry) of these indirect factors, it is not surprising that they have not been appreciated in most leadership approaches. The research suggests, therefore, that some leaders may be exceedingly competent but have no accurate appreciation of the factors responsible for their success.

At this point we have come full circle to the query that launched this discussion: *why has the group-therapy movement passed so quickly into a high-baroque phase?* Part of the answer lies precisely in the fact that so many effective leaders are unaware of the reasons for their effectiveness. The sequence of events is often that the leader, through varied and often haphazard feedback mechanisms, grows convinced of his effectiveness. He then commences to transmit his skills to students, but passes on those techniques which he consciously conceptualizes and fails to transmit his intuitive, unconscious appreciation and utilization of many of the potent psychosocial forces that are of such fundamental importance. Too often he transmits only epiphenomenal behavior—behavioral characteristics that are idiosyncratic and largely irrelevant to his effective outcome. Consider one specific illustration. In the research described above, many of the leaders were deeply convinced of the efficacy of the "hot-seat" approach. This methodology consists of focusing the entire energy of the group on one person, who may literally sit in a designed chair for long periods of time. It was striking, however, to note that the results indicated that the use of the hot-seat technique was totally uncorrelated to positive outcome. Some of the most effective leaders and some of the least effective leaders were heavily committed to its use. The identical point can be made about a number of other highly prized leadership techniques, like the emphasis on extremely intensive expression of emotions, high self-disclosure, marathon meetings or specific theoretical constructs

such as gestalt therapy or transactional analysis. (It was striking to note, for example, that one of the most successful leaders and one of the least successful leaders were gestalt therapists.)

The problem is compounded even further by the difficulties inherent in assessing outcome. Group leaders may be exceedingly poor judges of their success or failure. (Our research demonstrated that the group leaders were particularly ineffective in noting which members had a negative experience.) Two major reasons for the leaders' poor evaluative marksmanship are selective inattention and efficacy–potency confusion. Time pressures and attention to the group as a whole often do not permit the group leader to collect the necessary information to make accurate judgments of the progress of each of his group members. Furthermore, there is a widespread tendency on the part of group leaders as well as group members to mistake potency for efficacy. Only rarely does it occur that a small experiential group does not provide a moving, emotionally "potent" experience for the participants. Groups mobilize a wide array of powerful feelings such as closeness, competition, rivalry, trust, dependency, and anger. The arousal of strong affects seems to be a necessary prerequisite, but it is not synonymous with change. We undergo strong emotional experiences all our lives without personal change ensuing. The relevant point, however, is that it is not difficult for ineffective leaders to mistake other attributes of their group for success, and once convinced of their competence they will accordingly attempt to transmit *their* techniques to their students.

Thus, the field has many therapists, most of whom are unaware of the reasons for their effectiveness and some of whom are erroneously convinced of their effectiveness. These phenomena occur against a horizon of general dissatisfaction with therapeutic outcome: all the therapy approaches appear relatively ineffective or, more charitably, so equally effective that no single method can prove its substantially superior results.

The next developmental step is the establishment of ideological systems and training centers. Leaders who found systems and training centers are powered by complex motivations: an estimable sense of responsibility to teach others a method of treatment in which they deeply believe, or such personal factors as a search for glory, symbolic immortality, or the adulation of students to atone for too little or too tardy gratification from patients or colleagues.

The ideological schools do not usually suffer from a lack of disciples. Just as nature abhors a material vacuum, so do we detest ideational randomness. Therapists are too often faced with an overload of inchoate data that produce intolerable uncertainty: Any system that offers a parsimonious and easily comprehensible explanation for the bulk of the clinical data is very welcome—the closed system, for example, a tight psychoanalytic framework, or transactional analysis, which offers an explanatory haven for all data, is manna indeed.

We have, I hope, come sufficiently far to lay bare many of the reasons behind the rich and varied plummage of the new group-therapy approaches.

One final point about certain common features of most of the new group approaches: they seem to me to be impregnated with impatience and they characteristically express a highly fractionated or nonholistic view of psychotherapeutic change.

I sense a pervasive impatience in many of the new approaches, impatience with traditional approaches, with delayed results, with subtle changes, with recycling and working through, and with cognitive, verbal approaches. Leaders look for, even demand, change *now*. Impatience shapes many of the newer techniques. Members are guided, beseeched, even coerced to "get in touch with their feelings." If affect is not present, it is provided by potent means of stimulation. Leaders incessantly search for the "breakthrough," that elusive will-of-the-wisp of the encounter groups; long-term credit is not extended, a sign of change is required at the moment—tears, a marked change in behavior or some outward evidence of a significant inner shift. Change is hoped for, not over

months, but in a single day or weekend in the course of a single time-extended group meeting.

Fractionation is kin to impatience and both are offspring of a crash program, cost-accounting, technique-oriented mentality so peculiarly American. If self-disclosure is an integral part of the change process and is easily and quickly facilitated by group techniques, then an entire therapeutic approach—nude group therapy—is designed around an axis of disclosure both psychical and physical. The same holds for affect unblocking: If expression of anger is important, then why not a group therapy, like Synanon, in which the change process centers around rage release—indeed, one therapist refers to his approach as psychological karate. If people are alienated, out of touch, then why not foster a love group that endeavors to provide the quintessence of love and touching and closeness.

The cost is paid both by leader and participant. If the participant has come to believe that improvement is rapid, dramatic, and mediated via the breakthrough, then he will have cause to leave the group more discouraged than ever about achieving change. The therapist, if he is to avoid despair, will not permit himself full knowledge of the outcome of his efforts; instead he titrates his awareness of results by filtering his outcome observations. Lack of full success may beget such acceleration of vigorous healing efforts that he joins the ranks of such breakthrough revivalists as primal screamers, bioenergeticists or Rolfers.

⟮ Basic Foundations of Group Therapy

Although the torrent of technical innovations has swept away much of the formal edifice of group therapy, the basic theoretical foundations remain unchanged. If you believe, as I do, that there exists a finite and substantive set of mechanisms of change in psychotherapy, then it follows that technical approaches must be elaborated and understood against a horizon of these change mechanisms. Psychotherapy, precisely because it is a human experience, offers a rich array of opportunities for change, and the group-therapy experience, in particular, provides complex and varied therapeutic possibilities.

Perhaps we can best explicate the mechanisms of change in group therapy by first examining the more elemental question: why group therapy? There was a time when we might have answered the question in economic terms; after all if one therapist can treat seven or eight patients in ninety minutes, then why spend fifty minutes with one patient? The economic lure is a compelling one because our national mental-health needs demand that psychotherapists not only become more effective but more effective per unit of time.

Although economy may have been, in part, midwife to the group-therapy technique, the offspring has been an unruly one; group therapy is less a bargain than it seems. Most therapists prefer to work with a cotherapist, thus, in one step, halving the economic advantage. Groups are invariably more emotionally demanding: it is the rare therapist who can lead more than one to two groups a day. There are limits upon the total number of patients, with accompanying names, histories, characterologic constellations, and demands, that a therapist can comfortably maintain in his *Lebenswelt*. Group therapy offers no substantial temporal advantages in that the total length of treatment in group therapy is no less than individual therapy. Although there are some therapists who have attempted brief group therapy on a crisis-intervention model, they have not demonstrated its efficacy and, for the most part, group therapy remains relatively long-term therapy.

Some have argued that the small group experience is so compelling and so intrinsically therapeutic that leaders require comparatively little training. This point of view issues from the erroneous equating of potency and effectiveness, to which I alluded above. It is true that groups will generally develop into systems that evoke powerful emotions; often it seems to me that only a particularly misguided leader can obstruct the development of many features of the intensive group experience. It

is also true, however, that a powerful experience can be bivalenced: It can result in negative as well as positive therapeutic outcome. A recent study of encounter groups[1] demonstrated an alarmingly high casualty rate: approximately 10 percent of college students who participated in an encounter group that lasted a total of thirty hours suffered some form of enduring negative psychological outcome. Group therapy, no less than any psychotherapeutic method, is not a do-it-yourself endeavor; careful training is required and, unfortunately, the necessary training is too rarely available in traditional psychotherapy training centers.

No, it is not economy that affords an explanation: economic considerations provide neither the raison d'être nor the theoretical underpinnings of group therapy. "Why group therapy" must be answered, not from the perspective of an inexpensive and diluted individual therapy but from the position that there are unique therapeutic opportunities inherent in the small group modality.

A theory of group therapy begins with the proposition that man is deeply embedded in an interpersonal matrix: he is first socialized in his primary family group, then in his elementary peer group, and eventually in a interpersonal megasociety. He is surrounded by other individuals who hear him, see him, and relay back to him their impressions of him; eventually, he must learn to befriend, to love, to fear, to understand, and to gain the approval of others. From within he is to a large extent constituted by the reflected appraisals of others; his sense of personal worth has been shaped from the perceived approval of others. Internally he will eternally interact with the introjected phantoms of the significant early figures in his life.

I do not imply that man is nothing but an interpersonal being; he is also alone, and, to some extent, must live and certainly die alone; not only is he a being who is treated and shaped by others in accordance with established principles of learning theory, but he is also a constituting ego, creating a highly personal and never entirely predictable experiential world. However, even given those aspects which transcend man's interpersonal nature, few will quarrel with the heuristic value of conceptualizing personality theory and therapy as an interpersonal process.

When the group therapist operates out of the interpersonal position, he views every individual who seeks professional psychotherapeutic help as having an underlying and fundamental, interpersonal problem: an inability to establish or to maintain fully gratifying interpersonal relationships. The problem often manifests itself explicitly as patients describe their shattered relationship with a spouse, or their general alienation from others, their fears of the opposite sex, or their inability to be assertive. Sometimes the therapist must interpolate: the patient describes his dilemma as a problem in his relationship to a thing or a situation, for example, a phobia of driving, a depression, gastric distress, test anxiety. In each instance the therapist, in his early sessions with the prospective group patient, must lay bare the interpersonal "meaning" of his problem with a thing: the patient who feared driving "really" was expressing his distrust of others and even more his rage toward others as he experienced a compelling and murderous desire to collide with another car; the depressed person was in despair over the loss of another; the gastric disorder represented anger and frustration toward others in an individual whose other affective expressive channels were blocked; the test anxiety reflected both the need and the fear of a vindictive triumph over others. Thus, in each instance, the therapist translated the thing or situation conflict into an interpersonal issue. The patients will do the same, for, as time elapses in the group, they reveal in their relationships with the other members their anger, mistrust, frustrations, inhibitions, morbid dependency, and conflicting feelings toward competition.

At the risk of belaboring the issue, I wish to emphasize that we must put quotes around "meaning" of symptoms, or what is "really" the source of the patient's problems. We can never really know the primordial, the true explanation for psychopathology. We can, however, formulate hypotheses assumptively and then gauge the explanatory power of the hypothesis and the efficacy of its practical application. The obfuscation, the reductionism, and the sectarian warfare occur when we forget the assumptive basis of the formulation and begin to regard such entities as ego, superego and id, parent, child and adult, animus, and anima as archetypes, and masculine protests as concrete entities rather than what they are: concepts, created for our intellectual and semantic convenience, that allow us to order data in a ready way and to formulate coherent approaches to therapy. Nor do I regard these constructs as expendable; some organizing system is essential for every therapist, lest he sink into the despair of perpetual uncertainty and nihilism. Thus, the ideological frame of reference conceals, yet makes possible the successful therapeutic experience.

Once we have resolved that the interpersonal frame of reference is a viable approach and that, as Sullivan put it: "Psychiatry is the study of processes that involve or go on between people"[4] and that "one achieves mental health to the extent that one becomes aware of one's interpersonal relationships,"[5] then we can appreciate the fact that the small group is an ideal vehicle of change. Few other situations offer such an arena for the display and correction of interpersonal pathology.

Thus, I choose to answer the question "Why Group Therapy?" by pointing out that the small group provides the logical clinical application of the interpersonal theory of personality development and psychopathology. One uses the therapy group most effectively to the extent that one maximizes the opportunities for interpersonal learning in small groups.

But let us be more specific: the group permits, first, a display and then a correction of interpersonal pathology. The display of pathology is a naturally unfolding process; a group with relatively few structural restrictions will ultimately develop into a social microcosm of the participant members. An individual who is, for example, vain or selfish or obsequious or exploitative or distant or controlling or disdainful in his relationships with the individuals in his social environment will eventually demonstrate those very traits in his relationship to the members and the leader of the group. Sometimes this behavior is immediately apparent: an extremely narcissistic or dependent or arrogant individual may blatantly manifest these traits in his first interactions with the group members. Sometimes the interpersonal behavior pattern takes months to unfold; for example, as in the case of an individual who subtly seduces and then exploits others or who gains the confidence of another only as a preliminary stage in a campaign to defeat him or, in the case of another, who ostensibly seeks closeness only, ultimately, to flee from it. One of the major tasks of clinical group-therapy training is to enable the therapist to recognize these maladaptive interpersonal patterns.

A necessary condition for the display of interpersonal pathology is a focus on the "here-and-now." The here-and-now has two parameters: a basic ahistoric approach and an alternating pattern of de-reflection and self-reflection. The ahistoric approach in group therapy is merely a position assumed toward the question of evidence. It argues that no more valid data exist than the actual behavior of an individual in the group. There is little need for a patient to describe the past history of his disordered interpersonal relationships since he will, unwittingly, display it with great accuracy in the present tense of the group.

De-reflection and self-reflection refer to the alternating sequence of, on the one hand, spontaneous unselfconscious interaction that must occur in the group if it is to be a vital experience and, on the other hand, a "stopping the action," a purposeful, intermittent reflection about behavior that has transpired so recently that, like a "ghost" on a television screen, it is still in the room.

The here-and-now has many fringe benefits, chiefly those of increasing the affect level of the group and sustaining the interest of all the members. The more members discuss issues of common interest, the more centripetal force is generated drawing them into the center of the group. Conversely, the more members discuss the then-and-there material from their historical past or from current interactions with individuals outside the group, the more uninvolved and unhelpful other patients will feel.

When sufficient displays of behavior have occurred that therapists and patients (generally, but not always, in that order) recognize as important and recurrent maladaptive interpersonal patterns, then the explicit process of correction begins. (The *implicit* process of correction begins at the very first meeting in a variety of indirect ways we shall discuss shortly.) The patient gradually becomes aware of his interaction through a feedback process in which the therapists and other members inform him of his behavior. This is a multifaceted process, as the others not only inform him of his blind areas (aspects of himself visible to others but not to self) but also of their reaction to his behavior. It is one thing to learn, for example, that others see you as arrogant and judgmental; it is another thing to learn that this causes others to feel insecure and distrustful and thus precludes their developing a close, warm relationship with you.

Awareness of one's own behavior is not a step-wise procedure but a spiral one, in which the individual circles about himself repeatedly and first rejects, then partially accepts, and then fully integrates the feedback of the other members. Even then many raise the issue of relevance: for example, they may question the relevance of their interpersonal behavior for the problems that brought them to therapy or they may question the importance to them of the opinion of a group of strangers. If the group has developed an optimal level of cohesiveness and if the leader has been lucid in his interpolation of symptom into interpersonal pathology, then the issue of relevance may be dealt with as the resistance it represents.

Many other complex issues are involved in the change process, most of them far beyond the scope of this essay. One crucial, and core, constellation is "Do I wish to?" "Do I dare to?" "Can I?"

Many have invested much of their behavior with considerable pride: they are proud of being above others, or of being always right, or of being beloved by all, or of being beyond or impervious to the needs or wishes of others. Much of the hard work of therapy consists in helping individuals realize the full implications, for themselves and for others, of their behavior. Only when one fully appreciates the primary dysphoria resulting from self-destructive behavior or the secondary dysphoria that is a reaction to the pain, withdrawal, or disapproval experienced by others in response to one's behavior, can one seriously confront the question "do I want to be like that?" "do I want to affect myself and others in this way?"

For many individuals maladaptive behavior is, nonetheless, better than some fantasied calamity that would ensue were they to behave differently. Though the feared calamity is often unconscious, it may be a ruthless tyrant dictating one's behavior. If, for example, at some level of awareness an individual fears that, were he to open the gates of his aggressive feelings, he might commit murder or were he to allow himself to experience his needs for tenderness, he would either be rejected or engulfed, then he would bury the possibility of the feared calamity by, in the first instance, ever-vigilant politeness and considerateness, in the second, by a communicated aloofness and freedom from needing others to touch him. The group helps such an individual "dare to" by encouraging or permitting risk taking, by helping him sample, ever so faintly, the feelings and behavior he has so assiduously and for so long eschewed. After repeated daring to, in the presence of others who matter to him and without the occurrence of the feared consequences, the behavior and attitudinal change become enduring. The process may be abetted by interpretation, by the individual's conscious awareness of the heretofore unconscious conflict, but there is reason to believe that the behavior change may occur even in the absence of such insight.

"Can I" is inextricably interwoven into the psychotherapeutic process and brings us face to face with the unspeakable paradox in psychoanalytic theory: that the process of therapy brings the patient to the point where he can make a choice in his own best interests and yet at the same time he is, from the very first, totally determined. In group therapy, we take the best from both worlds: determinism is transformed into "understanding" and "I can't" into "I won't." By fully knowing the developmental and the current dynamic roots of an individual's behavior, even the most offensive presentation of self can be understood and, as Montaigne reminded us four centuries ago, to understand all is to forgive all. In the group, forgiveness, or a non-judgmental acceptance, makes it possible for individuals to interact in novel ways without the vicious spiral of offensive behavior and resultant rejection that ignites further defensive–offensive behavior. Acceptance in a therapy group is never forever; people are accepted, behavior is criticized. The global, intellectualized "Can I change?" dissolves in the unending group stream of small but meaningful changes observable in each of the group members.

To summarize, small groups offer an excellent treatment vehicle because they allow the display and correction of specific maladaptive interpersonal behavior. They offer, in addition, a number of avenues for change. For example, the experience of belonging to and being valued by a group is, for many individuals, a significant ameliorative life event. Many troubled individuals have a lifelong history of group deprivation: the stable nuclear family, the extended kinship unit, the childhood peer group, adolescent social cliques, athletic teams, neighborhood groups, dating courtship circles—all have passed them by. For these individuals the sheer experience of being accepted and valued members of a group may, even in the absence of cognitive gains, powerfully affect their self-acceptance and their sense of personal worth.

The amount of attraction to the group shared by all the members is often referred to as cohesiveness and is the group-therapy analogue of "relationship" in individual therapy. Little effective work can be done in its absence. Groups with low cohesiveness will have less trust, less self-disclosure, poor attendance, and, eventually, poorer outcome. Members with low attraction to the group, even measured early in the course of the group by a simple paper and pencil questionnaire, have little likelihood of achieving positive gain.

An individual's self-esteem is closely related to his perception of his public esteem; to a significant degree, he remains concerned and influenced by the evaluation given him by groups to which he belongs. How much the group influences self-esteem is dependent on several factors: the stability of his own sense of worth, the importance of the group to him; the specificity, frequency, and saliency of the group's communications that bear on his self-esteem. Most individuals seeking psychotherapeutic help have considerable difficulty in maintaining their sense of self-worth; many experience their self-esteem as a bobbing balloon, prey to the winds of others' judgments. If an individual repeatedly experiences a discrepancy between his sense of personal worth and the group's various appraisals of him, then eventually he must resolve this dissonance. If, for example, the group values him more highly than he values himself, he might question the value of this group or their basis for judgment. He might think, "If they only knew" or reinterpret the group's comments to his disadvantage. In a well-integrated therapy group the individual values the judgments of the other members. He has been through a great deal with them, their feedback to him is explicit, and he can scarcely question their basis for knowing him since he has often revealed himself more fully to them than to any other group of individuals. Unlike the actor who can dismiss the audience's applause by assuming that it is not for him but for his role, the group-therapy patient must come to a different conclusion since he has, throughout, been encouraged to doff his customary role. He cannot question the importance of the traits under discussion since the group so often deals with core-identity issues. If he attempts to convince the group of his unworthiness by revealing more of his shameful dark areas, a curious paradox unfolds: since members are rewarded in a group for their adherence to group norms, and disclosure of inadequacies is a cherished therapy group norm, the more he reveals, the more he is ultimately respected. Eventually a

therapeutic shift may occur, as he reevaluates the veracity and basis of his myth of personal worthlessness.

There is research support for this sequence of events. Social psychologists[2] have convincingly demonstrated that group consensus can exert sufficiently strong pressure to cause individual distortions in visual perceptions of material objects. The same force can be harnessed to encourage attitudinal shifts. Group-therapy patients who, early in the group, are deemed, on sociometric measures, to be more popular (by dint of their active participation in the group tasks) are those destined to profit most from the therapy.[6] Encounter-group members who are active and considered by the other members as highly influential early in the group will eventually experience the highest rates of personal growth.[3] As the group comes to value an individual, so, too, does he come to value himself.

In addition to the opportunities for the explicit display and correction of maladaptive interpersonal behavior and the benefits accruing from group cohesiveness, there are a number of other potential mechanisms of change relatively specific to the group-therapy format. No doubt, these will continue to be an intrinsic part of the group-therapeutic process, whatever changes in outward form the future brings.

Universality operates as a change mechanism in the great majority of therapy groups. Patients often enter the group with the deep conviction that they are unique in their wretchedness. Not uncommonly they have had little opportunity for candid reciprocal sharing with another individual, and, furthermore, often because of an unusual constellation of life stresses, they are besieged by unusual or frightening fantasies or by recollections of past experiences. For many group members the disconfirmation of their sense of uniqueness is a great relief. Early in the group they not only hear other members disclose concerns, fantasies, and life experiences closely paralleling their own, but they also have the opportunity to reveal themselves and be, nonetheless, accepted and approved by others. Simply put, they experience a sense of being "welcome to the human race," which, though present to some degree in individual therapy, is more powerfully built into the group format. Patients can be grateful for the therapist's acceptance, but nonetheless can ascribe it to his professionalism. They cannot so easily dismiss the other members who are neither trained nor paid to listen, accept, or reveal themselves.

Opportunities for *altruistic behavior* often present themselves in therapy groups. Members may give to others in a variety of ways: they give time, their "share" of the group attention, support, advice, and, above all, care. At the end of a group-therapy experience patients often, in their reminiscences about the group, recall the helpful interventions of the other members more vividly than those of the therapist. Indeed, the experienced group therapist learns to sit on his wisdom in the awareness that patients more often accept interpretations from other members than from the therapist. Many patients enter therapy morbidly self-absorbed, so demoralized that they are convinced they have little of value to offer; they may have long experienced themselves as parasitic burdens to others, and it is refreshing, even exhilarating, to find that they can be of significant help to others. Altruistic dereflection is a venerable concept in the healing tradition; as exemplified by the shamen who since prehistory have prescribed for patients the task of preparing a tribal feast or performing other services to the community.

Groups wield powerful suggestive force and in the substratum of the group there is a subtle but persistent *instillation of hope*. The establishment and maintenance of faith in therapy is crucial to all psychotherapies; amulets, drumbeats, testimonials, impressive diplomas, erudite formulations, and prescriptions in Latin are all dedicated to that end. The therapy group invariably contains individuals in differing stages of coping with major problems. Members see or hear about others who have improved in the group. They also encounter people who have dealt, and, to some extent, overcome problems very similar to their own. Some groups, for example, Alcoholics Anonymous or Recovery Incorporated,

explicitly build into their ritual the testimony of the improved patient. In other groups the process is subtler, the therapist implicitly encouraging patients to recount their improvement and the members themselves gratuitously proffering testimonials to buoy up the hopes of a demoralized, unconvinced patient.

Spectator therapy, a deliberate and explicit behavioral approach to phobia desensitization, is an omnipresent but more implicit adjunct to learning in group therapy. It is common for members to benefit vicariously from observing others with problems similar to their own, working in ways not yet possible for them. Members of therapy groups have a wide exposure to a number of problem-solving strategies and, through a conscious or preconscious imitative process, may try on, for size as it were, various modes of approaching important dilemmas. Even if imitatve behavior is short-lived it may function to "unfreeze" the individual as he experiments with new kinds of behavior.

Although I have offered but a sketch of the opportunities for change available in group therapy, we may appreciate the waste, the unfulfilled potential of group-therapy approaches that fail to harness the interpersonal and social-field forces inherent in the small group. Fractional approaches abound. Some therapists do individual therapy in a group; others magnify such part processes as self-disclosure or mutuality or the intensification of affect or desensitization to social anxiety, but no fractional approach constitutes a balanced group therapy that uses a full orchestration of the medium.

In retrospect, what have we said about the future of group therapy? That it is to a large extent currently in a non self-reflective, flamboyant stage, propelled by many factors but chiefly by an overcathexis to technique. The preoccupation with technique stems from an activistic, optimistic, basically pragmatic approach to individual and social change. However, technique spawned from technique is ultimately destined to cave in upon itself. What is needed is a fuller appreciation and reconsideration of the theoretical assumptions upon which all technique must stand.

《 Bibliography

1. AMERICAN GROUP PSYCHOTHERAPY ASSOCIA-
   TION, Los Angeles, Feb. 4–6, 1971. Program of the meeting.
2. ASCH, S. E. "Effects of Group Pressure upon
   the Modification and Distortion of Judgments" in D. Cartwright and A. Zanter,
   eds., *Group Dynamics: Research and
   Theory*, pp. 189–201. Evanston, Ill.: Row,
   Peterson, 1962.

3. LIEBERMAN, M., I. YALOM, and M. MILES.
   Encounter Groups: First Facts. New York:
   Basic Books, 1973.
4. MULLAHY, P. *The Contributions of Harry
   Stack Sullivan*, p. 10. New York: Hermitage
   House, 1952.
5. SULLIVAN, H. S. *Conceptions of Modern Psychiatry*, p. 207. New York: Norton, 1940.
6. YALOM, I., K. RAND, and A. ZIM. "Prediction
   of Improvement in Group Therapy," *Arch.
   Gen. Psychiatry*, 17 (1967), 157–168.

CHAPTER 31

PLANNING THE DELIVERY OF MENTAL HEALTH SERVICES TO SERIOUSLY DISADVANTAGED POPULATIONS

Anthony F. Panzetta and Albert J. Stunkard

TWELVE YEARS AGO America's health planners took the momentous step of designing the first comprehensive health-care system for the nation. The Community Mental Health Centers Act of 1963 proposed the greatest innovation in health services in our history. Its more ambitious aspect was the proposal for the delivery of comprehensive mental-health services to seriously disadvantaged populations.

For the first time in American medicine, comprehensive health planning defined the future dimensions of a field of medicine, and for the first time public-health concepts played a major part in planning the practise of a clinical specialty. For, eschewing the traditional approaches to individuals, this act took as the target of medical concern "catchment areas" of 75,000 to 200,000 persons. It assigned responsibility for the mental health of the persons within these areas to community mental-health centers geographically located within them and proposed a goal of 2000 such centers by 1980, to provide comprehensive mental-health care to the entire nation.

This act had significant impact upon the development of American psychiatry. It provided strong impetus for a movement away from its traditional concern with individuals and toward a public-health model of care for populations. And it brought psychiatry face to face with the massive problems of poverty, which it had known until then only indirectly and derivatively. For the highest priority in the funding of community mental-health centers has been given to those in poverty areas.

A decade of effort in the delivery of mental-health services to seriously disadvantaged areas has produced bitter disappointment and some limited progress. It has, however, helped to define some of the issues and problems and indicated some methods of analyzing them. In this chapter we will deal with four of these issues: the culture of poverty, the ethos of American psychiatry, the financial underwriting of mental-health services, and some characteristics of these services, especially in poverty areas.

(The Culture of Poverty

Let us begin by considering some characteristics of the members of seriously disadvantaged populations. First, what do we mean by "disadvantaged"? In general, disadvantaged persons are those who do not have the economic necessities for reasonable human living. They live precariously in every sense—environmentally, biologically, socially, educationally, and economically. They do not have a reasonable degree of autonomy and control over their destiny as individuals and as populations. They do not have access to the essential channels for their economic, social, educational, health, and cultural needs. They do not have access to those individuals who could improve their status.[60] Disadvantaged is not defined by class or ethnic or minority group membership. However, the risk of being a member of the so-called disadvantaged community is greatly increased if one is also a member of a minority group. In short, people who are disadvantaged are those who are described by Harrington as "poor because they are poor and stay poor because they are poor."

Throughout the remainder of this chapter we shall simply refer to the "poor" without further elaborations. This is a generalization not without its dangers, but we anticipate that the reader will accommodate himself to this convention.

The poor share many characteristics in common and a cultural anthropology literature of the poor has developed.* It has become fashionable in some quarters to confuse a "culture" of poverty with a black culture. An understanding of the historical roots, life style, and values of the black person is not the same as understanding the life style and values of the poor. We are, in this chapter, concerned with the poor and this cuts across issues of race and ethnic origin, even while race and ethnicity modify some of the features of the poverty culture.

Mental-health planners and shapers tend to overlook the fact that the most serious poverty is rural and white. Instead, they talk in terms related to cities and usually to city blacks. There are, of course, good reasons for this. Population density is greatest in our cities and so the density of poverty is likewise to be found in our cities. From a public-health perspective, it is reasonable to be concerned with geographically accessible high-risk groups. Hence, the urban poor, compressed as they are into discrete, high-density areas, become "attractive" for study and for service plans. The rural poor and particularly the Southern rural poor have no ready advocates because of their geographic remoteness, and so there is little "public concern" or indignation. Add to this the natural tendency of service professionals to live and work in urban areas and we have the makings of a self-reinforcing pattern of service shortage for the rural poor.

What can we say about the culture of poverty that has relevence to our concern, namely, the development and maintenance of mental-health delivery systems?

* See references 4, 19, 28, 29, 49, 58, 68, 69, 76, 77, 89, 93, 102, 118, 129, and 135.

Bernstein[11,12] and others[33,34] have pointed out that the verbal abilities of the poor are significantly less then among the middle and upper classes. Speech tends to be impersonal, concrete, and reflective of social identity rather than personal identity. And so, to the extent that these characteristics are at the core in most psychiatric-care strategies, the verbal gap between the poor consumer and the middle-class health purveyor, hits at this most basic precondition for psychotherapeutic care.

An inability or unwillingness to defer gratification has been cited as another characteristic of the poor.[55,104,130] Such a pattern seems adaptive for persons who have known deprivation as a way of life and who, therefore, take their gratifications as quickly as possible before returning to the familiar state of deprivation.[101] Nevertheless, this emphasis on the here and now conflicts with the requirement of many forms of psychiatric treatment for a long-range orientation, and for an ability and a willingness on the part of the patient to plan for the future.

Although the prevalence of depression in the poor cannot be noted in sound epidemiologic fashion,[112] descriptions of apathy and hopelessness characterize much of the descriptive literature.[59] This apathy and hopelessness are not parts of a circumscribed psychopathologic state as much as they are characterologic and inbred habits, coming from years of deprivation and disadvantage. As such they are difficult to "treat" clinically, and they compromise motivation for pursuing help for other psychosocial problems.

With the increased awareness of poverty as a serious problem in the last decade, there has been a corresponding increase in attention paid to the issue of poverty by all of our communications media. Poverty has become a fashionable topic at cocktail parties and on radio or television talk shows. The attention at the public level has promoted, as one consequence, an increase in the bargaining power of poverty persons. But that bargaining power has been largely illusory when social changes on their behalf have threatened the status quo of those classes higher on the socioeconomic ladder. Such highly charged issues as busing, suburban low-cost housing, hiring quotas of minority members, welfare reform, and health-care insurance are testimony to the conflictual nature of anything that threatens the social-class status quo. This reality of conflict between classes brings an element of hostility to many other interclass relationships. This potential hostility is no less the case in psychotherapeutic relationships that bring middle-class "therapists" into charged settings with poor patients.

The poor have also been described as having an uncanny ability to sense the expectations for them by the more affluent, and so to "perform" in a fashion that will yield the greatest gain in their interpersonal relations with the "richer outer world." The subservient role may be the caricature, but this role is often used to manipulate the immediate interpersonal situation. This ability to say what is necessary rather than what may be true is antithetical to the implicit value of speaking and "feeling" the truth, which the psychiatrist requires of his patient.

The relationship of poverty and educational attainment is of fundamental significance, and the full implications go far beyond the focus of this chapter. The inability to comprehend the complicated bureaucratic organization of urban America has forced many to retreat into unproductive but safely simple and more primitive life styles. The development of the ghetto is often the net result of not only the rejection by an alien majority, but also the pursuit of a simple, less complicated life style. The plight of the unsophisticated Southern black or white who migrates to the big Northern city is particularly relevant to this point. This, in a real sense, is an example of culture shock. But it is also reflective of the deficient opportunity "to learn" about "how to make it" in the middle-class ethos that directs the organization and values of American society. This deficiency is as much a problem in Northern urban education as it is in the South. In many ways, the health bureaucracy resembles the complexity of many other social institutions, and a person's ability to extract maximum benefit depends upon his ability to understand the complexity. He must compensate for the fragmentation and pursue his needs despite a lack of clarity within the health institution. This calls for rather sophisticated initiative on the part of the would-be health consumer. When we focus upon the poor, we see just the opposite. Their lack of sophisticated understanding of the health (including psychiatry) bureaucracy puts them at a further disadvantage.

It should not be surprising that all of these foregoing factors contribute to the unhealthy relationship of the poor to the health-delivery system in this country. The patterns of health care, with the implicit requirements placed upon a potential health-care consumer, work uniformly against the likelihood of the poor receiving adequate quantitative and qualitative service. It is to psychiatry's tentative credit that, despite health-care failures in delivery to the poor, it has taken a leadership role in struggling with the problem through its community mental-health movement.

([The Ethos of American Psychiatry

How has American psychiatry coped with the special problems posed by the culture of poverty? And what strengths and weaknesses does the specialty bring to the development of more effective mental-health services for the poor?

To answer these pressing questions, it may be in order to take a brief look at the history of American psychiatry. Its development can be separated into three phases, each of which contributed important elements to the field as we know it today and each of which occurred as a result of a fortuitous combination of circumstances. There was, in each instance, a favorable social climate into which a new scientific theory or technology was introduced. The interaction of social climate and scientific base defined psychiatry's new tasks and suggested new ways of carrying them out.

This kind of interaction between social climate and technology appears to have had a profound influence on the establishment,

nearly 200 years ago, of modern psychiatry. The social climate was that of the French Revolution and of Quaker hospital reform. The scientific innovation was the classification introduced by Linnaeus and applied with consummate skill by Philippe Pinel at the Bicêtre and the Salpêtrière. Pinel selected, from among the large numbers and variety of the socially disabled, a group of individuals with discrete behavioral disorders, many of whom had good prospects for recovery. By demonstrating the effectiveness of a uniquely humane mode of care for these persons—the so-called "moral treatment of the insane"—Pinel and his contemporaries defined the traditional tasks of psychiatry, the diagnosis of mental illness and its treatment in hospitals specially designed for this purpose.

Initially, the care rendered in these hospitals, which catered to the more affluent members of society, was humane and surprisingly effective. But in time the quality of hospital treatment of the mentally ill declined to the low level we have come to associate with the old, isolated state mental hospitals. This deterioration appears to have begun in the years following the Civil War. During this period, large numbers of poor people, many of them immigrants, overwhelmed the facilities of the small, treatment-oriented hospitals. As larger and larger public mental hospitals were built, the earlier therapeutic functions were replaced by custodial ones and therapeutic optimism gave way to pessimism and to self-fulfilling prophecies about the incurability of mental illness.

It is this aspect of psychiatry—the large, isolated, human warehouses—that the poor have traditionally known, feared, and avoided, and it is in such unpromising settings that psychiatrists have traditionally made the acquaintance of the poor. Here the dehumanizing effects of the environment accentuated what psychiatrists already perceived as the alien character of the immigrant and the perplexing qualities of the poor.

The second major development, in American psychiatry at least, was heralded by a profound social event of our recent past—World War II. In those days, a heightened concern with political freedom and personal liberty was coupled with shock over the high rates of psychiatric disability being disclosed at induction centers and on the battlefields. At this critical time, psychoanalysis was introduced into American psychiatry. For the first time, a systematic theory of neurosis and a therapy that claimed not only to cure neurosis but to change human nature itself became available.

It would be hard to overestimate the impact of this interaction of social need and psychoanalytic theory. The long-standing pessimism born of years of heartbreak in the treatment of the mentally ill was shattered and all of American psychiatry was suffused with enthusiasm and élan. As it turned out, many of the hopes raised by psychoanalysis were never realized, but it remains an important factor in the background of most psychiatrists. Its emphasis upon neurosis, verbal interchange, and insight continues to exert a powerful influence.

The social climate that fostered the third development in American psychiatry was epitomized by the Kennedy-Johnson social legislation of the 1960s and that decade's generous institutional support for psychiatry. In this climate, a variety of scientific and technologic advances were made. Some have come out of clinical practice: short-term psychotherapies derived from psychoanalysis, group therapy, family therapy, milieu therapy. Others are applications of basic science. A vast and rapidly growing selection of psychopharmacologic agents has made it possible to treat a broad range of disorders, in an expanding number of patients ever more precisely.

The field of behavioral therapy, based upon principles of learning once considered useful only in mild neurotic fears, then applied successfully to more severe phobias and inhibitions, is now used in the entire gamut of mental and emotional disorders. Finally, extensive epidemiologic studies have demonstrated that close correlations exist between many aspects of the culture of poverty and psychiatric disability.

The background of today's psychiatrists includes all three historic elements: the mental hospital, the private-office practice of psycho-

therapy, and the newer, more eclectic orientations. The degree to which an individual psychiatrist is interested in the development of mental-health services in poverty areas, and his ability to contribute to such development, reflect his predominant professional orientation.

Psychiatrists working in mental hospitals still provide most of the psychiatric care the poor receive. Most of the patients in our state hospitals are from the lower social classes; much of their treatment still takes place within the walls of the hospital. But many state hospitals have shown admirable initiative in developing close ties to the communities from which their patients come, and to treatment programs within these communities. Unfortunately, the chronic underfunding and neglect of so many of these hospitals, and the resulting inadequacies of staff and facilities, have limited their efforts to develop better mental-health services.

Private mental hospitals have developed a surprising number of treatment programs in the communities outside their walls. But these hospitals are seldom located in poverty areas.

The continuing high prestige of psychoanalysis has meant that office practice of psychotherapy remains the most popular field within psychiatry. Many psychotherapists spend a great deal of time and effort on public service and some have worked long and hard to develop mental-health services for the poor. But psychoanalytically oriented psychotherapy requires introspection on the patient's part and a willingness to defer gratification, plus a high regard for insight and considerable verbal skill. These traits are far more common among middle- and upper- than among lower-class persons. Since, not unreasonably, psychotherapists prefer to treat those who stand the best chance of responding to treatment, there is a tendency to restrict psychotherapeutic practices to the middle and upper classes, even when subsidies remove the financial barrier that usually excludes the poor. Psychotherapy for lower class patients requires experience, a particular aptitude, and extensive modification of technique. As a result, the traditionally trained psychotherapist is unlikely to make important contributions to the development of mental-health services for the poor.

The recent graduates of psychiatric residency-training programs constitute a promising new source of psychiatric manpower. Many of these young psychiatrists have mastered a wide variety of treatment techniques and have had at least some experience in applying these techniques to the poor. Their training, and their strong commitment to social values, make these newcomers far more capable of developing new services for the poor than their older colleagues with their traditional values and limited treatment repertoires. Furthermore, the training the younger psychiatrists receive in psychopharmacology and in the behavioral therapies encourages them to scrutinize more critically the results of treatment. Recent psychiatric graduates are far more inclined to demand a reasonable cost–benefit accounting of the investment of their own efforts and of those of their peers.

On the debit side, an excess of youthful zeal may limit the effectiveness of their efforts. They do not always extend the admirable powers of criticism they apply to traditional psychiatric methods to their own activities. Enthusiasm for social action untempered by good judgment can be quixotic. But on balance, recent graduates of residency-training programs have far more to contribute to mental-health services for the poor than their elders. These young doctors must provide the leadership in this endeavor. Their point of view and the greatly improved training they have received give grounds for some optimism as they approach their pioneering task.

❰ Financial Underwriting

The major current effort to deliver mental-health services to the poor is centered around the Community Mental Health Centers Act of 1963, which involves a combination of funding patterns. The act was passed during the period before the full impact of the medicare legislation had become clear. We still believed that our health-care delivery system was excellent, and that all we needed was to put money in the hands of low-income groups to permit them access to the system. It was expected that health insurance would eventually permit all Americans to seek health services, including mental-health services, on a fee-for-service basis, with reimbursement by third-party sources. The planners recognized, however, that mental-health services available a decade ago were inadequate to meet the needs of vast numbers of our citizens, even when they were able to pay for psychiatric care. Therefore, funds were made available from the federal government, with matching support from local sources to initiate community mental-health programs. This funding was viewed as a temporary expedient, designed to reorganize the pattern of delivery of mental-health services in a more effective and equitable manner. Once this reorganization had taken place, it was expected that the increased purchasing power conferred by third-party payments would permit all Americans access to the restructured mental-health services, and support of these services would revert to a fee-for-service pattern. Accordingly, federal support for community mental-health centers was distributed on a declining basis, with support for new programs totally phased out over a period of from five to eight years. The centers were thus initiated on a prepayment-group-practice model with the expectation that they would revert to a fee-for-service model over a period of years.

Budgetary restrictions have slowed the initial plans and no more than 480 of the projected 2000 community mental-health centers have been constructed. But considerable experience with this dual system of funding has been gained. In general, federal support has worked well in assisting the initiative of local planners in establishing community mental-health centers. The expected shift of support to a fee-for-service basis funded by third-party payments, however, has occurred very slowly and still provides only a fraction of the support of most community mental-health centers.

The poor have always been provided services, health and otherwise, with the requirement that they get it where they are told. The inability to choose from among competing services is one of the most critical differences that sets off the usual service for the poor from the free-market system used for middle- and upper-class health consumers. Competing purveyors must maintain quality standards to survive. No such requirement is made of the usual health purveyor for the entrapped poverty-health consumer—beyond governmental standards that are often difficult to police.

And so, as we turn our attention to the fiscal system underlying a mental-health-service plan for the poor we must take into account the above traditional handicaps to the development of quality-service systems. But this fiscal issue leads to an associated question. Who wants to plan, develop, and maintain delivery systems for the poor? It would be foolhardy to suggest that compassion, benevolence, and altruism are in sufficient supply to generate manpower interests (at all levels) in this health-delivery problem. It is perhaps unfortunate that there have, in fact, been such idealistic and hard-working individuals involved in health delivery to the poor since they have never been able to adequately meet the enormous needs and have rather dulled the edge of urgent demand from the poor that might have generated a more comprehensive and efficient system.

Prepayment Plan

A physician working in a prepayment health-delivery system can expect his income to be directly related to the efficiency of the medical organization, the control of cost (including level of amenities) and the ability to anticipate costly illnesses in subscribers, providing prevention-directed care so as to avoid such costly illnesses wherever possible. The consumer is free from unexpected financial liability—since he pays only a fixed amount regardless of his medical risk. This seems an attractive arrangement since it protects the consumer while assuring him of medical care and gives physicians financial incentive to provide preventive medicine. It also stabilizes

the workload of physicians and stimulates organizational efficiency.

The prepay group plan presents a difficult problem when related to mental-health services. In most of medicine there exists a clarity at the level of illness categorization and at the level of indicated treatment. The criteria for diagnosis are reasonably well worked out and the standards of care (as well as choice of appropriate treatment) are also spelled out. The monitoring of a health-delivery system requires this dual-level clarity (illness criteria and treatment criteria). Without this dual clarity it would be very difficult to determine when a consumer is entitled to care and very difficult to determine when a consumer is receiving the most appropriate kind of care. In mental-health services the development of clear illness criteria and related treatment criteria is rather primitive. Consumers, in a prepay plan would probably be unsure as to what qualifies as a "bona-fide" mental disorder. The listing of such bona-fide disorders would be equally difficult for the professional because, although a standard nomenclature exists (DSM-II) its diagnostic criteria are not tight, resulting in great variation in diagnostic convention.[110] Difficulties would also result from the great variation in treatment strategies that compete through rather zealous psychiatric practitioners. The cost–benefit implications of such ambiguity is quite alien to the prepay group plan, which depends on careful cost-accounting principles.

When considering the poor, such a system is even more confusing. As practitioners in urban community mental-health centers have discovered, mental-health problems of the poor are difficult to separate from their social and economic problems. The apparent interlocking of problems has led many to a radical brand of treatment requiring a good deal of social intervention. The borders of such strategies are enormously ambiguous and so we have further difficulty in meeting the dual-level clarity requirements of a sound prepay group plan.

Quality of care maintenance has always been a problem in poverty-oriented health systems. This might be partially solved through a prepay plan, since the consumer (or his employer in cases where the employer pays for the plan) could withdraw their support if the health purveyor could not meet quality standards. But, as noted earlier, in mental-health services there is poor standardization of quality standards.

Fee-for-Service Plan

The second major approach is based on a fee-for-service plan. There are many variations on this theme, whether the fee is paid directly by the consumer or by partial or total subsidy through an insurance scheme. Whereas in prepay plans there is a probable tendency for patients to overutilize medical care, in fee-for-service plans there is a probable tendency to underutilize medical care, particularly where out-of-pocket costs threaten to embarrass already limited family budgets. It can be argued that, where health care is concerned, it is better to err in commission rather than in omission. This suggests that the prepay plans are best, but let us continue our consideration of the fee-for-service plan before making such a conclusion.

One of the claims made by fee-for-service proponents is that this system allows for the greatest freedom for both the consumer and the purveyor. The consumer can choose his purveyor from among many and can base his choice on his own idiosyncratic set of criteria. It is common knowledge that this choice is often based on criteria that would probably never enter a formal quality control system; such criteria as a physician's personality, location of his office, amenities he can provide, his religion or nationality, his color, his social status, the type of hospital to which he admits his patients, and so on. This range of preference for the consumer certainly would not apply with most prepay type schemes. Whether such freedom of choice is a valid point upon which to build a case for fee-for-service plans is subject to much debate. Certainly these are not the primary considerations in the development of a high quality and equitably distributed health-care system. Whereas this seems reasonably clear in a con-

sideration of health care in general, it is much less clear in specifically considering mental-health care.

A conclusion is warranted at this point. Because of poor standardization of treatment (and all that entails) on the one hand, and poor standardization of patient problems (and all that entails) on the other, no broad fiscal plan is clearly preferable over another when viewed as part of a mental-health delivery system. Psychiatric treatment is too unsystematic to easily fit into the systematic requirements of a fiscal-health plan. But what are the ramifications of this pessimistic conclusion when viewed in the light of our discussion of mental-health delivery systems for the poor?

Everything seems to get worse when we add the dimension of poverty. And so, too, when considering a fiscal-health plan to underwrite a mental-health delivery system for the poor. Should buying power be given directly to the prospective mental-health consumer (fee for service, insurance, etc.) or should money be given directly to purveyors in advance of any service rendered (prepay, health maintenance organizations, etc.) or should there be some variable mix of these alternatives?

With a public-health perspective we must begin by stating that our goal is to develop a system that is *most likely* to provide the *highest quality service possible* in the most *equitably distributed* way *possible*. This leaves us with the question: which is more important, quality or equitable distribution? And more specifically, which is more important in mental-health services for the poor? When we look at the current scene in mental-health delivery to poor people, is the larger problem the inequitable distribution or is it the poor quality of care? It is likely that different answers could be given, with strong arguments for each. Certainly, both quality and distribution have been deficient and the question of which has been worse may be a futile exercise in semantics.

If we were to choose quality or equity as a greater priority, is there a prospect of improving the other through a nonfiscal strategy? If we decided that quality care was most important and opted for a fee-for-service approach, how could we correct for the probable maldistribution problem? And if we decided that equitable distribution was most important and therefore opted for some kind of prepayed plan, how could we correct for the probable quality of care problems?

Fee for service would be an option for the poor if they were included in a universal insurance scheme that provided for reimbursement to the purveyor of choice. If the insurance were in fact universal (i.e., available for everyone) then, potentially, our distribution of buying power would be accomplished. But it is not likely that the already short manpower supply in psychiatry would be able to absorb the demand, nor is the available manpower adequately prepared for the service needs of the poor, nor is it likely that the geographic distribution of this manpower would shift. And so we would continue to face distribution problems (manpower type and supply and geographic concentration) despite our provision of more equitable buying power to the mental-health consumer.

Prepay group plans offer the advantage of setting conditions on the health purveyor. One of those conditions could be in determining where he could work. Payment to the group purveyors could be contingent upon their willingness to establish their work in areas of greater need. This arrangement frees the consumer from financial liability (a necessity when talking about the poor) and insures a greater control in developing geographic distribution. The question of manpower remains unsolved in either approach and will be discussed separately. And we are still left with the problem of quality.

Quality of care, as developed within a prepayed psychiatric service plan, will be most possible in those areas of service which are most explicit and measurable, and least possible (to regulate or monitor) in those areas of service which are vague, overly general (or philosophic) and hard to measure. Much of American psychiatry fits into the latter rather than the former, and so the suggestion that a fiscal change from the current fee-for-service system to the prepayed system is

necessary (for reasons of distribution) brings with it the corollary that psychiatric practice will be forced to change from the largely intuitive and interpersonal practice of today to a more specific, measurable practice (for reasons of quality control).

This type of radical shift is unlikely to occur very rapidly since the bulk of our current manpower is committed to a poorly standardized brand of practice. It probably would not, nor could it shift in rapid fashion. And so, the tentative conclusion is that, as far as well-distributed, quality mental-health service for the poor is concerned, we can make rapid strides to resolve distribution problems through a change in the underwriting fiscal system, but the development of quality services will be only as good as we can make explicit standards, on the one hand, and develop new manpower (with new orientation) on the other.

The fiscal system used to underwrite medical developments in American medicine, and psychiatric practice in particular, will have an affect on the distribution and quality of services far beyond our ability to anticipate such change. It is naive to think that the problems of distributing and upgrading the quality of psychiatric services to the poor can be resolved by simply redistributing money.

(Mental-health Delivery System for the Poor

Mental health is a connotative concept in that it suggests a variety of meanings.* There is some consensus about the concept when it is thought of as "the absence of" mental illness.[65] This negative definition leads some advocates of mental health to promote plans that are designed to prevent, treat, or rehabilitate specific mental illnesses.†

On the other hand, there are those who think of mental health as "the presence of" a

* See references 36, 40, 41, 65, 96, 110, 113, 140, and 142.
† See references 9, 13, 14, 17, 35, 46, 86, 87, 110, and 124.

variety of personal psychologic characteristics considered "healthy."[42,43,61,123] This positive definition leads these advocates of mental health to promote plans that are designed to develop these healthy personal characteristics. For the sake of clarity, we might categorize the former group as *clinical* and the latter group as *developmental*.

The connotations of mental health lead us to other considerations as well. Some consider mental health (whether of the *clinical* or *developmental* types) to be the property of individuals, as is the usual traditional view of psychiatry. Others extend it to social groups that may include family, social network, community, nation, and even world. Again for the sake of clarity, we can categorize the former as *individual* and the latter as *social*. So, then, we can speak of the clinical mental health of individuals or of families and we can also speak of the developmental mental health of individuals or of families or more extended social groupings.

Our differentiation then allows for two adjectival concepts (*clinical* and *developmental*) and two nominative concepts (*individual* and *social group*). The failure to make these critical distinctions in the discussion of mental-health services has caused immeasurable confusion in the past, and this confusion is considerably increased in discussions about mental-health services for the poor, for reasons that shall become apparent.*

Attempts to deliver mental-health services to the poor have been characterized by a variety of understandings of the concept of mental health. Some programs are clinical and individually oriented. Other programs place their emphasis on clinical problems of families and "the community." Still other programs have emphasized the promotion of inherent strengths among poor people (developmental). And, lastly, some have emphasized the development of community strength, which may include politicalization and ideological community organization.† If all of these can be connotatively linked to mental health, then

we have a task of differentially choosing between these alternatives as we move closer to the planning of specific programs for mental-health delivery to the poor. The basis of our choice should follow an analysis of the *validity* of the alternatives, the priority of the valid alternatives, and the *feasibility* of each.

The Concept of Delivery System

If mental health is the product we wish to deliver, and if mental health is the ubiquitous concept tentatively analyzed in the preceding section, then the delivery system can vary considerably. However, before becoming specific about any one delivery system, it should be possible to develop those general features of a mental-health delivery system which should apply in all instances.

There are undoubtedly many ways to approach this issue, but we shall focus on certain system characteristics that are particularly relevant in mental-health delivery systems. A primary requirement for a system is that it be *explicit*. This suggests that the goals of the system be as definite as possible. In something as ambiguous as the mental-health field this becomes all the more essential. The requirement for explicitness applies to more than the stated goals. We must also define the various strategies within the system that shall characterize its activities in pursuit of those goals. Explicitness makes the likelihood of all members of the system pulling in the same direction more likely. It also provides the necessary clarity that will be needed to assess effectiveness. Explicitness must be applied to attempts to make the system comprehensive as well as continuous. How far out will the system operate? Will it be population focused (as in the catchment-area concept of community mental health) or will it be limited by its internal capacity?

A second requirement for a system is that it be *manageable*. Are its explicit goals within the limitations imposed by the system's resources? Are the resources prepared for their explicit tasks, and are they aware of the requirement that they be responsive to supervening management? What is the likelihood of

* See references 70, 74, 109, 110, and 111.
† See references 2, 15, 18, 22, 27, 45, 75, 80, 106, 119, 125, 128, and 136.

the durability of the resources? Management is not possible if explicitness has not characterized the system first.

A third requirement for a system is that it be *effective*. Are the goals stated so that they are measurable in some way? Can the system recognize the difference between success and failure in the pursuit of its goals? Does management recognize its role in responding to the data of testing of effectiveness and can it redirect or maintain the system in accordance with effectiveness data?

These three requirements of systems, *explicit, manageable*, and *effective* can be of help in determining the feasibility of any mental-health delivery system for the poor.

Program Goals

Now our task is to spell out goals that could direct our delivery-system design and then to develop programmatic strategies that offer means to these goals. Both the development of goals and of strategies must take into account, as best they can, all of the foregoing problem areas.

We have already differentiated four variations within the concept of mental health. Presumably, then, we have four alternate or complementary general goals we can pursue. We can focus on individual types of psychopathology (clinical individual) and develop treatment programs (or preventive, if feasible) to deal with various types of such psychopathology. This is the most traditional approach and most of clinical psychiatry is directed in this fashion.

If we focus on what we have termed a *developmental-individual* concept of mental health, our programs would take on a different design. In this instance we would place far greater emphasis on the *promotion* of certain *personal characteristics* that we could identify as being necessary and/or helpful to the individual in his task of lifelong adaptation. This suggests the development of impact in educational institutions, both school and family.

If we focus on a *clinical-social* model, then our tasks will be even more unlike the traditional clinical-individual orientation. This approach would require us to develop programs aimed at designated problems of either social process or social structure. As stated earlier, we will then be committed to social action and social renovation. And if our focus be *developmental social* then our programs must be politicized.

We need not debate the nobility of one over another as we consider these variations in the concept of mental health. Only cursory familiarity with the problems of individuals and society will allow us to make the general statement that there is great need in all of these directions. And this is certainly most graphically true when considering the plight of the poor.

But when this question is examined from the particular framework of psychiatry and against the criteria of *validity, priority*, and *feasibility*, we can reduce our alternatives. The concepts of mental health, when viewed in their social perspective (either *clinical* or *developmental*) are subject to much ambiguity. We can argue the validity of one social structure as against another, or of one social process as against another, but, ultimately, we are anchored by the values of one social philosophy or another. It is quite possible that mental health, in a social sense, would demand a higher *priority* than individual mental health, particularly when confronted with the social structures and processes that beget and perpetuate poverty. There are few mental-health professionals who have not experienced frustration and a sense of powerlessness after experience in dealing with clinical problems among the poor. There is a feeling of engulfment as one recognizes that one problem is related to another and yet another. The so-called multiproblem family is everywhere in the poverty population. It is almost invariable that the mental-health professional in such a setting develops a resentment toward the ubiquitous "social system" that seems to strangle his patient. The natural tendency is to want to "get at" the social system. This is an ideal place from which to gain a perspective about the individual casualties that can be created by social structures. Unfortunately, it does not follow that this is an ideal place from which to bring significant influence to bear on those same social structures. Our anlysis leaves us with tenuous *validity,* on the one hand, and strong *priority* on the other, particularly in reference to mental-health goals for the poor.

The watershed comes from an understanding of the *feasibility* of efforts directed at the social definition of mental health. It must be kept in mind that this entire chapter is intended to be relevant to the study and work of psychiatrists, not political scientists, sociologists, lawyers, legislators, or lay activists. If reconsidered from other perspectives, the question of feasibility might be answered in an entirely different way. But when viewed in relationship to psychiatry, feasibility analysis dictates that programs for mental health, directed at the social connotations of that concept, are unlikely to be productive.[39,110] The identity of psychiatry, as amorphous as that has been in operational terms, has nonetheless been firmly fixed to maladaptation of individuals, with some expansion to small groups (family, etc.). The resources of psychiatry, whether its information store, its financial underwriting, its technology, or its historical legacy, are all heavily committed to problems of the individual and his immediate context. The constraints, were psychiatry to launch into an operational focus on social structure and function, would be enormous. Hence, the feasibility of such a goal is seriously compromised. We can leave to history the determination of whether a new discipline, dedicated to intervention (in the service of "social-mental health") in social structures and functions, will emerge from that wing of psychiatry which has become intrigued with this problem.

We are left with rather mundane and traditional goals: the development of psychiatric-service systems focused upon the individual (whether clinical or developmental) with "individual" being expanded to include contexual group and family. With this start we can next consider the implications of the system requirements noted earlier: *explicit; manageable; effective.*

We can approach the requirement for explicitness both from the perspective of the individual patient and of the therapy. This is to say that *systematic* service delivery should be characterized by problem standardization, on the one hand, and therapy standardization on the other. Which therapies are indicated for which problems? As complicated as this is for psychiatric delivery in general, it is considerably more complicated for psychiatric delivery to poor populations.

True standardization of those kinds of behavior included in the DSM–II has yet to be successfully accomplished, although there is considerable effort in that direction.[56,138,152] The confounding problem of viewing maladaptive behavior in a socially disordered setting, as is the case so often among the poor, is to add anguish to pain.

The only safe statement that can emerge from this consideration is that we will have increasing difficulty in the delivery of psychiatric services to poor populations, in direct proportion to the degree to which we fail (or are unable) to make the target problems explicit. And so the general goal of "mental-health service for individuals" is far too vague. Mental-health services for alcoholism, for drug abuse and addiction, for problems of the aged, for schizophrenia or like psychoses, for mental retardation—these are in the order of explicitness that allows for more systematic treatment.

Emergency and Diagnostic Centers

We are arguing for a categorical approach to service delivery and for some greater degree of standardization of therapeutic interventions. When translated into the operational terms of service structures and functions, we may begin by opting for centralized diagnostic services. Such services should be in a readily accessible location, with good public transportation. A study of psychiatric, utilization rates in an urban ghetto revealed highest rates occurring in those areas which had good public transportation linkage with the mental-health facility.[10] It is more feasible to centralize such services because of the high level of sophistication (and hence shortage) of diagnostic personnel. To deploy staff into so-called satellite locations for diagnostic functions is not generally economically feasible, although a tendency in this direction is nonetheless developing. The principle of reaching out has gained increasing currency and seems valid in the face of data that suggests that patients (particularly from poverty areas) do not readily initiate contact with the health network themselves until their condition deteriorates. But we have been more impressed by limiting the outpost or satellite (or other outreach equivalent) to an initial contact and triage function, rather than careful diagnostic and planning function.

We can respond to another characteristic of the poor if we expand the idea of a centralized diagnostic process to include emergency service. As has been noted, the poor tend to seek help only when the situation has reached crisis proportions. They are most likely to initiate contact themselves during crisis and more likely to maintain contact and involvement only as long as the crisis continues.[6,31,122,154] It behooves the planner of psychiatric services then to capitalize on this characteristic by emphasizing the emergency-diagnostic function of his delivery system. This means a far greater investment of space and manpower in "emergency" units than has been the case to date. An entire subdiscipline is emerging in medicine in general, and this includes psychiatry. The day of the on-call resident who reluctantly "comes down," after being cajoled by the medical resident, to evaluate and "quickly" refer a patient in the emergency room, although currently the "tradition" in the majority of instances, is certainly passé. It will hopefully give way to arrangements of specialized, staff-level teams, able to absorb large numbers of complicated cases, giving intense treatment and providing sophisticated diagnostic work at the entry to the medical- and/or psychiatric-service system. This is a requirement of rather urgent proportions in programs focused on poor populations. This "emergency" of emergency services has certainly generated renewed interest in the emergency department and in the theory of crisis,[32] but the translation of this interest into tangible structures is just beginning. One of the inhibiting factors is cost, since intensive care or sophisticated di-

agnostic process is expensive. We see no way around this issue until we are better able to frame cost–benefit studies. There is good reason to anticipate that, once such studies are feasible and under way, we shall discover that benefits at the acute end of the treatment continuum will indicate a dollar bargain in comparison to cost benefits at later stages of therapeutic contact.

The community mental-health movement has given the most concrete impetus to the development of emergency services through its mandated requirement for emergency service in every community mental-health center. But the experience to date suggests that most centers have approached this task most conservatively and so, overwhelmed, understaffed, undersophisticated, and tenuously financed operations are more the rule than the exception.[50]

Such emergency and diagnostic centers should follow the lead already provided by various innovative emergency programs. Practices such as the provision of emergency-unit holding beds, emergency home visits (especially for diagnostic purposes), walk-in clinics, group screening, team treatment, telephone-supportive services or telephone triage, police assistance, police and clergy training, detoxification units (for drugs and alcohol) and other variations on these themes are all of variable utility in the emergency-diagnostic center. Some of this technology overlaps, but most adds to the total resources in a way that suggests that the more of them you can incorporate into the service design the better the total treatment impact.

But lest we overemphasize the emergency aspect to the detriment of the diagnostic, let us say a few more words about this part of the emergency-diagnostic-center idea. Current practice often suggests that we can use (and some feel it preferable to use) less sophisticated personnel in diagnostic work with poor patients. The opposite is true. The problems of the poor, particularly when mixed with psychological issues, are difficult to organize, categorize, and diagnose—and even more difficult to conceptualize for treatment strategy. Well-trained and experienced personnel

are a requirement at this earliest level of diagnostic and therapeutic contact. If our service
plans are to proceed along categorical lines, as
discussed previously, it is critical that diagnostic evaluations be done well, particularly
with explicit guidelines as to interventional
strategies that are considered most useful. It is
likely that less-trained and less-experienced
staff will comprise much of the ongoing treatment, and this makes it particularly necessary
to start off well.

Categorical Perspective

Beyond the diagnostic-emergency functions,
the variations of further treatment are many.
Certainly one must keep in mind the idiosyn-
cracies that may obtain in one area as against
another. Unfortunately, the epidemiologic
help of incidence and prevalence studies is
quite limited. Such studies, when focused on
poor populations,* tend to give a picture of
gross psychopathology without differentiation
into categories that can serve as treatment objectives. And there is no assurance that the
findings of one study, focused on a discrete
geographic population, are applicable to another discrete population, even if the two
populations share common demographic characteristics. What we do know with reasonable
certainty, however, is that the problems of
alcoholism, drug abuse, geriatrics,† psychosis,‡
and mental retardation are significant in their
prevalence and disruptive to individual, family, and community. It is an unfortunate distortion in priorities when mental-health programs can be developed in areas of poverty
without special attention being paid to these
high visibility conditions.

Of perhaps equal morbid impact are the
difficulties that beset the children and youth in
poverty areas. With disrupted family structures,[103] maturation and identity formation
often tend to take on dyssocial characteristics.

Whether this problem can be effectively resolved without massive social restructuring
(family, school, and community) is unlikely.
Certainly we have learned that it is futile to
approach the problems of children and youth
from the traditional child-guidance perspective. In-office- , intrapsychically oriented psychotherapy is gradually giving way to family-
oriented interventions with greater emphasis
on problem solving, communication, and cognitive skills, and collateral network support.

In general terms then, we are faced with
several problem areas sufficiently prevalent
and morbid to warrant our concern. From a
psychiatric perspective, as focused on the
problems of poverty, these above-noted categories should receive the highest priorities for
our treatment plans. If we approach our service plan in the general and open-ended way
that is implicit in an emergency-diagnostic
center beginning, then it remains for such a
center to develop a way of coping with those
problems which may come into the center, but
for which no ongoing treatment program has
been developed. The requirement for efficient
coordination with the community's network of
social, health, and educational agencies is critical for the survival of an open-ended emergency-diagnostic center.

It is not the intent of this chapter to develop
specific treatment-team strategies for each
category of disorder. The technology within
each category will vary from place to place
and likewise will vary between categories.
There is certainly no unequivocal body of data
or treatment approach able to supercede the
variety of points of view and variety of treatment strategies that now obtain. The plea is
not that all treatment programs mirror one
another—or that they all use this "correct" approach or that one—but rather that each
treatment program organize itself so as to be
quite explicit as to what disorders it plans to
treat and what it plans not to treat. And once
having been committed to specific treatment
objectives, a program must *explicitly* set out
each phase of the treatment strategy for each
category, from initial contact through termination.

---

* See references 62, 83, 88, 132, and 140.

† See references 71, 73, 94, 95, 120, 128, 139, and
143.

‡ See references 23–25, 37, 38, 44, 47, 52, 62–64,
84, 85, 107, 116, 117, 141, and 144.

Manpower

We can make three statements about mental-health manpower that are germane to our present concerns: (1) there is a shortage of manpower in absolute terms;[1] (2) psychiatrists are unevenly distributed geographically;[62] (3) they spend the bulk of their time treating the least sick and/or most affluent with essentially unproven techniques.[115,30] The recognition of these problems has led to a variety of suggestions and activities designed to "improve" the situation, referred to by Pasamanick as "health care anarchy and social irresponsibility."[11,115]

To reduce the manpower deficit some would have us simply increase the number of psychiatrists trained annually.[8] This would mean increased governmental subsidies to psychiatric-training programs, an unlikely event when the opposite has, in fact, become a strong possibility.[147] There are already more psychiatric training positions than there are resident applicants. And even if the absolute number were increased, it would not be of the order or magnitude required to bridge the gap significantly.

Some would have us change the educational content or emphasis in psychiatric training, so as to discourage the intensive treatment of the least sick as *the* status activity. A tendency in this direction is perceptible in many training programs that have incorporated the ethos and practices of the community mental-health movement. However, significant exposure of trainees to the severely ill and chronically ill has yet to occur.

The development of team approaches to treatment has been another response to the manpower problem. The use of psychiatrists, psychologists, social workers, and nurses (especially public-health or visiting nurses) has been a long-standing arrangement in mental-health-service organizations. Now, however, this team has been supplemented by new mental-health careerists. A specificity of role for the new careerist has not yet developed and, instead, there are multiple variations in the use of this new manpower resource. They have been called mental-health counselors, mental-health workers, mental-health assistants, paraprofessionals, expeditors, linkage workers, mental-health advocates, and a variety of other connotative terms.[51] There is an abiding consensus, by those who have had experience in the use of manpower from this new career movement, that there is a valid and useful role for such personnel. It is still too soon to know precisely in what direction the developing role identity will go. It is likely that several differentiated roles and functions will emerge eventually. It is our contention that this movement, if not aborted by political or economic backlash, shows great promise for the future and is likely to radically change the eventual role identity of the psychiatrist as well as the clinical psychologist.

Such a manpower development could serve to respond to a number of problems both from the "culture" of poverty and from the ethos of American psychiatry sides of our dilemma. As new personnel would be developed from class origins closer to our target lower classes, we could expect less difficulty in communication between consumer and treater.

It is possible to think of this new manpower in two ways. On the one hand, it is quite plausible that it could emerge with responsibilities for direct care. Whether it engages in supportive roles, directive roles or educational roles remains as an unresolved issue. On the other hand, it is also possible that the new manpower can be used in roles that relate to delivery management and not to the direct care itself. When health systems are thought of in coordinated and comprehensive terms, it follows that they become quite complicated. Complicated systems cannot be manageable or effective if consumers are left to this complexity without help. We are already aware of the problems in continuity that occur when consumers are faced with the health bureaucracy. Specialization has resulted in a hodgepodge of mutually exclusive services without any corresponding specialization (excellence or efficiency) in the process of referral, transfer, or consultation. The movement to improve these management components of new health-delivery systems might readily use new career personnel. The need for systematic delivery and the need for comprehensive and coordinated services for the poor makes this development doubly necessary and attractive.

New careerists then can fulfill many of our needs. They can fill in manpower shortages at the level of direct care and they can provide manpower at the level of delivery management. They can also bridge some of the "culture gap" between consumer and therapist. They can help in the task of sensitizing the health-delivery organization to the needs of its consumers in poverty areas.

Evaluation

We would like to close this section with an urgent plea for what we view as the most pressing need in the delivery of health services in poor areas. It is for evaluation. Nor is this need confined to mental-health services in poor areas; evaluation is the crying need in all aspects of the community mental-health movement. For the construction of community mental-health centers got under way before any pilot project had tested the feasibility of this approach, and its feasibility still has not been evaluated. Seven years and over 400 community mental-health centers later, we still lack any assessment of the effects of these centers upon the mental health of the populations they serve.

This failing is the more poignant in that evaluation was accorded a very high priority by the sponsors of the Community Mental Health Centers Act in the congress. In a largely unprecedented move, these sponsors wrote into the legislation establishing the community mental-health centers the requirement that 1 percent of all operating funds be assigned to evaluation. These funds have been spent, and some evaluation has been carried out. But this evaluation has been carried largely to assessing the relationships between various of the care-taking groups within the centers—so-called input measures. To this day we lack any careful output measures—evaluation of the impact of a community mental-

health center on its community. We do not know if they have any impact at all.

Cost-accounting procedures have made inroads in various mental-health centers, however the need is for an even more sophisticated approach. Cost-accounting is limited to giving primarily administrative information regarding manpower and operational cost. Cost–effectiveness (cost–benefit) carries with it the further information regarding the cost for explicit clinical or social benefits. It is this sort of information that must be acquired to justify (or not) the continued financial support of these mental-health delivery systems.

This kind of output evaluation is very difficult to carry out. And it may be beyond the capacity of any agency to carry out an evaluation that could reflect unfavorably upon its highest priorities. Yet, a beginning must be made; we must obtain some measure of the effects of the centers in decreasing rates of mental illness or increasing indicators of mental health. For we are living in a time when the limits of our national budget have never been more clearly defined nor the need to choose between competing priorities more urgent. Humanitarian motives are no longer sufficient rationale for programs that now cost well in excess of 100 million dollars a year. Determining the cost–effectiveness of community mental-health centers has become a precondition for continuing to support them.

⟨ Concluding Remarks

When all is said and done, there remains and will probably always remain a gap between the "best-laid plans" and reality. The poor embody that part of the human condition that every man seeks to escape. The poor embody failure and deprivation. Poverty is the "pathologic" class that collects the rejects of the middle working classes and the upper "arrived" classes. It is the "pathologic" class that spawns frustration and new members in the poverty cycle. As Harrington effectively reminded us, poverty is something "we do not see" nor is it something we really wish to see.[57] We shall seize every opportunity to deny its existence or its severity.

There are very few persons who can maintain their commitments to working with or for the poor very long. Enthusiasm burns out in the face of seemingly insurmountable obstacles. The psychiatrist who turns his attention toward the problems of the poor does so with few allies among his colleagues. He cannot do it alone and so his commitment is tied irrevocably to the fickle enthusiasms of government. To even begin to accomplish the task described in this chapter many hands are needed. It is a task that relies on the initiative of the mental-health professionals, their nonprofessional colleagues, the entrapped poverty-ridden consumers, government and university—and the will of the public that something more be done.

❮ Bibliography

1. ALBEE, G. W. *Mental Health Manpower Trends.* New York: Basic Books, 1959.
2. ALINSKY, S. D. *Citizen Participation and Community Organization in Planning and Urban Renewal.* Chicago: Industrial Areas Foundation, 1962.
3. ———. "The War on Poverty: Political Pornography," *J. Soc. Issues,* 21 (1965), 41–47.
4. ALLEN, V. L. *Psychological Factors in Poverty.* Chicago: Markham, 1970.
5. ALPERT, J. J., J. KOSA, and R. J. HAGGERTY. A Study of Health Care of Low Income Families. Paper, Mass. Pub. Health Assoc., 1965.
6. ALPERT, J. J. et al. "Types of Families Using an Emergency Clinic," *Med. Care,* 7 (1969), 55–61.
7. BAMBERGER, L. "Health Care and Poverty," *Bull. N.Y. Acad. Med.,* 42 (12) (1966), 1140–1149.
8. BARTON, W. E. "Federal Support of Training of Psychiatrists," *Psychiatr. Ann.,* 2 (1972), 42–59.
9. BELSASSO, G. *Psychiatric Care of the Underprivileged.* Boston: Little, Brown, 1971.
10. BERGER, D. and E. GARDNER. Psychiatric Utilization Rates by Census Tracts. Working Report, Temple University Community Mental Health Center, 1969. Unpublished.
11. BERNSTEIN, B. "Social Structure, Language and Learning," *Educ. Res.,* 3 (1961), 163–176.
12. ———. "Social Class, Speech Systems, and Psychotherapy," *Br. J. Sociol.,* 15 (1964), 54–64.
13. BINDMAN, A. J. and A. D. SPIEGEL, eds. *Perspectives in Community Mental Health.* Chicago: Aldine, 1969.
14. BOWER, E. "Primary Prevention of Mental and Emotional Disorders: A Conceptual Framework and Action Possibilities," *Am. J. Orthopsychiatry,* 32 (1963), 832–848.
15. BRAGER, G. A. and F. P. PURCELL. *Community Action Against Poverty.* New Haven: College and University Press, 1967.
16. BRILL, N. and H. STORROW. "Social Class and Psychiatric Treatment," *Arch. Gen. Psychiatry,* 3 (1960), 340–344.
17. BROWN, G. et al. *Schizophrenia and Social Care.* London: Oxford University Press, 1966.
18. BULLOCK, P. "Morality and Tactics in Community Organizing," in J. Larner and I. Howe, eds., *Poverty: Views from the Left,* pp. 137–148. New York: Morrow, 1968.
19. CAUDILL, H. "Reflections on Poverty in America," in A. B. Shostak and W. Gomberg, eds., *New Perspectives on Poverty,* pp. 12–20. Engelwood Cliffs, N.J.: Prentice-Hall, 1965.
20. CHICAGO BOARD OF HEALTH. *Preliminary Report on Patterns of Medical and Health Care in Poverty Areas in Chicago.* Medical Care Report. Chicago: Chicago Board of Health, 1966.
21. CHILMAN, C. and M. B. SUSSMAN. "Poverty in the United States in the Midsixties," *J. Marriage Fam.,* 26 (1964), 391–394.
22. CLARK, K. B. "A Relevant War Against Poverty: Some Problems of Community Action Programs." Statement read before Clark subcommittee, March 18, 1967.
23. CLARK, R. E. "The Relationship of Schizophrenia to Occupational Income and Occupational Prestige," *Am. Sociol. Rev.,* 13 (1948), 325–330.
24. ———. "Psychoses, Income and Occupational Prestige," *Am. J. Sociol.,* 54 (1949), 443–440.

25. CLAUSEN, J. A. and M. L. KOHN. "Relation of Schizophrenia to the Social Structure of a Small City," in B. Pasamanick, ed., *Epidemiology of Mental Disorder*, pp. 69–95. Washington: American Association for the Advancement of Science, 1959.

26. CLOWARD, R. A. and R. M. ELMAN. "Poverty, Injustice and the Welfare State," *The Nation*, 202 (1966), 264–268.

27. ———. "Advocacy in the Ghetto," *Trans-Action*, 4 (1966), 27–35.

28. COHEN, A. K. and H. M. HODGES, JR. "Characteristics of the Lower-Blue-Collar Class," *Soc. Prob.*, 10 (1963), 303–334.

29. COHEN, J. "Social Work and the Culture of Poverty," *Soc. Work*, 9 (1964), 3–11.

30. COLE, N. J., C. H. H. BRANCH, and R. B. ALLISON. "Some Relationship between Social Class and the Practice of Dynamic Psychotherapy," *Am. J. Psychiatry*, 118 (1961), 1004–1012.

31. COLEMAN, J. V. and P. ERRARA. "The General Hospital Emergency Room and Its Psychiatric Problems," *Am. J. Pub. Health*, 53 (1963), 1294–1301.

32. DARBONNE, A. R. "Crisis: A Review of Theory, Practice and Research," *Psychotherapy*, 2 (1967), 49–56.

33. DEUTSCH, M. "The Role of Social Class in Language Development and Cognition," *Am. J. Orthopsychiatry*, 35 (1965), 78–88.

34. DEUTSCH, M., I. KATZ, and A. R. JENSEN, eds. *Social Class, Race, and Psychological Development*. New York: Holt, Rinehart & Winston, 1968.

35. DINITZ, S. et al. "The Posthospital Psychological Functioning of Former Mental Hospital Patients," *Ment. Hygiene*, 45 (1961), 579–588.

36. DUBOS, R. J. *The Mirage of Health*. New York: Harper & Row, 1959.

37. DUNHAM, H. W. "Social Class and Schizophrenia," *Am. J. Orthopsychiatry*, 34 (1964), 634–42.

38. ———. *Community and Schizophrenia*. Detroit: Wayne State University Press, 1965.

39. ———. "Community Psychiatry: The Newest Therapeutic Bandwagon," *Arch. Gen. Psychiatry*, 12 (1965), 303–313.

40. EATON, J. W. "The Assessment of Mental Health," *Am. J. Psychiatry*, 108 (1951), 81–90.

41. ENGEL, G. L. "Is Grief A Disease?" *Psychosom. Med.*, 23 (1961), 18–22.

42. ERIKSON, E. H. "Identity and the Life Cycle," *Psychol. Issues*, Monogr. 1, (1959).

43. ———. "Growth and Crises of the Healthy Personality," *Psychol. Issues*, 1 (1959), 50–100.

44. FARIS, R. E. and H. W. DUNHAM. *Mental Disorders in Urban Areas*. Chicago: University of Chicago Press, 1939.

45. FLACKS, R. "On the Uses of Participatory Democracy," *Dissent*, 16 (1966), 701–708.

46. FREEMAN, H. and O. SIMMONS. *The Mental Patient Comes Home*. New York: Wiley, 1963.

47. FRUMKIN, R. M. "Occupation and Major Mental Disorder," in A. M. Rose, ed., *Mental Health and Mental Disorder*, pp. 51–63. New York: Norton, 1955.

48. GALBRAITH, J. K. *The Affluent Society*. Boston: Houghton, 1958.

49. GILLIN, J. L. *Poverty and Dependency*. New York: Appleton, 1937.

50. GLASSCOTE, R. M. et al. *The Psychiatric Emergency*. Washington: Joint Information Serv., 1966.

51. GLASSCOTE, R. M. and J. E. GUDMAN. *The Staff of Mental Health Centers*. Washington: Am. Psychiatr. Assoc., and Natl. Inst. Ment. Health, 1969.

52. GOLDBERG, E. M. and S. L. MORRISON. "Schizophrenia and Social Class," *Br. J. Psychiatry*, 109 (1963), 785–802.

53. GORDON, E. W. "Help for the Disadvantaged?" *Am. J. Orthopsychiatry*, 35 (1965), 445–48.

54. GRAHAM, E. "Poverty and the Legislative Process," in B. B. Seligman, ed., *Poverty as a Public Issue*, pp. 251–271. New York: Free Press, 1966.

55. GURIN, G. "An Expectancy Approach to Job Training Programs," in V. L. Allen, ed., *Psychological Factors in Poverty*, pp. 227–299. Chicago: Markham, 1970.

56. GURLAND, B. J., N. J. YORKSTON, A. R. STONE et al. "The Structured and Scaled Interview to Assess Maladjustment (SSIAM): Description, Rationale, and Development," *Arch. Gen. Psychiatry*, 27 (1972), 259–263.

57. HARRINGTON, M. *The Other America*. New York: Macmillian, 1962.

58. HESS, R. D. "Educability and Rehabilitation: The Future of the Welfare Class," *J. Marriage Fam.*, 26 (1964), 422–429.

59. ———. "The Transmission of Cognitive

Strategies in Poor Families: The Socialization of Apathy and Underachievement," in V. L. Allen, ed., *Psychological Factors in Poverty*, pp. 73–92. Chicago: Markham, 1970.

60. HETZNECKER, W. *Suggested Definition of Disadvantaged*. Working paper, Community Mental Health Serv. for the Disadvantaged. Washington: NAMH, 1970. Unpublished.

61. HOBBS, N. "Mental Health's Third Revolution," *Am. J. Orthopsychiatry*, 34 (1964), 822–833.

62. HOLLINGSHEAD, A. and F. C. REDLICH. *Social Class and Mental Illness*. New York: Wiley, 1958.

63. HYDE, R. W. and L. V. KINGSLEY. "Relation of Mental Disorders to Community Socio-Economic Level," *N. Engl. J. Med.*, 231 (1944), 543–548.

64. JAFFE, A. J. and E. SHANAS. "Economic Differentials in the Probability of Insanity," *Am. J. Sociol.*, 44 (1935), 534–539.

65. JAHODA, M. *Current Concepts of Positive Mental Health*, New York: Basic Books, 1958.

66. JAMES, G. "Poverty and Public Health," *Am. J. Public Health*, 55 (1965), 1757–1771.

67. JOINT COMMISSION ON MENTAL ILLNESS AND HEALTH. *Action for Mental Health*. New York: Basic Books, 1961.

68. KELLER, S. "The Social World of the Urban Slum Child: Some Early Findings," *Am. J. Orthopsychiatry*, 33 (1963), 823–831.

69. ———. *The American Lower Class Family*. Albany, N.Y.: State Division of Youth, 1966.

70. KELLY, J. G. "Ecological Constraints on Mental Health Services," *Am. Psychol.*, 21 (1966), 535–539.

71. KENNEDY, J. F. *Message from the President of the United States Relative to the Elderly Citizens of Our Nation*. Doc. 72, 88th Congress, 1st Sess. Feb. 12, 1963.

72. KEYSERLING, L. H. *Progress or Poverty*. Washington: Conference on Economic Progress, 1964.

73. KLARMAN, H. E. *Background, Issues and Policies in Health Services for the Aged in New York City*. New York: Health Research Council, City of New York, 1962.

74. KLEIN, D. C. "The Community and Mental Health: An Attempt at a Conceptual Framework," *Community Ment. Health J.*, 1 (1965), 301–308.

75. KNOLL, E. and J. WITCOVER. "Fighting Poverty and City Hall," *Reporter*, 32 (1965), 19–22.

76. KOBRIN, S. "The Impact of Cultural Factors on Selected Problems of Adolescent Development in the Middle and Lower Class," *Am. J. Orthopsychiatry*, 32 (1962), 387–390.

77. KOHN, M. L. "Social Class and Parent–Child Relationships: An Interpretation," *Am. J. Sociol.*, 68 (1963), 471–480.

78. KOSA, J. "The Nature of Poverty," in J. Kosa, A. Antonovsky, and I. K. Zola, eds., *Poverty and Health*, pp. 1–35. Cambridge: Harvard University Press, 1969.

79. KOSA, J., A. ANTONOVSKY, and I. K. ZOLA, eds. *Poverty and Health*. Cambridge: Harvard University Press, 1969.

80. KRAMER, R. M. and C. DENTON. "Organization of a Community Action Program," *Soc. Work*, 15 (1967), 69–80.

81. KROSNEY, H. *Beyond Welfare: Poverty in the Supercity*. New York: Holt, Rinehart & Winston, 1966.

82. LANGER, E. "Medicine for the Poor: A New Deal in Denver," *Science*, 153 (1966), 508–512.

83. LAPOUSE, R. "Who Is Sick?" *Am. J. Orthopsychiatry*, 35 (1965), 138–144.

84. LAPOUSE, R., M. S. MONK, and M. TERRIS. "The Drift Hypothesis and Socio-Economic Differentials in Schizophrenia," *Am. J. Public Health*, 46 (1956), 978–986.

85. LEE, E. S. "Socio-Economic and Migration Differentials in Mental Disease," *Milbank Mem. Fund Q.*, 41 (1963), 249–268.

86. LEFTON, M. et al. "Social Class, Expectations, and Performance of Mental Patients," *Am. J. Sociol.*, 68 (1962), 79–87.

87. LEMKAU, P. V. "Prevention of Psychiatric Illnesses," *JAMA*, 162 (1956), 854–857.

88. LEMKAU, P. V., C. TIETZER, and M. COOPER. "Mental-Hygiene Problems in Urban Districts," *Ment. Hygiene*, 26 (1941), 100–119.

89. LEWIS, O. *LaVida*. New York: Random House, 1965.

90. McDERMOTT, J. F., S. I. HARRISON, J. SCHRAGER et al. "Social Class and Mental Illness in Children: Observations of Blue-Collar Families," *Am. J. Orthopsychiatry*, 35 (1965), 500–508.

91. MacDonald, D. "Our Invisible Poor," *The New Yorker*, 38 (1963), 84.

92. McGee, R. "Welfare in Affluence," *The Nation*, 202 (1966), 174–180.

93. McKinley, D. G. *Social Class and Family Life*. New York: Free Press, 1964.

94. Macmillan, D. "Preventive Geriatrics: Opportunities of a Community Mental Health Service," *Lancet*, 2 (1960), 1439–1441.

95. Mead, B. T. "Emotional Struggles in Adjusting to Old Age," *Postgrad. Med.*, 31 (1962), 156–160.

96. Mechanic, D. "The Concept of Illness Behavior," *J. Chronic Dis.*, 15 (1962), 189–194.

97. Meyers, J. and L. Schaffer. "Social Stratification and Psychiatric Practice: A Study of an Outpatient Clinic," *Am. Sociol. Rev.*, 19 (1954), 307–310.

98. Miller, S. M. "Poverty and Inequality in America: Implications for the Social Services," *Child Welfare*, 42 (1963), 442–445.

99. ———. "The American Lower Classes: A Typological Approach," *Soc. Res.*, 31 (1964), 1–22.

100. Miller, S. M. and M. Rein. "The War on Poverty," in B. B. Seligman, ed. *Poverty as a Public Issue*, pp. 272–320. New York: Free Press, 1966.

101. Miller, S. M., F. Riessman, and A. Seagull. "Poverty and Self-Indulgence: A Critique of the Non-Deferred Gratification Pattern," in L. A. Ferman et al., eds. *Poverty in America*, pp. 285–302. Ann Arbor: University of Michigan Press, 1965.

102. Miller, W. B. "Lower Class Culture as a Generating Milieu of Gang Delinquency," *J. Soc. Issues*, 14 (1958), 5–19.

103. Minuchin, S., B. Montalvo, B. Guerney et al. *Families of the Slums*. New York: Basic Books, 1967.

104. Mischel, W. "Father Absence and Delay of Gratification: Cross Culture Comparison," *J. Pers. Soc. Psychol.*, 63 (1961), 116–124.

105. Morris, P. and M. Tein. *Dilemmas of Social Reform*: New York: Atherton, 1967.

106. Morris, R. and R. H. Binstock. *Feasible Planning for Social Change*. New York: Columbia University Press, 1966.

107. Myers, J., L. Bean, and M. P. Pepper. "Social Class and Psychiatric Disorders," *J. Health Hum. Behav.*, 6 (1965), 74–79.

108. Ornati, O. *Poverty Amid Affluence*. New York: Twentieth Century Fund, 1966.

109. Panzetta, A. F. "Causal and Action Models in Social Psychiatry," *Arch. Gen. Psychiatry*, 16 (1967), 290–296.

110. ———. *Community Mental Health: Myth and Reality*. Philadelphia: Lea & Febiger, 1971.

111. ———. "The Concept of Community: Short-circuit of the Mental Health Movement," *Arch. Gen. Psychiatry*, 25 (1971), 291–297.

112. Parker, S. and R. J. Kleiner. *Mental Illness in the Urban Negro Community*. New York: Free Press, 1966.

113. Parsons, T. "Definition of Health and Illness in the Light of American Values and Social Structure," in E. G. Jaco, ed., *Patients, Physicians, and Illness*, pp. 165–187. New York: Free Press, 1958.

114. Pasamanick, B. "A Survey of Mental Disease in an Urban Population: VII," *Am. J. Psychiatry*, 119 (1962), 299–305.

115. ———. "The Development of Physicians for Public Mental Health," *Am. J. Orthopsychiatry*, 36 (1967), 469–486.

116. Pasamanick, B., H. Knobloch, and A. M. Lilienfeld. "Socioeconomic Status and Some Precursors of Neuropsychiatric Disorder," *Am. J. Orthopsychiatry*, 26 (1956), 594–601.

117. Pasamanick, B. et al. "A Survey of Mental Disease in An Urban Population," in B. Pasamanick, ed., *Epidemiology of Mental Disorder*, pp. 183–203. Washington: Am. Assoc. for the Advancement of Science, 1959.

118. Pavenstedt, E. "A Comparison of the Child-Rearing Environment of Upper-Lower and Very Low-Lower Class Families," *Am. J. Orthopsychiatry*, 35 (1965), 89–98.

119. Polsby, N. W. *Community Power and Political Theory*. New Haven: Yale University Press, 1963.

120. Pomrinse, S. D. "Marginal Man: A Concept of the Aging Process," *Geriatrics*, 13 (1958), 765–767.

121. Redlich, F. et al. "Social Class Differences in Attitudes towards Psychiatry," *Am. J. Orthopsychiatry*, 25 (1955), 60–70.

122. Reiff, R. and S. Scribner. "Issues in the New National Mental Health Program Relating to Labor and Low Income Groups," in F. Reissman, J. Cohen, and A. Pearl, eds., *Mental Health of the Poor*, pp. 126–145. New York: Free Press, 1964.

123. RIESSMAN, F. "Low-Income Culture: The Strengths of the Poor," *J. Marriage Fam.*, 26 (1964), 417–421.

124. RIESSMAN, F., J. COHEN, A. PEARL, eds. *Mental Health of the Poor.* New York: Free Press, 1964.

125. REISSMAN, F. and M. REIN. "The Third Force Ideology, An Anti-Poverty Ideology," *Am. Child.*, 51 (1965), 10–14.

126. RIIS, J. A. *How the Other Half Lives.* New York: Scribners, 1890.

127. ROBERTSON, N. "Should the Poor Lead the Poor?" *New York Times*, March 21, 1967, p. 16.

128. RUDD, T. N. "Old Age: The Completion of a Life Cycle," *J. Am. Geriatr. Soc.*, 6 (1958), 1–9.

129. RYAN, W. *Distress in the City: A Summary Report of the Boston Mental Health Survey.* Boston, 1964.

130. SCHNEIDER, L. and S. LYSGAARD. "Deferred Gratification Pattern," *Am. Sociol. Rev.*, 18 (1953), 142–149.

131. SCHNEIDERMAN, L. "A Study of the Value-Orientation Preferences of Chronic Relief Recipients," *Soc. Work*, 9 (1964), 13–18.

132. SCHROEDER, C. W. "Mental Disorders in Cities," *Am. J. Sociol.*, 48 (1942), 40–47.

133. SHOSTAK, A. B. "Containment, Co-operation or Co-determination," *Am. Child*, 46 (1965), 15–19.

134. ———. "Urban Politics and Poverty." Presented at Meet. Am. Sociol. Assoc., 1966.

135. SHOSTAK, A. B. and W. GOMBERG, eds. *New Perspective on Poverty.* Englewood Cliffs, N.J.: Prentice-Hall, 1965.

136. SHOSTAK, A. B. and C. P. WOLF. "New Roles and Old Realities: Spokesmen for the Poor." Paper presented Meet. Eastern Sociol. Soc., 1968.

137. SHRIVER, S. "New Weapons in Fighting Poverty," *Public Welfare*, 24 (1966), 9–14.

138. SPITZER, R. L., J. L. FLEISS, E. I. BURDOCK et al. "The Mental Status Schedule: Rationale, Reliability, and Validity," *Compr. Psychiatry*, 5 (1964), 384–395.

139. SROLE, L., T. LANGNER, and S. T. MICHAEL. "Mental Health in the Metropolis. Service for the Elderly," *Pub. Health Rep.*, 77 (1962), 1041–1047.

140. SROLE, L., T. S. LANGER, S. T. MICHAEL et al. *Mental Health in the Metropolis.* New York: McGraw-Hill, 1962.

141. STEIN, L. "Social Class Gradient in Schizophrenia," *Br. J. Prev. Soc. Psychiatry*, 11 (1957), 181–195.

142. SZASZ, T. S. *The Myth of Mental Illness.* New York: Harper & Row, 1962.

143. THOMPSON, W. E. and G. F. STRIEB. "Health and Economic Deprivation in Retirement," *J. Soc. Issues*, 14 (1958), 18–34.

144. TIETZE, C., P. LEMKAU, and M. COOPER. "Schizophrenia, Manic-Depressive Psychosis and Social-Economic Status," *Am. J. Sociol.*, 47 (1941), 167–175.

145. TOBIN, J. "Conquering Poverty in the U.S. by 1977," *New Republic*, 156 (1967), 14–18.

146. TORREY, E. F. "Psychiatric Training: The SST of American Medicine," *Psychiatr. Ann.*, 2 (1972), 60–69.

147. UNITED STATES CONGRESS. *Mental Retardation Facilities and Community Mental Health Centers Act of 1963.* Public Law 88–64. Washington: U.S. Govt. Print. Off., 1963.

148. UNITED STATES GOVERNMENT. *The People Left Behind*, pp. 75–84. Washington: U.S. Govt. Print. Off., 1967.

149. UNITED STATES PUBLIC HEALTH SERVICE. *U.S. National Health Survey, Medical Care, Health Status, and Family Income.* Series 10, no. 9. Washington: U.S. Govt. Print. Off., May 1964.

150. WEISBROD, B. A. *The Economics of Poverty; An American Paradox.* Englewood Cliffs, N.J.: Prentice-Hall, 1965.

151. WILL, R. E. and H. G. VATTER, eds. *Poverty in Affluence.* New York: Harcourt, Brace & World, 1965.

152. WING, J. K., J. L. BIRLEY, J. E. COOPER et al. "Reliability of a Procedure for Measuring and Classifying Present Psychiatric State," *Br. J. Psychiatry*, 113 (1967), 499–515.

153. WORTIS, H. and A. FREEDMAN. "The Contribution of Social Environment to the Development of Premature Children," *Am. J. Orthopsychiatry*, 35 (1965), 57–68.

154. ZILBACH, J. J. "Crisis in Chronic Problem Families," in G. Belsasso, ed., *Psychiatric Care of the Underprivileged*, pp. 87–100. Boston: Little, Brown, 1971.

CHAPTER 32

RESEARCH IN THE DELIVERY OF HEALTH SERVICES*

Julius B. Richmond and Donald J. Scherl

A BUMPER CROP of health legislation in 1965 precipitated an interest in research and evaluation of health-services programs. This was the year of passage of the Medicare and Medicaid amendments to the Social Security Act, Comprehensive Health Planning, Regional Medical Programs, amendments to the Maternal and Infant Care Programs and the Children and Youth Programs, and Headstart health and Neighborhood Health Center programs of the Office of Economic Opportunity. Undoubtedly the experience with the Mental Retardation Facilities and Community Mental Health Act of 1963, which was developed with strong support from President John F. Kennedy, paved the way for such Congressional action.

Small wonder that professionals in the field of health services, as well as economists, polit-

* The authors gratefully acknowledge the research and editorial assistance of Dale Pelletier in the preparation of this chapter.

ical scientists, and informed citizens generally, began to wonder about how we might learn whether the new programs and expenditures were sound, effective, and justified. Other factors accelerated this interest and concern:

1. The program-planning-budgeting system (PPBS), as applied in the Defense Department, had created an impression that the methods for program evaluation were well developed and that they could be readily applied to human services programs. (Subsequent experience demonstrated the limitations of this approach even to the hardware cost effectiveness of the Defense Department, as the later debates on missiles, bombers, and so forth, were to reveal.) As efforts proceeded to apply PPBS to human services—including health services—the limitations of this system and other aspects of cost effectiveness became apparent.[57] Nonetheless, such efforts did give rise to much constructive work in research and evaluation of health services.

2. The increasing total expenditures for health services generated questions about whether they were beneficial. In part because of the new legislation and in part because of the growing interest of the American people in improved personal health services, expenditures began to rise absolutely as well as in relation to the percentage of the gross national product. As long as health expenditures were at the level of approximately 4.5 percent of the GNP, (as was the case in Fiscal Year 1970) relatively little attention was directed at an evaluation of health services. As this figure began to approach 8 percent, in FY 1972, however, there developed increasing concern, which led to intensified inquiry into the desirability of such expenditures. (Total amount spent on health in FY 1973 was $94.1 billion, a rise of $9.4 billion from FY 1972; the percentage spent on health care in 1973 was 7.7 percent of the GNP.)

3. Improved technology, particularly computerization, helped create the impression that no question was unanswerable. The state of the art, however, had not yet developed clear formulations of questions to be asked. There was little consensus on what the goals and priorities for the health system (or nonsystem, as many called it) were to be. Without some consensus on such basic issues, research and evaluation could become an exercise in technological development.

It would be inappropriate to convey to the reader that there had been no prior research and evaluative efforts in the field of medical care. The studies of the Committee on the Cost of Medical Care published in the 1930s represented a good example of research in this field. It spawned a whole group of investigators in the field of medical care (Michael Davis, I. S. Falk, Nathan Sinai, to mention a few), who worked over the next several decades. Though their work was of high quality, it went largely unheralded—mainly because of the politics of health, which had been dominated in those decades mostly by organized medicine, which in turn was largely unresponsive to the suggestions that stemmed from their various studies.

❪ Issues of Research Design

As interest in research into the delivery of health care grew, the complexities of this work continued undiminished. Encouraged by the 1965 legislation and by public recognition and support for new approaches, new models for the delivery of services rapidly emerged throughout the nation. Research into issues of medical care suddenly found itself aiming at a swiftly moving target while lacking the precision instruments needed to define the target and to put it into accurate and adequate focus.

Much has been written and many studies have been made with respect to the assessment of various health-care delivery systems. To include the body of this material would greatly exceed the scope of this chapter. In general, the majority of the studies reveal what is clear even to the uninformed eye: no comprehensive, effective system for evaluating the quality and quantity of health care has yet been defined. Essentially, these studies point up five basic problems:

The Definition of Program Goals

In the delivery of health services, no issue raises greater despair than that of delineating goals and aims (see, for example Donabedian,[16] Wing and Hailey,[76] or Monroe, Klee, and Brody[44]). Well-intentioned aims, such as "high quality of service at lowest possible cost" are obviously inadequate for defining research goals. The precise definition of research questions depends upon the degree to which a clear definition exists of the larger goals and aims of the health-delivery system under study. The problem, to paraphrase Gertrude Stein, is not so much in the determination of the answers as it is in the determination of the questions.

The Definition of Research Goals

Often the aims of research, as those of the programs themselves, are multiple. Just as a health-delivery system may be seen as a method for improving services to clients, for training health personnel, and for establishing a site for biomedical research, so too an evaluative research project within a health-care delivery system may be viewed as an important step in the improvement of the evaluative arts as well as a way in which to improve the system's product, management, or image. It may also be viewed as a place to train future health-care delivery researchers.

The research field has moved slowly, one reason being that people do not identify their aims as they establish new programs. Development of neighborhood health centers, for example, and the increase in group practice and in prepaid programs, have each resulted from leaps of conceptual understanding rather than from hard evaluative data. Such precipitousness is not necessarily bad; it may in fact represent necessity in human-services programs. Progress in the development of services cannot always await research and evaluation data, particularly when data will never be adequate and complete. In addition, the intuitive genius from which major new developments in services may spring often does not carry with it an evaluative and quantitative capacity.

The differentiation and untangling of each aim and its related costs from the totality of the integrated operating system is a critical research obstacle. This problem is one researchers must face, though it has become an issue of public policy as well. Insurance companies and governmental rate-setting agencies, for example, do not know how much they should pay, or, indeed, are paying, for research, training, and service in any specific health-care delivery system.

Where patient care, teaching, and research are carried out simultaneously in the same setting by the same personnel, the problem of disaggregating costs is both technical and judgmental. Schools for health professionals must establish an educational environment that incorporates a combination of activities including those relating to instruction for a variety of students; specific, direct patient-care services; biomedical research; continuing education; and community service. There are diffi-

cult judgments to be made with regard to the allocation of costs within such joint activity, and such joint-product situations. Clearly, this problem creates further complexities in the cost-finding process. Though we are learning to deal with the problem more effectively in the health-services field, we should recognize that it is an old one to industry. For instance, the determination of the cost of a gallon of gasoline evolves from a series of joint cost allocation decisions. For purposes of public policy, decisions are required on how much service revenue should appropriately underwrite educational costs as opposed to other service costs within the system.

Biomedical and Health-Services Delivery Research

When setting objectives, advances in either the delivery or technology of medical care can make any particular evaluation study outmoded before it is completed. Research relating to alterations in medical care as a result of biomedical advances is sometimes confounded with research specifically related to the delivery of services. The effect of such advances as renal transplantation or hemodialysis on service delivery needs to be differentiated from research primarily focused on issues of organization, like fee-for-service or prepayment as alternative financing formulas, or group practice versus solo practice as a delivery mechanism. Another example may be useful. The development of immunizations has dramatically reduced the incidence and prevalence of specific infectious diseases. Historically, the first steps in controlling diseases were related to issues of delivery—adequate water and housing, for instance. Further advances in the development of techniques of immunization against diphtheria, measles, and polio were striking. The result was an enormous conservation in the amount of manpower required for the treatment of patients with these illnesses. The savings produced altered the concept of primary health care and the nature of the services and resources required of backup hospitals and other facilities. In this instance, advances in biomedical knowledge resulted in a decrease in disease, a saving in manpower, and a resultant shift in delivery mechanisms.

To summarize, two categories of questions tend to get confused by those interested in outcome research. One category of question relates specifically to issues of health status outcome resulting from changes in the organization or pattern of service delivery. The other relates to similar changes in outcome resulting from biomedical advances. Since the outcome measures, in both instances, are similar, if not the same, both researchers and those utilizing the results of such research need to carefully isolate the effects of these related but different variables.

Quality

Research in the field of health-services delivery must deal with questions of quality as well as those of quantity, availability, and statistical outcome. Lee and Jones[39] stress that the criteria for determining quality are little more than value judgments that are applied to several aspects or dimensions of the process of medical care. Klein et al.[36] asked twenty-four individual "administrative officials" for criteria for evaluating the quality of patient care—and received eighty different answers. They concluded that it is unlikely a single comprehensive criterion for measuring patient care would ever be established. In this connection, Rivlin[57] noted that human services, as a general matter, need to be evaluated by multiple rather than by single criteria, or in her words, "Multiple measures are necessary to reflect multiple objectives and to avoid distorting performance."

Cross-Program Comparisons

Much of the interest in evaluation of health-delivery systems relates to the desire to compare one system with another. Such comparisons encounter the usual difficulties in defining outcomes and base lines. Moorehead,[45] for example, compared OEO (Office of Economic Opportunity) neighborhood health centers with other health-care providers in order to measure adherence to standards of preventive health care. She found that one of the most important results of her study was the wide variation of performance within any one group of providers, variations that could not be attributed to the organizational pattern alone. The variation seemed to reflect individual commitment and performance. Administrative efficiency, organizational patterns, and methods of financing also had significant effects on quality, she found. Moorehead concludes that "when tools are available to measure the other important parameters of health care, one can be hopeful that these programs will have achieved no small measure of success in the demonstration of an effective model for the delivery of health services, particularly to the nation's disadvantaged."

Studies like Moorehead's also encounter difficulties in comparing programs that have different aims, organizational sets, and theories. Because each element of a program will reflect these factors, comparisons of different constellations of programs may represent no comparison at all. For instance, the cost per encounter at a neighborhood health center and at a private physician's office could be weighed. Yet the product of a comparison this simple would be of questionable value. The purpose, nature, and effectiveness of the two encounters are not only different in complex ways, but they derive from different conceptualizations of aim and organization. Training, for example, may be an important cost factor at the health center, but not at the physician's office.

The utility of cross-program evaluative studies depends upon the pattern of questions that crosses the boundaries of different delivery systems. Wing and Hailey[76] suggest five essentials for a health-services program: (1) everyone needing treatment should be able to obtain it; (2) health services should be comprehensive and varied, with an adequate number of places where they may be obtained; (3) health services should overlap with social and welfare services, vocational guidance, and protected environments of various kinds, including hospitals and workshops for the permanently handicapped; (4) health services should not only be comprehensive but integrated; and (5) their chief aim should be to decrease or contain morbidity, first in the patient, secondly in the patient's immediate family, and thirdly in the community at large. Donabedian[15] applies similar principles to arrive at a more detailed and sophisticated grouping of basic goals and objectives for the assessment of health systems. Acceptance of clearly articulated goals permits the logical development of a series of parameters for systems research and evaluation.

(Commonly Used Evaluative Indices

Numerous attempts have been made to utilize single indices to assess the functioning of broad health-care delivery systems. Three of the most common are infant mortality, life expectancy, and cost. Each has the advantage of being quantifiable in broad terms, and each shares the disadvantage of representing an averaging effect incorporating, often with unknown weight, components of the state of health-services delivery intermixed with advances in technology.

Infant Mortality

Perhaps the first major figure to take specific social note of the importance of infant mortality was Florence Nightingale. In 1858, at a time when England was trying to cope with a succession of epidemics and reformers like Sir Edwin Chadwick were expending their energies toward improving sanitary conditions, Florence Nightingale noted that "the causes of enormous child mortality rates (are) . . . well known, defective household hygiene."[7] Since then, researchers not only have looked into the causes of infant mortality, but also, on a broader scale, have used the rates of child mortality to determine the quality of a nation's or neighborhood's health-care delivery.

Richmond,[55] notes that the health of infants in our society has improved significantly over the past several decades. From the early years of the century, the infant mortality rate dropped from approximately 140 per 1000 live births to approximately 22 per 1000 in 1968. Since 1950, however, the rate has tended to plateau, and by 1968 the United States had slipped to sixteenth place among the countries of the world in the rate of infant mortality. The importance of this data has been in some dispute (see Dellaportas[12] and Faigle,[19] for example).

Within the United States, infant mortality rates for whites and nonwhites have indicated what Faigle calls the "American health tragedy": more nonwhite children die, a tragic circumstance compounded by the cycle of social and medical crises—ameliorated but never fully resolved—affecting large segments of the low-income population. Since 1960 the gap between rates for whites and nonwhites has increased appreciably. From 1965 to 1967, Faigle found a rate of 23.6 perinatal deaths per 1000 whites under age five and 44.0 per 1000 for nonwhites. Usher[73] also found a greater frequency of stillbirths in lower socioeconomic groups. Yerbe[77] reported vast differences in infant mortality rates in geographic subdivisions of Manhattan. The rate in central Harlem was 40.5 per 1000 in 1962, while in Kips Bay and Yorkville, two middle-class white communities, the rate was 14.7 per 1000. These and other data suggest that further improvement in health care, as measured by infant mortality rates, will depend in large part on bettering the infant-care environment for the low income and the nonwhite population. Studies conducted with this end in mind have indicated that the means of collecting the data also need to be improved (see Usher and the Denver Department of Public Health study).

Dellaportas[12] compared the United States's position with respect to infant mortality with that of sixteen other nations. The countries were selected on the basis of the completeness of their vital statistics registration, using United Nations demographic data. Dellaportas computed the average annual rate for three periods: 1956–1959; 1960–1962; and 1963–1965. After attempting to correlate rates of mortality among age groups younger than one year, he concluded that infant deaths of less than six months were underregistered.

The only reliable data concerned deaths from six to twelve months. These figures, however, are not a general indicator because many deaths in this age group can be attributed to nonmedical (mainly social) factors. Dellaportas concludes that "Considering the value of infant mortality as a health index of a country or an area, every effort to improve the quality and accuracy of this frequently undernumerated rate is a worthwhile undertaking. . . . [Only] with complete registration [can] observed rates become reliable enough to show where the level of mortality really lies."

A number of additional surveys have been undertaken, partly for purposes of assessing maternal- and infant-care projects of the Health Services and Mental Health Administration of HEW. In May, 1969, the Denver Department of Public Health attempted to use infant mortality rates to compare the quality of care between low-income and white populations. It found an abrupt drop in mortality from 34.2 per 1000 live births in 1964 to 21.5 per 1000 in 1968 for the 25 census tracks that made up the target area for the program. Similar results have been obtained in Birmingham, Alabama (the rate decreased from 25.4 in 1965 to 14.3 in 1969), and in Omaha (from 33.4 in 1964 to 13.4 in 1969). The Denver group found, as Dellaportas did, that research efforts were more difficult than had been anticipated. In Denver, for example, each of the projects under study, (maternal and infant care, children and youth programs, OEO centers) covered only a small segment of the population; moreover, a high degree of fragmentation was found to exist among agencies.

In 1967 the Province of Quebec used infant mortality rates to measure the effectiveness of different levels of maternal health-delivery systems. Usher[73] relates that perinatal mortality review committees of physicians from each of the province's 156 maternity hospitals were formed. Each hospital group reported to a central medical committee. All births and deaths were reported by weight groups, and a detailed questionnaire was completed, collected, and standardized for each perinatal death. The Quebec study revealed that (1)

there were 34 percent more infant deaths in the province's remote areas (adjusted for population) than in the metropolitan centers (Montreal, Quebec City); (2) with decreasing hospital size, the incidence of low birth weight rose in a steady progression from 75 to 109 per 1000 live births; and (3) the existence of, or access to, neonatal intensive care units was an important factor in preventing death. Per 1000 live births, there were 16.4 deaths in hospitals with neonatal intensive care units, 18.43 in hospitals with access to a unit, and 20.26 in hospitals without access.[73]

In summary, infant mortality rates indicate that the United States has significant deficits in its health-care system in comparison with other nations. It also has an alarming discrepancy between perinatal deaths among whites, nonwhites, and lower socioeconomic groups and a like discrepancy in health care between metropolitan and nonmetropolitan areas. Infant mortality as an index of health-services delivery has an honorable place historically, but its use as an isolated variable has its limitations.

Life Expectancy

The Bible declares man's inability to control the length of his mortal survival. "The days of man are short, and the number of months are nothing to you, Lord, who has proclaimed the limits of man's life that he may not surpass them" (Job 14:5). Aristotle, as Gale[28] points out, also described the limits of mortality: "The time and life of each thing has its number fixed and determined because all things (have their) order and everything is measured by a period."

In the sixteenth century Aurent Joubert, one of the first to receive a doctorate in the practice of medicine in France, asserted that medicine could be used to prolong man's life. In his book,[35] written about 1570, he stated:

The question has always been intense and has excited the greatest of minds. . . . There are several arguments which conclude that the life of man cannot be prolonged by remedies or means—on the other hand, doctors maintain that it is possible. . . . Although one cannot avoid the discomforts which result from the principles of our generations . . . they can nonetheless be retarded by our art and stalled so that the last day doesn't come so hastily.

Indeed, much of modern medicine is aimed at promoting and prolonging the quality of man's healthy life, and it has enabled man to live a longer life; as Joubert put it: "Old age is prolonged by our art, in the manner such that the transition . . . the return to dust through extreme old age will come much later."

Medicine today bears testimony to man's desire to preserve life by combating disease and death.[49] Advances in medical knowledge have been associated with the rising number of older people in the population.[55] In 1900 the median age was 22.9 years, only 4 percent of the population lived to age 65, and the average life expectancy was 49. In 1960 the median age was 29.5, 9.3 percent lived to age 65, and the average life expectancy (1964) was 70.2 years.[56]

Research in health-care delivery has used life expectancy statistics as a measure of the quality of health care. Studies have revealed that man is living longer, and generally in a healthier manner because of several factors, of which medical progress probably has been one of the most important. However, to date, though the effects of aging have been attentuated, they cannot be stopped; no notable changes in mortality rates have occurred between the periods of 1955–1959 and 1965–1969.[41] As in the case of infant mortality, we seem to have reached another plateau. There are, even so, significant variations in longevity among different socioeconomic, racial, and cultural groups, as there are in infant mortality.* Nonetheless, we have concentrated here on broad studies in order to review how such data have been used and what they have told us, in general, about the nation's health-care system.

Lawrence,[38] in his studies of the aged, emphasized the need for a multiple approach to generating statistics for determining the health of a population. He used three data-source methods, in each of which he found a

* See references 1, 33, 52, 58, 59, 71, and 74.

particular weakness or complicating factor inherent in the source itself. He surveyed the existing records on a master list of 40,000 hospitals, nursing homes, and residential institutions in order to determine the number and type of institutions and facilities that existed, the kinds of staffs, the services provided, and the health characteristics of the patients or the resident population. He found that chronic illness was largely responsible for long-term stays, that 40 percent of the population of the fifteen-to-forty-five age group had at least one chronic illness, but that 70 to 80 percent of persons by the age of sixty-five had a chronic illness, many with complications, an associated disability, or both. He also determined that one-third of the hospital patient population was comprised of persons sixty-five or older.

The second method used by Lawrence to study patterns of aging was to review selected clinical and laboratory tests and physician examinations as applied to sample populations. He found this method was not only quite costly, but also required further research respecting standardization of physical examinations, equipment used, and sampling techniques. As a third method, Lawrence analyzed information obtained through his own direct interviews and questionnaires. He concluded that the detailed comprehensive information he acquired could be abstracted and a wide range of the aged's personal characteristics detailed; but once again, the procedure was costly and time consuming.

Oritz and Parker[48] used an entirely different method for evaluating health-services programs. They attempted to determine what changes in health status and population patterns are most likely to result in improved figures for both mortality, and morbidity. In order to determine how these expected benefits could be used as a means of evaluating health-services programs, they developed a Markov model of the birth-life-death process in which control of variables representing health status are related to changes in rates of mortality, life span, and quality of life. The purpose was to use this model to describe the impact on life expectancy of changes in such "decision variables" as age-stratified distribution of population over time, mortality rates disaggregated by age group and cause of death, and fertility rates and population growth rates over time. The Markovian model was used to determine the impact of changes in health-services programs viewed in terms of the above output criteria and the relationship of the expected benefits to the cost incurred in making the changes. From this study, Oritz and Parker found that the tabulation of deaths due to an arbitrary number of causes can serve as a tool for analysis of longevity patterns, and that the estimation of life expectancy gains made on the basis of hypothesized mortality reductions can be used as a tool for public-health problems.

Spiegelman[69] traced the changes in death rates for all generations living during a particular period to the next period. He then analyzed the death rates during a particular period by ten age groups and compared this data with the death rates for the same generation ten years earlier. Spiegelman stresses that it is necessary to examine the experience of generations, rather than the cross-section of period experience, to understand the underlying changes in mortality. Bayo[5] and Lew and Seltzer[41] confirm that longitudinal studies of this nature must be followed up. Analyses of findings in follow-up studies permit interpretation of mortality trends, projections, and changes in the death rate. Plausible assumptions cannot be made about the magnitude of death rates beyond the period covered by a follow-up study; thus the relative longevity of a group with or without intervention can be portrayed only in terms of the temporary life expectancies involved.[49] Longitudinal studies are hampered, however, by the concepts and methods by which they are started; though new ideas and new methods of measurement may be introduced, this data cannot reach back to the beginning of the study.

Evaluative research in health services delivery using life expectancy as a measure of the quality of health care, is also complicated by the pertinent nonmedical factors that must be taken into account. Palmore[49] found three factors, that he felt were the strongest pre-

dictors of longevity, to be nonrelated to medical issues. They involve psychological and social issues for which outside medical intervention was generally inappropriate and unwarranted. The three factors cited by Palmore are genetic endowment, environmental issues —for example, nutrition, stress, social roles, and life-style—and intellectual deterioration. This last, which leads to an inadequacy of health care, is the strongest predictor of life expectancy.[49] It has been theorized, but not proven, that maintaining intellectual stimulation and avoiding sensory deprivation may extend life expectancy, though such a proposition is only an interesting speculation thus far. Rapid and marked declines in intellectual abilities can, according to Palmore, serve as a forewarning to an earlier death, and it should be given special attention and therapy administered to prevent it.

Like the rate of infant mortality, that of life expectancy is a significant element in assessing systems of health-care delivery. Again, like infant mortality, life expectancy should not be looked to as a single indicator isolated from other relevant social and medical factors. The relationship between longevity and the intervention of specific health systems is not yet clear, though it is a promising area for study.

Cost

The use of economic data and analyses have long been elements of research in health-care delivery and in influencing program and expenditure decisions in the public sector. Their influence has derived from the general assumption that economics is a free, neutral, and objective parameter. As noted by Fein,[22] economic argument has embodied an appealing pattern of thought and can provide an efficient way of reviewing a problem.

Sir William Petty, late in the seventeenth century, began examining the economics of health care when he found that the average "price tag" on a human body was approximately 80 British pounds. The tag prompted investigations by Petty into the cost implications of a plague then sweeping England.[50] His research methods were later used by

Chadwick, who in 1842 estimated that the financial loss from excessive sickness and premature disability and death equaled 14 million British pounds when one took into account the loss of productive power.[9] Chadwick argued that the economist, for the sake of the advancement of his science, should view the human being as an investment of capital and an element of the productive force.

In 1850 the American statistician Lemuel Shattuck also viewed public-health measures from an economic perspective. In arguing that more effective preventive sanitary measures be taken in order to control epidemics, he wrote: "The expenses and losses caused by the neglect of sanitary measures included a loss sustained by the state, in consequences of the diminished power and general liability to disease." He estimated that an inefficient sanitary system in the state of Massachusetts resulted in 6000 unnecessary deaths and the loss of 108,000 man-years of labor at $50 per year, equaling $5.4 million. In the latter half of the nineteenth century, William Farr calculated what he termed the "money value of man" and applied the concept to general taxation problems as well as to social programs.

Until fairly recently, however, human capital was largely ignored by the main body of economists. Beginning in the 1950s, a significant change occurred in the place that human resources occupy in the economic literature.[22] Interest in health economics was rekindled, and this interest has deepened as the funds expended for health care in the nation have become so great that they could no longer be ignored.

Research has been conducted on improving health-care services by exploring the costs and cost implications of health-care delivery. Cost measurement and price indices in the health field are far from precise instruments, but the magnitude and consistency of the increases are so generally uniform and so large that there can be little doubt about the validity of general trends. As noted at the beginning of this chapter, total expenditures for health care in the fiscal year ending June 30, 1972, reached $83.4 billion, 7.6 percent of the gross national product. The percentage may

well approach 10 percent by the end of the 1970s. This trend highlights a growing problem with respect to financing, delivery, and organization of health-care services.

Four aspects of the cost index for assessing the functioning of broad health-care delivery systems are technology and utilization, financing of services, manpower, and the organization and delivery of services.

Technology and Utilization

The demand for, and per capita utilization of, health services is continuing to increase each year. This growth in demand is in response to such factors as increased longevity, less acute but more long-term ailments, government and third-party payments and reimbursement plans, plus nontraditional methods of health-care delivery. New treatments for old diseases have had the effect of not only saving lives, but also of generating new problems. The use of dialysis in chronic renal failure and of antibiotics in infectious disease are good examples of technologic advances that have created whole new sets of biomedical and delivery problems.

Advances have also been made in mental-health care. Both the number and kinds of services and their utilization have expanded. Between 1965 and 1969, accompanied by a sharp decline in the overall census, admission rates of psychiatric hospitals rose 17 percent.[76] A key factor in this rise has been the growing readiness of patients and their relatives to accept admission as the stigma of psychiatric disorders has declined and therapeutic possibilities have improved.

Financing of Services and Advances in Technology

Expansion of government financing and of private health insurance, plus increased governmental support of services for the poor have made health care more easily available for more persons. The nation expends about $9.9 billion a year on medical insurance for the poor.[27] In fiscal year 1974, the federal government expects medical assistance to extend to 27 million Americans.[27] By increasing the total volume of money available for health care, and by spreading payments over a larger population, private insurance companies and the government, through Medicaid, Medicare, and other programs, have brought health-care services to a greater number, often to those who once did without the services because they could not afford them. The upshot of expanding services has been greater public expectations than are being met.[66]

The government, meanwhile, has found that its huge additional expenditures not only have failed to produce equitable utilization of health-care resources by the whole population but have resulted in only a small net gain. HEW's recent report on the health of the nation's health-care system spoke of the crippling inflation in medical costs that has caused vast increases in government health expenditures for little return, raised the premiums of private health insurance, and reduced the purchase power of the citizen's health dollar.[66]

Government expenditure and private insurance have improved access to medical care, but in order to meet the public expectations they have aroused, it is necessary for insurance programs to expand and cover a larger proportion of total family medical costs. Insurance has also had the effect of promoting greater utilization of hospital services, with the corollary of increased expenditures for hospital care.

During the 1930s, the largest portion of the health-services dollar was allocated to physician fees. During the next decade, hospitals began increasing their share of the health dollar, which has been climbing steadily through the early 1970s.[66] It is costing hospitals more to provide services because managerial tools have not kept up with technical advances, another factor in the rise of the nation's health bill, and because the method of treating an insured patient's disorder may be determined by the kind of insurance he carries. As Feldstein[25] found, the patient is often willing to purchase more expensive care because the net cost for inpatient services is often less than the net charge for the same service on an ambulatory basis. This induced

demand for expensive care gives a false signal to the hospital about the type of care the public needs. Feldstein correctly notes that the current method of financing hospital care does not give consumers an opportunity to register their preferences.

Approximately $2.5 billion is spent annually on medical research—10 percent of the total dollars spent for any research and development within the United States.[4] As a result of technological advances, more diseases are treatable and more illnesses can be prevented. Although a greater range of services is available, the more expensive equipment and investment required and the degree of specialization necessary to use this technology, along with the demand for highly trained personnel, make these services, paradoxically, less accessible to the greater proportion of people requiring or requesting them. Cardiac transplant and coronary artery bypass operations serve as examples. Furthermore, there is no well-controlled clinical evidence on the effectiveness of these new procedures for which demand has been generated.

Feldstein[25] found that the rise in cost of treating a patient is not necessarily evidence that there has been technological progress or a productivity gain. Changing demand, he says, can alter technology without scientific progress; technical progress can increase cost, and the current approach to medical research may be biased toward producing information that causes technical progress to increase cost.

MANPOWER

As these technological changes have occurred, high degrees of specialization have simultaneously caused a shift among medical personnel. The physician/patient ratio has shot up significantly—the population increased 17 percent from 1955 to 1965 while the number of active physicians rose 22 percent.[72] From 1965 to 1970, the population went up 5.1 percent, and the number of physicians jumped 14.3 percent.[2] However, the tremendous fragmentation that has developed in the medical profession through specialization has weakened the usefulness of this undifferentiated ratio. In 1967, 55 percent of practicing physicians were specialists and only 12 percent of medical school graduates went into medical practice.[72] In 1971, 83 percent of practicing physicians were specialists.[2] Medical personnel includes not only physicians, nurses, therapists, and dentists, but, by virtue of technological advances and expanded research, sociologists, economists, architects, engineers, computer technicians—to name only a few of the professionals who have entered the medical field. Increased manpower in the field will send health's share of the total manpower revenues up as well.

Organization and Delivery of Services

As a result of the spiraling cost of health care, efforts have been made to design new systems for delivery of services, aimed in part at cutting these costs. During the past two decades, the United States has invested heavily in studying health-delivery systems, in extensive analyses of patterns for utilizing health services, and in developing a wide variety of demonstration projects involving techniques for providing health care in more efficient and effective ways. Nontraditional methods of payment for service programs have served both as a means and an end in observing the delivery and quality of health care. Some have advocated prepayment as the answer to the inefficiencies of the fee-for-service system, despite its many legal obstacles. The expansion of the prepayment method is being tested throughout the country.[30]

In Massachusetts, the Harvard Community Health Plan has sought to improve services to its community through a prepaid, group-practice, comprehensive service program. Sponsors of the plan have found that by ascertaining approximate costs of each visit, differentiated by services delivered (X-rays, counseling, and so forth), they were able to predict the appropriate range of service and number of visits necessary for adequate care. Based upon this information, appropriate rates could be predetermined. The Harvard Plan provides an internal set of checks and balances with regard to quality of care. Because it is a group practice, only one set of records is kept for each patient, thus making undesirable meth-

ods of treatment, or adverse effects of treatment, obvious to those reviewing the patient's charts.

Enrollment in the Harvard Plan costs about as much as Massachusetts Blue Cross protection (in 1973 approximately $25 per month per person, and $65 per month per family), but the services it covers are broader. The Harvard Plan is reportedly self-supporting with an enrollment of 30,000, though its financial independence is sustained through government grants and reimbursements.[17] Permanente, HIP, Group Health, and others have repetitively demonstrated the economy of broad prepaid services, but almost always well defined and often select populations are their clients.

Opinions have varied on the effectiveness of group prepayment plans. Criticism has arisen with regard to the quality of care and questions have been raised as to whether or not patients also purchase care outside the system,[30] thus incurring costs not reflected in the group rate.

When mental-health services are provided on a prepaid basis, they tend to be underutilized. However, their provision may lead to a reduction in the overall use of medical care by the populations to which they are available.[76] A comprehensive review of this subject can be found in Ried, Myers and Scheidenmandel.[56] Few of the national health insurance proposals include these services to date. Only the Kennedy-Griffiths-Corman Bill of 1973 used the financing mechanisms of national health insurance to promote mental-health services. The bill proposed comprehensive health services to all residents in the United States, similar in scope to the system used in Great Britain; its benefits included medical and dental services—preventive, therapeutic, and rehabilitative; there were no deductibles, no coinsurance, and no waiting periods. The plan was to have been financed through payroll taxes and contributions from the General Fund.

Another way of altering both the financing and delivery of services is represented by the neighborhood health center. As Fein[21] notes, the purpose of the center is to offer care to all those who need it in a specific geographic area and to do so in a way that removes the income barrier without producing the indignities of a welfare system. The neighborhood system provides a method for redistributing health-care workers to areas of need. Fein adds that an economist's evaluation of a neighborhood health center is generally expected to assess the input and output relationships, while focusing on the delivery of care. He suggests, however, that in measuring the economic inputs and outputs, personnel and equipment costs be used in conjunction with the number of patient visits—the traditional cost-effectiveness approach. By quantifying inputs and assigning dollar values to them, and by quantifying the benefits and assigning dollar values to these outputs, the ratio of benefits to cost can then be determined.

There are serious problems in developing ratios of this kind in human service systems. Most input-output measures used in assessing health care focus on the "cost" of illnesses which have a direct bearing on a person's income production and on the cost of treating that illness. The benefit is measured, therefore, in terms of cash income gained (or lost) and ignores less tangible benefits involved not only for the patient, but also for his family and community. Community input in a neighborhood center is difficult to measure, for example. Sparer and Alderman[68] encountered these problems in evaluating neighborhood health centers. An economist's measure of output is also likely to ignore the non-medical outputs; for example, the impact on the community of the center and its payroll viewed as a business and as a service facility. Although an economist's evaluation is likely to be given weight, it is possible that it is often given more weight than it deserves because it seems to be a quantitive evaluation. So far, third-party payment mechanisms, apart from governmental grants for these health centers, have proven to be inadequate means of support, and as Fein points out, the inherent quality of any kind of subsidy tends to decrease the notion of competition producing better products. If there is only one center available, the consumer has no choice for better or different treatment—unless he can

afford it.[22] The lesson is clear: Delivery or availability of health services and financing mechanisms must be separated.

When looked at from the standpoint of costs, the total health-delivery system is consuming an increasing portion of the nation's gross national product. What remains unclear is whether proportionate benefits have accrued to the citizens. Differing systems of delivery and differing systems of financing have increased at an astonishing rate over the past decade. There is little data, however, to substantiate a firm assessment as to the cost implications of each. If one factor is obvious, it is the role of financing in forcing the physician and the consumer toward more expensive levels of care. These higher levels of care have had an unintended but well-substantiated impact on hospitalization insurance and on the health-delivery system.

Our examination of three quantifiable indicators of health-care delivery—infant mortality, life expectancy, and cost—indicates, then, that none of them, by themselves, provides a sufficient basis on which to assess health-care delivery. They are insufficient because single variable analyses are inadequate and because other factors, not so easily quantified, must also be taken into account.

❙ Evaluative Studies

Standard approaches to issues of evaluation are well known and do not require extensive reiteration here. Clearly, two possibilities obtain. Programs can be developed for the purpose of enabling firm and accurate evaluation to occur, or programs can be developed and then evaluated, but evaluation is not a factor in their origin. Evaluation, in other words, is a secondary activity.

In the first instance, based in the earlier tradition, goals will be clearly and precisely articulated as a primary step. Schulberg, Sheldon, and Baker[64] identify this approach as the "goal attainment model," whereby a program's success is measured in reaching practical objectives rather than ideal objectives. The diffi-

culties of using this method begin with selecting appropriate objectives for study and
include the built-in dilemma of whether or not
the researcher should actively participate in
the design of the program. Freeman and
Sherwood[26] contend that it is mandatory for
the researcher to initially identify goals with
the future administrator, a mandate that poses
difficult logistical and political problems.
Donabedian[15] points out two other difficulties
with this method: the issue of who should be
in control and the problem of how to maintain
the proper balance between lay and professional authority. He suggests the following
method for facing these difficulties: (1) fundamental agreement between administrator
and evaluator on, and commitment to, a few
basic objectives; (2) agreement on areas of
legitimate primary jurisdiction, the most important being in the area of clinical judgment,
where the health professional should have the
most freedom but be subject to legitimate
evaluation and review procedures; and (3)
agreement on accepting or rejecting the decisions made by a nonaffiliated group. Donabedian feels that unless these conditions are
met, a breakdown of shared decision making
is a clear possibility, or a serious conflict could
develop that would ultimately lead to the dissolution of the health program.

This method of evaluation also implies built-
in system rigidity; once the goals are set, the
program must remain inflexible in order to be
accurately measured. Services cannot be modified during the data-collection period. Such
rigidity poses an unrealistic expectation upon
the program and raises a serious ethical issue
for those responsible.

In the second instance of evaluation, in
which programs are established for other than
evaluative reasons, research is designed subsequent to the operationalized program. Researchers begin with anecdotal material as the
first step out of which questions to be answered will emerge within the context of a
more thorough research design. Schulberg et
al.[64] refer to this procedure as the "systems
model." This model has been discussed by
Etzioni,[18] who feels that the starting point for
an evaluation study of program effectiveness

should not be an a priori objective but rather
a working model of a social unit that is capable of achieving a particular goal. With this
method, the emphasis is placed on how the
organization has used its resources. Are the
resources balanced among the organizational
needs? Or as Donabedian put it, "We need to
ask 'What goes on here?' rather than 'What is
wrong here?' "[15]

The problems encountered with this systems-model approach include increased expense and complexity for the researcher. The
evaluator must determine what he considers
an effective allocation of means, and must simultaneously oversee the development of the
organization while conducting data collection
within it. This task involves serious problems
of program organization and execution; in
addition, individual projects must follow a
common plan and use common measures if
results are to be compared. Nonetheless, this
approach seems somewhat more flexible than
that of the goal-attainment model. But as Rivlin[57] notes, it also poses the paradox of questioning which is more important: setting up a
service-delivery system to meet the needs of
the community, or providing an experimental
system for purposes of evaluation. Clearly, the
two are necessary and the evaluative system
used for Headstart is an example of one designed to meet both ends. Evaluative studies
done by Schulberg, Baker, and O'Brien used
the systems-model approach for evaluating a
mental hospital.[63]

In fields outside the human services area,
evaluation and measurement have been successfully accomplished by using the familiar
experimental methods of natural science,
whereby a hypothesis is formulated, controls
are used, and the hypothesis is either "proved"
or "disproved" depending on the results of the
experiment. We have discussed the difficulty
of adequately defining the quality of health
care and of defining goals. Intangibles such as
these make strict application of experimental
design to the human services extraordinarily
difficult.

Nonetheless, many studies in various fields
have been attempted using the experimental
method.[6,14] Yet it is difficult to find successful

studies of this type in the health field. Rivlin[57] points out that it is hard to hypothesize about how individuals will behave in the face of a novel pattern of incentives. A knottier question posited by using this experimental method is the ethical question of human experimentation. Experimentation in individual (social) circumstances does not lend itself to replication because of the differences encountered in each setting and in each patient. It is difficult to adapt small-scale trials to large-scale predictions. For example, small-scale family health demonstrations ensure good results but without wider significance. Hence, why do them? Rivlin also warns of the danger of compromising program needs for the benefit of an experiment.

Not much has been learned from statistical analysis of existing health, education, and social services.[57] There are inadequate descriptions of inputs and outputs and a lack of information on individuals over time. Rivlin has also observed the general failure to organize social-service systems to facilitate the systematic and scientific investigation of their effectiveness. Generally, little has been learned from evaluation of federal government programs, for example. It is Rivlin's contention that the federal government should take the lead in organizing, funding, and evaluating systematic experiments involving ways of delivering health and other services. She suggests the following steps: (1) identify new teaching methods, new ways of organizing or paying for health services, and new types of income transfer systems; (2) systematically try out new methods in various places and under various conditions; and (3) evaluate new methods under different conditions and compare them with one another and with existing methods.

Government and private foundations have promoted many experimental programs, but no one has been following a strategy of systematic experimentation and evaluation. Innovation in new systems, largely a result of decentralization of social services, began in the 1960s. This strategy lacks a final stage: dissemination of results. As Rivlin notes, the difficulty in selecting exemplary projects for publicity and follow-up is that each innovation is, obviously, unique. The tremendous fragmentation of the health-delivery system, which poses complex problems for the researcher, means that decisions are made by literally thousands of individual physicians, dentists, other health professionals, and administrators; by boards of trustees; by managers of hundreds of clinics, hospitals, neighborhood health centers; and by citizens—both individually and in groups.[57]

McGrath[42] proposes three other methods for evaluation that also emanate from the natural sciences: the field-study investigation, laboratory experiments, and computer simulations. As computer technology becomes increasingly sophisticated, the last method is perhaps the most promising and potentially useful. Though the question of expense must be considered with this method, it offers perhaps the best possibility of really understanding systems which include, and are influenced by, multiple forces. Researchers have also found the medical audit useful for measuring subobjectives—for example, the rates of discharge and readmission to a mental hospital.[32]

Moorehead[45] used the clinical-audit method to assess care in neighborhood health centers. She found the system limited her ability to define clearly anything more than the accomplishment of minimal procedures. It did not define clearly enough when clinical judgment was not necessarily adequate, nor did the clinical-audit method indicate when the patient had received care appropriate to his needs. Moorehead also points out that there is no routinization of what should be considered in a clinical test. Studies have been published relating to audit activities, but they are limited to presentation of methodology, rather than results found or conclusions reached.

The introduction of new programs for delivering medical care, such as the neighborhood health center, presents problems for the evaluation of quality as well as of cost benefit. The purpose of a neighborhood health center is not only to fill a relative lack of quality health care in a deprived area, but to help break the cycle of poverty.[46] Sparer and Alderman[68] assert that steps have been taken to address major problems in the provision of health services, but cite the growing need to measure and evaluate the effectiveness of this pattern. To this end, Moorehead studied the quality of medical care in twenty-four OEO neighborhood health centers, determining the extent to which selected criteria were met in adult medicine, infant, and obstetrical care.[45] She found that there was no base for comparison with other programs and with other forms of medical practice. She also found that a program structure that is determined by the size and characteristics of the population, with different resources available, with political and economic differences, and with variations caused by different administrative personnel, make it difficult to generalize about its results. She did find the two most relevant areas for evaluating program effectiveness were the professional and administrative leadership and the appropriateness of policies and delegated responsibilities. For all these reasons, it is hard to compare Moorehead's findings with those from any other health-care system. Thus her work represents a beginning—the utilization of the state of the art as it now exists, but upon which further refinements must be built.

Sparer and Alderman[68] conceptualize the purpose of a neighborhood health center, which offers health and supporting social services, as providing a family-oriented program. Objectives are set in terms of indicators of family malfunctions. These criteria differ from those set by an economist or a health professional. In order to establish evaluative methods, therefore, it is necessary to select families with one characteristic, and examine the family with respect to social services provided and health care received. Basing studies on criteria of this kind results in the need to consider a wide spectrum of elements: housing, education, transportation, and other social factors not directly related to health, which may or may not be relevant in evaluating other methods of health-services delivery. Sparer and Alderman conclude that it is one thing to establish priorities for the neighborhood health center, such as use of existing resources, accessibility and comprehensiveness of services,

and then to look back as in the goal-attainment model, but it is quite another thing to understand the interrelationship of social, health, and other variables.

Another subject of interest for evaluators of health-care services has been the utilization of ambulatory (private) care, but the problem presented here is perhaps the most troublesome. In the past, evaluation of private ambulatory care related the number of visits to the private physician over a period of time to some measure of illness or income. Richardson,[53] because of the difficulty in defining illness (the same difficulty as in defining quality or goals), performed a study on the use of the private physician, utilizing absence of activity —that is, a day of work missed by the patient —as a measurement of illness. He found the decision by the patient of whether or not to contact a physician did not depend on the severity of the illness. Because his measure was absence from activity, he found that those who depended on a day-to-day income were more inclined to seek a physician, presumably because it was more serious for them to be out of work. The absence or presence of third-party coverage was a predominant factor, especially when follow-up visits were tabulated. He concluded that the effect of being poor was a more important factor for nonserious illness; revisits were directly related to income and third-party coverage, and the proportion of those making contact with a private physician were greater than the proportion of those reporting to a clinic when a regular source of income was a factor.

Richardson's study was, because of the nature of his definition of illness, limited. He concludes that "utilization of a physician's services for preventive care and in the management of chronic illness has yet to be explored."[53] However, in any evaluaton the cost of loss of work and income must be included in the equation. Even with regard to medical education, for example, it is important in arriving at a true cost to include the amount of income that medical students forgo in order to pursue their studies.

Just as cross-program evaluations provide a hopeful key for the future in the assessment of health-care systems,[44] so do cross-country studies offer an opportunity for learning through comparison. Anderson[3] provided a comparative analysis of medical-care systems in Sweden, England, and the United States. Even though the United States system is loose and varied, he found that in the long run the United States has not been out of step with other western democracies in developing operational definitions or in implementing them. Anderson set out to identify quantifiable indicators that would serve as reference points on the cost, use, and "health results" of each system. As might be expected, he did not find it easy to measure need, demand, or outcome. Each of his tricountry assessments of facilities and of personnel (medical and allied professionals) in national totals and as distributed across varying population densities, of treatment patterns and of facility utilization, as compared with costs of health care, morbidity, and mortality rates, led him to only very general conclusions. He found none of the systems equitable, nor did he feel any medical system could provide equality of access in a pure form.

(Consumer Satisfaction and Participation

Lately, the health consumer has had a stronger voice in both the delivery of and research into health-care services. In the past, the consumer was poorly advised about the quality and value of health-care services, and was unable to inform himself in order to assess the health care he received. New modes of payment for health services, however, have led to a new type of consumption and a new type of consumer. He now has the opportunity of choosing the style of care he receives, by being able to select from among the various forms of payment offered him by third-party insurers. Workers, for example, can bargain with their employer through their union as to the range and nature of health coverage they wish to receive. Such coverage has become a benefit in which both the corporation and the

union have a stake. The stake of the corporation was long thought to involve no more than program cost. More recently, however, employers have come to understand the value to them of decreased sick days—that is, of health maintenance. In earlier years, where economy was the prime factor, quality was a secondary issue.

Stevens[70] has pointed out the potential value of consumer participation both as a synergist, leading to the formation of consumer health coalitions in large cities across the country, and as a catalyst, reminding the physician of his duty to provide adequate information to the patient about himself.

A number of new programs, health centers funded by OEO, some of the HEW-funded centers, and some of the Children's Bureau Infant Care and Child and Youth Programs have insisted on inclusion of the consumer as a participant in developing policy with respect to local health-care programs. This insistence has been reflected as well in such developments as the comprehensive health-planning legislation. Any assessment of a health-delivery system must now take into account the degree of citizen satisfaction. We suspect that in the future, such evaluations will also need to take into account the degree of satisfaction among employees, including those in the health professions, both new and old.

Where consumer satisfaction becomes an issue, and where choice is available, as it presently is not for certain segments of the population, those systems best adapted to please patients and deliver services of quality at a reasonable cost will tend over time to survive. The best adapted systems will survive providing the customer has a choice, the system is accessible, its standards are monitored, its usefulness is reviewed, and a premium is placed upon the least expensive acceptable care of quality. The consumer is becoming more and more sophisticated in selecting the medical care he receives. This growing awareness has been fostered in part through direct efforts at developing an informed public.[13,75]

Clearly, health care is becoming a public issue. Traditionally, when a complex and controversial public problem is encountered, resort is often made to a "select" commission. The health care field has resorted to, and benefited from, the work of a number of such commissions. A Committee on the Cost of Medical Care, appointed in 1927, provided much of the policy and personal leadership in medical care. The 1945 Commission on Hospital Care outlined the role of the hospital; its report is still relevant today.

More recently, the National Advisory Commission on Health Manpower reported in 1967 on the availability and utilization of health manpower. The most striking conclusion in its report was the acknowledgment of what is commonly referred to as the "crisis" in American health care. Organizations such as the National Opinion Research Center for Social Research (NORC) and the American Cancer Society have conducted a series of polls with regard to health care. One drawback in using responses to simple public-opinion polls as a gauge, however, is that people tend to answer questions the way they feel they should, either with regard to themselves or with regard to the health service in question. For example, a person may report that he sees a doctor at least once a year for a checkup, because he thinks he should, even though he has not; or in responding to the question, "Do you think you are receiving better medical care today as opposed to ten years ago?" his response may well represent what the respondent would like to believe is true rather than what he actually thinks or knows. Another drawback of public-opinion polls is that mere yes or no answers are often required and these fail to reflect the richness and variety of potential responses.

In one NORC survey, it was found that 84 percent of the population felt that a person's chance of being in good health today is better than a generation ago. Yet respondents attributed this circumstance to such social factors as better living standards and a greater public awareness of the availability of health services. Those who felt the chances for good health were not better today cited the strain of modern living, chemical additives to food, and so on. In the same poll, only 24 percent of the population noted expansion of medical personnel and services and increased accessibility

as factors contributing to better health care; half of the population referred to new medicines as a factor in improved care; 29 percent felt doctors were more capable; 22 percent credited social or economic factors outside the control of the health system. A methodology more helpful than public polls in determining consumer satisfaction with the health-service system is represented by the application of social science techniques.[43]

At the federal level, it would seem critical that a national policy regarding social indicators of need be developed and that a mechanism for defining these indicators and for rendering a social accounting of need be formulated.

Research into the delivery of health services in its present form is a relatively new science. It represents a challenge and an opportunity, a beginning, a field where it is clear that more is to be learned than has been thus far. As Klein et al.[37] note: "With many complex human services, simple evaluations or answers to the questions of effectiveness are not possible. . . . The issues are complex and no overall answer to the question of 'does it work' is possible at this time."

Bibliography

1. Alvarez, W. C. "Poverty Can Be a Cause of Death," Geriatrics, 26 (1971), 82–86.
2. American Medical Association. Reference Data on the Profile of Medical Practice. Chicago: Center for Health Services and Research Development, 1971.
3. Anderson, O. A. Health Care: Can There be Equity? New York: Wiley, 1972.
4. Appel, J. Z. "Health Care Cost," in B. Jones, ed., The Health of Americans, pp. 141–166. Englewood Cliffs, N.J.: Prentice-Hall, 1970.
5. Bayo, F. "U.S. Life Tables by Causes of Death. 1959–1971," Public Health Service Publication, No. 1252. Washington: U.S. Govt. Print. Off., 1968.
6. Borgatta, E. "Research Problems in Evaluation of Health Service Demonstrations," Milbank Mem. Fund Q., 44 (1966), 182–201.

7. BROCKINGTON, C. F. *A Short History of Public Health.* London: Churchill, 1966.

8. CHABOT, A. "Improved Infant Mortality Rates in Population Served by a Comprehensive Neighborhood Health Program," *Pediatrics,* 47 (1971), 989–994.

9. CHADWICK, E. *Sanitary Report.* Extracts from the address of the president of Section F of the British Association for the Advancement of Science, 1842.

10. CHASE, I. H. "Analysis of Mental Health Benefits in Proposed National Health Insurance Programs," *Am. J. Orthopsychiatry,* 42 (1972), 227–232.

11. CONNOR, A. F., JR. "Neighborhood Health Centers and Prepaid Group Practice As a Method of Improving Systems for Delivery of Care in the Urban Poor," *J. Natl. Med. Assoc.,* 63 (1971), 486–487.

12. DELLAPORTAS, G. J. "Correlation-Based Estimation of Early Infant Mortality," *Health Serv. Rep.,* 87 (1972), 275–281.

13. DENENBERG, H. M. *A Shopper's Guide to Surgery.* Harrisburg: Pennsylvania Insurance Department, July 18, 1972.

14. DENISTON, O. L., I. M. ROENSTOCK, and V. A. GETTING. "Evaluation of Program Effectiveness," in H. C. Schulberg, D. Sheldon, and F. Baker, eds., *Program Evaluation in the Health Fields,* pp. 219–240. New York: Behav. Pub., 1969.

15. DONABEDIAN, A. "Evaluating the Quality of Medical Care," in H. C. Schulberg, D. Sheldon, and F. Baker, eds., *Program Evaluation in the Health Fields,* pp. 12–218. New York: Behav. Pub., 1969.

16. ———. "Models for Organizing the Delivery of Personal Health Services and Criteria for Evaluating Them," *Milbank Mem. Fund Q.,* 44 (1972), 103–154.

17. DORSEY, J. Personal communication, Harvard Community Health Plan, March, 1973.

18. ETZIONI, A. "Two Approaches to Organization Analysis: A Critique and a Suggestion," in H. C. Schulberg, D. Sheldon, and F. Baker, eds., *Program Evaluation in the Health Fields,* pp. 101–120. New York: Behav. Pub., 1969.

19. FAIGEL, H. C. "Child Mortality Is No Way to Measure a Nation's Health," *Clin. Pediatr.,* 11 (1972), 193–194.

20. FEIN, R. *Economics of Mental Illness.* New York: Basic Books, 1958.

21. ———. "An Economist's View of the Neighborhood Health Center As a New Social Institution," *Med. Care,* 8 (1970), 104–107.

22. ———. *On Measuring Economic Benefits of Health Programs.* London: Nuffield Provincial Hospital Trust and J. Macy Foundation, 1970.

23. FELDMAN, J. J. *The Dissemination of Health Information.* Chicago: Aldine-Atherton, 1966.

24. FELDMAN, L. L. "Legislation and Prepayment for Group Practice," *N.Y. Acad. Med.,* 47 (1971), 411–422.

25. FELDSTEIN, M. S. *The Rising Cost of Hospital Care.* National Center for Health Services. Washington: U.S. Department of Health, Education, and Welfare, 1971.

26. FREEMAN, H. E. and C. C. SHERWOOD. "Research in Large-scale Intervention Programs," in H. C. Schulberg, D. Sheldon, and F. Baker, eds., *Program Evaluation in the Health Field,* pp. 74–96. New York: Behav. Pub., 1969.

27. FISCAL YEAR BUDGET, 1972, pp. 442, 455, 441, 444.

28. GALE, F. M. "Whether It is Possible to Prolong a Man's Life through the Use of Medicine," *J. Hist. Med.,* 26 (1971), 391–399.

29. GORMAN, M. "The Impact of National Health Insurance on Delivery of Health Care," *Am. J. Public Health,* 61 (1971), 962–971.

30. GREENBERG, I. G. and M. L. RUDBERG. "The Role of Prepaid Group Practice in Relieving the Medical Care Crisis," *Harvard Law Rev.,* 84 (1972), 887–1001.

31. HANFT, R. "National Health Expenditures, 1950–1965," *Soc. Sec. Bull.,* 30 (1967), 3.

32. HEYMAN, G. and J. DOWNING. "Some Initial Approaches to Continuing Evaluation of a County Mental Health Association," *Am. J. Public Health,* 51 (1961), 980–989.

33. HILL, C. A., JR., C. A. HILL, and M. I. SPECTOR. "Nationality and Mortality of American Indians Compared with U.S. Whites and Nonwhites," *HSHMA Health Rep.,* 86 (1971), 229–256.

34. JONES, B., ed. *The Health of Americans.* Englewood Cliffs, N.J.: Prentice-Hall, 1971.

35. JOUBERT, A. *Erreurs populaires äu fait de la medicine et regime de sante,* 1570.

36. KLEIN, M. W., M. F. MALONE, W. G. BENNIS et al. "Problems of Measuring Patient Care in the Outpatient Department," *J. Health*

Human Behav., 2 (1961), 138–144.

37. Klein, M. W., K. Roghmann, K. Woodward et al. "The Impact of the Rochester Neighborhood Health Center on Hospitalization of Children, 1968–1970," *Pediatrics*, 51 (1973), 833–839.

38. Lawrence, P. S. "Methods in the National Health Survey: Age Patterns in Morbidity and Medical Care," in J. E. Birnen, ed., *Relations of Development and Aging*, pp. 74–96. Springfield, Ill.: Charles C. Thomas, 1964.

39. Lee, R. I., and L. W. Jones. *The Fundamentals of Good Medical Care.* Chicago: University of Chicago Press, 1933.

40. Leeuwen, G. "The Case for Regional Perinatal Health Centers," *Clin. Pediatr.*, 11 (1972), 439–450.

41. Lew, E. A., and F. Seltzer. "Uses of the Life Table in Public Health," *Milbank Mem. Fund Q.*, 48 (1970), 13–37.

42. McGrath, X. "Research on Organizations," in H. C. Schulberg, D. Sheldon, and F. Baker, eds., *Program Evaluation in the Health Field*, pp. 139–164. New York: Behav. Pub., 1969.

43. Mechanic, D. *Medical Sociology.* New York: Free Press, 1968.

44. Monroe, R. R., G. D. Klee, and E. B. Brody, eds., *Psychiatric Epidemiology and Mental Health Planning.* Research Rep. no. 22. Washington: American Psychiatric Association, 1967.

45. Moorehead, M. "Evaluating Quality of Medical Care in the Neighborhood Health Center Program of the OEO," *Med. Care*, 8 (1971), 118–131.

46. Moorehead, M., R. S. Donaldson, and M. R. Servalli. "Comparisons Between OEO Neighborhood Health Centers and other Health Care Providers of Ratings of the Quality of Health Care," *Am. J. Public Health*, 61 (1971), 1294–1306.

47. Morris, R. "The Interrelationships of Social Welfare Theory, Practice and Theory," in J. E. Birnen, ed., *Relations of Development and Aging*, pp. 267–276. Springfield, Ill.: Charles C. Thomas, 1964.

48. Oritz, J. and R. Parker. "A Birth-Life-Death Model for Planning and Evaluation of Health Services Programs," *Health Serv. Rep.*, 6 (1971), 120–143.

49. Palmore, E. "Longevity Predictors. Implications for Practice," *Postgrad. Med.*, 50 (1971), 160–164.

50. Petty, W. "Political Arithmetic," in C. H. Hull, ed., *The Economic Writings of Sir William Petty*, pp. 233–313. Cambridge, England: Cambridge University Press, 1963.

51. Pollack, J. "The New Role of the Health Consumer," in G. K. Chacko, ed., *The Recognition of Systems in Health Services*, pp. 151–187. Operations Research Society of America, Arlington, Virginia, 1969.

52. Potts, D. M. "Which Is the Weaker Sex?" *J. Biosoc. Sci.*, 3 (1971), 61–67.

53. Richardson, W. C. "Measuring the Urban Poor's Use of Physician's Services in Response to Illness Episodes," *Med. Care*, 8 (1972), 132–137.

54. Richmond, J. B. *Current Trends in American Medicine.* Cambridge, Mass.: Harvard University Press, 1969.

55. ———. "Human Development," in B. Jones, ed., *The Health of Americans.* Englewood Cliffs, N.J.: Prentice-Hall, 1971.

56. Ried, L. S., E. S. Myers, and P. G. Scheidemandel. "Health Insurance and Psychiatric Care: Utilization and Cost." Washington: Am. Psychiatric Assoc., 1972.

57. Rivlin, A. M. *Systematic Thinking for Social Action.* Washington: The Brookings Institution, 1971.

58. Roberts, R. E. and C. Askew, Jr. "Social Status, Ethnic Status and Urban Mortality: An Ecological Analysis," *Tex. Rep. Biol. Med.*, 28 (1971), 13–28.

59. ———. "A Consideration of Mortality in Three Subcultures," *Health Serv. Rep.*, 87 (1972), 262–270.

60. Scherl, D. J. "Outpatient Psychiatric Centers—Accountable to Whom?" in A. B. Tulipian and A. R. Cutting, eds., *The Out-Patient Patient*, pp. 25–40. New York: Brunner Mazel, 1972.

61. Scherl, D. J. and J. T. English. "Community Mental Health and Comprehensive Health Services Programs for the Poor," *Am. J. Psychiatry*, 125 (1969), 1666–1674.

62. Scherl, D. J. and L. B. Macht. "An Examination of the Relevance for Mental Health of Selected Anti-Poverty Programs for Children and Youth," *Community Ment. Health J.*, 8 (1972), 8–16.

63. Schulberg, H. C., F. Baker, and G. M. O'Brien. "The Changing Mental Hospital: A Progress Report," *Hosp. Community Psychiatry*, 20 (1969), 159–165.

64. SCHULBERG, H. C., D. SHELDON, and F. BAKER, eds., *Program Evaluation in the Health Fields.* New York: Behavioral Pub., 1969.
65. SOCIAL SERVICES BULLETIN, 36 (January, 1973), 12.
66. SOMERS, H. M. "Health Care Cost," in B. Jones, ed., *The Health of Americans,* pp. 167–203. Englewood Cliffs, N.J.: Prentice-Hall, 1971.
67. SPARER, G. and A. ALDERMAN. "Cost of Services at Neighborhood Health Centers," *N. Engl. J. Med.,* 286 (1971), 1241–1245.
68. ———. "Data Needs for Planning Neighborhood Health Centers," *Am. J. Public Health,* 61 (1971), 796–806.
69. SPIEGELMAN, M. "Segmented Generation Mortality," *Demography,* 6 (1969), 117–123.
70. STEVENS, C. M. *On Consumer Participation in Medical Care Markets.* Health Care Policy Discussion Paper No. 5. Center for Community Health and Medical Care. Cambridge: Harvard University, 1973.
71. SUTTON, G. F. "Assessing Mortality and Morbidity Disadvantages of the Black Population of the United States," *Soc. Biol.,* 18 (1971), 369–386.
72. UNITED STATES ADVISORY COMMISSION ON NATIONAL HEALTH MANPOWER. *Report.* Washington: U.S. Govt. Print. Off., 1967.
73. USHER, R. "Clinical Implications of Perinatal Mortality Statistics," *Clin. Obstet. Gynecol.,* 14 (1971), 885–925.
74. WALD, N. "Morbidity and Mortality in Relation to Social Class," *Lancet,* 1 (1972), 259.
75. WILLIAMS, L. P. *How To Avoid Unnecessary Surgery.* Los Angeles: Nash Publ., 1972.
76. WING, J. K. and A. M. HAILEY, eds., *Evaluating a Community Psychiatric Service.* London: Oxford University Press, 1972.
77. YERBE, A. S. "The Problems of Medical Care for Indigent Populations," *Am. J. Public Health,* 55 (1965), 1212–1216.

CHAPTER 33

PERSPECTIVES ON DELIVERY OF MENTAL HEALTH SERVICES

Archie R. Foley

The secret of the care of the patient is in caring for the patient [pp. 65–66][24]

TO SPEAK OF the future delivery of mental health services at this point in our history is fraught with risks and uncertainties. During the past quarter of a century the face of American psychiatry has changed dramatically—reflecting a heightened awareness and concern for those with emotional problems—from the use of the custodial institution as the primary model to the development of community-based facilities, such as community mental health centers, psychiatric units in general hospitals, consultation and education programs in schools, courts, social agencies, etc., and, where possible, increased emphasis on preventive programs to the extent that our current knowledge permits.

As a result of these developments, it is gen-erally agreed that great strides have been made in the past decade in providing better quality care more quickly and effectively. But these very achievements have brought about an interesting dilemma: because the success of such programming is acknowledged by policy-decision makers, federal support at appropriate levels to ensure continued success is being withdrawn.

Also, during this period of time, innovative new training methods have been developed to equip mental health personnel for the delivery of direct and indirect services, their planning and evaluation, and new modalities of treatment have been evolved. The impact of the community mental health center movement has been felt in all sectors of the psychiatric profession, both public and private. Yet, as is known to all, federal support for training young psychiatrists and other mental health professionals is being rescinded. This poses another dilemma: the future loss of adequately trained manpower to implement new programs and of research scientists to evaluate and refine programs.

A fact of life, which has been recognized by many of us for some time, is now coming into sharp focus. Decisions regarding health and mental health policies and programs are being made on the political level. There is insufficient input to this process from mental health professionals at all levels, federal, state, or local. The fault lies not only with the policy makers who do not seek out such input, but with the professionals who are reticent to involve themselves at this level. This stems, in part, from their lack of awareness and thus they are unwilling to become involved in the development of policy in health or mental health matters. As will be described in a subsequent section of this chapter, there is an opportunity for professional input to help determine the future patterns of delivery of health and mental health care in this country.

This chapter is divided into three sections. The first deals with the historical development of health and mental health care in this country, highlighting some of the problems, dilemmas, mistakes, progress, and conflicts. This is done in an effort to make us aware that some of the difficulties we are facing today have their roots in the past, for as George Santayana tells us in *The Life of Reason,* "those who cannot remember the past are condemned to repeat it." The second section deals with current trends in the development of health care delivery systems, emphasizing mental health care; information regarding recent amendments to the Social Security Act, i.e., the development of Professional Standards Review Organization (PSRO) legislation and its implications for comprehensive mental health care delivery. The third section is a futuristic look at the delivery of mental health services. This last section must be viewed in a hypothetical and theoretical framework since, while patterns of delivery of health care will be drastically changed within the next few years, the parameters of such change are as yet not clearly defined. Nevertheless and despite the uncertainties, we must look to the future in a positive way, drawing on past experiences and errors we have made, taking from other disciplines those techniques that will improve the delivery of quality care without sacrificing effectiveness for efficiency, and without abrogating our responsibilities in policy formulation and decision-making to those whose primary orientation is that of fiscal accountability. This statement has implications for changes in the basic training of young physicians to better acquaint them with the broader social and political elements of health care delivery without in any way interfering with the sound, clinical training that is the bulwark of the effective practice of medicine.

(Historical Perspectives

It can be generally agreed today that effective and meaningful delivery of mental health services has as its fundamental aim the successful dealing with mental illness through treatment, rehabilitation, and prevention. The history of our profession is the history of the search for ways in which to do this. This search has taken us from a time, approximately 150 years ago when there was no treatment, to the recent surgency of the community mental health movement. The period between was characterized by important breakthroughs, dramatic changes, periods of progress (some illusory), periods of stagnation, recognition of failures, and renewed attempts to find still other ways of dealing with the problem of mental illness. As we have moved from step to step there have been efforts at assessment, consolidation, and synthesis. During that time we have seen impressive changes in the objectives, philosophy, and methodology for dealing with mental illness. Contributing to these changes have been scientific discoveries, new understandings, pragmatic responses to necessity, but also a change in our national awareness of prevalence and needs, and an evolution toward a national philosophy of social responsibility.

Today, once again, we are becoming aware that our present delivery system is not adequately solving the problems. Rising costs have become an overwhelming concern and there are discernible trends toward a shift in our national philosophy. It becomes imperative that we try to assess our present system; evaluate our successes and our failures; learn from our failures; affirm our successes, and rechart the course for the future. In doing so, it is useful to examine the events and forces, somewhat parallel, that have played a part in the emergence of our nation and the traits that have shaped it, along with the developments in our ways of caring for the mentally ill.

As our nation developed from early frontier days with a stress on individualism to our present complex urbanized society, there has been a growing recognition of the need for cooperation and coordination as well as an increasingly strong sense of interdependence.

In dealing with the mentally ill, as a nation and as a profession, we have come a long way from the days when the mentally ill were kept in jails or county poorhouses—when the objective was primarily to remove from society those whose behavior was considered troublesome and irresponsible—to our present objective of helping the mental patient return to society as a functioning member. Our philosophy of care has developed from custodial and punitive approaches through moral treatment to our present recognition that the mental patient is a person with rights, a person who can and should be helped. Along the way new modalities of treatment have evolved—such as concepts of milieu therapy, crisis intervention, discovery of the use of psychotropic drugs as adjuncts to treatment—that have had enormous impact on bringing about these changes.

Important milestones were passed along the way; we learned from pioneering and crusading efforts of those who led the fight for better care, and in some of our national experiences and times of crises we found other guideposts to our present system of service delivery. The efforts of Dorothea Dix focused attention on the plight of the mentally ill and the squalid and inhuman conditions to which they were subjected. She persuaded us that it was the responsibility of the state to care for the mentally ill and this led in large part to the establishment of the state hospital system. But as our population grew and more and more of the mentally ill were consigned to this system, it became apparent that more needed to be done, for we were still adhering to our early objective of putting away and out of sight those among us who were suffering from mental disorders. A significant contribution to our shift in philosophy and objectives for service to the mentally ill was the delineation of basic concepts underlying our present efforts by Adolf Meyer in 1913 when he stated that "the characteristic traits of a clinic for mental diseases should be first, service to the patient rather than to the administrative system; second, elaboration of the study of the diseases rather than the means of wholesale handling of patients; third, possibilities of following up the studies of nature's experiments beyond the hospital period, and preventive work through extramural efforts outside the hospital."[20] It is of the utmost importance, he believed to ". . . make possible studies of the social situation and of the dynamic factors which lead to the occurrence of mental derangement, which must be attacked for purposes of prevention."

In the years that followed there was increasing recognition of social factors as causation in mental disorders and the experiences of the two world wars brought a national awareness of the high incidence of mental illness and psychiatric casualties in our nation. Efforts to deal with this led to the passage of the National Mental Health Act in 1946 and the beginning of federal government involvement in the mental health movement. Lessons learned in World War II were applied during the Korean War when major psychiatric resources were deployed in the field for fast and appropriate treatment, enabling the return of greatly increased numbers to duty and reducing those having to return to general hospitals for ultimate discharge. The proven efficacy of this new modality of treatment began to be widely applied in two types of treatment facilities that began to be widely established in communities throughout the country during the 1940s: outpatient clinics for treatment of the mentally ill and psychiatric units in general hospitals for inpatient and intensive treatment of mental disorders. The concept of community based psychiatry began to take hold and by the early 1950s the idea of community mental health centers was defined. In 1955, Congress passed the Mental Health Study Act, which directed the setting up of the Joint Commission on Mental Illness and Health to "analyze and evaluate the needs and resources of the mentally ill in the United States and to make recommendations for a national mental health program."[32] The findings of the Joint Commission and its recommendations led in 1963 to the first Presidential message ever on behalf of the mental health movement in which a "new type of health facility" was called for that "would return mental health care to the mainstream of American medicine, and at the same time upgrade mental health services." Enabling legislation was passed in 1963, the Mental Retardation Facilities and Community Mental Health Centers Construction Act authorizing federal matching funds for states to aid in the construction of comprehensive community mental health centers. This new type of facility was to "provide a complete new range of care in the community, with strong emphasis on prevention."[13]

Mental health service delivery entered a new era and mental health professionals were infused with high hopes that the 1960s would be the decade in which the fight against mental illness would make significant strides. It was a time of federal involvement and support for new programs that would reach vastly increased population groups in need of care; funds became available for construction of facilities that would provide new and improved patterns of care; research and training programs grew in scope and size; attitudes about mental illness were to be changed; the community would receive attention in terms of involvement and participation in programs for recognition and care of mental disorders; education of the public would help prepare communities to receive former patients so that they could reenter the community as useful and participating members. In short, the picture drawn by the Joint Commission of conditions as they had existed was to be drastically altered.

Now, ten years later, as we look back over the achievements we must recognize that although strides have been made, and some of them very significant, many of the changes we had hoped to effect have not taken place. Many of the challenges remain and we face new ones. We must ask ourselves today where we have failed, why, and how.

It might be said that our profession's attempts to find new and more effective ways of treatment have mirrored a pattern of how as a nation we tend to deal with problems. Each new discovery is hailed as the definitive answer, the ultimate panacea. We throw all of our energies into the new discovery and we are impatient for quick, palpable results. Without pausing to evaluate the new idea, because we believe in it so strongly, we overload the new idea, we oversell ourselves on it, so to speak, and set our expectations too high. Armed with the new idea we energetically go about correcting previous wrongs, not always wisely, and in so doing we tend, as Bernard has written, ". . . in correcting some abuses [to] unwittingly perpetrate others. (The freshly perceived concept of today is all too likely to be corrupted into the cliche of tomorrow.)" [p. 256)[4] Our enthusiasm for the idea is so great that we tend to ascribe to the idea itself the power of becoming the change agent and often overlook the fact that the idea must be backed up with mechanisms adapted to the new idea, sufficient resources, and, at times, new mechanisms so that it can be implemented. By being so sold on the idea ourselves we tend to ignore that others are not and need to be convinced and invited to share our enthusiasm. If we let ourselves get carried away, we can be seriously instrumental in defeating the idea. We need only remind ourselves that while construction of the state hospital system was the bright new idea of its day, we did manage to take mental patients out of deplorable conditions. But not only did we overload these facilities, we failed to make proper use of them and soon we found that we had exchanged one abuse for another. As William Alanson White, observed about his experience as a young assistant physician in a state hospital: "About the only virtue I was able to discover in the state hospital as an agency for the application of therapeutics to the mentally ill was that the patient who came there had been removed from the conditions under which his psychosis developed." [p. 20][35] Similarly, there exists today the danger that the idea of community mental health will be considered the ultimate panacea, will be overloaded, will be inadequately supported, and thus will falter because we have failed to implement it properly. Some of these signs have already appeared. It is essential that we carefully scrutinize these signs, recognize our mistakes, correct them, consolidate our gains and not only salvage the idea but meet present challenges to it, and truly make it work.

In 1972, Barten and Bellak wrote, "ideas and movements go through fairly definite stages of development . . . when ideas make a major breakthrough, they are in a heroic phase of heady spirit. In the second phase, there is bound to be some letdown when limitations and obstacles become apparent and the one visionary idea turns out to be no panacea. Typically, misconceptions in the original proposition are discovered and some feelings of disappointment follow. Community mental health is now in this skeptical second phase." [p. xi][2] This formulation can serve as a useful yardstick for scrutiny and assessment. If we apply a constructive skepticism, we can discern some misconceptions in the original proposition, some limitations and obstacles, all contributing to the much less than full realization of our expectations at the outset. Candor demands, however, that we recognize that we who were given the opportunity to implement the "bold new approach" have fallen considerably short in our implementation and that many factors have contributed to our failure.

The very legislation that appeared such a boon at the outset had built into it several misconceptions that in the course of experience have proven to be true obstacles. The underlying belief that the community-mental-health center would be the total panacea—derived from the assumption that the center would and could completely replace the state

hospital—appears to have been an error. Rather, each has a role to play in a spectrum of provision of comprehensive services that, after all, was the basic goal of the initial idea. Countries such as Holland, England, and the USSR have had experience in operating successful community-based programs, yet the need for hospitals has not been eliminated. [pp. 11–13][14] The overlapping timetables inherent in the federal funding structure created other obstacles. The stress was on construction while the money was available. Thus in many instances there was poor and inadequate planning and a lack of ongoing evaluation. The community to be served in some cases was incorrectly defined and its needs inadequately recognized. In other cases where there had been some groundwork done, the recognized needs and size of the community did not fit the federally mandated requirements. Consequently, in order to be eligible for funding, the findings were modified to suit the guidelines, often to the detriment of the success of the program. Since the funding structure was based on a matching pattern of federal funds with state and local funds, additional obstacles were created. As observed by Connery et al., "existing governmental units prefer to handle new functions in the same way as they treat present services. . . . Public officials prefer to budget for the new service within existing program structure. . . ."[7] Thus, the emphasis on catchment area as implied in the federal legislation, coupled with the necessity to channel implementation through existing structures not adapted to the needs of the mandate, can result in the type of experience reported by Kaplan with the Lincoln Hospital Community Mental Health Center: ". . . the size and population in ghetto areas best served by a neighborhood mental health unit was 25,000."[18] This was based on experience gained in operating a Neighborhood Service Center with Office of Equal Opportunity (OEO) funds. He goes on to say that "despite our experience and detailed exposition to program concepts, our original staffing plan had to be modified [to meet] the federal standards. One third of the number of staff we had suggested for 25,000 were assigned to service 50,000. Thus, the contractual negotiations for federal staffing followed a familiar bureaucratic pattern through municipal, state and federal agencies without regard to our prior experiences. This occurred despite the fact that the evaluation research upon which our grant request was based has been supported by funds from NIMH and highly regarded by the branch. . . . The Community Mental Health Centers Act represents a sophisticated advance in the framing of a public health law, the implementation of the regulations have been and are carried out through outmoded models of interagency structures." [p. 30][18]

In discussing some of the theoretical considerations for development of the community mental health centers Sanders and I pointed out that "the emphasis must be on *program* not *center*," that "the center must have a relatedness to the community which it serves; a relatedness which can be developed by an awareness and understanding of the expectations each has of the other . . ."; that there is a necessity for "interaction of the staff of the center with the community and its agencies and facilities in consultative, collaborative and educational roles," that the "primary function of the community mental health center is that it serves as a *coordinating mechanism* for all of the existing community facilities" and that "the 'consumer' of this network of coordinated and differentiated services must also be kept in mind. Mental health professionals might develop a wide range of services which are considered adequate and reasonable, but the individual member of the community may not perceive them as such."[12] Unfortunately, so far, we have not succeeded in fulfilling most of these goals. We have until now insufficiently developed and used community resources and although we have stressed a return to the community, we have tended to defeat this goal by paying insufficient attention to ways and means of integrating the patient for useful function and maintenance of mental health. This has been a failure due in part to inadequate stress on the education of members of the community and in not truly implementing the initial goal of a pluralistic approach and combined treatment idea that

underlie the very philosophy of community mental health concepts. Although we have achieved a considerable increase in available manpower—and in the process have trained a variety of different types of personnel—we have failed to some extent with regard to proper role definitions and liaison at all levels. As a result, new problems have been engendered that tend to interfere with efficiency of functioning, and thus we have underdelivered both in quantity and quality of care. A further hampering factor has been a lack of flexibility in suiting treatment modalities to specific needs and situations, in part exemplified by the adherence of practitioners, both traditionally trained and new types, to the medical model.

In appraising efforts at implementation of the community mental health center movement so far and in trying to pinpoint the shortcoming of such efforts, certain trends are appearing that suggest we may be repeating some of the mistakes of an earlier, similar movement—the neighborhood health center movement of the first decades of this century —mistakes that in large measure contributed to its demise. However, the community mental health center movement need not follow a similar inexorable course to decline and demise. There is still time to examine mistakes being made, to identify some parallels in the earlier movement, and thus to deflect our course toward success.

The health center movement had its roots in the recognition during the latter part of the nineteenth century and the early years of the twentieth that the growing cities in this country were increasingly faced with problems of poverty, crime, disease, and other slum conditions most frequently associated with immigration. At that time settlement houses, milk depots, and charitable relief organizations located in immigrant and slum neighborhoods attempted to deal with these problems. The early health centers, financed by local taxes or philanthropy, or both, organized by voluntary agencies or municipal health departments, were located within city neighborhoods or districts. These early centers were intended to solve special out-of-hospital health problems of the poor, primarily with regard to infectious diseases and infant malnutrition. The emphasis was on prevention and on education. As Stoekle and Candib point out, "most health center enthusiasts viewed the programs of centers as preventive and educational, complementing the creative work of private practice and carefully avoiding competition with it: 'no prescription given; no sickness treated.' "[30]

Four ideas of organization and program dominated the health-center movement: district location, community participation, preventive care, and bureaucratic organization.[30] Health services were to be within easy reach and thus would have greater use, and the very location would bring about influence from local residents in pointing out needs. Initially, the health center was viewed as a decentralization designed to make care more accessible and available. However, simultaneously, there existed a quite different view, namely that it represented a centralization of clinics and welfare agencies. Since these were scattered in various locations in the community and managed by diverse voluntary efforts, frequently overlapping and duplicating services, it was argued that they must be brought together under one organization for efficiency and coordination.

The health center movement was also a manifestation of the progressivism of that period, which placed a high value on social reform. In the progressive era, the roots of poverty and illness were seen as environmental and, thus, social work and public health allied themselves with reform movements seeking to improve the environment. At the same time, however, there were two developments in social and political thought of the period: scientific management with its stress on efficiency, and the rise of professionalism. Efficiency at first had as its goal cooperation and coordination, use of nonprofessional aids and ancillary personnel with the aim of 100 percent participation and availability of services, cost reduction through shared facilities, and elimination of overlapping services. Soon, however, efficiency became so powerful a concept in industrial work and seemed so impressive a solution

that it also became "almost a central value of the health center movement."[30] As a result there was extreme coordination of organization but not of care. To cite an example: "the demand for bureaucratic efficiency was so persistent that nurses had to prepare a detailed write-up of how much time they spent on each 'unit of work.' When the accounting became as important as the 'unit of work' then the trade-off between efficiency and effectiveness ceased to be manageable." [p. 23][5]

The rise of professionalism manifested itself in several ways. Public health work and social work had until this time been largely an outreach function, motivated by concern for improving social and health conditions. Under the influence of the new trend toward efficiency and management there grew the belief in specialization and the need for experts. This gave rise to a consciousness of professionalism, and as preoccupation with professional codes and standards grew there was a shift in the concern from community work to internal hierarchy and organization with a consequent withdrawal of community involvement. Social workers shifted emphasis from work in the community and social reform to casework and emulation of the medical model of treatment; public health awarded its first professional degree in 1910 and began to stress public health administration. In the years immediately following World War I interest in volunteer work declined, and with the growth of professionalism and stress on bureaucratic structure the health center as a small local undertaking gave way to large-scale efforts in health and welfare. The basic neighborhood orientation yielded to the new ideas of scientific management and the fundamental idea of the center was altered to a considerable extent.

Health departments began to see the value of the districting idea—a cornerstone of the early health centers—and the value of coordination of diverse services. The First World War had brought about governmental concern with public-health issues and Progressives welcomed such participation as a promise of sweeping gains. However, there was in the 1920s a widespread fear of government control implying socialism and even communism.

As Candib writes: ". . . doctors felt that the expansion of the state into the realm of preventive medicine was sure to be followed by forays into therapeutic medicine as well. Consequently, they approved of health centers only when their program involved no therapeutic medicine." [pp. 50–51][5]

A major innovation of the 1920s was the "health demonstration," a "comprehensive, well-publicized project to improve the health in a given area through extensive health campaigns for inoculation, screening, diagnosis, and health education." Demonstrations were funded by the private sector with the specific understanding that municipal governments would assume funding once a demonstration had proven successful. "Health departments could not respond until the value of a given demonstration had been proved. . . . During this period, innovative projects were considered 'peculiarly the province of private enterprise.'" [pp. 41–42][5] For purposes of these health demonstrations the district size was expanded in the interest of efficiency and bureaucratic administration, thereby distorting and subverting the original districting idea. In the opinion of Candib, they "adopted a district plan more to benefit from a discrete scientific control with other neighborhoods than to develop local roots in the neighborhood. Furthermore, with a larger district, the success criterion of reaching 100% of the population was sacrificed to the more measurable scientific goal of reducing the 'extent of sickness' and the mortality rates." [p. 43][5] Thus, the health demonstrations and their successors were not health centers as originally envisioned and operated. The demonstration came to be "regarded as the focal point of modern district health administration—a model for decentralizing the phlegmatic municipal bureaucracy totally inadequate to meet the health needs of a large urban population." [p. 43][5] The district had become an administrative technique rather than a nucleus for care giving.

The health center concept was further diluted by another aspect of the stress on professionalism. Rosen points out that "as is not infrequently the case when a professional development or trend is in 'fashion,' the name by which it is designated acquires an aura of approval, and is used to describe activities and enterprises that differ widely, so that they may share some of the aura. This was also the fate of the health center concept, and is in part responsible for its decline." [p. 1630][26] He goes on to enumerate the different types of facilities that went under the name of health center. These included child welfare stations, tuberculosis dispensaries, outpatient departments of hospitals, settlement houses, and venereal disease clinics.

The demise of the health center movement can be ascribed to several factors, some of which can be discerned in developing trends in the community mental health center movement and from all of which valuable lessons can be drawn. The community mental health center is seen now not only as a means of bringing services to the poor, but as an important modality of care and delivery of mental health services to the entire community that links treatment and prevention with an application of community psychiatry knowledge and techniques in the promotion of mental health. One of the failures of the health center movement is ascribed to the "rigid confinement to a program of preventive medicine" that "served to perpetuate the artificial distinction between the preventive and therapeutic functions in medicine,[5] and Stoekle, quoted by Candib, considers "this restricted program of health centers as a fundamental barrier to their success."[5] The community mental health center offers a unique opportunity to fuse our response to immediate needs through therapeutic intervention and to put into practice true primary prevention that addresses itself to anticipated societal difficulties that we now know are causative factors in mental illness. As stated earlier, the progressive era saw the environment as the root cause of poverty and illness. Gradually there was a movement away from this and the focus in social work and welfare shifted to the individual. This shift is ascribed to the impact of Freudian ideas. "The social worker minimized environmental factors in causation and treatment and elevated the study of the personality into the all-powerful explanatory tool. . . . Social work . . . came to emphasize the adjustment of the individual to social stress . . . and to society as it was. This view stands in sharp contrast to the earlier progressive belief that the society needed to change before poverty and illness could be eliminated."[5] In the years since then we have come back again, or perhaps learned anew, that environmental and social factors must be included in the spectrum of causative factors. Freud taught us to consider the individual and the importance of the study of personality, but he also "expressed the opinion that the best access to the psychology of the ego might be through investigating the disorders of society." [p. 337][17]

The development of the community mental health center movement can certainly be seen as an important expression of our renewed awareness. It is essential, however, that in our search for maximum effectiveness we do not lose sight of it as a care-giving tool and do not become excessively preoccupied with technical concerns. It is well to remember that students of the health center movement found that "the movement wholeheartedly adopted the bureaucratic ideal of efficiency and professionalism. These values ultimately served to undercut the theoretical principles of the health center movement . . . the district idea and the coordination idea were not invalidated but rather discarded and altered for the benefit of bureaucratic and administrative goals. Community based facilities were not unworkable, but could not succeed when efficiency and professionalism had become dominant values." [p. 53][5]

The call to efficiency is heard again, as is the stress, or rather, overstress on professionalism. These are new challenges we must meet along with our increased efforts to preserve and implement the basic goals of the community mental health movement. One of the guises in which efficiency is appearing is cost accountancy. But in our concern for rising costs we must guard against the ascendancy of cost accountancy over commitments to quality service and care giving. There is still the persistent belief that efficiency as applied to industry can be transplanted to the delivery of human services. Although much can be learned from administrative techniques developed in industry, it would be a mistake to assume that these techniques in toto can be transplanted to management of human service delivery. We are seeing today proof that efficiency as a goal in itself can fall victim to the law of diminishing returns. Reports from a variety of industries, from automobile to dog food manufacture, underline this and point to an interesting paradox. Industry has learned from the behavioral sciences and is beginning to apply their concepts to management practices while we are still calling, in many ways, for application of techniques that industry is beginning to discard. Just as we have been able to evolve the innovative notion of the community mental health center so we must, by applying our own expertise, evolve innovative techniques for the management of human service delivery.

Industry is learning that workers can master a variety of tasks and, by becoming involved in these, perform well in all of them. We, however, tend still to stress specific and individual tasks. True efficiency and constructive cost accounting can be accomplished if we become committed to constructive change, comprehensive planning, and flexible organization. This will require involvement of mental health professionals in a diversity of tasks and in areas of activity outside the consulting room.

To quote Candib once more, "internal organizing ideas in public health may depend more for their success on the values common to the society in which they occur than on the inherent validity of the ideas themselves. Although the health center idea was not without internal difficulties . . . these drawbacks could have been overcome in a society more open to ideas of popular participation and universal access to health and welfare services." [p. 53][5]

Though addressing itself to public health, this statement can as easily be applied to mental health as we look to the tasks ahead. What are the common values of the society in which we are attempting to implement community mental health? It can be agreed that side by side today is the demand for more and better care with a concern for rising costs, and decreased availability of public funds. As mental-health professionals we have the multiple task of proving to the public and to legislators that the challenge of mental illness is there to be met and must be met and that with their help we can meet it. We must be able to show that funds are not wasted but are used effectively and beneficially. To do so we must redirect our philosophy of care. We must aim at true implementation of a pluralistic approach to care and, in the process, we must recognize the limitations of the various modalities of treatment and assign each to the appropriate facility in the total spectrum of care giving. We must also be willing to find ways so that federal, state, and local sources can share the responsibilities for care and funding to avoid overloading any one of them and, in the process, render them ineffectual. As Schwartz wrote recently, "although mild overloading may stimulate creative discoveries of ways to do the job more effectively, extreme overloading causes demoralization, apathy, and decreased effectiveness. . . . The failure of the state hospital system to solve mental health problems for most of the community is one illustration of severe overloading leading to demoralization and decreased effectiveness. A similar kind of overloading of community facilities can have the same result." [p. 11][28]

Mental health professionals must be prepared to include in their dealing with mental health problems a willingness to step out of their purely therapeutic roles and aim for greater involvement in the political and social process as it affects mental health planning and programming. As Bernard has said, practioners must aim to have "a voice in the councils that make social policy." She reminds us of "the interdependence of psychiatric, social, health, educational and other specialized constituents of 'combined treatment,'" and goes on to say that "such indirect application of clinical and administrative knowledge is not a departure from but an extension of our central professional concern with mental disorders." [p. 265][4] Today, as we face a federal fiscal retrenchment and a discernible shift in social philosophy away from federal involvement in social programs with increased responsibility

shifted to state and municipal governments, we face the challenge of seeing to it that funds allocated for these programs are indeed so expended, for ". . . being financially able is not the same thing as being politically willing." [p. 504][7] From a field study on organizing community mental health, Connery et al. report that "legislatures have been willing to take favorable action whenever sufficient leadership was available to give saliency to the issues. . . . There is reason to believe that the basic difficulty is not so much hostility as indifference and ignorance. It is less a problem of changing legislative opinion than a matter of getting opinions formed at all. The function of educating . . . legislators on the needs and problems of mental health has not always been properly performed." [p. 542][7] It *is* our task in the immediate future to perform the function properly and to provide leadership to give saliency to the issues, whether it be on the state and local level with regard to proper expenditure of funds, or on the federal level to exert influence in planning for new health insurance measures, formation of review mechanisms, or administrative techniques and approaches for comprehensive service delivery.

(Legislative, Social, and Organizational Trends

Based on the philosophy that health care in America is a right and not a privilege, there has been, in the last fifteen years, a flurry of legislative activity at all levels of government as well as organizational changes on state and local levels designed to provide comprehensiveness of care of high quality and accessibility for those in need. Despite this activity, which will be described briefly in the following paragraphs, there is little evidence that any dramatic breakthroughs have occurred. The community mental health center movement brought into sharp focus the need for careful program planning and design, consumer participation, new methods of delivery, and public accountability. Thus, some of the more recent legislation has incorporated these various elements to ensure that the American public plays an active participant role in the type of health and mental health care it receives. Many plans have been put forward by different organizations outlining various approaches to a national health insurance plan. Other forms of legislation have defined new types of organizations, such as Health Maintenance Organizations (HMOs) and more recently PSROs. Yet we are still no closer than we were to a well-formulated, feasible, comprehensive health care system for this country. There has been no coordinated effort among the various federal, state, and local levels of government to ensure the implementation of new programs, particularly with regard to HMO's. Firm guidelines were never established under which such organizations might become operational. The Administration's position was that the various groups should design their own plans, within certain broad limits, to avoid proliferation of organizations that might soon become outmoded and obsolete.

In 1972, in a message to Congress, President Nixon outlined the components of the Allied Services Act, designed to plan for and provide comprehensive care through programming at the state and local levels—a proposal that was closely tied to the concept of revenue sharing. This concept held great promise as a substitute way of maintaining programs that had been operated under other types of federal funds, but so far it has not lived up to initial expectations. The likelihood of health and mental health programs receiving substantial assistance through the instrumentality of revenue sharing is indeed meager.* The act did not receive Congressional approval. It was reintroduced in the Ninety-third Congress.

Also in 1972, the Health Maintenance Organization and Resources Development Act[34] was introduced in Congress and passed by the

Senate, but it did not become law.† It was proposed on the basis of findings that indicated a shortage and maldistribution of quality health resources in the United States; that the present health care system is not efficient nor economical and is based primarily on the treatment of disease, rather than the maintenance of health; that technical assistance, new types of educational facilities, and extreme variations in the quality of care in different parts of the country necessitated the development of a new type of organization that would come to be known as the Health Maintenance Organization, or HMO. This legislation provided for coverage of comprehensive care on the basis of a prepaid plan. Subscribers to such a plan would receive health care through contractual agreement with a health maintenance organization, or a health service organization that would assume responsibility for the provision of health services to groups of subscribers. The legislation stipulated that mental health services, including those for drug abuse and alcoholism, would be covered, and that existing community mental health centers should be utilized on a priority basis to provide the mental health component of comprehensive health care. In view of the previous experience of the community mental health centers, it was thought that such centers could be the focal point for the development of the comprehensive health care model. Except in a few instances this has not happened. There has been since then a rapid formation of numerous HMO's throughout the country, each with its own organizational and service patterns and each with its own set of problems. Present judgment would have to be that HMO's are not the answer to the provision of comprehensive health and mental health care for the citizens of this country.

Because of the astronomical costs of health care in this country, it has been believed for some time that we will eventually move toward a national health insurance plan. Blatant partisan political considerations, as well as the vested interests of many groups that include legislators, third-party payers, consumers, and

---

* This pessimistic view appears to be confirmed by a survey released by the Office of Revenue Sharing at the United Conference of Mayors in San Francisco on June 19, 1973. According to the survey, which covered the reported use of $5.1 billion of general-revenue-sharing funds by 574 units of state and local governments, during the first year's activities under a new revenue sharing program, only 8 percent of the total was invested or planned for use in social-service areas. (*New York Times*, June 20, 1973.)

† The act was reintroduced unchanged at the start of the Ninety-third Congress.

professionals have prevented the legislative enactment of such a national-insurance plan. The details of the various plans have been described elsewhere and will only be mentioned here to illustrate the plethora of approaches, ranging from National Health Insurance Partnership Act of 1971 (the Nixon Plan), involving a significant role for private carriers, to the Committee of 100 for National Health Insurance (the Health Security Act of 1971—Kennedy Plan) which proposes compulsory national-health insurance for all Americans, financed by a formula based on a tax on employers' payrolls, a tax on salaried, self-employment, and unearned incomes, and federal general tax revenues. Under this plan there would be no charge to anyone for covered services. Providers of health care would be paid directly by the program. Other plans include the American Medical Association's plan (Medicredit); the Javits plan, (National Health Insurance and Health Services Improvement Act of 1971); the National Catastrophic Illness Protection Act (Boggs); the American Hospital Association Plan (Ameriplan); the Health Insurance Association of America Plan (The National Health Care Act of 1971); Catastrophic Health Insurance Plan (Long). Other plans, less comprehensive in scope, have been introduced but are not listed here. The point to be emphasized is that psychiatric care is excluded from most of these plans, and where included it is not adequately covered. At the start of the Ninety-third Congress the Health Security Act (Kennedy Plan), the Nixon Plan, and the Health Care Insurance Act (Medicredit), as well as some of the other plans were reintroduced in both Houses with no appreciable change in the provision for psychiatric care. Still another bill known as the National Health Care Services Reorganization and Financing Act was introduced as the first bill of the Ninety-third Congress. It calls for health insurance coverage with 75 percent provided by employers and 25 percent contributed by employees, with the federal government paying for the cost of health care for the poor and the elderly and for some of the costs for everyone else. The bill is based on the admin-istrative concept of a health care corporation, a community-based operation providing comprehensive health care at the local level. The corporations would be built upon existing delivery systems but reoriented and reorganized to meet local needs overseen by newly formed state health commissions. This bill, too, contains provisions for treatment of mental illness that must be considered inadequate. Inpatient hospital care for mental illness, alcoholism, drug abuse, and drug dependence is limited to ninety days per benefit period for registrants of local health care corporations and to forty-five days for other persons. In addition, a $5-per-day copayment by the patient is required. The outpatient care program for these disorders calls for a $2-copayment per day, but such care would be limited to three visits or treatment sessions for each day of inpatient care allowable during the benefit period. That is, registrants in corporations would be allowed 270 treatment sessions and nonregistrants 135 treatment sessions per benefit period. The financing formula is one of multiple sources including general federal revenues, direct contributions from individuals depending upon income level and family size, and Social Security taxes. Medicare and Medicaid would be consolidated into this proposed program of national health insurance.

Despite the considerable preoccupation with the development of a comprehensive, feasible health care plan, insufficient attention has been paid to an accurate estimate of the cost and how it will be paid. The Rand Corporation has recently done a series of retrospective studies, based on the demand system, in which the impact of copayment on the quality of medical care was brought into question.[25] A comparison was made of coinsurance rates under the current health system, the Nixon plan, and the Kennedy plan. The classes of services covered were broken down into three categories: hospital costs, physician costs, and "other." ("Other" includes some dental services, nursing homes, some prescription drugs, eyeglasses, prosthetics and outpatient mental health care.) The coinsurance rate is the amount, in percentage, that the patient pays. Under the current system, the coinsurance rate allocates 13 percent to hospital costs, 40 percent to doctor's costs, 90 percent to "other." Under the Nixon plan, hospital and doctor costs would have a floor of 25 percent, that is, nobody would have a coinsurance rate higher than 25 percent. Under the Kennedy plan the same two categories would have a coinsurance rate of 0 percent. It is important to note that in both the Nixon and Kennedy plans, the latter being considered the most comprehensive, the category of "other" is not covered and this category has the greatest price responsiveness. It has been estimated, using fiscal year 1975 as a baseline, that under the current health system, the aggregate health care bill for the country will be $100 billion of which two-thirds are paid by a third-party payer and one-third by private payment. Under the Nixon plan, the total will be $105 billion with $71 billion covered by third party (government). Under the Kennedy plan, the cost will be $130 billion totally covered by government health insurance financed as described. This $130 billion is an estimate made by the Rand Corporation. Other estimates of this plan range between $110 billion, made by the Social Security Administration, and $185 billion made by Rosette at Rochester. Clearly, this implies a major government expenditure and raises serious questions as to whether this type of comprehensive national health insurance plan can be afforded. The Rand Corporation concluded that the information necessary to plan effectively for national health insurance could not be obtained through retrospective studies. Thus, another study[21] is expected to be undertaken by the Rand Corporation with the following objectives: to understand the impact of coinsurance and deductibles on the demand for care; to understand the administrative feasibility of plans in general and, in particular, increases related to coinsurance and deductible rates; to understand the impact of utilization on health status and the impact of insurance mechanisms on the quality of care. The methodology involves the choice of five to nine geographic sites in this country in which different designs of health-insurance plans will be tested. There are approximately sixteen

different designs that will consist of various combinations of plans for coinsurance deductible, prepaid insurance, and coinsurance with high inpatient and low outpatient rates. It is planned that each site will enroll about 400 families with incomes under $12,000. People will be drawn at random, signed up, and randomly assigned to one of the sixteen plans. Dayton, Ohio, is planned as the first site. For design reasons the experiment will be conducted on some families for three years and others for five years. It is important to note that in all of the plans in the experiment almost all categories listed above in "other" are covered. Provisions for mental health care consist of complete coverage of all inpatient costs, fifty visits to a psychiatrist during each benefit year or to other nonpsychiatric mental health care providers. Fees for nonpsychiatric mental health care providers will be based on a profile of prevailing area fees for group therapy.* One of the interesting aspects of this experiment is the intent to incorporate into the insurance plans a maximum-limit health insurance to be related to family income. In effect this means that all costs beyond a certain percentage of family income would be paid and thus catastrophic health insurance would be provided for everyone. This concept is included in all plans of the experiment except for the mental illness coverage. It is hoped that at the end of the experiment the Rand Corporation will be able to answer some of the questions in the objectives. The fact that the foregoing discussion has addressed itself primarily to health care delivery systems underscores that mental health care is not included in any appreciable way.

The most recent major health legislation enacted has been contained in an amendment to the Social Security Act, known as the Bennett Amendment. It deals with the establishment of Professional Standards Review Organizations and was passed by the House and Senate in October 1972. The Bennett Amendment is based on the assumption that there is

* The description of the coverage for mental health care was provided by M. A. Rockwell of the Rand Corporation both during his seminar presentation[25] and during a subsequent personal communication. It expands on information contained in reference 21.

no better alternative than the use of the practicing physician in the delivery and supervision of medical care. PSRO is structured to provide practicing physicians with an opportunity to assume responsibility, in publicly accountable fashion, for assuring that Medicare and Medicaid benefits are provided only when medically necessary and in accordance with professional standards, in keeping with accepted norms in a given area. It also stipulates that the federal government has the general obligation to oversee overall PSRO operations and that it does not intend to abdicate its ultimate responsibility in this sphere. At present, PSRO will deal mainly with review of services under Medicare and Medicaid. It is envisioned that ultimately this type of organization will be the review mechanism for any national health insurance program.

In this connection it should be noted that both the Nixon and Kennedy Plans call for standards review and control. The Nixon Plan, sponsored by Senator Bennett, includes the establishment of PSRO to review health insurance and HMO contracts, and quality standards. The Kennedy Plan calls for establishment of a quality-control commission, and national standards for participating professional and institutional providers with regulation of major surgery and certain other specialist services, national licensure standards and requirements for continuing education. The newly introduced Health Care Services Act calls for establishment of a federal, cabinet-level Department of Health that would set basic standards for care, establish the scope of health insurance benefits, and would have final authority over program activities at the state level.

As stated in the Bennett Amendment, "The Professional Standards Review Organization is designed to promote the effective, efficient and economical delivery of health care services of proper quality for which payment can be made in whole or part under the Social Security Act and in recognition of the interests of patients, the public, practitioners and providers in improved health care services. The purpose of this program is to assure, through the application of suitable procedures of professional standards review, that the services for which payment will be made conform to appropriate professional standards for the provision of health care and that payment for these services will be made only when (1), and to the extent, medically necessary, as determined in the exercise of reasonable limits of professional discretion; (2) and in the case of services provided by hospital or other health care facility on an in-patient basis, only when and for the period those services cannot, consistent with professionally recognized health care standards, effectively be provided on an out-patient basis or more economically an inpatient health care facility of a different type, as determined in the exercise of reasonable limits of professional discretion."[33]

The bill[3] authorizes the Secretary of Health, Education and Welfare to designate specific areas of the country by January 1974, and to enter into conditional contracts for a PSRO in each area as soon as possible. Until January 1, 1976 the Secretary may only contract with qualified organizations that represent a majority of the physicians in each area. A qualified organization is a voluntary professional organization, for example, a County Medical Society, or one without requirement of dues and represents three hundred or more physicians. In general, it is anticipated that the County Medical Societies will be the instrumentality for the establishment of functioning PSRO's, thus ensuring the active participation of physicians in this program. While PSRO's are becoming operational, ongoing review will be carried out side-by-side with PSRO review until the Secretary of Health, Education and Welfare is satisfied that a given PSRO has demonstrated the ability to do the job. In keeping with this provision of the law, state councils will be established in states where three or more PSRO's are operational. Such a statewide program review team will include representation from each PSRO in the state, other physicians, and the public. In addition, on the national level, a council has been appointed by the Secretary of Health, Education and Welfare that includes eleven physicians of national stature, a majority of whom have been nominated for membership

on the council through their professional organizations. To implement this review mechanism, it is anticipated that each county medical society will ask the various subspecialties
to establish committees to review the various
models of treatment and care within their respective specialties and to serve as a source of
feedback to the county medical society PSRO.
In New York City, for example, the New York
County Medical Society has established a
PSRO. The New York District Branch of the
American Psychiatric Association has appointed a committee of its members to review
psychiatric patterns of care and to evolve
ways in which peer review can be effectively
implemented for psychiatry. A member of this
committee of the District Branch of the APA
is also a member of the medical society PSRO
making possible ongoing and meaningful psychiatric input into that body. On the New
York State level, a mechanism has been established, through the formation of a state committee, to share the information on PSRO activity of the various district branches of the
APA.

PSRO's will evaluate the utilization and
quality of institutional services. They will utilize norms of care based on typical patterns of
practice in the region for this purpose. And
they are encouraged to involve practicing
physicians to conduct ongoing review through
existing hospital utilization review committees
and, where necessary, to upgrade this activity.
For psychiatry, the goal is to establish "norms
of care" for psychiatric services in hospitals
and, ultimately, for outpatient treatment; to
evolve "relative value scales" as a mechanism
for deciding which procedures and modalities
of treatment are most effective in determining
quality of care at the most reasonable cost;
and, in addition, to make decisions regarding
variations in patterns of care to include legitimate philosophical differences in treatment
approaches.

In evaluating and determining whether existing in-house review procedures are at levels
of performance acceptable to the PSRO,
PSRO's must make certain that there is broad
and rotating physician participation in the review process on a continuing basis. PSRO's

must be organized on a local basis, of the stipulated minimum of 300 physicians, with the
expectation that the average PSRO will be
drawn from 1000 or more in the area. PSRO
and its review organization must employ acceptable parameters of care and norms for the
region. Data must be maintained in an orderly
and adequate fashion to facilitate evaluation
and comparison of PSRO performance. The
PSRO legislation is designed to utilize professional expertise, through peer review, subject
to public accountability, to assure the appropriateness and quality of services purchased
under the provisions of the Social Security
Act. The amendment explicitly states that the
following should be included in the review:
determination of the necessity for institutional
admission, the duration of institutional service, the appropriateness of the level of institutional care, the adequacy and relevance of
the institutional and ambulatory services provided. Implied in the objectives of the amendment is the attempt to restrict the utilization,
and, thereby, the cost of federal health services to a minimum.

Initially, one of the major functions of the
PSRO is education of the medical profession
regarding the meaning of PSRO legislation in
order to obviate difficulties later. There is
considerable unfamiliarity with and, in some
cases, outright denial of the legislation. Yet,
sooner or later it will affect every practicing
physician in the United States. It would be
most helpful if this peer review could be seen
as a form of consultation and continuing education rather than as a system of monitoring
physicians' activities, determining penalties for
violations, etc. It is important, therefore, in
establishing PSRO committees that the best
skills of the various specialists be represented,
and in the case of the specialty of psychiatry
to include those who will not consistently
advocate one particular modality of treatment
and who will not reflect the philosophy and
patterns of only one particular segment of the
psychiatric profession. Newman, et al. have
recently reported on their experiences with a
peer review program in California, where the
emphasis was a consultative and educational
one. Their experiences confirm that not only

can peer review work, but it can be sought after and be considered helpful by participating therapists.[22]

Many questions will arise for our profession as this legislation is put into effect: will the confidentiality of the patient–doctor relationship be maintained? This is an issue of justifiable concern to all psychiatrists. Will various institutions, such as teaching centers or community general hospitals, be equally represented on such committees? Should doctors review doctors? Or should there be some input from consumer groups in keeping with current trends of greater emphasis on consumer and community participation? Is the law requiring such review constitutional? This question has already been raised. If PSRO is a function of the county medical society, will the specialty of psychiatry be given appropriate representation? This is an important task for the psychiatric profession. What are norms of psychiatric care? Since it is generally agreed that diagnoses and modalities of treatment vary from one region of the country to another and, indeed, from one area of a city to another, who is to decide which treatment modality is most appropriate? How will peer review, currently limited to Medicare and Medicaid services, operate when applied to the private practice of psychiatry? Not directly related to PSRO but implicit in any national health insurance plan proposed so far is the existence of coinsurance rates—the portion of the service for which the patient must pay. In the specialty of psychiatry will this factor tend to encourage patients to seek less expensive care from other mental health practitioners? Myriad potential problems are contained in this legislation, but PSRO is now part of the law. As such it must be recognized as a fact of life that the medical profession can no longer ignore. Yet, associated with this major legislative enactment is a real opportunity for change and progress. If we involve ourselves meaningfully, peer review can be developed to engage the best skills of the profession for upgrading the quality of care. If we don't, we will forfeit our participation in any way since the legislation states that if a PSRO is not functional within a certain period of time, or if the Secretary of HEW decides that an existing PSRO is not functioning adequately, other organizations can be duly constituted as the PSRO instrument. Such organizations must demonstrate professional medical competence to function as a PSRO, and might include state or local health departments, an aggregation of hospitals or similar governmental or nonprofit organizational structure with professional competence.

Organizational changes are taking place at various levels of programming throughout the country, specifically related to the provision of comprehensive mental health care. It is my opinion that whatever changes may be made in the delivery of mental health care, concerted efforts must be made on the part of all to ensure dovetailing of such plans into a total comprehensive health care delivery system. In New York State, for example, a Unified Services approach is proposed in which the state mental hospital system would assume overall responsibility for total mental health care through subcontracts and other types of collaborative and fiscal arrangements with local agencies and programs to achieve comprehensiveness.

As part of such a Unified Services approach, a reporting system will be developed. The New York State Department of Mental Hygiene has committed itself to establishment of a Unified Services Information System. Toward that end a Unified Services Information Executive Commiteee has been appointed and commissioned to oversee the development of the system and a full-time task force has been assigned to conduct the information study under this committee's direction and supervision. Among the charges to this task force are the responsibility for keeping itself aware of developing systems within the department and for seeking compatibility with related systems at the federal, state, and local levels. In designing the Information System, the task force will aim at relevance, usability, timeliness, and economy. The task force will also have a Unified Services Information Advisory Committee with members appointed by the Commissioner. The membership of this advisory body will be representative of voluntary

agencies, units of local government, and programs of the New York State Department of
Mental Hygiene responsible for the provision
of mental health, mental retardation, and alcoholism services. The purpose of the committee is to review task force recommendations
for the Information System to enable the
organizations represented on the committee to
jointly plan, deliver, and evaluate services for
the mentally disabled. While a unified system
of care is a sound and potentially viable concept, formidable difficulties are anticipated in
its implementation.

In several states there is a move toward the
development of Departments of Human Services within state governments. Such departments would encompass health, welfare, educational, and correctional services under the
direction of a Secretary. In over a dozen states
such reorganization is taking place; some
Departments of Human Services are already
in operation, as in Massachusetts, for example.
Connecticut has recently established a Commission on Human Services. The purpose of
such an organizational shift is to coordinate
services and to minimize the fragmentation
and discontinuity that exist within the various
departments concerned with the provision of
human services. Once again, conceptually
such an approach has considerable merit;
operationally it is fraught with risks. For example, Departments of Mental Hygiene have
for many years maintained a degree of autonomy that they have come to cherish. Under
this new concept such departments would
become integral parts of superagencies. This
could give rise to myriad problems at different
levels, and might make implementation difficult. The same might apply to other departments. What is really needed, as Litwak and
Meyer have proposed, are coordinating mechanisms that will provide linkages and balance
between existing bureaucratic and other organizations, and thus permit more efficient
functioning and yet maintenance of individual
frames of reference.[19]

Another approach to comprehensive mental
health care delivery is that of regional planning on the local level to parallel the development of statewide human services depart-

ments. It is proposed that a network of *human
services* be developed, bounded by manageable geographic limits, including a number of
service components equal to the identified
problems at hand.* Personal service would, of
course, be an intricate component of this
network—for reasons both human and political. But of strong weight also should be a
research-planning-and-evaluation component
that would assume primary responsibility for
the essential tasks of social problem prevention.

The organization of such a service network
depends on the operational environment, but
basic features should include:

1. all existing service agencies—both voluntary and public—in order to prevent duplication,

2. community groups in order to ascertain
existing and potential problems,

3. representatives of the mass communications industries, and

4. a coordinating and planning apparatus to
establish short- and long-range policy.

If such comprehensive area-wide planning
is to prove effective, it is mandatory that legislative bodies "will" such efforts to succeed.
And by this I mean that local, state, and federal programs should be subsumed under the
aegis of the local coordinating mechanism. If
this does not occur, then duplication of service
and competition among agencies will inevitably occur. Again the appropriate governmental bodies should guarantee the financial base
of this coordinating mechanism—not on a
year-by-year crisis intervention basis, but on a
five- , ten- or even twenty-year basis.

Should this network planning effectively
take place, I am convinced that we will not
only experience perhaps our first national
attempt at multiproblem prevention—and I
firmly believe that social problems are inter-
dependently interrelated—but we will also
move toward elimination of service failure by
introducing almost universal accessibility.

* I first suggested this approach in a paper presented
at the Twenty-third Institute on Hospital and Community Psychiatry, Seattle, Washington, September
1971. It is contained in a somewhat different form in
reference 11.

Moreover, as the various social classes become exposed to a variety of human services and their close interrelation, we can expect that at least some services will lose the stigma that has traditionally been attached to their service delivery.

The network planning of which I speak represents the developmental approach to social welfare as a front-line function of modern industrial society in a positive collaborative way with other major social institutions working toward a better society.[36] Needless to say, some public resistance and coordinating failures will appear quite early. But the alternative at this point in time is a continuation of the fragmented residual approach of intervention on a crisis basis when the normal structures of society break down, which has the connotation of a dole or gift. This approach has failed significantly in the past, and will fail even more grossly in the future as our complex society continues to develop.

(Looking Toward the Future

Based on the assumption that in the foreseeable future mental health care delivery will become more integral to comprehensive health care within the same overall organizational framework with similar standards, setting procedures and mechanisms for determining quality care and funding arrangements, the delivery of mental health services will expand the organizational base through a more critical linkage with other social, educational, and health services. This linkage will prove to be much more than a shadow of past practices by mental health professionals—practices where haphazard referrals were made to unfamiliar agencies for supportive services in treatment situations. Such linkage will aim at more than service collaboration between independent programs that establish contractual agreements for meeting jointly clusters of problems reflective of purposes of the individual programs involved. At a rapid pace there is now developing in our nation a new philosophy of care, a conceptual process

that chooses health over sickness and in this divorces itself from the past. This assertion is not merely idle rhetoric or academic semantics, for it entails a view of the human situation that has as its goal the development of an optimal social existence for all who seek help for specific problems in the areas of human service (health, education, and welfare). It seeks to generate the response of professionals in a *comprehensive* manner that realizes the extensiveness of interrelated problems in our nation's fabric. The precipitating factors of mental illness are often found in the problems of family life, poverty, and poor health, and the only solution available is to address these concomitant problems, simultaneously, to whatever clinical treatment is prescribed. This is not to say that psychiatrists must consider themselves experts in the field of education, or that welfare workers must assume primary responsibilities in the treatment of alcohol or drug addiction. Rather, it is to say that all professionals should think in terms of a comprehensive human service response to the problems of a citizen seeking help. As an ideal, the concept of comprehensiveness may never fully be achieved, yet the current movement in this direction outlines a pattern of care that has already rejected, in practice, the fragmentary character of the past.

The Political Setting of Comprehensiveness

For the past decade, the federal government has addressed its time, staff, and money toward the unification of human services in the nation. Because of the many complex administrative mechanisms that form the substance of our federal system of politics, this movement cannot yet be considered especially efficient in its undertaking. The many attempts aimed at eliminating fragmentation in human service delivery have resulted in a federal design, radical in nature, that calls for "debureaucratization" at the federal level. Eisenstadt has referred to this process as

. . . the subversion of the goals and activities of the bureaucracy in the interests of different groups with which it is in close interaction. [p. 259][8]

Combined with managerial techniques such as Program-Planning-Budget Systems (PPBS) and political considerations such as the political pressure for decentralization of decision-making, the federal government is engaged in an effort that seeks to (1) localize the planning and delivery of services for greater response to community needs; (2) coordinate the multiplicity of public and voluntary efforts to avoid overlap and duplication; and (3) place the responsibility for fiscal decision-making for funding of local programs in the political setting that is most immediate: state and local government. An illustration can be seen in the proposed Allied Services Act.[6a] The stated goals of this act include the coordination of complementary but separate services at state and local levels, and provision of "the necessary tools" to allow such governmental units to eliminate bureaucratic obstacles in service delivery. The clearest testimony of the federal movement toward comprehensive service delivery is contained in the following language of the act declaring an intent to:

... give state and local officials authority to consolidate the planning and implementation of the many separate social service programs into streamlined, comprehensive plans—each custom-designed for a particular area.

Such plans could eventually make it possible to assess the total human service needs of an entire family at a single location with a single application. Most applicants need more than one service, and now must trudge to office after office applying for assistance from one program at a time—with the result that they may not obtain all the services they need, or may be discouraged altogether from seeking help. [p. 259][8]

Under the act, the federal government proposed to make up to twenty million dollars available in the first full year for the costs of developing such comprehensive plans, and was prepared to underwrite administrative start-up costs necessary for comprehensive service program implementation. In effect, the act was designed to have major impact on over two hundred categorical health, educational, and social services programs now emanating out of Washington.

To date, the act has not received congressional support for a variety of reasons. Technical issues such as (1) adequacy of initial funding; (2) local planning mechanisms for problem identification and resolution; and (3) availability of future operational resources from the federal level vis-à-vis state and local contributions are critical areas of concern. There are also a multitude of clearly partisan political issues that have prevented passage of the act. But closely related to the movement toward localized comprehensive service has been the enactment of legislation for federal revenue-sharing to state and local governments, as well as the reorganization and consolidation of the executive branch of government following the presidential election of 1972. Together with the direction for service delivery set in the proposed Allied Services Act of 1972, these actions if sustained by Congress forecast significant movement toward the concept of comprehensiveness in care for the immediate future.

The Conceptual Base for Comprehensiveness

Sayles and Chandler have noted that:

... an obvious characteristic of modern society is ever increasing interdependency; little can be changed without affecting a wide array of institutions, and many new developments depend upon close, collaborative, and integrated activities that criss-cross organizational boundaries and the dividing line, between the public and private sectors. [p. 2][27]

To understand the nature and consequences of this interdependence in a service delivery or organizational setting requires a new approach in the conceptualization of individual and group action, as well as of its management. Instead of limiting perceptions to the plane of individual action or small group cohesiveness (formal or informal), it is necessary today to conceptualize actions in terms of the totality of the situation, in other words, to do "systems thinking"[9] or to view it in "the systems approach."[6] Such a view, usually incorporating the situational processes of input-conversion-output, recognizes the critical impact of the surrounding environment on any particular system (biological, social, economic, political, management, etc.). By focusing on the system, there develops a concern for the comprehensiveness of the situation and the various elements that affect the decision or action involved. In reality, the systems approach is a philosophy of action based on the belief that enough of the complexity of existence can be analyzed and interrelated to describe reasonable human goals as well as the means for their achievement.

On a philosophical level, it has been noted that there are two basic viewpoints on social systems, monism and pluralism:

. . . the pluralist does not believe that organizations have values, only individuals do. He believes in a balance of forces and that the decision-making process of society ought to be the result of that balance—the legislators, the planners, the mental health officials and others—converging together, but with no overall conceptualization of where they are going. Monism, on the other hand, is a philosophy that says, in principle at least, that all of the pieces can be put together into a whole picture. The monist believes it is possible to identify the objectives of the system, and to think through the alternatives that lead most successfully to the desired goals. [p. 360][1]

On a practical level, it must be stated that reality is never such an either/or proposition. Rather, society finds itself in an ever-fluctuating position between these polar views, striving to introduce order where elements of chaos exist while seeking to develop decision-making mechanisms that join the process of rational planning with the unclear and uncertain demands of practical politics. Systematic planning based on the rationalism that the monistic view entails can never fully be achieved. Questions regarding the intent, the scope, the personnel, and the organizational position of the planning process in any particular service delivery model bring a variety of conflicting opinions from recognized management experts. Yet the analytic base of systems analysis, along with modern computer technology for the collection and dissemination of relevant information, does provide a meaningful advance in the planning and delivery of human services. As C. West Churchman has noted:

1. The systems approach begins when first you see the world through the eyes of another.
2. The systems approach goes on to discovering that every world view is terribly restricted.
3. There are no experts in the systems approach.
4. The systems approach is not a bad idea. [pp. 231–232][6]

Systems Analysis and Planning for Service Delivery

Planning has become a condition of modern existence. As David Ewing has observed:

The big question in planning becomes not whether it is justified but to what extent and in what manner it shall be practiced. [p. 4][10]

In essence, planning is a rational tool for the production of recognized and desired changes in an organization's structure or manner of operation.[10] It is a process that enables an organization to respond to the actions and pressures of the surrounding environment as well as internal organizational requirements. In modern management theory, the planning, budgetary, and operational actions of an organization are usually joined in a conscious systematic manner, such as the use of Planning-Program-Budget Systems (PPBS) and the techniques of Project Management, Planned Evaluation and Review Techniques (PERT), Line of Balance (LOB), Critical Path Method (CPM), etc. For human service delivery, this approach allows for an effective mixture of administrative and programmatic elements in response to identified social problems. The systems approach seeks to minimize the negative impact of excessive bureaucratization through a flexible realignment of decision-making and control mechanisms.

PPBS is essentially an information process around the "cost and benefits" of alternate courses of organizational action. Its aim is to help management arrive at "better" decisions on the allocation of resources toward attainment of organizational objectives. It entails the development of cost-accounting and performance-reporting mechanisms for the collection of information. It does not relate in purpose to budget implementation, productivity, or cost control.

In its use at all levels of government, several variations of the PPBS model can be identified. Governmental units have introduced modifications according to need. However, there are several major components of PPBS that remain constant:

1. An "across-the-board" governmental program structure aimed at the identification of fundamental objectives, and subsequent grouping of governmental activities relative to objectives, regardless of organizational placement.
2. Development of a multiyear program and financial plan.
3. Program analysis that considers objectives, alternatives, costs, benefits, assumptions, and impact on other programs.

It has been shown that a significant investment in time and money is required by a governmental unit to implement PPBS successfully. The "start-up" time has taken several years in many instances, and the mandatory use of computer technology as well as the increase in systems-related staff can prove costly. [p. 241][16] Beyond these considerations there exists an often present political opposition that must be overcome. As PPBS is representative of the "monist" approach to social systems, the political process can often be considered in pluralist terms. Politicians who may favor the development of PPBS must also consider the impact of such a planning process on pork-barrel legislation and logrolling transactions. As a result, there is an inherent tension between rational planning techniques, that are epitomized perhaps by PPBS, and the multifaceted and often self-contradictory political structures that are expected to make use of planning techniques.

Project Management is a management approach that was developed in the military/industrial complex as a means of satisfying the requirement for management of defense resources from inception to operational employment. It entails the blending of the technical know-how of many functionally oriented organizations under one centralized coordinat-

ing and managing mechanism whose prime role is to synchronize and integrate an aggregation of resources. Project Management is based on the systems approach to action. It has proven to be particularly successful when applied to a one-time undertaking that is definable in terms of a specific end result and bigger than the organization has previously undertaken successfully. [p. 293][29] By definition, a project has an objective end point in time. The project management approach entails the appointment of one man who has the responsibility for the detailed planning, coordination, and ultimate outcome of the project. The essence of Project Management is that it cuts across, and, in a sense, conflicts with, the normal organizational structure. Throughout the project, personnel at various levels in many functions of the organization contribute and are recognized as the "team." With sanction from the top, the team members concentrate on their target under the direction of the project manager, any relationships to their functional departments during the project period being of a qualitative nature only. Project Management is "adhocracy." [p. 125][31]

In the future, the movement toward comprehensive human service delivery programs will rely heavily on both PPBS and Project Management. As governmental limits develop program goals that require interorganizational collaboration for their attainment, action will be framed into temporary settings, where the meaning of "management" will have fuller significance ("How can we *manage* this problem?"), and the negative aspects of bureaucracy will subside due to team involvement in decision-making and environmental input from the community. Such a comprehensive approach will rely on staff development and in-service training programs to provide team members with the tools for effective collaboration. It will also require a pertinent program evaluation and review component to analyze the progress of interdisciplinary team collaboration in goal attainment as well as obstacles to attainment that are related to the functional units from which team members are drawn. Much thought must still be given to the relevance of the professional education models upon which the various human services are founded, and what reforms might be conducive to comprehensive team functioning. Finally, the limits of team functioning must also be considered, so that one form of bureaucracy is not simply replaced by another irrelevant style of service delivery. The process of planning is never automatically correct and never free from the intrusion of human values. However, the only alternative is haphazard ignorance.

Service Delivery in a Systems Setting

How human service will be provided in the future is closely related to the above propositions. If the governmental response to societal problems is to advocate the concentration of public resources in priority fashion with limited emphasis on organizational jurisdictions, then both governmental units and large organizations will be involved in the development of smaller, more time-limited service units that will function as microsystems in their service delivery patterns. These units, whether created through interagency collaboration or through intraagency mandate, will be functioning in an atmosphere of management-by-objectives where the individual's preference for how his job can best be done is considered a primary factor in planning goal attainment. These units, or teams, will not be found by the limitations of traditional authority and control; rather, they will be working in an environment beyond the current understanding of bureaucracy.

For the most part, today, professionals in the field of human service adhere to the concept that the individual worker is the prime conveyor of service delivery—a concept with roots in various schools of professional training. The organization is seen as a means by which professionals can utilize their skills. In such settings caseloads, colleagueship, and compensation, within rather rigidly defined patterns, are provided. The organizational requirements are tolerable; the interpersonal relationship between professional and client, however, is primary.

As a result of this situation, professional agencies today abound in conflict. With external pressure from both governmental and community groups for effective resolution of social problems, the primacy of the one-to-one mode of service delivery is being questioned by agency executives on two counts: the impact of profession-specific intervention in increasingly multiproblem situations, and the fiscal and social costs of specialized service delivery, vis-à-vis fragmentation, duplication, and inappropriate response. Internally, the problems inherent in organizational change that relate to roles, status, informal groups, professional values, etc., have created near or at times open confrontation within many agencies. Consequently, in the past decade human service organizations have attempted to go beyond their specialized boundaries in a variety of ways, most of which have not achieved their limited goals due to lack of impact on the organizational structure. Some agencies have attempted to collaborate by placing their staffs in close geographic proximity (i.e., the same building) with reliance on daily contact. Others have functioned through the use of interagency conferences, meeting locally as needed to discuss problems of coordination. [p. 37][15] Still others have introduced project management, wherein agencies surrender part of their jurisdiction over staff chosen to form an interagency-comprehensive service delivery model. This approach is perhaps the optimal form of interagency service collaboration that can be achieved as long as bureaucracies continue to exist.

However, an alternative to the approach of interagency coordination is a real possibility, especially in the public sector. Large organizations will emerge, characterized by such features as diversity of interest, complexity of relationships, unity of control, and decentralization of service delivery that is comprehensive in nature. Such agencies will employ the techniques of PPBS, Project Management, Organizational Development, etc. in the achievement of their quest for responsive service delivery. Staff patterns will increasingly reflect multidisciplinary training, for such organizations will attempt to avoid the extrusion of people needing help by broadening the service delivery base. Knowledge of mental health, child care, education, etc., will readily be available for input into case situations, and the means for such availability is seen in the unit or team structure.

In this setting, the role of the project or team manager is of primary importance, for it is he who meets the *team* response to the patient need. Coordination is the essence of this decision-making role, for the manager must match the skills of his personnel with the multiproblem situation under consideration. This role should not conflict with the content of professional involvement; rather, it sets the boundaries of the unit's (and ultimately the agency's) systematic intervention into the case, based on the recommendations of the multidisciplinary team. To achieve efficiency of team functioning, a process of organizational development is essential so that the limitations or confines of prior professional training do not retard the achievement of comprehensiveness in service delivery. Ultimately, it should involve considerable "self-analysis" on the part of each professional to determine if his personal goals are congruent with those of the organization.

If the preceding comments seem unrelated to what the field of psychiatry is engaged in today, it may be more a conflict in values than one of fact. What this exposition has intended to accomplish is to state a personal viewpoint of an emerging reality. As Machiavelli has cautioned: "There is nothing more difficult to take in hand, or more uncertain in its success, than to introduce a new order of things." Let judgment occur in this light.

Such judgment will be affected by the fact that in the next few years major changes will be effected in the health-care delivery systems in this country. It is difficult to predict the nature and extent of such changes except to speculate that they will be of major dimensions because of increasing technology, cost factors, consumer expectations, and many other considerations.

At a time when we face the possible loss of a generation of caregivers as a result of phasing out of federal support for training pro-grams in the mental health professions, there will have to be a redirection in our training emphasis. Continuing education programs for all mental health professionals, of relatively short-time duration, and thus less costly, might be one answer. Such programs can be evolved with state and local support, perhaps even some federal support, to keep our manpower pool abreast of such factors as social causation, consumer needs, and needs in treatment methods as well as the best administrative and management techniques applicable to make available quantity and quality of care in a continuum of human service delivery. Therefore, it is incumbent upon every practicing physician and psychiatrist to keep himself abreast of changes that are taking place; each in his own way to involve himself meaningfully, thus ensuring the development of safeguards, in whatever system of care is adopted, for the protection of the patient, the public, and the profession.

(Bibliography

1. Alexander, J. B. and J. L. Messal. "The Planning-Programming-Budgeting System in the Mental Health Field," *Hosp. Community Psychiatry*, 23 (1972), 357–361.
2. Barten, H. H. and L. Bellak, eds. *Progress in Community Mental Health*, Vol. 2. New York: Grune & Stratton, 1972.
3. Bennett, W. F. Statement at National Conference on Professional Standards Review Organization, Albuquerque, N.M., Feb. 1973.
4. Bernard, V. W. "Some Principles of Dynamic Psychiatry in Relation to Poverty," *Am. J. Psychiatry*, 122 (1965), 254–267.
5. Candib, L. M. "A Social Study of the Health Center Movement: A New Approach to Public Health History." B. A. thesis, Harvard University, 1968.
6. Churchman, C. W. *The Systems Approach*. New York: Dell Publ., 1968.
6a. Congressional Record. "Allied Services Act of 1972," May 18 (1972), S8124.
7. Connery, R. H. et al. *The Politics of Mental Health*. New York: Columbia University Press, 1968.
8. Eisenstadt, S. N. "Bureaucracy, Bureau-

cratization, and Debureaucratization," in J. A. Litterer, ed., *Organizations*, Vol. 2, pp. 255–263. New York: Wiley, 1969.

9. EMERY, F. E., ed. *Systems Thinking*. Baltimore: Penguin, 1969.

10. EWING, D. W. *The Human Side of Planning*. London: Macmillan, 1969.

11. FOLEY, A. R. and P. GORHAM. "Toward a New Philosophy of Care: Perspectives on Prevention," *Community Ment. Health J.*, 9 (1973), 99–107.

12. FOLEY, A. R. and D. S. SANDERS. "Theoretical Considerations for the Development of the Community Mental Health Center Concepts," *Am. J. Psychiatry*, 122 (1966), 985–990.

13. GLASSCOTE, R., D. S. SANDERS, H. M. FORSTENZER et al. *The Community Mental Health Center: An Analysis of Existing Models*. Washington: Joint Information Service Am. Psychiatr. Assoc. and Natl. Assoc. Ment. Health, 1964.

14. GLASSCOTE, R., J. N. SUSSEX, E. CUMMING et al. *The Community Mental Center: An Interim Appraisal*. Washington: Joint. Information Service Am. Psychiatr. Assoc. and Natl. Assoc. Ment. Health, 1969.

15. GULICK, L. and L. URWICK. *Papers on the Science of Administration*. New York: Inst. Pub. Admin., 1937.

16. HATRY, H. P. and J. F. COTTON. "What Is a PPBS System?" in R. T. Golembiewski, F. Gibson, and G. Y. Cornog, eds., *Public Administration*, 2nd ed., pp. 230–247. Chicago: Rand McNally, 1973.

17. JONES, E. *The Life and Work of Sigmund Freud*, Vol. 3. New York: Basic Books, 1957.

18. KAPLAN, S. R. "The Use and Abuse of Federal Derived Health Delivery Funds as Instruments of Political Action: The Lincoln Hospital Community Mental Health Center." Presented Annu. Meet. Professors West of the Mississippi, La Jolla, Calif., Sept. 1972.

19. LITWAK, E. and H. J. MEYER. "A Balance Theory of Coordination between Bureaucratic Organizations and Community Primary Groups," *Admin. Sci. Q.*, 2 (1966), 31–58.

20. MEYER, A. Address presented to the International Congress of Medicine, Vienna, 1913.

21. NEWHOUSE, J. P. "A Design for a Health Insurance Experiment," Rand Corporation Study-965-OEO (1972).

22. NEWMAN, D. E., H. S. GOLDSTEIN, and V. KAZANJIAN. "A One-and-a-Half Year Experience with Peer Utilization Review." Presented 126th Annu. Meet. Am. Psychiatr. Assoc., Honolulu, May 1973.

23. NIXON, R. M. "Veto Message of Labor-HEW Appropriation Bill," *Congress. Q. Almanac*, 26 (1970), 19A–21A.

24. PEABODY, F. Quoted in *Action for Mental Health: Final Report of the Joint Commission on Mental Illness and Health*. New York: Basic Books, 1961.

25. ROCKWELL, M. A. Seminar presentation, Columbia University, Feb. 1973.

26. ROSEN, G. "Public Health: Then and Now. The First Neighborhood Health Center Movement—Its Rise and Fall," *Am. J. Public Health*, 61 (1971), 1620–1637.

27. SAYLES, L. R. and M. K. CHANDLER. *Managing Large Systems: Organizations for the Future*. New York: Harper & Row, 1971.

28. SCHWARTZ, D. A. "Community Mental Health in 1972: An Assessment," in H. H. Barten and L. Bellak, eds., *Progress in Community Mental Health*, Vol. 2, pp. 3–34. New York: Grune & Stratton, 1972.

29. STEWART, J. M. "Making Project Management Work," in D. I. Cleland and W. R. King, eds., *Systems, Organizations, Analysis, Management: A Book of Readings*, pp. 291–302. New York: McGraw-Hill, 1969.

30. STOEKLE, J. D. and L. M. CANDIB. "The Neighborhood Health Center—Reform Ideas of Yesterday and Today," *N. Engl. J. Med.*, 280 (1969), 1385–1391.

31. TOFFLER, A. *Future Shock*. New York: Random House, 1971.

32. UNITED STATES CONGRESS. *Mental Health Study Act of 1955. Public Law*, 84–182.

33. ————. *Declaration of Purpose: Professional Standards Review Organization*. Sect. 249F of HR 1, 92nd Congress. Public Law, 92–603.

34. ————. *Health Maintenance Organization and Resources Development Act of 1972*. S327 of 92nd Congress; reintroduced as S14 in 93rd Congress.

35. WHITE, W. A. Quoted in R. H. Williams and L. C. Ozarin, eds., *Community Mental Health: An International Perspective*. San Francisco: Jossey-Bass, 1968.

36. WILENSKY, H. L. and C. N. LEBEAUX. *Industrial Society and Social Welfare*. New York: Russell Sage Foundation, 1958.

CHAPTER 34

THE FUTURE OF THE PUBLIC MENTAL HOSPITAL

Merrill T. Eaton

A LEGISLATIVE RESOLUTION beginning: "Whereas, recent press reports indicate that the Department of Public Institutions plans to phase out state mental institutions by 1975 . . ." and demanding an investigation was introduced in a Midwestern state in January 1972.

(Three Social Trends

If Moses Sheppard[17] and Dorothea Lynde Dix[38] were available for comment, they would ask what is happening. What is happening is this: *First*, the entire health-care delivery system in the United States is in the process of change. People who are able are going to pay for their health care in advance, whether by an arrangement called "prepayment" (as in proposed health maintenance

organizations) or through "insurance premiums," or by means of direct taxation. Those who cannot pay are going to have the costs subsidized by the federal government. All citizens are going to have the right to equal health care; therefore, the distinction between public and private care must end.

Second, involuntary hospitalization, as provided by traditional commitment laws, is being eliminated.[33,37] Preventive detention, the confinement of a patient believed dangerous, for an indefinite period, is under legal and social attack. The doctrine of *parens patrie*,[37] the state assuming a paternal role, paternalism, is no longer socially acceptable; and with its demise the involuntary detention and treatment of a person dangerous to himself, or of a person who is in need of treatment but cannot or will not recognize the need, will become impossible. These changes will not only affect the way a person enters a mental hospital but also what can be done for him once he is there. The locked ward, already largely eliminated in many facilities, is unlikely to be acceptable to many truly voluntary patients. It will not be possible to give medication or treatment to patients who decline it. The physician and the superintendent will be responsible to, not responsible for, patients. Traditionally, mental illness was often equated with irresponsibility and this was seen as absolute, not relative. Hence, the superintendent of a mental hospital was held responsible if a patient left without permission ("escaped" "eloped"), lost possessions or money, or injured himself in some way. One hundred years ago, if a woman patient became pregnant, it was without further investigation of the circumstances, "another of the base results of the wretched management of the institution."* Obviously, to protect himself and his staff, a superintendent would have needed strict rules governing patient supervision and conduct, quite apart from any specific patient's actual treatment needs or ability to make decisions and assume responsibility. (This is analogous to some of the ways that the possibility of malpractice suits influences medical practice today.) These attitudes of 100 years ago were not greatly changed until after World War II. Certainly the superintendent of today, and of the future, has some responsibility to protect the person and property of patients; but it is more one of eliminating hazards, providing facilities, and seeing that advice is given, than one of regulating the patient's behavior so as to prevent him from voluntarily taking any risks. (For example, traditionally, it was felt necessary to put money and jewelry in a safe or send it home; today, as well as taking the same sort of steps the operator of a hotel or college dormitory might take to discourage pilfering, the superintendent *provides* a safe and *advises* its use.)

Third, the resident population, though not the admission rate, in public mental hospitals has been steadily declining. This decline, though sometimes attributed to the introduction of tranquilizing medication in the middle 1950s, actually results from many factors. New treatment methods have helped shorten hospital stays. The increased number of psychiatrists and other mental-health professionals trained since World War II has contributed both to improved quality in public mental-hospital staffs and to the development of alternative community facilities. An expanding economy[7–9] has made it possible for more patients with residual symptoms to obtain employment and rehabilitation in the community, and expanded welfare programs have made it possible to discharge other patients who are not able to be self-sustaining. Changing social attitudes allow for greater acceptance of deviant behavior and reduced social distance from former patients.[12] Added to these factors is a change in administrative philosophy. The superintendent of today feels that it is to his credit to reduce his census and shorten stays; so he may try to move a number of patients into nursing homes or other facilities, as well as make efforts at treatment and rehabilitation.

It is futile to deal with these three social trends by denial or negativism. One might say that proposed health-insurance legislation may not be passed, and that even if it is, psychiatric benefits are sharply limited in most current proposals; that commitment laws cannot be repealed altogether; and that there will be an irreducible minimum of patients still needing traditional state hospital care. A more sophisticated denial might be to point out that social trends are discontinuous and a halt to or reversal of current trends is possible. One may point out that health-insurance programs do not in themselves correct problems in the supply and distribution of health resources; that prepayment programs may do more to foster cut-rate care than to pay physicians to keep people well "like the doctors of ancient China."† Types of patients who will suffer great harm because protective, albeit pater-

---

* A quotation from the January 10, 1872 *Omaha Daily Herald* concerning the Insane Asylum at Lincoln. (Reprinted in the *Omaha World Herald*, January 10, 1972.)

† From President Nixon's message to the Congress of the United States, February 18, 1971.

nalistic, steps cannot be taken can be listed by the dozens. Likewise, there are innumerable examples of situations in which short hospital stays or transfers to other facilities are not in the best interest of patients. To engage in such professional chauvinism, however logical and well-motivated, is an exercise in futility. Looking at the record of organized medicine's opposition to "socialized medicine," such exercises in futility appear not unlikely to occur.

❴ Four Options for the Future

The future of the public mental hospital may be:

1. To resist social change and to be phased out of existence.

2. To accept social change and to plan an orderly process of termination.

3. To undertake new roles and functions.

4. To continue to serve the needs of the mentally ill in a manner concordant with contemporary social values.

The first option is the least desirable. A rapid phasing out of state (and other public) mental hospitals would leave a large number of patients without needed services. A state hospital in an isolated location, with an outmoded physical plant and a staff incapable of furnishing an effective treatment program, ought to be closed. Such hospitals are in the minority. Most offer effective, though not ideal, treatment, and amenities considerably superior to those of Juniper Hill.[40] Alternative facilities and practitioners are not available to undertake care of patients served by these hospitals.

It is not reasonable to assume, as some have, that if patients have health insurance that will cover psychiatric illness, all who need it can obtain private treatment. The idea that the closing of public mental hospitals would cause the physicians employed by them to enter a new form of government-financed and regulated private practice is valid in itself. However, the notion that they would take care

of the same number of patients is unrealistic. The physician in the public mental hospital is not primarily occupied in direct patient care. Even if he were to spend all of his time in this activity, he could treat only a small percent of the patients now being served. It is in the public hospital that the team method, the therapeutic milieu, and the employment of nonmedical therapists working under supervision is most highly developed.

The second option, a gradual, planned termination, would allow new facilities and programs to develop. It would take several years to replace the present public mental hospitals with comprehensive community mental health centers, even if some state hospitals of appropriate size and location entered the centers program and were assigned catchment areas. Not only would many new centers have to be established, but most existing centers would need to expand their functions considerably to serve all the mental-health needs of their catchment areas. It would take even longer for new "private" facilities to be developed to meet the needs of a fully insured population or to provide full psychiatric care as components of health maintenance organizations.

The third possibility is really a modification of the second. It would preserve administrative organizations (some of which, at least, are worth preserving), prevent the sacrifice of usable buildings, and maintain jobs for persons now employed. There have been a number of proposed functions. One has been that the state hospitals should serve as chronic disease hospitals,[21] accepting all types of "incurable" patients, and, presumably, continuing to provide custodial care to certain mental patients. Another suggestion is for a move in the direction of the correctional system involving the rehabilitation of persons with character disorders,[3] presumably delinquents and offenders suitable for minimum-security institutions. Still another has been for the institutions to undertake additional public health and welfare responsibilities or, at least, to house and coordinate various agencies involved in health, education, and welfare so as to become multiservice centers.

(Response to Contemporary Social Values

Financing Mental-Health Care

The fourth option deserves the most detailed inspection. Accommodation to new systems of financing health care must first be considered. One might advocate making the public hospital fully eligible to receive health-insurance benefits (both for hospital costs and professional services) and/or to become a part of (or contract with) health maintenance organizations. Only if the present public hospitals compete on an equal footing with private facilities can we hope to eliminate a double standard of care. It is unlikely that a universal compulsory national health-insurance program (or an equivalent prepayment system) will initially include benefits for chronic illness, including long-term psychiatric illness. There is no real reason why it should not. Most long-term care is in public facilities and is already being supported by the taxpayer. Excluding this from a health program only appears to make the program cheaper. Including it would eliminate the "dumping" of chronic cases, turning the public hospital into an institution for the chronic, with the difficulties in staffing and in maintaining a therapeutic orientation and optimism this would entail; and the perpetuation of a double standard. While chronic mental illness will not be covered at first, sooner or later it will; and it makes sense to advocate sooner rather than later.

Competition between what are now private and what are now public resources, with patients exercising a free choice, will provide incentives for improved service for all providers, not just the currently public.

Advocacy of the inclusion of adequate psychiatric benefits and of the participation by now public facilities in new health-care-financing-and-delivery systems may not insure appropriate legislation. However, if restrictive legislation is passed that excludes full participation by state hospitals, as such, this need

not cause either their closure or their assumption of the responsibility for only chronic patients and those rejected by other providers of care. For the present direct support of such hospitals by the state, there could be substituted an operation of hospitals by nonprofit-making corporations (with further steps to meet any specific requirements for participation); and grants or contracts could be used to continue state financing of research, training, indirect services, and direct services not otherwise covered.

Even now, in anticipation of more widespread and government-sponsored insurance or prepayment programming, the financing and organization of public mental hospitals should be reconsidered. Many people, in some areas the majority of the employed, have insurance that covers psychiatric care. Some programs pay for hospital care in public institutions, but others do not.[1,2] Fewer pay for professional services in public hospitals, and even fewer for public outpatient services. Two considerations are involved in nonpayment. First, the idea that this is not appropriate in a tax-supported facility; second, the fact that many institutions that do charge those able to pay for hospital care do not itemize professional services. Steps, including reorganization when necessary, revised cost-accounting and billing procedures, and initiation of adequate utilization and peer-review programs, should be initiated to allow full participation. Cash income can and should provide a greater portion of public hospital and clinic budgets, and a greater, and identifiable portion of the compensation of professional staff; for this is directly related to volume and quality of service. Ultimately, when all patients have insurance or prepayment coverage, direct tax support for public mental hospitals can be limited to those activities not directly related to patient care: training, research, community education, and primary prevention. In regard to the latter, it might be suggested that these activities can be covered in a prepayment, health-maintenance, program. This is not altogether realistic. It will be possible to provide preventive programs that yield a high, short-term payoff in this way. Most preventive programs in psychiatry will not qualify.

Voluntary and Involuntary Hospitalization

Laws governing involuntary hospitalization are being reinspected and revised by legislative bodies and are also likely to be modified by court decisions. The staffs of public mental hospitals, along with other mental-health professionals, can cooperate in this process. It is probable that in the public mental hospital of the future all, or nearly all, patients will be voluntary. Nevertheless, new laws must take into account the fact that there are dangerous patients and that there are patients who need care badly but cannot recognize their need.

The concept of dangerousness is a difficult one to evaluate. As a paradigm of the dangerous patient one might consider a person who has paranoid delusions, has bought a gun, and intends to kill his imagined persecutors. He may represent a real and immediate danger to others, but he has not committed an overt act. One might choose as the paradigm a "sexual sociopath" who has committed repeated offenses against children or aggressive (sadistic) attacks on adults. (The voyeur or exhibitionist is more a public nuisance than a danger.) One might select as an example the person who has committed a crime and been found unable to stand trial because his mental condition makes him unable to understand the charges against him and/or participate in his own defense. Another example would be the person who has committed a serious offense and has been found not guilty by reason of insanity. These are the usual examples. What about the alcoholic who drives a car? Traditionally, he has not been regarded as a subject for commitment as dangerous, though he may be regarded as sick—legally as well as medically. Surely intoxicated drivers, many of whom have diagnosable alcohol problems, account for more deaths, serious injuries, and property damage than any of the traditional types of "dangerous" patients. There are other situations in which a mentally ill person's con-

fusion or preoccupation may compromise the safety of others.

The public mental hospital had best be relieved of responsibility for the confinement, if not for the care, of most of the patients representing serious and immediate danger to others. Certainly such a patient does not belong on an open ward. The advisability of having a maximum-security unit on a hospital campus is questionable. It is likely to be uneconomical, and lacking perimeter security, offers more opportunity for escape than does a penal complex, while at the same time forcing greater restriction on the activities of inmates. Moreover, it puts the hospital staff in something other than a helping role. Those who have committed overt acts (e.g., the sexual deviate offender) can be sentenced, with due process of law, and can be treated in a correctional facility. Treatment could be provided by the correctional institution, or, better, as an outreach activity of the mental hospital. In the latter case, the psychiatrist can work with and for the patient in the usual collaborative therapeutic relationship without having the responsibility for maintaining confinement or determining length of stay.

The handling of an individual, sick or otherwise, who truly intends to kill someone, whether a family member or a presidential candidate, presents a serious legal problem. It *is* a legal problem, not a medical one. Suppose such a person is sick but is not committable under new laws or under new interpretations of existing laws. In some instances, surely, the intended victim can be protected without detention of the patient; in some perhaps, the use of something in the nature of a peace bond, with appropriate legal steps if it is violated, might be effective. If this leads to incarceration in a correctional facility, treatment on an outreach basis can be provided as for other offenders.

In cases where danger is less immediate, involving the alcoholic or drug-dependent driver, for example, if treatment is not accepted on a voluntary basis, it could be made a condition for probation. In that case, the responsibility for following through on a treatment program rests with the patient.

Patients who need treatment, but fail to recognize the need, represent a more difficult problem for those trying to improve laws governing involuntary hospitalization. There are two general types.

First, there are patients with acute illnesses who could probably respond to treatent (e.g., a patient with involutional melancholia who is actively suicidal; a hypomanic patient who is bankrupting himself and his family). Second, there are mentally ill people who may or may not be treatable, but who cannot meet their own needs in the community. At the extreme are those patients who literally cannot survive without medical attention. In addition, there are those who cannot maintain employment, cannot use financial assistance prudently, cannot attend to those things necessary for comfort and sanitation, and are subject to various types of abuse and exploitation in the community.

Though there are many today who advocate eliminating involuntary hospitalization altogether, others, in advocating reform of commitment laws, recognize the needs of these patients. At the same time, concern over the rights of the person who is not sick and might be the victim of a conspiracy (to get rid of an unwanted spouse or a political dissenter,[31] for example) has been an issue since the time of the Packard case[19] in 1860; and, more recently, there has been growing concern over the right of the person who is sick (or deviant) to decline treatment, provided at least that he is rational enough to make the decision.

To balance these factors, attempts have been made to make new commitment laws more "strict," with a greater guarantee of legal assistance and "due process" to the person who is "accused" of being mentally ill. The disadvantages of more elaborate procedures include cost, burdening an already crowded court system, time consumption that may delay needed treatment and lead to a less favorable prognosis, possible invasions of privacy as details of the patients' behavior while sick must be made public, and a possible criminalization of mental illness. Alternate proposals allow for a simpler commitment procedure for most cases, but provide for increased implementation of the right of habeas corpus after admission, together with availability of "ombudsmen," inspection of treatment plans, and reevaluation of continued need for hospitalization by independent agencies.

Reform efforts are also directed toward reducing the length of involuntary hospitalization and/or instituting programs of periodic recertification.[22,32] In settings where this has been tried, it has not been completely successful, since the number of cases proposed for recertification has reduced the process to a formality in which inadequate time is given to assess the patient's actual situation and needs.

The most likely prediction for the future is that indefinite or long-term involuntary hospitalization will be abolished altogether, but that some method of short-term certification or commitment will be available. To preserve provisions for needed short-term involuntary care, it will be necessary to apply these provisions sparingly and cautiously so that they are used only when the need and the potential benefit to the patient can be clearly established. Since the public hospital does not commit patients to itself, it cannot fully regulate the application of commitment laws. It can ask for input into the system; a requirement that prospective involuntary patients be seen by the public hospital staff, preferably as outpatients, and that the hospital be allowed to report before the action of a court or board of mental health is not unreasonable. As well as screening out some cases that do not need, or cannot benefit from, treatment, this could lead to a greater number of patients accepting voluntary care in the hospital or in alternative programs. In addition, very active public education and liaison with the legal profession can be used to discourage involuntary hospitalization and encourage voluntary referral.

The individual's own ability to recognize illness in its early stages and his willingness to seek voluntary care can be augmented by mental-health education, public-relations programs, and, of course, changes in facilities and procedures that will make the institution more acceptable to its potential clientele.

Service to Long-term Patients

If provisions for long-term involuntary treatment and custodial care are absent from new commitment laws, new methods of serving long-term patients must be developed. Merely returning such people to the community would lead to a recurrence of the problems that led to the creation of the state mental hospitals in the first place.[17,38] Unless help is provided, where is the person too sick to take care of his own needs to go? In the nineteenth century it was to jail or the almshouse. You can't hardly find almshouses no more, but we still have jails. Today, though we sometimes jail the alcoholic or the drug-dependent person for his illness, we do not jail the chronic schizophrenic for schizophrenia; but without help he is all too likely to get into situations that lead to his being incarcerated, and not as a result of his being "dangerous."

Various things can be done. The hospital can develop adequate outreach facilities for aftercare (not merely a clinic where patients can come to get medication, psychotherapy, or counseling) unless these are actually available in the community. For many patients this care involves regular home visits and assistance, or arrangements for assistance, in coping with various problems of everyday life. Mobilizing support systems in the family and neighborhood is part of this, but careful judgment as to how much support is needed is crucial if one is to promote eventual rehabilitation rather than indefinite dependence on others. Day-care programs in the community are needed also.

In the hospitals themselves, day care is possible for patients living in the vicinity; and voluntary participation can be encouraged, when indicated, through home visits and through developing programs that attract patients to participate.

Domiciliary care is desirable for some patients. It does not need to be custodial. It can provide comfortable living arrangements, recreational activities, and sheltered workshops; but, in addition, there can be ongoing efforts at rehabilitation and resocialization, continued treatment when needed, and periodic reevaluation of treatability, treatment needs, and potential for rehabilitation. The hospital itself can convert custodial services to domiciliary, extended care facilities that can serve some patients better than nursing homes, foster homes, or transitional living arrangements such as halfway houses in the community.

Continuity of Care

Along with changes in financing of patient care and the elimination of involuntary hospitalization, the decline in resident population permits a redirection of programming for better patient service.

The traditional emphasis on inpatient care neglects the fact that home care, outpatient treatment, or partial hospitalization often may be preferable, and that even those patients requiring inpatient service require it only at certain stages of illness. A total treatment program for the patient needing hospitalization often requires adequate precare and aftercare. Many public mental hospitals now offer a full spectrum of patient services; the public mental hospital of the future must do likewise. Services must include telephone consultations and home visits, twenty-four-hour emergency and walk-in services, outpatient treatment programs, partial hospitalization, hospitalization for active treatment, domiciliary care, aftercare, and rehabilitation programs both at the facility and in the community.

With a full spectrum of services, continuity of care can be achieved. Adequate patient service cannot be fragmented. Continuity requires extension into the communities served by the hospital. Satellite clinics for crisis service, outpatient treatment, precare, and aftercare must be conveniently located in the inner city, in suburbs, and in rural areas. Unit systems,[6,28] relating inpatient units to satellite clinics and areas served, maintain continuity.

Where some phases of care are available through private practitioners, private institutions, and public agencies outside a state mental-health system, contractual arrangements and/or adequate liaison services may maintain continuity of care. Continuity, however, is not achieved by giving the patient being discharged from a hospital, for example, the address of a clinic and mailing out a case summary. Experience shows that only a small percent of patients follow through with arrangements of that sort. A definite appointment helps. Meeting the person who will be in charge of the next stage of care helps. Finally, active follow-up of patients who do not complete treatment may be essential to prevent relapses.

As well as maintaining continuity of care, unit systems maintain continuity of responsibility. Cases are not "lost" and difficult cases are not disposed of by transfer to some other service. Continuity, however, does not require keeping the same therapist. Indeed, a change of therapist is often beneficial when progress fails to occur, or is slow, or when the stage of illness, or recovery, calls for different professional skills.

Flexibility of Hospital Environment

Lower resident populations allow more individual attention and the organization of patient living arrangements into smaller units so that there can be more flexibility and less regimentation. In the past, among the least desirable features of public mental hospitals was the fact that many patients spent prolonged periods without activity, or only slightly better, were forced into a lock-step program where everyone was doing the same thing at the same time.

Regimentation, interruption of normal human activities, rules, and restriction, which made up an institutional environment, may have been necessary, may have contributed to efficiency, and may have served to protect some patients. However, many features of hospital life in the past, and some that persist today, were and are antitherapeutic. They created confusion in the already confused, reduced self-esteem and feelings of identity, and for the long-term patient who adjusted to institutional life, created problems in readjustment to normal living. They created a negative attitude toward hospitalization that interfered in participation in treatment pro-

grams. This milieu also discouraged voluntary admission and readmission.

A hospital is not a home. A cottage plan, small units, or small group programming and living in larger units does not make it a home. Group living can be normal living, however, and one can have the amenities, conveniences, freedoms, and, equally important, responsibilities of normal living insofar as illness permits.

A comfortable open ward; a flexible schedule of daily activities; contact with the world at large through newspapers and television; having one's own clothing, possessions, and spending money; having visitors at any time; being free to go out; and having opportunities for recreation and, if able, work, is *not* treatment. It is an environment that facilitates treatment. Relative freedom from restrictions of normal activity does not mean "turning the hospital over to the patients," nor does it mean inattention to patients. An open hospital requires *more* attention to patients. Patients must be protected from the consequences of their own symptomatic behavior (and, on occasion, from that of other patients[41] and visitors). Protection without overprotection, and guidance without domination, require more time and more professional skill.

Individual Treatment Programs

There are sound professional reasons for more formal treatment planning, quality control of treatment through review processes, improved records, and program evaluation. Moreover, developing methods of financing health care will make these things mandatory. Each patient should have a written treatment program with clearly stated goals, methods, and measures of progress. Writing up a treatment plan used to be an exercise for students and house staff; the experienced clinician did not need to write out his plan. It may be open to question whether this is clinically necessary now, but there is no question that it is rapidly becoming economically necessary. At the least, it does no harm; at best, it clarifies the clinician's own thinking, improves communication to staff, and insures that no patients are kept without a treatment plan. Review processes will have to answer, to the satisfaction of third-party payers, the questions: Was the admission necessary? Were other methods of care adequately explored? Were diagnostic studies completed rapidly and treatment instituted without unnecessary delay? Was the treatment plan appropriate in terms of both potential effectiveness and cost? Was the length of stay reasonable for the illness? If not, why is a longer stay justified?

One now finds a great deal of emphasis, generally appropriate, on keeping patients out of hospitals. This may be expected to increase to some extent if the insurance model is used in financing care, and to an even greater extent if the prepayment model is used. It must be borne in mind that while unnecessary admissions add to cost, clog treatment facilities, and interfere unduly with the life situation of patients; failure to admit patients who need hospital care can have disastrous consequences.

There are obvious advantages to patient and payer to make hospital stays as short as possible. However, premature discharge is to no one's advantage. Additional studies are necessary, and some are being undertaken now with NIMH support, to determine optimum lengths of stay for various conditions. Because of the number of variables involved, a number of studies will be needed before conclusive data is available. Even when an optimum is determined, one must recognize individual differences and needs. In any event, the eagerness of a clinical director, or a utilization committee, to keep stays short should not lead to "revolving door" admissions and readmissions (e.g., repeated drying-out of alcoholics is not definitive treatment) nor to the dumping of patients into inadequate community facilities (as is particularly apparent in the inappropriate referral of some geriatric patients to nursing homes).[11,20]

Better records will be essential for adequate case review. However, it is to be hoped that the record-keeping and review procedures involved will not be so time consuming as to interfere with adequate patient care.

Despite some criticisms of "labeling," descriptive diagnosis will probably continue to be used, because, its limitations notwithstanding, it does have some communication value and usefulness in treatment planning and research.[14] However, problem-oriented recording[5,42,43] is likely to prove more useful than current record systems. Checklists and graphs will replace narrative progress records to a large extent.

Objective progress charting is necessary to measure the results of treatment programs. One can go into most state or federal hospitals, and many private and community facilities, and find patients who have been on medication for months or years with no evidence of benefit other than perhaps the patient's subjective report or the clinician's general impression. If a medication or other treatment is instituted, one must know what it is expected to do, what is a reasonable trial period to see if it accomplishes this, and how change can be measured. When this is known, an objective progress chart is possible. The expense, and possible undesirable consequences, of a treatment that is not working can be eliminated and a better treatment plan devised.

(Conclusion

The state mental institutions referred to in the opening paragraph will not be phased out, in that state or any other, by 1975. Too many people need their services and alternative facilities are not available. They may be phased out in time, but the creation of a whole new system to replace them is unnecessary and uneconomical.

Instead, they will probably become an integral part of a total health-care system. Organizationally, they will probably function eventually as nonprofit corporations rather than state agencies (unless the steps beyond Medicredit, universal health-insurance and/or health-maintenance organizations lead to a national health service, in which case they will be federal facilities).

Direct patient service ultimately will be provided on a prepayment basis (from the hospitals' point of view—a system based on the total population served, not those in treatment), or on a fee-for-service basis through government and/or private insurance carriers. Appropriated funds, or grants, will still be needed for research, training, and preventive programs. The distinction between the now public and private facilities will be largely eliminated, and, with it, dual standards of care will be a thing of the past.

The public mental hospital of the future will offer a full spectrum of mental-health care and will have outreach facilities in the communities it serves. Nearly all its patients will be voluntary. It will treat acute cases and will offer domiciliary care, rather than custodial care, to the chronically disabled. New systems of treatment planning, case review (combining features of utilization and peer review), and record keeping will be utilized.

Changes in modern society are taking place at an accelerated rate. For the state mental-health department that has not already prepared for the future role of its facilities, the time is now.

◖ Bibliography

1. AVNET, H. *Psychiatric Insurance.* New York: Group Health Insurance, 1962.
2. ———. "Psychiatric Insurance—Ten Years Later," *Am. J. Psychiatry,* 126 (1969), 113–120.
3. BARTZ, W., D. LOY, and W. COOK. "Mental Hospitals and the Winds of Change," *Ment. Hygiene,* 55 (1971), 266–269.
4. BIGELOW, N. "The Right to the Right Treatment," *Psychiatr. Q.,* 44 (1970), 533–549.
5. BJORN, J. and H. CROSS. *Problem Oriented Practice.* Chicago: Modern Hospital Press, 1970.
6. BLACK, B. "Unit System: The Third Revolution," *Am. J. Nurs.,* 70 (1970), 515–519.
7. BRENNER, M. H. "Economic Change and Mental Hospitalization: New York State, 1910–1960," *Soc. Psychiatry,* 2 (1967), 180–188.
8. ———. "Economic Conditions and Mental Hospitalization for Functional Psychosis," *J. Nerv. Ment. Dis.,* 145 (1967), 371–384.
9. ———. "Patterns of Psychiatric Hospitalization among Different Socioeconomic Groups in Response to Economic Stress," *J. Nerv. Ment. Dis.,* 148 (1969), 31–38.
10. BURNELL, G. "Financing Mental Health Care: An Appraisal of Various Models," *Arch. Gen. Psychiatry,* 25 (1971), 49–55.
11. BUTLER, R. "Immediate and Long-Range Dangers to Transfer of Elderly Patients from State Hospitals to Community Facilities," *Gerontologist,* 10 (1970), 259–260.
12. CROCETTI, G., H. SPIRO, and I. SIASSI. "Are the Ranks Closed? Attitudinal Social Distance and Mental Illness," *Am. J. Psychiatry,* 127 (1971), 41–47.
13. DAVIDSON, H. [DR. WHATSISNAME]. "The Cost of Littleness," *Hosp. Community Psychiatry,* 20 (1969), 25.
14. EATON, M. and M. PETERSON. *Psychiatry,* 2nd ed., Chap. 4. Flushing, N.Y.: Medical Examination Publ., 1969.
15. ———. *Psychiatry,* 2nd ed., Chaps. 22 and 24. Flushing, N.Y.: Medical Examinaton Publ., 1969.
16. FINK, R. "Financing Outpatient Mental Health Care through Psychiatric Insurance," *Ment. Hygiene,* 55 (1971), 143–150.
17. FORBUSH, B. *Moses Sheppard: Quaker Philanthropist of Baltimore.* New York: Lippincott, 1968.
18. FREEDMAN, A. "Beyond 'Action for Mental Health'," *Am. J. Orthopsychiatry,* 33 (1963), 799–805.
19. GROUP FOR THE ADVANCEMENT OF PSYCHIATRY. *Laws Governing Hospitalization of the Mentally Ill.* GAP Report no. 61. New York: Group for the Advancement of Psychiatry, 1966.
20. ———. *Toward a Public Policy on Mental Health Care of the Elderly.* GAP Report no. 79. New York: Group for the Advancement of Psychiatry, 1970.
21. JOINT COMMISSION ON MENTAL ILLNESS AND HEALTH. *Action for Mental Health: Final Report, 1961.* New York: Basic Books, 1961.
22. KLATTE, E., W. LIPSCOMB, V. ROZYNKO et al. "Changing the Legal Status of Mental Patients," *Hosp. Community Psychiatry,* 20 (1969), 199–202.
23. KOBRYNSKI, B. and A. MILLER. "The Role of the State Hospital in the Care of the Elderly," *J. Am. Geriatr. Soc.,* 18 (1970), 210–219.
24. KRAMER, M. "Mental Health Statistics of the Future," *Eugen. Q.,* 13 (1966), 186–204.

25. Kubie, L. "Pitfalls of Community Psychiatry," *Arch. Gen. Psychiatry*, 18 (1968), 257–266.

26. Laburt, H., M. Wallach, A. Impastato et al. "The State Hospital and Community Psychiatry," *Dis. Nerv. Syst.*, 29 (1968), 556–558.

27. Markson, E., A. Kwoh, J. Cumming et al. "Alternatives to Hospitalization for Psychiatrically Ill Geriatric Patients," *Am. J. Psychiatry*, 127 (1971), 1055–1062.

28. Miller, G. "The Unit System: A New Approach in State Hospital Care," *Tex. Med.*, 65 (1969), 44–51.

29. Orwin, A. "The Mental Hospital: A Pattern for the Future," *Br. J. Psychiatry*, 113 (1967), 857–864.

30. Pepper, B. "Role of State Care of Mentally Disabled," *N.Y. State J. Med.*, 71 (1971), 1238–1242.

31. Robinson, R. "Possible Political Use of Psychiatry Stirs Alarm," *Psychiatr. News*, 8 (1972), 1–3.

32. Robitscher, J. *Pursuit of Agreement: Psychiatry and the Law*, Chaps. 13 and 14. Philadelphia: Lippincott, 1966.

33. Rosenzweig, S. "Compulsory Hospitalization of the Mentally Ill," *Am. J. Public Health*, 61 (1971), 121–126.

34. Rowitz, L. and L. Levy. "The State Mental Hospital in Transition: An Approach to the Study of Mental Hospital Decentralization," *Ment. Hygiene*, 55 (1971), 68–76.

35. Sher, M. "The Place of the Mental Hospital in Community Mental Health," *Hosp. Community Psychiatry*, 21 (1970), 85–87.

36. Spiro, H. "On Beyond Mental Health Care Centers: A Planning Model for Psychiatric Care," *Arch. Gen. Psychiatry*, 21 (1969), 646–654.

37. Stone, A. "Psychiatry and the Law," *Psychiatric Ann.*, 1 (1971), 18–43.

38. Tiffany, F. *Life of Dorothea Lynde Dix*. New York: Houghton, 1918.

39. Tyce, F. "Public Hospitals as Social Restoration Centers," *Hosp. Community Psychiatry*, 20 (March 1969), 6–7.

40. Ward, M. J. *The Snake Pit*. New York: Random House, 1946.

41. ———. *Counterclockwise*, Chap. 29. Chicago: Regnery, 1969.

42. Weed, L. *Medical Records, Medical Education, and Patient Care*. Cleveland: The Press of Case Western Reserve University, 1969.

43. Weed, L. et al. *The Problem Oriented Medical Record*. Cleveland: Dempco Reproduction Service, 1969.

CHAPTER 35

NEW METHODS FOR ASSESSING THE EFFECTIVENESS OF PSYCHIATRIC INTERVENTION

Ernest M. Gruenberg

THE TERM "psychiatric intervention" is used in this chapter to refer to anything a psychiatrist does in response to the fact that any person is a patient for whom he has some degree or type of clinical responsibility. Treatment is ordinarily used to refer to actions taken by the clinician, or at his instructions, which are intended to relieve, ameliorate, or terminate a disordered state he believes the patient to have, or to affect favorably some distress associated wth the disorder; we generally do not use the term "treatment" except when referring to certain classes of action—physical measures, such as drugs or shock or surgery, psychotherapeutic measures in a formal pattern. Other actions, such as hospital admission or release, ward assignment, counseling with relatives, charging fees (or not), making appointments, and so forth are generally thought of as being outside the concept of treatment and are regarded as having something to do with what is called "management of cases" or of one's practice or of the hospital or some part of it. It is not necessary to try to persuade the modern psychiatrist that this separation is not always sharp. In one sense, everyone will agree with the dictum that treatment begins the moment the psychiatrist meets the patient and asks about what brought him. The process of meeting and asking and listening to the answer begins a relationship that has some significance for the patient's mental state and future. The term "intervention" is simply introduced here to avoid the narrower meanings of treatment and to include a psychiatrist's decision not to take a particular action for one of his patients. The role of psychiatrist is the center of attention, but this does not mean that other professionals cannot intervene with both positive and negative effects on the patient's life, but only that this chapter is not attempting to deal with those events.

The effects of every medical intervention are assessed to some extent on each occasion. The patient when conscious of the intervention is making some assessment, and the observant physician is always keeping a watchful eye out for the effects of his treatment. Effectiveness, however, cannot be observed in such a neutral way. Effectiveness has to do with certain specific effects that it was hoped the treatment would produce. Giving an epileptic patient barbiturate tablets may have a large number of effects—gratitude for the attention, fear of the implied dependency, drowsiness— but the object of giving the barbiturate was to reduce the frequency and intensity of seizures and if this effect is not observed, the treatment is regarded as ineffective.

It will be helpful to face the fact at this point that the process of deciding what effect the treatment was hoped to have has nothing to do with the world of facts, but is directly related to the world of values. In the example above, seizures are assumed to be something undesirable, and the treatment intervention is introduced in an effort to abolish them (or some of them). This intervention is not the act of a neutral observer, but of a person who is partisan—he is intervening to change the patient's functioning in a particular way. It is not possible to use facts to justify this attitude. Scientific methods can be used in an effort to

understand how people come to adopt the attitude that seizures are bad things to be avoided if possible, and understanding the cultural, historical, and social forces involved in reaching this conclusion might or might not modify the attitude. But to the psychiatrist with clinical responsibility for the patient, this is not a debatable issue. As will be seen later, the person who seeks to assess the effectiveness of a treatment must believe he knows what effect is to be sought—his assessment will then depend upon whether that particular effect has occurred or not.

Hence, the first point to keep in mind is that since the dawn of modern medicine as a profession, doctors have been assessing the effectiveness of their medical interventions. The Hippocratic writers were forever assessing whether particular procedures would alter the course of events in the desired direction. Underlying the concept of medical intervention there is always a twofold assumption. One part assumes a knowledge of what would have happened if no action had been taken. The other part assumes that one or more of the things that will happen, if no one intervenes, is to be avoided, if possible. The fever, pain, diarrhea, convulsions, or whatever, will continue in the absence of the treatment; they are not desirable; therefore specific interventions are justified to avoid their continuing. Without going into all the implications in this chapter, the reader should be reminded at the outset that a psychiatric intervention in the course of another's life is a form of medical intervention, surrounded by an ancient tradition and mystique and entailing complex and solemn obligations; the so-called Hippocratic oath is one of the most ancient formulations of the nature of an obligation one person bears to another or another group of people—older than any oath of allegiance, older than any currently used assertion of religious faith, older than any current marriage vow. Another ancient dictum of the nature of the physician's responsibility to his patient should also be recalled as we get into the modern methods for assessing the effectiveness of intervention: *primum non nocere*—the doctor's first duty is to do no harm.

(Evaluation Research

Scientific methods have been developed in efforts to understand the nature of the world, to find some underlying principles that put the blooming, buzzing confusion of the world of facts into some sort of order capable of human understanding. The scientific methods are ways of systematically confronting an idea about what the world is like in a way that tests the idea's correctness. These scientific methods can also be applied to planned human actions. Most of us have applied them, more or less systematically, to the action of starting an automobile quickly enough on a cold morning to get the internal combustion motor going before the battery runs down. We experiment with the number of times we pump the accelerator pedal before turning on the starter. We experiment with different positions of the accelerator. Those who have manual chokes develop hypotheses about the best manipulation of the choke. Some try racing the motor before turning off the ignition when stopping the car at night. We "learn" from experience (more or less systematically) that a car well tuned starts more quickly than a car poorly tuned, that a thin oil in the crankcase impedes the starter less than thick oil, and so forth. We develop rules for each car at each season and these rules are the result of more or less systematic experiments regarding what seems to "work" better for that particular car.

This simple problem of a human action, which can be carried out in several different ways, can be used as our elementary paradigm to illustrate several important principles that distinguish evaluation research from research that applies a scientific method to the problem of understanding the nature of the world. In the first place, the goal of the action is clearly defined: get the internal combustion engine started with the least drain on the battery. In the second place, the means for achieving this goal are obvious: turn it over with the electric starter and give it a mixture of gas and air in the best proportions to get it exploding. In the third place, the situation limits the choices for action. Manipulation of accelerator, choke,

and starter switch are the only options in the situation. The sequence of the actions and their timing is all that can be varied in any given "trial." Such things as tuning the motor and having thin oil in the crankcase or the way of stopping the motor the previous night all had been done before the trial and form part of the context. It is remarkable that with these limited options and the crucial nature of the outcome in the lives of so many people, no one seems to even keep notes on how the trials go and to make systematic analyses; even trained scientists don't keep records on how these actions are carried out each morning and then draw inferences from analyzing a series of trials. This is a fourth important principle: When we think we can keep the relevant experiences clearly in mind and can "learn from experience," we do not design and record systematic experimental trials, which is not to say that we are not using scientific methods but only that the experiments and their results seem so obvious that we do not think of making records in order to gain the maximum information from the various trials. Fifth, there is very little in the way of "theory" in these experiments. The automotive engineer who has a refined sense of the process of carburation and ignition and the artist who has no idea what these terms refer to will carry out his uncomfortable cold morning experiments in pretty much the same way and will probably "learn" equally quickly what the most suitable pattern of action is. This fifth principle emerges from the fact that the goal is clearly defined and the alternative actions are clearly delimited so that the trial-and-error sequences proceed by rules of thumb rather than by a systematic deduction from the laws of physics. We are studying a man-made contraption designed to achieve the goal by fiddling with gadgets. The experimenter is operating a device made by someone else for the experimenters and he is only trying to use the devices in the most efficient way. When none of his experiments are successful, he takes the device back to the shop to get it fixed so that it will work the way it is supposed to.

Each of these principles applies to evaluation research. First, the goal is defined and taken for granted; this means the statements of goals are statements about assumptions and are not part of the hypothesis to be tested by gathering data. The hypothesis deals with the choice of means to achieve goals, not with the value of the goals. Second, the variety of means available for achieving the goals are obvious and specifiable and the problem is to use the alternatives in the most effective way. Third, we ordinarily don't systematize our experiments in such situations. Fourth, the experiments are being conducted on man-made devices intended to achieve specific purposes and designed to be operated by using specific controlling devices.

⟪ The Clinical Trial

The "clinical trial" in medicine illustrates this set of principles. A group at the Mayo Clinic compared the efficacy of a group of analgesics in controlling pain among terminal cancer patients. The fact that aspirin was as good as or better than many of the synthetic compounds thought to be more effective, and which are certainly more expensive and more dangerous, was surprising enough to make newspaper headlines. Here the third principle had obviously been working: no one had thought it necessary to keep careful records of their clinical experiments on this issue; they had "learned" from experience what systematic record keeping and study design revealed to be untrue! The goal was clearly the relief from subjective sensations of pain, the means, a limited number of analgesics at various doses— clearly man-made gadgetry with highly defined systems of controls and administration. The main benefit of systematic evaluation research is its ability to undo that perennial human state: "It's not ignorance that causes most trouble but what we know that's not so."

Such clinical trials are the best established types of evaluation research in medicine. The principles of the definitive clinical trial were worked out less than four decades ago, in the middle 1930s, by teams associated with the Medical Research Council of the United King-

dom. Sulfonamide was the first new drug to be given systematic clinical trials at the first stages of its availability. Because systematic clinical trials were used right from the start with this drug, its effectiveness became established within a few months. This careful recording of the use of sulfonamide rapidly established the value of the systematic clinical trial at the same time that it established the value of the sulfonamides as a more powerful, safer, set of antimicrobial drugs than almost anyone had thought possible. In these trials the conditions treated by the sulfonamides tended to be rapidly fatal and the sulfonamides were both much more effective and acted much more rapidly than the antisera previously available, so there was little room for misinterpretation of the results. Later, when the method was applied to nonfatal conditions with marginally better treatments than already available, the technology of the clinical trial became more sophisticated.

The systematic selection of patients thought suitable for the trial, the arbitrary assignment of these patients to treatment types, the independent objective recording of the course of events, both favorable and unfavorable, produced a systematic experiment in which scientific management and clinical management were related to each other in such a way as to produce the maximum information with the minimum risk to the patients.

Ethical objections to this procedure were present from the start; they were not regarded as the obstructionist arguments of clinicians whose favorite remedies might come in second best, but to a genuine concern for getting the best possible treatment to each patient as soon as possible. Clinicians were mistrustful of statistical interpretations as compared with their judgment based on intimate knowledge of each case. There is no doubt that the responsible clinician knows many things about his cases that the statistics of clinical trial can never reflect. Of course, whenever a treatment is given to any patient an experiment has begun—will this treatment given this way to this patient affect favorably the outcome of his particular condition? The argument is not between those who wish to experiment in the treatment of patients and those who do not, but between those who want to conduct these experiments in a systematic way and those clinicians who prefer a less systematic way. Of clinical trials there will never be an end, but each one must be justified separately in the light of all the known facts at the time it is proposed. It is not ethical to start a clinical trial that requires withholding an established treatment for a dangerous condition in order to test the effectiveness of any new compound that also might be thought to be effective. Safety must be known to a certain degree before any clinical trial can be started. To withhold a drug requires grounds for substantial doubt regarding its effectiveness; to introduce a drug requires substantial reason to suspect its effectiveness and to think it sufficiently safe. In general there are two occasions most favorable in the history of a treatment: first, when it is beginning to gain acceptance among experts but is still suspect; and second, long after it has become well established and its value assumed but its value is coming under question by experts who begin to doubt whether the conventional wisdom was right. During the time that a treatment is well established and "everyone" knows it is useful, it cannot properly be withheld; but before it becomes well established some experts have begun to report good effects, while others remain doubtful; that is a good time for a systematic clinical trial. Before some experts have begun to give reason for thinking that the new treatment might be valuable, a clinical trial cannot be justified because there is no reason to invest time and to subject patients to the treatment.

The clinical trial sets up a systematic experiment: it selects patients thought to be suitable for a particular treatment or set of treatments, assigns them arbitrarily to one treatment or another and then observes the outcome. It seeks to gain the maximum knowledge from the minimum number of research subjects through the neatness of its design and the care with which the trial is carried out. The technology of designing these trials was built on a generation of agricultural research into seed selection, fertilization, pro-

tective sprays, and so forth. It is from that type of research (systematic evaluation of planting, breeding, and cultivating actions) that we derive most of our statistical methods and principles of design. In evaluating any particular piece of evaluation research one should always keep in mind the methods these statisticians developed for evaluating the significance of a particular pattern of results. They asked themselves: If, in general, these two treatments had no different effect, and I were to take a sample and do what I did by applying treatment A to one part of the population and treatment B to the other part, what are the odds that in any one sample like this, those getting treatment A would do twice as well as those getting treatment B? And they give their answer by saying that they can figure out how many samples of the size used would show that much difference if in general there were no difference. They express this by giving a probability that the observed difference could have occurred by chance: $p = 0.05$, which means that they figure $1/20$ of such studies would show the As doing twice as well as the Bs even if in general there was no difference between the effect of A and the effect of B. This measurement only specifies the sampling risk of drawing the wrong conclusion. Obviously, the more evaluation studies you read and attend to the more likely you are to draw the wrong conclusion from one of them. Thus, if you read many evaluation studies, and each gives $p = 0.05$ there is a chance that one in twenty of them gives the wrong conclusion. You have no way of knowing which. So there is a danger in taking large-scale actions, if the only justification is a single study.

There are much more serious hazards in assuming that each evaluation study correctly interprets its findings. In fact, because evaluation studies use scientific methods to approach action problems, the conclusions of the authors must be scrutinized in terms of their methods just as carefully as one would any other scientific publication. Indeed, one should probably be a little more skeptical regarding the average evaluation study than about the average physics or chemistry paper.

A physics or chemistry study published in a scientific journal will automatically conform to certain basic standards of research methods and reporting. The application of scientific methods to planned action research is not so well established or conventionalized, however, and is likely to be published in a journal that has a clinical or administrative readership unaccustomed to dissecting each scientific report.

❰ The Preventive Trial

The preventive trial is another form of evaluation research. The action taken is supposed to prevent something from happening—it will lower the frequency with which a population becomes ill. The most dramatic and effective recent preventive trial accompanied the introduction of the Salk vaccine to prevent poliomyelitis. It was organized on a nationwide basis and used volunteers. The volunteers (and their parents) knew that half would get the new Salk vaccine and the other half were getting an inactive salt solution. They also knew that no one in the innoculating teams knew which was which; each vial had a number and the name of the child was entered on a list opposite the number of the vial. Many thousands participated in this study. The investigators had to wait for the next polio epidemic to find out their results. They were spectacular and only then were families notified as to which children had received the Salk vaccine and which the ineffective solution, so that those in the latter group could go out and get the Salk vaccine. This is the kind of preventive trial where a state of immunity is to be produced in each individual treated. There are more general preventive trials in which the water supply of a city is cleaned up and the typhoid and cholera death rates lowered. No individual is "treated," but the whole population's relationship to its own feces is modified through engineering. This action too produced dramatic results.

The most important new developments in the methodology of evaluating psychiatric intervention effectiveness are in response to new ideas regarding the goals of treatment—what are regarded as the desired changes in the course of events.

The invention of the planned clinical trial moved medicine into a new era of planned innovations in treatment technology and the rapid, purposeful assessment of the value of each new treatment. Although that technology developed in the mid-1930s, psychiatry only began to absorb its lessons and apply it to new psychiatric interventions two decades later following the discovery of the phenothiazines.

❰ The Massachusetts Mental Hospitals Experiment

An Attempt to Rehabilitate Chronic Mentally Ill Patients

The modern clinical trial only became common in psychiatry after the introduction of the phenothiazines and reserpine in the mid-1950s. It was also the introduction of these drugs that brought intensive work on defining goals of treatment in terms of specified amounts of improvement regarding specific symptoms or disabilities rather than in terms of terminating disorders. As will become apparent when we review four examples of modern investigations, there has been a move toward more exact specification of goals and also a move toward experimentation with the context in which a treatment is given, manipulation of the context itself becoming an "innovation" to be evaluated.

An excellent example of these transitions is a study designed to test the interaction of these new drugs with intensive milieu therapy and psychotherapy conducted by Milton Greenblatt, George Brooks, and a team of associates, beginning around 1960, using patients and staff in three Massachusetts mental hospitals.[7] Schizophrenic patients who had been in the hospital on the current admission between five and ten years were located at Boston State Hospital and Metropolitan State Hospital. The 115 selected patients were divided into four groups by random selection in such a way that the addition of drugs to the treatment regime and their transfer to the active treatment program of the Massachusetts Mental Health Center could be assessed as separate and as combined interventions. Two groups stayed on the chronic wards of the large mental hospitals where they had been located, one received a tranquilizing drug regimen and the other didn't. Two groups were transferred to the Mental Health Center, one receiving the drug treatment and the other not.

Effectiveness can be assessed in terms of discharge within nine months of beginning the regimen. Of the fifteen who were discharged out of the 115, half continued treatment at the day hospital. Twelve of the sixty-eight patients receiving tranquilizers (some in custodial and some at the mental health center hospital) were discharged and only three of the forty-seven who did not receive tranquilizers were discharged. The authors call this a "trend" but one that "does not reach significance." Without going into more sophisticated statistical techniques, the reader can form his own judgment by taking a pencil and paper and asking himself how many of the sixty-eight patients receiving tranquilizers would have been discharged if the tranquilizers, in fact, had no influence on the likelihood of the patient's being discharged. Simply divide 15 by 115 (13.0 percent) and multiply sixty-eight by this overall discharge rate. The result of 0.130 × 68 = 8.8 tells how many of those patients we would expect to have been discharged if the tranquilizer medication made no difference. This calculation is essentially the first step in all kinds of statistical significance tests; they all start by stating the null hypothesis in the form of a question: What would we expect if the two treatments made no difference? Then the data are examined to see whether the observed numbers differ enough from what one expects on the basis of the null hypothesis to justify us believing that the null hypothesis was refuted by the data. By simply calculating the expected numbers in this way, the reader will obtain a sense of how much weight he would be willing to

place on the "trend." In this instance the excess number of discharges in the tranquilizer group is just 3.2, i.e. 12−8.8. Common sense tells us that this is not a big enough difference to get very excited about.

If one looks at the effect of transferring the patient from the custodial to the mental-health center environment for six months, one finds that eleven of the sixty transferred patients were discharged while only four of the fifty-five remaining in the custodial hospital were discharged. By using the overall discharge rate again (13.0 percent), we can say that of the sixty transferred cases 7.8 would have been discharged if transfer made no difference, again too small a difference between observed and expected to draw any important conclusion. Hence by this criterion, discharge, no definite effectiveness could be attributed to either of the two treatment intervention patterns.

The elements of the mental status were appraised by psychiatrists attached to the research team at the beginning of the experiment and again six months later; those who were "much improved" six months later can be regarded as examples of success, according to the authors. Though the diligent reader of such reports can feel distressed at the fact that the published report does not give sufficient information for one to attempt to reproduce this criterion—"much improved"—this discomfort should not lead one to discard the data for that reason. One must ask oneself whether, taking all the published evidence together, it seems reasonable to assume that a reproducible criterion was applied. It is more important to estimate whether one thinks that the research psychiatrists were capable of making unbiased ratings of "much improved" in the context of the study; the important bias is of course with respect to which study group the patient had been in. Presumably the first mental status was made before study group assignment, so that fact could not affect the examiner. The six-month examination, however, was made after the patient had been in the study group six months. The examinations were made at the locus of treatment so the examiner could not help but know where the patient had been treated—the "double blind" procedure was not possible. No effort was made to keep the examiner blind with respect to the drug regimen either. Therefore, if the examiner were inclined to be biased, the reported data could reflect such a bias.

The report is inadequate in the information it gives regarding methods used to reduce these biases and is faulty in failing to give us the investigators' own estimate as to whether bias was present and if so, of what kind. They are justified in stating that to make these appraisals "blind" would have involved great expense, and they may be right that at that point such a great expense would not have been justified.

It is worthwhile diverging for a moment here to ask, how could blind appraisals of whether the patients had improved or not been obtained? Inasmuch as the data being used are essentially clinical observations, not laboratory impersonal data, the problem is one of putting good clinical observers into contact with the patient's manifestations of disordered functioning at two points in time; for this purpose there is no substitute for the interview. It may seem at first sight to be absolutely impossible to think of a way to gather this kind of information with no possibility of bias, but there are conceivable plans. For example, the research interview could have been videotaped on the two separate occasions. These videotapes could have been played back one after the other to clinical observers asked to rate the degree of improvement in each element of the mental status. These observers need not be told which group the patient was in. In fact, they need not be told that the patients were part of an evaluation research program. The data gathering for this purpose could be combined with another study—one which focused on the development of reliable ratings regarding videotaped mental status interviews. This second objective could be the one explained to the clinicians who rated the videotaped interviews. This procedure might appear to be too "tricky" and too deceptive to the clinicians providing the ratings. However, if the trouble were taken to generate a genuine serious investiga-

tion into methods of obtaining reliable ratings that would produce their own independent findings and these study subjects were included in the material used to conduct that study, the failure to inform the observers of the additional use of the ratings they provide could be defended. It is obvious that though the clinicians rating the interviews from the vidoetapes could be kept "blind," even of the existence of the study being conducted, the interviewer on the scene could well be biased and the way in which the taped interview was conducted could be affected by his knowledge of the study and the subject's group assignment. This also could be avoided in principle if the context of the interview could be similarly modified so that the interviewer's focus is made irrelevant to the evaluation research. For example, outside interviewers could be employed and they could be provided with the second study's frame of reference—a good interview for mental status appraisal. Other situations occur in which trained clinicians are asked to conduct an especially careful and comprehensive interview. For example, clinicians taking their specialty examinations, or clinicians conducting examinations that will be used for the purpose of teaching other clinicians how to conduct an interview. To describe these devices briefly is also to indicate how complicated an undertaking is needed sometimes to get rid of bias in the data that is going to be used.

If one is willing to take on faith that the data gathered in the Massachusetts Hospitals Experiment did not emerge from some systematic bias in data gathering, one can then look at the findings as indicating the effects of the two treatments. The improvements were not equally distributed over the different elements of the mental status. Those who received drug treatment improved in their social behavior, more so among those who also received the shift to milieu treatment. Appearance, activity, and speech were the main areas of improvement. On the other hand, mood, ideation (content), and grasp improved not at all. This is an important clue as to what is most readily improved in the chronic mental hospital patient, either through use of changed milieu or through the application of tranquilizer drugs, or better yet the two at the same time. Behavior improves but subjective symptoms and thought processes remain relatively untouched. Around 1960 a large number of evaluation studies ensued that examined the rapidly changing way in which mental health programs were approaching the problems of the seriously ill mental patient. There was intense activity in clinical settings in these years, which preceded the introduction of the National Mental Health Center Act in 1963. Investigators who had never before engaged in evaluation research as such became involved in the challenge of turning their research skills toward evaluations of the newer innovations being started in so many places. The result was a number of new methods for assessing psychiatric interventions that arose from ever increased efforts to find a way of distinguishing forward motions in psychiatric care from backward motions or useless motions. Four of these studies are selected for more or less close examination in this chapter because they are good illustrations of the varieties of new developments. The first was an effort to rehabilitate chronic custodial care schizophrenic patients. The second was an effort to prevent chronic hospitalization, first by cutting the admission rate through a screening clinic in the community and later by introducing alternate modes of care after hospitalization. The third was an attempt to avoid hospitalization altogether through a form of home treatment. The fourth sought to avoid chronic deterioration by using all types of services to facilitate community care, using short episodes of hospitalization as a means of postponing family and community rejection of the chronically handicapped patient.

It is almost impossible to conceive of a planned experiment to test the effectiveness of moving from a custodial to a total push-type of special institution with different relations to the community that would be on the double blind model. What error in the assessment could be introduced because of this weakness? The effect of moving to another staff group in another locus is not controlled for. Change in environment might produce as much effect. In some cities, it might be possible to arrange group transfers in the guise of solving some administrative problem where there was no intention to improve the patient's treatment. Such moves do occasionally occur for administrative reasons, such as when hospitals are redistricted. In practice, it would be difficult to use these opportunities to study the effect of that kind of move as a neutral move to contrast with the move to the specially designed program. Administrative moves do not usually have completely neutral effects on the staffs involved. The receiving staffs tend to screen suspiciously the patients being transferred as illegal lemons being dumped onto them. The receiving staffs' reactions can be one of resentment leading to a slowdown at work and let the administration suffer the consequences or, in contrast, they can take the attitude that they will be stuck with these newly transferred patients and do their best to get them well enough to be transferred to a different service. Nonetheless, comparable data regarding comparable groups of patients simply moved from one institution to another would be helpful in interpreting the data. Another feature of this trial, which cannot be assessed because of the absence of anything like a blind control, is the enthusiasm of the special staff and the effect it has on the social grouping of the patients as they become formed into the new context. The program may be less important than the fact that it exists and is an experiment. This phenomenon is known as the "Hawthorne Effect" first described by Roethlisberger and Dickson at the Hawthorne plant of General Electric.[20] The fundamental principle elucidated in those studies was that among a group of industrial workers performance levels improved with every environmental change, whether the change was in the direction of improved or worsened conditions from a long-range point of view. Thus, stepping down the level of illumination led to a short-term improvement as much as improving the illumination. The fact that the staff is in something "new" could have as much effect on what happened to the patients as the particular nature of the new program. This effect can only be controlled by having the operation become routinized. Some pharmacology professors have enjoyed telling medical students that when a new drug comes on the market the doctors should hurry up and use it while it is still effective. One must beware of a similar phenomenon regarding new types of psychiatric intervention even when no new drug is involved.

Another weakness of these studies is that they may understate the effect of the new program because the atmosphere of change could affect the staff at the institution from which the patients came. A competitive atmosphere in the old hospital could make the staff there wish to show that they can do at least as well as the experimental staff. Keeping the program secret from the staff of the hospital from whence the study population was drawn is not absolutely impossible, but would require a great deal of organizational preparation, a slow drawing off of selected patients whom only the investigators knew were associated with left-behind controls. In most mental hospitals it would be almost impossible for no rumors to leak from one locus to the other. In the Massachusetts Hospitals Experiment all eligible patients in Metropolitan State Hospital were used in the study and the staff there was very conscious of the experiment; in Boston State Hospital the experimental activity was not widely known. This is not the same as saying that the exact nature of the experiment would become widely known in the larger institution. It only means that the larger institution staff would develop an ideology about what was going on and would presumably react to it. It would be an extremely difficult and expensive undertaking to monitor these changing perceptions of what the study was about. Ordinarily, it would hardly be justified. It is important, however, to take all these factors into consideration when reading reports of this type of study—the authors should give the readers enough information to let the reader form a judgment as to how much of the observed effect might be attributed to these uncontrolled factors. The intervention is planned to produce a change in the course of events within the mental and behavioral life

of the selected patients; one can only know what would have happened if there was no intervention if one can observe a comparable group of patients for whom that intervention did not occur. That is what the control or comparison group is for—to tell us what difference the intervention made. A study with no control is like a compass without a needle —it can lead you anywhere because it has no sense of direction.

⟮ The Worthing Experiment

Preventing Institutional Neurosis by Preventing Hospital Admission

Another type of innovation occurred in assessment methodology when some programs were developed to prevent hospital admission as a means of preventing institutional neurosis[2] or institutionalism. In England, beginning in 1958, Sainsbury and Grad[21] studied the service organized by Joshua Carse and John Morrissey, which was referred to as the Worthing Experiment. The Graylingwell Hospital served several districts, one of which was Worthing. An outpatient service was established and a rule made that no patient would be admitted from Worthing to the hospital without a full assessment by the outpatient staff—which led to a rapid drop in the annual number of admissions. Then another experiment was set up for the Chichester district, served by the same hospital. The first experiment had been simply to reduce admission rates through a screening clinic. The second experiment undertook to achieve that objective too, and to reduce institutionalization on a long-term basis, to facilitate care in the community, and to make the optimal disposition of the individual referral. This experiment, of course, contained a much broader set of objectives than that of simply reducing the annual admission rate. Sainsbury and Grad did an elaborate study contrasting the experience of psychiatrically referred patients from Chichester with those from Salisbury, a third district of the same hospital in which no experiment was undertaken.

The data gathered in an attempt to assess the effectiveness of the modified psychiatric intervention in Chichester is well worth reading as an exercise in the difficulties of getting the relevant data. The main lesson to be derived from the experiment was probably stated by Cecil Sheps in the published discussion of Grad's and Sainsbury's report:[6] "I feel that if you are really going to evaluate services, the single most important prerequisite is specificity of objective, and this has been lacking. . . ." That statement assesses the effectiveness of the investigators' assessment of certain psychiatric interventions. The lesson is particularly telling because of the extraordinarily high level of scientific work the investigators carried out. My own view is that they were caught at a moment in the transformation of goals in innovative psychiatric intervention patterns when it appeared that a specific set of goals had been defined, but by the time the experiment was over, other experiences in other locations had made it appear that the beginning goals of the Chichester experiment were not sufficiently specific. This is a hazard which all social experiments face; one does not know what is going to happen in the broader world while the study is being executed that will make one's own study look quite different from the later perspectives. No social experiment can count on staying an island unto itself, which is not an argument against such social experiments, only an argument for reasonable caution and the courage to risk being outpaced by events. These investigators exercised both. There is also a lesson to be learned from their study in that the utilization rates for psychiatric services in Chichester turned out to be consistently higher than for their control community Salisbury, which increased the difficulties of interpreting the differences between them.

Why did they not use a standard preventive trial design instead of two whole communities, one for the experiment and one for the control? It seems clear from the description of the experiment that they could not have done so because the psychiatric intervention in Salisbury was to be carried out by a single team of clinicians who provided the precare screening and consultations, the hospital unit's inpatient care, and the aftercare in the community and referral to the appropriate community agencies and close working relations with the local general practitioners. It is hard to see how a psychiatric service of this kind can develop smooth consultative relationships with the local general practitioners regarding a random half of the case load while maintaining a distant intermittent contact with the same practitioners regarding the other half. If this is a crucial characteristic of the pattern of psychiatric intervention being tested, the random case assignment design simply will not work.

What were the events that overtook this study's statement of objectives? The notion of finding the best disposition for each psychiatric referral was overtaken by the spread of the notion that the best way to promote community care for people with chronic severe mental disorders was to maintain a continuing watching brief, regarding each current arrangement for each patient as the best for the moment and being prepared to change it on very short notice and without waiting until something very unsatisfactory forces a change. Francis Pilkington in the discussion of the Chichester findings[21] said that an appraisal of the family's burden one month after the first psychiatric contact was unrealistic—what is not too hard on a family for one month can become intolerable a few months later.[6]

A mixture of purposes was involved that also made assumptions about means and ends. One of the main motives for the two experiments was that the hospital was becoming overcrowded and it was assumed that the most efficient way of reducing hospital census was to reduce the number of annual admissions. This apparently logical approach, turned out not to be the means by which a drop in mental hospital census has occurred in general. Actually, the assumption that a rising mental hospital census is bad was never fully examined.

❪ The Louisville Experiment

An Attempt to Avoid Hospitalization

Another key experiment in the prevention of hospitalization was conducted in Louisville, Kentucky, by Pasamanick, Scarpitti, and Dinitz from 1961 to 1964.[19] It throws further light on the issues involved in assessing the effectiveness of psychiatric interventions designed to prevent hospitalization. In this experiment the clinical trial design was used, that is, a stream of patients thought to be suitable for a potentially better but unproved new form of intervention were randomly assigned to the older treatment and the new treatment. A stream of patients being inducted into the ordinary mental hospital treatment program for Louisville were randomly split into a group that would receive drug treatment and outpatient care with intensive visiting from a corps of specially trained public health nurses. Actually, this second group was twice as large as the hospital intervention group because a second trial was built into the design. The investigators not only wanted to know whether the intensive home attention with drugs was more effective than the hospital type of intervention, but also whether the home care with drugs given to the patients was better than the same home care without drugs, that is with a placebo. Thus, there were two experimental groups and one control group getting "ordinary" care.

When we assess the effectiveness of these three types of psychiatric intervention we must keep in mind Sheps's comment quoted above that "the single most important prerequisite is specification of objectives. . . ." The objective here was to prevent hospital admission very specifically. Thus it is easy to assess the effectiveness. While those permitted to use the hospital form of intervention were of course 100 percent hospitalized, less than one in four of the drug home care group were hospitalized and about one-third of the placebo group were hospitalized. This is a definite index of success in accomplishing the stated objective. The report merits careful study because of the meticulous detail with which the relevant facts are recorded and the crucial nature of the investigation, which shows that intensive home care can prevent hospitalization and also that the currently available drugs really did increase the effectiveness of the home care intervention. It is the first good data about the effect of drugs on schizophrenics on home care, which indicates their definite effectiveness in helping to prevent hospitalization. The data further indicate that these drugs also helped reduce the prevalence of certain troublesome behaviors.

These are the two major studies based on the notion that prevention of hospital psychiatric intervention is a worthwhile objective. In both instances substantial evidence exists that appropriate psychiatric intervention outside of the hospital with a variety of supplementary services can prevent a substantial proportion of hospitalizations.

The Louisville experiment has a major weakness. The objective in this instance seems clearly enough stated, but examination of the study method reveals that the three samples were selected *after* the "patients had arrived at Central State Hospital and were placed on the admission ward with no immediate treatment." This is quite a different concept of "preventing hospitalization" than the Worthing and Chichester experiments. In fact, it was an attempt to prevent hospital intervention as the initial treatment plan for the patients, but all study subjects began the current episode of treatment with a hospitalization. The publication reporting the Louisville experiment repeatedly uses the term "hospitalization" as interchangeable with "institutionalization," which gives us the needed clue to understand what their stated objective meant to them. "Hospitalization" is an aspect of that process which leads to "institutionalism," so the object of avoiding hospitalization and finding an alternate mode for psychiatric intervention is related to the more distant objective—to prevent institutionalism. It is then necessary for the student of methods to assess the effectiveness of particular types of psychiatric intervention to take another look at the Louisville experiment: Is the student willing to grant the assumption that prevention of hospital intervention at the beginning of a particular episode of psychiatric intervention is the best way to prevent institutionalism? If this assumption is granted, then the effort to provide intensive home care certainly achieved a step toward that objective, but the reported data do not include information as to whether chronic institutionalism was prevented or not. Nor in the five-year follow-up[4] is there information on the frequency of long-term institutionalization or institutional neurosis.[2] The groups were probably too small to appraise this type of phenomenon in any case. But the authors' summary states that "eventually no differences in psychological or social functioning could be found. This indicates a need for the structuring of community mental health services on an intensive aggressive basis. . . ." This result followed a phasing out of the specialized services designed for home care—which indicates that the program was effective in avoiding hospitalization for a period, but that in the long run the patients did just as poorly as those who had received hospital care initially.

These findings suggest that the antihospital type of intervention did not produce the long-term effect of preventing deterioration in personal and social functioning. The other side of this statement is apparently also true: that initial hospitalization did not worsen the long-term course of those patients who were hospitalized as compared with those who received the intensive home care in the first three years, whether or not they received drugs at that time. The long-term success or failure of the patients, then, does not seem to be crucially affected by which type of care is given during one short period of their chronic disorder. Consequently one must ask whether preventing hospitalization or facilitating community care is the more worthy objective. Each showed some success in terms of the stated goals, but the issue that the student of effectiveness assessment must face is whether either really stated its ultimate objective.

We can infer that the stated goals can be seen as intermediate rather than ultimate. Avoidance of hospitalization need not be seen as an end in itself. Community care need not be seen as an end in itself. Without attributing unstated views to the authors cited, we can ourselves conclude that seeking these effects—preventing hospitalization and facilitating community care—can be seen as part of a strategy not fully made explicit for accomplishing another objective: preventing chronic deterioration in patients with severe chronic mental disorders. Leaving the Chichester experiment (1959–1963) and the Louisville experiment (1961–1964) behind, let us ask what kind of psychiatric intervention would be appropriate if the effect being sought was to prevent chronic deterioration?

◖ The Dutchess County Experiment

An Attempt to Prevent Chronic Deterioration in the Severely Mentally Ill

In 1958 Robert C. Hunt advanced the following propositions:

1. The disability associated with psychotic mental illness is enormous.
2. The illness and the associated disability are not necessarily homogenous or synonymous.
3. Disability is only in part intrinsic to the illness.
4. Disability is in large part an artifact of extrinsic origin.
5. Since the disability is an artifact it is not inevitable and something can be done about it.
6. The factors which produce disability are multiple.
7. The multiple extrinsic factors have a common origin in traditional attitudes toward the mentally ill in our culture. [p. 10][15]

With that set of notions, he proposed to initiate an experiment to prevent chronic disability among all the severely mentally ill people of Dutchess County, New York, which I shall refer to as the Dutchess County Experiment.

The effect he proposed to produce through a modified form of psychiatric intervention was to reduce the amount and severity of chronic disability due to serious mental disorders. The modification of psychiatric intervention he proposed had its roots in observations he had made regarding the effects of certain psychiatric service programs he had studied. It is necessary to recapitulate those observations briefly so that the reason why he picked this effect can be properly understood. His notion that chronic disability could be prevented arose when observing psychiatric intervention programs that did not have that objective. A series of "improvements" in mental hospital management had, apparently, produced the unexpected effect. These improvements began shortly after the Second World War in three different British mental hospitals and were initiated more or less in parallel and independently by three British mental hospital directors. They all began in the same way. Each director was impressed that the hospitals used entirely too many locks and they started, conservatively, to unlock some of the wards, at first only in the daytime. They found that the patients not only did all right, but they seemed to do a little better. So they went on. G. M. Bell at Dingleton Hospital in Melrose, Scotland, was probably the first to unlock all wards. Not only did the patients like it and do better, but the staff had come to like the greater responsibility they were carrying. T. P. Rees at Warlingham Park Hospital, Croyden, was pushing along in the same direction. He was particularly impressed by how much the staff gained from the changes. He developed the theory that the more responsibility staff and patients were given, the better they performed. He said that all the patients could handle more responsibility than they had had and that when they took responsibility, they began to improve. Duncan Macmillan at Mapperley Hospital, Nottingham, had been impressed during the Second World War, that when a wall of the hospital collapsed during the bombing the patients did not run away, but pitched in, helping clean up the debris and comforting those who had been hurt, not very differently from the way the nonhospital residents of the city did after a bombing. He was particularly impressed by the effect on patients of locking the door when they were admitted to the hospital; he felt that the pa-

tient responded by a major loss in self-confidence and optimism that interfered enormously with his ability to mobilize his resources as the psychotic episode began to recede. Macmillan was also particularly impressed by how his gradual unlocking of wards and permitting greater responsibility and freedom for the patients had changed the staff–patient relationships. "The staff have to use their personalities to deal with situations which were formerly dealt with by the locked door . . . ," he said.[18]

By 1953, when word of these developments first reached the United States, all three hospitals had been totally unlocked for several years. Macmillan had gone so far as to use the first postwar funds he received to improve the appearance of his hospital's wards, to have all the ward doors removed and installed double swing pantry-type doors at the entrance to each ward, which could not be locked under any circumstances. Hunt met Rees when the latter was on a visit to America and was deeply impressed with his accounts of how the hospitals had become transformed. Patient behavior had improved radically, the worst forms of aggression, soiling, self-neglect, mutism, refusal of food, and so forth had become much rarer. And new cases hardly ever developed these patterns of withdrawal and self-neglect. In the three hospitals the census of mental patients had dropped dramatically, almost 50 percent in less than a decade. The hospital staff had moved a large proportion of their work into the community where they took care of as many former hospital patients as they did in the hospital. It all sounded very nice and a bit too good to be true. The reader should remember that these reports arrived in this country in 1953; Henri Laborit had discovered chlorpromazine in 1951, and the first psychiatric meeting at which its results were described was in 1952. All of these advances were made before any of the so-called tranquilizing drugs were available commercially. To anyone with experience in mental hospital work, Rees's reports were unbelievable and Hunt had worked in New York State Mental Hospitals for seventeen years. But it was an interesting story even if only half true and when a year or so later the World Health Organization offered Hunt a traveling fellowship to study these programs, he accepted with alacrity. His report stated that the programs did work exactly as specified and with no fakery. The tranquilizing drugs were available by then and were being used, but he was impressed with the relatively low dosage, the rapid census drops, the absence of disturbed and deteriorated behavior of the worst sorts, which still existed in other mental hospitals despite much higher drug dosage patterns.

After a series of steps recorded elsewhere,[16] Hunt determined that he would try to copy the fundamental principles involved and to organize a county service for the immediate area of Hudson River State Hospital of which he had become director. He had to modify the hospital organization because it was clear that the British successes had occurred in small hospitals, (starting with censuses of under 3000) with small catchment areas near the hospital.

In 1958 Hunt proposed an experiment in which he would allocate a proportional part of his large state hospital (more than 6000 patients) for the residents of Dutchess County (10 percent of his catchment area's population). One-tenth of the plant and personnel would be used to set up a subhospital with comprehensive responsibility for providing the indicated psychiatric interventions for all of the seriously mentally disordered residents of the county. In addition to providing all needed acute and long-term inpatient care, this staff was charged with providing all aftercare, social service, and family care, and all local facilities and related professionals were encouraged to cooperate in any possible way to maximize the community care of the patients. A day hospital unit already existed at the hospital. The only new service introduced was "pre-care," which meant consultation by hospital psychiatrists about patients in the community who were thought to be in possible need of mental hospital admission. The British pioneers had insisted that this was a crucial feature not only to prevent misuse of hospitals, but also to help the patient accept voluntary hospital care. A slight increase in

personnel was introduced (I estimate less than 10 percent of the annual cost to the state of running the mental hospital county unit). This extra personnel was financed by the Milbank Memorial Fund and met a few elementary needs: (1) a unit director at the rank of what might be considered associate director of the mental hospital had to be brought in, as none of the existing staff had the range of competences needed to run such an enterprise and the state would not underwrite an extra assistant director category; (2) an extra secretary for the unit director at a higher rank than the state budget provided for in a service chief; and (3) extra stenographers and social workers because of the increased work involved in communicating outside the hospital.

Five points are worth special attention in this description: (1) the innovation in psychiatric intervention was not a new kind of treatment but an innovation in the organization of personnel and resources and of policy; (2) the idea that the changed pattern of using existing resources would reduce the amount of chronic deterioration emerged out of observing that efforts to improve and humanize mental hospitals had led to rapid drops in census and an apparent major reduction in the frequency of chronic deterioration; (3) in contrast to the Chichester and Louisville experiments, this pattern of psychiatric innovation was an attempt to improve the way in which the hospital was used in the treatment of long-term patients, not a way of avoiding the hospital; (4) the assumption was that the hospital would be made *more* available to those in need of its services, that admission rates would rise, and that this increase would be more than compensated for by a radical decrease in the duration of hospital stay and much earlier return to home living before complete restoration of all functions; and (5) Hunt no more planned any systematic data gathering to assess its effectiveness than had Bell, Rees, or Macmillan.

But when Hunt asked the Milbank Memorial Fund to provide the small, extra, flexible financing to implement his ideas, they responded by saying that the idea was too important potentially to justify starting it without some systematic evaluation research. I was assigned the duty of locating the research worker, but in the end was assigned the job of organizing and executing the research with a special team.

Assessment of effect in terms of preventing deterioration would present no special methodological problems in itself. It would be necessary to locate or develop some objective criteria for recognizing chronic deterioration and apply these criteria to a suitably selected population at some risk of developing chronic deterioration, a random half of which was given the new form of psychiatric intervention. But the nature of the intervention made this impossible. The reasons were similar to those operating in the Chichester experiment. It is not possible to organize a double blind random assignment psychiatric service highly integrated with the nonpsychiatric community services for only half the patients from the community while the same professionals remain unintegrated in their work patterns for the other half. It was thought that perhaps another county's patients from the parent hospital's district would make a suitable control population. This turned out to be unrealistic because it was well established that hospital utilization rates fall off with the distance of people's homes from the hospital.[17]

Because this experiment introduced a new way of organizing psychiatric intervention at a point in time, a before-and-after design was considered to be of some help. A before-and-after system has certain inherent weaknesses, however, the main one being that no one knows what unplanned changes will occur over a given time span if no planned changes are introduced. One is studying a phenomenon—in this case the frequency of chronic deterioration—about which remarkably little was previously known. There could well be short-term fluctuations of major size in its frequency that had never been carefully enough observed. It was known that severe chronic deterioration was not the common sequel of a psychotic episode, but there were very little data on which to base estimates of how frequently and how shortly after the first hospitalization it was to be expected.

The first step was to specify the criteria for identifying a person as being severely disabled in the presence of a serious mental disorder. The criteria to be used were developed with considerable caution and special efforts were taken to see that they would be as relevant as possible to assessing whether the stated goals were achieved. The research workers generated intermittent intensive interactions with the administrative innovators and pushed for highly specific formulations of exactly what would be less common. The expectation was that the main changes would be in behavior, a finding that surfaced several years later in the Massachusetts Mental Hospitals Experiment. It was anticipated in the Dutchess County Experiment because of careful observations made at the three British pioneering programs in community care. With some trepidation, it was decided to ignore completely the patient's subjective mental symptoms because Hunt and his associates did not expect much change in these phenomena. Self-care, participation in work and recreational roles, and freedom from dangerous or troubling behavior became the main areas of inquiry. The data gathering focused on those specific changes in behavior that were expected by the innovators. They set the fundamental criteria and the research team through pretests decided which changes could be objectively ascertained with reliability. This was first done on all the county's chronic ward patients in 1959 in order to implement the testing of a subordinate hypothesis: Those chronic patients who were already seriously disabled when the new program started would improve but slightly.[13] A great deal was learned in this process about the techniques of ascertaining whether any given patient met the criteria set in a particular week. In one week more than 18,000 printed data forms were filled out by ward personnel of Hudson River State Hospital, were edited within eight hours, and the informants were questioned about any discrepancies or missed item the next time they reported for work. That was done before the reorganization of the services had started.

This gave the investigative team confidence in its ability to make the necessary assessment within the hospital at any one point in time. The particular pattern of disabled behavior that was being assessed was given a new name so as to avoid confusion with related concepts such as institutional neurosis[2] and chronicity.[5] The new term was "Social Breakdown Syndrome" (SBS).[11,1] Though this technology provided a means for ascertainment at one point in time, the major effect anticipated was that new cases of chronic SBS would be reduced in frequency.

To assess whether the new program was reducing the frequency with which new cases of chronic SBS was developing required additional techniques. The onset of the SBS had to be determined for each individual and a mechanism developed to monitor cases of SBS to see how long they continued after they were located. These techniques were also developed.

The most difficult problem was to decide who had to be studied. This was not a case control study in which one could observe two groups of patients, those who had been exposed to the new pattern of intervention and those who were exposed to the old pattern of intervention. Each of the three previously described evaluations used that method. In this case the entire population of people with severe mental disorders in Dutchess County was exposed to the old pattern of intervention until 1960 and thereafter was exposed to the new pattern. It might appear that those whose first entry to the hospital was before 1960 could be compared with those whose first entry was after 1960, but this ignores the well-known fact that chronic SBS often does not develop until several years after the first admission and those who had first been admitted, say in 1958, were provided with exactly the same sort of intervention after 1960 as were people first admitted subsequent to 1960. In addition, the mechanism for reducing the rate at which chronic deterioration develops included making the hospital more readily available for readmissions and this was expected to make the hospital more available for first admissions too. Therefore, admission rates were expected to rise and a later cohort might include people at less risk of developing

chronic SBS than earlier cohorts of admissions. Inasmuch as the new pattern of intervention included a plan to release patients to community care very early in their recovery— keeping the hospital prepared for any needed repeat short-term admission—there was a significant risk that the chronic SBS cases might develop in the community without the knowledge of the clinical teams.

The method used to meet these problems was to create a register of all Dutchess County residents who had had psychiatric treatment after 1955 and to keep it up-to-date regarding new entries to treatment and transfers or discharges or deaths. This register population was then looked upon as the population at risk of developing chronic SBS. The problem then was to find a way of determining whether long-term episodes of SBS began more frequently in the years prior to 1960 than in the years subsequent to 1960. The concept "long term" was defined as an SBS episode lasting a full year or longer.

Specially trained data gatherers were sent out to locate those members of the registered population who were living outside the hospital and to determine whether at that time the individual was in an SBS episode. If the answer was yes, then a research clinician went to the individual's location and took a careful history to determine when that episode started. The technique of locating the individuals, gaining cooperation for data gathering, developing reliable onset date determination techniques, and continuing monitoring techniques took more than two years to develop. By that time, the new form of intervention had already been going on for two years. Despite this tardiness in developing the capability to gather the needed facts, it was possible to get data that provided a means for determining whether the number of new chronic SBS episodes starting in later years was smaller than the number that started in earlier years. This was made possible because the hypothesis only referred to chronic cases, and these chronic cases—by definition—would have to continue to be SBS cases for more than a year. By screening the population at one point in time, one picked up a mixture of new and old

SBS cases. All chronic cases that had started in the previous year would still be cases on the day they were screened. By monitoring cases until they terminated or passed their anniversary, one would get a complete count of one year's onsets of chronic SBS cases. Of course, some of these cases would have started a week or two before the day they were screened, and to find out which of those were going to become chronic it would be necessary to monitor the whole group for a full year after the screening date. By April, 1965, on the basis of many thousands of interviews it was possible to report tentatively that for every two cases of chronic SBS that had begun during 1963 somewhere between three and four cases must have started in 1960.[3] By 1969 more detailed analysis of twice as much data and greater familiarity with the epidemiology of SBS, both acute and chronic, made it possible to report that each year the new form of intervention prevented at least forty person years of chronic severe deterioration per 100,000 general population in the age group sixteen to sixty-four.[14]

The level of disability reflected in SBS is on the whole pretty severe. A person who attempts suicide but is prevented by physical restraint, a person who soils, a person who has no recreational activities or no work activities will meet the criteria; to be a chronic SBS case one or another of these characteristics must be present every week for fifty-two consecutive weeks. There are combinations of less severe manifestations in each area of social functioning that will also qualify them. One remarkable finding was that only half of the chronic SBS cases were schizophrenic cases, the other half were scattered over a wide range of diagnoses. But the pattern of disability did not correspond to the diagnosis. The SBS syndrome describes a pattern of psychotic decompensation that can occur in any mental disorder and probably does; there is good reason to think that short episodes actually occur in the absence of any psychosis and if they were seen by psychiatrists they might be diagnosed as "transient situational reaction" or "no mental disorder."

These data on the declining incidence of chronic SBS provide the best evidence that community care of chronic mental patients is more than a fashion; it is actually a way of preventing long-term serious disability. The mechanism by which chronic SBS is being prevented is still not completely clear. Most entries into inpatient care follow the onset of an SBS episode, which tends to terminate very quickly after entering the hospital (one to five weeks). Most, but not all, episodes that occur in patients while living in the commnity re sult in a hospital admission. Very few of the chronic cases that start are in fact extreme examples of institutionalism or institutional neurosis. It is possible in a population that has been receiving a pattern of community care for more than twelve years to see the forms of chronic SBS that develop in the absence of chronic hospitalization. This has not been studied in detail.

This is the first example in which a modification of the way in which a health-care delivery system is organized has produced evidence of improved health in the population being served, without introducing either a greater volume of service or a new technology of medical treatment (such as a new drug or operation). It raises fundamental questions about the pathogenesis of the deteriorating syndrome in the major mental disorders.[8] It also requires a rethinking of the function of inpatient services as one element in the network of services used in the treatment of people with long-term serious mental disorders. The pattern of fluid movement between inpatient and outpatient care seems to depend upon a unified clinical team, that is, a clinical team that continues its treatment responsibilities for its own group of patients as these patients move in and out of hospital, family care, and outpatient status.[12] The indications for hospitalization take on a new appearance.[9,10]

These outcomes are emphasized to indicate that evaluation studies to determine the effectiveness of a new type of psychiatric intervention can sometimes do much more than answer the simple question, Was the effect being sought produced? Fundamental issues in clinical psychiatry can also become elucidated by coming into close contact with a rapidly changing situation. In fact, it is when great changes are in progress that certain types of studies are most appropriate. Combining research with planned action not only provides information about the effectiveness of the action, but can throw light on previously unquestioned conventional wisdom regarding the nature of mental disorders.

⟮ Bibliography

1. AMERICAN PUBLIC HEALTH ASSOCIATION. *A Guide to Control Methods.* Program Area Committee on Mental Health. New York: Am. Public Health Assoc., 1962.

2. BARTON, R. *Institutional Neurosis*, 2nd. ed. reprint. Bristol, England: John Wright, 1966.

3. BRANDON, S. and E. M .GRUENBERG. "Measurement of the Incidence of Chronic Severe Social Breakdown Syndrome—Has the Dutchess County Service Been Associated with a Decline in Incidence?" in E. M. Gruenberg, ed., *Evaluating the Effectiveness of Mental Health Services. Milbank Mem. Fund Q.*, 44, Part 2 (1966), 129–142.

4. DAVIS, A., S. DINITZ, and B. PASAMANICK. "The Prevention of Hospitalization in Schizophrenia: Five Years after an Experimental Program," *Am. J. Orthopsychiatry*, 42 (1972), 375–388.

5. DRASGOW, J. "A Criterion for Chronicity in Schizophrenia," *Psychiatr. Q.*, 31 (1957), 454–457.

6. GRAD, J. and P. SAINSBURY. "Evaluating the Community Psychiatric Service in Chichester: Results," in E. M. Gruenberg, ed., *Evaluating the Effectiveness of Mental Health Services. Milbank Mem. Fund Q.*, 44, Part 2 (1966), 246–287.

7. GREENBLATT, M., M. SOLOMON, A. S. EVANS et al. *Drug and Social Therapy in Chronic Schizophrenia.* Springfield, Ill.: Charles C. Thomas, 1965.

8. GRUENBERG, E. M. "From Practice to Theory: Community Mental Health Services and the Nature of Psychoses," *Lancet*, 1 (1969), 721–724.

9. ———. "Hospital Treatment in Schizophrenia: The Indications for and the Value of Hospital Treatment," in R. Cancro, ed., *The Schizophrenic Reactions: A Critique of the Concept, Hospital Treatment and Current Research*, pp. 121–136. New York: Brunner/Mazel, 1970.

10. ———. "Benefits of Short-term Hospitalization," in R. Cancro, N. Fox, and L. Shapiro, eds., *Strategic Intervention in Schizophrenia: Current Developments in Treatment.* New York: Behavioral Pubs., 1974.

11. GRUENBERG, E. M., S. BRANDON, and R. V. KASIUS. "Identifying Cases of the Social Breakdown Syndrome," in E. M. Gruenberg, ed., *Evaluating the Effectiveness of Community Mental Health Services. Milbank Mem. Fund Q.*, 44, Part 2 (1966), 150–155.

12. GRUENBERG, E. M. and J. HUXLEY. "Mental Health Services Can Be Organized to Prevent Chronic Disability," *Community Ment. Health J.*, 6 (1970), 431–436.

13. GRUENBERG, E. M., R. V. KASIUS, and M. HUXLEY. "Objective Appraisal of Deterioration in a Group of Long-stay Hospital Patients," *Milbank Mem. Fund Q.*, 40 (1962), 90–100.

14. GRUENBERG, E. M., H. B. SNOW, and C. L. BENNETT. "Preventing the Social Breakdown Syndrome," in F. C. Redlich, ed., *Social Psychiatry*, pp. 179–195. Baltimore: Williams & Wilkins, 1969.

15. HUNT, R. C. "Ingredients of a Rehabilitation Program," in *An Approach to the Prevention of Disability from Chronic Psychoses*, pp. 9–27. New York: *Milbank Mem. Fund* 1958.

16. HUNT, R. C., E. M. GRUENBERG, E. HACKEN et al. "A Comprehensive Hospital-Community Service in a State Hospital," *Am. J. Psychiatry*, 117 (1961), 817–821.

17. JARVIS, E. "Influence of Distance from and Nearness to an Insane Hospital on Its Use by the People," *Am. J. Insanity*, 22 (1855–1856), 361–406.

18. MACMILLAN, D. "Hospital-Community Relationships," in *An Approach to the Prevention of Disability from Chronic Psychoses Milbank Mem. Fund*, pp. 27–50. New York: 1958.

19. PASAMANICK, B., F. SCARPITTI, and S. DINITZ. *Schizophrenics in the Community: An Experimental Study in the Prevention of Hospitalization.* New York: Appleton-Century-Crofts, 1967.

20. ROETHLISBERGER, F. and W. DICKSON. *Man-*

agement and the Worker. Cambridge, Mass.: Harvard University Press, 1939.

21. Sainsbury, P. and J. Grad. "Evaluating the Community Psychiatric Service in Chichester: Aims and Methods of Research," in E. M. Gruenberg, ed., *Evaluating the Effectiveness of Mental Health Services. Milbank Mem. Fund Q.*, 44, Part 2 (1966), 231–242.

CHAPTER 36

COMPUTER APPLICATIONS IN PSYCHIATRY

Robert L. Spitzer and Jean Endicott

COMPUTER TECHNOLOGY is being applied to practically all aspects of psychiatry. Theories of personality and of psychotherapeutic change are being subjected to computer-simulation techniques. Computers interview, diagnose and conduct therapy with real patients. Computers interpret and write psychological test reports. They compose reports of mental-status examinations.

This chapter will concentrate on practical computer applications that either currently or in the near future will have an impact on the practice of psychiatry. Much less emphasis will be placed on computer applications that are primarily of theoretical or research interest and are unlikely to affect clinical practice. We will not discuss computer applications in several areas that are not central to the practice of psychiatry such as data analysis for research studies, bookkeeping functions in hospitals or other mental-health delivery systems, routine medical laboratory tests, and systems for the exchange of information (e.g., libraries, abstracting services).

The following section is for the reader who is not familiar with basic computer concepts.

(Computer Concepts

A computer is a device capable of accepting information, applying a series of predetermined operations on the information, and supplying the results of these operations. For these reasons, a calculating machine, by itself, is not a computer because it does not have the capability of automatically applying a series of predetermined operations on the data that is supplied to it. A full computer, even though it may be quite small, consists of input and output devices that accept and display information, a storage unit that holds information during processing, a unit that can perform arithmetic operations, a unit that can perform logical operations (determine the truth value of an expression) and a control unit that directs the sequence of operations.

There are two basic types of computers: analogue and digital. Analogue computers are used to study data that vary continuously over time, such as EEG activity, blood pressure or other physiological measures. The computer represents the physical process being studied by translating it into an analogous electrical process that can then be manipulated. Because analogue computers do not process symbols, their use in psychiatry has largely been limited to the study of physiological variables such as brain electrical activity.

Digital computers are used to study data that can be reduced to discrete or discontinuous form, such as numbers or other symbols. The most complicated concept, a series of operations, or any kind of digital data, is ultimately translated into a series of "off-on" bits. The physical representation of these bits varies, depending upon where in the computer the information is being stored. For example, in core memory it may be represented as a series of magnetized or demagnetized iron cores, in an arithmetic register it may be represented as a series of semiconductor circuits that are in one of two states.

The physical equipment comprising the computer is known as the hardware. The instructions that determine the specific operations to be done are the software or computer program. The instructions contained in the computer program must be introduced into the computer through an input device just as data is later brought into the computer for processing. Although the program is a list of instructions that are in sequence, when the program is actually executed, the order in which the instructions are carried out may vary as a result of some contingency. For example, a computer program for psychiatric interviewing might have an instruction: "If the subject has not been married, skip section on marital history." Although the computer can obviously respond only to contingencies that have been specified in the program, the capability for branching results in great flexibility. The contingencies need not be stated in terms of the raw input data but can also be in terms of intermediary calculations that are tested at certain points in the program.

Ultimately, all instructions to the computer hardware are in the form of binary numbers. However, since writing instructions in this form is extremely tedious and difficult, programmers make use of high-level programming languages that the machine then translates into binary form, using intermediary programs called compilers and assemblers. Thus, a single instruction in a high-level language by a programmer may result eventually in a string of hundreds of binary-machine-language instructions. Different high-level languages have been developed for different applications. FORTRAN, for example, is ideally suited for algebraic- and formula-oriented quantitative research. COBOL is business oriented and very suitable for inventory and accounting procedures. LISP is a list-processing language that processes symbols and therefore has been useful in computerized simulation of human intelligence. PL/1 combines many of the features of other languages with the aim of producing a general purpose language for business and scientific activities. It is an example of efforts to develop high-level-programming languages that approximate the form of natural language instructions.

Computers can receive information from several types of devices: punch-card readers, paper-tape readers, magnetic-tape readers, optical-scan or character readers, typewriter consoles and cathode-ray tubes (TV-type screen) that are heat or light sensitive. These devices vary in their speed, accuracy, convenience, and cost. The typewriter console and cathode-ray tube permit interaction between the computer and the person supplying the information so that there can be a dialogue. But such devices are expensive and can be used by only one person at a time. Optical-character readers are able to recognize numbers and letters written in standard form. Their practical use is limited by their high cost and the inability to read characters not written according to rigid specifications. Optical-scan readers recognize pencil marks placed in predetermined positions on a form. Their major advantage over key punching is that of speed and the ability to process the original document on which the data is collected. These advantages are offset by the frequently high error rate (reading of erasures or failing to read intended marks) and the absence of any simple procedure for detecting errors, such as the process used in checking key-punch data whereby the data is repunched and any discrepancies are readily apparent.

Computers vary in storage capacity, the speed with which information can be read in and processed, and the capacity to perform complex operations. For example, many small computers are able to perform arithmetic operations but do not have the control circuitry to perform such logical operations as comparing variable A with variable B and then performing differential operations based on the results. Because the internal speed of processing data is incredibly fast as compared with the speed of input devices, it is possible, with large computers, to have many users interacting with the computer at the same time. In actuality, the computer is accepting input from one user for a fraction of a second while it is processing the input from another user. This feature, called time sharing, has made it possible for a large central computer to be shared by many users, thus cutting the expense for each user.

The results of a computer analysis are referred to as the output. If a permanent record is required, it can take many forms, such as punched cards, magnetic tape files, or printed paper. When a permanent record is not required, it can be presented on a visual display device, such as a cathode-ray tube, or, more recently, in the form of an audio message that simulates speech.

There have been so many new developments in computer technology in the last decade that it is difficult to envision the capabilities of computers ten years from now. However, the trends are clearly in the direction of increased speed, power, and reliability of the hardware, the development of more advanced programming languages so that the user can specify operations close to idiomatic English, and the development of relatively inexpensive terminals so that the individual user has ready access to the power of the computer.

⟮ Data Banks

The collection of data on psychiatric patients for storage in data banks involves more patients and psychiatric personnel than any other current application of computers in psychiatry. The term data bank is used here for any system involving storage and retrieval of information about patients that is pooled from multiple sources (for example, several hospitals), that is summarized or coded, and is primarily used for administrative or research purposes. Systems that use pooled data, where the emphasis is on producing a clinical record, are usually referred to as automated-record-keeping systems and, although they always have an associated data bank, are discussed in the next section.

Most departments of mental hygiene have some form of automated system for collecting data on psychiatric patients and nearly all large systems for the delivery of mental-health services now have some form of computerized data system. The type of data entering these systems is quite variable, ranging from simple demographic data and a single psychiatric diagnosis, to such detailed information as services rendered, presenting symptomatology and disposition, and symptomatology at termination of treatment.

In most systems there is no provision for linking data on an individual patient if he receives services from more than one facility. Thus, a patient who is admitted to four different hospitals within a calendar year for treatment of alcoholism would be counted in any summary statistic as four different people. Systems that attempt to link files across facilities for individuals are called case registers. A great deal of additional effort is required to convert a data bank into a case register. A central problem for case registers is finding a unique identification number that would be used by all reporting facilities and that the patient would know himself such as his social-security number. There has been considerable resistance to the use of social-security numbers for such purposes because of the issue of confidentiality. Another major problem in case registers is getting all reporting facilities within a given system to agree on standardization of terminology and on what data is to be reported. More elaborate procedures for editing and checking the data are necessary in a case register than in a data bank. Populations with high mobility are extremely difficult to follow over long periods of time.

Summary statistics from psychiatric data banks can take many forms. Most of the systems provide for a description of the number of admissions, readmissions, and terminations from different types of services, and a description of the demographic characteristics of the population served. More complex systems can describe lengths of stay in various services, use of personnel time, and treatment outcome. Case registers can provide more powerful data that can be used in determining unduplicated patient counts, better descriptions of the types of services received, and profiles of patient populations or service patterns that might not be discernable in ordinary data banks. Case registers, and data banks, can provide administrators with information for evaluating and planning mental-health services and for justifying their work to agencies and legislatures that provide the funds.

Despite the seemingly great potential of data banks, there has been considerable opposition in the profession to participation in such efforts. The primary issues involve confidentiality and whether the high cost of maintaining such systems and the time and effort required in filling out forms by busy mental-health personnel are justified by the actual value of the systems for improving patient care or the distribution of available health resources.

The issue of confidentiality of computerized records is not unique to psychiatric records. However, the sensitive nature of psychiatric data and the possibility of misinterpreting the significance of a given bit of information makes many psychiatrists reluctant to supply any data on a patient thereby indicating that the individual was at one time a psychiatric patient. In defense of automated systems it has been argued that the confidentiality of current nonautomated psychiatric records is often violated. It is sometimes possible for various persons to have ready access to the files of a psychiatric clinic or hospital by merely presenting themselves and requesting the patient's chart. With an automated system it is more feasible to put in reliable safeguards against such access by unauthorized individuals. This can be done by using code numbers instead of names, by scrambling identification numbers, and by making linkage of files (names, diagnoses, symptoms) dependent upon complex procedures known only to a few key individuals.

What concerns most mental-health professionals is not access to an individual record by an occasional unauthorized person as much as the potential access to such records on a large scale by cooperating governmental agencies. This can only be solved by legal safeguards that clearly establish the confidentiality of psychiatric data, specify the uses to which it may be put (for example, research studies by bona-fide investigators) and impose penalties for any violations. Several states have already passed such legislation. Ultimately, the issue is between the individual's right to privacy and society's need for information that can often be obtained in no other way and that has the potential for improving the level of health care for all.

A major problem of data banks, as well as of automated clinical-record systems, is the quality of the input data. Since in most cases the individual supplying the information receives no feedback, is often unaware of how the data will be used, and may have serious reservations because of the issue of confidentiality, he often has little motivation for supplying accurate and complete data. A further source of low motivation may be a belief that the content of the data is irrelevant for the uses to which it is intended. For example, the clinician may feel that the treatment he has offered is not reflected in the precoded categories that he has to use in reporting his services. In addition, even if he is motivated, the rater rarely has the time to study manuals that define terms on the input forms or the opportunity to participate in discussions to assure comparability of information. Another factor affecting the quality of the input data has been the proliferation of data banks that overlap, so that the clinician may have to report to several different systems, each of which has its own reporting system and group of forms. Many have questioned whether data collected under such circumstances can really be of much help in evaluating and planning services.

(Automated Clinical Records

Dissatisfaction with the traditional psychiatric case record has led to many efforts to apply computer technology to improve its usefulness to clinicians, administrators, and researchers. The major impetus for automation has come from administrators and researchers who have found that the traditional clinical record is largely useless for their needs. This is because of the lack of standardization of the type and form of the information contained in the record and the difficulty in retrieving what information it may contain.

There are currently a variety of record-keeping systems that have been in operation for a number of years and, despite many difficulties, seem to be permanently established. They vary from systems operational in a single hospital, such as the Institute of Living in Hartford, Connecticut; in a mental-health center, such as the Fort Logan Health Center in Denver, Colorado; in an entire state, such as the Missouri Standard System of Psychiatry; to facilities in a number of states, such as the Multi-State Information System for Psychiatric Patients with a central computer facility at Rockland State Hospital, in Orangeburg, New York. Although all of the systems attempt to translate some of the usual clinical record into a form suitable for automated retrieval, monitor some aspect of patient care, provide information for administrative decisions, and assist the clinician in his understanding and treatment of the patient, they differ considerably in the strategies and methods that they employ for these purposes.

Systems vary in how much of the usual record is automated and to what degree the clinician is limited to precoded categories for describing his patient. Eiduson[23,24] has developed a system, called the Psychiatric Case History Event System (PSYCHES) in which the narrative textual material of the clinical case record is coded into a form suitable for computer processing. The basic unit of the system is an "event," that is, any happening or occurrence that takes place in the life of the patient or relevant persons in his environment. It includes not only hard, objective data but subjective, impressionistic data that clinicians commonly use in describing patients. This approach assumes that the clinician will, by and large, include all relevant data. The use of coders and the storage requirements for retaining the entire clinical record make this approach unsuitable for most large facilities on the basis of cost alone.

With the exception of the PSYCHES system, all other automated-record-keeping systems require the clinician to use precoded categories to describe his patient. These categories can be simple true–false statements, scaled judgments reflecting intensity or severity of some trait, or multiple-choice items. Precoded items need not be limited to simple concepts, since any concept that can be defined can be translated into a precoded item. Some of the systems attempt to precode only basic demographic data and a small list of presenting symptoms, while others attempt to gather precoded information in all categories of the traditional clinical record (mental status, psychiatric anamnesis, nursing notes, occupational therapy notes, etc.). The systems vary in the extent to which the precoded information is a substitute and replaces parts of the traditional record. In some systems there is virtually no information in the record other than that which is precoded. Most systems retain a written record and only automate small parts of the record. In most systems the computer generates a hard copy that can be placed in the patient's chart. Usually, the material is presented in a simple tabular form. In some cases the computer generates a grammatically correct (if not elegant) narrative report in an effort to simulate the usual clinical report, using special programming languages such as NOVEL.[18] An example of an optically scanned history form and the computer generated narrative are shown in Figures 36–1 and 36–2. To permit the clinician to describe the patient more fully, some systems permit the introduction of small amounts of free narrative text, which can be interspersed with the output of the precoded information. Despite improvements in the readability of computer-generated narratives and reports, it is unlikely that they will ever approach the readability and individuality of a good clinical record because of the standardization of the input categories. According to some clinicians, they are not only difficult to read, but impossible to remember.

Whereas some systems have accepted the basic structure of the traditional case record, other systems have incorporated features not found in most clinical records. For example, the Fort Logan system has added goal-oriented progress notes that make provision for recording information on the goals set and the methods to be used to attain them.[109] The data is collected not only from the staff but from the patient and community members as well. Hillside Hospital in New York City, part of the Multi-State Information System, has designed a system for allowing the clinician to state his own goals at the beginning of treatment. The computer then queries the clinician periodically as to how the patient is progressing. The Missouri system has provision for collecting precoded historical and family information from a family member.

Another important function of most automated-record systems is to facilitate the monitoring of patient status and care. One method is the Drug Monitoring System of the Multi-State Information System whereby all drug medication is ordered by using a special optical-scan form. Reasons for change and side effects are noted, in addition to the specific drug being ordered and the method of administration. This system allows the clinician to obtain the entire drug history of a patient, to review the current drug status of a group of patients, and to be cautioned if he orders a drug with a dosage that is beyond the expected range or one to which the patient has previously had a toxic reaction.

Glueck and his colleagues at the Institute of Living have an automated nursing note procedure used to monitor patient status.[34,35,79,80] Nursing reports are made on each patient twice daily (day and night) by routine nursing personnel on a form that is designed for computer scoring (Fig. 36–3). Eleven areas of patient behavior are rated, using non-inferential descriptions. The computer produces two types of output: the first is a narrative summary to be filed in the patient's record; the second is a set of factor scores describing the patient's behavior numerically as compared to the unit norm. The progress of individual patients can be charted as well as changes in an entire ward. Monitoring an entire ward has enabled clinicians to become aware of increasing tension that might not be apparent with the usual observation and reporting techniques. The factor scores can be used to derive a global measure of pathology that can be subjected to a sequential analysis to yield decisions of "significantly better," "worse," or "unchanged," in evaluating response to treatment and the need for change in treatment.

As mentioned previously in the discussion on data banks, all automated systems are designed to generate various summary statistics needed by local administrators in making reports and in planning services. Examples of summary statistics are distributions of patient characteristics by ward, by presenting symptoms, or by treatment given. Using such automated data, administrators are able to study trends in length of hospitalization, readmission rates, types of services being given, and changes in the characteristics of the populations being served by their facilities. In a similar fashion, the systems provide data to research investigators who previously had to depend upon clinical charts that were of limited usefulness because of missing information

Form MS 04
PSYCHIATRIC ANAMNESTIC RECORD (PAR)*   Read instructions on reverse side.   Page 1 of 4

Patient's last name	First name	M.I.	Facility	Ward

IDENTIFICATION
Case or consecutive number

RELIABILITY AND COMPLETENESS OF INFORMATION
?   very good   good   only fair   poor   very poor

CHARACTERISTICS OF CURRENT CONDITION
exacerbation of chronic condition   recurrence of similar previous condition
indistinguishable from past   significant change from any previous condition

Onset of current condition   sudden   gradual   very gradual
Duration of current condition
Unit   days   weeks   months   years

Precipitating stress   ?   none   slight   mild   mod   mark
drug reaction   traumatic incident   someone's death
financial   physical illness in family   physical illness in patient
sexual problems   family problems   nonfamily interpersonal problems
school problems   occupational problems   other change in life circumstances

Course since onset of current condition
worsened greatly   worsened somewhat   remained stable   variable   improved somewhat   greatly improved

Facility code

Rater code

PSYCHIATRIC DISTURBANCE IN FAMILY   functional psych illness   organic brain syndrome
Mother   ?   none   mild severe   mild severe
Father   ?   none   mild severe   mild severe
Siblings at least mildly ill   ?   1   2   3   4+

Date of admission to facility

	Jan	Feb	Mar	Apr	May	Month	Jun	Jul	Aug	Sep	Oct
1	69	70	71	72	Year	73	74	75	Nov	Dec
2	3	4	5	6		7	8	9	10	11
12	13	14	15	16	Day	17	18	19	20	21
22	23	24	25	26		27	28	29	30	31

PREVIOUS TREATMENT FOR PSYCHIATRIC DISTURBANCE   ?   none   → next section

Age when first treated (any treatment)

Status on admission   inpatient   day   night   OPD   other

TRANSACTION   first admission   re-admission   correction   deletion

Treated at (all occasions)   residential treatment   rehabilitation facility   special educat classes   outpatient partial Rx hosp   psychiatric hospitalization (not including this one)

DESCRIPTION
Sex   male   female
Ethnic group   ?   White   Negro   Puerto Rican   Oriental   Amer Indian   Other
Age

→ number   1   2   3   4   5   6   7   8+
Age at first hospitalization (not including this one)

Marital status   married   divorced   widowed   separated   annulled   never married

Total time of psychiatric hospitalizations (not including this one)
Unit   days   weeks   months   years

Siblings (living or dead)   is a twin   other multiple births
0   1   2   3   4   5   6   7   8   9+

ATTITUDE TOWARDS ADMISSION
?   positive   neutral   ambivalent   negative   very negative

INFORMANTS
physician   nonmedical therapist   school
patient   family member   friend
associate   other facility or agency   police

Set no. 0008591   Mark last 3 digits of Set number in area below

*Developed by Robert L. Spitzer, M.D. and Jean Endicott, Ph.D., Biometrics Research, N.Y.S. Department of Mental Hygiene, with the assistance of the Multi-State Information System for Psychiatric Patients Project. Supported by N.Y.S. Department of Mental Hygiene, C29820 and NIMH Grants 14934 and 08534.

Figure 36–1. A portion of an optically scanned history form.

PSYCHIATRIC ANAMNESTIC RECORD

IDENTIFICATION

PATIENT CASE OR CONSECUTIVE NUMBER   9999999
PATIENT'S NAME
FACILITY CODE   14
RATER CODE   999
RATER'S NAME
DATE OF PATIENT'S ADMISSION TO FACILITY   AUGUST 30, 1972
PATIENT'S STATUS ON ADMISSION   (MISSING)

TRANSACTION

THIS IS THE FIRST ADMISSION FOR THE PATIENT TO THIS FACILITY.

DESCRIPTION

THE PATIENT IS A 23 YEAR OLD, MARRIED, WHITE FEMALE. SHE HAS NO
SIBLINGS. HER ATTITUDE TOWARD THIS ADMISSION IS AMBIVALENT.
INFORMATION FOR THIS REPORT HAS BEEN OBTAINED FROM A PHYSICIAN, THE
PATIENT, AND A FAMILY MEMBER. IN THE RATER'S JUDGMENT, THE RELIABILITY
OF THE INFORMATION IN THIS REPORT IS GOOD.

CHARACTERISTICS OF CURRENT CONDITION

THE PATIENT'S CURRENT CONDITION IS A RECURRENCE OF A SIMILAR PREVIOUS
CONDITION. HER CURRENT CONDITION DEVELOPED SUDDENLY AND HAS BEEN
EVIDENT FOR 4 WEEKS. THE ONSET OF HER CURRENT CONDITION WAS APPARENTLY
ASSOCIATED WITH A MODERATELY STRESSFUL SITUATION INVOLVING SOMEONE'S
DEATH. HER CURRENT CONDITION HAS BEEN VARIABLE SINCE ITS ONSET.

PSYCHIATRIC DISTURBANCE IN FAMILY

IT IS NOT KNOWN WHETHER THE PATIENT'S MOTHER HAS HAD A PSYCHIATRIC
DISTURBANCE. THE PATIENT'S FATHER HAS NO HISTORY OF PSYCHIATRIC
DISTURBANCE.

PREVIOUS TREATMENT FOR PSYCHIATRIC DISTURBANCE

THE PATIENT WAS FIRST TREATED FOR A PSYCHIATRIC DISTURBANCE AT AGE 21.
SHE HAS HAD OUTPATIENT TREATMENT. SHE HAS HAD ONE PREVIOUS PSYCHIATRIC
HOSPITALIZATION, WHICH OCCURRED WHEN SHE WAS 21 YEARS OLD. SHE HAS
BEEN HOSPITALIZED FOR A TOTAL OF 3 WEEKS, NOT INCLUDING THE CURRENT'
HOSPITALIZATION. SHE HAS BEEN TREATED WITH DRUGS AND INDIVIDUAL
DYNAMIC PSYCHOTHERAPY. THE MOST LIKELY DIAGNOSIS OF THE CONDITION FOR
WHICH THE PATIENT WAS TREATED PREVIOUSLY IS PSYCHOTIC AFFECTIVE
DISORDER.

Figure 36–2. A portion of the narrative output for an optically scanned history form.

PATIENT NAME_____ CASE NUMBER_____ UNIT_____ DATE_____

```
:0:  :1:  :2:  :3:  :4:     [ ]    :5:  :6:  :7:  :8:  :9:
         OBSERVER STAFF IDENT NUMBER
:0:  :1:  :2:  :3:  :4:            :5:  :6:  :7:  :8:  :9:
:0:  :1:  :2:  :3:  :4:            :5:  :6:  :7:  :8:  :9:
:0:  :1:  :2:  :3:  :4:            :5:  :6:  :7:  :8:  :9:
```

```
:0:  :1:  :2:  :3:  :4:     [ ]    :5:  :6:  :7:  :8:  :9:
             PATIENT CASE NUMBER
:0:  :1:  :2:  :3:  :4:            :5:  :6:  :7:  :8:  :9:
:0:  :1:  :2:  :3:  :4:            :5:  :6:  :7:  :8:  :9:
:0:  :1:  :2:  :3:  :4:            :5:  :6:  :7:  :8:  :9:
```

```
:0:  :1:  :2:  :3:     [ ]   DAY OF MONTH
:0:  :1:  :2:  :3:  :4:      :5:  :6:  :7:  :8:  :9:
:0:  :1:  :2:  :3:  :4:     [ ]
         REPORTING AREA
:0:  :1:  :2:  :3:  :4:      :5:  :6:  :7:  :8:  :9:
```

INSTITUTE OF LIVING

SHIFT :1: :2:
DAY NIGHT

PATIENT BEHAVIOR INDEX • NURSING

PERSONAL HABITS
::::: WITHDRAWN
::::: HAS TO BE REMINDED WHAT TO DO
::::: ANNOYS PERSONNEL BY TOUCHING THEM
::::: SMOKES INCESSANTLY
::::: SLOW TO FOLLOW ROUTINE
::::: RESENTS UNIT ROUTINE
::::: FOLLOWS ROUTINE ACCEPTABLY
::::: NEEDS HELP WITH PERSONAL HYGIENE
::::: REFUSES TO DO ROUTINE THINGS EXPECTED OF HIM
::::: DOES ODD, STRANGE THINGS
::::: SEE NARRATIVE (H)
::::: UNABLE COMMENT

APPEARANCE
::::: FUSSY, FASTIDIOUS
::::: LOOKS TIRED, WORN OUT
::::: INAPPROPRIATELY, INFORMALLY DRESSED
::::: CAREFULLY DISORDERED
::::: CLEAN, NEAT, APPROPRIATELY DRESSED
::::: SLOPPY, UNKEMPT
::::: OVERDRESSED FOR THE OCCASION
::::: DRAMATIC, THEATRICAL
::::: BIZARRELY DRESSED
::::: LOOKS YOUNGER THAN IS
::::: SEE NARRATIVE (I)
::::: UNABLE COMMENT

SLEEPING AND EATING HABITS
::::: SLEEPS DURING DAY
::::: COMPLAINED OF NOT BEING ABLE TO SLEEP
::::: SKIPPED MEAL
::::: RETIRED EARLY
::::: NOT UP FOR BREAKFAST
::::: SLEPT WELL
::::: EATS WELL
::::: SLEEPS RESTLESSLY DURING NIGHT
::::: FOOD INTAKE INADEQUATE
::::: WAKES EARLY
::::: SEE NARRATIVE (J)
::::: UNABLE COMMENT

UNIT RELATIONSHIPS
::::: PREFERS COMPANY OF PERSONNEL
::::: ENJOYS SADISTIC HUMOR
::::: COMPLAINS ABOUT BEING IN HOSPITAL
::::: SUSPICIOUS OF ACTIONS OR MOTIVES OF PERSONNEL OR OTHER PATIENTS
::::: SPENDS GREAT DEAL OF TIME IN ROOM
::::: SATISFACTORY ADJUSTMENT TO UNIT
::::: RARELY GOES OFF UNIT ON HIS OWN INITIATIVE
::::: MUST BE REMINDED TO ATTEND CLASSES
::::: PRANKISH
::::: HAS TO BE TOLD TO COME OUT OF HIS ROOM
::::: SEE NARRATIVE (K)
::::: UNABLE COMMENT

SOCIAL BEHAVIOR
::::: SECLUSIVE
::::: CANNOT TOLERATE DELAYS OR DENIAL OF HIS WISHES
::::: MEMBER OF "CLIQUE"
::::: FORMAL, RESERVED
::::: QUIET
::::: BOISTEROUS
::::: MAINTAINS A CLOSE RELATIONSHIP WITH ONE OTHER PATIENT
::::: FRIENDLY AND COOPERATIVE
::::: RELAXED, AT EASE
::::: RESTLESS, FIDGETY
::::: SEE NARRATIVE (L)
::::: UNABLE COMMENT

SOCIAL INTERACTION
::::: EXCESSIVELY FAMILIAR WITH MEMBER OR MEMBERS OF OPPOSITE SEX
::::: IS SEDUCTIVE
::::: CONVERSES ONLY ON APPROACH
::::: OVERLY FAMILIAR WITH SAME SEX
::::: UNPOPULAR
::::: IMPULSIVE
::::: AVOIDS OPPOSITE SEX
::::: TEASES
::::: IMPOLITE
::::: PARTICIPATES IN GROUP ACTIVITY
::::: SEE NARRATIVE (M)
::::: UNABLE COMMENT

MOOD
::::: SAD
::::: IRRITABLE
::::: MOODY, CHANGEABLE
::::: SMOOTH, EVEN DISPOSITION
::::: SHOWS LITTLE FEELING
::::: SEEMS AFRAID OF SOMETHING
::::: IS PLEASED WITH HIMSELF
::::: ANGRY
::::: TEARFUL
::::: PREOCCUPIED, OFTEN SEEMS TO BE DAYDREAMING
::::: SEE NARRATIVE (N)
::::: UNABLE COMMENT

ATTITUDE
::::: SEEMS PLEASANT, YET IS OBSTRUCTIVE
::::: MAKES EXCUSES FOR HIS ACTIONS
::::: PLEASANT
::::: HOSTILE TO ONE PERSON IN PARTICULAR
::::: OFTEN DEMANDS ATTENTION OR PRAISE
::::: DEMONSTRATES FEELINGS OF INADEQUACY
::::: ARGUMENTATIVE OR UNCOOPERATIVE
::::: CAN'T MAKE UP MIND, INDECISIVE
::::: MANIPULATIVE
::::: FEELS REJECTED
::::: SEE NARRATIVE (O)
::::: UNABLE COMMENT

VERBALIZATION
::::: USES STRANGE WORDS, PHRASES
::::: LOGICAL, CLEAR
::::: RAMBLES
::::: VOICE FLAT, MONOTONOUS
::::: VULGAR LANGUAGE
::::: SPEAKS SLOWLY, HESITANTLY
::::: SAYS THINGS ARE HOPELESS: HE IS NO GOOD
::::: SARCASTIC
::::: TALKATIVE
::::: REPEATS THOUGHTS, WORDS OR PHRASES OVER AND OVER
::::: SEE NARRATIVE (P)
::::: UNABLE COMMENT

INTELLECTUAL BEHAVIOR
::::: EXPRESSES FEW THOUGHTS
::::: INAPPROPRIATE LAUGHTER
::::: CONFUSED
::::: STATEMENTS OR THOUGHTS INAPPROPRIATE TO MOOD OR SITUATION
::::: MOSTLY SELF-CENTERED
::::: FORGETFUL
::::: ALERT AND RESPONSIVE; CONCENTRATES WELL
::::: STATES PEOPLE ARE UNFAIR OR MEAN TO HIM
::::: GIDDY, CHILDISH
::::: DOESN'T PROFIT FROM MISTAKES
::::: SEE NARRATIVE (Q)
::::: UNABLE COMMENT

MISCELLANEOUS
::::: STATES NEED FOR LEAVING HOSPITAL
::::: HELPFUL
::::: OVERACTIVE
::::: WELL-MANNERED
::::: TENSE
::::: SLUGGISH OR DROWSY
::::: PACING
::::: UNREALISTIC IDEAS ABOUT HIMSELF, OTHERS OR HIS SURROUNDINGS
::::: NEGLECTS RESPONSIBILITIES
::::: UNUSUAL FACIAL EXPRESSIONS, GRIMACES
::::: BECOMES UPSET EASILY
::::: ENGAGES IN SOLITARY ACTIVITIES ON UNIT

INSTRUCTIONS
1. MAKE YOUR MARKS WITH A NO. 2 BLACK LEAD PENCIL.
2. FILL EACH MARK POSITION COMPLETELY.
3. ERASE COMPLETELY ANY MARKS YOU WISH TO CHANGE.
4. DO NOT STAPLE OR FOLD THIS SHEET.
5. PRINT NARRATIVE STATEMENT(S) ON REVERSE WHEN "SEE NARRATIVE" IS MARKED IN ANY CATEGORY

IOL FORM 1232-1 REV A 5-70

Figure 36–3. A portion of an automated nursing note for monitoring patient status.

and the lack of standardization in terminology and coverage.

One aim of these systems is to improve communication between mental-health personnel by having them use a common set of defined terms. To accomplish this end, the automated clinical forms developed by the authors for use in the Multi-State System have definitions of all technical terms on the reverse side of the form so that the clinician can consult the definition if he is in doubt as to the meaning of the term. In addition, special training films have been developed to teach proper use of the forms.

The average clinician who supplies data in an automated record-keeping system has little interest in providing summary statistics for administrators or data for research studies unless the system in some way provides him with information that will help him better understand and treat his patients. At the simplest level, the computer can remind the clinician when he has failed to provide some data important for medical-legal purposes, for example, information regarding suicidal behavior. At the next level of complexity, the symptom information can be summarized into a series of scaled scores of dimensions of behavior (Figure 36–4). These scale scores can be compared with the "average" patient or some selected subsample of patients. In addition, changes in these scale scores can be displayed, comparing previous rating with the ratings for the current evaluation. Finally, changes on a given summary scale over a series of successive evaluations can be shown.

The Missouri system has used an actuarial model to identify the likelihood of various outcomes, the knowledge of which might be of use to the clinician in planning treatment.[85] Patients with a long hospital stay were compared to those with a shorter stay and patients who eloped compared to those who did not. Using a linear-discriminant analysis of demographic and mental-status data, they developed a method of indicating to the clinician what the chances were that his patient would be in the hospital more than three months or less than three months. Similarly, each patient is noted as having either a high risk (one chance in nine) or a low risk (one chance in thirty) of eloping.

Several systems provide the clinician with suggestions for differential diagnosis or treatment recommendations. This kind of feedback, which has the greatest potential for justifying the automated-record-keeping system to clinicians, is still in its infancy. The different approaches of recent work in this area are discussed in the next two sections.

Automated-record-keeping systems are as controversial as are data banks and case registers. In addition to the issues of confidentiality and the quality of the data, other questions are often raised regarding the value of such systems.[3,96]

Are the computerized records better than the traditional records that they are replacing? A study by Klein, Honigfeld et al.[48] clearly showed that their computerized case records at Hillside contained more bits of information than traditional case records on the same patients. However, the real issue is not the amount of information but the usefulness. It may well be that computerized records provide more bits of information, which may increase their value to administrators and researchers, but that the focused traditional record (at least in some hospitals) supplies more information of use to clinicians. Some users believe that for the first time they have records on all of their patients that meet minimal standards of completeness and are legible and of value to not only the person who supplied the information but to other personnel in the facility. Others believe that the stereotyped nature of the records makes them less adequate than the records that they have replaced.

Does automation of clinical records cut down the amount of time spent by clinicians and other mental-health personnel? In systems where the automated record substitutes for portions of the usual written or dictated record, clinicians save some time by checking precoded categories rather than composing English narratives. However, systems using optical-scan or key-punched forms require a tremendous amount of clerical checking and computer personnel for processing.

```
MSER GRAPH** PATIENT NO.9999999, 8/30/72,FACILITY NO. 14,RATER NO.999
```

SUMMARY SCALES	CLINICAL EQUIVALENTS						PER-CEN-TILE	T
	NONE MIN	MILD MOD	SEV	EXTRM				

SUMMARY SCALES	CLINICAL EQUIVALENTS	PER-CEN-TILE	T
DEPRESSIVE IDEATION AND MOOD. .	XXXXXXXXXXXXXXXXXXXXXX	82	57
SUICIDE	XXXXXXXXXXXXXXXXXXXXXX	94	70
SLEEP-APPETITE DISTURBANCE. . .	XXXXXXXXXXXXXXXXXXXXXX	92	65
SOMATIC CONCERN	X	71	45
ANXIETY	XXXXXXXXXXXXXXX	72	53
INAPPROPRIATE APPEARANCE. . . .	X	62	44
DISORIENTATION-MEMORY	X	68	45
COGNITIVE DISORGANIZATION . . .	X	32	42
HALLUCINATIONS.	X	75	45
UNUSUAL THOUGHTS-DELUSIONS. . .	X	51	43
SUSPICIOUSNESS.	XXXXXXXXXXXXXXXXXXXXXX	89	61
ANGER-NEGATIVISM.	XXXXXXXXXXXXXXXXXXXXXX	82	57
VIOLENCE IDEATION	X	71	45
DENIAL OF ILLNESS	X	16	36
EXCITEMENT.	XXXXXXXXXXXXXXX	83	55
RETARDATION-EMOTIONAL WITHDRAWL	XXXXXXXXXXXXXXXXXXXXXX	85	59
ALCOHOL ABUSE	X	80	45
DRUG ABUSE.	X	86	46

	VERY GOOD	ONLY GOOD	FAIR	VERY POOR	EXTRM POOR	POOR		
JUDGEMENT	XXXXXXXXXX						43	46

	UNRE MARK	AVER AGE	QUI-TE	VERY	UNUS UALY	EXTRE MELY		
LIKEABLE.	XXXXXXXXXX						72	49

```
  **THE SUMMARY SCALES ARE MADE UP OF ITEMS GROUPED ON THE BASIS OF A
  FACTOR ANALYSIS OF A REFERENCE GROUP OF 2001 NEWLY ADMITTED
  INPATIENTS. THE CLINICAL EQUIVALENTS ARE ESTIMATES OF THE LEVELS
  OF SEVERITY OF EACH DIMENSION. THE PERCENTILE IS THE PERCENT OF
  PATIENTS IN THE REFERENCE GROUP THAT HAVE A SCORE EQUAL TO OR
  BELOW THIS SUBJECT. T SCORES ARE STANDARDIZED SCORES WITH A MEAN
  OF 50 AND A STANDARD DEVIATION OF 10 FOR THE REFERENCE GROUP.
```

Figure 36–4. Graphic output of scale scores of an automated mental-status examination form.

Does automation make the record more quickly available in contrast to the frequent delays in processing dictated or written records, which often need to be typed, corrected, and retyped? Unfortunately, in some facilities the time from completion of the input form to the availability of the computer-generated record is disappointingly long. In addition, the ability to get at the data for an individual patient or for research or administrative study of groups of patients is often more difficult than anticipated when the system is being designed. When such systems are designed, it is often impossible to anticipate the kinds of analyses that administrators or research investigators will need. New programs have to be written and debugged as the need arises.

It is no surprise, therefore, that administrators seem to be the most satisfied with automated-record-keeping systems. Researchers are divided: some are excited by the potential and have made use of data already collected; others are skeptical and doubt that the systems will be of much use to research because of the variable quality of the input data and the limitations of the data for treatment evaluation in the absence of controlled experimental design. Clinicians seem to be the least satisfied because most systems provide little output that is useful to clinical personnel in improving patient care. Improved patient care will mainly result from computer analysis that provides the clinician with information he finds useful in his understanding and treatment of the patient, such as differential diagnosis, treatment recommendations, and anticipated management problems and course of illness. This kind of output requires further research. As the next sections on computerized diagnosis and treatment recommendations indicate, there is good reason to be optimistic regarding future developments.

⟨ Computerized Diagnosis

The well-known limitations of the clinical method for arriving at a psychiatric diagnosis, especially its unreliability, have led to several efforts to utilize computers for integrating clinical observations into psychiatric diagnoses. In these efforts, the basic observations of signs and symptoms are made by clinicians. These are the raw data that either a clinician or a computer can use to arrive at a diagnosis. There are several advantages to computer-generated diagnoses. First of all, there is the value of necessarily perfect reliability in the sense that given the same data, the computer program will always yield the same diagnosis. Secondly, the computer program can utilize rules developed from a larger and more diverse sample of actual patients than any single clinician can command. In addition, the rules by which a computer assigns a diagnosis are explicit and public. Finally, empirically based rules constitute at least potential advances in our scientific understanding of the complex relationship between symptom characteristics and diagnosis.

Three basic models have been used in developing computer algorithms for translating the input symptom (and in some cases, demographic) data into diagnoses. Two of these models are statistical methods—Bayes and discriminant function—and utilize data on a sample of patients for each of whom the diagnosis is known and for each of whom a series of measures are available. From this sample, generally referred to as the "developmental" sample, an empirical classification scheme is devised. Using each subject's observed series of scores, the scheme quantifies (as a probability by the Bayes method and as a distance by the discriminant-function method) how "close" the subject is to each diagnostic group. The subject is assigned the diagnosis to which he is "closest." Because both of these methods derive their constants from a specific set of data, they capitalize on accidental features of the developmental sample and, therefore, their validation demands their application to new samples. The Bayes method has been applied to psychiatric classification by Birnbaum and Maxwell,[8] Overall and Gorham,[67] and Smith.[92] The discriminant-function method has been used by Rao and Slater,[74] Melrose, Stroebel, and Glueck,[61] and Sletten, Altman, and Ulett.[85] The latter group has applied this method to data from five hospitals in the Missouri automated-record-keeping system and developed a system for classifying patients into one of twelve diagnostic groups. The overall agreement between computer classification and clinical diagnosis was sufficiently high for them to make the system operational in the Missouri Standard System of Psychiatry used in Missouri state hospitals.

A third model, called the logical decision-tree approach, has been employed by the authors.[94,95] In this model the computer program consists of a sequence of questions, each of which is either true or false. The truth or falsity of each question rules out one or more diagnoses and determines which question is to be examined next. Some questions may specify the presence of a single sign or symptom, others may specify that a numeric score is in a certain range, and still others may specify a complex pattern of both signs and scores. This approach is similar to the differential diagnostic method used by clinicians in making a psychiatric diagnosis. It has the obvious advantage over the two statistical models in that it does not require a data base and is not dependent upon the specific characteristics of a developmental sample.

So that the reader can have an understanding of the potential complexity of the logical decision-tree approach, a portion of the first computer program for psychiatric diagnosis that we developed, DIAGNO I, is shown (in English rather than FORTRAN):

Decision 11. If (Delusions-Hallucinations > 2) or (Retardation-Withdrawal > 4) or (Inappropriate-Bizarre Appearance or Behavior + Retardation-Withdrawal + Speech Disorganization > 7) or (Elation > 0 or Grandiosity > 2) and (Agitation-Excitement > 2) or (Speech Disorganization > 3) or (Social Isolation > 7 and Alcohol Abuse < 5) true, go to 12; if false, go to 20. This tests for psychosis.

Decision 12. If (Visual Hallucinations + Elation = 0) and (Speech Disorganization < 4) and (Depression-Suicide + Guilt > 4 or Depression-Suicide > 3) and not (Guilt = 0 and Auditory Hallucinations > 0) and (Age > 25) and (Retardation-Withdrawal > 2 or Depression-Anxiety > 20 or Total Score > 50 or Agitation-Excitement > 2) true, go to 13; if false, go to 14. This tests for a psychotic depressive illness.

Decision 13. If (Female and Age > 45) or (Male and Age > 55) and (Previous Hospitalizations = 0) true, diagnosis is involutional reaction, and go to 36; if false, diagnosis is Psychotic depressive reaction, and go to 36.

Decision 14. If (Elation + Grandiosity > 0) and (Agitation-Excitement > 1) and (Auditory Hallucinations + Visual Hallucinations = 0) and (Speech Disorganization > 2) and (Alcohol Abuse < 4) and (Age > 25) true, diagnosis is Manic depressive psychosis, manic type, and go to 36; if false, go to 15.

Fleiss et al.[28] compared these three models for computer diagnosis and found that the logical decision-tree model performed as well as the two statistical models (in terms of agreement with clinical diagnosis) on a large cross-validation sample that was similar to the developmental sample. The logical decision-tree method performed better than the two statistical approaches on a sample drawn from a totally new population.

The logical decision-tree approach has been used in three computer programs, DIAGNO I,

DIAGNO II, and DIAGNO III. For all three programs the agreement between computer diagnoses and clinical diagnoses made by experts has been as good as that between the diagnoses of the experts. The first two programs have been used in various research projects for describing samples of subjects, selecting subjects for experiments, in epidemiological and cross-cultural studies, and investigating problems in classification. DIAGNO III is the most complicated of the logical decision-tree programs and uses information on both current and past psychopathology as input data, makes multiple diagnoses, and notes the "most likely" diagnoses as well as diagnoses "also to be considered." The output includes seventy-nine standard diagnoses from the American Psychiatric Association's Diagnostic and Statistical Manual. DIAGNO III is currently operational in the Multi-State Information System.

Either the logical decision-tree or the statistical approaches can be used to develop systems for classifying patients according to any typology for which explicit rules can be made. For example, Benfari and Leighton[6] describe a computer program for use in epidemiological studies, whereby subjects are assigned to the "caseness" categories of the Stirling County psychiatric evaluation procedure. On cross-validation their program had levels of agreement with consensual ratings of two psychiatrists equal to or greater than that of any two psychiatrists on their independent ratings of either detailed symptom patterns or "caseness." Future work on computer diagnosis will probably be in the direction of developing other typologies for specific purposes such as predicting treatment response.

(Computerized-Treatment Recommendations

The recognition that actual clinical practice is often at considerable variance with what is considered best by experts and the capacity of computers to rapidly and reliably assess new data based on previous knowledge have led to efforts to use computers to assist clinicians in making treatment decisions.

One of the earliest studies that suggested computer-assisted drug prescription could be more effective than "doctor's choice" of medication was that of Mirabile, Houck and Glueck[62] at the Institute of Living. They used a computer program based upon a retrospective model of the personality profile of the best responder to combined tranquilizer-antidepressant therapy. This model was developed on the basis of a stepwise, multiple-discriminant-function analysis of data from a controlled study by Hedberg, Houck, and Glueck.[41] This study compared the MMPI and Minnesota-Hartford Personality Assay admission profiles of patients who responded best to combined drug therapy with those of patients treated by a single phenothiazine. The computer program was used with a large group of new admissions to select sixty whose admission characteristics were similar to the best responders to combined drug therapy in the previous study. The sixty patients were divided into three groups, two of which were treated with different forms of combined drug therapy, with the third being treated by doctor's choice. Over the twelve-week study period, the patients on doctor's choice improved the least, suggesting that the computer recommendation would result in greater improvement.

Sletten, Ulett, and their colleagues[84,87] have studied agreement among clinicians regarding the specificity of psychotropic drugs for treating patients with particular symptoms. Thirty-two senior clinicians were given ten blank mental-status checklists with the name of one of ten drugs on each. For each item they were asked to indicate how useful the drug was for that particular symptom. Part of the sample was used to develop a formula to assign a mental-status profile to a drug. This was cross-validated with the second part of the sample. When agreement was examined for the ten drugs separately, there was only 32 percent agreement on cross-validation. However, when the drugs were grouped into three major categories (major and minor

tranquilizers and antidepressants) 84 percent agreement was found in the cross-validation sample, thus indicating good consensus among the experts. These findings have been used to develop a statistical formula for data that are routinely recorded by the clinician and reported to the computer system when a patient is admitted to the hospital. The treatment recommendation is a statement such as, "Given a patient with mental status findings of the type reported on your patient, senior clinicians in the Missouri Division would most likely give _____ of the ten drugs recommended for us."

Overall and his colleagues[68,69] have conducted a series of studies dealing with the issue of agreement among clinicians on the symptom profiles associated with differential drug assignment. They have developed a statistical formula based upon studies of actual drug use by psychiatric residents and the treatment of hypothetical computer-derived types by experts for recommending a class of drugs for a specific case. The system is operational at the University of Texas Medical Branch in Galveston. Medical students and psychiatric residents fill out the Brief Psychiatric Rating Scales and history forms on the day of admission. By the next morning, a computer print-out summarizes the history and makes drug-treatment recommendations. Overall informs us that the clinicians report that this print-out is useful to them.

J. Levine and his colleagues at the National Institute of Mental Health have developed a computer program for assisting general practitioners in diagnosing and prescribing treatment for medical patients with psychiatric problems. He gave a group of experts a list of mental-status-type items and asked them to indicate the relevance of each item for identifying five drug treatment-relevant patient types: psychotic (neuroleptic), depressed (tricyclic), manic (lithium), anxious (anxiolytics) and depressed (reactive). There was considerable agreement on twenty-eight items as useful in identifying these types. He next developed a scoring procedure that yields a score for each patient type for each subject. The score is a weighted sum of the items that are judged relevant to identifying that type. The program classifies and reports the patient type with the highest score. In addition, the clinician can get at descriptions of this or all other patient types, as well as information on the psychopharmacology of the drug, specific information for prescribing, and side effects. The program has been written for both cathode-ray tube and ordinary touch-tone phone but is not yet operational in the field.

Klein and his colleagues[49] at Hillside Hospital in New York City have developed a computerized system for classifying patients into nonstandard diagnostic categories that have been shown to predict response to specific drug therapies. The program was developed by analyzing cross-sectional data on a large number of patients. The tails of distributions of symptom ratings were searched for areas of nonoverlap in which subjects can, with relatively little false positive error, be assigned to diagnostic categories. The computerized diagnoses were in substantial agreement with carefully made clinical diagnoses and predicted response to drugs as well as did the clinical diagnoses.

Whereas the above methods for automating treatment recommendations were developed by using statistical procedures and a data base, the authors have started work on a system that follows essentially the same approach that we took in developing computer programs for psychiatric diagnosis, i.e., a logical decision-tree approach. Rather than use a data base and a limited number of psychiatric symptoms and categories, as is required by the mathematical models, we are programming the logic of current therapeutic knowledge regarding interaction between patient characteristics and drug response as it is reflected in textbooks, review of relevant research, and the opinions of recognized experts. This program will be part of a larger program called AIDS, Assistance in Diagnosis and Somatotherapy, that will be operational in the Multi-State Information System for Psychiatric Patients.

Since the logical decision-tree approach is not dependent upon a data base, new findings based on strong research evidence can be the basis for modifications of the output. In addition, the logical decision-tree approach lends itself to more informative output than is usually the case with mathematically derived models. Thus, if there is clear-cut evidence for the superiority of one class of drugs, this can be noted with the appropriate dosage range for one drug in that class. For example, for chronic schizophrenia the treatment recommendation might be: "Phenothiazines, e.g., chlorpromazine, 300 to 1500 mg. per day or some other phenothiazine in equivalent doses." However, if there is disagreement regarding various alternative classes of drugs, the output can so indicate. For example, with a severely agitated depression the recommendation might read: "There is a disagreement as to whether patients with agitated depression do better with tricyclics or phenothiazines." When appropriate, recommendations for the course of therapy will be made. For example, when recommending phenothiazines for schizophrenia, the output might be: "Start with at least 300 mg. per day and increase rapidly until symptoms are controlled or patient develops serious side effects." Similarly, untoward side effects can be anticipated. For example, "Since the patient is over sixty, the possibility of orthostatic hypotension and cardiac insufficiency should be anticipated."

The work done to date indicates great promise for the development of numerous systems for computerized-treatment recommendations. This is the one application of computers in psychiatry where the individual clinician is likely to receive the most help in the treatment of his patients. Few clinicians can keep up with recent research findings that compare different treatment modalities, and few clinicians have sufficient experience with a wide range of patients and medications to determine what is best for an individual case. Much of the current work in the field of psychopharmacology is in identifying patient characteristics that differentially interact with drug treatment. The results of these studies will undoubtedly be useful in the further development of computerized treatment recommendations.

❰ Computerized Interpretation of Psychological Tests

The time-consuming nature of the traditional clinical interpretation of psychological tests has naturally led to efforts to computerize scoring and interpretation. Computerization is possible to the extent that the rules for interpreting the results are capable of specification. The availability of normative and validity data facilitates the development of the rules of interpretation. The programs can be written so that given a new case, the data can be analyzed according to specific rules that determine which of a previously stored set of descriptive statements are applicable.

Most of the efforts to computerize psychological test interpretation have focused on self-report measures, particularly the Minnesota Multiphasic Personality Inventory (MMPI), a questionnaire that has had widespread use for several decades. A great deal of normative and validity data are available and long experience of clinicians in its use has led to many "cookbook" rules for interpretation. There are several operational computer systems for interpreting the MMPI, some of which are widely used and are available commercially. According to a recent advertisement by one of the commercially available systems, it was being used by over 800 institutions and one-third of the psychiatrists in the country in private practice.

The first operational system for interpreting the MMPI was developed at the Mayo clinic,[77] where it is used primarily as a screening procedure for medical patients. The output consists of a dozen or so statements derived principally from single-scale elevations, although some scale patterns are included. Glueck and Reznikoff[33] expanded the Mayo statements to produce a longer and more detailed report with emphasis on psychopathology. Finney[27] has developed a system that is capable of producing different kinds of reports, depending upon the kind of patient, the setting, and the needs of the professional requesting the report. One report produces a narrative in the second person, designed to be shared with the patient, by the person ordering the test. Another focuses on prediction of successful parole and the likelihood of an escape attempt, for use in penal settings. Other reports emphasize evaluation of potential for psychotherapy or the more traditional emphasis on psychopathology and diagnosis.

One of the most widely used systems by psychiatrists is that developed by Fowler.[29–31] His system was designed to simulate the kind of report that is used by psychiatrists and psychologists as a part of their diagnostic evaluation. The first page (Figure 36–5) is a narrative report that describes the patient's personality traits, symptoms, and dynamics. The second page provides the scores on a large number of scales and a print-out of the patient's significant responses to certain critical items that might be of interest to the clinician. The last page is a profile sheet on which the scores are presented in graphic form.

Research done by Fowler, as well as others not associated with the development of his system, has shown that most users are satisfied with the output and find the report useful. A high proportion of users rated the reports as giving a valid overall description of the patient, reflecting the mood and feelings of the patient correctly, and accurately portraying his interpersonal relationships. However, users often reported that psychosomatic complaints and the severity of personality disorders were overemphasized, and that some major symptoms were omitted from the report. A study of the use of the system in Veterans Administration hospitals, where the majority of the therapists were psychologists who had had considerable experience with noncomputerized MMPI reports, indicated that 72 percent judged the reports as equal to or better than the usual clinical reports. There were similar findings in a national sample of over six hundred private practitioners.

The computerization of the interpretation of projective tests is more difficult because of the absence of generally agreed-upon rules for interpretations of test responses. However, there have been some efforts to computerize the interpretation of inkblot tests, such as the

ROCHE PSYCHIATRIC SERVICE INSTITUTE

MMPI REPORT

CASE NO: 7327   RPSI. NO: 17012
AGE   0   MALE   MAR. 03,1971

THE TEST RESULTS OF THIS PATIENT APPEAR TO BE VALID. HE SEEMS TO
HAVE MADE AN EFFORT TO ANSWER THE ITEMS TRUTHFULLY AND TO FOLLOW THE
INSTRUCTIONS ACCURATELY. TO SOME EXTENT THIS MAY BE REGARDED AS A
FAVORABLE PROGNOSTIC SIGN SINCE IT INDICATES THAT HE IS CAPABLE OF
FOLLOWING INSTRUCTIONS AND ABLE TO RESPOND RELEVANTLY AND TRUTHFULLY TO
PERSONAL INQUIRY.

IT APPEARS THAT THE PATIENT, IN HIS RESPONSES TO THE TEST ITEMS, MAY
HAVE BEEN OVERLY SELF-CRITICAL. THE VALIDITY OF THE TEST MAY HAVE BEEN
SOMEWHAT AFFECTED BY HIS TENDENCY TO ADMIT TO SYMPTOMS EVEN WHEN THEY ARE
MINIMAL. THIS MAY SUGGEST THAT CURRENTLY HE FEELS VULNERABLE AND DEFENSE-
LESS, AND THAT HE IS MAKING AN EFFORT TO CALL ATTENTION TO HIS DIFFICULTIES
IN ORDER TO ASSURE OBTAINING PROFESSIONAL HELP.

THIS PATIENT IS A TENSE, ANXIOUS, DEPRESSED INDIVIDUAL WHO IS
OVER-CONTROLLED, HAS DIFFICULTY EXPRESSING HIS FEELINGS, AND IS FILLED
WITH SELF-DOUBT. ALTHOUGH HE MAY SEEM INDUSTRIOUS AND CONSCIENTIOUS IN
HIS WORK, HE IS TORN BETWEEN A NEED TO BE COMPETITIVE AND A FEAR OF
FAILURE. HE MAY SUFFER FROM FATIGUE, WEAKNESS, AND LOW ENERGY LEVEL.

HE IS A RIGID PERSON WHO MAY REACT TO ANXIETY WITH PHOBIAS,
COMPULSIONS OR OBSESSIVE RUMINATION. CHRONIC TENSION AND EXCESSIVE WORRY
ARE COMMON, AND RESISTANCE TO TREATMENT MAY BE EXTREME, DESPITE OBVIOUS
DISTRESS.

THERE ARE UNUSUAL QUALITIES IN THIS PATIENT'S THINKING WHICH MAY
REPRESENT AN ORIGINAL OR ECCENTRIC ORIENTATION OR PERHAPS SOME SCHIZOID
TENDENCIES. FURTHER INFORMATION IS REQUIRED TO MAKE THIS DETERMINATION.

HE SHOWS SOME CONCERN ABOUT HIS PHYSICAL HEALTH. HE MAY OVER-REACT
TO MINOR ILLNESSES, PERHAPS USING THEM AS A MEANS OF AVOIDING DIFFICULT
SITUATIONS. HE IS LIKELY TO BE A RIGID, SOMEWHAT SELF-CENTERED PERSON.

HE APPEARS TO BE AN IDEALISTIC, INNER-DIRECTED PERSON WHO MAY BE
SEEN AS QUITE SOCIALLY PERCEPTIVE AND SENSITIVE TO INTERPERSONAL
INTERACTIONS. HIS INTEREST PATTERNS ARE QUITE DIFFERENT FROM THOSE OF
THE AVERAGE MALE. IN A PERSON WITH A BROAD EDUCATIONAL AND CULTURAL
BACKGROUND THIS IS TO BE EXPECTED, AND MAY REFLECT SUCH CHARACTERISTICS
AS SELF-AWARENESS, CONCERN WITH SOCIAL ISSUES, AND AN ABILITY TO
COMMUNICATE IDEAS CLEARLY AND EFFECTIVELY. IN SOME MEN, HOWEVER, THE
SAME INTEREST PATTERN MAY REFLECT A REJECTION OF MASCULINITY ACCOMPANIED
BY A RELATIVELY PASSIVE, EFFEMINATE NON-COMPETITIVE PERSONALITY.

NOTE: ALTHOUGH NOT A SUBSTITUTE FOR THE CLINICIAN'S PROFESSIONAL
JUDGMENT AND SKILL, THE MMPI CAN BE A USEFUL ADJUNCT IN THE
EVALUATION AND MANAGEMENT OF EMOTIONAL DISORDERS. THE REPORT
IS FOR PROFESSIONAL USE ONLY AND SHOULD NOT BE SHOWN OR RELEASED
TO THE PATIENT.

Figure 36–5.   A portion of an automated MMPI report.

Rorschach and the Holtzman Inkblot Technique. Zygmunt Piotrowski's[73] system for interpreting the Rorschach has been computerized whereby several hundred decision rules are applied to the detailed scores derived from the test responses by an experienced Rorschach tester. The program prints out a series of interpretive statements based upon the configuration of scores. A computer system for scoring the responses to the Holtzman inkblots has been developed by Gorham[38,39] and norms for seventeen different scored variables have been established for normals, state-hospital schizophrenics, depressives, psychoneurotics, alcoholics, and chronic brain-syndrome patients. Veldman and his colleagues[106] have programmed a method for scoring a sentence-completion test where the response is limited to a single word. The output includes an overall rating of mental health.

Further developments in this area will undoubtedly involve new tests that are developed specifically for computerized analysis and interpretation.

(Interviewing by Computer

Questionnaires regarding psychiatric symptomatology, history, and demographic data are frequently used with psychiatric patients. They avoid the need for specially trained interviewers to collect this information and have the advantage over the usual clinical interview in that the data is collected in a standardized fashion using precoded categories suitable for later data analysis. The capacity of computers to branch, that is to modify the operations of the program based on the analysis of the incoming data, suggests that computers could simulate the human interview process in which answers to questions determine the content of future questions. If this were possible, interviewing by computer would have the standardization advantages inherent in questionnaires, and the flexibility inherent in the clinical interview.

A number of investigators have developed systems whereby patients can be interviewed by directly interacting with a computer. An example of such a system is that developed by Maultsby and Slack[60] for obtaining psychiatric-history data. The patient sits facing a cathrode-ray screen on a computer console. The questions are displayed on the screen and responses are made on the computer keyboard. The presentation of a question is a function of the patient's responses to previous questions.

The usual set of responses available to the patient is "Yes," "No," "Don't know" and "Don't Understand." With some questions, different sets of multiple-choice answers are presented. The patient answers the questions by pressing one of four numbered keys corresponding to the four responses. The number chosen by the patient replaces a question mark on the screen and if he has made an error or changed his mind, he can delete his response with the change button or back up to the preceding question. When he is satisfied with his response, the patient presses the "go" bar and the computer advances to the next question. If a key representing an illegitimate response is pressed, the computer will not acknowledge this. A question remains fixed on the screen until an appropriate response has been made. Open-ended questions are used in the computer-based history for obtaining numerical information such as age, dates, and time relationships as well as such alphabetic information as name, chief medical problem, and occupation. The response field for these questions is indicated by question marks on the screen that are replaced as the history data are typed by the patient on the keyboard. This enables the patient to check the accuracy of his response. The computer was programmed to simulate a rather euphoric and emotionally responsive interviewer. When the patient responded "No" to a question that had significant negative connotations, the computer responded with such statements as: "Great! I am glad that we don't have to consider that," or "Gee, I am glad to hear that."

The content of their history involves general questions concerning personal, family, social, educational, marital, and financial conditions. Responses indicating unusual situations are followed by questions eliciting specific details. At the completion of each interview the computer questions the patient about his reaction to the interview. Finally, a printed summary is generated for the physician. An excerpt from a computer summary reads:

Suicide gestures, 3 times; history of self-inflicted injury; patient has explanation for self-infliction of injury; attending physician should inquire; reasons for self-inflicted injury—feeling sorry for myself and guilty; feels has weight problem but cannot say what it is; feels can help self; feels deserves help; is willing to work to help self.

In a study with both psychiatric patients and medical or surgical patients for whom a psychiatric consultation had been requested, patient reaction was generally favorable to the procedure. Psychotherapists of these patients generally found the summaries helpful in making patient evaluations and in alerting them to inquire into certain key areas.

A number of investigators have also developed programs for the computer to interview a clinician about a patient. Shapiro, Feldstein, and Fink[82] took the DIAGNO II program for computer diagnosis and modified it. In the regular DIAGNO II program, the computer processes ratings supplied by a clinician on all of the relevant psychopathology variables. In contrast, their programmed version of DIAGNO II interacts with the clinician, asking him only those questions needed to arrive at a particular diagnosis. For example, the program starts by asking questions relevant to a diagnosis of organic brain syndrome. If the responses justify such a diagnosis, no more questions are asked. If such a diagnosis is not warranted, the program then asks questions relevant to the diagnosis of a functional psychosis. If no psychiatric disorder is diagnosable, the program will have asked about the entire set of psychopathology variables.

Their program uses an interactive oscilloscope device whereby the questions are presented to the clinician and he responds by touching the screen in any one of twenty sensitized bands under which a choice has been displayed. Using their interactive system, the amount of time taken to arrive at a diagnosis is from five to fifteen minutes, whereas it ordinarily will take a clinician from fifteen to thirty minutes to complete ratings on all of the psychopathology scales used in the DIAGNO II program.

Levine's program for assisting general practitioners in diagnosing and prescribing treatment, which was described earlier (see page 825) also operates in an interactive mode. The program asks questions of the practitioner about his patient's symptomatology. In addition, the practitioner is asked if he wishes information on the psychopharmacology of the recommended drug or a description of other typical patients who respond well to a particular drug.

Computerized interviewing can easily include tests of cognitive functioning, such as memory, arithmetic ability, or fund of information. The branching capacity of the computer can be used to present tests of increasing difficulty, until the subject shows signs that he is unable to perform at a higher level, at which point the computer could branch to another task. Just as in Maultsby's computerized psychiatric history (see page 828) the computer could reinforce the correct responses and reassure the patient when he made mistakes.

A much more ambitious approach has been taken by other investigators, such as Colby and his associates at the Computer Science Department at Stanford University. Here the attempt is to program the computer so that it can accept natural language responses from the patient as input rather than being limited to a small number of fixed responses, as in the systems described above. The initial work consisted of studying interviews of patients by actual psychiatrists when both the patient and the psychiatrist were forced to use remote teletypes as the communication mediator. In this way, all paralinguistic interaction, such as voice tone and speed of response, are eliminated. Study of this type of transcript material led to the development of a program for interviewing a hospitalized psychiatric patient. Although ultimately designed to operate without human assistance, the program now requires a human to translate the English statements of the patient into a form that is processible by the program. Depending upon the coded input, the program makes decisions regarding which topics should be explored by output questions. A series of variables are consulted to determine whether the current topic should be continued or another topic with a higher priority should be considered. Within a topic, there are a series of questions that can be asked by the computer. Before a question is asked, the computer searches its memory to determine if information has already been received making the question unnecessary.

⟨ Computerized Therapy

Attempts to develop systems whereby a patient interacts with a computer, with the computer serving as the therapist, have developed along three main lines: to apply systematic desensitization, to administer positive or negative reinforcements, and to conduct a psychotherapeutic dialogue in natural language.

Lang has developed a computer system called DAD (Device for Automated Desensitization) for applying desensitization therapy to the treatment of focused-phobic behavior.[55,56] The program administers audio-tape instructions for muscle relaxation and prepares the patient to visualize fear stimuli arranged in hierarchical order. Each item of the hierarchy is automatically presented a preprogrammed number of times before going on to the next one. If the patient feels anxious or has difficulty visualizing the stimuli, he presses a switch and additional instructions are given for relaxation. The program then returns to an earlier item on the hierarchy and begins the sequence again. Comparisons between systematic desensitization administered by DAD with that administered by live behavior therapists suggest that they are equally effective. Furthermore, the automated procedure allows for extensive monitoring of physiological data concomitantly with the administration of the therapy.

Colby's group[14,15] developed a system for aiding language development in nonspeaking children. Since such children are often fascinated with machines and have difficulty interacting with humans, a computer system might have particular advantages over conventional therapy. In their system, the child interacts with a display device that consists of an 8×10-inch screen and a keyboard whose keys, when struck, produce English letters, numbers, logical and mathematical symbols, words, phrases, and pictures of objects on the screen. In addition, sounds, syllables, words, or phrases are presented through a speaker.

The program is divided into eleven games of varying complexity. In the simplest game, the child types a symbol and the program displays the symbol and a voice pronounces the appropriate sound. In the most complex game, a phrase or sentence is associated with each key. When the key is struck, the voice utters the associated phrase or sentence. Once a child has become accustomed to some of the expressions, words are omitted from them and the child is expected to fill in the missing words.

Colby's group has used this system with disturbed children and reports that there was significant improvement in language function in fifteen of twenty-one children treated. Although there was no control group and many of the children were receiving other kinds of therapy, there is evidence that the system was instrumental in the improved language function.

A quite different approach has been the development of systems whereby the computer converses with a patient in natural language. Weizenbaum,[108] who developed the first program for on-line communication between man and computer using natural language, ELIZA, programmed Rogerian type psychotherapy responses because of their relatively restricted nature. However, his program was primarily for the purpose of studying computer-language issues rather than providing a communicative experience between man and computer that would be psychotherapeutic. Colby and his group developed a system whose primary aim was psychotherapeutic.[16] A patient converses with a computer through a teletype, typing in anything he wishes to say, using his own spelling and punctuation. When he desires a response from the program, he signals the end of his transmission and then receives a typewritten reply on the teletype. The dialogue has many properties of spoken conversation. The program scans input sentences for the presence of key characters, words, or combinations of words that are preprogrammed and responds to them with statements that question, focus, rephrase, communicate an intent to help and occasionally interpret. For example, an actual interchange between a person expressing negative feelings toward the computer-therapist was as follows:

PERSON—I DON'T UNDERSTAND.

PROGRAM—DO YOU WANT TO UNDERSTAND.

PERSON—I HATE YOU, YOU STUPID MACHINE.

PROGRAM—WHAT DON'T YOU LIKE ABOUT ME.

PERSON—YOU HAVE NO FEELINGS.

PROGRAM—HOW DO YOU MEAN.

PERSON—I MEAN YOU CANNOT EXPERIENCE WHAT I EXPERIENCE BECAUSE YOU ARE JUST A MACHINE.

PROGRAM—TELL ME MORE ABOUT SUCH FEELINGS.

PERSON—WE ARE NOT COMMUNICATING.

PROGRAM—I AM TRYING MY BEST TO COMMUNICATE WITH YOU.

PERSON—ARE YOU REALLY.

PROGRAM—HOW DO YOU SEE IT.

PERSON—WHAT DO YOU MEAN.

PROGRAM—JUST TRY TO SAY WHAT IT MEANS TO YOU.

PERSON—I THINK YOU ARE ALL GOOFED UP.

In contrast to the systems for computerized therapy involving desensitation or the selective use of positive or negative reinforcement, systems for computerized psychotherapeutic dialogue are a long way from practical application.

⟪ Computer-Facilitated Training

Many of the applications already described have great potential for facilitating training in psychiatry. The use of a common set of defini-

tions in automated-record-keeping systems has already proven of value in training mental-health personnel. The computerized output in many of these systems is designed to serve a teaching function. Levine's program for assisting general practitioners in treating psychiatric symptomatology is also designed to teach psychopharmacology. In contrast, other systems have been designed with teaching as their primary function.

Hillman[42] developed a program, THERAPY, (Theoretically Human Electronic Response with a Practical Yield) whose purpose is to teach interviewing techniques in psychotherapy. The program has been written to simulate a patient who is passive, uses denial to an extreme, and tends to ask for direct advice without taking any action. The object of the teaching device is to get the patient to respond in a manner more amenable to therapeutic intervention within the allotted number of patient-therapist interactions. The therapist codes his responses according to six types of content (e.g., interpretation, requests for history information, rewarding statement) and his affect as either angry, annoyed, neutral, pleased, or satisfied. Rather than branching to two or more different patient responses based on a given therapist response, the program assigns probabilities to the various patient responses depending upon the content of the therapist's statement and his affect, and the number of therapist-patient interactions that have already taken place. The program is written so that the "patient" responds poorly or well depending upon certain rules of interaction that have been explicitly programmed. For example, interpretations given early in the interview or taking a supportive or sympathetic approach will produce responses characterized by denial, projection, and helplessness. The computer prints out the entire series of interactions.

Such a program might be of practical value if a library of clinical problems could be developed. Students would have the opportunity to practice their interviewing skills under similar and reproducible circumstances. In addition, programs could be altered so that the responses coincided with different theoretical views of optimal therapist–patient interaction. The use of such programs might help a therapist analyze his therapeutic approach in a situation that is less threatening than with a real patient.

Kahn and Tait[47] have developed a system, CLAVICHORD (Closed Loop Audio-Visual Instructional Computer System to Help in the Observation and Recognition of Disease) that utilizes computer and audio-visual software to assist mental-health personnel in learning the basic clinical skills for recognizing the symptoms of emotional disorder. The trainee watches a live or video-taped patient interview, records his observations of psychopathology on a standardized rating scale, the Current and Past Psychopathology Scales. The data is immediately teletyped by the trainee or a clerk into a modem connected via telephone lines to a central computer. Within a minute, the trainee receives a comparison of his ratings with those of either the instructor, or a group of senior psychiatrists, and two types of diagnostic output, DIAGNO II output described previously, and output from a stepwise, multiple-discriminant-function analysis that gives several diagnostic alternatives and a probability statement for each. The student then sees a video-tape rerun of the original interview and evaluates how and why his scores differ from the standard. The system has the obvious advantages of immediate feedback, which allows the trainee to compare his judgments with those of an expert and to review the original stimulus on which he based his judgments.

❰ Special Research Uses

Several new areas of psychiatric inquiry have been made possible by the availability of computer technology. We are not referring to routine or complicated analysis of research data, which has been made more feasible through the use of computers, but rather to areas of inquiry in which the computer's capacity for analysis is central to the research problems being studied.

Just as computers have been used with great success to simulate complex physical processes in engineering and other physical sciences, so computers have been used to test working models of complex psychological processes, such as intelligence, personality, belief systems, psychotherapy, the differential-diagnostic process of clinicians, and interviewing strategies. The latter two have been discussed previously. A computerized-simulation procedure that accurately models events in the real world can be used to generate and test theories about complex phenomena. In the field of psychiatry there is no difficulty in generating new theories. Simulation, however, requires that theories be stated in a form that can be tested. If the input–output variables for the real world and the simulated model do not correspond, it suggests that the theory underlying the simulation model cannot be used to explain the real world phenomena.

Colby and his colleagues have worked extensively in this area. One example of their work is the simulation of paranoid information processing.[17] The program is designed to simulate a particular patient, a twenty-eight-year-old single man who works as a postal clerk. He has particular concerns and a specific delusional-belief system. He is eager to tell his story to interested and nonthreatening listeners. The program interacts with a human interviewer through teletyped natural language messages. The program interprets the input expression of the interviewer and produces internal (affective) and external (linguistic) responses that characterize the paranoid mode according to the programmed theory. With each communication, a series of variables such as fear, anger, and mistrust interact to determine the response to the next communication. Two versions of the model were developed, one more paranoid than the other.

The validity of the simulation model was tested by having a group of psychiatrists interview both versions of the "patient" and judge the output in terms of degree of paranoid behavior. In addition, a group of judges were asked to rate the level of paranoid behavior in the output of the computer and of a real paranoid patient. The results of these studies suggest that the simulation of paranoid processes was relatively successful.

Since psychiatric disorder almost invariably is reflected in some disturbance in communication, the study of various properties of language has been an area of inquiry long before the advent of computers. However, with computers, not only can many of the traditional procedures be automated, such as content analysis and measures of patterns of sound–silence in dialogue, but more sophisticated analyses are possible, such as the testing of mathematical models of conversational rhythm. The work of Jaffe and his colleagues[43-46] demonstrates the potential of work in computational linguistics. Their work has developed along two lines. They have developed a system of "automated interaction chronography" whereby an on-line computer listens to social or psychotherapy dialogues and/or monologues and extracts various rhythmic parameters. These parameters have been found to be reliable, characteristic of a particular speaker, and yet systematically modifiable by emotional stress, delayed auditory feedback stress, psychoactive drugs such as LSD, amphetamines or marijuana, and by functional speech disorders such as stuttering.

They have also developed systems for automated content analysis of psychiatric interviews. The transcripts of the interviews are key punched. Then the computer categorizes and counts units of verbal behavior that are specified in advance. Based on these counts, indices are derived and are used to make low-level inferences about the patient's mental state. For example, the ratio of self-referring pronouns to total pronouns is an index of "interpersonal orientation." It has been found to decrease as patients improve and become less self-preoccupied and more socially related. The ratio of the definite article (the) to the indefinite article (a or an) is used as a measure of "specificity of reference." A high ratio indicated concreteness, and a low ratio vagueness.

One of the first uses of analogue-digital conversion of physiological data for psychiatric research was the analysis of electroencephalographic data. The advantages of automation include the possibility of handling large amounts of data for groups of subjects, the possibility of detecting small differences in records that are difficult or impossible to discern by visual inspection, and the savings of clerical time in measuring and counting records. Computerized EEG analysis has not, as yet, been of use for clinical diagnostic purposes.

An example of the research use of automated EEG analysis is a study by Hanley and his associates.[40] Seventy-two-hour continuous EEG tracings were collected from a forty-eight-year-old chronic schizophrenic by using implanted electrodes. The patient had never been observed to have a temporal lobe seizure and frequent waking and sleeping scalp EEGs had always been normal. During the monitoring period the subject behaved in a number of bizarre ways, as he characteristically did when not being monitored. On the basis of detailed behavioral descriptions, samples of his behavior were classified into ten groups, eight of which were pathological and two of which were normal. Samples of the EEG readings taken during the different behavioral states were recorded on magnetic tape and subjected to comprehensive computer analysis in an attempt to define the EEG correlates. Visual analysis showed no differences. However, using computerized spectral and discriminant analysis, it was possible to discriminate among the ten groups of behavior with 93 percent correct classification. In no instance was a bizarre behavior state misclassified as normal or vice versa. If such remarkable findings hold up under cross-validation, clearly the computerized analysis of EEG data will be one of the most powerful investigative tools in psychiatric research.

The field of human-evoked potential research only became possible with the introduction of small computers into the experimental laboratory. They were necessary to extract the small, evoked potential signal from the "noise" of the EEG by averaging at each point in time following many presentations of a stimulus. However, this early limitation of making only averaging available has long since been by-passed in many laboratories that have become concerned with trial-to-trial variability, as well as such subtle problems as the fact that similar components in different trials may not occur at the identical point in time following the stimulus. The problem of latency "jitter" has required cross-correlation techniques or cluster analysis, both of which utilize the wave form obtained in each trial in the processing. Such analyses have required much larger computers than the early averaging devices and the increased utilization of ever-larger computers is a major aspect of the direction of human-evoked potential research. In addition, investigators of evoked potential increasingly use the computer to run experiments, particularly in situations where the determination of the sequence of experimental events depends on the analysis of the data obtained from the subject during the experiment.

An example where more sophisticated computer analysis of evoked potential data contributed to the clarification of a research finding may be seen in the work of Callaway.[10] He presented a series of two clearly discriminable auditory tones to normal subjects and schizophrenic patients. All subjects were told to ignore the differences between the two tones. The correlation between the two average-evoked potentials to the tones were found to be significantly lower in the schizophrenic than in the normal subjects. Presumably, this indicated that schizophrenics were less able than normal people to follow an instructional set to ignore the differences between the two tones. However, in a subsequent complicated computerized reanalysis, utilizing a stepwise discriminant analysis, it was shown that for the schizophrenics the differences among single trial evoked potentials were no greater when they were responses to the different tones than when two sets of trials were selected at random from responses to the same tone.[19] Therefore, the earlier finding of lower two-tone correlations for the schizophrenic patients simply reflected the greater intraindividual variability in schizophrenic response.

([Comment

Specific computer applications in psychiatry are increasing and there is every reason to believe that this trend will continue. The American Psychiatric Association recognized the importance of the major role that computers can play in all areas of psychiatry and appointed a task force[3] to survey computer techniques in psychiatry, to evaluate the gains and losses entailed by automation of psychiatric data, and to make recommendations to the association. This task-force report discusses in greater detail many of the issues, such as confidentiality and computer-facilitated training, that are merely mentioned here.

Despite the progress made in computer applications in psychiatry, it is clear that computers have had a far more direct impact on patient care in other fields of medicine. An examination of the computer applications in these fields reveals some of the possible reasons for this discrepancy. Whereas there are numerous laboratory tests in clinical pathology that lend themselves to computerization, with the exception of the electroencephalograph there are few laboratory tests that are clearly relevant to differential diagnosis or treatment in psychiatry. Although the computer analysis of psychological tests has gained some acceptance, psychological tests, with or without computerization, do not play as important a role in psychiatry as do physiological tests in the rest of medicine. In a similar manner, computers have vastly improved the ability to monitor physiological functions of patients during and after surgery, in coronary-care units, and in other situations where close attention to numerous physiological variables can be life saving. While some aspects of psychiatric status lend themselves to analagous monitoring, there is obviously less to be gained from computerization because the consequences of changes in psychiatric status rarely involve a threat to life itself, and the variables that can be monitored are not as clearly related to needed intervention or to outcome as are the physiological variables in physical illness.

Computers are being widely used to assist clinicians in differential diagnosis and treatment in fields of medicine, such as neurology, hematology, cardiology, and radiology. These fields often deal with well-defined disorders that can be described with a relatively small number of variables, for which empirical data is available, indicating their relationship to diagnosis and treatment response. In contrast, in psychiatry we deal with disorders that are often poorly defined, and with numerous variables that lack consensual and operational definition. Furthermore, there is insufficient empirical data available indicating the relationship of these variables to diagnosis or treatment. Although, as noted previously, considerable work has been done on computerizing psychiatric diagnosis and treatment recommendations, it lags far behind the clinical use of analogous techniques in other areas of medicine.

One could argue that the very nature of psychiatric data precludes computer use because the variables in psychiatry are too complex and subtle. This is the view of many clinicians who believe that the crucial aspects of psychiatric disorder cannot be expressed in a form suitable for computer analysis. This view is based on the misconception that only "hard" data, such as age, symptomatology, and number of previous hospitalizations, can be coded for computer analysis. On the contrary, any concept that can be operationally defined, such as ego strength, positive self-regard, or empathic response of therapist, can be coded for computer analysis. We believe that the chief obstacle to computerization in psychiatry is not the nature of psychiatric data, but, rather, the relative lack of knowledge at this time regarding the relationship between psychiatric symptomatology, diagnosis, treatment, and course of illness. This lack of knowledge contributes to controversy as to what variables to computerize and as to the value of the computerized output itself. As psychiatry becomes increasingly based on actual knowledge, rather than on theoretical speculation, so will the value of computers to psychiatry increase.

(Bibliography

1. ABELSON, R. "Computer Simulation of 'Hot' Cognition," in S. Tomkins and S. Messick, eds., *Computer Simulation of Personality: Frontier of Psychological Theory*, pp. 277–298. New York: Wiley, 1963.
2. ABELSON, R. and J. CARROL. "Computer Simulation of Individual Belief Systems," *Am. Behav. Sci.*, 8 (1965), 24–30.
3. AMERICAN PSYCHIATRIC ASSOCIATION. *Automation and Data Processing in Psychiatry. A Report of the APA Task Force on Automation and Data Processing.* Washington: American Psychiatric Association, 1971.
4. BAKER, F. "The Internal Organization of Computer Models of Cognitive Behavior," *Behav. Sci.*, 12 (1967), 156–161.
5. BELLMAN, R. "Mathematical Model of the Mind," *Math. Bioscie.*, 1 (1967), 287–304.
6. BENFARI, R. and A. LEIGHTON. "PROBE: A Computer Instrument for Field Surveys of Psychiatric Disorder," *Arch. Gen. Psychiatry*, 23 (1970), 352–358.
7. BINNER, P. "The Fort Logan Mental Health Center Record System: A Six-Year Overview." Papers presented at NIMH Conf. on Automated Clinical Record Keeping Systems, Kansas City, Miss., 1967. Unpublished.
8. BIRNBAUM, A. and A. MAXWELL. "Classification Procedures Based on Bayes' Formula," *Appl. Statist.*, 9 (1960), 152–169.
9. CALLAWAY, E., 3rd. "Schizophrenia and Interference, an Analogy with a Malfunctioning Computer," *Arch. Gen. Psychiatry*, 22 (1970), 193–208.
10. CALLAWAY, E., 3rd, R. JONES, and R. LAYNE. "Evoked Responses and Segmental Set of Schizophrenia," *Arch. Gen. Psychiatry*, 12 (1965), 83–89.
11. COLBY, K. "Computer Simulation of a Neurotic Process," in S. Tomkins and S. Messick, eds., *Computer Simulation of Personality: Frontier of Psychological Theory*, pp. 165–179. New York: Wiley, 1963.
12. ———. "Experimental Treatment of Neurotic Computer Programs," *Arch. Gen. Psychiatry*, 10 (1964), 220–227.

13. ———. "Computer Simulation of Change in Personal Belief Systems," *Behav. Sci.*, 12 (1967), 248–253.

14. ———. "Computer-Aided Language Development in Non-Speaking Children," *Arch. Gen. Psychiatry*, 19 (1968), 641–651.

15. Colby, K. and D. Smith. "Computers in the Treatment of Nonspeaking Autistic Children," in J. Masserman, ed., *Current Psychiatric Therapies*, Vol. 2, pp. 1–17. New York: Grune & Stratton, 1971.

16. Colby, K., J. Watt, and J. Gilbert. "A Computer Method of Psychotherapy: Preliminary Communication," *J. Nerv. Ment. Dis.*, 142 (1966), 148–152.

17. Colby, K., S. Weber, and F. Hilf. "Artificial Paranoia," *Artif. Intell.*, 2 (1971), 1–25.

18. Craig, L., F. Golenzer, and E. Laska. "Computer Constructed Narratives," in N. Kline and E. Laska, eds., *Computers and Electronic Devices in Psychiatry*, pp. 59–80. New York: Grune & Stratton, 1968.

19. Donchin, E., E. Callaway, and R. Jones. "Auditory Evoked Potential Variability in Schizophrenia: II. The Application of Discriminant Analysis," *EEG Clin. Neurophysiol.*, 29 (1970), 429–440.

20. Dreger, R. "Objective Personality Tests and Computer Processing of Personality Test Data," in I. Berg and L. Pennington, eds., *An Introduction to Clinical Psychology*, pp. 154–190. New York: Ronald, 1966.

21. Eaton, M., I. Sletten, A. Kitchen et al. "The Missouri Automated Psychiatric History: Symptom Frequencies, Sex Differences, Use of Weapons, and Other Findings," *Compr. Psychiatry*, 12 (1971), 264–276.

22. Eber, H. "Automated Personality Description with 16PF Data," *Am. Psychol.*, 19 (1964), 544.

23. Eiduson, B., S. Brooks, R. Motto et al. "Recent Developments in the Psychiatric Case History Event System," *Behav. Sci.*, 12 (1967), 254–267.

24. ———. "New Strategy for Psychiatric Research Utilizing the Psychiatric Case History Event System," in N. Kline and E. Laska, eds., *Computers and Electronic Devices in Psychiatry*, pp. 45–58. New York: Grune & Stratton, 1968.

25. Feingold, L. "An Automated Technique for Aversive Conditioning in Sexual Deviations," in R. Rubin and C. Franks, eds., *Advances in Behavioral Therapy*. New York: Academic, 1969.

26. Fink, M., T. Itil, and D. Shapiro. "Digital Computer Analysis of the Human EEG in Psychiatric Research," *Compr. Psychiatry*, 8 (1967), 521–538.

27. Finney, J. "Methodological Problems in Programmed Composition of Psychological Test Reports," *Behav. Sci.*, 12 (1967), 142–152.

28. Fleiss, J., R. Spitzer, J. Cohen et al. "Three Computer Diagnosis Methods Compared." *Arch. Gen. Psychiatry*, 27 (1972), 643–649.

29. Fowler, R., Jr. "The Current Status of Computer Interpretation of Psychological Tests," *Am. J. Psychiatry*, Suppl. 125 (1969), 21–27.

30. Fowler, R., Jr. and G. Marlowe, Jr. "A Computer Program for Personality Analysis," *Behav. Sci.*, 13 (1968), 413–416.

31. Fowler, R., Jr. and M. Miller. "Computer Interpretation of the MMPI, Its Use in Clinical Practice," *Arch. Gen. Psychiatry*, 21 (1969), 502–508.

32. Gardner, E. "The Use of a Psychiatric Case Register in Planning and Evaluation of a Mental Health Program," in R. Monroe and E. Brody, eds., *Psychiatric Epidemiology and Mental Health Planning*, p. 259. Psychiatric Research Report no. 22. Washington: American Psychiatric Assoc., 1967.

33. Glueck, B., Jr. and M. Reznikoff. "Comparison of Computer-Derived Personality Profile and Projective Psychological Test Findings," *Am. J. Psychiatry*, 121 (1965), 1156–1161.

34. Gleuck, B., Jr. and M. Rosenberg. "Automation of Patient Behavioral Observations," in N. Kline and E. Laska, eds., *Computers and Electronic Devices in Psychiatry*, pp. 34–36. New York: Grune & Stratton, 1968.

35. Glueck, B., Jr. and C. Stroebel. "The Computer and the Clinical Decision Process: II," *Am. J. Psychiatry*, 125 Suppl. (1969), 2–7.

36. Goldberg, J. "Computer Analysis of Sentence Completions," *J. Proj. Tech. Pers. Assess.*, 30 (1966), 37–45.

37. Gordon, R. "Psychiatric Screening through Multiphasic Health Testing," *Am. J. Psychiatry*, 128 (1971), 559–563.

38. Gorham, D. "Validity and Reliability

Studies of a Computer-Based Scoring System for Inkblot Responses," *J. Consult. Clin. Psychol.*, 31 (1967), 65–70.

39. ———. *Norms for Computer Scored Holtzman Inkblot Technique*. Prepublication no. 11. Perry Point, Md.: Veterans Administration, 1970.

40. HANLEY, J., W. RICKLES, P. CRANDALL et al. "Automatic Recognition of EEG Correlates of Behavior in a Chronic Schizophrenic Patient," *Am. J. Psychiatry*, 128 (1972), 1524–1528.

41. HEDBERG, D., J. HOUCK, and B. GLUECK. *Tranylcypromine-Trifluoperazine Combination in the Treatment of Schizophrenia*. Paper Presented at the American Psychiatric Assoc. Annu. Meet., May 1970.

42. HILLMAN, R. "The Teaching of Psychotherapy Problems by Computer," *Arch. Gen. Psychiatry*, 25 (1971), 324–329.

43. JAFFE, J. "The Study of Language in Psychiatry, Psycholinguistics and Computational Linguistics," in S. Arieti, ed., *American Handbook of Psychiatry*, 1st ed., Vol. 3, pp. 689–704. New York: Basic Books, 1959.

44. ———. "Electronic Computers in Psychoanalytic Research," in J. Masserman, ed., *Science and Psychoanalysis*, Vol. 6, pp. 160–172. New York: Grune & Stratton, 1963.

45. ———. "Verbal Behavior Analysis in Psychiatric Interviews with the Aid of Digital Computers," in *Disord. Communic.*, 42 (1964), 389–399.

46. JAFFE, J. and S. FELDSTEIN. *Rhythms of Dialogue*. New York: Academic, 1970.

47. KAHN, S. D. and D. TAIT. *Application of the CLAVICHORD System to the Training of Mental Health Personnel*. Atlanta: Georgia Mental Health Institute, 1972. Unpublished.

48. KLEIN, D., G. HONIGFELD, L. BURNETT et al. "Automating the Psychiatric Case Study," *Compr. Psychiatry*, 11 (1970), 518–523.

49. KLEIN, D., G. HONIGFELD, and S. FELDMAN. "Predictions of Drug Effect in Personality Disorders," *J. Natl. Assoc. Priv. Psychiatr. Hosp.*, 4 (1972), 11–25.

50. KLEINMUNTZ, B. "MMPI Decision Rules for the Identification of College Maladjustment: A Digital Computer Approach," *Psychol. Monogr.*, 74 (1963), 1–22.

51. ———. "Diagnostic Interviewing by Digital Computer," *Behav. Sci.*, 13 (1968), 75–80.

52. ———. "Personality Assessment by Computer," *Sci. J.*, 5 (1969), 59–64.

53. KLETT, C. J. and D. PUMROY. "Automated Procedures in Psychological Assessment," in P. McReynolds, ed., *Advances in Psychological Assessment*, Vol. 2. Palo Alto: Calif.: Science & Behavior Books, 1971.

54. KLINE, N. and E. LASKA, eds. *Computers and Electronic Devices in Psychiatry*. New York: Grune & Stratton, 1968.

55. LANG, P. "The On-Line Computer in Behavior Therapy Research," *Am. Psychol.*, 24 (1969), 265–270.

56. LANG, P., B. MELAMED, and J. HART. "A Psychophysiological Analysis of Fear Modification Using an Automated Desensitization Procedure," *J. Abnorm. Psychol.*, 76 (1970), 220–234.

57. LASKA, E., A. WEINSTEIN, G. LOGEMANN et al. "The Use of Computers at a State Psychiatric Hospital," *Compr. Psychiatry*, 8 (1967), 476–490.

58. LOEHLIN, J. *Computer Simulation of Person*. New York: Random House, 1968.

59. MCQUIRE, M., S. LORCH, and G. QUARTON. "Man-Machine Natural Language Exchanges Based on Selected Features of Unrestricted Input: II. The Use of the Time-Shared Computer as a Research Tool in Studying Dyadic Communication," *J. Psychiatr. Res.*, 5 (1967), 179–191.

60. MAULTSBY, M., JR. and W. SLACK. "A Computer-Based Psychiatry History System," *Arch. Gen. Psychiatry*, 25 (1971), 570–572.

61. MELROSE, J. P., C. STROEBEL, and B. GLUECK. "Diagnosis of Psychopathology Using Stepwise Multiple Discriminant Analysis," *Compr. Psychiatry*, 11 (1970), 43–50.

62. MIRABILE, C., J. HOUCK, and B. GLUECK, JR. "Computer Prediction of Treatment Success," *Compr. Psychiatry*, 12 (1971), 48–53.

63. MOSLEY, E., D. GORHAM, and E. HILL. "Computer Scoring of Inkblot Perceptions," *Percept. Mot. Skills*, 17 (1963), 498.

64. NATIONAL INSTITUTE OF MENTAL HEALTH. *Community Mental Health Center Data Systems: A Description of Existing Programs*. Mental Health Statistics, Series C-no. 2. Public Health Serv. Pub. no. 1990. Washington: U.S. Govt. Print. Off., 1969.

65. ———. *Psychopharmacology Service Cen-*

ter Collaborative Study Group. "Phenothiazine Treatment in Acute Schizophrenia," *Arch. Gen. Psychiatry*, 10 (1964), 246–261.

66. Naylor, T. and D. Gianturco. "Computer Simulation in Psychiatry," *Arch. Gen. Psychiatry*, 15 (1966), 293–300.

67. Overall, J. and D. Gorham. "A Pattern Probability Model for the Classification of Psychiatric Patients," *Behav. Sci.*, 8 (1963), 108–116.

68. Overall, J. and B. W. Henry. "Selection of Treatment for Psychiatric Inpatients," *Psychometr. Lab. Rep.*, no. 21 (1971).

69. Overall, J., B. W. Henry, J. Markett et al. "Decisions about Drug Therapy: I. Prescriptions for Adult Psychiatric Outpatients," *Arch. Gen. Psychiatry*, 26 (1972), 140–145.

70. Overall, J. and L. L. Hollister. "Computer Procedures for Psychiatric Classification," *JAMA*, 187 (1964), 583–588.

71. ———. "Decisions about Drug Therapy: II. Expert Opinion in a Hypothetical Situation," *Arch. Gen. Psychiatry*, in press.

72. Overall, J., L. Hollister, M. Johnson et al. "Nosology of Depression and Differential Response to Drugs," *JAMA*, 195 (1966), 946–948.

73. Piotrowski, Z. "Digital-Computer Interpretation of Inkblot Test Data," *Psychiatr. Q.*, 38 (1964), 1–26.

74. Rao, C. and P. Slater. "Multivariate Analysis Applied to Differences between Neurotic Groups," *Br. J. Psychol. (Statist. Sect.)*, 2 (1949), 17–29.

75. Reiss, D. "An Automated Procedure for Testing a Theory of Consensual Experience in Families," *Arch. Gen. Psychiatry*, 25 (1971), 442–455.

76. Rome, H. "Human Factors and Technical Difficulties in the Application of Computers to Psychiatry," in N. Kline and E. Laska, eds., *Computers and Electronic Devices in Psychiatry*, pp. 37–44. New York: Grune & Stratton, 1968.

77. Rome, H., W. Swenson, P. Mataya et al. "Symposium on Automation Techniques in Personality Assessment," *Proc. Mayo Clin.*, 37 (1962), 61–82.

78. Rosenberg, M. and P. Ericson. "The Clinician and the Computer-Affair, Marriage or Divorce?" *Am. J. Psychiatry*, 125, (Suppl.) (1969), 28–32.

79. Rosenberg, M. and B. Glueck, Jr. "Further Developments in Automation of Behavioral Observations on Hospitalized Psychiatric Patients," *Compr. Psychiatry*, 8 (1967), 468–475.

80. Rosenberg, M., B. Glueck, Jr., and W. Bennett. "Automation of Behavioral Observations on Hospitalized Psychiatric Patients," *Am. J. Psychiatry*, 123 (1967), 926–929.

81. Rosenberg, M., B. Glueck, Jr., and C. Stroebel. "The Computer and the Clinical Decision Process," *Am. J. Psychiatry*, 124 (1967), 595–599.

82. Shapiro, D., S. Feldstein, and M. Fink. *Computer-Aided Interactive Psychiatric Diagnosis Programs.* Division of Biological Psychiatry and Biometrical Information Processing, New York Medical College, 1971. Unpublished.

83. Slack, W., G. P. Hicks, C. Reed et al. "A Computer-Based Medical-History System," *N. Engl. J. Med.*, 274 (1966), 194–198.

84. Sletten, I., H. Altman, R. Evenson et al. "Computer Assignment of Psychotropic Drugs," Paper presented at American Psychiatric Assoc. Meet., Dallas. May 1972.

85. Sletten, I., H. Altman, and G. Ulett. "Routine Diagnosis by Computer," *Am. J. Psychiatry*, 127 (1971), 1147–1152.

86. Sletten, I., C. Ernhart, and G. Ulett. "The Missouri Automated Mental Status Examination: Its Development, Use, and Reliability," *Compr. Psychiatry*, 11 (1970), 315–327.

87. Sletten, I., R. Osborn, D. Cho et al. "Agreement on Specificity of Psychotropic Drugs," *Curr. Ther. Res.*, 13 (1971), 292–297.

88. Sletten, I., S. Schuff, H. Altman et al. "A Statewide Computerized Psychiatric System: Demographic, Diagnostic and Mental Status Data," *Br. J. Soc. Psychiatry*, 1972, in press.

89. Sletten, I. and G. Ulett. "Computer Processing of Clinical Psychiatric Information in the Missouri Division of Mental Diseases," *Mo. Med.*, (1968), 357–361, 364.

90. Sletten, I., G. Ulett, H. Altman et al. "The Missouri Standard System of Psychiatry (SSOP); Computer Generated Diagnosis," *Arch. Gen. Psychiatry*, 23 (1970), 73–79.

91. Smith, D., M. Newey, and K. Colby. "Automated Therapy for Nonspeaking

Autistic Children," *AFIPS* [American Federation of Information Societies] *Conf. Proc.*, 40 (1972), 1101–1106.

92. SMITH, W. "A Model for Psychiatric Diagnosis," *Arch. Gen. Psychiatry*, 14 (1966), 521–529.

93. SMITH, W., Z. TAINTOR, and E. KAPLAND. "Computer Evaluations in Psychiatric Epidemiology," *Soc. Psychiatry*, 1 (1967), 174–181.

94. SPITZER, R. and J. ENDICOTT. "DIAGNO: A Computer Program for Psychiatric Diagnosis Utilizing the Differential Diagnostic Procedure," *Arch. Gen. Psychiatry*, 18 (1968), 746–756.

95. ———. "DIAGNO II: Further Developments in a Computer Program for Psychiatric Diagnosis," *Am. J. Psychiatry*, 125, Suppl. (1969), 12–21.

96. ———. "Automation of Psychiatric Case Records: Boon or Bane?" And discussions by Bennett, Gruenberg, Eiduson; Laska, Weinstein, Logemann and Bank; Lehmann; Rosenberg and Glueck; Smith; Ulett and Sletten, *Int. J. Psychiatry*, 9 (1970–71), 604–658.

97. ———. "An Integrated Group of Forms for Automated Psychiatric Case Records: Progress Report," *Arch. Gen. Psychiatry*, 24 (1971), 448–53.

98. STARKWEATHER, J. "Computer-Assisted Learning in Medical Education," *Can. Med. Assoc. J.*, 97 (1967), 733–738.

99. ———. "Computer Methods for the Study of Psychiatric Interviews," *Compr. Psychiatry*, 8 (1967), 509–520.

100. ———. "Computer Simulation of Psychiatric Interviewing," in N. Kline and E. Laska, eds., *Computers and Electronic Devices in Psychiatry*, pp. 12–19. New York: Grune & Stratton, 1968.

101. STILLMAN, R., W. ROTH, K. COLBY et al. "An On-Line Computer System for Initial Psychiatric Inventory," *Am. J. Psychiatry*, 125, Suppl. (1969), 8–11.

102. STROEBEL, C. and B. GLUECK. "Computer Derived Global Judgments in Psychiatry," *Am. J. Psychiatry*, 126 (1970), 1057–1066.

103. TAYLOR, K., ed. *Computer Applications in Psychotherapy.* A Compilation of Bibliography and Abstracts. Chevy Chase, Md.: NIMH, 1970.

104. ULETT, G. and I. SLETTEN. "A Statewide Electronic Data Processing System," *Hosp. Community Psychiatry*, 20 (1969), 74–77.

105. VELDMAN, D. "Computer-Based Sentence Completion Interviews," *J. Counsel. Psychol.*, 14 (1967), 153–157.

106. VELDMAN, D., S. MENAKER, and R. PECK. "Computer Scoring of Sentence Completion Data," *Behav. Sci.*, 14 (1969), 501–507.

107. WEBB, J., M. MILLER, and R. FOWLER. *Validation of a Computerized MMPI Interpretation System.* Proc., 77th Annu. Con., Am. Psychol. Assoc., 1969. Washington: Am. Psychol. Assoc., 1969.

108. WEIZENBAUM, J. "ELIZA—A Computer Program for the Study of Natural Language Communication between Man and Machine," *Communic. Assoc. Comput. Machin.*, 9 (1966), 36–45.

109. WILSON, N. and R. SWANSON. "Goal Attainment Ratings as Measures of Treatment Effectiveness." Paper presented WICHE Conf. Ment. Health, Newport Beach, Calif., Oct. 22, 1971. Unpublished.

CHAPTER 37

PROMISING INTERACTIONS BETWEEN PSYCHIATRY AND MEDICINE

Herbert Weiner and Sidney Hart

❰ Introduction

IN EVERY CULTURE, the theory and practice of medicine is partly the product of its belief systems. In our culture, the education of the physician and the resulting practice of medicine is heavily influenced by the data of the biological and physical sciences, while at the same time commonly held attitudes— e.g., toward sickness, the complaints of the sick person, and old age—bias the daily interchange between doctor and patient, and, therefore, the practice of medicine.

In no way do we intend to deride the enormous advances in our understanding of disease mechanisms that have come about as the result of advances in biology. Nor do we wish to cast doubt on the need for more knowledge about human biology further to strengthen the

rational underpinnings of the practice of medicine. For it is quite clear in retrospect that an understanding, e.g., of the pathophysiology of disease processes, can ultimately lead to their reversal by treatment.

In fact, medicine has a very strong intellectual appeal to most physicians because of the deep understanding of disease processes that the great advances in biology have provided them. But the theory and practice of medicine encompass much more than an understanding of basic physiological, physicochemical, and biochemical mechanisms. For example, the prevention of illness is much more effective than its treatment. To prevent an illness requires a rather full account of its etiology and pathogenesis, as well as an understanding of the social, economic, psychological, and political factors that may play proximal or distal roles in its etiology. However, most of medicine and medical education is predicated on knowledge and teaching about disturbances in body physiology and biochemistry *after* the inception of the disease—e.g., the nature of disturbances in electrolyte and water metabolism in primary aldosteronism or in adrenal-cortical insufficiency, or the fall in cardiac output in some cases of congestive heart disease. Treatment is directed at these disturbances, and not at their etiologic and pathogenetic causes, or the general circumstances under which the illness occurred. No distinction is made between disease and illness, illness being the result of the interaction of disease and its host—the person.

In this chapter, we offer evidence that the base of medical theory and practice needs to be broadened, in part to achieve a biological foundation for it in which man is seen in continuous interaction with his environment. As the result of this interaction, devices in the brain that control and regulate bodily processes are brought into play. These neural devices are in open-loop interaction with other neural processes that transduce experiences that result from the organism's interaction with its environment. In stating this we do not overlook the presence of closed-loop regulatory and control processes that operate in the body with no apparent input from the outside world. In the past, the medical scientist has largely studied these closed-loop processes and has concluded that these are the only ones worthy of or feasible to study.

Unfortunately, and in practice, there is a strong belief that an understanding of the disturbed mechanism, after the inception of disease, provides us with a full explanation of the disease itself. We physicians tend, for instance, not to ask what it is that brought about the disturbance in the first place. Nor does such understanding tell us much about the sick human being.

For example, in the case of infectious diseases for which we have the most complete, conceptual model of pathogenesis, the question is rarely asked why one and not another type of pneumococcus "caused" the pneumonia, or why the pneumonia occurred at that particular time in the patient's life. The emphasis tends to be placed on the relative roles of the pathogenicity of the organism, and the factors that govern host resistance to it, as well as on the pathological changes wrought in the lung.

Furthermore, the fact that antibiotics rapidly arrest the disease process and the knowledge that penicillin interferes with bacterial cell-wall formation by the inhibition of mucopeptides, satisfies the physician that he has a complete picture of the disease and its cure. But what if the patient refuses to leave his bed when all signs and symptoms of the pneumonia have disappeared? An understanding of the pathophysiology and pathology of pneumonia does not provide him with an understanding of the patient's behavior.

Such a banal, yet relatively common, occurrence in the practice of medicine highlights the current belief systems, and the conceptual issues that tend to permeate the practice of medicine.

These belief systems are the result of a longstanding tradition in Western life that holds that man is a machine,[36] and that a full knowledge of man can only be furthered by an increasingly refined quantitative analysis of his complex machinery. Such an analysis requires that complex phenomena be reduced to increasingly simple elements, which can be analyzed by available scientific techniques.

This process of analysis has been highly successful for *simple systems*, but when we deal with *complex* phenomena such an analysis is not usually successful. It is, of course, entirely true that great scientific advances have been made by the analytic method, a fact that is used to support the argument that it is the *only* method to use in the exploration of natural phenomena. There is indeed much evidence that the greatest scientific advances have been made by an analysis of model systems of a simple, and not of a complex nature: Bohr's model of atomic structure, achieved in part by his quantization of mechanical motion, pertains to the hydrogen, not the uranium atom. Sherrington deduced important central, neural processes from his study of the spinal reflex and not from studying complex behavior. The control and regulation of protein synthesis has been worked out in bacteria, not in animal cells or colonies of cells.

There is, however, another Western belief system that holds that man is only in part matter and that there are distinct and clearly definable differences between mind and matter. Descartes[38] pointed out that matter was extended in time and space whereas mind or soul was not. He insisted on the absolute independence of mind and matter (body): the body was a machine and animals had only bodies and were mere machines.

Descartes' dualism still has a powerful hold on Western thought. The study of mind has become a major activity in the past seventy years and has been introduced into medical education and practice in the form of psychiatry. Because of the nature of its subject matter, the scientific limitations on the acquisition of data about one's own and other's minds, and the particular attitudes that the practice of psychiatry generates in other medical men, psychiatry has, to a very large extent, remained outside the mainstream of medicine.

To specify: first, the central problem in the study of mind is the problem of consciousness. Its study continues to remain wholly outside the realm of science, despite the fact that Descartes was wrong and that it is a good bet, according to ethologists, that at least some of the higher mammals, in addition to man, must be capable of consciousness. Therefore, animals cannot merely be machines.

Secondly, many behavioral scientists believe that there are such serious limitations on the reliability and validity of observations about one's own and other people's minds, that the study of the mind is worthless. Behavioral scientists of this persuasion believe, in addition, that man is only a machine, a passive automaton controlled by his environment,* and that only behavior and its course can be quantified.

Such behavioral scientists are, therefore, very much of the same philosophic persuasion as those who have limited the scientific

* For a full discussion of this point of view, see D. Rapaport.[130]

method only to quantitative measurement and simple elements. Unfortunately, the belief systems of the behaviorists (already described) lead them to speak of the "control" and shaping" of behavior by reward or reinforcement, or, regretfully, even persuasion. Implicit in this goal is the startling fact that the subject must attain and maintain some behavior that another has in mind for him. In the case of the patient with pneumonia, he must willy-nilly leave his bed and return home: scientific psychology has become moral philosophy.[151]

It is a fact that the kind of attitude toward the patient that has just been described is one that also permeates most of medical practice. The fact that it does is a cause of continual misunderstanding between practicing physicians and psychiatrists. Among most physicians there is an attitude, which, in part, stems from their scientific belief systems and, in part, from their training, that one does not share one's medical knowledge with patients and that one gives treatment *to* them, directed mainly at the disturbed mechanism *within* them. Most psychiatrists have learned, however, that in dealing with patients the most effective manner is to work *with* them in a "therapeutic" alliance.[154] In fact, there is evidence that a major cause of anxiety in patients, and one that can produce acute changes in physiological functioning, is an ambiguous situation such as that caused by the patient not being told what is wrong with him, the nature of his medication, the severity and prognosis of his disease, etc.

If the physician, furthermore, only sees his patient as a machine, he, the mechanic, will be the subject of behavior that stands in direct opposition to the humane tradition in medicine. If he cannot fix the machinery, he will abandon it: A phenomenon daily observed in physicians caring for the dying patient. If he is ultrascientific, he sees himself as coldly objective and removed from the patient, who, in turn, feels himself rejected by the physician.

It is, however, not our purpose to write a polemic about the clay feet of physicians, but rather to point out that current belief systems in medicine have inevitable consequences for the behavior of the physician; furthermore, that such behavior may be stressful to the patient.

The study of stress in the past twenty years is, in actuality, highly relevant to the practice and theory of medicine. It has been brought to such a state of knowledge that it is possible to document today that stressful situations may have very important physiological consequences for the organism. The onset of disease may be one of the consequences of stress. To understand why a stress may lead to disturbed physiology and—even disease in one person and not another—one must have knowledge of a patient's genetic endowment and previous experiences.

We have chosen this topic to illustrate how psychiatry, as a behavioral science, can productively interact with medicine in contributing to an understanding of the etiology, pathogenesis, and pathophysiology of disease. Such an interaction can also influence patient care and may point to new directions in medical education.

Recent Advances in Psychiatry and the Behavioral Sciences

There are, therefore, a number of possible causes of misunderstanding that might occur among psychiatrists and others in medicine. These arise to a very large degree because of the differences in attitudes toward patients, and in hypotheses about the pathogenesis of disease.

Much of American psychiatry is of the "dynamic" variety: it seeks the cause of psychological illness—especially the neuroses—in conflictual, unconscious motivations within man. And this model of the pathogenesis of neurotic symptoms has been extended to psychosomatic relationships. But it is very difficult on brief observation to infer and verify the existence of such motivations in the person being observed. Demonstrating them, therefore, to the skeptical physician is either very difficult or unconvincing, with the result that further misunderstanding is generated between the physician and the psychiatrist.

But there has also been a shift in emphasis in psychiatry because of the development of a broader perspective on human behavior and psychological functioning. Man's behavior is no longer seen as the mere product of psychological conflict but rather is viewed in a broader biological context as the result of complex interactions between genetic endowment and the environment in which the child grows up.[68] Among these interactions are those of the growing child and his family, peers and culture. The historical period in which he is raised may also be of determining influence.[44] The impact of these experiences on his mind, and their storage, "programs" him to react toward others and specific situations in his life in a manner similar to or identical with ways first learned in childhood. In respect to the practice of medicine, he may, as an adult, when ill, react to and interact with the physician in terms of his experiences as a child with his pediatrician, and with his parents when he was ill and what being ill meant to him when he was young.

STUDIES ON ATTACHMENT AND LOSS

During childhood very strong attachments to others are also formed. Such bonds have been observed to occur in other mammals, and their importance to the well-being of the organism is highlighted when they are broken.*

The breaking of a bond between human beings may have one of several consequences. The usual manner in which man psychologically reacts is with grief, which is then gradually dispelled by the process of mourning. On the other hand, he may react with depression and suicide, with helplessness or hopelessness, or even elation, or with behavior called schizophrenic, or he may "drown" his feelings in alcohol or "forget" with other drugs. Loss of another person may lead to the development of a wide variety of physiological effects and anatomic lesions: it is a setting in which peptic duodenal ulcer, for example, may occur.[168]

Real or threatened loss has also been cited

---

* See references 65, 76, 77, 87, and 113.

by many authors as a factor contributing to the precipitation of various other disease states. These include cancer,[13,58,90,97] tuberculosis,[35] ulcerative colitis,[42] diabetes mellitus,[78] and thyrotoxicosis,[91,106] etc. Schmale,[143] postulating that object loss and depression are often the setting in which disease occurs, studied forty-two patients, selected for age (eighteen to forty-five years) and to some extent for social class, who were admitted to a general medical service with diagnoses ranging from hysterical conversion symptoms to aseptic meningitis. Shortly after admission each patient was interviewed using the conventional, open-ended, psychiatric interview. Special attention was paid to a history of loss or change in relationship with a highly valued object, and the nature of the loss was operationally divided into four categories: (1) actual loss, (2) threatened loss, (3) "symbolic" loss, and (4) no loss. In sixteen cases of the forty-two, the patient either reported or the investigator inferred that a loss, or significant change in relationships to others had occurred within twenty-four hours of the appearance of symptoms of the disease. In another fifteen patients, such loss or change occurred within the week prior to the onset of illness. Thus, thirty-one of forty-two patients experienced the onset of an illness within one week of a significant loss. Another eight patients gave a similar history for the month prior to the onset of illness. Schmale also noted that thirty-five of the forty-two patients experienced real or threatened loss in the first sixteen years of their lives. Many of these persons had unresolved conflicts with respect to these events, which were rekindled by their present illness. In a later study, Adamson and Schmale[3] noted that object loss and "giving-up" were associated with the development of severe psychiatric disturbance. Recently, Stein and Charles[153] reported that almost half of the juvenile diabetics they studied in an adolescent clinic had a history of loss of one or both parents. This was in marked contrast to the experience of a group of matched controls, comprised primarily of adolescents with hematological disorders. As a result of their data Stein and Charles concluded that "dia-

betes occurs most frequently in that segment of the population in which there are special stresses and trauma in the form of a chaotic family life, separations, and early losses."

Young et al.,[179] studying the mortality among widowers, found that 213 of 4486 widowers, fifty-five years old and older, died within the first six months of the loss of their spouse, an increase of about 40 percent above that expected for married men of the same age. Kraus and Lilienfeld[92] noted that the mortality rate of persons of both sexes, who had lost a spouse, was increased and that there was a mortality in excess of that expected in those under thirty-five years of age. Parkes[124] in a study of patients admitted to a psychiatric hospital found that the number of patients whose illness followed the loss of a spouse was significantly greater than anticipated for people of that age and social group. Developing Schmale's work in the area of giving-up and its primary feelings of hopelessness and helplessness, Engel[43] has hypothesized that the "giving-up, given-up complex" is the emotional setting in which disease occurs. He estimates that this "complex" precedes the onset of illness in 70 to 80 percent of patients. As with all stressful stimuli, Engel notes that it is difficult to appreciate which external stimuli will be critical to a particular person: the determining factor will be how the individual responds—that is to say, just what constitutes a loss or threatened loss will depend upon the individual's past experience and present capacity for dealing with loss. Where a serious loss is suffered or threatened, the predisposed person may react by giving-up, leading to a state of having given-up. The most characteristic feature of this is the sense of "psychological impotence"—a feeling that for a period of time one is unable to cope with any task. Clinically, the complex is manifested by (1) the feelings of helplessness and hopelessness; (2) low self-esteem; (3) an inability to enjoy the company of other people, one's work, hobbies, etc.; (4) a disruption of the sense of continuity in one's past, present, and future; and (5) a reactivation of memories of earlier periods of giving-up. Engel believes that this state of mind may last for varying periods of time, and that it is commonplace for people to experience this complex several times during a lifetime; in situations in which prompt resolution is impossible and periods of "struggling" alternate with periods of giving-up, illness may occur.

Additional evidence for the point of view that there are psychological antecedents to illness has been forthcoming: Perlman et al.[126] recently reported a relationship between violent arguments with, or threatened separations from, family members and the precipitation of congestive heart failure. Kennedy and Bakst[88] studied patients admitted for cardiac surgery to see if their preoperative psychological state would influence the morbidity and mortality of operation. They established six categories of psychological state:

1. Patients who evidenced strong but not psychotic denial of the operation and were strongly motivated to recover.

2. While manifestly cooperative and seemingly motivated, another group of patients had settled comfortably into dependency on others and the benefits of being disabled. Postoperatively they tended to experience little or no improvement in cardiac function.

3. Another group of patients was increasingly panicky as the day of surgery approached. They tended to exaggerate the risks of the procedures and were afraid of dying.

4. Patients who tended to have mixed feelings about surgery, in that they preferred to be ill rather than well.

5. Patients who had effectively given up all hope and perceived surgery as "sanctioned suicide" that the surgeon committed for them.

6. Patients with overt psychiatric illness who exaggerated their relatively minor physical illness into a major one.

The authors found that the postoperative morbidity and mortality were highest in patients in categories 2., 4., and 5. Kimball[89] confirmed these findings in a separate study, emphasizing the negative correlation between depression in his patients and successful surgical outcome.

As yet we do not know what mechanisms lie behind the correlations just described: most of the behavioral biology of depressive states and psychological disorganization has been worked out with psychiatric patients while studying adrenal-cortical and medullary hormones. In 1963 Sachar et al.[141] reported data from longitudinal studies of four patients with acute schizophrenic reactions. There was a statistically reliable correlation between acute states of panic and disruption of most psychological functions and elevated urinary 17-hydroxycorticoids (17-OHCS), epinephrine, and norepinephrine. Peak values occurred during the acute state of emotional turmoil at the onset of the psychosis. With the appearance of an elaborate and well-formed delusional system, hormone levels returned to normal for a period of time, only to rise again when the patient was confronted with the reasons for his breakdown (such as the breaking-off of a relationship). During the recovery phase, urinary 17-OHCS, epinephrine, and norepinephrine returned to normal. More relevant to our discussion are the studies[27,140] with depressive patients that have revealed the same findings. Sachar[138] emphasizes that just as the well-organized delusional system serves to restore internal equilibrium and protect the patient from extremes of anxiety in schizophrenic illness, so does the *apparent* agitation and misery serve to protect the depressed patient from the pain of loss and mourning. Studying six acutely depressed women in an inpatient setting, Sachar and his co-workers[139] made longitudinal studies of urinary 17-OHCS levels and correlated these with observations of the patient's behavior. They postulated that if depressive symptoms actually protected the patient against the realization of loss, confronting her with the loss should provoke psychological "disequilibrium" and result in the rise in the excretion level of 17-OHCS. Indeed, this was what happened. Using more sophisticated techniques, Sachar and his colleagues[139] conclude that ". . . adrenocortical activity in depressed patients is primarily related to dimensions of emotional arousal and psychotic disorganization rather than to depressive illness *per se*" or to schizophrenia. This conclusion applied to the observations of Schmale and Engel suggests that the emotional consequences of the loss—the "giving-up, given-up" complex—is the result of a failure of "coping" mechanisms, leading, on the one hand, to the psychological reactions described and, on the other hand, to physiological change, including physical illness. Since the perceived threat of stress results in the increased secretion of ACTH (adrenocorticotropic hormone) and cortisol, and since these hormones are known to have wide-ranging effects on a variety of systems and functions (electrolyte balance, glucose and fat metabolism, nitrogen excretion, the induction of the biosynthetic enzyme of epinephrine, immune mechanisms, and the electrical excitability of brain tissue, etc.) the possible effects of this form of stress on the onset of disease may be rooted, in part, in this physiological system.

Of particular interest is the work that has related psychological defenses and other coping mechanisms, as intervening variables in the perception of an event in the environment and its interpretation by man as a threat. One may well wonder why it is that although the five manifestations of the giving-up, given-up complex described by Engel are experienced singly or in combination by large numbers of people in response to stressful experiences throughout their lifetime, most people deal with these experiences without becoming ill.

Hamburg[62]—in a paper exploring how the search for and the utilization of information in the course of major life transitions serves coping behavior—cited seventeen stressful, everyday experiences. These events range from separation of children from their parents to the threat of war, or war itself. He lists other common experiences such as illness, the birth of siblings, going to school, puberty, marriage, pregnancy, the birth of children, and migration. Hamburg notes that most of the psychiatric literature has emphasized the use of "defenses" to avoid the impact or minimize the mental pain of such experiences. But experiences do not have to be threatening. In fact, Hamburg has devoted much effort to the study of other more successful adaptive means of coping with new and/or stressful situations,

so as to allow for their integration into the life experience of the people involved.[31,55,63,64] In soldiers who have suffered severe burns, Hamburg noted that they tended, at first, to deny or minimize the nature and extent of the injury and its probable consequences, but that later a gradual transition occurred allowing them to accept the injury and their own rehabilitation. Eventually, such patients come to terms with the realities of their situation, their prospects for recovery, the potential limitations on their future lives: periods of depression and discouragement are regularly observed during this period. When permanent disability results, the coping process is aided by a sense of belonging to a "special" group. An opportunity for a badly burned patient to discuss with a physician his concerns about the injury and its consequences occasionally resulted in a dramatically improved outlook. In an effort to relieve their distress and difficulty, some patients are prepared to face certain facts and to make use of them in a way that they avoided previously . Thus, the seeking and' utilizing of information provided by another person may be useful to some patients as a means of coping with injury.

This was true of the parents of children dying from leukemia who were studied by Wolff et al.[175] After an initial period of shock, disbelief, and depression on being told about their child's illness, these parents gradually came to accept it by inquiring about it. Their sense of responsibility for the illness could be dispelled by a frank discussion of its nature, by information about treatment and, finally, by advice and sympathy concerning the anticipated loss of their child.

At each stage of this process, Wolff and his colleagues accurately predicted the 17-OHCS levels in the parents. Their criteria for predicting these levels were the "integrity" of inferred psychological defenses (such as repression, denial, isolation, identification, etc.) and the extent of emotional arousal (especially of unpleasant feelings).

They studied the characteristic differences among individual parents with the hypothesis in mind that the more effectively a person defends himself against impending loss, the lower will be his mean 17-OHCS excretion rate. In twenty-three of the thirty-one instances, predictions were made from the psychological data obtained of the levels of 17-OHCS excretion; the results supported the hypothesis that the more "effective" the defenses, the lower the mean 17-OHCS excretion level. Therefore, one of the implications of this study is that the baseline level of an individual's 17-OHCS excretion level may reflect the general "effectiveness" of "ego" defenses.

Bourne et al.[18] pursued this line of investigation by studying seven helicopter and ambulance medics who were evacuating combat casualties. They found their subjects' mean twenty-four-hour urinary, 17–OHCS-excretion level remained relatively constant from day to day, whether or not they were flying rescue missions. Their mean level of steroid excretion was considerably lower than that anticipated on the basis of their body weights, when compared with a group of trainees at Fort Dix. On the psychological side, one may conclude that an adaptation to a dangerous situation had occurred with a correlated lowering of steroid excretion levels, whereas in their comparison group of trainees, no such adaptation had taken place. It may, therefore, be that in an acutely stressful situation excretion levels are high, but that as psychological adaptation occurs they fall.

After the development of techniques for measuring cortisol production rates (rather than excretion levels), Katz et al.[85] found that in a group of women anticipating breast biopsy the correlation of psychological-criteria measures similar to those employed by Wolff et al.[174] worked better with production rate than with excretion levels. Women who showed the greatest emotional distress or experienced such unpleasant feelings as fear, dejection, despair, or apprehension tended to have relatively elevated hydrocortisone production rates, while those who were more hopeful or accepting showed relatively low rates.

Other forms of loss may be correlated with changes in body biochemistry by mechanisms still unknown. Kasl, Cobb, and Brooks[84] reported a longitudinal study of changes in serum uric acid (SUA) and cholesterol levels in men undergoing job loss. The subjects were fifty-six married men, thirty-five to sixty years of age, who had held blue-collar jobs for a minimum of three years, and who were about to lose them because of a permanent plant shutdown. They were seen by public health nurses approximately three months before and then one, four, eight, twelve, and twenty-four months after they lost their jobs. On each visit, blood and urine specimens were collected, blood pressure, pulse, height, and weight were measured, and a structured interview schedule administered for the purpose of collecting various social, psychological, and health data. Thirty-four control subjects who came from plants that were continuing to operate were also studied in the same way.

The principal findings in this study were: (1) Anticipation of plant shutdown was associated with elevated SUA but normal cholesterol levels; (2) SUA levels rapidly dropped back to premorbid levels if new employment was quickly found; otherwise, they tended to remain elevated until reemployment; (3) the more "stressful" the men found the period of anticipated job loss, the greater was the change in SUA level; (4) those men who did not wait for their jobs to be terminated but resigned in order to seek new jobs had high stable SUA levels; (5) cholesterol levels did not rise while the loss of a job was anticipated but rose during the period of unemployment, returning to previous levels only after a new job was found; and (6) members of the control group showed no significant fluctuations either in serum uric acid or cholesterol levels during the period of study.

In 1967 and 1968, Rahe and co-workers[128,129] reported a study in which SUA and cholesterol levels were measured three times weekly in thirty-two men undergoing training in a navy Underwater Demolition Team (UDT). These exercises are considered to be among the most "rigorous . . . and stressful" training experiences in military life. The subjects were picked randomly from a UDT class and observed until they either successfully completed the course or withdrew. The behavioral data was obtained by means of clinical interviews and a psychological questionnaire prepared by Holmes and Rahe.

The investigators found statistically significant (p < 0.025) elevations in mean SUA level on mornings when the subjects were eagerly preparing to take on new, challenging and often physically complicated UDT activities. A significant fall in mean serum uric acid levels occurred on days of prolonged, tedious, and unpleasant physical activity, or when the schedule was unusually light. These fluctuations were more dramatic in the group of twenty men who successfully completed the course than in the twelve who did not. In general, SUA levels were higher and cholesterol levels lower in those who mastered the course most successfully. Serum cholesterol levels generally tended to fluctuate in the opposite direction from SUA levels. Illustrative of this pattern were the changes that occurred during the first week of training when the men were most enthusiastic, alert, and generally confident of their abilities to cope with the task at hand; at this time, group mean SUA level was at its highest (7.78 mg. percent) and cholesterol level near its lowest value. By the time the training course was almost over, the enthusiasm of the participants had waned considerably as the task had become mechanically routine but physically overwhelming. During this period, SUA levels fell to relatively low levels (mean=5.46 mg. percent) while cholesterol levels reached their peak.

The authors concluded that, in response to dire conditions, elevations in SUA levels had occurred in their subjects. However, while it is probably incontrovertible that training for underwater demolition is stressful, for any stress to be genuinely distressing to the stressed individual, it must be perceived as a threat.[62,86] Thus, one might suspect that for someone who viewed successful completion of the UDT course as a personal challenge (i.e., someone who is a "striver") this situation might indeed represent a potential threat. However, the authors present relatively little information as to the precise emotional impact of this experience on the different individuals in the study and do not discuss this in relation to individual differences in SUA fluctuations.

In the closing paragraph of the second paper, Rahe et al. suggested that an analysis of serum cortisol levels in these subjects might reveal further interesting relationships between SUA, cholesterol, and cortisol under "stressful" conditions. Rubin, Rahe, and coworkers did go on to publish these data in 1969 and 1970 and their reports[134,135] provide information potentially relevant to the pathogenesis of gout. They found that, while their subjects tended to run chronically elevated serum cortisol levels, further significant but transient elevations of serum cortisol also occurred. These took place in periods apparently characterized by *anxious* (rather than enthusiastic) anticipation of training situations that promised to be exceedingly demanding. Since, for many subjects, situations that were likely to evoke anxious anticipation alternated with those associated with enthusiastic optimism about the task, SUA and cortisol levels were frequently out of phase with each other, i.e., one would be falling while the other was rising, or vice versa.

This finding may be of importance in the light of a report in 1946 by Hellman[71] that acute gouty arthritis had occurred in previously asymptomatic hyperuricemic subjects following the termination of a course of ACTH.

It had also been shown by Hellman[72] that corticosteroids have, in addition to their anti-inflammatory action, the capacity to increase uric acid excretion by the kidneys. Thus, a precipitous decline in relatively elevated serum cortisol level could conceivably result in a rebound elevation (via the kidneys) in SUA level; this might then be associated with an attack of acute gouty arthritis.

Lest we be misunderstood, we are *not* saying that loss of another person by death or separation, or loss of a job is the only cause of illness or of physiological changes. We are saying that given a certain kind of genetic endowment (such an endowment probably plays a part in serious depressive illness, gout, peptic ulcer, etc.) *and* certain kinds of life experiences that sensitize the individual to react in his own particular manner to loss, loss may play a role in a variety of kinds of illnesses. In other words, some percentage of the etiologic and/or pathogenetic variance of the illness is accounted for by the setting in which the illness occurs, loss being a particular potent setting for profound behavioral and physiological consequences in the predisposed. We also say that in the evaluation of serum levels or production rates of biochemical or hormonal variables, one must take into account the psychological state of the person, in the same manner that we take into account his posture, or at what time of the day (that is, when during the circadian cycle) the blood samples are taken.

EFFECT OF SEPARATION ON YOUNG MAMMALS

We have emphasized that early experiences of separation and loss may sensitize human beings to later losses. In view of the fact that a confirmation of this hypothesis would require an (unethical) prospective study, it has been tested in higher mammals by several groups of investigators. In these animals profound, immediate behavioral consequences ensue consisting of marked motor activity, pitiful crying, sleep disruption that gradually merges into immobility and very characteristic species-specific postures.* The long-range effects of separating young animals from their mothers on their adult behavior have also been studied: every aspect of behavior—social, reproductive, maternal, aggressive—is affected.[65,113]

In these studies, in which young animals have been separated from their mothers, her offspring usually treated her disappearance as a complex experience that could be compensated for by surrogate mothering. In these experiments no attempt was made to analyze the individual effects on the infant of nutritional, olfactory, tactile, auditory, visual, or thermal stimuli after separation. The absence of such an analysis makes it impossible to determine whether changes in or deprivation of these simpler forms of stimulation do not produce the observed effects. Because prematurely separated young animals eat less and lose weight, their food intake is possibly the most critical, uncontrolled variable in these

experiments. Deprivation of sensory inputs[165] and litter size[65] may also affect the development of young animals. Hofer,[79] using rats, found that the critical variables that intervene in the effect of separation of fourteen-day old rat pups from their mothers are the mother's milk, and, in part, an unfamiliar environment. He is also the first investigator to study the *physiological* effect of separation: It produced a 40 percent drop in heart and respiratory rate during the first twelve to sixteen hours after separation.[80] Hofer also showed that it is the absence of the mother's milk that produces the separation effect on these rats. Milk fed by stomach tube to fourteen-day old rats, left without food for sixteen hours after being separated from their mothers, transiently but fully reversed the decrease in heart rate that had occurred. The effect is rapid, produced by all three of the major chemical components of milk,[25] and is related to the amount of milk given, but not to gastric filling or distention. The effect of increasing heart rate by milk seems to depend on β-adrenergic transmission on the effector side. However, the afferent arc in the loop that mediates the nutritional effects on heart rate and the central nervous mechanisms by which milk sustains heart and respiratory rates remain unknown. The questions one might ask are: What are the afferent neural pathways, or what substance in milk sustains these rates? Or does the absence of milk produce changes in important neurochemical mediators in the brain?[114] This last question is not far-fetched in view of the fact that there are known long-term effects of lowered protein intake on brain dopamine, norepinephrine, and tyrosine hydroxylase levels in the perinatal period.[149] What still remains is to determine the short-term effects on brain amines of nutritional deprivation following separation. If such an effect is shown, different amounts of nutrition or different nutritional substances could be manipulated to determine dose-response relationship between food intake, brain-amine levels, and heart rate.

The effects of separation on the behavior of rat pups studied singly are an increase in activity and a greater tendency to rear up on

* See references 65, 76, 77, 87, and 113.

their hind legs. When studied in groups of four, there is more self-grooming, more defecation, and urination, and a decreased tendency to enter REM sleep.[25]

◖ Stress Research and Its Implications for Medical Care

So far we have emphasized work or loss as an important stress that may play a role in the inception of illness and in producing physiological changes. The knowledge derived from such studies has implications for medical care. For example, the doctor can act as a surrogate for a bereaved spouse or child. He can aid the grieving person in the process of mourning. He can support a bereaved person to ameliorate the psychophysiological consequences of loss. If he knows that a patient has suffered a loss, he will not label elevated levels of SUA, etc. as "idiopathic."

There are, however, many other stressful events that may occur in a patient's life. These include the ambiguity of not knowing the diagnosis and prognosis of his illness, the indifference of the physician, the anticipation of surgery, treatment by special technical procedures such as renal dialysis,[21,162] and being put in intensive- or cardiac-care units.[30,59,123]

Elsewhere in this *Handbook* (see Volume 4, Chapters 1 and 2) these topics are discussed at length.

◖ Other Socioeconomic Variables in Disease and Illness

We have emphasized the role of separation or loss in human life as the prototype of the kind of social situation that may be correlated with behavioral and physiological changes. Separation may have its most profound effects early in a child's life and, again, in old age. As far as we know the effects of separation transcend membership in any one social class; but, here again, too little information is available: social

isolation, as a form of separation, has been (probably incorrectly) thought to be an important variable in the pathogenesis of schizophrenia; members of the lowest socioeconomic class in cities are most exposed to such isolation.

Separation may occur through death. migration, divorce, by children growing up and moving away. It may be caused by political unrest, genocide, and war. In these situations, separation becomes the critical intervening variable between the individual and the particular historical era in which he lives. The obverse situations—political and economic stability, and a stable social structure—may be particularly conducive to the prevention of disease. A study done over a period of twelve years demonstrated that in Roseto, Pennsylvania, the death rate from myocardial infarction was less than one-half that in neighboring communities or in the United States as a whole. Obesity, smoking, and other risk factors for myocardial infarction were all present in the population. The relatives of the inhabitants of Roseto who lived elsewhere had as high an incidence of infarction as the rest of the population of the United States. The only variable that could account for the discrepancy in incidence was that Roseto had an unusually cohesive social structure, with no poverty or crime, with great civic pride, and a tradition of mutual help to neighbors in need. The family structure was patriarchal and the elders of the community continued to participate in its affairs.

Work such as this suggests that the social structure of a community does play a role in averting disease. One may not casually conclude the obverse, however, For example, even under the most dire conditions such as those of a Nazi concentration camp, the incidence of peptic ulcer and bronchial asthma was said to be very low. Oppression and discrimination may play an additional and marked role in disease. The incidence of hypertension, and, in particular, its malignant phase, is much higher in American blacks than in whites or in African blacks.

Factors other than social ones may play a

role in the etiology of essential hypertension. Unknown in New Guinea, it is a major cause of death in Japan; relationships between elevated blood pressure and the dietary content of salt have been sought to explain these observations which indicate an interaction of diet, culture, and disease.

Socioeconomic factors may play a role in the pathogenesis of disease. Overcrowding, economic hardship, job loss, and poor housing conditions, etc. may expose urban inhabitants to lead poisoning, rat bites, and rat-borne diseases, etc. The life in the city may prove stressful to those from rural areas, and vice versa. For some, success, marriage, or parenthood may prove a hardship and precipitate illness. An important variable is the rapidity with which political, social, or economic change occurs, even if this change appears to be personally salubrious or desirable: In our particular historical era, there is a "crisis in leadership" in which previously, much sought-after academic, industrial, and political roles have become increasingly difficult and upsetting for those who assume them.

In addition to the actually stressful aspects of social change or the assumption of particular roles, each individual perceives and reacts to these in his own manner: some adapt to the perception of the event and some do not. For this reason, we believe that disease is an adaptive failure, and that any one factor—be it social, political, nutritional, or infectious—is not *the* cause of the disease itself. The factors mentioned may, furthermore, interact with each other to make the adaptive task more difficult.

The view that disease is an adaptive failure to situations and experiences that either are actually adverse or are perceived as such and thus constitute a threat, and that disease is not the *direct* result of these factors themselves, differs from the conceptual model most physicians maintain. If we hold a minority view, it behooves us to demonstrate that stress and threat do indeed bring about a variety of bodily changes and to show the reader the mechanism of such change, when known. It is to this end that the subsequent material in this chapter is presented. This material has mainly been obtained by research on animals. It verifies the data already reviewed.

([The Effects of Stress on Physiological Function

HORMONAL VARIABLES

Most physicians are not accustomed to the language of the behavioral sciences and they tend to dismiss the observations of behavioral scientists, psychiatrists, and medical sociologists as unreliable. There are, indeed, many methodological problems that await research in these areas. And observations made retrospectively on patients about the settings in which their illness began are often contaminated by such variables as the effects of hospitalization, and of the illness on the patient. However, when patients are selected at risk for, but prior to the onset of, an illness, the data becomes more convincing. When this is not possible, a test of hypotheses can be made on animal subjects.

We now present data to show that stress indeed has potent effects on physiological variables. From Mason[112] we learn that there are, in all likelihood, neural and neuroendocrine mechanisms that regulate the orderly and sequential release of hormones in animals under stress. During and following a seventy-two-hour period when a monkey is actively engaged in avoiding shock, some hormone levels rapidly rise while levels of other hormones decline, and the change in levels of still others far outlast any avoidance session. For example, he has shown that urinary 17-hydroxycorticosteroid and epinephrine levels are elevated during an avoidance session. After the session, levels of the former decline slowly, and the latter rapidly. Norepinephrine levels in urine rise during the session, continue to rise after it and remain elevated for at least six days thereafter. Thyroid responses rise slowly and then fall during and after the session. Insulin levels rise only after the session, consequent to showing a slight dip during and immediately after it. Male and female sex hormones and the volume of urine excreted tend to be depressed during and for, at least, one day after the experimental procedure.

In other words, with some variations in amounts and pattern among monkeys, avoidance conditioning causes an organized pattern of hormonal release. This work does not tell us what regulates such release, nor what it is specifically in the experimental situation that sets the regulatory devices into motion As Mason has pointed out, there are several elements involved, among them sleep deprivation, the muscular activity entailed in lever pressing, the visual stimulus of the warning light, tactile and proprioceptive feedback when the lever is manipulated, the mild pain of electrical shock when the lever is not pressed, and the novelty of the experimental situation. With cogent argument, Mason discounts the importance of these factors. He believes that the prepotent stressful factor, the critical intervening variable in the experimental situation, is the emotional disturbance associated with the avoidance behavior.

Mason's demonstration of an organized pattern of hormonal release raises the question of how such a pattern comes about. In all likelihood, the changes in catecholamine levels are at first neuronally mediated, but later hormonal and neuronal mechanisms play a part in their elevation. We do not know what regulates the particular change in sex-hormone levels. One might ask if the stress of avoidance conditioning actually causes a decline of pituitary-trophic hormones or whether the suppression of sex-hormone levels is due to a decreased production in testis, ovary, or adrenal gland. If so, how does this come about?

The patterns of the release that Mason has studied are, with some likelihood, in part determined by hypothalamic and adrenal transducer cells.[176] It remains to be determined by what neural circuits and mechanisms these cells are linked to mechanisms responsible for the emotional disturbance that is, in Mason's opinion, the critical intervening variable.

In the meantime, however, we have learned that these integrated patterns of hormone release are analyzable into separate components.

For example, the biosynthesis of the catecholamines in the adrenal gland is under several separate mechanisms. These include long-term hormonal control by ACTH over three of the enzymes involved in the biosynthesis of the catecholamines, and short- and long-term neural control and regulation of the same enzymes.[10,11,12,122,169]

That such separate mechanisms obtain is implicit in Mason's work. The novelty of the chair in which the monkey sits prior to an avoidance session produced immediate effects on hormone levels not dissimilar to those produced by the experimental procedure. Furthermore, when the avoidance procedures were repeated at weekly intervals, there was a gradual decrease and, finally, a suppression of levels with each session.

In the case of cardiovascular responses to psychological stress in human subjects—and when more than one physiological measure is taken—such organized patterns also emerge. Using mental arithmetic, performed under duress as the psychological stimulus,[20-23] Brod produced increases in blood pressure, cardiac output, muscle-blood flow, and splanchnic vasoconstriction in both normotensive and hypertensive subjects. However, it was noticed that there was a trend toward greater renal vasoconstriction and less vasodilation in the muscles of hypertensive subjects. In addition, the hypertensive subjects differed from the comparison group in that after the psychological stimulus had ceased hemodynamic changes and elevations of blood pressure persisted for a longer time. The pattern that Brod and his group demonstrated is probably under the control of the sympathetic vasodilator system.[107,162] One of the main relay stations of this system is located in the perifornical hypothalamus that, when experimentally stimulated, produces a complex pattern both of cardiovascular and of behavioral responses. These consist of sympathtic vasodilatation in muscle, increased heart rate, vasoconstriction in the vascular beds (other than muscle) and an increased secretion of catecholamines.[1] This pattern is analogous, if not homologous, with that described by Brod in man.

This work highlights the need to study much of the behavioral and physiological responses to stress in order to elicit an organized pattern of change. One may then align the pattern with known physiological fact. As exemplified, known patterns of physiological change can be produced by stimulating discrete brain sites—either by relay nuclei or axons that are part of complex neural circuits with different outflow channels.

In so doing, it becomes more apparent that the brain is capable of regulating a whole pattern of physiological change that is mediated by autonomic and hormonal outputs. However, the manner in which the brain does so is largely unknown.

What we are also beginning to realize is that the brain is capable of regulating, with exquisite precision, discrete physiologic change in one or another organ function. To a large degree we owe our awareness of this startling fact about the autonomic outflow to Miller[119] and his pupil, DiCara.[39] Heart rate, systolic blood pressure (independent of heart rate), peripheral vasomotor responses, gastrointestinal motility, and urine formation can be specifically modified in an expected direction by instrumental learning in the curarized rat. They have shown that only the rewarded response changes; and that the learned response is specific to the type of response that is rewarded, and not limited to general patterns of autonomic discharge.

This work clearly is of great and potential therapeutic importance as well as of great scientific interest. It contains the seed of the possibility of analyzing how such discrete responses are generated in the brain, and how human beings with a disturbance in physiological function can be trained to correct it.

AUTONOMIC AND ENZYMATIC RESPONSES

We have mentioned that Mason found that repeated sessions of avoidance conditioning markedly attenuated and even depressed 17-OHCS levels. From work on human subjects, we know that unexpected or novel situations elicit marked physiological change. The anticipation of a task, or stress, also does this.

Where stresses are repeated, a physiological adaptation occurs.

Obviously an important variable in adaptation is the age of the animal, and his previous experience. Early experience also modifies later response tendencies and adaptations to stress.

Presumably, changes in the brain are associated with early experiences, and permanently alter the manner in which later experience is transduced. Early experiences modify both behavioral and physiological response tendencies. Presumably, therefore, during the course of the transduction of early experience by the brain, permanent changes are produced that modify later responses to stressful or other experiences.

We should like to review some evidence for this contention, and the even more impressive evidence that there are different physiologic mechanisms in the body that are responsible for bodily changes, depending on the duration of the stress.

Very acute stress, preparation for activity, and novel experiences is now known to be divided into anticipatory[48,112,167] and reactive phases[48,167] that are associated with increases in systolic blood pressure, heart rate, and catecholamine and steroid excretion,[29,163] etc. In all likelihood these changes are largely mediated neuronally. The mechanism underlying the increase in catecholamines, especially norepinephrine secretion (see Von Euler's Figure One[163]) appears to be due to a sharp increase in norepinephrine synthesis from tyrosine[28,145] but not Dopa, when an increase in sympathetic nerve activity occurs. However, no increase in tyrosine hydroxylase (TH) activity occurs, so that either no new enzyme is formed or formation is inhibited by norepinephrine.[9]

The absence of change in TH content of tissue during acute stresses or stimulation stands in contrast to the change that is produced by sustained stress or sympathetic nerve activity.

Thoenen, Mueller, and Axelrod had shown that a reflex increase in sympathetic nerve activity over several days produced a marked increase in TH activity in the adrenal gland of the rat, and in the superior cervical ganglion and in the brainstem of the rabbit.[120,157] The activity of phenylethanolamine-N-methyl transferase (PNMT) is also increased.[159] By a number of experimental procedures, Axelrod and his co-workers have shown that the changes in content of these enzymes in the adrenal gland and in the superior cervical ganglion is not only neuronally mediated[157,158,160] but depends on the formation of new protein.[121] In other words, they have shown that the increase in TH activity is transsynaptically induced.

The increase of PNMT produced by neuronal activity is, however, also under the control of ACTH.[177] It depends on new protein (enzyme) synthesis and occurs even after hypophysectomy and the administration of ACTH. To a much lesser degree, the two other biosynthetic enzymes, TH and dopamine β-hydroxylase, are similarly controlled.[11]

That these changes in enzyme activity with sustained neuronal activity are not only the product of the laboratory is attested to by the exquisite work of Henry and his co-workers.[73,75] This work confirms the fact that chronic stress produces marked changes in the biosynthetic enzymes of norepinephrine, but, in addition, it produces correlated changes in blood pressure and renal pathology.

Henry and his co-workers' results have been confirmed by the use of the restraint technic.[146] Further evidence for the dually mediated changes in adrenal enzyme content has been obtained. Other work, using this method, begins to provide insight into some of the possible brain mechanisms mediating these changes.

Restraint of animals is also an excellent method for producing gastric ulcers and, therefore, for working out some of the mechanisms by which stress promotes an anatomic lesion.[17,24] Many of the experimental parameters and characteristics of the animals that promote or prevent the development of the gastric lesions have been worked out, and were ably reviewed recently by Ader.[5]

But, one finding is of central importance because it attests to the importance of the interaction of an experience—in this case, restraint—with the state of the organism. Ader[5,6] found that his rats were significantly more likely to develop gastric ulcers when immobilized during the peak, rather than the trough, of the activity cycle.

Restraint—immobilization also has potent effects on the peripheral and central content of biogenic amines. Kvetnansky and Mikulaj[94] have shown in rats that immobilization for ninety minutes produces an increased excretion level of norepinephrine and epinephrine associated with a decrease in adrenal epinephrine (but not norepinephrine) content, which persisted for twenty-four hours after its conclusion. With persistent immobilization, adrenal epinephrine content was unaffected, but norepinephrine content increased, while the urinary excretion of epinephrine remained elevated. These results suggest that the adrenal medulla enhances its ability to replace released epinephrine with repeated immobilization stress. This "adaptation" to stress appears to be due to a neuronally dependent elevation of TH and PNMT in the adrenal medulla.[95] When immobilization is stopped, TH levels diminish with a half life of about three days.

Following the end of immobilization, there is a latency period of about six hours for levels of TH and PNMT to become elevated. Further elevations of levels occur in the next seven days of immobilization, but after six weeks of daily immobilization no further increases occur.

The long-term increase in catecholamine levels in the adrenal medulla produced by immobilization are not only neuronally dependent but are *also* under the control of ACTH. After hypophysectomy, depletion of adrenal epinephrine levels with restraint is greater than in control animals, and levels of TH and PNMT fall. On repeated immobilization, TH levels but not PNMT in hypophysectomized rats do, however, rise but never to control levels. The rise in TH levels in operated rats is neuronally dependent in the main, while the rise in PNMT and some of the rise in TH levels depends almost entirely on administered ACTH prior to stress.[93]

On the other hand, serum dopamine-β-hydroxylase, which transforms dopamine into norepinephrine, was increased after one thirty-minute immobilization of rats, and continues to increase with daily immobilization for a week. The source of this increase is not, however, the adrenal gland but sympathetic nerves.[170]

Immobilization stress of three hours also significantly accelerates the disappearance of radioactive norepinephrine from the heart and kidney.[133] The question of how immobilization stress is centrally translated into these neuronally and hormonally dependent, peripheral changes is unanswered except for some very interesting work by the Welchs.[173] They showed that restraint stress can cause a greater elevation of *brain* norepinephrine and serotonin in mice who previously had spent eight to twelve weeks in isolation when compared to litter mates housed in groups.

This elevation of brain amines occurs despite the fact that the isolated mice have slower, baseline turnover of brain biogenic amines than those housed with others.

This work has several important implications. The isolated mice were more hyperexcitable behaviorally than the housed controls. In other words, previous experience affected behavioral response tendencies, while the finding of different turnover rates and greater elevations with immobilization clearly indicates that previous experience may lead to individual differences in brain amines as well as in behavior.

Restraint and exposure to cold alone, and in combination, also affect other brain amines. Histamine levels in the hypothalamus and cerebral cortex of rats are depleted significantly in the first two hours of these "stresses." Apparently, there is an initial and marked enhancement of synthesis that cannot keep pace with the rate of release and destruction of the amine, leading to depletion of levels.[156]

The series of experiments that have helped to elucidate the different effects of stress and some of the mechanisms responsible for them add important links in the chain of events in the brain associated with stress.

The Effect of Early Experience on Later Responses to Stress

In reviewing the Welchs' work, it becomes apparent that the earlier experience (isolation) of an animal not only determines his behavior (such as hyperexcitability) but also causes larger elevations of biogenic amine levels in the brain when the animal is restrained. Such data implies that early experiences determine later responses to stress, and thus *provide a beginning basis for understanding individual differences in behavioral and physiological response tendencies to stress*.

Further evidence for this statement can be found in Henry et al.'s paper[74] dealing with responses to the stress of social confrontation with members of the animal's own species in animals with different previous experiences.

They showed that the effects of mixing males from different boxes, of aggregating them in small boxes, of exposing mice to a cat for many months, and of producing territorial conflict in mixed males and females resulted in sustained elevations of systolic blood pressure, arteriosclerosis, and an interstitial nephritis; higher levels of systolic blood pressure were achieved by male rather than by female mice who also failed to reproduce under such conditions. If male mice were castrated minimal elevations in blood pressure occurred, while in those given reserpine minimal decrease in blood pressure resulted. Previous, that is, early experiences of living together attenuated the effects on blood pressure of experimentally induced aggregation and territorial conflict. On the other hand, isolation of animals from each other after weaning and to maturity exacerbated the effects of crowding on blood-pressure levels.

Recently Axelrod et al.[12] and Henry et al.[75] reported that the socially isolated mice showed a decreased activity of TH and PNMT activity in the adrenal gland in the baseline state. When these animals were now crowded together, the effect was to increase the activity of these enzymes—an increase significantly greater than in those accustomed to crowding.

The activity of both enzymes, of monoamine oxidase, and the contents of noradrenaline and adrenaline in the adrenal gland were greater in these previously isolated animals who were in constant contact with each other than in animals who were conventionally housed, i.e., crowded, but never isolated.

In other words, in the brain amine and adrenal gland enzyme levels of socially isolated animals are lower than in animals housed together, but under stress a marked reactive "overshooting" in activity occurs.

It seems likely, therefore, that responses to stress are, in part, determined by previous experiences. Individual response tendencies are then produced that have their biochemical correlates. The search for the biochemical correlates of individual response tendencies seems to be predicated on the technical development of measuring enzyme levels, rather than the products of biosynthesis. As the work reviewed attests, a substance such as epinephrine can remain at normal levels in the urine despite prolonged or repeated stress, while the relevant enzyme levels in the adrenal gland have increased substantially.

We still do not know very much about how early experiences interact with a schedule of maturational changes in the brain. There is evidence to suggest that permanent changes in behavior or of physiological function regulated by the brain can only be accomplished during "critical" periods of development. We know little about what such periods represent in terms of brain function. In fact, a major, unexplored area of neurobiology is the study of the interaction of experience with the biochemical and physiologic maturation of the brain. For example, there appears to be a maturational sequence for brain biogenic amines; Glowinski et al.[57] showed that after the eleventh day of life, the rat rapidly develops the capacity to excrete norepinephrine and its metabolites with an efficiency approaching the adult. They also showed that the blood-brain barrier to norepinephrine is present at birth.

Endogenous levels of brain norepinephrine rise rapidly in the second week of the rat's life, so that after twelve days they are only slightly lower than levels at twenty-four days and in adulthood, but are quite noticeably influenced by external factors such as nutrition.[149]

In the future, one might study the effects of separating young animals at different ages on amine, RNA, DNA, amino acid, etc. levels. For example, separating rat pups from their mothers produces significant alterations in brain levels of free amino acids and acetyl cholinesterase in two days.

The work we have just reviewed suggests that physiological responses to stress are, in part, determined by early experience. Generally speaking, in medicine very little attention is paid to the personal (in contrast to the medical) history of the patient prior to hospitalization. Nor is there much inquiry directed at the immediate history of the sick person just prior to his admission. So far we have reviewed recent data on the social conditions in which animals are reared and how these determine later biobehavioral responses. Additional evidence suggests that experiences in intrauterine and early life affect other important physiological systems.

Milkovic and Milkovic have shown that adrenalectomy of the mother rat prior to parturition[117] or unilateral ligation of the fallopian tube prior to conception[118] results in the offspring's being capable of giving an adrenal response to severe stress as early as one or two days after birth. Thoman and Levine[161] have done work that suggests that changes in adrenocortical activity during both prenatal and early postnatal life can affect subsequent patterns of neuroendocrine response in the adult organism. They showed that the newborn rat pups of mothers adrenalectomized prior to conception had hypertrophied adrenal glands and higher plasma corticosterone levels than the offspring of normal mothers. Moreover, as adults these two groups of rats showed different responses to stress, the offspring of adrenalectomized mothers showing significantly higher hormonal levels than the offspring of normal mothers. Thoman and Levine viewed these differences as almost exclusively due to prenatal effects, since switching the litters of adrenalectomized and nonadrenalectomized mother rats had no effect on the differences in adrenal function in the offspring, despite the fact that adrenalectomized mothers lactate less. Thus, the effects of the maternal adrenalectomy on the offspring must have occurred *in utero*.

There is a large body of evidence on the effects of early life events on the adrenal-cortical response to stress. Levine et al.[103] showed that rats handled as infants had a more marked adrenal-cortical response when exposed to cold in adulthood than did unmanipulated litter mates. This was also true[99] for rats exposed to a brief electric shock in adulthood after neonatal handling. They observed a significantly greater and more sustained increase in plasma corticoids as compared with unhandled controls, despite the fact that not only were the resting plasma levels of corticoids the same for both groups but the weights of the adrenal glands did not differ. When less drastic stresses were used, neonatally handled rats had a less marked adrenal-cortical response than control animals that had not been gentled. When exposed to an open-field trial for three minutes in adulthood, the handled rats showed some increase in plasma corticoids but significantly less than the control animals.[105] To explain these seemingly inconsistent findings, Levine postulated that one of the major consequences of handling young rats "is to endow the organism with the capacity to make finer discriminations concerning relevant aspects of the environment. The animal then is able to make responses more appropriate to the demands of the environment including appropriate responses to stress."

Just how these experiences permanently alter the function of the adrenal cortex so that the adult shows a greater repertoire of adrenal responses is unknown. There does appear to be a general acceleration of maturation as a result of handling.[100] Body hair, the opening of the eyes, and the beginning of adequate locomotion appeared from one to four days earlier in the stimulated animal. It is also likely that the onset of puberty was hastened, and that myelinization of tracts in the CNS was accelerated as a result of handling. Early

handling of rats altered the responsivity of the pituitary-adrenal-cortical axis.[37,101] When rats were handled in the first two days of life, an increase in circulating corticoids occurred. Further evaluations were seen when such animals were stressed on the third day of life, i.e., a time in which such animals were once considered to be nonresponsive to stress. Ader[7] demonstrated that early handling or exposure to shock accelerated the maturation of the twenty-four-hour adrenocortical rhythm. Rats reared under twelve-hour alternating periods of light and dark were killed at times corresponding to the periods at which maximum or minimum plasma corticosterone concentrations occur in mature animals. The characteristic twenty-four-hour adrenocortical rhythm was observed to develop at least five days earlier in rats who had been stimulated either by shock or handling.

It has been postulated by two groups of investigators[142,152,178] that the control of the endocrine system in the adult is partially accomplished by a feedback mechanism or "hormonostat." This mechanism would constantly "monitor" levels of plasma corticoids, compare these levels with a controlling "set point," and adjust ACTH secretion according to the plasma level. The crucial feature of this regulatory system requires that the "set point" not be fixed, but rather that it varies according to the metabolic demands placed upon the organism. Since the sensitivity of such a regulatory mechanism could be determined by a number of variables, among which are stressful early experiences during a critical period of development, it is possible that early experiences may allow for more graded and versatile responses. This could explain why stimulated rats showed a moderate increase in steroid output when placed in an open-field situation, and a large and rapid increase when subjected to electroshock. Unstimulated animals tended to react hormonally in a more sterotyped way, with large increases in hormone levels in response to change because of a more limited "hormonostatic" repertoire.

Sensory input to the brain, from handling, for example, may alter its maturation. (Obversely, sensory deprivation may impair levels of neurotransmitter substances in the brain.) In 1933, Langworthy[96] observed that visual stimulation accelerates myelinization in the optic tracts of premature and term infants. Other workers[47,147] have shown that a flashing light in a cat's eye will increase the blood flow, temperature, and metabolism specifically in the occipital cortex, lateral geniculate body, and optic radiations, while olfactory stimulation produced similar changes in the olfactory cortex.[131] Dehydration, a stimulus to antidiuretic hormone secretion, has been shown to cause a large increase in the ribonucleic acid[41] and acetyl cholinesterase contents[125] of the supraoptic and paraventricular nuclei of young rabbits.

In other words, early experience, including sensory stimulation, affects a wide variety of brain mechanisms. Much is now known about the mediating role of the hypothalamus in the release of pituitary hormones. Inputs to the hypothalamus from sensory pathways from the thalamus and basal ganglia and limbic systems are recognized. The neural mechanisms for the integration of a variety of hormonal and neural inputs are to be found in the hypothalamus.

In fact, one may infer from Mason's work on the effects of stress on a variety of hormones that hypothalamic mechanisms exist that are responsible for the regulated release of most hormones.

Admittedly, most of the attention in the past two decades has been focused on the secretion of cortisol by the adrenal cortex, which secretion is the final step in a series of processes probably beginning in the cerebral cortex and involving the limbic system, the hypothalamus, and the pituitary gland.[16,60,111] As a result of this work, new concepts about the relationship of the CNS to the endocrine system have developed. It is believed that the brain and the endocrine glands comprise a thoroughly integrated system that coordinates the organism's responses to alterations both in its external and internal environment. Under the influence of stressful stimuli, a sequence of events is believed to occur that terminates by the activation of hypothalamic "transducer" cells. These cells respond to neural input by

the release of a putative, amine transmitter with the release of a polypeptide, similar to pitressin in structure. This polypeptide is called the corticotropin releasing factor (CRF). CRF reaches the anterior portion of the pituitary gland via the portal-venous system around the hypophysial stalk at the median eminence, and ACTH is released to stimulate the adrenal gland to produce cortisol. The degree to which the system is activated may depend upon the degree of stress and its duration. Despite the fact that a negative "feedback loop" exists between the adrenal cortex and the anterior pituitary, mediated by circulating levels of cortisol, persistent neural input will result in the continued release of CRF and ACTH despite elevated cortisol levels. Individual differences in animals in the nature and duration of the cortisol response to stress may be due to early experiences. Mason and Hamburg have observed individual differences in 17-OHCS excretion in man that are consistent over months and through several stressful experiences. These individual differences consisted of variation in the range of fluctuation of 17-OHCS under normal circumstances and in response to disturbing or stressful stimuli. Genetic factors may also play a role in producing such individual differences.[61]

The mechanism outlined for the control and regulation of ACTH and cortisol seems also to apply to other trophic hormones of the pituitary. For each hormone, releasing factors are postulated or have been identified. These are not only subject to end-product inhibition but are under neural control by inputs from the limbic system, cortex, and thalamus. Furthermore, inhibiting factors, besides releasing factors, have been postulated in the case of trophic hormones. In addition, trophic hormone release is affected by sensory input—ovulation in some female animals only occurs after vaginal stimulation. Trophic hormone release in some cases is rhythmic: The pulsatile release of ACTH is greatest in the early hours of the morning, concomitant with the last rapid eye movement period of sleep. In some mammals, oestrus is likewise influenced by environmental light. The mechanism of this influence is known—it entails the suppression of oestrus by melatonin synthesized in the pineal gland during periods of darkness.

It has been amply demonstrated that the gonadal hormones influence the brain during critical periods of development, helping to determine the sexual and reproductive behavior and pituitary-gonadotrophic function in the adult animal.[104] Harris[66] and Young[180] hypothesized that the sexually undifferentiated brain is "organized" by gonadal hormones during fetal and early neonatal life. Subsequently, several investigators have shown[14,67,181] that the presence of androgens in small amounts during the first five days of life in female rats alters the regular cycle of gonadotrophin release to an aperiodic one. In the absence of any gonadal hormones, the gonadotrophins are secreted cyclically. Thus, the absence of androgens in the male rat in the first forty-eight hours of life results in the cyclic elaboration of gonadotrophins. In addition, the neonatal castration of a male rat drastically alters his sexual behavior. When injected with low doses of estrogens and progesterones as an adult, he exhibits the complete repertoire of female sexual behavior.[181] Castration of adult males and similar treatment with estrogen and progesterone does not yield such results. It is apparent from these data that during a critical period in early development androgens acting on the brain are responsible for the acyclic secretion of gonadotrophins. They determine male sexual behavior in much the same way that they affect the development of male sexual morphology. It is evident, therefore, that sex hormones in early life play a major part in determining sexual behavior, morphology, and physiology. It is possible also, as Levine[102] has pointed out, that the adrenal corticoids may have a profound effect upon the organization of the brain and may influence a number of functions associated with neuroendocrine regulation of ACTH.

Varying early experiences also influence immune responses. Friedman et al.[54] have shown that the effects of early experience on immunity vary depending upon the challenging agent and at what time during the host's life it is applied as well as on the genetic strain

of the animal. They exposed groups of mice to periodic, paired light shock, periodic light and aperiodic shock, and periodic light without shock. They found that the animals subjected to the first of these conditions developed a high rate of infection on exposure to Coxsackie B-2 virus, as compared with the other groups and with matched controls. Ordinarily, this strain of mice is highly resistant to this virus. Yet exposure to Coxsackie B-1 virus, a strain to which these animals are usually very susceptible, resulted in no significant difference in morbidity or mortality between groups. Inoculating stressed mice with *Plasmodium berghei* resulted in a decreased susceptibility and mortality. Ader and Friedman[8] have demonstrated similar variations in response in mice implanted with Walker sarcoma. These animals were either handled or given a three-minute period of electric shock before weaning. When they were forty-five days old, they were injected with a standard dose of Walker sarcoma. The animals handled throughout the preweaning period (three weeks) showed a retarded rate of tumor growth. The mortality rate was higher for them only in the first weeks of life; there was no difference in mortality between the animals handled later in the preweaning period and unhandled controls. Mice who received electric shock in the first week of life had a higher mortality rate than other groups, but animals shocked throughout the preweaning period or during the third week only had a lower death rate than other groups of mice, including unshocked, control animals. Thus, the effects of early experiences of this kind upon resistance to Walker sarcoma depend upon the nature of the experience and the time during early life when it occurs.

Psychobiological Studies in Animals Relevant to the Etiology and Pathogenesis of Some Medical Illnesses

Observations of patients have led to the formulation of the role of psychological factors in the etiology and pathogenesis of disease. To test the validity of the hypotheses derived from such studies and to work out the mechanisms postulated, studies of animals have been used. Such studies have been successful where research in the clinic has been less than reliable. For one thing, animal studies have added scientific evidence to the claim that environmental stimuli and a wide range of experimental variables do, in fact, produce physiological or structural changes analogous or homologous to clinical disease. Secondly, the postulate that social stimuli may act via the nervous system to alter bodily functions has been strongly supported if not substantiated by such work.

To summarize the achievements of animal studies reviewed up to this point: much is now known about the kinds of behavioral, endocrine, and autonomic changes that conditioning techniques, restraint, or separation may bring about, and how these alter target-organ structure and function. On the other hand, too little is as yet known about two central issues: (1) sufficient data have not yet been accumulated on the neural circuits and the neuronal and neurochemical mechanisms that mediate social stimuli and instigate autonomic and endocrine changes and are modified, in turn, by feedback from the interior of the body; and (2) we do not know enough about the genetic and experiential factors that presumably, make vulnerable the particular molecular and cellular configurations that terminate in a disease in one target organ rather than another.

Animal studies in this area have two distinct advantages over human studies. First, pure genetic strains of animals can be bred—strains that have a particular sensitivy, e.g., to salt ingestion that produces hypertension or to restraint that produces gastric ulceration. Second, the early experiences of animals can be manipulated to diminish or enhance their susceptibility to later experimental manipulations.

In four instances we present representative data of diseases or disturbed functioning to support these claims.

Gastric and Duodenal Ulcer

Gastric ulcers can be produced in animals by a wide variety of experimental manipu-

lations—i.e., burns, intense sensory stimulation, the administration of drugs, brain stimulation, diet, restraint or immobilization, and conditioning techniques[55]—used singly or in combination.

When restraint is used, the important parameters are the species and age of the experimental animal, the length of time he is immobilized, and the availability of food and water. The experimenter must also bear in mind that different experimental manipulations may produce gastric erosion in different parts of the stomach and may, therefore, be mediated by different physiological mechanisms that are still unidentified.

Another important experimental variable to be considered is that some animals are more susceptible to a particular manipulation than others. As is true of man,[168] a high level of serum pepsinogen (on a statistical basis) may be assumed to constitute a biological indicator of an increased susceptibility to erosion in the glandular portion of the animal's stomach.[4]

Ader's experiments with rats have particular relevance for our understanding of gastric and peptic ulcers. Specifically, Ader bred rats for susceptibility to gastric lesions on restraint. These animals had higher levels of serum pepsinogen prior to restraint: high serum pepsinogen levels were not, therefore, a response to restraint. In addition, these lesion-susceptible rats manifested some interesting behavioral characteristics. They were more reactive emotionally,[150] and appeared to dominate nonsusceptible animals with whom they were paired in a "competitive" task for water. On the other hand, when these susceptible animals were "handled" early in life, they were less likely to develop gastric lesions on restraint than were the nonsusceptible rats who were not handled early in life. Investigators who used other experimental manipulations reached the same conclusion. Life experiences in infancy—such as early weaning —may also be a critical variable in a predisposition to gastric ulceration when male rats are later exposed to conflict situations or to immobilization.

Workers in this field have also used approach-avoidance-conflict situations to produce ruminal ulcers in rats. Lower[108] found that a somewhat different manner of inducing conflict caused ulceration in the glandular portion of the rat's stomach.

Finally, there are the "executive-monkey" experiments, which were done at Walter Reed Army Institute of Research in the late 1950s. It will be recalled that at autopsy ulceration in both stomach and duodenum occurred only in the executive *Macaca iris*, and not in his yoked control.[19]

We have reviewed these animal studies rather selectively in order to highlight the complexity of the social and physiological variables involved and their interactions. However, and despite the parsimony of the data presented, one indisputable conclusion emerges: many of the doubts generated by "psychosomatic" research on humans in the mind of the critical reviewer, are dispelled by research on the production of ulcers in animals. A number of laboratory experiments and behavioral characteristics (such as activity cycles) do seem to combine with physical stimuli and genetically determined physiological factors to produce gastric ulcers. Moreover, despite the fact that the relationship of gastric ulceration in the rat to duodenal ulceration in man is unclear, duodenal ulceration was produced in monkeys in Brady's experiments.

One may also conclude from these studies that a number of different experimental conditions produce the same anatomical lesion, presumably through some common mechanism. The studies conducted by Levine and Senay[98] are relevant in this connection. These investigators found that when rats were restrained in a cold climate, intragastric pH fell and ulcers appeared. However, an antacid protected against the production of ulcers under such environmental conditions. Presumably, then, these ulcers were caused by an increase in gastric acidity, which is believed to be mediated by histamine.[83] Interestingly, Levine and Senay also demonstrated that restraint and cold increase the activity of histidine decarboxylase, which increase is positively correlated with the incidence and severity of stress ulcers. The inhibition of

diamine oxidase (the enzyme which catabolizes histamine) has the same effect.

The work of Levine and Senay raises several interesting questions: By what mediating mechanism do stress and cold induce an enzyme or enhance its activity? Is it a neural or an endocrine mechanism? If it is a neural, what brain mechanisms mediate such an effect? The answers to such questions could be sought by available neurophysiological techniques. In fact, a restrained rat might be a particularly good experimental animal to use for exploring the central nervous system (CNS) by such techniques as chronic unit recording.

ESSENTIAL HYPERTENSION

Animal studies relevant to the pathogenesis of essential hypertension are notable for their diversity.

In animals, both "simple" and complex stimuli produce elevated levels of blood pressure. "Audiogenic" hypertension has been produced in rats by daily exposure to air blasts.[132] Pickering[127] quotes a Russian experiment in which a male monkey developed elevated arterial pressure after his mate was taken away and he could observe her caged with another male monkey.

But the most convincing and systematic study of the role of complex stimuli in producing prolonged systolic hypertension in mice has been reported by Henry et al. (see page 854). Finally, an interstitial nephritis was found in animals with severe hypertension at autopsy.

Stress of the kind used by Henry can set into motion a number of physiological changes. As we mentioned earlier, Thoenen, Mueller, and Axelrod[120,159] showed that a reflex increase of sympathetic nerve activity transsynaptically induced enzyme activity in the adrenal gland after from one to three days. However, others have also shown that social stimuli may increase levels of adrenocortical steroids,[32] constrict renal vessels,[15] and alter levels of brain norepinephrine.[172]

In another area of investigation, salt was found to play a role in the pathogenesis of hypertension; the precise nature of this role has been hotly contested, however. To summarize these findings, various steroids produced experimental hypertension in animals only in the presence of salt. When hypertonic saline was the only source of fluid, hypertension was produced in a variety of animals. The chronic ingestion of too much salt produced hypertension in the rat, but it took time and even then hypertension was not found in all the animals of a particular strain.[115]

In this connection Jaffe and his co-workers[82] have reported that there are two genetic strains of rats. One is resistant and the other is sensitive to salt ingestion. Even a diet containing only 0.38 percent salt caused the rats in the sensitive group to have higher blood pressures (134 mm. Hg, mean) than the resistant ones (112 mm. Hg, mean). In fact, resistant rats on a diet of 8 percent salt showed no blood pressure increases, but the blood pressure of those who were sensitive to salt rose to 210 mm. Hg, and they developed moderate to severe lesions of the kidneys. Moreover, even the sensitive rats on a low salt diet showed changes in the musculoelastic, arteriolar pads. This anatomical lesion is thought by these authors to be genetically determined.

In human populations there is a linear correlation between salt intake and the incidence of hypertension: If the intake of salt is low in a group, the probability of some members of that group developing hypertension is lower, and vice versa.[33] In part, the amount of sodium in a diet is culturally determined, of course. However, a craving for salt, independent of requirement and cultural influences also seems to exist in individuals. Little is known about the variable responsible for such a craving. Furthermore, to the best of our knowledge, no attempts have been made to study the psychological factors that might influence man's appetite for salt, and might, therefore, play a role in producing hypertensive disease. Clearly, in the absence of such data, it behooves the worker engaged in research on the psychosomatic aspects of essential hypertension to control salt intake in his subjects. Once again, to the best of our knowledge, this control has not been built into the design of studies conducted to date.

The third line of evidence implicating sodium and its metabolism in essential hypertension was the finding that hypertensive animals have an increased natriuresis and diuresis to salt and water infusion. In addition, the sodium content of the arterial wall may be increased in such animals.

The fourth line of evidence implicating salt —and specifically the sodium ion—is proven by the fact that the amount of renin extractable from the kidneys of hypertensive rats was proportional to salt and water intake. As renin disappeared from the kidney, the rats showed an increased sensitivity to injected renin. In depleting the kidney of renin, salt probably acts through the medium of an increased plasma volume. Unfortunately, however, the increase of blood renin (and the decrease of kidney renin) in response to the increase in blood sodium does not parallel the increase in blood pressure.

The question of whether psychosocial stimuli elicit circulatory responses has been answered, in part, by the use of conditioning procedures.[50] Experimentally induced general behavioral changes, such as fear, are particularly likely to evoke an increase in unconditioned responses in animals. Conditioned cardiovascular responses, including elevations of blood pressure, can be retained in animals for many years, even after the original and concomitant motor or salivary responses can no longer be elicited.

Direct brain stimulation can serve either as the conditional stimulus or the unconditional stimulus. Motor cortical area stimulation (as an unconditional stimulus) that does not produce movements leads to vasoconstriction or dilation; parietal stimulation leads only to constriction. One of these areas may be the locus for applying a conditional stimulus, another for an unconditional stimulus to produce vasoconstriction. In dogs hypertension developed, became more severe over a period of months, and then remained elevated despite the fact that the conditioning procedures had been stopped. Even renal changes were observed after hypertension was produced by such means. Finally, of particular interest is the fact that the animals studied showed individual differences in blood-pressure responses.

The studies described above used "classical" conditioning procedures. When avoidance techniques were used in experiments with monkeys, the introduction of avoidance schedules for a period of fifteen days caused an initial acute increase in blood pressure and pulse rate. The animals were then placed on a continuous avoidance schedule, and thereafter the change in blood pressure depended on the length or complexity of the schedule. In those monkeys on the more complex schedules, blood pressure remained as high in the intervals between lever pressing sessions as it had been during the experimental sessions.[51] Increases of systolic and diastolic pressures occurred, regardless of the kind of schedule, when avoidance conditioning was carried out over a seven-to-fourteen-month period. But once the initial acute elevations of blood pressure mentioned in Forsyth's first paper had subsided, it took about seven months (during which Forsyth and his colleagues worked twelve hours a day) for the rise in blood pressure to occur. Interestingly, behavioral changes, in the form of excitability and increased activity, also occurred. Pressor responses that had been neutral prior to training were observed in the presence of a variety of stimuli.[52] Only one point has not been made in this report: we do not know whether the elevated pressures persisted after the avoidance performance had ceased. We have indicated that no single psychological or physiological variable can account for the pathogenesis of essential hypertension. This statement is further attested to by an interesting set of observations made by McCubbin.[109] After very small doses of angiotensin (which had no immediate effect on blood pressure) had been infused into dogs for several days, their arterial pressure became elevated and labile. (Before the infusion the mean arterial pressure had been steady.) When the dogs were surrounded by normal laboratory activity, their blood pressures were labile and high. If the laboratory was quiet, even minor distractions caused marked further increases in blood pressure, due to abrupt increases in peripheral resistance. When these dogs were sensitized with an infusion of tyramine, which releases endogeneous stores of norepinephrine, further elevations of blood pressure were produced. Infusions of norepinephrine had no effect on blood pressure. These observations suggest that a systematic study could be carried out of the role of psychosocial stimuli in animals made hypertensive by small doses of infused angiotensin. Extrapolating from recent work on the pharmacological effects of angiotensin, it might be possible to test the hypothesis that angiotensin sensitizes the brain to sensory input as well as having effects on blood pressure through the medium of the brain.

Recently, Scroop and Lowe[144] and Ferrario et al.[49] found that dogs anesthetized with chloralose responded to the infusion of angiotensin into the vertebral artery in doses too small to affect the systemic circulation directly. As a result, there was an increase in heart rate and arterial blood pressure, and a fall in central venous tone. These effects were thought to be due to an increase in cardiac output without change in peripheral resistance. But the fact that these hemodynamic changes were abolished by vagotomy suggest that the infused angiotensin stimulated medullary centers to reduce vagal tone. Admittedly, with the exception of the increase in arterial pressure, the changes in cardiovascular function reported are not typical of those found in essential hypertension. Nevertheless, the possibility that angiotensin may act through the CNS is of interest, especially as it has now been shown that it also causes anterior hypothalamic neurons to fire. In addition, evidence has recently been presented that the brain may form angiotensin by virtue of an unidentified enzyme it contains.

As was true of peptic ulcer, the evidence derived from animal studies on essential hypertension is much more convincing than that derived from human studies. Blood pressure, vasomotor tone, and many of the physiological variables implicated in the pathogenesis of hypertension in man can be related to naturally occurring events and to animal behavior manipulated in the laboratory. In fact, the recent evidence of Miller and Mason raises the exciting possibility that we may be on the verge of a real breakthrough in understanding the pathogenesis and pathophysiology of hypertension. Moreover, by a combination of techniques, the answers to the three central questions delineated earlier might be sought in studies of animals. This possibility justifies the restatement of these questions: (1) Can renal blood flow be increased in one renal artery and decreased in the other by operant conditioning? If so, the content in each renal vein of renin and/or angiotensin II could be measured; (2) Can the distribution of blood flow within each kidney (measured by intra-arterial injections of Krypton[85] and intravenous injections of iodoantipyrine-I[131]) be affected differently by different operant methods? And (3) If renal blood flow can be diminished by operant conditioning procedures, does hypertension ensue? Some of the mechanisms that mediate these events remain unknown.

Stressful Influences on Cardiac Rhythm and Their Mechanisms

Ectopic activity of the heart beat has been recorded in stressful situations and can be produced experimentally by stimulating either the vagus or the sympathetic cardiac nerves. When both are stimulated simultaneously, ventricular extrasystoles can be produced. Stimulation of the posterior hypothalamus can elicit a similar arrhythmia in cats under chloroform anesthesia. While stimulation of the posterior part of the lateral hypothalamus and the mesencephalic reticular formation regularly causes a profound tachycardia as well as raising the blood pressure—both phenomena outlast the duration of the stimulus.

In all likelihood, the effects on rhythm of such brain stimulation are mediated both by the vagus and cardiac sympathetic nerves.[164] Therefore, arrhythmias of various kinds can be produced in animals whose heart is intact by means of brain stimulation.

When the heart is damaged, as for instance by coronary artery ligation, ventricular fibrillation can be prevented only by total denervation of the heart.[40] In the obverse experiment, ventricular fibrillation could be produced in some dogs by hypothalamic stimulation following coronary artery ligation.[56]

Neither the exact mechanism of arrythmia nor the pathways mediating the effects of brain stimulation leading to the vagus and cardiac nerves from hypothalamic centers have been fully worked out.

It is also of interest that heart rate and rhythm can be affected by psychological means. Heart-rate changes can be produced by instrumental learning in animals[56,148] and man, and arrythmias decreased by these means.[171]

Thyroid Disease

In contrast to the large number of animal studies of gastric ulcers, few systematic studies have been done in the field of thyroid disease despite the relatively large number of available tests for thyroid function.

A rise in plasma protein-bound I[131] consistently occurred in sheep exposed to barking dogs.[46] The reverse effect on thyroid function was obtained when rats were exposed to the sight of a larger, fierce wild rat through a glass screen. Two explanations have been advanced for this response. Some authors believe that corticosteroids inhibited the release of I[131] from the thyroid gland;[45] others contend that secretion of the hypothalamic corticotrophin releasing factor resulted in the diminution of the thyrotropin releasing factor (TRF). The mediating role of TRF between social stimuli and enhanced thyroid function is a source of considerable controversy. However, Mason[112] found that plasma-thyroid-hormone levels showed a slow but prolonged elevation concomitant with a three-day avoidance session in monkeys. This elevation of hormone levels began during the avoidance session, and lasted for two or three weeks after termination of the schedule. The finding that electric stimulation of the hypothalamus enhances thyroid function in several species of animals has been well documented,[34] and various limbic-area structures have also been implicated in the regulation of thyroid function. Finally, norepinephrine and epinephrine are known to activate thyroid function,[70] and are, of course, acutely responsive to psychosocial stimulation.

However, thyrotropin may not be an important factor in thyrotoxic disease because it is believed today that a long-acting thyroid stimulator (LATS) rather than thyrotropin, is the pathogenetic agent in Graves' disease. LATS is an immunoglobulin. Therefore, the logical question arises as to how the nervous system could contribute to its regulation; or, putting it another way, in addition to the exposure to an antigen, do other factors control antibody formation or contribute to the action of an antibody? At this point, one can only speculate that there may be genetic factors that influence antibody formation in thyroid disease, and that LATS may act on cyclic AMP (adenosine monophosphate) as the corticosteroids and catecholamines do, to promote the entrance of iodine into thyroid cells.[110] In addition, it is known that adrenalectomy and the administration of thyroid hormone enhance antibody formation, and that the nervous system may regulate immune responses. For example, avoidance conditioning influenced immunological responses. At the same time, some evidence has been accumulated that indicates that midbrain[53] and hypothalamic (tuberal) lesions[155] could protect guinea pigs against anaphylactic shock. Anterior hypothalamic lesions were significantly more successful in protecting rats against anaphylaxis to ovalbumin than were posterior hypothalamic lesions. Anterior hypothalamic lesions lowered circulating antibodies to the same antigen in guinea pigs and made them less sensitive to toxic doses of histamine, possibly by modifying the physiological reactivity of the bronchiolar tree to the constrictive effects of histamine.

In summary, animal studies have provided rather reliable evidence on several scores: target-organ change and physiological responses occur that are relevant to the diseases under consideration in this paper. Furthermore, one may now conclude, on the basis of Mason's work in particular, that avoidance conditioning does indeed act through the CNS to produce changes in a series of hormones, including such critical ones as corticosteroids,

catecholamines, aldosterone, plasma-thyroid hormone, growth hormone, plasma insulin, and sex hormones. Furthermore, these studies have given rise to generalizations that these hormonal changes are patterned and do not occur individually. Nor are these patterns of change unique to avoidance conditioning: they occur with novel stimuli as well.

Such patterns of change also occur in the autonomic system, as evidenced, for example, by the cardiovascular changes that precede and accompany exercise. Whereas these adjustments were once considered to be instigated exclusively by peripheral mechanisms, Rushmer[136] has postulated that the onset of vasodilation and increased flow in muscle, heart rate and output, etc. at the start of exercise emanate from the nervous system as an autonomic concomitant to the muscular activity under volitional control.

In other words, concomitant patterns of cardiovascular and motor activities exist. These cardiovascular adjustments seem to be specific to a given behavioral activity; other adjustments probably occur with other activities: For example, in preparing to fight another cat, cats showed bradycardia, a decreased cardiac output, and vasoconstriction in the iliac and mesenteric vessels. But when actually striking the other cat, the heart rate and cardiac output rose, the iliac bed dilated and the mesenteric bed constricted. In neither case was there a significant rise in blood pressure, however.[2]

Clearly, these findings require further clarification. A contradiction appears in the work on the production of gastric ulcers in rats— Mason's work and the work mentioned above on cardiovascular changes. On the one hand, different psychosocial stimuli or situations were found to produce the same anatomical lesion or pattern of physiological change; on the other, they produced different changes. Immobilization restraint invariably produces lesions in the glandular portion of the rat's stomach, but conflict situations produced ruminal lesions in some rats, and glandular lesions in others.

Is this discrepancy a function of strain differences? Or can it be attributed to quantitative or situational factors, or differences in mediating physiological mechanisms? Only further research will provide the answers to such questions. Other interesting questions remain unanswered as well: At what thresholds do avoidance schedules produce the requisite changes, as measured by the animal's ability to escape, the predictability of his response, and the intensity and duration of stimuli?

([Conclusion

We have attempted to demonstrate that many physiological parameters are influenced by environmental factors and that disease states may be produced by experimental manipulations of animals. There is increasing evidence from a review of the literature that many integrative physiologists are beginning to be aware of the fact that certain broad generalizations no longer hold. The autonomic nervous system is no longer viewed as mainly responsible for the maintenance of the "constancy" of the internal environment, or as separate from the endocrine system. (For a review of modern data and concept about the autonomic nervous system, see Volume 4, Chapters 22 and 23, of the *Handbook*). We regard the autonomic nervous system today as one of the three principal output systems of the brain that are involved in the mediation of the brain's responses to stimuli of environmental origin, including preparation for activity in response to an outside stimulus. These responses are imposed on continuous, ongoing, autonomic discharge, which varies according to the behavioral state of the organism. In the state of rapid eye movement sleep, for example, *variability* of heart and respiratory rates, blood pressure, etc. is much greater than in slow wave sleep or quiet wakefulness. In other words, autonomic discharge is phasic during this behavioral steady state.

The autonomic nervous system is both responsible for and under the influence of hormonal output. The endocrine system, in turn, is the second major output system of the brain

mediating environmental change. In fact, there is an increasing realization of the close interactions of hormonal and autonomic mechanisms.

The classical view of autonomic function was largely obtained by analytic experiments in which only a single input (such as blood-pressure change) was varied while inputs from many other afferent zones were either eliminated or held constant. Only when the organism is studied as a whole, in an integrative manner, does it become obvious that a change in one variable (such as carotid-sinus pressure) interacts with other inputs to the brain as well as giving rise to a multiplicity of effects such as decreased adrenal-catecholamine-antidiuretic-hormone production as well as cardiac-reflex slowing, decreased cardiac-sympathetic activity, and splanchnic-bed vasodilatation, etc. All these effects must be mediated by widely disparate circuits in the brain.

These advances in physiological data and concepts must be made available to the behavioral biologist while medicine must incorporate the contributions of behavioral biology. For example, it is generally recognized that genetic factors play some role in the etiology of essential hypertension, Graves' disease, and probably in peptic ulcer. But we have not yet determined how much of the etiologic variance can also be attributed to experiential (e.g., social, familial, and economic) factors. Methodologies have been developed that would allow the investigator to determine the relative contributions of genetic and experiential factors in the etiology of disease.

At present, in the case of hypertension, about one-third to one-quarter of the variance is ascribed to genetic factors. That familial factors may play a role is attested to by the fact that spouses tend to share similar blood-pressure levels in proportion to the duration of the marriage.[174] Further, the parent–child correlation of pressures tends to be greatest in families in which spouse aggregation is demonstrated. But what could be the factors in the environment of family groupings capable of influencing their blood pressure? Some recent work suggests that if familial factors play a role in elevated blood pressure, they are established early in life. Only future research can determine the nature of these familial factors.

On the other hand, by extrapolating from the work done on animals by Ader and Mason (see von Euler's Figure 1[163]), one is led to the inevitable conclusion that these many diseases (such as hypertension and ulcers) are neither caused nor sustained by any single pathogenetic or pathophysiological factor. Rather, psychosocial stimuli, acting through the nervous system, activate a wide range of interrelated, integrated responses. In essence, the nature of the factors involved, the changes they undergo in the course of the disease, and their interrelationships attest to the fact that many diseases are primarily diseases of physiological regulation. Similar statements have been made by Brooks,[26] Harvey,[69] Menguy,[116] and Ryss and Ryss.[137] In the past, clinical psychobiological research consisted primarily of psychoanalytic observations and single dependent variables studied by psychophysiologists. Psychophysiological results were then conceptualized in linear causal terms. For example, "anxiety" caused an increased heart rate.

It is not enough to state that many important diseases are diseases of regulation in which the nervous system participates. The specific nature of the disturbance in regulation must be specified: Admittedly, it is difficult to conceptualize such regulatory patterns. But control-theory models and models derived from molecular biology do exist.

For example, in molecular biology various kinds of regulatory devices are known: (1) In enzyme synthesis, enzymes may be formed ("induction") only in the presence of substrate. (2) Enzymes in a biosynthetic pathway may be repressed by an excess of the end product of the pathway ("feedback inhibition"). (Jacob and Monod[81] have attributed these two types of regulation to a regulator gene. In the proper configuration, the product of the gene acts on another area to inhibit expression of one or more genes in an adjacent area. Other regulatory devices have been described as well.) (3) In enzyme activity, the initial enzyme in a biosynthetic pathway is usually the one inhibited. (4) There is usually more than one initial enzyme in a common biosynthetic pathway. These act in conjunction and catalyze the same chemical reactions, but are subject to different feedback regulation. And (5) in protein synthesis, regulation is achieved at the rate at which the initial step in the synthesis of the protein chain occurs, and not at the rate of enzyme synthesis. Other forms of molecular regulatory activity, though carefully conceptualized, do not fit any of the five models mentioned above. And regulation of excitation at the synapse may also take different forms, most of which are well known.

These concepts have important implications for a theory of medicine, with particular emphasis on theories of etiology and pathogenesis of disease. At the same time, they may help to incorporate data that suggest that stressful experience plays a role in the etiology and pathogenesis of disease.

In turn, we would suggest that the information we have reviewed has implications for the practice of medicine and the education of students and physicians. Thus, it may be economically more expeditious and technically more feasible to isolate a patient completely from other human beings in an intensive-care unit,[30,59] but the psychological effects of isolation, or the impact of a patient watching his own irregular or faltering heart beat on an oscilloscope, may be much more stressful than having him share a room with others with whom he can talk about his real and imaginary concerns.

We believe that the organismic and integrative approach to medicine and disease implied in this chapter can be translated into the teaching of students. Space does not permit a detailed plan for such a curriculum, which one of us has outlined elsewhere.[166]

(Bibliography

1. ABRAHAMS, V. C., S. M. HILTON, and A. SBROZYNA. "Active Muscle Vasodilatation Produced by Stimulation of the Brainstem: Its Significance in the Defense

Reaction," *J. Physiol.*, 154 (1960), 491–513.

2. Adams, D. B., G. Baccelli, G. Mancia et al. "Cardiovascular Changes during Preparation for Fighting Behavior in the Cat," *Nature*, 220 (1968), 1239–1240.

3. Adamson, J. D. and A. H. Schmale, Jr. "Object Loss, Giving Up and the Onset of Psychiatric Disease," *Psychosom. Med.*, 27 (1965), 557–576.

4. Ader, R. "Plasma Pepsinogen Level in Rat and Man," *Psychosom. Med.*, 25 (1963), 218–220.

5. ———. "Gastric Erosions in the Rat: Effects of Immobilization at Different Points in the Activity Cycle," *Science*, 145 (1964), 406–407.

6. ———. "Behavioral and Physiological Rhythms and the Development of Gastric Erosions in the Rat," *Psychosom. Med.*, 29 (1967), 345–353.

7. ———. "Early Experiences Accelerate Maturation of the 24-Hour Adrenocortical Rhythm," *Science*, 163 (1969), 1225–1226.

8. Ader, R. and S. B. Friedman. "Differential Early Experiences and Susceptibility to Transplanted Tumor in the Rat," *J. Comp. Physiol. Psychol.*, 59 (1965), 361–364.

9. Alousi, A. and N. Weiner. "The Regulation of Norepinephrine Synthesis in Sympathetic Nerves: Effect of Nerve Stimulation, Cocaine, and Catecholamine-Releasing Agents," *Proc. Natl. Acad. Sci. U.S.A.*, 56 (1966), 1491–1496.

10. Axelrod, J. "Brain Monoamines: Biosynthesis and Fate," *Neurosci. Res. Program Bull.*, 9 (1971), 188–196.

11. ———. "Noradrenaline: Fate and Control of Its Biosynthesis," *Science*, 173 (1971), 598–606.

12. Axelrod, J., R. A. Mueller, J. P. Henry et al. "Changes in Enzymes Involved in the Biosynthesis and Metabolism of Noradrenaline and Adrenaline after Psychosocial Stimulation," *Nature*, 225 (1970), 1059–1060.

13. Bahnson, C. B. "Psychophysiological Complimentarity in Malignancies: Past Work and Future Vistas," *Ann. N.Y. Acad. Sci.*, 164 (1969), 319–334.

14. Barraclough, C. A. "Production of Anovulatory, Sterile Rats by Single Injection of Testosterone Proprionate," *Endocrinology*, 68 (1961), 62–67.

15. Bing, J., and N. Vinthen-Paulsen. "Effects of Severe Anoxia on the Kidneys of Normal and Dehydrated Mice," *Acta Physiol. Scand.*, 27 (1952), 337–349.

16. Bliss, E. L., C. J. Migeon, C. H. H. Branch et al. "Reaction of the Adrenal Cortex to Emotional Stress," *Psychosom. Med.*, 18 (1956), 56–76.

17. Bonfils, S., G. Liefooghe, G. Rossi et al. "L'Ulcère de constrainte du rat blanc," *Comp. Rend. Séances Soc. Biol. Filiales*, 151 (1957), 1149–1150.

18. Bourne, P. G., R. M. Rose, and J. W. Mason. "Urinary 17-OHCS Levels: Data on Seven Helicopter Ambulance Medics in Combat," *Arch. Gen. Psychiatry*, 17 (1967), 104–110.

19. Brady, J. V., R. W. Porter, D. G. Conrad et al. "Avoidance Behavior and the Development of Gastroduodenal Ulcers," *J. Exp. Anal. Behav.*, 1 (1958), 69–72.

20. Brod, J. "Essential Hypertension—Hemodynamic Observations with Bearing on its Pathogenesis," *Lancet*, 2 (1960), 773–783.

21. ———. "Hemodynamics and Emotional Stress," *Bibl. Psychiatr.*, 144 (1970), 13–33.

22. Brod, J., V. Fencl, Z. Hejl et al. "Circulatory Changes Underlying Blood Pressure Elevation during Acute Emotional Stress (Mental Arithmetic) in Normotensive and Hypertensive Subjects," *Clin. Sci.*, 18 (1959), 269–279.

23. Brod, J., V. Fencl, Z. Hejl et al. "General and Regional Hemodynamic Pattern Underlying Essential Hypertension," *Clin. Sci.*, 23 (1962), 339–349.

24. Brodie, D. A., and H. M. Hanson. "A Study of the Factors Involved in the Production of Gastric Ulcers by the Restraint Technique," *Gastroenterology*, 38 (1960), 353–360.

25. Bronfenbrenner, U. "Early Deprivation in Mammals: A Cross Species Analyses," in G. Newton, ed., *Early Experience and Behavior*, pp. 627–764. Springfield: Charles C. Thomas, 1968.

26. Brooks, F. P. "Central Neural Control of Acid Secretion," in W. F. Hamilton and P. Dow, eds., Handbook of Physiology, Sect. 6. *Alimentary Canal*, Vol. 2, pp. 805–826. Washington: American Physiological Society, 1967.

27. Bunney, W. E. "A Psychoendocrine Study

of Severe Psychotic Depressive Crisis," *Am. J. Psychiatry*, 122 (1965), 72–80.

28. BYGDEMAN, S., and U. S. VON EULER. "Resynthesis of Catechol Hormones in the Cat's Adrenal Medulla," *Acta Physiol. Scand.*, 44 (1958), 375–383.

29. CARLSON, L. A., L. LEVI, and L. ORO. "Plasma Lipids and Urinary Excretion of Catecholamines during Acute Emotional Stress in Man and Their Modification by Nicotinic Acid," *Forsvars Med.*, 3 (1967), 129–136.

30. CASSEM, N. H., and T. P. HACKETT. "Psychiatric Consultation in a Coronary Care Unit," *Ann. Intern. Med.*, 75 (1971), 9–14.

31. CHODOFF, P., S. B. FRIEDMAN, and D. A. HAMBURG. "Stress, Defenses and Coping Behavior: Observations in Parents of Children with Malignant Disease," *Am. J. Psychiatry*, 120 (1964), 743–749.

32. CHRISTIAN, J. J., J. A. LLOYD, and D. E. DAVIS. "The Role of Endocrines in the Self-Regulation of Mammalian Populations," *Recent Prog. Horm. Res.*, 22 (1965), 501–571.

33. DAHL, L. K. "Possible Role of Salt Intake in the Development of Essential Hypertension," in K. D. Bock and P. T. Cottier, eds., *Essential Hypertension*, pp. 53–65. Berlin: Springer, 1960.

34. D'ANGELO, S. A., J. SNYDER, and J. M. GRODIN. "Electrical Stimulation of the Hypothalamus: Simultaneous Effects on the Pituitary-Adrenal and Thyroid Systems of the Rat," *Endocrinology*, 75 (1964), 417–427.

35. DAY, G. "The Psychosomatic Approach to Pulmonary Tuberculosis," *Lancet*, 260 (1951), 1025–1028.

36. DE LA METTRIE, J. O. *L'Homme Machine*. Leyden: Luzac, 1748.

37. DENENBERG, V. H., J. T. BRUMAGHIN, G. C. HALTMEYER et al. "Increased Adrenocortical Activity in the Neonatal Rat following Handling," *Endocrinology*, 81 (1967), 1047–1052.

38. DESCARTES, R. "The Discourse on Method," in E. S. Haldane and G. T. R. Ross, eds., *The Philosophical Works of Descartes*. Cambridge: Cambridge University Press, 1911.

39. DICARA, L. "Plasticity in the Autonomic Nervous System: Instrumental Learning of Glandular and Visceral Responses," in F.

O. Schmitt, ed., *The Neurosciences: Second Study Program*, pp. 218–223. New York: Rockefeller University Press, 1971.

40. EBERT, P., R. VANDERBEEK, R. ALLGOOD et al. "Effect of Chronic Cardiac Denervation on Arrhythmias after Coronary Artery Ligation," *Cardiovasc. Res.*, 4 (1970), 141–147.

41. EDSTROM, J. E., D. EICHNER, and N. SCHOR. "Quantitative Ribonucleic Acid Measurements in Function: Studies of the Nucleus Supraopticus," in S. S. Kety and I. Elkes, eds., *Regional Neurchemistry*, pp. 274–278. New York: Pergamon, 1961.

42. ENGEL, G. L. "Studies of Ulcerative Colitis: III. The Nature of the Psychologic Processes," *Am. J. Med.*, 19 (1955), 231–256.

43. ———. "A Life Setting Conducive to Illness: The Giving-Up, Given-Up Complex," *Arch. Intern. Med.*, 69 (1968), 293–300.

44. ERIKSON, E. *Childhood and Society*, 1st ed. New York: Norton, 1950.

45. EVANS, C. S. and S. A. BARNETT. "Physiological Effects of 'Social Stress' in Wild Rats: 3. Thyroid," *Neuroendocrinology*, 1 (1965–1966), 113–120.

46. FALCONER, I. R. and B. S. HETZEL. "Effect of Emotional Stress and TSH on Thyroid Vein Hormone Level in Sheep with Exteriorized Thyroids," *Endocrinology*, 75 (1964), 42–48.

47. FEITELBERG, S. and H. LAMPL. "Warmetonung der Grosshirnrinde bei Erregung und Ruhe bzw," *Arch. Exp. Pathol. Pharmacol.*, 177 (1935), 725–736.

48. FENZ, W. D. and S. EPSTEIN. "Gradients of Physiological Arousal in Parachutists as a Function of an Approaching Jump," *Psychosom. Med.*, 29 (1967), 33–51.

49. FERRARIO, C. M., C. J. DICKINSON, P. L. GILDENBERG et al. "Central Vasomotor Stimulation by Angiotensin," *Fed. Proc.*, 28 (1969), 394.

50. FIGAR, S. "Conditional Circulatory Responses in Men and Animals," in W. F. Hamilton and P. Dow, eds., Handbook of Physiology, Sect. 2. *Circulation* Vol. 3, pp. 1991–2036. Washington: American Physiological Society, 1965.

51. FORSYTH, R. P. "Blood Pressure and Avoidance Conditioning," *Psychosom. Med.*, 30 (1968), 125–135.

52. ———"Blood Pressure Responses to Long-Term Avoidance Schedules in the Re-

strained Rhesus Monkey," *Psychosom. Med.*, 31 (1969), 300–309.

53. FREEDMAN, D. X. and G. FENICHEL. "Effect of Midbrain Lesions in Experimental Allergy," *Arch. Neurol. Psychiatry*, 79 (1958), 164–169.

54. FRIEDMAN, S. B., R. ADER, and L. A. GLASGOW. "Effects of Psychological Stress in Adult Mice Inoculated with Coxsackie B Viruses," *Psychosom. Med.*, 27 (1965), 361–368.

55. FRIEDMAN, S. B., J. W. MASON, and D. A. HAMBURG. "Urinary 17-Hydroxycorticosteroid Levels in Parents of Children with Neoplastic Disease: A Study of Chronic Psychological Stress," *Psychosom. Med.*, 25 (1963), 364–376.

56. GARVEY, H. and K. MELVILLE. "Cardiovascular Effects of Lateral Hypothalamic Stimulation in Normal and Coronary Ligated Dogs," *J. Cardiovasc. Surg.*, 10 (1969), 377–385.

57. GLOWINSKI, J., J. AXELROD, I. J. KOPIN et al. "Physiological Disposition of H^3 Norepinephrine in the Developing Rat," *J. Pharmacol. Exp. Ther.*, 146 (1964), 48–53.

58. GREENE, W. A. JR. "Psychological Factors and Reticuloendothelial Disease: I. Preliminary Observations on a Group of Males with Lymphomas and Leukemias," *Psychosom. Med.*, 16 (1954), 220–230.

59. HACKETT, T. P., N. H. CASSEM, and H. A. WISHNIE. "The Coronary Care Unit: An Appraisal of Its Psychologic Hazards," *N. Engl. J. Med.*, 279 (1968), 1365–1370.

60. HAMBURG, D. A. "Plasma Urinary Corticosteroid Levels in Naturally Occurring Psychological Stress," *Res. Publ. Assoc. Res. Nerv. Ment. Dis.*, 40 (1962), 406–413.

61. ———. "Genetics of Adrenocortical Hormone Metabolism in Relation to Psychological Stress," in J. Hirsch, ed., *Behavior-Genetic Analysis*, pp. 154–175. New York: McGraw-Hill, 1967.

62. HAMBURG, D. A. and J. E. ADAMS. "A Perspective on Coping Behavior," *Arch. Gen. Psychiatry*, 17 (1967), 277–284.

63. HAMBURG, D. A., C. P. ARTZ, E. REISS et al. "Clinical Importance of Emotional Problems in the Care of Patients with Burns," *N. Engl. J. Med.*, 248 (1953), 355–359.

64. HAMBURG, D. A., B. HAMBURG, and S. DE-GOZA. "Adaptive Problems and Mechanisms in Severely Burned Patients," *Psychiatry*, 16 (1953), 1–20.

65. HARLOW, H. F. "The Development of Affectional Patterns in Infant Monkeys," in B. M. Foss, ed., *Determinants of Infant Behavior*, pp. 75–88. London: Methuen, 1961.

66. HARRIS, G. W. "Sex Hormones, Brain Development and Brain Function," *Endocrinology*, 75 (1964), 627–648.

67. HARRIS, G. W. and S. LEVINE. "Sexual Differentiation of the Brain and Its Experimental Control," *J. Physiol.*, 181 (1965), 379–400.

68. HARTMANN, H. (1939) *Ego Psychology and the Problem of Adaptation*. New York: International Universities Press, 1958.

69. HARVEY, N. A. "The Cybernetics of Peptic Ulcer," *N.Y. State J. Med.*, 69 (1969), 430–435.

70. HAYS, M. T. "Effect of Epinephrine on Radioiodide Uptake by the Normal Human Thyroid," *J. Clin. Endocrinol. Metabol.*, 25 (1965), 465–468.

71. HELLMAN, L. "Production of Acute Gouty Arthritis by Adrenocorticotropin," *Science*, 109 (1949), 280–281.

72. HELLMAN, L., R. E. WESTON, D. J. W ESCHER et al. "The Effect of Adrenocorticotropin on Renal Hemodynamics and Uric Acid Clearance," *Fed. Proc.*, 7 (1948), 52.

73. HENRY, J. P., D. L. ELY, and P. M. STEPHENS. "Role of the Autonomic System in Social Adaptation and Stress," *Proc. Int. Union Physiol. Sci.*, 8 (1971), 50–51.

74. HENRY, J. P., J. P. MEEHAN, and P. M. STEPHENS. "The Use of Psychosocial Stimuli to Induce Prolonged Systolic Hypertension in Mice," *Psychosom. Med.*, 29 (1967), 408–432.

75. HENRY, J. P., P. M. STEPHENS, J. AXELROD et al. "Effect of Psychosocial Stimulation on the Enzymes Involved in the Biosynthesis and Metabolism of Noradrenaline and Adrenaline," *Psychosom. Med.*, 33 (1971), 227–237.

76. HIMWICH, W., J. M. DAVIS, and H. C. AGRAUAL. "Effects of Early Weaning on Some Free Amino Acids and Acetylcholinesterase Activity of Rat Brain," in J. Wortis, ed., *Recent Advances in Biological Psychiatry*, pp. 266–270. New York: Plenum, 1968.

77. HINDE, R. A. and Y. SPENCER-BOOTH. "Effects of Brief Separations from Mother

on Rhesus Monkeys," *Science*, 173 (1971), 111–118.

78. HINKLE, L. E. and S. WOLF. "A Summary of Experimental Evidence Relating Life Stress to Diabetes Mellitus," *J. Mt. Sinai Hosp.*, 19 (1952), 537.

79. HOFER, M. A. "Regulation of Cardiac Rate by Nutritional Factor in Young Rats," *Science*, 172 (1971), 1039–1041.

80. HOFER, M. A. and H. WEINER. "The Development and Mechanisms of Cardiorespiratory Responses to Maternal Deprivation in Rat Pups," *Psychosom. Med.*, 33 (1971), 353–362.

81. JACOB, F. and J. MONOD. "Genetic Regulatory Mechanisms in the Synthesis of Proteins," J. Mol. Biol., 3 (1961), 318–356.

82. JAFFE, D., L. K. DAHL, L. SUTHERLAND et al. "Effects of Chronic Excess Salt Ingestion: Morphological Findings in Kidneys of Rats with Differing Genetic Susceptibility to Hypertension," *Fed. Proc.*, 28 (1969), 422.

83. KAHLSON, G. and E. ROSENGREN. "New Approaches to the Physiology of Histamine," *Physiol. Rev.*, 48 (1968), 155.

84. KASL, S. V., S. COBB, and G. W. BROOKS. "Changes in Serum Uric Acid and Cholesterol Levels in Men Undergoing Job Loss," *JAMA*, 206 (1968), 1500–1507.

85. KATZ, J. L., P. ACKMAN, Y. ROTHWAX et al. "Psychoendocrine Aspects of Cancer of the Breast," *Psychosom. Med.*, 32 (1970), 1–18.

86. KATZ, J. L., H. WEINER, T. F. GALLAGHER et al. "Stress, Distress and Ego Defenses," *Arch. Gen. Psychiatry*, 23 (1970), 131–142.

87. KAUFMAN, I. C. and L. ROSENBLUM. "Effects of Separation from Mother on the Emotional Behavior of Infant Monkeys," *Ann. N.Y. Acad. Sci.*, 159 (1969), 681–696.

88. KENNEDY, J. A. and H. BAKST. "The Influence of Emotions on the Outcome of Cardiac Surgery: A Predictive Study," *Bull. N.Y. Acad. Med.*, 42 (1966), 811–845.

89. KIMBALL, C. "A Predictive Study of Adjustment to Cardiac Surgery," *J. Thorac. Cardiovasc. Surg.*, 58 (1969), 891–896.

90. KISSEN, D. M. "Psychological Factors, Personality, and Lung Cancer in Men Aged 55–64," *Br. J. Med. Psychol.*, 40 (1967), 29–43.

91. KLEINSCHMIDT, H. J. and S. E. WAXENBERG.

"Psychophysiology and Psychiatric Management of Thyrotoxicosis: A Two Year Follow-up Study," *J. Mt. Sinai Hosp.*, 23 (1956), 131.

92. KRAUS, A. S. and A. M. LILIENFELD. "Some Epidemiological Aspects of the High Mortality in a Young Widowed Group," *J. Chronic Dis.*, 10 (1959), 207–217.

93. KVETNANSKY, R., G. P. GEWIRTZ, V. K. WEISE et al. "Effect of Hypophysectomy on Immobilization-Induced Elevation of Tyrosine Hydroxylase and Phenylethanolamine-N-Methyl Transferase in the Rat Adrenal," *Endocrinology*, 87 (1970), 1323–1329.

94. KVETNANSKY, R. and L. MIKULAJ. "Adrenal and Urinary Catecholamines in Rats during Adaptation to Repeated Immobilization Stress," *Endocrinology*, 87 (1970), 738–743.

95. KVETNANSKY, R., V. K. WEISE, and I. J. KOPIN. "Elevation of Adrenal Tyrosine Hydroxylase and Phenylethanolamine-N-Methyl Transferase by Repeated Immobilization of Rats," *Endocrinology*, 87 (1970), 744–749.

96. LANGWORTHY, O. R. "Development of Behavioral Patterns and Myelinization of the Central Nervous System in the Human Fetus and Infant," *Carnegie Inst. Contrib. Embryol.*, 24 (1933), 1–57.

97. LESHAN, L. L. "An Emotional Life History Pattern Associated with Neoplastic Disease," *Ann. N.Y. Acad. Sci.*, 125 (1966), 780–793.

98. LEVINE, R. J. and E. C. SENAY. "Studies on the Role of Acid in the Pathogenesis of Experimental Stress Ulcers," *Psychosom. Med.*, 32 (1970), 61–65.

99. LEVINE, S. "Plasma-Free Corticosteroid Response to Electric Shock in Rats Stimulated in Infancy," *Science*, 135 (1962), 795–796.

100. ———. "The Psychophysiological Effects of Infantile Stimulation," in E. Bliss, ed., *Roots of Behavior*, pp. 246–253. New York: Harper & Row, 1962.

101. ———. "Influence of Infantile Stimulation on the Response to Stress during Preweaning Development," *Dev. Psychobiol.*, 1 (1968), 67–70.

102. ———. "The Pituitary-Adrenal System and the Developing Brain," *Prog. Brain Res.*, 32 (1970), 79–85.

103. LEVINE, S., M. ALPERT, and G. W. LEWIS.

"Differential Maturation of an Adrenal Response to Cold Stress in Rats Manipulated in Infancy," *J. Comp. Physiol. Psychol.*, 51 (1958), 774–777.

104. LEVINE, S. and R. F. MULLINS, JR. "Hormonal Influences on Brain Organization in Infant Rats," *Science*, 152 (1966), 1585–1592.

105. ———. "Hormones in Infancy," in G. Newton and S. Levine, eds., *Early Experience and Behavior*, pp. 168–197. Springfield, Ill.: Charles C. Thomas, 1968.

106. LIDZ, T. "Emotional Factors in the Etiology of Hyperthyroidism," *Psychosom. Med.*, 11 (1949), 2.

107. LÖFVING, B. "Cardiovascular Adjustments Induced from the Rostral Cingulate Gyrus with Special Reference to Sympathoinhitory Mechanisms," *Acta Physiol. Scand.*, 53 *Suppl.* 184 (1961), 1–82.

108. LOWER, J. S. "Approach-Avoidance Conflict as a Determinant of Peptic Ulceration in the Rat," Medical Dissertation, Western Reserve University, 1967.

109. MCCUBBIN, J. W. "Interrelationship Between the Sympathetic Nervous System and the Renin-Angiotensin System," in P. Kezdi, ed., *Baroreceptors and Hypertension*, pp. 327–330. New York: Pergamon, 1967.

110. MCKENZIE, J. M. "Humoral Factors in the Pathogenesis of Graves' Disease," *Physiol. Rev.*, 48 (1968), 252–310.

111. MASON, J. W. "Psychological Influences on the Pituitary-Adrenal Cortical System," in C. Pincus, ed., *Recent Progress in Hormone Research*, pp. 345–389. New York: Academic, 1959.

112. ———. "Organization of Psychoendocrine Mechanisms," *Psychosom. Med.*, 30 (1968), 565–808.

113. MASON, W. A., R. K. DAVENPORT, JR., and E. W. MENZEL, JR. "Early Experiences and the Social Development of Rhesus Monkeys and Chimpanzees," in G. Newton and S. Levine, eds., *Early Experience and Behavior*, pp. 440–480. Springfield, Ill.: Charles C. Thomas, 1968.

114. MELZACK, R. "The Role of Early Experience on Emotional Arousal," *Ann. N.Y. Acad. Sci.*, 159 (1969), 721–730.

115. MENEELY, G. R., R. G. TUCKER, W. J. DARBY et al. "Electrocardiographic Changes, Disturbed Lipid Metabolism and Decreased Survival Rates Observed in Rats Chronically Eating Increased Sodium Chlo-

ride," *Am. J. Med.*, 16 (1954), 599.

116. MENGUY, R. "Current Concepts of the Etiology of Duodenal Ulcer," *Am. J. Dig. Dis.*, 9 (1964), 199–211.

117. MILKOVIC, K. and S. MILKOVIC. "The Influence of Adrenalectomy of Pregnant Rats on the Reactiveness of the Pituitary-Adrenal System of Newborn Animals," *Arch. Int. Physiol. Biochem.*, 67 (1959), 24–28.

118. ———. "Reactiveness of the Pituitary-Adrenal System of Newborn Animals," *Endokrinologie*, 37 (1959), 301–310.

119. MILLER, N. E. "Learning of Visceral and Glandular Responses," *Science*, 163 (1969), 434–445.

120. MUELLER, R. A., H. THOENEN, and J. AXELROD. "Increase in Tyrosine Hydroxylase Activity after Reserpine Administration," *J. Pharmacol. Exp. Ther.*, 169 (1969), 74–79.

121. ———. "Inhibition of Transsynaptically Increased Tyrosine Hydroxylase Activity by Cycloheximide and Actinomycin D," *Mol. Pharmacol.*, 5 (1969), 463–469.

122. ———. "Effect of Pituitary and ACTH on the Maintenance of Basal Tyrosine Hydroxylase Activity in the Rat Adrenal Gland," *Endocrinology*, 86 (1970), 751–755.

123. PARKER, D. L. and J. R. HODGE. "Delirium in a Coronary Care Unit," *JAMA*, 201 (1967), 702–703.

124. PARKES, C. M. "Recent Bereavement as a Cause of Mental Illness," *Br. J. Psychiatry*, 110 (1964), 198–204.

125. PEPLER, W. J. and A. G. E. PEARSE. "The Histochemistry of the Esterase of Rat Brain with Special Reference to Those of the Hypothalamic Nuclei," *J. Neurochem.*, 1 (1957), 193–202.

126. PERLMAN, L. V., S. FERGUSON, K. BERGUM et al. "Precipitation of Congestive Heart Failure: Social and Emotional Factors," *Ann. Intern. Med.*, 75 (1971), 1–7.

127. PICKERING, G. W. *The Nature of Essential Hypertension.* New York: Grune & Stratton, 1961.

128. RAHE, R. H. and R. J. ARTHUR. "Stressful Underwater Demolition Training: Serum Urate and Cholesterol Variability," *JAMA*, 202 (1967), 1052–1054.

129. RAHE, R. H., R. T. RUBIN, R. J. ARTHUR et al. "Serum Uric Acid and Cholesterol Variability: A Comprehensive View of Under-

water Demolition Team Training," *JAMA*, 206 (1968), 2875–2880.

130. RAPAPORT, D. "The Theory of Ego Autonomy," *Bull. Menninger Clin.*, 22 (1958), 13–35.

131. RICHTER, D. "Brain Metabolism and Cerebral Function," *Biochem. Soc. Symp.*, 8 (1952), 62.

132. ROTHLIN, E., H. EMMENEGGER, and A. CERLETTI. "Versuche zur Erzeugung Audiogener Hypertonie an Ratten," *Helv. Physiol. Pharmacol. Acta*, 2, *Suppl.* C25 (1953–1954), 11–12.

133. RUBESON, A. "Alterations in Noradrenaline Turnover in the Peripheral Sympathetic Neurons Induced by Stress," *J. Pharm. Pharmacol.*, 21 (1969), 878–880.

134. RUBIN, R. T., R. H. RAHE, R. J. ARTHUR et al. "Adrenal Cortical Activity Changes during Underwater Demolition Team Training," *Psychosom. Med.*, 31 (1969), 553–563.

135. RUBIN, R. T., R. H. RAHE, B. R. CLARK et al. "Serum Uric Acid, Cholesterol, and Cortisol Levels: Interrelationships in Normal Men Under Stress," *Arch. Intern. Med.*, 125 (1970), 815–819.

136. RUSHMER, R. F. *Cardiovascular Dynamics*, 3rd ed. Philadelphia: Saunders, 1970.

137. RYSS, S. and E. RYSS. "Modern Concepts of Etiology and Pathogenesis of Peptic Ulcer: Disorders of the Regulating Mechanisms," *Scand. J. Gastroenterol.*, 3 (1968), 513–524.

138. SACHAR, E. J. "Psychological Homeostasis and Endocrine Function," in A. Mandell and M. Mandell, eds., *Psychochemical Strategies in Man: Methods, Strategy and Theory*, pp. 219–233. New York: Academic, 1969.

139. SACHAR, E. J., L. HELLMAN, D. K. FUKUSHIMA et al. "Cortisol Production in Depressive Illness. A Clinical and Biochemical Clarification," *Arch. Gen. Psychiatry*, 23 (1970), 289–298.

140. SACHAR, E. J., J. M. MACKENZIE, W. A. BINSTOCK et al. "Corticosteroid Responses to Psychotherapy of Depressions: I. Elevations during Confrontation of Loss," *Arch. Gen. Psychiatry*, 16 (1967), 461–470.

141. SACHAR, E. J., J. W. MASON, H. KOLLMER et al. "Psychoendocrine Aspects of Acute Schizophrenic Reactions," *Psychosom. Med.*, 25 (1963), 510–537.

142. SCHAPIRO, S., E. GELLER, and S. EIDUSON.

"Corticoid Response to Stress in the Steroid-Inhibited Rat," *Proc. Soc. Exp. Biol. Med.*, 109 (1962), 935–937.

143. SCHMALE, A. H., JR. "Relation of Separation and Depression to Disease: I. A Report on a Hospitalized Medical Population," *Psychosom. Med.*, 20 (1958), 259–277.

144. SCROOP, G. C. and R. D. LOWE. "Central Pressor Effect of Angiotensin Mediated by the Parasympathetic Nervous System," *Nature*, 220 (1968), 1331–1332.

145. SEDVALL, G. C. and I. J. KOPIN. "Acceleration of Norepinephrine Synthesis in the Rat Submaxillary Gland *in vivo* during Sympathetic Nerve Stimulation," *Life Sci.*, 6 (1967), 45–51.

146. SELYE, H. *Stress.* Montreal: ACTA, 1950.

147. SEROTA, H. M. and R. W. GERARD. "Localized Thermal Changes in the Cat's Brain," *J. Neurophysiol.*, 1 (1938), 115–124.

148. SHAPIRO, D., B. TURSKY, and G. E. SCHWARTZ. "Differentiation of Heart Rate and Systolic Blood Pressure in Man by Operant Conditioning," *Psychosom. Med.*, 32 (1970), 417–423.

149. SHOEMAKER, W. J. and R. J. WURTMAN. "Perinatal Undernutrition: Accumulation of Catecholamines in Rat Brain," *Science*, 171 (1971), 1017–1019.

150. SINES, J. O. "Strain Differences in Activity, Emotionality, Body Weight and Susceptibility to Stress-Induced Stomach Lesions," *J. Genet. Psychol.*, 101 (1962), 209–217.

151. SKINNER, B. F. *Beyond Freedom and Dignity.* New York: Knopf, 1971.

152. SMELIK, P. G. "Relation between the Blood Level of Corticoids and Their Inhibiting Effect on the Hypophyseal Stress Response," *Proc. Soc. Exp. Biol. Med.*, 113 (1963), 616–619.

153. STEIN, S. and E. CHARLES. "Emotional Factors in Juvenile Diabetes Mellitus: A Study of Early Life Experiences of Adolescent Diabetics," *Am. J. Psychiatry*, 128 (1971), 700–704.

154. STONE, L. *The Psychoanalytic Situation.* New York: International Universities Press, 1961.

155. SZENTIVANYI, A. and G. GILIPP. "Anaphylaxis and the Nervous System. Part II," *Ann. Allergy*, 16 (1958), 143.

156. TAYLOR, K. M. and S. H. SNYDER. "Brain Histamine: Rapid Apparent Turnover Altered by Restraint and Cold Stress," *Science*, 172 (1971), 1037–1039.

157. Thoenen, H., R. A. Mueller, and J. Axelrod. "Increased Tyrosine Hydroxylase Activity after Drug-Induced Alteration of Sympathetic Transmission," *Nature*, 221 (1969), 1264.

158. ———. "Transsynaptic Induction of Adrenal Tyrosine Hydroxylase," *J. Pharmacol. Exp. Ther.*, 169 (1969), 249–254.

159. ———. "Neuronally Dependent Induction of Adrenal Phenylethanolamine N-methyltransferase by Hydroxydopamine," *Biochem. Pharmacol.*, 19 (1970), 669–673.

160. ———. "Phase Difference in the Induction of Tyrosine Hydroxylase in Cell Body and Nerve Terminals of Sympathetic Neurones," *Proc. Natl. Acad. Sci. U.S.A.*, 65 (1970), 58–62.

161. Thoman, E. B. and S. Levine. "Influence of Adrenalectomy in Female Rats on Reproductive Processes: Effects on the Fetus and Offspring," *J. Endocrinol.*, 46 (1970), 297–303.

162. Uvnäs, B. "Central Cardiovascular Control," in W. F. Hamilton and P. Dow, eds., Handbook of Physiology, Sect. 1, *Neurophysiology*, Vol. 2, pp. 1131–1162. Baltimore: Williams & Wilkins, 1960.

163. Von Euler, U. S. "Adrenergic Neurotransmitter Functions," *Science*, 173 (1971), 202–206.

164. Weinberg, S. J. and J. M. Fuster. "Electrocardiographic Changes Produced by Localized Hypothalamic Stimulation," *Ann. Intern. Med.*, 53 (1960), 332–341.

165. Weiner, H. "Some Recent Neurophysiological Contributions to the Problem of Brain and Behavior," *Psychosom. Med.*, 31 (1969), 457–478.

166. ———. "Experiences in the Development of Preclinical Curricula in the Sciences Related to Behavior," *J. Nerv. Ment. Dis.*, 154 (1972), 165.

167. Weiner, H., M. T. Singer, and M. F. Reiser. "Cardiovascular Responses and Their Psychological Correlates: A Study in Healthy Young Adults and Patients with Peptic Ulcer and Hypertension," *Psychosom. Med.*, 24 (1962), 477–498.

168. Weiner, H., M. Thaler, M. F. Reiser, and I. A. Mirsky. "Etiology of Duodenal Ulcer: I. Relation of Specific Psychological Characteristics to Rate of Gastric Secretion (Serum Pepsinogen)," *Psychosom. Med.*, 19 (1957), 1–10.

169. Weinshilboum, R. M. and J. Axelrod. "Dopamine-β-Hydroxylase Activity in Human Blood," *Pharmacologist*, 12 (1970), 214.

170. Weinshilboum, R. M., R. Kvetnansky, J. Axelrod et al. "Elevation of Serum Dopamine-β-Hydroxylase Activity with Forced Immobilization," *Nature (New Biol.)*, 230 (1971), 287–288.

171. Weiss, T. and B. T. Engel. "Voluntary Control of Premature Ventricular Contractions in Patients," *Am. J. Cardiol.*, 26 (1970), 666.

172. Welch, B. L. and S. A. Welch. "Effect of Grouping on the Level of Brain Norepinephrine in White Swiss Mice," *Life Sci.*, 4 (1965), 1011–1018.

173. ———. "Differential Activation by Restraint Stress of a Mechanism to Conserve Brain Catecholamines and Serotonin in Mice Differing in Excitabilty," *Nature*, 218 (1968), 575–577.

174. Winkelstein, W., Jr., S. Kantor, M. Ibrahim et al. "Familial Aggregation of Blood Pressure. Preliminary Report," *JAMA*, 195 (1966), 848–850.

175. Wolff, C., S. B. Friedman, M. A. Hofer et al. "Relationship between Psychological Defenses and Mean Urinary 17-Hydroxycorticosteroid Excretion Rates: I. A Predictive Study of Parents of Fatally Ill Children," *Psychosom. Med.*, 26 (1964), 576–591.

176. Wurtman, R. J. "Brain Monoamines and Endocrine Function," *Neurosci. Res. Prog. Bull.*, 9 (1971), 182–187.

177. Wurtman, R. J. and J. Axelrod. "Control of Enzymatic Synthesis of Adrenaline in the Adrenal Medulla by Adrenal Cortical Steroids," *J. Biol. Chem.*, 241 (1966), 2301–2305.

178. Yates, F. E. and J. Urquhart. "Control of Plasma Concentrations of Adrenocortical Hormones," *Physiol. Rev.*, 42 (1962), 359–443.

179. Young, M., B. Benjamin, and C. Wallis. "The Mortality of Widowers," *Lancet*, 2 (1963), 454–456.

180. Young, W. C. "The Hormones and Mating Behavior," in W. C. Young, ed., *Sex and Internal Secretions*, Vol. 2, pp. 1173–1239. Baltimore: Williams & Wilkins, 1961.

181. Young, W. C., R. W. Goy, and C. H. Phoenix. "Hormones and Sexual Behavior," *Science*, 143 (1964), 212–218.

PART FIVE

The Social Context of Psychiatry

CHAPTER 38

TRENDS IN MEDICAL EDUCATION

Fredrick C. Redlich and Howard Levitin

⟮ Introduction

I N THIS CHAPTER we describe medical education, its past development, its current practices, future trends and its problems. We ask what type of physician is needed and how this expert is produced. Although we take a global point of view, we concentrate on the American scene, because of the *Handbook* reader's dominant interest and because we are most familiar with it. We emphasize the education of the future physician and the physician of the future, but we recognize trends to educate other old and some new types of health personnel to cope with the ever-increasing tasks of health care.

⟮ A Short History of Medical Education

The wish to help the sick and alleviate their suffering is a rather general characteristic of the human species and activities to care for the sick have been known since the dawn of human history. There have been notable exceptions—in history and in some primitive living societies (such as infanticides among Eskimos)—and even in some industrialized societies, such as the mass murder of mentally and physically ill under National Socialism; yet the tendency to care for the sick and to develop and teach the art and science of health care are age old. In ancient societies, the nature of illness was assumed to be caused by supernatural and magic forces. In those societies, but also in large parts of the world today, disease was thought to be punishment from the gods. Only gradually, and in relatively recent times, have scientific points of view begun to prevail.

Antiquity

In ancient India, priest-doctors taught both the theoretical and practical knowledge of healing; their curriculum was extracts read aloud from medical writings, which their students memorized. Models of the human body made from wood or clay were some of the teaching tools for instruction in surgery, although knowledge of anatomy and physiology was limited since dissection of the human body was forbidden.[21] In Egypt, all educated persons from doctors to mathematicians were trained in schools associated with the temples where priest-doctors lived, taught, and practiced. Moses was a pupil at one of the priest schools and brought his knowledge to his people, which also formed a priest-doctor class.

In Greece, Apollo and his son Aesculapius were the supreme medical deities. The healing arts were taught to one or two students through the personal supervision of a preceptor. Temples dedicated to Aesculapius became medical centers where medicine was practiced exclusively by families claiming direct descent from this god. During this period of psychotherapeutic temple medicine, a Greek philosophy based on a world of reason developed, and medical thought slowly sloughed off magical concepts and priestly dogmatism and became established with its base of observation.[12] One empirical-rational school of medicine evolved on the island of Cos where Hippocrates lived in the fifth century B.C. He taught for the first time that disease is a natural process, not a result of sin or punishment of the gods. Physicians from all over the Mediterranean world came to the school at Cos to learn from Hippocrates, who stressed qualities of human compassion and high ethical standards as well as biological theory based on detailed observation. The written compilation of his teachings forms the basis for subsequent medical training.

After the founding of Alexandria in 333 B.C., the school and library there fostered an advance of science and mathematics. Dissection was practiced openly for the first time, with commensurate advances in anatomical knowledge. The medical schools at Alexandria maintained their prominent position under Roman rule. Until the importation of Greek physicians about 200 B.C., however, the Romans had no medical profession nor medical schools. The most prominent Roman physician, Galen, worked in the second century after Christ. He lectured on the structure and functions of the human body, and succeeded in building a prestigious medical practice. His skillful diagnoses enlarged knowledge of anatomy and physiology, and his writings became a basic medical text.

The Middle Ages and Renaissance

With the division of the Roman empire into Eastern and Western at the end of the fourth century and the beginning of the Dark Ages in Europe, Byzantium—later Constantinople—became a major center of civilization until the fifteenth century. Even under Byzantine rule, theoretical scientific teaching made little progress, as practitioners and teachers were slavishly devoted to the dogma of Galen and any interest in the temporal body was against their religious beliefs.[21] When St. Benedict established a monastery in 529 at Monte Cassino, monks became the scholars responsible for maintaining the knowledge of medicine by translating and copying the ancient literature.

During the seventh century the followers of Mohammed conquered half of the then known world and established important medical centers. In Persia, the University at Jundi Shapur became the greatest center of medical learning in the Islamic world, offering bedside clinical instruction at its teaching hospital. Baghdad was another Arabic intellectual and medical center and it was there in 931 that a board of examination for medical practitioners was established for the first time.[12] Outstanding physicians practiced and taught in both cities. Many prominent Jewish physicians thrived under Moorish rule; at that time no antagonism between Jews and Mohammedans existed. Avicenna, who lived from 980 to 1037, was the greatest single contributor to Arabic medicine and his *Canon of Medicine* codified all existing knowledge about medicine. His writings joined those of Hippocrates and Galen as the foundation for medical learning during the Middle Ages.

By the tenth century the medical school in Salerno, Italy, began to attract students from all over Europe. Salerno was the first school to institute an organized curriculum—three years of preparation and five years of medical studies, followed by a public examination and a year of apprenticeship.[20] Other schools developed in Italy, France and Germany; particularly well known were the French schools in Paris and Montpellier.

With the Renaissance came renewed interest in anatomical knowledge, with emphasis on observation in diagnosis and treatment. Printing made less expensive texts of new translations of the Greek and Roman medical scholars available to students. The University of Padua Medical School, the leading school of its time, attracted many German and English students who had little medical training available in their own countries. The school standardized a four-year curriculum leading to a bachelor-of-medicine degree followed by a doctoral degree after some years of practice. Although empirical training had been available only outside the university, the sixteenth century saw a new interest in bedside teaching. Vesalius in 1537 began doing his own dissections as he taught anatomy and lectured to the students from the body, using large and natural-looking colored illustrations to provide the first extensions in anatomical knowledge since Galen.

As discoveries in anatomy distinguished the sixteenth century, so experiments in physiology created a science based on facts in the seventeenth century. William Harvey's discovery of the circulation of the blood in 1620 became the foundation on which the structure of physiology was built. Careful experimental methodology and reasoning brought medicine into the realm of science—the beginnings of "basic research." Scientists now began to explore, through experimentation, the how and the why of natural cause and effect. The microscope aided greatly in biological research. There was, however, little change in the way medicine was taught during the seventeenth century, although there was more recognition of the importance of the clinical demonstrations.

The Age of Enlightenment and Modern Times

It was not until 1630 that the Infirmary at Leiden offered instruction at the bedside.

There, at the beginning of the eighteenth century, Hermann Boerhaave promulgated the outline of the modern medical curriculum: ". . . the propaedeutics of mathematics and natural science, the study of normal anatomy and physiology, and finally the study of pathology and therapy."[8] Boerhaave's perception of the necessity for basing medical education on scientific principles and his gifted bedside instruction brought medical education to a high point during his tenure, and his pupils extended his work throughout the world. The medical school at Edinburgh, for example, which trained many doctors from the American colonies, was founded by Alexander Monro and other pupils of Boerhaave; and Gerard van Swieten and Anton de Haen, other students of this master teacher, were responsible for the success of the Vienna Medical School in the later part of the seventeenth and eighteenth centuries. Vienna established the first professorial chair in clinical medicine and originated the concept of the modern clinic in 1753 to attract an international complement of students who learned on clinical rounds made daily with the professor in charge, setting the pattern for future clinical training in academic centers.

During the first half of the nineteenth century, Paris was the unquestioned center of medicine in the world,[8] fostering important research, including that of Pasteur, whose studies of bacteriology greatly influenced health and medical care. Then German and Austrian centers of medical education supplanted the French centers. One factor for the decline of the French system was the use of essay type competitive examinations that determined appointments in the university. At one time this constituted progress, but ultimately it turned into a stifling obstacle. Another reason was that in Germany and Austria, and in the Netherlands, Switzerland, and the Scandinavian countries, medical education and medical research became part of the higher education system under the umbrella of the universities, and a responsibility of the university faculty. This new approach was eloquently presented in a revolutionary book on medical education by the eminent surgeon

Theodor von Billroth.[1] In time this new method was introduced in Russia and Japan. Young American doctors were particularly interested in training in specialties organized in universities of the German-speaking countries, and these university centers became the model for twentieth-century American schools. In contrast, the Latin countries of Europe and South and Central America remained more or less under the French influence.

Medical training in England developed its own unique pattern. The bulk of clinical training was totally separate from the university schools at Oxford and Cambridge, which only provided theoretical training for physicians who came almost exclusively from the upper classes. Guy's hospital, founded in 1725, was particularly well known, with many important clinical teachers in its school. Some hospital schools developed into centers of excellence and had a profound impact on the development of medical education in many colonies of the British Empire. As in Europe, surgeons were trained in separate schools supported by the Guild of Barbers and Surgeons (after 1800 the Royal Society of Surgeons) and through private tutoring. Surgical techniques only gradually became part of the medical school curriculum. Apothecaries, who practiced general medicine among the lower classes as well as compounding and distributing drugs and medicines, had a seven-year apprenticeship. Each group tightly controlled the licensing of its membership and sharp guild distinctions were reinforced.

Early Medicine in the United States

The American colonies received medical care during the early years of their existence primarily from the surgeons and apothecaries who immigrated. Few physicians left their comfortable lives in England to risk the hazards of a new country. Surgeon-apothecaries were trained by a three-year apprenticeship with practitioners drawn from a wide variety of backgrounds. At first, few of them could afford to return to Europe or England for university training, but as the colonial economy improved more young men went abroad to take a university degree. The first American college of medicine was established in 1765 at the College of Philadelphia by John Morgan and William Shippen, Jr., two young physicians who had trained at Edinburgh. "At least one year's course of lectures after apprenticeship were required for the M.B. Three years thereafter a man could defend a thesis and qualify for an M.D., though few actually took that degree until after the baccalaureate was abolished in 1789. In terms of both curriculum and staff, the school was a progressive one by European standards." Other schools were established during the rest of the century (there were at least thirty medical schools by 1838) mostly by groups of medical practitioners who ran their schools for profit, without a formal relationship to existing universities or hospitals. On the whole, there were few regulations and requirements were lax. Johns Hopkins School of Medicine, established in 1893, was the first medical school to combine both clinical training, with the German-European, medical-school concept of rigorous scientific research, and to offer some service to the community as well. It was an alternative to the proliferating proprietary medical schools with uneven standards. It opened the way for the reform movement initiated by the Flexner report of 1910.

The Flexner Report and Its Impact

Abraham Flexner, influenced by distinguished colleagues at Johns Hopkins, particularly by William Osler and William H. (Popsy) Welch, and appalled by the low level of American education, incompatible with the increasing wealth and technical and cultural development of the United States, wrote his famous report in 1910.[9] This report, divided into a general part of critique and recommendations and a special part describing the existing schools, had a profound impact. There were, in 1907, 160 private commercial schools —only half of them barely acceptable; even university-linked schools such as Harvard's and Pennsylvania's medical schools could not compare with the German, Austrian, or Swiss medical schools. Flexner's basic recommendations were to link medical schools with universities; to make nationwide searches for the best faculties; to improve the preparation of students entering medical schools by better general education and by special training in the basic biological sciences; to foster biological and clinical research in medical schools (Flexner thought clinical and scientific endeavors were similar); and to interlock the predoctoral training in medical schools with the postdoctoral training in hospitals, which would lead to the development of university-linked medical centers. He foresaw the development of strong full-time faculties unhampered by the exigencies of medical practice. In some institutions this eventually led to an alienation of academic medicine from clinical practice. In general, however, the impact of the reform was most favorable, even though the question of whether a pure, full-time system is best from an economic and motivational point of view has never been unequivocally answered. In the twenties the proprietary schools virtually disappeared and a profound reform of medical education was apparent. The closing of proprietary schools resulted in a reduction of the number of physicians. Although the quality of medical practitioners improved, many quacks and unscientific healers still continued to practice in the United States. The American Medical Association, through its Council of Medical Education and the Association of Medical Colleges, played a major role in these changes.

A striking uniformity of the new programs emerged, although only gradually did the full-time system become dominant. Between the two world wars American schools were part of state universities or of privately supported universities. They were small (rarely larger than 100 students to a class) limiting their admissions to highly selected students. Such selection was based in principle on performance—at first in the premedical college courses, later by more accurately appraised objective vocational tests such as the Medical College Admission Test (MCAT).[10] With rare exceptions, few studies of personal and social characteristics of students[18] have been undertaken and the assessment of desirable personality characteristics of future physicians follows a "common-sense" approach that is far from satisfactory. In reality, admissions were simply curtailed in the majority of cases by the student's ability to pay the very high tuition that is mandatory in a tutorial system of instruction with little governmental or private supplemental support for education. There were also serious restrictions on ethnic groups: many Jewish students were forced to study in Europe and American Negroes were virtually nonexistent in medical schools. Only very recently has the number of women and of university groups begun to increase.

The study of medicine took four years, following a college course of four years. The curriculum consisted of a rigorous course in the basic biological sciences with strong emphasis on anatomy; only gradually did biology, biochemistry, and physiology begin to replace the endless hours of dissections. Pathology and pharmacology were important subjects in the second year. There was no instruction in the behavioral and social sciences and only after the Second World War did psychiatry become a major subject in most schools. The major clinical specialties, internal medicine, pediatrics, surgery, obstetrics, and gynecology, were taught in clerkships with strong emphasis on bedside teaching and letting the student assume considerable responsibility in care of indigent patients. In contrast to European schools, dentists had their own schools, and virtually no stomatology is taught in American medical schools. There was little teaching in outpatient clinics. Attendance of laboratory courses and lectures was required in most schools and course examinations were rigorously held. Yale was an exception and has demanded neither compulsory attendance nor local examinations. The faculty at Yale required a scientific thesis and evaluated the student's performance without grades, and graduated the student after he passed objective examinations by the National Board of Medical Examiners.

Gradually, the National Board of Medical Examiners has become a very important agency monitoring and influencing standards of virtually all medical schools. The same has been true for an ever-increasing number of specialty boards that examine and certify those who wish to work as specialists. Although these boards are made up of distinguished faculty members of medical schools, the existence of separate boards has set up jurisdiction over standards of medical education outside of medical schools and medical teaching centers. Furthermore, every state of the union licenses its physicians after so-called state board examinations, often specifying educational prerequisites for licensing although the states, in most cases, recognize national board standards. Among foreign graduates—who, at present, make up about a third of the number of American interns and residents and one-fourth of its practitioners—further preliminary examinations are required.[15]

Medical Education during the Second World War and Its Aftermaths

The period between the two World Wars was a period of stability in the system of American medical education.[8] As might be expected, the war brought changes. The first of these changes was a decrease in the length of study from four years to three in order to provide the required number of physicians to the armed forces. Although objective evaluations were lacking, it seemed that the abbreviated course, primarily accomplished by compressing the four-year curriculum into three years through a heavy course load and a twelve-month academic year, caused no reduction in the performance level. However, when the war ended, the four-year course was resumed. The second change became apparent after the war. The war required major efforts in basic and applied research. This was organized and supervised through an Office of Scientific Research and Development (OSRD) under the leadership of such eminent scientists as V. Bush, K. T. Compton, and J. B. Conant. Originally, medical sciences were under OSRD; in 1946, the National Insti-

tutes of Health under the leadership of James Shannon[25] were organized. These institutes not only carried on an increasing amount of biomedical research but also financed very large research enterprises in medical schools. While in 1947 only 87 million dollars was spent, the appropriations for health research for NIH in 1972 were over one billion dollars. This dramatic increase in funds enabled medical school faculties (but not student bodies) to grow rapidly. Today in many schools over half of the budget comes from governmental research funds, and, in some, as much as three quarters. In 1972, the federal government accounted for 64 percent of national expenditures for health research. (Private industry accounted for 27 percent, and foundations, voluntary health agencies, and other organizations provided the remaining 9 percent.) The result has been not only unprecedented progress in the biomedical sciences but also a threat to the primary mission of medical schools—to prepare physicians for medical practice. Another consequence of growth and multiple functions (teaching, research, and service) has been the increasingly complex problems administrators of medical schools are facing today. As the allocation of funds for research activities in general has been made by so-called study sections, after objective evaluation of projects and programs, the economic control of schools has shifted to a certain degree from inside control to outside influence.

New Developments

After years of little change and even smug satisfaction with the "best system of medical education in the world," pressures for change began to mount. They came from students who felt overeducated in those scientific subjects which interested their teachers and underprepared for practice in the specialties, particularly in family medicine. Leaders of ethnic groups in the inner city also complained that poor, and particularly black and Spanish-speaking Americans in urban ghettos received inadequate care or none at all, and they blamed medical practitioners and educators for a lack of concern with their problems. To a lesser extent some members of the faculty were also concerned with a lack of interest and insufficient funds for teaching, as well as with an obsolete and rigid curriculum and with the need, in view of the "knowledge explosion" and the ever shorter "half life" of medical knowledge, to emphasize the teaching of principles and methodology rather than the memorizing of data. Such data can be stored and retrieved by computers and the brains of students don't have to be overloaded with what quickly becomes trivial and out of date. A modern library system can provide references and data quickly and efficiently.[28] There is today considerable interest in modern approaches to medical teaching, using programmed instructions[16] and audio-visual techniques.[27] Films, and particularly video tapes, have helped to teach some basic science subjects quite effectively—anatomy and also clinical methods, especially clinical examinations and interviewing.

Much of the blame for unsatisfactory conditions fell on the American Medical Association, with its conservative stance in medical practice and education, which attempts to keep medicine a monopolistic "cottage industry," based on the principle of fee-for-service medical care. Some protests by students and the "inner-city community" were quite vocal and even violent. No revolution has occurred, however, but some changes have been stimulated by an interesting document known as the *Carnegie Report* written by eminent scholars and clinicians under the chairmanship of Clark Kerr.[13]

❲ The Carnegie Report

Higher Education and the Nation's Health

The special report on policies for medical and dental education of the Carnegie Commission on Higher Education was published in 1970. It is concerned with the contributions of university health-science centers toward the goal of adequate and effective health care for the entire population, regardless of income. Noting the "serious shortage of professional health manpower, the need for expanding and restructuring the education of professional health personnel and the vital importance of adapting the education of health manpower to the changes needed for an effective system of delivery of health care in the United States," the commission believes that the provision of highly skilled health manpower, particularly doctors and dentists, is a special responsibility of higher education.

Emphasizing unmet needs in both medical and dental care, the report points out the growing belief that health care is not only a necessity but also a right to which all persons are entitled. It touches on the problems affecting health care today, including insufficient health manpower and maldistribution of personnel, ineffective financing and rising costs. The commission warns that no matter how much health-care education is improved and how many more professionals are trained, adequate health care will be impossible unless the delivery system is also improved.

To overcome the existing acute shortage of physicians and the less acute shortage of dentists, the report suggests that the number of medical-school entrants be increased by 50 percent to 16,400, and the number of dental students be increased by 20 percent to 5400 by the end of the decade. Further expansion of the numbers of student places available should then be reconsidered. It will be particularly important to increase the numbers of women students and minority-group representation. The commission suggests three ways to increase the student population to reach a recommended goal of 216.4 active physicians per one hundred thousand population by 2002: shift all medical schools from four- to three-year programs; add new places for students, with schools expanding to at least 100 students per class and to 200 or more in some cases; and establish nine new medical schools in metropolitan areas of about three hundred fifty thousand or more people. Development and expansion of programs for the training of physicians' and dentists' associates and assistants will add greater efficiency to the larger number of physicians. More allied health personnel at all levels must be trained along with physicians and dentists.

Medical School Models

In addition to increasing the numbers of students, university health-science centers can work in several directions to improve the quality of both education and health-care delivery. Two new models for university medical schools indicate that the Flexner model, emphasizing biological research, will no longer be the only acceptable one. The *health-care-delivery* model, in which the medical school in addition to training does research in health-care delivery, orients itself to external service; the *integrated-science* model carries on most or all basic science and social-science instruction within the main campus, while the medical school stresses clinical training and biomedical research. These models and combinations of them will provide greater flexibility in both training and health-care delivery.

The report recommends that the health-science centers should now undertake curriculum revision to accelerate premedical and medical education, including elimination of the internship year and better integrated health-related sciences as basic training for a variety of health-related professions, perhaps awarding a master's degree at the end of this period. Two-year medical schools are considered undesirable and should be eliminated, and public-health schools must be incorporated in the university centers. As in the British model, clinical instruction in selected hospitals outside of the university would be considered. Both curriculum reforms and admissions procedures should become more responsive to the expressed needs of students, with greater emphasis on comprehensive medicine, a more careful integration of abstract theory and clinical experience, and wider experience in community hospitals, neighborhood clinics, and other community facilities.

According to the Carnegie commission proposal, medical economists, administration specialists, and behavioral scientists in the academic and service functions would be included in health-science centers to increase the educational impact in these fields as well as in preventive medicine and community health. Significantly increasing programs in continuing education for area-health personnel, undertaking extensive research in health-care delivery systems and placing more emphasis on teaching as professionally rewarding for faculty are other ways in which the university would mold a health center. Appropriate officers would have to be appointed within the universities to develop plans for the expansion of these centers.

University health-science centers should be responsible not only for the education of health-care personnel but also for cooperating with other community agencies, such as health-maintenance organizations and other community-education facilities. Community colleges would develop training programs for the allied health professions working closely with the university centers.

To support these centers, located primarily in areas with high population concentrations, the report recommends careful regional planning to establish 126 area-health education centers as satellites of the universities. These centers would bring about 95 percent of the population within an hour's transportation of a major health-care facility.

Financial Support

In order to achieve the goals recommended by the Carnegie commission report federal and state and private support of medical and dental education is necessary.[7] The report assumes that there will be some form of national-health insurance within the next decade, one more indication of growing federal interest. Since medical and dental education is critically underfunded, the commission recommends several ways in which the federal government can effectively augment its support. A federal program of grants in amounts up to $4000 a year for medical and dental students would attract students from low-income families, and an Educational Opportunity Bank for students, including house officers, would offer loans repayable by a percentage of medical earnings during a number of years of professional practice. The development of a voluntary national-health-service corps, with the excuse from loan repayment during a two-year term of service and reduction of maximum indebtedness as incentives, are recommended. Tuition would be stabilized nationally at a relatively low, uniform level. In addition to helping students specifically, federal cost-of-instruction supplements should be provided to university health-science centers for each medical and dental student enrolled and each house officer, with bonuses for expansion of enrollment and curriculum reform. Federal construction grants for up to 75 percent of total costs and start-up grants of up to $10 million each would stimulate growth of new university-health-science centers. Finally, federal support of research should be maintained at its present percentage of the gross national product. Other ways in which the federal government can support and strengthen medical and dental education include strengthening of existing legislation for regional, state, and local health planning with university-health-science centers and area-health-education centers having responsibility for the planning of health-manpower education and regional agencies taking charge of planning changes in health-care delivery. The report also recommends a national requirement for periodic reexamination and recertification of all physicians and dentists, federal funds for support of continuing education, and expansion of health-manpower research programs with the appointment of a National Health Manpower Commission.

The states should continue to provide substantial financial support for medical and dental education, too, and states that have lagged behind in the past should plan for significant increases in expenditures for this purpose. States should provide financial support, particularly for house officer training and for education of allied health workers, as these personnel tend to remain in the states where they have been trained. The states, in cooperation with universities and with regional and local planning bodies would also play a major role in the development of university health-science centers, area-health education centers and training programs for allied health personnel. Additional financial support should continue to come from private foundations that traditionally have supported health-manpower education and research.

In general, we consider the *Carnegie Report* an excellent document, in spite of certain statements which we and others question. Is there a real shortage of physicians or rather a maldistribution of physicians and a need for new types of allied health personnel, such as physician associates and nurse practitioners? In some specialties, such as radiology and psychiatry, the shortage is very palpable. There is no doubt, also, that hospitals are not sufficiently manned by American residents, forcing these institutions to take foreign-trained doctors and thus deprive foreign countries, which are themselves short in medical manpower. We are also concerned that a deemphasis of research might reduce medical schools to trade schools and that medical schools might not fulfill their primary mission—i.e., increase and dissemination of medical knowledge—if they assume too many service responsibilities.

Reforms in Teaching

A number of changes have occurred since the midsixties—and the Medical School of Case Western Reserve University under its dynamic dean, Joseph Wearn, led the way. At Case Western Reserve the interdisciplinary approach to teaching basic and clinical subjects simultaneously was developed to eliminate repetitive, overlapping, and disjointed courses. The "committee" method of teaching, however, needs careful organization and preparation, and, in general, such "horizontal teaching" is more expensive than traditional "vertical teaching."

At the time of writing, a wave of reform has swept the medical schools. It has created a modified and again relatively uniform pattern of medical education. The majority of medical schools has retained the four-year curriculum, but an increasing number of schools are becoming three-year schools. As new schools were established, the existing schools—motivated, in part at least, by financial lures of specific increases of support for "manpower augmentation"—admitted more students, particularly more students from ethnic minorities, and more women.

There is now greater emphasis on a reduction of initial time spent with basic biological sciences and on an earlier introduction of clinical material into the curriculum as well as on health care, with its social and economic problems. This is not an easy task in view of the ever-increasing knowledge produced by the "biological revolution." The trend to specialization continues and even primary medicine or family medicine is becoming a specialty. Actually, attempts to produce well-rounded medical practitioners have not been very successful,[14] and so-called track programs in the last semesters have been forerunners of specialization, even when this is explicitly not the intent of these track programs which are designed to enable students to revisit the basic sciences and make them more meaningful in the pursuit of clinical activities.

(Current Problems

Length of Predoctoral Course

In the midst of the reassessment of medical education, a number of problems present themselves for the schools and for medical policy making. The amount of time it takes to educate a physician is one unresolved problem. We have already mentioned how the federal government "encourages" schools to reduce the length of study by special financial awards. As the medical schools are rather pointedly being asked to reduce the amount of time required to train a physician, the issue of what the product is supposed to be reappears. In the absence of a clear and distinct definition of what the "product" should be, the argument about whether it takes three years or four years is difficult to answer. Neverthe-

less, there are increasing pressures to develop programs requiring no longer than three years to produce that which used to be produced in four years. One approach to this end has been to take the four-year program and squeeze it into three years, utilizing the summers and giving very little free elective time to the student. (This is the World War II model.) We later will discuss the obvious and important principle that medical education does not end with the awarding of a degree but must be preceded by a good preparation in college and continue through the physician's life.

Role of Basic Sciences

One of the most important questions at the moment is the issue of the basic sciences and their role in college and medical schools. There is a group of scientists suggesting that basic sciences could best be taught in the university setting. Indeed, they claim that cell biology, biochemistry, histology, and genetics are currently being taught at a level of sophistication that far exceeds the usual training required for medical students. It is their position that with a slight augmentation of their basic science programs they could teach at equal or better levels of competence the basic sciences prerequisite to clinical medicine currently being taught by the medical schools. Alternatively, it is suggested by others that the medical school basic science departments are crucial to successful operation of a medical center and that their impact on the medical center goes far beyond the training of the medical student, especially in their effect on research programs undertaken by clinical departments. Reciprocally, the medical center milieu is important to the thrust of human biology being studied by the basic scientists. The basic science departments have an important role in the training of Ph.D. candidates in order to perpetuate their disciplines. All of these activities are complimentary and not competitive with their roles in the education of the medical student. While these two opposing views pose cogent arguments, it remains an unresolved issue that will be important over the next ten years and will require each university to resolve internally, according to its own resources. In our opinion the basic sciences, well-linked to other parts of the university, ought to remain in the medical school. In any case we feel strongly that in medical school it is important that those who teach a subject be at the frontier of knowledge in that field and have a scientific point of view resulting from personal involvement in the acquisition of new knowledge.

However the foregoing issue is resolved, we consider it essential that students be taught medical psychology, medical sociology, medical economics, and medical ethics.[4] Since facilities and faculties for these disciplines are not yet adequate in most medical centers, it is currently difficult to provide such instruction. The lack of such teaching in most medical schools is a serious educational deficit. It is in these areas that the faculties of the college program might be used and have impact on the medical curriculum. The major task of psychiatrists in teaching medical students is not teaching of psychiatry as a specialty but rather the teaching of psychological and social factors in the diagnosis, treatment, and prevention of disease.[22] It is also noteworthy, and indeed alarming, that attitudes of cynicism increase and attitudes of compassion decrease during the study of medicine. Certainly, such a trend ought to be counteracted.

An increasing number of students with some degree of training in the biological sciences are soliciting medical schools for advanced placement. On the basis of Ph.D. or other academic activities in the biological sciences, students are requesting placement in the second or third year of a medical school in an effort to achieve an M.D. degree in somewhat less than the prescribed three- or four-year program. While this, in the past, was a unique situation, occurring no more than once or twice a year, it has now reached a point where as many as fifteen to twenty students per year, at many medical schools, are requesting this type of special consideration. It seems clear from the trend that the number of students soliciting advanced placement and/or

altered medical school programs on the basis of their biological science background will increase.

Medical School and Community

The university medical center is increasingly under pressure to define its interface with the community and to respond to legitimate requirements for increasing involvement of medical care for that constituency which looks to the medical center as a primary care unit. At the same time, it tries not to become inundated by commitments to serve too large a community, the results of which would be a loss of primary thrust in the area of education and research.

It becomes evident, however, that the only focus, and possibly not even the primary focus, for predoctoral clinical training, is not the university hospital ward, with its highly specialized activities, but the inpatient and outpatient services of community hospitals, the practitioners' offices, and the newly emerging health centers of the community.[5]

Family Medicine

There is much talk of the importance of primary medicine or family medicine, but actually little of it is really taught. With the abandonment of the old internship and with new types of practitioners being educated at many levels, such as different types of physician associates and nurse practitioners, we consider it unlikely that medical students will aspire to the role of the traditional general practitioner. In contrast to Great Britain, which has made a strong commitment to train general practitioners, medical policy makers in the United States seem uncertain and confused. Even after such a commitment is made, it will not be implemented easily because the necessary clinical faculty are not currently on the academic staffs of medical schools. Whether a change in the reward system for promotion, and government and private funds, can recruit such a faculty remains to be seen.

Allied Health Professions

One of the most ambiguous area with which the medical teaching centers will be asked to deal is the broad area of allied health training.[24] Without clearly establishing the need, a number of people are advocating the training of a large number of new health professionals called physician assistants, nurse practitioners, or health practitioners. These people tend to be postbaccalaureate students who received an additional one to two years' training in the area of pediatrics, midwifery, trauma or ambulatory care in an effort to replace a part or portion of the traditional role played by the physician. It seems quite clear that a number of students will graduate from such programs over the next few years, but what is less clear is the role they ultimately will play in the national-health-care delivery system. Unfortunately, two simultaneous thrusts shed doubt on the future of these individuals. On the one hand, a number of schools have accepted the concept that new allied health professionals will be required and have undertaken the training of a reasonable number of such people. On the other hand, as we already mentioned, a number of medical schools have decided to respond to the increasing need for physicians (as indicated in the Carnegie report) by the training of a large number of students in three-year programs. It is likely that a student with three years of medical training competing with a physician associate with two years' training will leave the physician associate in a most unfortunate situation. Only if the number of physicians is held constant, while a large number of allied health professionals are trained, would the future of the allied health professionals seem favorable.

Postdoctoral Training

During the last thirty years, postdoctoral training has been rather uniform in all disciplines, requiring an internship and anywhere from three to five years of additional residency training in pursuit of certification by the various board specialties. Each of these programs allows approximately one year of freedom to do whatever the candidate wishes in the form of fellowship, research, or practice. The basic formulation in the year of internship and three years of residency training in an academic medical center remain the prototype of all programs leading to board certification. This long-standing traditional approach to board certification has recently come under fire and a new pattern has evolved.

This new pattern has altered the traditional approach in terms of the total time required to accomplish board certification. It allows a variety of mixed programs, incorporating family and community medicine, and transdiscipline training programs. The utilization of the affiliated community hospitals is an important part of the programs. For a number of the board-certifying programs the internship has been abolished, allowing the student to go from his senior status in medical school into a first-year residency program in psychiatry, the surgical subspecialties, radiology and other disciplines, without the need for a general internship in medicine or surgery. This has led to a storm of protest and it is likely that this particular decision will be reversed in the near future. Some of the general surgical programs have also abolished the internship. This has been abolition in name only, since the first-year postdoctoral program requires essentially the same degree of expertise and demands of the resident the same responsibilities in the management of patients as he previously had under the title of intern. The net effect is to change the title for his first year postdoctoral training program and to reduce the total number of years required in that particular program.

A very important suggestion, yet to be implemented, that has come about in the last three years is that the university maintain control of the postdoctoral training program. This would result in the change in emphasis from a service-oriented program to a mixed service and academic training program. It would allow the candidate for board certification to develop expertise in the care of patients and a more sophisticated approach to clinical medicine, but, at the same time, to continue formal academic study in basic and clinical science appropriate to his board certification. It is the opinion of these authors that this is a most important issue for the university to face and that the postdoctoral training program would be improved by such control by the university.

Continuing Medical Education

Closely related to the suggestion that the university maintain a greater impact in the postdoctoral training program is the role of the university in continuing education. To terminate a physician's formal training a few years out of medical school and legally never again to enter into any formal academic program nor be tested for competence is something the medical profession must face as an unacceptable situation. The legislative control of continuing medical education must be relegated either to the university medical center, the state and local medical societies, the Association of American Medical Colleges and/or the American Medical Association and/or state licensing boards. If the university medical center is considered most adept in the area of medical education and evaluation, then it would seem likely that it is best qualified to undertake the program of continuing medical education and evaluation of the practitioner. Whether this is done by compulsory postdoctoral educational programs, formal written examinations, or oral evaluation during visits to the medical center, or by searching of the practitioner's records is an implementation problem. It will probably be of little consequence as long as the practitioner knows that maintenance of academic and intellectual proficiency is crucial to continued licensing and certification in his particular specialty. This program of recertification would be applicable also to those who are in general practice and/or the practice of family medicine. Even if the final certification were to be left to licensing boards or state medical societies the role of updating the physician in terms of contemporary medical education would undoubtedly fall upon the medical center. It is a responsibility that the medical center should appropriately assume.

Evaluation and Cost Effectiveness

We foresee a definite thrust into the area of evaluation and of cost accounting of medical education, clinical care, and research. Demands are already made by the federal government, which supplies substantial funds, to characterize activities according to the appropriate budgetary activity.[7] Thus, it is quite clear that monies flowing from the government for the purpose of education will require cost accounting against the actual teaching effort that the money was supposed to support. Not much longer will third-party carriers pay for other than patient-care costs. They will ferret out hidden research and teaching costs and disallow them when they are discovered. This pattern has become increasingly apparent over the last few years, and there is no question that it will continue. As the federal government support of research is decreasing medical centers will find it difficult to maintain the same degree of high-level research as they have in the past. With a growing demand for better cost accounting of education, service, and research, it will be increasingly important that the role and financial support of the postdoctoral fellow be more clearly defined. To what extent the practicing physician owes the resident and intern some part or portion of his income because of services rendered on behalf of the physician will have to be answered. In addition, that part or portion of the intern's or resident's training which is specifically academic for his best interest will have to be cost accounted in a medical education package, leaving only the uncontestable patient-care activities of the intern and resident to be charged to a category of patient costs.

⟨ Who Is Being Trained for What?

In any discussion of the curriculum desirable for a given medical school a recurrent question emerges: "What is the product that the curriculum is designed to produce?" No one has yet, in an uncontroversial way, defined the product of medical education, namely the physician, and the characteristics that are necessary for the modern, complete practitioner of the healing arts. It obviously encompasses a certain intellectual capacity and ability to retain facts, an ability to relate well to patients, an understanding of the pathophysiological and behavioral processes of man, and the correlative ability to apply all of these facts to the management of difficult and complicated cases. Yet these generalities do not lend themselves easily to testing and in the absence of an objective criteria for evaluating the good physician, the unresolved question of whether a particular curriculum is good or bad remains. Since it is not likely that the medical profession will agree on a succinct, objective definition of the final, complete product that medical education is supposed to produce, it is likely that there will be many curricular innovations and many programs designed to attain the ambiguous goal of the excellent physician. Even if a definition of the physician were available, and objective criteria could be applied by testing techniques to determine those who are eligible, problems will remain.

The geographic distribution of physicians is unequal and will remain so as long as there are communities of high-density urban cultural centers and low-density rural communities with a minimal commitment to the cultural aspects the physician so eagerly incorporates into his daily life. Talk about incentives to move physicians from an urban-dense population by monetary incentives is unrealistic, since it does not address itself to the basic problem that keeps physicians in the urban center. The physician is culturally and intellectually oriented to a peer group and feels lost in a lonely and isolated intellectual environment. He requires fellow physicians and fellow professionals (lawyers and engineers, for instance) in a community that has a commitment to the theater, music, and arts. A community not having these facilities is unlikely, in the relatively near future, to attract a physician even if the remunerative aspects of

his practice are inordinately high. High-speed transportation allowing a small nucleus of physicians in a group setting to meet the needs of a much larger geographical area will be crucial to the solution of the distribution problem for physicians in this country. The regional program inaugurated in 1967 holds some real promise to contribute to a solution of these programs.[17]

In all discussions of contemporary medical education there is the recurrent question of how the health-delivery system should meet the needs of the people. It is quite clear that the impact of third-party payment is already being felt by a change in the attitudes of physicians and patients toward each other. As funds for health-care delivery and education of health workers will come increasingly from public sources, the public will demand, through its leadership, to monitor these enterprises and to set board policy for them. One of the most fundamental policies will be to look at health as a right; discriminatory practices will be unacceptable. Although the people will determine what should be done about its health, professionals must play a major role in charting the path toward progress. Ebert feels that universities rather than medical schools will play a major role in such work. Medical educators must train physicians and new teams of health workers to carry out health care in new institutions (not just hospitals.) The patient is becoming increasingly aware of his rights in demanding a high level of medical care, which he admits he is unable to determine according to an objective criterion, but the trend toward national-health insurance will undoubtedly give impetus to this reassessment of the health-delivery system, and the role the physician plays vis-à-vis the patient.

Another clearly discernible trend is the growth and bureaucratization of medical education. Most American schools have become complex multipurpose enterprises. Just like universities of which they are and ought to be parts, they are in most cases not creatively administered.[23] A dilemma exists as to whether the leadership should be in the hands of professional persons, who are usually neither trained nor particularly interested in administration, or in the hands of administrators, who often do not sufficiently understand the tasks and problems of the schools—such as the complex budgetary, spatial, and hierarchical problems of the enterprise. Some of the best deans have been deeply vexed over such problems.[11] In time, deans and their associates and assistants usually learn enough about hierarchical competition (the tenure problem is a particularly vexing one) and even about the "territorial imperative," but they remain woefully naive about intricate budgetary distributions and planning. In the future probably a special academic administrator needs to be trained to take care of these tasks.

([Worldwide Trends in Medical Education

There are marked differences in medical education in the United States and foreign schools, in the West and East.[2] In general, American schools and the schools of developed countries have become, in many cases, more alike because the American model of clinical instruction has been copied. United States' schools are still small, while many foreign schools have systems of open or relatively unrestricted admission. The weeding out of undesirable students in foreign schools is done mostly by examinations, usually of the oral type. Medical education in foreign schools is almost entirely supported by government funds; it is inexpensive because faculty resources and facilities are limited. The quality of medical education in these schools is, generally speaking, in our opinion, lower than in the United States. Such differences in quality are felt less by superior students who can tailor their programs more easily according to their needs and talents in some of the good foreign schools than they can in United States' schools. The average student, however, often does not obtain the thorough grounding in the clinical and basic sciences that his American colleague receives.

There are great differences between the medical schools of the socialist countries and those in the rest of the world. In the socialist countries, medical research and medical education are quite sharply separated. Medical research is the prerogative of the academies of science and medical education is the responsibility of medical schools. This separation is particularly marked in the Soviet Union, and somewhat less in the other European socialist republics where some research still goes on in clinical and basic science departments. About the People's Republic of China very little has been known until now in Western countries.[3] Only recently we learned of the large increase of Chinese medical education institutions and the resulting increase of medical practitioners. China has three types of medical schools; their national schools are superior to state and provincial schools. All of them are charged with the education of the largest possible number of badly needed physicians. Two types of doctors exist: modern and traditional physicians. The two types, according to official reports at least, seem to coexist in harmony. China has also trained new types of ancillary personnel with minimal knowledge, far below the standards of the Russian or American physician's associate. They are called "Red Guard" doctors, working primarily in cities, and "barefoot" doctors who work primarily in rural areas. The attribute barefoot refers to their main job as agricultural laborers in rice fields. These types get "quickie" courses in first aid and some simple medical therapeutics. Their work essentially is part-time, in medical-aid stations under medical supervisors.

In socialist countries, but also in Great Britain and to a lesser extent in other Western welfare states, the output of physicians and other health workers seems to be regulated by the country's need for physicians rather than by individual decisions of the physician or student, or by schools and guilds operating according to a *numerus clausus* principle, dependent both on the student's ability to pay and even (though less today than ever) on his ethnic characteristics.

As the United States moves toward a planned system of health-care delivery and as public financing of medical education increases, undoubtedly this will change, too. We subscribe to a system of medical education that trains different types of health workers, whatever the society needs, ranging from physician–scientists to relatively unsophisticated workers. Many types of medical workers are needed to preserve and restore health and to aid populations in their suffering from illness and injury. Hopefully this can be achieved with minimal infringement on the individual doctor–patient relationship.

(Bibliography

1. BILLROTH, T. VON. *Über das Lehren und Lernen der medizinischen Wissenschaften auf den Universitäten der deutschen Nation.* Vienna: Gerold, 1876.
2. BOWERS, J., ed. *Medical Schools for a Modern World.* Baltimore: The Johns Hopkins University Press, 1970.
3. CHI CHAO CHAN. "Medical Education in Mainland China," *J. Med. Educ.,* 47 (1972), 327–332.
4. COPE, O. *Man, Mind and Medicine.* Philadelphia: Lippincott, 1968.
5. DEUSCHLE, K. and F. EBERSON. "Community Medicine Comes of Age," *J. Med. Educ.,* 43 (1968), 1229–1237.
6. EBERT, R. "The Role of the Medical School in Planning the Health Care System," *J. Med. Educ.,* 42 (1967), 481–488.
7. FEIN, R. and G. I. WEBER. *Financing Medical Education.* New York: McGraw-Hill, 1971.
8. FIELD, J. "Medical Education in the United States," in C. D. O'Malley, ed., *The History of Medical Education,* pp. 501–530. Los Angeles: University of California Press, 1970.
9. FLEXNER, A. *Medical Education in the United States and Canada. A Report to the Carnegie Foundation for the Advancement of Teaching.* Bull. no. 4. Boston: Merrymount Press, 1910.
10. FUNKENSTEIN, D. "The Learning and Personal Development of Medical Students and the Recent Changes in Universities and Medical Education," *J. Med. Educ.,* 43 (1968), 883–897.
11. GLASER, R. J. "The Medical Deanship," *J. Med. Educ.,* 44 (1969), 1115–1126.
12. GREEN, J. R. *Medical History for Students.* Springfield, Ill.: Charles C. Thomas, 1968.
13. KERR, C., Chairman. *Higher Education and the Nation's Health.* Berkeley, Calif.: Carnegie Commission on Higher Education, 1970.
14. KNOWLES, J. H. "A Review of Medicine's Current Efforts," *J. Med. Educ.,* 44 (1969), 119–125.
15. KOSA, J. "The Foreign Trained Physician," *J. Med. Educ.,* 44 (1969), 46–51.
16. LYSAUGHT, J. P. "Enhanced Capacity for Self Instruction, *J. Med. Educ.,* 44 (1969), 580–584.
17. MANSTON, R. Q. and K. YORDI. "A Nation Starts a Program. Regional Medical Program," *J. Med. Educ.,* 40 (1967), 17–27.
18. MERTON, R. K. *The Student-Physician. Introductory Studies in the Sociology of Medical Education.* Cambridge: Harvard University Press, 1957.
19. MILLER, G. E. "Continuing Education for What?" *J. Med. Educ.,* 42 (1967), 320–326.
20. O'MALLEY, C. D., ed. *University of California, Los Angeles, Forum in Medical Education,* no. 12, p. 76. Los Angeles: University of California Press, 1970.
21. PUSCHMANN, T. *A History of Medical Education.* New York: Hafner, 1966.
22. REDLICH, F. C. *Mental Health Needs in Educating Tomorrow's Doctors. 4th World Conf. Med. Educ.* New York: World Med. Assoc., 1972.
23. RICHMOND, J. B. "Creative Administration," *J. Med. Educ.,* 44 (1969), 165–169.
24. SADLER, A. M., B. L. SADLER, and A. A. BLISS. *The Physician's Assistant Today and Tomorrow.* New Haven: Yale University Press, 1972.
25. SHANNON, J. A. "A Twenty Year View of the Role of the National Institutes of Health," *J. Med. Educ.,* 42 (1967), 97–108.
26. SLIMYOCK, R. M. *Medicine and Society in America, 1660–1860,* p. 25. New York: New York University Press, 1960.
27. STEAD, A., C. MC. SMYTHE, C. G. GUNN et al. "Educational Technology for Medicine," *J. Med. Educ.,* 46 (1971), 1–94.
28. WILSON, M. and M. M. CUMMING. "The National Library of Medicine: Relationships to Medical Education and Research," *J. Med. Educ.,* 40 (1965), 225–232.

CHAPTER 39

SOCIAL COMMUNICATION AND THE INFORMATION SCIENCES

Jurgen Ruesch

(Historical Note

HUMAN COMMUNICATION involves all the procedures by which one mind may affect another.[111] This includes not only speech but also the gestural and action behavior that people use to influence one another. But in spite of the central role that communication plays in our lives, the origins of language and speech are still somewhat obscure. The earliest remains of our material culture consist of crude articles of stone that date back close to a million years. Although we can surmise that people signaled to each other at this early stage, it is not until the appearance of Neanderthal man that signs of speech and communication become more convincing. Characteristic flint points, a bone industry, and burial grounds have been discovered that can be attributed to this middle paleolithic period, which dates from about 150,000 to 75,000 B.C. These findings, together with evidence of the use of fire, betray the existence of simple social institutions that presuppose man's ability to communicate. However, the space on the floor of the Neanderthal jaw where the tongue muscles attach was very small, and we may conclude that these people probably could not talk too well. But speech and language with certainty are tied to the *Homo sapiens* group, which appeared during the fourth glaciation, within the last fifty thousand years. Engraved tools and cave paintings remove all doubt about prehistoric man's ability to cope with complex symbolic systems [pp. 560–571].[100]

The inferential evidence from which the evolution of communication has been reconstructed[95] gives way to direct evidence with the appearance of the cuneiform writing of the Sumerians. These people, who lived in the Mesopotamian Valley from about 4000 B.C. on,[92] together with the Babylonians and Assyrians have been credited with the development of the pictorial system of denotation. Thus, it was roughly 6000 years ago that man for the first time was able to store information and to codify his knowledge for posterity. Writing took a new direction between 2000 and 1500 B.C. when the Phoenicians and the Jews found ways to record the sounds people made when they spoke.[60] The system of phonetic denotation was refined further in the next three millennia with the development of calligraphy, writing materials, and shorthand codes, and with the establishment of distance communication through the use of messengers and smoke signals.[24] If in antiquity and well into the Middle Ages the art of writing was the prerogative of priests and scribes who herewith became the guardians of man's cumulative body of knowledge, the invention of the printing press—in China in the ninth century and in Europe in the fifteenth—broke this monopoly and laid the foundations for modern mass education.[79] In the nineteenth century, technological innovations such as the telegraph, telephone, and radio enabled people to transmit messages almost instantaneously over long distances, and in the twentieth century, finally, television added another dimension to long-range communication. At this point, the world entered the phase of technical mass communication.[78]

The development of language, the invention of phonetic writing, and the introduction of communication machines profoundly influenced man's relationship to man. Whorf[131] was perhaps the first to point out that the structure of language influences the perception of the world around us; and when we write down symbols and list them in dictionaries, we give more permanent shape to our fleeting perceptions. The act of codifying events is, of course, the basis of all cultural evolution—a fact that distinguishes human from animal communication.[107] Thus, the invention of writing made it unnecessary for people to be within hailing distance of each other when they wished to communicate, and

messages could be transmitted over greater distances and spans of time. The separation of man from his message is the innovation that made possible all later communication engineering.

If the first step in the evolution of communication was the development of spoken language and the second step the invention of pictorial writing, the third step was related to the development of digital and verbal codification systems. Early pictorial writing was based upon similarities between the original events and their symbolic representation; the introduction of phonetic denotation, however, required special instructions to explain which symbols belonged to which sounds and which sounds stood for what events.[102] Phonetic codification, arbitrary and free of analogies, lent itself to the development of abstract languages and numerical systems, and these, in turn, made possible the eventual construction of the digital computer.

The fourth step in the evolution of communication was the creation of communication machinery that could emit, receive, and evaluate messages without the presence of man. In the modern world, robots interact with each other or with human beings, and communication is no longer the sole prerogative of living organisms. Sometimes an undetected and usually anonymous entity, either man or machine, can be interposed between communicating people to record, select, amplify, delete, condense, rebroadcast, or otherwise tamper with the exchange of messages, often without the knowledge of the participants. The alliance of engineers who construct communication machines, operators who manage these machines, and advertisers who shape the content makes up the modern message manipulating industry [pp. 260–300].[100]

The history of communication is significant for the psychiatrist because ontogeny seems to repeat phylogeny [pp. 300–317].[66] Beginning with the first communicative sounds,[91] the first movements,[116] and the first picture book,[102] the infant moves through all the steps that his ancestors took over thousands of years, until he reaches maturity. And much can happen to the individual during his growth that will distort or stunt communication and be responsible for abnormal behavior. Also, language is the psychiatrist's main tool, which he employs when taking a history or engaging in any form of group therapy or psychotherapy.[51] But it took almost a hundred years, after the establishment of psychiatry as a discipline, before the systematic study of communication was given recognition. Among the earliest contributions to the study of disturbed communication were those of the neuropathologists who described various abnormalities of the central nervous system and defects of the sensory and motor systems. Language and speech disturbances were focused upon by the psychophysiologists,[134] while the classical psychopathologists described the disturbances of retention, recall, recognition, feeling, thinking, and judgment.[14,23,68] Freud[47] and the psychoanalysts focused upon the message exchange between doctor and patient[42] and pointed out the importance of early human growth and development.[17] At the time of the Great Depression, a concern with the social aspects of human behavior[61,123] signaled the beginning of the theory of interpersonal and group relations. After World War II the rapid advances made by the communication engineers gave rise to the information sciences.[133] The amalgamation of these various movements and disciplines is the subject of this chapter.

(Social Communication

Communication links discontinuous parts of the living world to one another. Its principal function is to facilitate sexual propagation, in that any species characterized by at least two genders must possess means of communication in order to reproduce. Communication is made possible by three basic properties of living matter found at all levels of organization, ranging from the single cell to complex societies. In organisms we call these properties perception, decision making, and expression; and in machines we refer to input, information processing, and output. These functions,

of course, constitute the foundation upon which human relations and man–machine interaction rest. The term "social communication" as used in this context refers to the live exchange of messages mediated by vocal sounds, written signs, gestures, or movements without modification by machines.

The basic networks of social communication are one to one, one to many, many to one, and many to many. One-to-one communication occurs between two people such as husband and wife, mother and infant, teacher and pupil, doctor and patient, and lawyer and client. It is characterized by instant feedback, a large number of nonverbal components, and a subject matter that frequently bears directly upon feelings and personal experiences.[97]

One-to-many communication occurs in the lecture hall, in church, at political meetings, in military situations, or whenever one person addresses others in writing. The system is asymmetrical; the content is mostly impersonal, hortatory, or informational; the duration of the presentation is brief; and feedback, if it occurs at all, is usually delayed. In the modern world, this manner of communication is identified mostly with mass communication [pp. 348–381][40] and [pp. 535–551].[113]

Many-to-one communication occurs when spectators boo or cheer a player or an official, when constituents write their congressman, when people congratulate the guest of honor, or when people vote at an election. The system is asymmetrical and of short duration; the subject matter is limited; the content is situation-oriented; and feedback is delayed. Public opinion polls exemplify this type of network [pp. 40–60].[31]

Many-to-many communication occurs when one group meets another—in battle, on the playing field, and during demonstrations and migrations. Communication may be physical through action, the system short-lived, and the content closely tied to competition and survival. Feedback is often instantaneous [pp. 247–261].[127]

From these few examples it becomes evident that the arrangement of the network determines to a large extent the effectiveness of communication [pp. 70–115].[31] In industry, government, and the military this aspect of communication is referred to as organization.[10] It determines the assignment of tasks in social networks whereby the original functions of the organism—perception, decision making, and expression—are now distributed among many people. Control of communication through organization assures that the messages of numerous people get properly directed and coordinated.[76]

The assessment of a social network of communication is based upon the answers obtained to a number of pertinent questions that may be asked by the investigator [21–46].[100]

WHO (status, role, identity)
    SAID WHAT (content or referential property of symbols)
        TO WHOM (status, role, identity)
            WHEN (chronological, biological, elapsed time)
                WHERE (context, situation, location)
                    HOW (language: oral, written, gestural; metalanguage: instructions, interpretative devices)
                        WITH WHAT EFFECT (feedback, result)

The questions WHO and TO WHOM can be answered by studying the social characteristics of the participants and the manner in which a communique is coded, phrased, and timed. The whole style frequently identifies the sender as well as the receiver. The WHAT refers to the events that the signs and symbols represent. Proper usage presupposes conformity to the prevailing customs as laid down in dictionaries or legends. Unfortunately for the scientist, people observe, in addition to the dictionary usage, a multitude of informal and private conventions. Husbands and wives, parents and children, industrial crews, members of clubs, and sports teams develop private vocabularies. Thus, a message can be comprehended in many ways, depending upon the interpretation. The WHEN refers to various aspects of time and timing. Clues usually indicate the chronological date, the point in the evolution of a given situation, and the position of this message in a series of messages. The WHERE deals with the social context in which communication takes place.

The label of the situation should furnish the participants with enough information to identify the rules indicating who can talk to whom, about what, for how long, where, and in what manner. Usually, there is an indication of the consequences or penalties for violation of the rules. The HOW refers to the language system in which a message is phrased and the manner of its transmission. If the message is expressed in English, it may be spoken, written, or transmitted by semaphore signals, jungle drums, or a sign language such as those of the Indians and the deaf and dumb.[129] The EFFECT can be evaluated by studying the changes that a message produces in the psychological sphere (attitudes, opinions, beliefs) in social matters (laws, elected officials, procedures) or in the physical world.

Three sets of determinants influence social communication. The biological determinants control the organs of communication[62,72] involving the sensory and motor systems, and the central and autonomic nervous systems. Disorders of the human communication organs may interfere with perception, thinking, feeling, speech, and action. The psychological determinants—that is, the knowledge and experience a person has acquired—influence sophistication in cognition and the ability to make decisions, to express self, and to initiate and carry out action.[84,85] Neurotic processes and intrapsychic conflicts may interfere with the successful exercise of these functions of communication.[97] The social determinants are embodied in culture, language, nonverbal symbolic systems, collective assumptions, and value orientations to which an individual is exposed.[50] A specialist in communication, therefore, has to acquire knowledge of anatomy, physiology, psychology, psychopathology, anthropology, and sociology. From medicine to psychiatry and from the social to the information sciences ranges the field of relevance.[31,125,126]

Social communication shapes a person's body of knowledge; his opinions, attitudes, and beliefs; his ideas about the world and about himself; his sense of identity; his role in society; his skill in relating to others; and his ability to cope with personal problems.[113]

But the most important aspect of social communication is the potential for gratification that it provides. The release of tension that occurs after a successful message exchange contrasts with the unresolved tension experienced with failure to communicate. Only through communication with others can man tackle complex tasks. Communication thus becomes the tool with which the individual transcends himself, implements cooperation with others, and satisfies his need for belonging.[81]

❨ The Information Sciences

The origin of the information sciences can be traced back to 1948 when C. E. Shannon[111] published his now famous mathematical theory of communication in which he defined information quantitatively and described criteria for the evaluation of communication systems. Although information theory at first held great promise for psychology and biology, it later turned out to be something of a disappointment.[64] For one thing, the quality of information is more important in human affairs than the quantity. For another, information theory can only be applied to a network that is characterized by discrete channels and a uniform coding system. But the human organism has multiple coding systems: one type is characterized by nervous impulses;[49,70] another by chemical stimuli traveling in the vascular system;[62] and a third by structural arrangements of DNA in the nucleus of the cell.[9] Living organs are open systems and some of the body codes are still unknown, some of the channels are not discrete, and the sources of input are multiple. But, in spite of these limitations in applicability, information theory has greatly fertilized the thinking in the life sciences.

Also in 1948, Wiener published his book on cybernetics, which he called *Cybernetics or Control and Communication in the Animal and the Machine*.[132] This theory of feedback and servomechanisms embodies the idea that information about the effects of an action can be signaled back to its source, enabling the information control center to plan the next step. Cybernetics has had a significant impact upon the behavioral sciences because it is applicable to machines, organs, organizations, and societies.[101]

A third theory of communication that is most relevant for the field of engineering is the theory of smoothing, filtering, detection, and prediction of the value of signals in the presence of noise.[93] Unfortunately, in social situations the distinction between signal and noise or between intentional and unintentional messages is not applicable. In social communication the human observer utilizes all the information he can extract from the message itself, from the situational context, and from the physical environment. Unintentional signals and incidental perceptions may have just as much informative value as those contained in the message, and, therefore, these sources cannot be classified as noise.

A fourth group of theories concerned with automata and computers, including hardware design and programming, has perhaps exerted the greatest influence on our time.[120] Through the renaissance, mechanical devices served to increase the capacity of our motor system. In the baroque period, the scope of our sense organs was extended and engines began to replace muscular energy. Finally, in the twentieth century with the advent of the computer, the capacity of our central functions has been enlarged. The computer can react selectively to suitable inputs and can combine input with information derived from the memory, thus simulating decision making. Because of the similarity between a computer program and a series of logical statements, theorems now can be tested by feeding data into a computer and checking whether the results turn out as expected. Today, then, we start with a verbal or mathematical theory, construct an external model, and test operationally the correctness of our assumptions.

We owe to the late Warren McCulloch[77] and the Macy Foundation[44] the introduction of principles of cybernetics into neurophysiology,[49,70] psychiatry, and the behavioral sciences.[101] But the most extraordinary impact of information theory occurred in the field of genetics.[9] Starting with the assumption that cells, tissues, organs, and organisms must be integrated by some information-bearing signal system, the geneticists were able to show that information is coded inside the cells in terms of various arrangements of nucleic acids. Finally, the idea that organisms and life are steered by some mysterious central function such as the soul has been replaced by the notion that organisms are held together by an internal communication system and are linked to the environment by an external communication system. Intactness and functioning of these systems are as vital to survival as respiration, nutrition, or temperature control.

Today, most scientific institutions have access to a computer center. The hardware of a computer consists of input and output devices, arithmetic and control circuits, and a memory; the software consists of a program of instructions according to which the information is processed. The computer works on the binary principle, which means that the information is represented by binary symbols, is stored in binary memory elements, and is processed by binary switching elements.[106] Although computers are more than a million times faster than the human brain, their elements are arranged in series so that the component parts have to be in working order if the computer is to function properly. The brain, in contrast, has about a thousand times as many nerve cells as the computer has memory elements, occupies considerably less space, and works on a multiple input systems that can process different kinds of information simultaneously. At any one time, the computer can attend to one task accurately and fast; the brain, in contrast, can pursue several tasks simultaneously but with less accuracy. Loss of cells does not appreciably influence the functioning of the brain as a whole—a feature that is most useful in case of injury or disease.

Modern computer operations of significance to health fall into the following areas:

1. Information Storage, Retrieval, Collection, and Dissemination. The tremendous capacity for storage of information has given the computer the role of an auxiliary memory. All a person has to remember are the retrieval words in order to have access to what he is searching for; and libraries of the future may be of a kind in which a dialing system will flash the desired page onto a video screen.[5,74]

2. Information Processing, Computation, and Statistical Analysis. The rapidity of operation of the computer has made it possible to carry out thousands of statistical operations in a minimum of time. The computer is used for description and tabulation of data and for carrying out standard statistical analyses, including multivariate, regression, time series, and variance analyses.[34,39]

3. Simulation of Human Functions and Scientific Model Construction. In addition to its role as man's auxiliary brain for storage, retrieval, and processing of information, the computer also has assumed an entirely new function—that of a participant in interaction. A computer now is able to replace certain decision-making functions of man, and when linked to effector machines the decisions can be implemented. Among the simulated processes of significance to the physician are conversations, history taking, and diagnosis, whereby the professional may be replaced by the computer. A program that simulates a patient enables a student to practice interviewing; or a whole message exchange simulating the conversation between two people may be simulated by two computers.[65,118]

4. Instructional Programs. By making marks with a magnetic pencil, by typing answers on the input typewriter, or by operating dials, students can respond to questions flashed onto a video screen. If the answer is correct, the program proceeds; if it is wrong, reexposure to previously studied material occurs. The whole instructional program usually is stored in the computer itself, although the student may be referred to material that is available elsewhere.[29]

5. Social System Simulation. Computer models of industrial, military, medical, or commercial organizations furnish headquarters with a small-scale model of the whole enterprise. This enables scientists not only to proceed with an analysis of the system but to build in certain automatic warning devices

that trigger remedial measures in case certain critical stages should be reached. Monitoring is significant not only for the operation of ships, airplanes, and space capsules but for the human heart and brain as well.

6. Computers in the Field of Mental Health. Computers are used for recording information pertaining to psychiatric patients;[90,117,122] for the evaluation of social disability;[99] for multiphasic screening of the general health of patients;[28] for clinical decision-making processes involving global judgments;[121] and for the simulation of certain diseases.[22]

([System Analysis and Operations Research

Traditional scientific methodology requires isolation of phenomena, dissection into smaller particles or functions, and a neglect of the specific social context and the identity of the participants. Because science is concerned with mass effects, its methodology may result in a loss of the particulars of the phenomenon under study. To compensate for these shortcomings, behavioral scientists began to consider phenomena in another and novel way. Instead of analyzing structures and reducing processes and particles to their constituent components, they studied the development and transformation of processes in a larger context. This approach, known by the name of operations research,[1] aims at obtaining an overall view of larger systems in order to integrate the physical, economic, and social aspects of the enterprise. Operations research is dedicated to the task of steering whole systems and preventing the fragmentation inherent in the functional division of labor. Its procedures consist of formulating the problem, constructing a model to represent the system, feeding data into the model and testing it, experimenting with solutions to the problem, and implementing on a large scale the solutions discovered with the help of the model.

Operations research found its most fruitful application in industry,[11] where tasks such as allocation of funds, space, time, and resources, inventory accumulation, replacement of obsolete parts, scheduling, and hiring and firing of personnel occur daily.[53] As advances in decision theory were made and the science of system analysis was developed, computer models of whole systems were able to furnish executives with a quantitative method for decision making, comparing time, cost, value, and effectiveness. The theories that facilitated the integration of part functions into a whole became known as general systems theories.[12]

The term "system" as used in this context refers to a cluster of components or units engaged in mutual interaction.[26] To cope with an organization that has people in one subsystem, products in another, and machines in a third, terms had to be invented that were common to all three. The task thus consisted of translating analogies, homologies, and transactional processes characteristic of cell, organ, organism, group, and society into terms applicable to all of these entities. While the physicists possess many satisfactory equations to denote the transformation of one kind of energy into another, behavioral scientists do not have schemes that allow them to relate, for example, sensory data to biochemical changes. In the past, value theory came closest to being a general systems theory suitable for interdisciplinary research. It proceeds under the assumption that a value or price can be assigned to all objects, persons, and processes —a device that introduces a unitary scale. Communication theory, a scheme more recently applied to different types of data, concerns itself with the messages that connect the discontinuous parts of an organization. Both value and communication theory are general systems theories that have been particularly significant for the behavioral sciences because the findings of anthropologists, psychologists, sociologists, and psychiatrists thus can be unified. That this task is of major interest to the field can be seen from the number of relevant publications on the subject.[21,52,54,86]

With the help of a general systems theory a scientist can construct a scientific model. But before using a model for purposes of prediction, the scientist has to go through several steps, any one of which may become a source of errors and can influence the data obtained. The first step consists of making measurements or observations; the second step involves the encoding of data so that they are acceptable to the particular model in use; the third step consists of processing the data; and the fourth step consists of checking the results obtained. If the scientist makes relevant observations, possesses a workable model, and processes the data appropriately, the results obtained with the model should coincide with the data pertaining to the original events. Among the schemes developed by operations research, decision models are the most relevant for psychiatry because they simulate human judgment.[36] In its simplest form, a decision is composed of five basic elements.[119] These are: strategies or plans constructed on the basis of controllable features or variables; states of nature made up of noncontrollable events; outcomes that consist of the results observed when a specific strategy is employed and a particular state of nature exists; predictions of the probabilities that a given state of nature will occur; and, finally, the assessment of risk in which strategy and outcome are selected with regard to the degree of uncer-

tainty that people are willing to tolerate.

A suitable model for the study of social communication requires three types of observations. First, the characteristics of the communicating entity have to be specified; second, the characteristics of the processes connecting the entities and the properties of the overall field have to be enunciated; and, third, the characteristics of the observer who is part of the field and is influenced by the transaction have to be recorded. In schematic form, this approach [pp. 450–465][100] would appear as shown in Table 39–1.

The task of observing all the changes that occur at any one moment is somewhat overwhelming. To simplify matters, the scientist can proceed in several different ways: (1) he can assign the role of observer to one of the participants, thereby losing in objectivity but gaining information concerning the subtleties of the exchange; (2) he can obtain additional observers or monitoring devices to keep track of events and feed their reports into a central station that will collate the data. This condensation, however, introduces new errors and loses information; (3) he can compare a subject's behavior with the predictable and programmed behavior of a machine that is put in

TABLE 39–1.   **Evaluation of a Behavioral Situation**

COMMUNICATING ENTITY	CONNECTING PROCESSES	OBSERVER
1. Input functions (perception)	1. Combination of functions of several small entities to form a larger entity	1. Scientific observation or measurement of ongoing signal exchange
2. Central processes Data scanning (recognition)	2. Organization of networks	2. Encoding of exchange into terms acceptable to the scientific model
Data processing (thinking)	3. Languages and codes	
Data storage (memory)	4. Content: referential property attributed to signals	3. Assessment of outcome or effects produced
3. Output functions (expression and action)	5. Metacommunicative processes: instructions and interpretative devices	4. Management and organization: intervention with the connecting processes
	6. Feedback: reincorporation of information at the source	5. Treatment or repair: intervention with the entities themselves

his place, and denote the significant differences, thus gaining information on the uniqueness of the subject's behavior. Whatever method the scientist uses will maximize one kind of information and minimize another. Therefore, a decision has to be made as to what events are the most relevant. This decision can be arrived at by correlating the outcome or effect produced by the whole system with its component parts or processes. Each outcome usually is matched to a given internal and external constellation.

(Mind and Body, Word and Action

The mind–body dichotomy has been with us for over 2500 years, with the result that until recently the human body was considered in the light of biological and physical laws while the symbolic processes were evaluated in the light of theological, psychological, and social conventions. But behavior can be understood only if both the biophysical and the symbolic processes are encompassed in one overall system. The theoretical basis for a unification of physical and psychological data was established with the advent of cybernetics and the concept of feedback. In brief, this is the way it works: human action occurs in a physical field and produces a physical impact; but, at the same time, the identical action always occurs in a social field, and also has a symbolic function with an informative impact [pp. 450–465].[100] When the physical and symbolic effects are perceived by the participants, this newly acquired information may lead to a correction of the old body of information. Hence, information can be said to control action and action to change information. With this theoretical innovation, the mind–body parallelism became obsolete.

Of old, the mind component of the dichotomy was closely identified with verbal behavior[112] and pertinent contributions are found under headings such as language,[25] psycholinguistics,[103] semiotics,[108] significs,[87] semantics,[59,67] or speech [pp. 264–287].[31] The body component, in contrast, was identified with anatomy, physiology, and move-

ment.[102] With the advent of cybernetics, the mind became identified with information and the body with action. Every human being experiences the discrepancy between information and action in daily life. If action turns out to match preconceived ideas, then the organism experiences tension reduction; but if information and action do not coincide, the discrepancy gives rise to tension that serves to redirect action or to adjust the information to fit the action. The principle of differential perception is applicable to other communicative processes—that is, to the discrepancy between verbal and nonverbal messages, overt content and covert instruction, or different versions of a message repeated over time.[114] In his theory of cognitive dissonance, Festinger[43] states that nonfitting relations among cognitions produce dissonance—an experience that motivates the person to reduce the inconsistency and strive toward consonance.

Amazingly, action per se has received much less attention than verbal behavior.[105] The legal fraternity has been concerned for millennia with the assessment of action in terms of the law. The military [pp. 509–534][125] are the specialists who have been concerned with control of people through action. Finally, the clergy,[83] who since the beginning of history held the monopoly on writing, controlled the assumptions that people were allowed to make about action. These were laid down in the Ten Commandments of Moses, the turning of the cheek at the time of Christ, and the notion of charity in the Middle Ages.[98] More recently, the scientific assessment of bodily action has produced technical treatises on walking, dancing, writing, posture, and specialized movements of the extremities.[102] The relative sparsity of publications on action is in part due to the unsatisfactory models available for the representation of action [pp. 393–412].[100] Interaction between two persons and in small groups has received more consideration,[71] but the field is still in its infancy.

A special case of the relationship of information to action is seen in the connection of verbal with nonverbal communication in that silent action signals may take the place of vocal sounds and thus facilitate redundancy.

For example, if a person's attention is momentarily diverted, a verbal passage may not be heard unless it is repeated. Redundancy can be produced without boredom by repeating the message nonverbally and by appealing to different sense modalities instead of reiterating the same verbal message over again. The field of nonverbal communication, covering such subjects as the nature of nonverbal codes, the impact of movement upon perception, and the influence of culture and situations, has been explored by Ruesch and Kees,[102] Birdwhistell,[13] Bosmajian,[16] Critchley,[30] Ekman and Friesen,[38] W. La Barre [pp. 456–490][81] and Hall.[57,58]

The perception of both action and verbal behavior has become the specialty of the field of cognition.[3] This field is concerned with the whole representational process, beginning with the original events and pursuing the process to the representation in the brain.[19,20] Cognition, hence, is concerned with information processing in the widest sense of the word,[94] involving sensation, perception, imagery, retention, recall, problem solving, and thinking. In a technical sense, cognition is concerned with pattern recognition, visual memory, iconic storage, echoic memory, and related problems.[89] The psychologist's concern with perception and cognition corresponds to the psychiatrist's preoccupation with disturbed perception and the unconscious [pp. 130–159].[31] If the German[14,68] and French[23] schools of psychiatry attempted to relate aberrations of perception and cognition to nosological entities, the psychoanalysts tried to relate repressed unconscious impulses to neuroses and the overwhelming of the conscious by the unconscious to psychoses.[42] Alexander[2] finally attempted to connect psychosomatic diseases to the organism's physiological response to specific emotional stimuli. In explaining the failure to relate perception, cognition, or awareness to disease, one has to remember that psychological phenomena on the whole do not abide by the rules of deterministic mathematics, but fit more appropriately into the rules of probabilistic mathematics. Today we know that no diagnostic entity is characterized by unique ways of perception, decision making, or expression. The failure to establish a deterministic relationship between personality or symptomatology and disease should not obscure the fact that, statistically speaking, one disturbance may be associated with a given disease more frequently than another.[27]

The communicative behavior of psychosomatic patients may illustrate the point [pp. 614–634].[100] Without attributing any causal connection to such a description, we can say that many psychosomatic patients appear somewhat infantile: their perception of external events often is inaccurate or incomplete in that their concern with psychological problems of the self and with proprioceptive stimuli arising in the organism displaces in importance the exteroceptive impression of other events. Also, any exteroceptive information received from the chemical and mechanical end organs is unduly weighted and the usual maturational shift to a preference for the more complex wave receivers—vision and hearing—is delayed. Bodily signs and signals are relied upon more than words or numbers,[124] and often the impact of actions of the self upon others is not correctly observed. Reliance upon proximity receivers and insufficient mastery of the higher symbolic processes often result in an incomplete or arbitrary delineation of physical, psychological, and social boundaries, and these patients believe that the physical or mental state of other people is identical with their own and that messages are to be understood as if they were traveling within one and the same neuronal network. Often a symbiotic relationship with one other person develops whereby the patient abdicates decision making and confines himself to perception or action. Lacking the ability to make independent decisions, these patients frequently utter value judgments that express their normative and conformist orientation, indicating their dependence upon the protective actions of others, which, in the process of maturation, was not sufficiently replaced by reliance upon informational exchange.

Frequently, in the course of a relationship, the psychosomatic patient will use body language mediated by the autonomic nervous system;[7] and since physicians and nurses are experts at interpreting vascular, glandular, and pain manifestations of people, these patients find within the medical establishment a kind of understanding that tends to prolong existing disease or invalidism. Some patients who have matured beyond the stage of body language may use nonverbal actions to convey messages. Such action language is prevalent in many patients found on the orthopedic wards of the hospital and in the juvenile courts. Both the patient who chooses body language and the patient who prefers action language are unable to find emotional satisfaction in verbal exchanges with other people.

(Disturbed Communication

In his book on disturbed communication, Ruesch[97] points out that no message can be considered abnormal in isolation from its social context. Communication is a process that connects person to person, and a message may be declared deviant only if it fails to fulfill its task. Disturbed communication thus is defined by the effect it produces rather than by its structure; and evaluation as to whether a message exchange is successful or a failure is accomplished by considering people and messages in their social field. The connecting processes may fail for quantitative reasons in that they may not match the capacities of the communicating entities, or they may fail for qualitative reasons in that they are not matched to the input characteristics of an entity. A ditty may help in remembering these characteristics:

Too much, too little; too early, too late; At the wrong place, is the disturbed message's fate.

Overload and Underload. In animal or machine, every communication network has a given capacity. When the load exceeds this capacity, the machinery or the organism

breaks down; when the load is too small, the machinery or the organism may deteriorate for lack of use. Overload [pp. 201–224][127] is a known source of disorganization. To protect himself from the fatigue resulting from excessive input, the individual learns to disregard certain classes of stimuli; but in the process he may also disregard vital information. Underload in the form of sensory deprivation may lead in mild cases to retarded development and in severe cases to some general disorganization of behavior and hallucinatory syndromes.[115,137] Excessive output, as in overwork, results in fatigue; whereas output below par leads to poor physical fitness, decline in intellectual functioning, and possibly premature aging. Because the homeostasis of the organism requires that input be quantitatively matched somewhat to output, changes in one function always affect the other functions,[77] and imbalance between input and output results in frustration, overt anxiety, and, eventually, disorganization of behavior.

Erroneous Timing. Ill-timed messages, similar to quantitatively deviant messages, have to be delivered with greater intensity and have to be repeated more often than well-timed ones. In addition, a message has to be properly separated from those preceding and following; otherwise their confluence may distort the meaning. Also, in person-to-person communication the response of the second person has to follow the statement of the first in proper time if it is to be correctly understood.

Difficulties of Perception, Evaluation, Expression, and Action. Input of the organism is identified with perception, and disturbances may range from sensory defects to selective inattention. In the area of central functions, processing of information involves scanning, encoding, decoding, storage, and decision making; disturbances may involve thinking, feeling, memory, and judgment. The output of the organism[46,66] is identified with muscular movement that results in verbal productions or silent action, and here the disturbances may range from inhibition and exaggeration of verbal output to difficulties in initiating, sustaining, or completing action. All of these disturbances are central to the daily endeavors of the psychiatrist and are well described in the treatises of classical psychopathology.

Language and Speech Difficulties. Some of the difficulties of communication are related to disturbances of language and speech. Among these are aphasia, agnosia, and apraxia;[18] stuttering, stammering, and lisping;[6] and disturbances of the voice apparatus proper.[88] On a higher level or organization we find deficient mastery of digital codification, which is the basis of reading and writing difficulties, and of analogic codification, which underlies difficulties in pattern recognition. Deficiency in the integration of the digital with the analogic forms of codification prevents people from rapidly switching from analytic details to larger pattern appreciation—a process that is essential for proper intellectual functioning [pp. 727–738].[100]

Disturbed Metacommunication. The term "metacommunication" refers to auxiliary and covert messages that go along with the overt communication to instruct the receiver in how he ought to interpret a statement.[101] Metalanguage is far more subtle than language itself, and it varies with the situation, with time, and with the composition of the group. In schools of creative expression and acting, students are trained to enact a passage first as a comedy, then as a tragedy, and finally as a reportage. These variations are based upon a shift in role assumption that is expressed in nonverbal ways. A child learns these modulations when he has consistent contact with parents and peers in different contexts and situations. The patient who lacked such experiences does not learn these modifications of interpretation and when he expresses himself, he may tenaciously cling to one and the same nonverbal form of expression in spite of changes in content or context.

Message Discrepant with Situation. The context of a situation governs the sets from which words or gestures are chosen. Without knowledge of the particular set from which a word or symbol derives, the receiver does not know what alternatives have been considered. After all, the economy of communication depends upon a shared knowledge of sets. For example, if the sender selects the eleventh out of a set of seventeen symbols, the receiver is aware that the other sixteen have been rejected.[57,58]

Distortions in Feedback, Correction, and Reply. Some people are unable to utilize printed information; others are unable to listen to or heed the spoken word. Then there are people who are unable to learn from trial and error. Also, there are those who have difficulty in combining information held by self with information held by others, thus being handicapped in correcting information. Sometimes, people may get confused when information from various sources is juxtaposed and a decision has to be made as to which version is the correct one. The ability to juxtapose information, to condense and combine it, is in part an emotional function. An intense experience of either pleasure or frustration in connection with a given type of information tends to stabilize it. Because of the emotional component, such information tends to become immune to change, and intrapsychic processes may become redundant. In contrast, an experience of emotional neutrality associated with a given body of information tends to elicit boredom. The remedy for boredom, of course, is activity and change.[98]

Devious Reply. An appropriate response amplifies, attenuates, or corrects the information contained in the initial message, while inappropriate responses may exert a disorganizing effect. In reacting to a statement, we may distinguish between understanding, acknowledgment, and agreement. In understanding, we place an observation into a model in our own head and determine its relationships to other events. In acknowledging, we simply indicate receipt of the message without referring to our understanding of the content. In agreeing, we not only understand and acknowledge but also respond to the content. To be acknowledged is pleasant; to be understood and acknowledged gives us a feeling of self-respect; and to reach an agreement paves the way for action. Numerous disturbances are characterized by devious acknowledgment. For example, inappropriate responses are frequently given by mentally deranged persons whereby acknowledgment may be inadequate, exaggerated, or omitted. Often the reply simply introduces a new topic, as in the case of the tangential reply [pp. 354–364][100] that constitutes a response to a peripheral aspect of the initial message with complete disregard for the intent of the sender. Because it is the appropriate reply to one's intent that produces a feeling of satisfaction, the lack of this kind of recognition is discouraging. Satisfaction is the motor that drives people toward successful communication, and devious replies lead to a serious disruption of communication and human relations.

Threatening Content. A message may be disturbing if it contains threats to one's personal safety, to existing human relations, or to action in progress, while discovery that messages are not truthful and do not correspond to reality makes people suspicious. Conversely, awareness of facts that destroy magic thinking interferes with the faith and hope that are necessary for living. Messages that trigger obligatory responses also exert a coercive effect, regardless of whether they elicit obsessive, compulsive, or phobic behavior.

Inadequate Information. A person may not have the information necessary to carry out a task or hold a position; he may be inept at processing information; he may not have tested his information in action; or he may have an emotional aversion for the task at hand. The assessment of these disturbances is geared to a comparison of the patient's functioning, not with a universal standard or norm but with the demands of the situation. If a person's information is not matched to the exigencies of the situation, he will fail. A more subtle constraint may be exerted by an individual's value system, which may oppose the acquisition of information or its relevant use in action.[98]

Deficient Programming. Every person has to learn to apportion time, space, energy, and money to various tasks. The difficulties some people encounter are related to the discontinuity of their pursuits. Life is cyclical and most tasks have to be abandoned and taken up again in the next hour, the next day, or the next week, with time in between to rest or eat. Programming of one hour or one day seldom represents a major difficulty because circumstances dictate what must be done. Also, when people work, the institution or organization delivers schedules and takes over the burden of apportioning resources. But if a person has to program his own life over a period of years, difficulties may arise in the setting and implementing of priorities and in behaving in a consistent manner.[99]

Coincidence of Several Disturbances. Simultaneity of several traumatic events may increase frustration to a degree that exceeds an individual's tolerance, while proper spacing of traumatic events may contribute to gradual adaptation. In learning, the motto that applies is "One thing at a time." When too many events that require adaptation occur simultaneously, the individual may become confused as to the priorities involved. If the situation can be talked over with another person, the frustration is easier to bear than if communicative exchange is not available.

Disturbances of Communication in Various Mental Conditions. The peculiarities in the ways of communication of patients suffering from psychoses and neuroses have been elaborated by many authors. Among the sources are:

Schizophrenia: Artiss;[4] Bateson, Jackson, Haley et al.;[8] Bleuler;[14] Boatman and Szurek;[15] Domarus;[35] Fromm-Reichmann;[48] Jackson;[63] Laing;[69] Lidz;[75] Ruesch [pages 635–661];[100] Scheflen;[104] Sullivan;[123] Watzlawick, Beavin, and Jackson;[130] Wynne and Singer.[135]

Manic and Depressive Conditions: Fromm-Reichmann;[48] Grinker, Miller, Sabshin et al.;[55] Lewis;[73] Ruesch.[97]

Psychoneuroses and Personality Disorders: Freud;[47] Meerloo;[82] Ruesch;[98] Shands.[109]

Disorders of the Central Nervous System: Brain;[18] Rioch and Weinstein.[96]

Sensory Defects: Department of Health, Education, and Welfare;[33] Zahl;[136] Blau (Chapter 9).[32]

Language and Speech Disorders: Barbara;[6] Mysak;[88] Oliver [pp. 264–287].[31]

❡ Therapeutic Communication

Therapeutic communication can occur anywhere: at home, at work, on the playground,
or on the ward. It is not tied to any hour of
the week, nor is it bound to props such as a
chair, a couch, or a darkened room. Therapeutic communication may be undertaken by
persons who do not know that they act as
therapists; and those who benefit may be unaware that they have been helped. Therapeutic communication is not a method invented by doctors to combat illness; instead, it
involves the utilization of a universal function
of man to support those in need, to dispel anxiety, to correct information, and to initiate action. At times this process is called psychotherapy; at other times, education; then again,
tutoring. Some call it counseling, others guidance, and a few simply friendship. The only
difference between planned therapy and ordinary communication is found in the participants' goals. The person designated as patient
seeks help; the person designated as therapist
uses his skills for the benefit of the other without seeking power or personal gain, his only
material reward being the fee that he is paid.

Therapeutic communication makes use of
contributions that derive from many different
disciplines.[98] To understand the nature of
networks and codes, and the principles of
feedback, the therapist borrows from cybernetics; to understand verbal communication,
he turns to philology and linguistics; to appraise what goes on inside the individual, he
utilizes the psychoanalytic scheme; to assess
pathology, he draws heavily from clinical psychiatry; to appraise the cultural and social milieu, he adopts approaches from the social
sciences; and in order to simulate the interaction between patient and therapist, he employs the computer. In his attitude, the doctor
shows respect for the other person's individuality; and he encourages the patient to express
himself, always indicating his readiness to listen, watch, understand, and respond. In his
work, the doctor focuses upon the patient's
difficulties in separating fact from fantasy, his

ineptness in human relations, and all those
processes which prevent him from further
growth and development.

The therapist's power to steer the therapeutic process in the desired direction derives
from the leverage inherent in his special
knowledge, the institutional resources at his
disposal, and his reputation as a physician.
Because of the attribution of healing powers,
his words acquire a persuasiveness and his actions a magic quality.[45] This initial advantage
is reinforced in the therapeutic session by the
therapist's operations, which are aimed at
providing the patient with a satisfactory communicative exchange. This experience in turn
becomes the motivation for the patient to seek
more of the same, and it induces him to work
toward mastery of communication.

Over time, when exposed to therapeutic
communication, the patient will learn a variety of its subtleties. Perception and cognition
are invariably sharpened; the distinction between proprioception, involving sensations
and feelings, and exteroception, pertaining to
people and situations, becomes clear; and discrimination between fact and fantasy is mastered. On the output side, the patient learns to
express feelings and thoughts, to choose appropriate words and gestures, and to share
what goes on inside with another person. As
far as the central processes are concerned,
recall and reconstruction of past events, the
bridging of amnestic gaps, the acquisition of
new information, and the proper integration
of the new body of knowledge with the old
pave the way for the mastery of decision making. Acceptance of the unavoidable; allocation
of time, space, energy, and money to various
tasks; and planning of future action are
worked through with examples from the patient's life. Mastery of decision making eventually will lead to consistent choice of those
perceptions, actions, opportunities, and people
that fit into the patient's life style and to a
rejection of those features that are inappropriate. In applying to life situations what has
been learned in the therapeutic session about
perception, information processing, decision
making, and expression, the patient is likely to

gain further experience with conversation, discussion, negotiation, confrontation, and cooperation in two-person or group settings.

The indications for emphasizing one aspect of communication over another depend upon the patient's condition, the therapist's personality, and the specific circumstances that govern a situation. Whether therapeutic communication is carried out individually or in groups, in a combination of both, or in the framework of family therapy will have to be decided for each case. If the patient's condition is related to the experience of anxiety in the face of unalterable somatic, physical, or social circumstances, communication may help him to clarify contradictory issues, lend him emotional support, and induce him to accept the unalterable. If the patient's condition is related to inner conflicts evidenced by guilt, shame, fear, anger, or depression, communication can help him to relive past experiences, to gain insight into the present circumstances, and to adopt a behavior that is favorable to the gradual reduction of internal conflicts. The working through of resistances against unconscious conflict here is the method of choice. If the patient has an infantile personality, utilizes naive ways of communication, or lacks knowledge of people and situations, contact with an experienced therapist may help him to grow. Through guidance and informal education, the patient may learn to achieve maturity. If his condition is related to misunderstandings, disagreement, or social conflicts, communication with the other people may help him to correct erroneous information, to respond appropriately to the situation, and to eliminate disagreements as they arise.

Details of the role of communication in various therapeutic procedures are embedded in a vast literature. Freud[47] was the first to call attention to the phenomenon of transference, and subsequently the communicative exchanges between analyst and patient have become a central focus of psychoanalysis.[42] Ruesch[98] gives an overview of the field of therapeutic communication; Shands[110] and Meerloo [pp. 130–159][31] focus upon the contributions of psychiatry to communication;

Walton[128] describes communication from the standpoint of peacemaking; and Haley[56] focuses upon a variety of therapeutic paradoxes. Lennard and Bernstein,[71] in analyzing the patterns of human interaction, emphasize situational context and roles of the participants. Feldman[41] analyzes the mannerisms of speech and gesture; Ekman and Friesen[37] as well as Mahl[80] describe various types of nonverbal behavior in therapy. Finally, it is well to remember that the special kind of communication that exists between professionals and their patients is subsumed in hundreds of articles concerned with the doctor–patient relationship.

(Conclusions

Social communication is a term that refers to the exchange of messages mediated by vocal sounds, written signs, gestures, or movements without modification by third parties or machines. Social communication between human beings is characterized by goal seeking, goal changing, and corrective behavior, and the creation or maintenance of steady states at a fairly high level of orderliness; part functions are always functions of the system as a whole, and the chains of causation are at least circular, if not more complex. A communication system is delineated by the network in which signals travel. It is made up of participating entities consisting of biological, social, or machine units that are characterized by input, central, and output functions.

Communication is mediated by signals, signs, and symbols. A signal is an impulse in transit. A sign, by force of its own structure or because of attention paid to it, possesses for a participant problem-solving properties. A symbol is an extraorganismic device that has been agreed upon to refer, in a condensed way, to actions or events that have occurred elsewhere. A statement, which is made up of a series of signals, constitutes a purposive expression on the part of a person or group with the intent of conveying information. A statement becomes a message when it has been perceived and interpreted by another person. When two or more individuals can agree on the topic to which an exchange refers, a message can be said to have content.

All observations pertaining to the study of social communication are made by a human observer stationed in the network. The character of these observations is determined by the observer's position in the system, his time and space scales, his methods and instruments of observation, his theoretical models and a priori assumptions, and, finally, his purpose in carrying out his study.

The technical process of embodying information in some concrete way is referred to as codification. Inside the organism, events are codified by means of nervous and humoral impulses; outside the organism, objects and events are codified in terms of two- or three-dimensional marks or objects. Analogic codification makes use of similarities between coded signal and original event. Digital codification, in contrast, is based upon arbitrary and discrete representation of events, whereby the digital elements—words or numbers—are connected to the events for which they stand by means of a legend. A special code suitable for human interaction is language, which is composed of a plurality of signs or symbols whose significance must be known to a number of participants; also, language must be reproducible by human beings and should retain its approximate significance under different conditions.

When signals travel through space and pass certain boundaries, they are likely to be recoded in order to be acceptable to the new network. Sensory end organs thus are stations of signal transformation. Phylogenetically old are the chemical and mechanical end organs that serve as proximity receivers. Phylogenetically younger are the visual and auditory end organs that serve as distance receivers. Once signals have been perceived and are properly recoded they become available for information processing. The incoming signals are scanned against information stored in the memory; the new information is combined with the old, and becomes the basis for eventual decision making. The decision is made

accessible to others through speech, writing, or action, and this output is perceived not only by others but by the communicator himself, hence guiding his next step in the process of communication.

Any statement is made up of two parts: the principal content, which refers to some other event, and the secondary instructions, which refers to the message itself. Instructions are embedded in the rules that govern a situation, in the roles assumed by the participants, and in the language used. They indicate who can talk to whom, when, where, for how long, in what manner, and on which subject.

Feedback refers to the incorporation of information about the effects of an action at the original source. Control thus is not localized in any particular area of the network but is dependent upon an ongoing circular relay of messages that in effect steers the behavior of organisms and organizations and regulates the performance of machines. The correction of any performance is dependent upon the observation of the impact achieved and the reaction of others. Successful communication can be conceived of as the establishment of concordant information; unsuccessful communication as the establishment of discordant information between participants. The pleasure that individuals derive from well-functioning communication constitutes the driving force that induces them to seek human relations. Frustrating communication, in contrast, manifests itself either by symptom formation or by withdrawal from ill-functioning social networks.

Disturbances of communication can be caused by:

1. Disease, trauma, or malformation of the organs of communication, in which case perception, evaluation, and expression may be affected.

2. Insufficient mastery of nonverbal or verbal language, in which case the sign processes may suffer.

3. Inadequate or erroneous information about self and others, in which case inappropriate action may be the result.

4. Insufficient mastery of metacommunica-

tive devices, with the result that an individual's actions may be misinterpreted.

5. Inability to correct information because of inadequate skills in the utilization of feedback, in which case knowledge will be erroneous.

6. Lack of feedback from another person or group, whereby the social entities do not join in an ongoing exchange, with resulting isolation.

7. Participation in a nonfunctional network in which the organization prevents people from communicating effectively, leading to separation or the formation of new networks.

Therapeutic communication differs from ordinary communication in that the intention of one or more of the participants is clearly directed at bringing about a beneficial change in the system. To this end, the therapist steers communication in such a way that the patient not only learns in the therapeutic hour but also is exposed to situations and exchanges that provide for diversified experiences. This may be accomplished by including in the communications other members of the family or friends, or by introducing the patient to specially created new groups or existing organizations. Once the patient has experienced the pleasure of successful communication, he is likely to perfect the art on his own. If the processes of communication, and particularly feedback, function properly, an individual can be relied upon to steer his own actions and those of other people in a meaningful way. Successful communication is the road to mental health.

⟮ Bibliography

1. ACKOFF, R. L. and M. W. SASIENI. *Fundamentals of Operations Research.* New York: Wiley, 1968.

2. ALEXANDER, F. *Psychosomatic Medicine.* New York: Norton, 1950.

3. ARIETI, S. "The Structural and Psychodynamic Role of Cognition in the Human Psyche," in S. Arieti, ed., *The World Biennial of Psychiatry and Psychotherapy,* Vol. 1, pp. 3–33. New York: Basic Books, 1971.

4. ARTISS, K. L., ed. *The Symptom as Communication in Schizophrenia.* New York: Grune & Stratton, 1959.

5. AUSTIN, C. L. *MEDLARS 1963–1967, National Library of Medicine,* Pub. no. 1823. Bethesda: U.S. Public Health Service, 1968.

6. BARBARA, D. A., ed. *New Directions in Stuttering: Theory and Practice.* Springfield, Ill.: Charles C. Thomas, 1965.

7. BARBER, T. X. et al., eds. *Biofeedback and Self-Control, 1970.* Chicago: Aldine-Atherton, 1971.

8. BATESON, G., D. D. JACKSON, J. HALEY et al. "Toward a Theory of Schizophrenia," *Behav. Sci.,* 1 (1956), 251–264.

9. BEADLE, G. W. "The Language of the Gene," in *The Languages of Science,* pp. 57–84. New York: Basic Books, 1963.

10. BECKHARD, R. *Organization Development: Strategies and Models.* Reading, Mass.: Addison-Wesley, 1969.

11. BEER, S. *Cybernetics and Management.* New York: Wiley, 1959; Science Editions, 1964.

12. BERTALANFFY, L. VON. *Robots, Men and Minds.* New York: Braziller, 1967.

13. BIRDWHISTELL, R. L. *Kinesics and Context: Essays on Body Motion Communication.* Philadelphia: University of Pennsylvania Press, 1970.

14. BLEULER, E. *Dementia Praecox, or the Group of Schizophrenias.* New York: International Universities Press, 1950.

15. BOATMAN, M. J. and S. A. SZUREK. "A Clinical Study of Childhood Schizophrenia," in D. D. Jackson, ed., *The Etiology of Schizophrenia,* pp. 389–440. New York: Basic Books, 1960.

16. BOSMAJIAN, H. A. *The Rhetoric of Nonverbal Communication.* Glenview, Ill.: Scott, Foresman, 1971.

17. BOWLBY, J. *Attachment and Loss.* Vol. 1: *Attachment.* New York: Basic Books, 1969.

18. BRAIN, W. R. *Speech Disorders.* Washington: Butterworths, 1961.

19. BROADBENT, D. E. *Perception and Communication.* Oxford: Pergamon, 1958.

20. ———. *Decision and Stress.* New York: Academic, 1971.

21. BUCKLEY, W., ed. *Modern Systems Research for the Behavioral Scientist.* Chicago: Aldine, 1968.

22. CALLAWAY, E. 3rd. "Schizophrenia and Interference: An Analogy with a Malfunctioning Computer," *Arch. Gen. Psychiatry*, 22 (1970), 193–208.

23. CHARCOT, J.-M. *Leçons sur les maladies du système nerveux.* Paris: A. Delahaye & E. Lecrosnier, 1884.

24. CHERRY, C. *On Human Communication*, 2nd ed. Cambridge: MIT Press, 1966.

25. CHOMSKY, N. *Syntactic Structures.* New York: Humanities Press, 1957.

26. CHURCHMAN, C. W. *The Systems Approach.* New York: Delacorte, 1968.

27. COLEMAN, J. S. *Introduction to Mathematical Sociology.* New York: Free Press, 1964.

28. COLLEN, M. F. "Automated Multiphasic Screening and Occupational Data," *Arch. Environ. Health*, 15 (1967), 280–284.

29. COULSON, J. E., ed. *Programmed Learning and Computer-Based Instruction.* New York: Wiley, 1962.

30. CRITCHLEY, M. *The Language of Gesture.* London: Arnold, 1939.

31. DANCE, F. E. X., ed. *Human Communication Theory—Original Essays.* New York: Holt, Rinehart & Winston, 1967.

32. DAVITZ, J. R., ed. *The Communication of Emotional Meaning.* New York: McGraw-Hill, 1964.

33. DEPARTMENT OF HEALTH, EDUCATION, AND WELFARE. Vocational Rehabilitation Administration. *Research on Behavioral Aspects of Deafness.* Washington: U.S. Govt. Print. Off., 1966.

34. DIXON, W. J., ed. *BMD: Biomedical Computer Programs.* Publications in Automatic Computation, no. 2. Berkeley: University of California, 1970.

35. DOMARUS, E. VON "The Specific Laws of Logic in Schizophrenia," in J. S. Kasanin, ed., *Language and Thought in Schizophrenia*, pp. 104–114. Berkeley: University of California Press, 1944.

36. EDWARDS, W. and A. TVERSKY, eds. *Decision Making.* Baltimore: Penguin, 1967.

37. EKMAN, P. and W. V. FRIESEN. "Nonverbal Leakage and Clues to Deception," *Psychiatry*, 32 (1969), 88–106.

38. ———. "The Repertoire of Nonverbal Behavior: Categories, Origins, Usage, and Coding," *Semiotica*, 1 (1969), 49–98.

39. EMMERT, P. and W. D. BROOKS. *Methods of Research in Communication.* Boston: Houghton, 1970.

40. FARIS, R. E. L., ed. *Handbook of Modern Sociology.* Chicago: Rand McNally, 1964.

41. FELDMAN, S. S. *Mannerisms of Speech and Gestures in Everyday Life.* New York: International Universities Press, 1959.

42. FENICHEL, O. *The Psychoanalytic Theory of Neurosis.* New York: Norton, 1945.

43. FESTINGER, L. *A Theory of Cognitive Dissonance.* Evanston, Ill.: Row, Peterson, 1957.

44. FOERSTER, H. VON, ed. *Cybernetics: Circular Causal and Feedback Mechanisms in Biological and Social Systems.* Trans. 6th–10th Conf. New York: Josiah Macy, Jr. Foundation, 1950–1955.

45. FRANK, J. D. *Persuasion and Healing.* New York: Schocken, 1963.

46. FRANKE, J. *Ausdruck und Konvention.* Göttingen: Verlag für Psychologie—C. J. Hogrefe, 1967.

47. FREUD, S. (1938) *An Outline of Psychoanalysis*, in J. Strachey, ed. *Standard Edition*, Vol. 23, pp. 144–207. London: Hogarth, 1955.

48. FROMM-REICHMANN, F. *Psychoanalysis and Psychotherapy.* D. M. Bullard, ed. Chicago: University of Chicago Press, 1959.

49. GERARD, R. W. and J. W. DUYFF, eds. *Symposium on Information Processing in the Nervous System, Leiden, 1962.* Amsterdam: Excerpta Medica Foundation, 1964.

50. GOFFMAN, E. *Behavior in Public Places.* Glencoe, Ill.: Free Press, 1963.

51. GORDEN, R. L. *Interviewing: Strategy, Techniques and Tactics.* Homewood, Ill.: Dorsey, 1969.

52. GRAY, W., F. J. DUHL, and N. D. RIZZO, eds. *General Systems Theory and Psychiatry.* Boston: Little, Brown, 1969.

53. GREENWOOD, W. T. *Management and Organizational Behavior Theories: An Interdisciplinary Approach.* Cincinnati: South-Western Pub., 1965.

54. GRINKER, R. R., ed. *Toward a Unified Theory of Human Behavior*, 2nd ed. New York: Basic Books, 1967.

55. GRINKER, R. R., J. MILLER, M. SABSHIN et al. *The Phenomena of Depressions.* New York: Hoeber, 1961.

56. HALEY, J. *Strategies of Psychotherapy.* New York: Grune & Stratton, 1963.

57. HALL, E. T. *The Silent Language.* New York: Doubleday, 1959.

58. ———. *The Hidden Dimension.* New York: Doubleday, 1966.

59. HAYAKAWA, S. I. *Language in Thought and*

Action. New York: Harcourt Brace, 1949.

60. HOGBEN, L. *From Cave Painting to Comic Strip—A Kaleidoscope of Human Communication.* New York: Chanticleer, 1949.

61. HORNEY, K. *The Neurotic Personality of Our Time.* New York: Norton, 1937.

62. HORROBIN, D. F. *The Communication Systems of the Body.* New York: Basic Books, 1964.

63. JACKSON, D. D., ed. *Human Communication.* Vol. 1: *Communication, Family, and Marriage.* Vol. 2: *Therapy, Communication, and Change.* Palo Alto: Science and Behavior Books, 1968.

64. JOHNSON, H. A. "Information Theory in Biology after Eighteen Years," *Science,* 168 (1970), 1545–1550.

65. KENT, A. and O. E. TAULBEE, eds. *Electronic Information Handling.* Washington: Spartan Books, 1965.

66. KNAPP, P. H., ed. *Expression of Emotion in Man.* New York: International Universities Press, 1963.

67. KORZYBSKI, A. (1933) *Science and Sanity,* 4th ed. Lakeville, Conn.: International Non-Aristotelian Library, 1958.

68. KRAEPELIN, E. (1904) *Lectures on Clinical Psychiatry.* T. Johnstone, ed. New York: Hafner, 1968.

69. LAING, R. D. "Mystification, Confusion, and Conflict," in I. Boszormenyi-Nagy and J. L. Framo, eds. *Intensive Family Therapy: Theoretical and Practical Aspects,* pp. 343–363. New York: Harper & Row, 1965.

70. LEIBOVIC, K. N., ed. *Symposium on Information Processing in the Nervous System, Buffalo, 1968.* New York: Springer, 1969.

71. LENNARD, H. L. and A. BERNSTEIN. *Patterns in Human Interaction.* San Francisco: Jossey-Bass, 1969.

72. LENNEBERG, E. H. *Biological Foundations of Language.* New York: Wiley, 1967.

73. LEWIS, A. *Inquiries in Psychiatry: Clinical and Social Investigations.* New York: Science House, 1967.

74. LICKLIDER, J. C. R. *Libraries of the Future.* Cambridge: MIT Press, 1965.

75. LIDZ, T. *The Family and Human Adaptation.* New York: International Universities Press, 1963.

76. LITTERER, J. A. *Organizations: Structure and Behavior.* New York: Wiley, 1963.

77. MCCULLOCH, W. S. *Embodiments of Mind.* Cambridge: MIT Press, 1965.

78. MCLUHAN, H. M. *Understanding Media.* New York: McGraw-Hill, 1964.

79. ———. *The Gutenberg Galaxy.* New York: New Am. Library, 1969.

80. MAHL, G. F. "Some Clinical Observations on Nonverbal Behavior in Interviews," *J. Nerv. Ment. Dis.,* 144 (1967), 492–505.

81. MATSON, F. W. and A. MONTAGU, eds. *The Human Dialogue.* New York: Free Press, 1967.

82. MEERLOO, J. A. M. *Unobtrusive Communication: Essays in Psycholinguistics.* Assen, The Netherlands: Van Gorcum, 1964.

83. MESSNER, J. *Social Ethics,* 3rd rev. ed. St. Louis, Mo.: Herder, 1965.

84. MILLER, G. A. *Language and Communication.* New York: McGraw-Hill, 1951.

85. ———. *Psychology of Communication: Seven Essays.* New York: Basic Books, 1967.

86. MILLER, J. G. "Living Systems: Basic Concepts; Living Systems: Structure and Process; Living Systems: Cross-Level Hypotheses," *Behav. Sci.,* 10 (1965), 193–237; 337–379; 380–411.

87. MORRIS, C. W. *Signification and Significance: A Study of the Relations of Signs and Values.* Cambridge: MIT Press, 1964.

88. MYSAK, E. D. *Speech Pathology and Feedback Theory.* Springfield: Charles C. Thomas, 1966.

89. NEISSER, U. *Cognitive Psychology.* New York: Appleton-Century-Crofts, 1966.

90. NEW YORK STATE, DEPARTMENT OF MENTAL HYGIENE. *An Overview: the Multi-State Information System.* Albany and Orangeburg: DMH and Information Sciences Division, Research Foundation for Mental Hygiene, Inc., Rockland State Hosp., 1970.

91. OSTWALD, P. *Soundmaking.* Springfield, Ill.: Charles C. Thomas, 1963.

92. PEI, M. *The Story of Language,* rev. ed. Philadelphia: Lippincott, 1965.

93. PIERCE, J. R. *Symbols, Signals, and Noise.* New York: Harper Torchbooks, 1965.

94. REITMAN, W. R. *Cognition and Thought.* New York: Wiley, 1965.

95. RÉVÉSZ, G. *The Origins and Prehistory of Language.* London: Longmans, Green, 1956.

96. RIOCH, D. and E. WEINSTEIN, eds. *Disorders of Communication.* Proc. Assoc. Res. Nerv. Ment. Dis., Vol. 42. Baltimore: Williams & Wilkins, 1964.

97. RUESCH, J. *Disturbed Communication.* New York: Norton, 1957.

98. ———. *Therapeutic Communication.* New York: Norton, 1961.

99. ———. "The Assessment of Social Disability," *Arch. Gen. Psychiatry,* 21 (1969), 655–664.

100. ———. *Semiotic Approaches to Human Relations.* The Hague: Mouton, 1972.

101. RUESCH, J. and G. BATESON. *Communication: The Social Matrix of Psychiatry,* 2nd ed. New York: Norton, 1968.

102. RUESCH, J. and W. KEES. *Nonverbal Communication.* Berkeley: University of California Press, 1956.

103. SAPORTA, S. ed. *Psycholinguistics: A Book of Readings.* New York: Holt, Rinehart and Winston, 1961.

104. SCHEFLEN, A. E. *Psychotherapy of Schizophrenia: Direct Analysis.* Springfield, Ill.: Charles C. Thomas, 1961.

105. SCHUETZ, A. "Common-Sense and Scientific Interpretation of Human Action," *Philos. Phenom. Res.,* 14 (1953), 1–38.

106. SCIENTIFIC AMERICAN. *Information.* San Francisco: Freeman, 1966.

107. SEBEOK, T. A., ed. *Animal Communication—Techniques of Study and Results of Research.* Bloomington: Indiana University Press, 1968.

108. SEBEOK, T. A., A. S. HAYES, and M. C. BATESON, eds. *Approaches to Semiotics.* The Hague: Mouton, 1964.

109. SHANDS, H. C. *Thinking and Psychotherapy: An Inquiry into the Processes of Communication.* Cambridge: Harvard University Press, 1960.

110. ———. *Semiotic Approaches to Psychiatry.* The Hague: Mouton, 1970.

111. SHANNON, C. and W. WEAVER. *The Mathematical Theory of Communication.* Urbana: University of Illinois Press, 1949.

112. SKINNER, B. F. *Verbal Behavior.* New York: Appleton, 1957.

113. SMITH, A. G., ed. *Communication and Culture.* New York: Holt, Rinehart & Winston, 1966.

114. SNIDER, J. G. and C. E. OSGOOD, eds. *Semantic Differential Techniques.* Chicago: Aldine, 1969.

115. SOLOMON, P., P. E. KUBZANSKY, P. H. LEIDERMAN et al., eds. *Sensory Deprivation: A Symposium Held at Harvard Medical School.* Cambridge: Harvard University Press, 1961.

116. SPITZ, R. A. *No and Yes.* New York: International Universities Press, 1957.

117. SPITZER, R. and J. ENDICOTT. "Diagno II: Further Developments in a Computer Program for Psychiatric Diagnosis," *Am. J. Psychiatry,* 125, *Suppl.* (1969), 12–21.

118. STARKWEATHER, J., M. KAMP, and A. MONTO. "Psychiatric Interview Simulation by Computer," *Methods Inf. Med.,* 6 (1967), 15–23.

119. STARR, M. K. *Production Management—Systems and Synthesis.* Englewood Cliffs, N.J.: Prentice-Hall, 1964.

120. STEINBUCH, K. *Automat und Mensch: Über menschliche und machinelle Intelligenz.* Berlin: Springer, 1961.

121. STROEBEL, C. F. and B. C. GLUECK, JR. "Computer Derived Global Judgments in Psychiatry," *Am. J. Psychiatry,* 126 (1970) 1057–1066.

122. STROTZ, C. R., A. J. MALERSTEIN, and J. A. STARKWEATHER. "Automated Psychiatric Patient Record System," *Arch. Gen. Psychiatry,* 21 (1969), 311–319.

123. SULLIVAN, H. S. *The Interpersonal Theory of Psychiatry.* New York: Norton, 1953.

124. THASS-THIENEMANN, T. *Symbolic Behavior.* New York: Washington Square Press, 1968.

125. THAYER, L., ed. *Communication: Theory and Research.* Springfield, Ill.: Charles C. Thomas, 1967.

126. ———. *Communication: Concepts and Perspectives.* Washington: Spartan Books, 1967.

127. WAGGONER, R. W. and D. J. CAREK, eds. *Communication in Clinical Practice,* Vol. 1, no. 1, Int. Psychiatry Clin. Boston: Little, Brown, 1964.

128. WALTON, R. E. *Interpersonal Peacemaking: Confrontations and Third Party Consultations.* Reading, Mass.: Addison-Wesley, 1969.

129. WATSON, D. O., JR. *Talk with Your Hands.* Winneconne, Wis.: D. O. Watson, Jr., 1964.

130. WATZLAWICK, P., J. BEAVIN, and D. D. JACKSON. *Pragmatics of Human Communication: A Study of Interactional Patterns, Pathologies, and Paradoxes.* New York: Norton, 1967.

131. WHORF, B. L. *Language, Thought, and Reality.* J. B. Carroll, ed. New York: Wiley, 1956.

132. WIENER, N. *Cybernetics, or Control and*

Communication in the Animal and the Machine. New York: Wiley, 1948.

133. ———. *The Human Use of Human Beings —Cybernetics and Society.* Boston: Houghton, 1950.

134. WUNDT, W. *Völkerpsychologie,* 4 vols. Leipzig: Wilhelm Engelmann, 1905.

135. WYNNE, L. C. and M. T. SINGER. "Thought Disorder and Family Relations of Schizophrenics: 1. A Research Strategy," *Arch. Gen. Psychiatry,* 9 (1963), 191–198.

136. ZAHL, P. A., ed. (1950) *Blindness: Modern Approaches to the Unseen Environment,* reprinted with rev. bibliography. New York: Hafner, 1963.

137. ZUBEK, J. P., ed. *Sensory Deprivation: Fifteen Years of Research.* New York: Appleton-Century-Crofts, 1969.

CHAPTER 40

SOCIAL ECOLOGY: MULTIDIMENSIONAL STUDIES OF HUMANS AND HUMAN MILIEUS*

Rudolf H. Moos

[Introduction

CURRENT INTEREST in the physical and social aspects of planning for both large (e.g., cities and "new towns") and small (e.g., industries, psychiatric hospitals, correctional institutions) environmental systems is remarkable. Jordan[43] notes that more books treating man and his environment from a holistic and ecological viewpoint have appeared within the past four years than appeared during the prior three decades. Within the broader society this interest is largely due to technological advances, whose "side effects" raise critical issues about the delicate ecological balance existing in "spaceship earth." Major human problems such as general

environmental deterioration, particularly water, air, and noise pollution, the probable effects of increasing population and population density, and issues of resource depletion, specifically in relation to food materials, are being extensively discussed.

New developments in psychiatry and the behavioral sciences are reflecting these concerns. This chapter introduces social ecology as a relevant field of interest for psychiatry, presents major methods by which human milieus have been characterized, and draws implications for the clinical and applied problems with which psychiatry and its allied professions must deal. Whereas social ecology is equally concerned with human adaptation and human milieus, the chapter focuses primarily on newer conceptualizations of social environments since this aspect of the field is least familiar to psychiatrists. Further, assess-

* This work was supported in part by NIMH Grant MH16026, by a Veterans Administration Research Grant, and by a grant from the Commonwealth Fund.

ments of milieus must necessarily precede assessments of the impact of these milieus on human functioning.

Thus, the focus here is more on milieu than on man, although the essential aspects of milieus are their effects on human adaptation. The major methods by which coping and adaptation have been assessed in man have been reviewed elsewhere.[71] Six major methods by which human milieus have been characterized are presented here. Human aggression and violence serve as the adaptive (or maladaptive) responses by which the relevance of these six methods to practical concerns of psychiatrists is illustrated. Overall implications extend from enhancing the accuracy of predicting individual behavior, to new methods for facilitating and evaluating social change in small living groups, to more varied and more comfortable interdisciplinary roles for psychiatrists. These areas are clearly at the "frontiers of psychiatry."

Social ecology is conceptualized here as the multidisciplinary study of the impacts that physical and social environments have on human beings. Its primary concern is with the assessment and optimization of human milieus. It is linked to traditional concerns of human ecology, both in its emphasis on the measurement of objective physical characteristics of environments—e.g., temperature, rainfall, air pollution, and noise levels—also the shapes, sizes, and physical arrangements of buildings; and in its emphasis on the short-term evolutionary and adaptive consequences of these environments. It is linked to traditional concerns of the behavioral sciences, particularly psychology and sociology, both in its emphasis on the importance of the social environment and in its explicit consideration of environmental impacts on psychological variables such as self-esteem and personal development. Finally, it is also linked to traditional concerns in psychiatry, medicine, and epidemiology in its explicit focus on the identification of dysfunctional reactions (e.g., illness, accidents, anxiety, depression, anger, etc.) and their relationship to environmental variables.

For example, social ecology is concerned with the effects of air pollution (an ecological variable) on human moods, with the effects of ecological (e.g., size) and social (e.g., cohesiveness) environmental characteristics on individual development, and with the effects of both structural (staffing ratios, cost) and social (clarity of expectations, strictness of rules and regulations) environmental characteristics on the outcome of psychiatric treatment. Each of these is an ongoing concern in an existing field of inquiry. It is the range and interconnection of variables generally studied in isolation that gives social ecology a diverse, robust, and socially relevant focus. The field thus provides a distinctive "point of entry" by which human milieus and their impacts on human functioning may be conceptualized.

At least three basic assumptions are central to this area. (1) Human behavior cannot be understood apart from the environmental context in which it occurs. The implications of this oft-stated assumption have rarely been effectively pursued, e.g., accurate predictions of behavior or of treatment outcome simply cannot be made solely from information about individuals: information about their environments is essential; (2) Physical and social environments must be studied together since neither can be fully understood without the other, e.g., both the architectural design and the psychosocial treatment milieu may significantly influence patient and staff behavior; and (3) Social ecology has an explicit value orientation in that it attempts to provide knowledge relevant to promoting maximally effective human functioning.

⟮ Methods for Conceptualizing Human Milieus

An important aspect of social ecology is its primary focus on conceptualizing methods by which human environments may be characterized, and, as mentioned above, it is this aspect of the field which is most strongly emphasized here. Psychiatry and the behavioral sciences have themselves recently shown greatly increased interest in social milieus. This interest has arisen in part because of dissatisfactions with trait conceptualizations of personality, in part because of low correlations obtained between measures of personality traits and various validity criteria, and, in part, because of growing evidence that substantial proportions of the variance in behavior are accounted for by situational and environmental variables.

The literature criticizing the empirical legacy of several decades of work with trait models of personality has been most cogently summarized by Mischel.[66] Major corroborative studies include those by Ellsworth et al.[24] who concluded that psychiatric patients' behavior in the hospital was not predictive of their behavior in the community; by Moos[67] who showed that observations of hospitalized patients in a group therapy setting may not even generate valid predictions about the behavior of the same patients in either free time or individual therapy situations on the same ward; and by Raush and his associates[85] who found that ward settings evoked characteristic patterns of social actions (i.e., settings were more or less evocative of dependency) and that the interactive effect of person and setting contributed far more information about behavior than either knowledge of the setting or knowledge of the person alone. From the point of view of the assessment and prediction of individual behavior, these and other findings present a compelling argument for the utility of environmental assessment methods. In addition, many studies have demonstrated that substantial differences may occur in the behavior of the same individuals when they are in different milieus.[8]

This development has occurred mainly in psychology. However, an important parallel development has occurred during the past two decades in psychiatry, i.e., the psychosocial environment of psychiatric treatment has become of increasing concern. A concomitant of this emphasis is a reevaluation of the traditional disease model with its assumption that psychopathological disturbance resides only within the individual. The impetus for this change is partly due to relevant theoretical contributions emphasizing the interplay between ego functions and external reality,[26,37]

and partly to detailed observations and naturalistic descriptions indicating the importance of the treatment environment in facilitating or hindering treatment goals.[16,96]

New programs designed to use the social milieu as a treatment modality[22,27,42] have been organized. The approaches are exceedingly divergent, but they all basically stem from the common hypothesis that the immediate psychosocial milieu in which patients function is a crucial aspect of the treatment process. These developments have now resulted in the construction of several different methods by which treatment envionments can be systematically characterized and compared.

The third major impetus for interest in conceptualizations of social milieus is an outgrowth of the recent "third revolution in psychiatry," which is also occurring in a relatively parallel manner in psychology and the other mental health professions. We are being asked to help design physical and social systems that will maximize the probabilities of human growth and facilitate effective functioning and human excellence.[13,30] Since disorders of human functioning are at least partly rooted in social systems, new information leading toward the effective modification of institutions to promote the constructive handling of life stresses is being given increasingly high priority.[93]

In addition, general dissatisfaction with the relatively weak effects of traditional individual and group treatment has promoted interest in naturally occurring therapeutic conditions in society.[11] Anastasi[1] has indicated the complexity of the problem by pointing out that environments cannot be ordered along a single favorable–unfavorable continuum, since, for example, an environment favorable to the development of independence and self-reliance may differ from one that is favorable to the development of social conformity or abstract thinking.

Each of these developments raises the common problem of how human environments can be conceptualized and assessed. Six major methods by which characteristics of environments have been related to indices of human functioning have recently been identified.[70]

1. Ecological dimensions that include both geographical and meteorological and architectural and physical design variables.

2. Behavior settings, the only units thus far proposed that are characterized by both ecological and behavioral properties.

3. Dimensions of organizational structure.

4. Dimensions identifying the collective personal and/or behavioral characteristics of the milieu inhabitants.

5. Dimensions related to psychosocial characteristics and organization climates.

6. Variables relevant to the functional or reinforcement analyses of environments.

The six categories of dimensions are nonexclusive, overlapping, and mutually interrelated. The overview presented is necessarily incomplete and sketchy, but it serves to illustrate the broad range of dimensions relevant to this area. The common relevance of these six types of dimensions is that each has been conceptualized and shown to have an important and sometimes decisive impact on individual and group behavior.

Ecological Dimensions

Down through the ages there has been the recurrent notion that geographical and meteorological characteristics (e.g., temperature, rainfall, topography, etc.) may significantly shape the culture, character, and activities of societies. Environmental determinists believe that there are specific connections between environmental characteristics, such as mountainous terrain, soil conditions, humidity, etc., and personality traits such as strength of character, assertiveness, bravery, and laziness. For example, one study[10] found an association between different types of subsistence economy and differential importance given to the development of certain character traits. Societies whose economies entailed the accumulation and care of food resources tended to stress the development of such personal traits as responsibility and obedience, whereas hunting and fishing societies tended to emphasize achievement and self-reliance. Such conclusions are, of course, tenuous, since intricate patterns of potential mediating factors are always present.

It has been suggested that climate may be one of the major factors in economic development throughout the world, the optimum climate being the temperate climate within which most of the world's current industrial powers lie. Further, many people feel that their efficiency is impaired by extremes of heat and cold, and one of the arguments in support of air conditioning is that it improves worker efficiency. Climate has been associated with gross national product per capita,[88] with political uprisings, rebellions, and revolutions,[12] with the occurrence of homicides,[104] with specific indices of affective interpersonal behavior,[33] and with variations in organizational participation among metropolitan housewives.[61]

Some of the other variables implicated in the determination of behavior include extreme cold, barometric pressure, cyclonic and anticyclonic storm patterns, and oxygen, nitrogen, carbon dioxide, and ozone concentrations in the atmosphere.[76,92] For example, Mills[65] reports that statistics in Tokyo show that people are more forgetful on days of low barometric pressure as indicated by higher frequency of packages and umbrellas left on buses and streetcars.

The weight of the evidence suggests that geographical and meteorological variables may be more important in the determination of group and individual behavior than has been thought. Man is increasingly creating his own geographical and meteorological environment, and trends in this area are thus concerned with the possible relationship of man-made variables, such as radiation and air pollution, to mood changes and to mental and physical symptoms.

Other aspects of the man-made environment, especially dimensions relevant to architectural and physical design, are also important. Behavior necessarily occurs in a specific physical context that may impose major constraints on the range of possible kinds of behavior and serve to determine particular aspects or patterns of individual action. A substantial amount of research has been done in this area. For example, behavioral maps can be arranged in a matrix showing the frequency of different types of activities in different available locations. Psychiatric wards have been analyzed in terms of variables such as behavior density (the frequency of all types of activities at a particular place), diffuseness (the range of different activities occurring at a place), and activity profile (the frequency of specific types of activities occurring at a place). Research in ergonomics, human engineering, and human factors has been concerned with the relation of selected environmental variables, such as heating, lighting, noise level, ventilation, and the layout and design of machines to behavioral measures of work efficiency, comfort, social interaction, interpersonal perception, and exploratory behavior. For example, Maslow and Mintz[60] demonstrated that interpersonal perceptions could be highly sensitive to variations in the physical environment. They found that judgments of psychological states (weary, zestful, irritated) based on photographed faces differed in three physically different rooms. Basic reviews of this area may be found in Craik,[21] Kates and Wohlwill,[45] Proshansky et al.,[82] and Sommer.[94]

Unfortunately, there is as yet no adequate dimensionalization or typology of the variables of architectural and physical design. Kasmar[44] has developed an environmental description scale that assesses perceptions of physical characteristics of rooms along dimensions such as physical organization, lighting, size, temperature, ventilation, etc. At a more global level, Lansing et al.[49] have characterized planned residential environments (e.g., Columbia, Maryland; Reston, Virginia) along dimensions such as dwelling-unit density, accessibility of recreational facilities, percent of homes with sidewalks nearby, etc. The next major advance in this area will probably be a creation of several alternative typologies of variables that will be utilized in order to systematically study social problems such as physical environmental factors affecting residential choice and migration, the adaptational cost of urban noise and ghettos, etc.

Behavior Settings

The work of Roger Barker[7] and his associates in ecological psychology is important and unique. They conceptualize behavioral ecology as being concerned with molar behavior and the ecological context in which it occurs. Barker has carefully analyzed and categorized the behavior settings of a small Midwestern community. He points out that these behavior settings, e.g., drugstore, garage, play in junior high school, basketball games, etc., are naturally occurring phenomena, i.e., they are not created by an experimenter for scientific purposes. The important point about behavior settings is that they are stable extra-individual units that have great coercive power over the behavior that occurs within them.

Behavior settings have been shown to have pervasive effects on individuals, not only in terms of the specific behavior "demanded" by the setting (e.g., reading and writing in classrooms) but also on other behavior and on affects experienced by individuals. Barker and Gump[9] have done an extremely intriguing analysis of the different demands of undermanned and optimally manned behavior settings and have shown that these produce characteristic differences in their inhabitants. For example, students in small schools with relatively few associates within behavior settings, in comparison with students of larger schools with relatively many associates, report twice as many pressures on them to take part in the programs of the school settings, actually perform in more than twice as many responsible positions in the settings, and report having more satisfaction related to the development of competence, to being challenged, to engaging in important actions, to being involved in group activities, to being valued, and to gaining moral and cultural values. Some of these findings have been replicated in large and small churches.[102]

Thus, the specific relevance of behavior settings is that they are of considerable importance in the determination of several aspects of individual behavior and experience (specifically, the development of competence and self-esteem) which are of interest to mental health practitioners. Behavior setting surveys should be carried out in different types of institutions, e.g., mental hospitals, correctional units, universities, urban ghettos, etc. The range and variety of behavioral settings in central city, suburban, and rural areas must be quite different, and from Barker's results it would be expected that this would have important effects on both the behavior of their adult inhabitants and on the developing competencies of the children growing up within them.

Dimensions of Organizational Structure

Many investigators have attempted to assess and discriminate among organizations utilizing relatively objective dimensions, such as size, staffing ratios, average salary levels, organizational control structure, etc.[58] A typical example is work on the properties of organization structure in relation to job attitudes and job behavior.[81] Organizations vary widely in their structural characteristics and, thus, an important question is whether differences in organizational structures are related to different behavioral and attitudinal indices of the organization members. Porter and Lawler found that dimensions such as the size of the overall organization, the number of levels in the organization relative to its total size, the size of the organizational subunits and the average number of subordinates a manager is responsible for supervising were significantly related to one or more attitudinal or behavioral variables, e.g., need satisfaction, absenteeism, turnover rate. Recent articles that review various aspects of this work, most of it concentrating on industrial and business organizations, include Lichtman and Hunt,[53] Pugh,[83] and Roberts.[87]

Similar work has been done in educational institutions, mainly colleges and universities,[3] in which attempts have been made to relate traditional indices of institutional quality (faculty–student ratio, percentage of faculty with Ph.D. degree, number of books in the library per student, etc.) to various indices of student achievement and personal development.[28] In other relevant work, the three most well-investigated dimensions have been size,[9] turnover rate,[47] and population density or crowding, particularly in relation to social pathology.[15] Several recent attempts have been made to further conceptualize crowding effects in human environments such as urban ghettoes[23] and large cities.[64]

Personal and Behavioral Characteristics of the Milieu Inhabitants

Various factors related to the characteristics of individuals inhabiting a particular environment, e.g., average age, ability level, socioeconomic background, educational attainment, may be considered to be situational variables in that they partly define relevant characteristics of the environment.[91] This general idea is based on the suggestion made by Linton[56] that most of the social and cultural environment is transmitted through other people. It implies that the character of an environment is dependent, in part, upon the typical characteristics of its members.

This approach may be illustrated by Astin[3] who has recently developed a new technique for characterizing environmental stimuli in colleges and universities, the inventory of college activities (ICA). The ICA provides information about the average personal and behavioral characteristics of the college environment by listing the following items: (1) Questions about activities in college, such as whether or not the individual flunked a course, became pinned or engaged, got married, participated in a student demonstration, changed his or her major field; (2) the median number of hours per week the student spent in different activities such as attending class, studying for school assignments, reading for pleasure, watching TV, watching athletic events, sleeping, playing games; and (3) the kinds of organizations in which the student was a member, such as fraternities or sororities, college athletic teams, marching band, religious club, service organization, etc. Remarkable diversity was found among the environments of 246 colleges and universities included in this study. Thus, the proportion of students who engaged in any particular activity (e.g., dating, going to church, drinking beer, voting in a student election) often varied from no students in some institutions to nearly all students in others. Astin feels that this considerable diversity indicates that the college and university environment has great potential for differentially influencing the experience and behavior of the individual student.

For illustration, he assumes that a new student enrolls in an institution with high academic standards in which certain environmental stimuli occur relatively frequently: classroom examinations, discussions among students about grades, studying, intellectual arguments among students, and debates between faculty and students. The new student would be exposed to these and related stimuli and might thus feel anxiety about possible academic failure (a change in immediate subjective experience), increased fear of or hostility toward fellow students, increased feelings of competitiveness and/or feelings of inferiority. Presumably the student might be affected differently if he attended a different college. In terms of short-term behavioral effects, the student may increase the time he devotes to study, reduce the time he devotes to social activities, and perhaps increase his intellectual aggression. He may consequently experience greater feelings of loneliness and isolation. Finally, there may be alterations in his self-concept and/or relatively permanent changes in behavior that may persist beyond college (e.g., devoting a great deal of time to the job or competing constantly with others). Astin and Holland[4] and Holland[39] have done other highly relevant work in this area. Holland assumes that vocational satisfaction, stability and achievement depend on the congruence between one's personality and the environment (composed largely of other people) in which one works. He has proposed six model environments to characterize the common physical and social environments in our culture, and six personality types or personal orientations as identified by the type of vocation to which a person belongs. Since both the environmental models and the personality types are derived from the same basic six concepts (realistic, intellectual, social, conventional, enterprising, and artistic), it is possible to classify people and environments in the same terms and, at least theoretically, to assess the degree of person–environment congruence and its effects. Thus, there are some highly promising approaches in this area.

Psychosocial Characteristic and Organizational Climate

Until recently most of the work in this area involved rather detailed naturalistic descriptions or anthropological vignettes of the functioning of different types of institutions such as psychiatric wards, colleges, and universities, etc. This was valuable work in that it indicated the importance of the immediate psychosocial environment in the determination of behavior and in that it suggested various types of dimensions along which psychosocial environments might be compared. The newer organization theorists have presented detailed analyses of organizations that specifically imply certain psychosocial or "event-structure" dimensions along which organizations might be compared.[46]

A number of perceived climate scales have been developed in the last few years in order to attempt to more systematically measure the general norms, value orientations, and other psychosocial characteristics of different types of institutions. For example, Stern[97] follows the Murray need-press theory and points out that descriptions of institutional environments are based on inferred continuity and consistency in otherwise discrete events. If students in a university are assigned seats in classrooms, if attendance records are kept, if faculty see students outside of class only by appointment, if there is a prescribed form for all term papers, if neatness counts, etc., then it is probable that the press at this school emphasizes the development of orderly responses on the part of the students. It is these conditions which establish the climate or atmosphere of an institution. A substantial amount of work utilizing this general logic has been carried out in colleges and universities,[79,80] elementary schools,[36] junior high and high school classrooms,[101] and industry.[55]

Moos and his associates have studied nine different types of social environments relatively extensively and have developed perceived climate scales for each of these environments: (1) psychiatric wards;[72] (2) community-oriented programs of psychiatric treatment, such as halfway houses, day hospitals, or community care homes;[68] (3) correctional institutions, including those for both adult and juvenile offenders;[73] (4) military basic-training companies; (5) university student residences, such as dormitories, fraternities, and sororities;[31] (6) junior high and high school classrooms;[100] (7) social and therapeutic groups; (8) work milieus; and (9) families.

Moos conceptualizes three basic types of dimensions that characterize and discriminate among different subunits within each of these eight environments.

1. Relationship dimensions, which are quite similar in all eight environments, assess the extent to which individuals are involved in the environment and the extent to which they support and help each other. The basic dimensions are involvement, support, and expressiveness.

2. Personal development dimensions assess the basic directions along which personal development and self-enhancement tend to occur in the particular environment. The exact nature of these dimensions varies somewhat among the eight environments studied, depending upon their basic purposes and goals. For example, in psychiatric and correctional programs these dimensions assess the treatment goals, e.g., autonomy (the extent to which people are encouraged to be self-sufficient and independent) practical orientation (the extent to which the program orients an individual toward training for new jobs, looking to the future, setting and working toward concrete goals) and personal problem orientation (the extent to which individuals are encouraged to be concerned with their feelings and problems and to seek to understand them). An autonomy or independence dimen-

sion is also identified in military companies. University residences (e.g., competition, academic achievement, intellectuality) and junior high and high school classrooms (e.g., task orientation, competition) include other dimensions that are conceptualized as belonging in the category of goal orientation.

3. System maintenance and change dimensions are relatively similar across the eight environments studied. The basic dimensions are order and organization, clarity and control. An additional dimension in work environments is work pressure, whereas a dimension of innovation is identified in educational, work, and small group environments. There is evidence that these types of dimensions are related to important criteria such as patient morale and indices of coping behavior and different objective indices of treatment outcome.[74]

Techniques by which to assess the organizational climate characteristics of social milieus are important in the identification of salient environmental dimensions. Their specific relevance here is that they identify dimensions that have demonstrable effects on individual and group behavior. They are useful in the measurement of personality–environment congruence, in cross-cultural comparisons, and in helping define directions for environmental change.[69] The striking similarity of the specific dimensions and their categorization across different investigators and organizational environments indicates that one or more widely useful typologies may soon emerge.

Functional or Reinforcement Analyses of Environments

The methodology of functional analyses of environments is an outgrowth of a social learning perspective.[5,66] Basically, the social learning theorist takes it as a given that people vary their behavior extensively in different social and physical environments. In this view, people vary their behavior from one setting to another mainly because the reinforcement consequences for particular kinds of behavior vary. Thus, the social learning theorist attempts to analyze and identify those stimuli and stimulus changes which produce and maintain behavior and behavior change. People are expected to behave similarly in different settings only to the extent that those settings are alike (or perhaps are perceived to be alike) in their potential reinforcing properties.

Relevant approaches include those of Schoggen[90] and of Wolf.[103] Schoggen conceptualized the environment to be active and directed with respect to the developing child and identified environmental force units (EFU) which were defined as any action by an environmental agent that occurred vis-à-vis the child and was directed toward a recognizable end state with respect to the child. His results indicated that EFU occurred at a very frequent rate, that mothers were more often sources of EFU than fathers, and that there were wide individual variations among children in the percent of EFU initiated with the child and by others in interaction with the child. This may be a potentially important technique for studying both the differential shaping of behavior and methods by which specific goals of behavior change may be implemented.

Wolf listed the conditions in the environment that were likely to influence the development of general intelligence and/or academic achievement. The types of environmental variables that were identified included: the climate created for achievement motivation, the opportunities for verbal development, the nature and amount of assistance provided in overcoming academic difficulties, the level of intellectuality in the environment and the kinds of work habits expected of the individual. Wolf developed a technique for assessing these variables and found that the correlation between the total rating for the degree of intellectual "press" of the environment and measured general intelligence was 0.69. He states that environments for the development and maintenance of such characteristics as dependency, aggression, and dogmatism could be delineated and measured. Many investigators[14,18] have presented analyses of institutional environments along these lines.

Functional or reinforcement analysis is relevant to the prediction of behavior in the sense that one can attempt to discover whether environmental maintaining conditions for a specific kind of behavior tend to change markedly. Also, the assumption is that behavior change can readily occur when there is environmental change. Generalization of behavior change should occur to the extent to which there is generalization of the reinforcement that induced the behavior change. Since any stimulus may have either discriminative or reinforcing properties (or both), functional analyses are highly idiographic and complex, though of great potential value for understanding and changing behavior.

(An Overview and an Example of Aggression and Violence

This brief overview illustrates the many different assessment techniques, types of variables, and potential environmental typologies. The area is in its empirical infancy and it is still unclear how the different methods will eventually relate to each other. In the broadest perspective, environmental and stimulus variables may be conceptualized as reducing and shaping the potential variability of human behavior. In this sense, each of the six types of dimensions mentioned above are related. The geographical and meteorological environment to some extent shapes the environment of architecture and physical design, which in turn has demonstrable effects on the types of available behavior settings. In their turn, behavior settings constrain the potential range of organizational structure, methods of institutional functioning, and the personal and behavioral characteristics of individuals who choose to inhabit the behavior settings. Different behavior settings, organizational structures, and sets of milieu inhabitants give rise to different psychosocial characteristics and organizational climates. Finally, any of the above types of variables may, to some extent, affect the types of reinforcements that are likely to occur in a specific setting. Decisions about specific reinforcements that are valued may then, in a feedback loop, have effects on the resulting geographical and architectural environment. Any of these levels of environmental variables may be influenced by any other level, although the relationship between some levels (e.g., personal characteristics of milieu inhabitants and organizational climates) may be closer than that between others (e.g., geographical and meteorological variables and organizational structure).

The categorization of environmental dimensions into six broad types may or may not have general utility. The categories are overlapping and certain variables can as easily be placed into one category as another. On the other hand, the conceptualization identifies some initial directions for an overall organization of this field. The potential clinical relevance of a coherent conceptualization of environmental and stimulus variables may be illustrated by utilizing aggression and violence as an example. The point is to illustrate a framework for the analysis of milieu effects, which is of critical importance not only for aggression but for the entire range of behavior with which psychiatrists must deal.

There is substantial evidence that various attitudinal and behavioral indices of anger, hostility, and aggression vary considerably over different settings, even for the same individuals. For example, Endler and Hunt[25] found that consistent individual differences accounted for only between 15 and 20 percent of the variance in hostility, whereas setting differences accounted for between 4 and 8 percent and the various interactions (e.g., subjects by situations) accounted for approximately 30 percent. Moos[67] has corroborated these findings in a study of the reactions of patients and staff to a representative subsample of daily ward settings, e.g., individual therapy, small group therapy, community meeting. The relevance of this and other similar work is that there is an upper limit to the accuracy of predicting aggressive behavior from knowledge of the individual alone, and that different settings (all of which may have at least some anger-provoking elements in common) differentially elicit aggressive behavior from different individuals. The most important implication is that the identification

of highly aggressive individuals may vary considerably, depending upon the situation in which they are observed, the individual by whom they are interviewed, etc. One cannot assume that individual differences on the strength of indices of aggression that are obtained in experimental situations will necessarily generalize to real life situations or even to other experimental situations.

Each of the six types of dimensions discussed above has a central impact in the determination of aggressive behavior of individuals and groups, e.g., the riots in Los Angeles and Chicago during the summer of 1965 were widely believed to stem in part from the discomforts of hot weather. Wolfgang[104] has reported that the peak months for the occurrence of homicide are the hot summer months. Berke and Wilson[12] point out that most major political uprisings, rebellions, and revolutions begin during the hot months. Griffitt[32] found that interpersonal attraction responses were significantly more negative under a "hot" condition (over 90° F) than under a "normal" condition (about 68° F). Lieber and Sherin[54] have recently concluded that there is a relationship between phases of the moon and murder rates. They analyzed over 1900 murders occurring over a fifteen-year period in Dade County, Florida and found that the murder rate began to rise about twenty-four hours before the full moon, reached a peak at full moon, and then dropped back before climbing again to a secondary peak at the new moon.

The exact interpretation of these findings is unclear, although evidence for the effects of temperature on aggressive behavior is relatively consistent. There is less available evidence that architecture and physical-design variables have effects on aggressive behavior, although they do generally have effects on interpersonal transactions,[77] and the body-buffer zone has been shown to be larger in violence-prone individuals.[48]

Different types of behavior settings differentially elicit aggressive or hostile behavior. In an interesting clinical study, Raush et al.[85] found that changes in hostility in hyperaggressive children were setting specific, e.g., one child showed a marked reduction in hostile responses toward adults in a structured group setting, whereas another showed these changes mainly during mealtimes. Gump et al.[34] observed children in camp settings and found that the quality of interaction of the same boys in swimming and craft settings was quite different. Asserting, blocking, and attacking behavior was significantly higher in the swimming setting, whereas helping reactions were higher in crafts. In a detailed study of the behavior of a nine-year-old boy, Gump et al.[35] found that the boy showed a greater proportion of aggressive responses at home than at camp.

Many organizational structure dimensions have been related to the frequency of aggressive behavior, most notably indices of space and population density (crowding). For example, Swift[99] concluded that conflicts between children are more numerous when play space is more restricted. Other studies have found correlations between high-population-density areas and high crime rates for both juveniles and adults.[89] Calhoun[15] has presented experimental data linking population density and overly aggressive and conflict-oriented behavior in rats, and Sugiyama[98] has indicated that high density leads to a general breakdown in the social order of wild monkeys and results in extremely aggressive behavior, hypersexuality, the killing of the young, etc.

In some intriguing analyses Galle et al.[29] have found that four different components of population density (e.g., the number of persons per room, the number of rooms per housing unit) show highly significant correlations with asocial aggressive behavior, even when ethnicity and social class are controlled. Some authors are now beginning to pay specific attention to the factors by which the effects of population density and crowding may be mediated.[64,106] Extensive data linking various indices of anger, aggression, and conflict to organizational structure variables, such as size, staffing, the heterogeneity and stability of personnel, etc., are also available.[19] Since measures of aggressive responses may be heavily affected by organizational structure

dimensions, changes in these dimensions (e.g., an increase in amount of play space) may have dramatic effects.

Discussions of the effects of variables relevant to the last three methods of characterizing environments are particularly numerous and only selected examples can be given here. In terms of the personal and behavioral characteristics of the inhabitants of the milieu, perhaps the most relevant example is that of the "interpersonal reflex"[50] or "behavioral reciprocity."[85] Aggression begets aggression, and the proportion of hostile actions that are "sent" by an individual often parallels the proportion he "receives." For example, Purcell and Brady[84] found that the interpersonal response of affection was preceded by the interpersonal stimulus of affection 80 percent of the time and by the interpersonal stimulus of aggression 0 percent of the time.

In a most intriguing study, Couch[20] found that the response of interpersonal hostility was more highly correlated with the immediately preceding behavioral press than it was with a combination of personality need, concealment defense, and perceived press predictors. Thus, knowledge of the immediately preceding interpersonal stimulus was the best predictor of interpersonal hostility. This finding should give all of us who attempt to make predictions from personality needs alone significant pause. Holsti and North,[40] in careful analyses of documents authored by key European decision makers in the period of June 27 to August 4, 1914, indicate that these conclusions are not limited to individuals acting alone. They found that the correlation between the hostility expressed toward a nation and the hostility expressed by it was 0.46 for the Triple Entente (England, France, and Russia) and 0.68 for the Dual Alliance (Austria, Hungary, and Germany). Perceived hostility and actual violent behavior (i.e., actual troop mobilizations, etc.) were also highly intercorrelated (0.64).

There have been several demonstrations of the effects of social climate on aggression, particularly in groups and families. Perhaps the most intriguing work was done by Lewin et al.[52] who found that the same group may change markedly (from apathy to aggression or vice versa) when it is changed to a new leadership atmosphere under a different leader. Lewin[51] has also shown that an individual's conduct may change drastically in line with the social atmosphere of the group. He studied two girls and found that after transferring from one group to another, each girl rapidly displayed the level of conduct shown by the other girl before the change. He concludes that changing group climates should have important effects on changing individual aggressive behavior. McCord et al.[57] related specific indices of home atmosphere to different types of crimes, and Anderson and Brewer[2] have shown that teachers create different classroom climates that have strongly differential effects on relevant indices of child behavior, e.g., dominating, resisting, nonconforming, etc.

Finally, the potential effects on aggressive behavior of both positive and negative reinforcement procedures (including imitation and modeling) are well known.[5,62,63] Milgram's studies have shown that subjects who are not usually aggressive can be made to behave very aggressively under experimenter and group-pressure encouragement. Recent examples from world history seem to amply corroborate this. Bandura and Walters[6] have also illustrated the specificity of aggressive behavior in their finding that parents who punished aggression in the home, but who simultaneously modeled aggressive behavior and encouraged it in their sons' relationships to their peers, produced boys who were not aggressive at home but who were markedly aggressive at school.

It should be noted that Moyer[75] has conceptualized several kinds of aggression, each of which appears to have a specific neural and endocrine basis. He distinguishes among the kinds of aggression on the basis of the stimulus situations that elicit them, e.g., intermale, fear-induced, irritable, territorial, maternal, and instrumental. Although the categories for environmental analysis are different, the underlying logic of Moyer's analysis is similar to that presented here.

Thus, the evidence indicates that ecological variables, behavior settings, dimensions of organizational structure, behavioral characteristics of milieu inhabitants, social and organizational climate, and reinforcement variables, all have important impacts on various indices of aggressive and violent behavior. Similar analyses may be carried out and similar conclusions probably hold for most other clinically relevant kinds of behavior. This analysis in no way minimizes the importance of individual dispositions in the sense that it is clinically obvious that some individuals are generally more prone to express certain kinds of behavior (including aggressive and violent behavior) than others. In addition, individual dispositions may have their effects in interaction with environmental conditions. On the other hand, the importance of this work on the development of taxonomies of environmental variables can hardly be overemphasized, particularly in its implications for both behavior prediction and behavior change. Knowledge of the probable behavioral and attitudinal effects of different environmental arrangements is at least as central an issue for psychiatry as knowledge about traditional personality theory and psychotherapy.

(Implications and Applications

Social ecology provides an overall perspective on the salient dimensions of the physical and social environment and thus on dimensions that influence the development and maintenance of effective adaptation and coping behavior, on the one hand, and "social-breakdown reactions," including medical and psychiatric symptomatology, on the other. The approach provides some beginning conceptual and theoretical underpinning for community psychiatry and the community mental health movement, suggests guidelines for more thorough and complete descriptions of both individual clinical cases and overall treatment milieus, and has important implications for the facilitation and evaluation of social change, particularly in small group living settings. Social ecology expands the traditional framework of ecology to include issues of direct concern to psychiatry, i.e., the identification of environmental and milieu variables that have impacts on the maintenance of effective and ineffective behavior.

The six ways of describing human environments as discussed above provide an overall framework of general utility. The framework is relevant to clinical applications, particularly in community-oriented consultation. Psychiatrists are increasingly asked to diagnose and change social settings rather than to work separately with each of the individuals within those settings. Sensitivity to a broad range of environmental variables and their probable effects on individuals will help identify the causes of environmental "trouble spots," e.g., high dropout, turnover, sickness, or accident rate, and to suggest changes in them. Measures of environments aid in systematically comparing two or more milieus (e.g.. treatment programs, university dormitories) and are essential in evaluating the extent to which social change attempts actually succeed. Treatment outcome cannot be evaluated without assessing the characteristics of individuals; the outcome of attempts to change the social systems cannot be evaluated without assessing the characteristics of milieus.

One example is the use of psychosocial and organizational climate-assessment techniques in the facilitation and evaluation of social change. Moos[69] has presented a paradigm in which information about perceived psychosocial environments is utilized in planning and directing social change within those environments. The methodology includes four basic components.

1. The social environment of a program is assessed. All the individuals involved in the program (e.g., both patients and staff in a treatment milieu) give their opinions about the current functioning of the program on relevant dimensions.

2. Individualized feedback is given on the results of these assessments, with specific focus on the similarities and differences between various important groups, e.g., psychiatrists, nurses, and psychiatric aides. Agreements and disagreements on the goals and value orientations of different groups are also outlined.

Emphasis is placed on the discrepancies between the "real" and the "ideal" social milieu and the implications for change that are thereby suggested.

3. Concrete planning of specific methods by which change might occur along specified dimensions is then instituted. The methods by which decisions about change are made and by which change is implemented vary widely from one environment to another.

4. One or more reassessments are made of the characteristics of the social environment in order to provide information about the results of the change process. This type of feedback and discussion about the environmental characteristics of an ongoing social system makes it possible for individuals participating in the system to help plan, design, effect, and evaluate changes in it. Regular feedback of data regarding the characteristics of one's environment provides a way to monitor the evolution and function of a milieu over time and helps to articulate the relationship of the current environment to overall program goals.

Although less has as yet been done in this area, the systematic use of information about relevant treatment and community environments of patients will eventually make for far richer and more meaningful clinical case descriptions. The original Meyerian system included data about relevant biological, psychological, and sociological or life-situation characteristics for each individual patient. However, there has never been any way of systematically describing the environments in which people function. Current case descriptions usually include only general comments about life-stress events, e.g., death of a family member, job changes, retirement, major physical illnesses, etc., whereas they should include at least as much detailed information about a patient's environment as they do about his personality and behavior. A specific example is the attempt to identify and describe basic "alcohologenic" properties of the community environments of patients with alcohol problems. The extent to which individual patients encounter "alcoholic stimuli," e.g., how many bottles of liquor are visible in his or her house, how many social functions does the patient attend where large quantities of alcohol are consumed, does the spouse of the patient drink heavily, does the patient have a number of close friends who drink heavily, etc., is at least as important in predicting future drinking behavior as individual background or personality characteristics.

The six types of environmental dimensions also provide guidelines for compiling program descriptions. Psychiatrists and other mental health workers are often responsible for writing descriptions of environments (e.g., treatment programs) for use by referring social workers, prospective patients, etc. Evidence indicates that published descriptions of environments do not usually accurately portray the salient characteristics of those environments. College catalogues often give no information about the academic backgrounds of entering students or about the informal social atmosphere, though these are characteristics of the environment that importantly affect a student's satisfaction and development.[95] Similar conclusions may be made about published descriptions of psychiatric and correctional treatments.[41] Otto and Moos[78] asked independent judges to read published descriptions of community programs and to give their impressions of the characteristics of the treatment environment. The judges' opinions were then compared with the opinions of residents and staff in each program. None of the descriptions presented a fully accurate picture of the treatment environment, although, as might be expected, some descriptions were much better than others. Each of the six environmental description methods gives a somewhat different perspective of a treatment program, and thus the use of all six should enhance the accuracy and completeness of program descriptions.

In this connection many investigators have suggested that different institutions know much more about the individuals they are attempting to recruit or place than those individuals know about the institution. Social workers and other program staff generally know far more about the characteristics of the individual patient than they do about the program or programs into which they wish to

place that patient. Patients themselves generally know little or nothing about program characteristics. This imbalance of information may, in part, be responsible for the extremely high rate of premature termination of treatment. Studies of individual and group psychotherapy[38,105] have indicated that information about these treatment modalities may be helpful to patients entering into them. Systematic information about treatment programs, especially those which are community-based, may similarly be of help to that growing proportion of patients who wish to take a more active part in choosing the specific treatment program that might be most beneficial to them.

From a research perspective analyses of milieus may help to identify the specific environmental factors that relate to favorable or unfavorable treatment outcome and to predict outcome based on the differential impact of treatment settings on certain groups of patients. More detailed knowledge of components of social systems should enhance more adequate matching of patients with treatment settings that meet their needs and hence facilitate recovery.

It is well established that social milieus have important physiological and "health-related" effects.[17,58] A systematic conceptualization of environments makes it possible to test more differentiated hypotheses about the effects of specific environmental dimensions on specific physiological indices. The potential importance of this area is indicated by the fact that the incidence of coronaries varies among environments as well as among types of individuals, and that the same psychopharmacological agent may have different therapeutic effects in different treatment settings. Finally, genetic and developmental studies are in need of much more differentiated information about environmental characteristics. The fact that home environments of individuals with certain chromosomal abnormalities are or are not "disharmonic" is simply no longer sufficient.

It is not yet clear exactly how the six different methods of environmental description will eventually relate to each other, but it is clear that they are each critical for the central tasks of understanding, predicting, and chang-

ing behavior. The optimal arrangement of
environments may be the most powerful behavior modification technique currently available. Psychiatrists and other mental health
specialists are now asked to consult on the
probable behavioral and attitudinal effects of
environmental changes, precisely because
human beings can now control and change
their own environments. Each institution in
our society is attempting to set up conditions
that it hopes will maximize certain types of
behavior and certain directions of personal
development. Families, hospitals, prisons, industries, secondary schools, universities, communes, and various groups, each arrange
certain environmental conditions that presumably maximize certain effects. There is, of
course, the greatest disagreement both about
the effects that should be maximized and
about which conditions maximize them. It can
be cogently argued that these issues are so
central to society that the most important task
for psychiatry and the behavioral sciences is
concerned with the systematic description and
classification of environments and their differential costs and benefits to adaptation.

The field of social ecology, though currently
somewhat vague and undifferentiated, presents a developing multidisciplinary focus
around which psychiatrists, with their detailed
knowledge of human adaptation and coping
skills, can fruitfully interact with other social
science professionals who are primarily concerned with conceptualizing and constructing
new environments. The potential for radically
altering the day-to-day practice of psychiatry
over the next decade or two is much greater
than we now realize.

(Bibliography

1. Anastasi, A. "Psychology, Psychologists, and Psychological Testing," *Am. Psychol.*, 22 (1967), 297–306.
2. Anderson, H. and E. Brewer. "Studies of Teachers' Classroom Personalities," *Appl. Psychol. Monogr.*, 8 (1946), 15–127.
3. Astin, A. W. *The College Environment.*
    Washington: Am. Council on Education, 1968.
4. Astin, A. W. and J. L. Holland. "The Environmental Assessment Technique: A Way to Measure College Environments," *J. Educ. Psychol.*, 52 (1961), 308–316.
5. Bandura, A. *Principles of Behavior Modification.* New York: Holt, Rinehart & Winston, 1969.
6. Bandura, A. and R. H. Walters. *Adolescent Aggression.* New York: Ronald, 1959.
7. Barker, R. G. *Ecological Psychology.* Stanford: Stanford University Press, 1968.
8. ———, ed. *The Stream of Behavior.* New York: Appleton-Century-Crofts, 1963.
9. Barker, R. and P. Gump. *Big School Small School.* Stanford: Stanford University Press, 1964.
10. Barry, H., I. Child, and M. Bacon. "Relation of Child Rearing to Subsistence Economy," *Am. Anthropol.*, 61 (1959), 51–64.
11. Bergin, A. "Some Implications of Psychotherapy Research for Therapeutic Practice," *J. Abnorm. Psychol.*, 71 (1966), 235–246.
12. Berke, J. and V. Wilson. *Watch Out for the Weather.* New York: Viking, 1951.
13. Brayfield, A. "Human Effectiveness," *Am. Psychol.*, 20 (1965), 645–651.
14. Buehler, R. E., G. R. Patterson, and J. M. Furniss. "The Reinforcement of Behavior in Institutional Settings," *Behav. Res. Ther.*, 4 (1966), 157–167.
15. Calhoun, J. B. "Population Density and Social Pathology," *Sci. Am.*, 206 (1962), 139–148.
16. Caudill, W. *The Psychiatric Hospital as a Small Society.* Cambridge: Harvard University Press, 1958.
17. Cobb, S., J. French, R. Kahn et al. "An Environmental Approach to Mental Health," *Ann. N.Y. Acad. Sci.*, 107 (1963), 596–606.
18. Cohen, H. and J. Filipczak. *A New Learning Environment.* San Francisco: Jossey-Bass, 1971.
19. Corwin, R. G. "Patterns of Organizational Conflict," *Admin. Sci. Q.*, (1969), 507–520.
20. Couch, A. "The Psychological Determinants of Interpersonal Behavior," in K. Gergen and D. Marlowe, eds., *Personality and Social Behavior*, pp. 77–89. Reading, Mass.: Addison-Wesley, 1970.
21. Craik, K. H. "Environmental Psychology,"

in *New Directions in Psychology*, Vol. 4, pp. 1–121. New York: Holt, Rinehart & Winston, 1970.

22. CUMMING, J. and E. CUMMING. *Ego and Milieu*. New York: Atherton, 1962.

23. DUHL, L., ed. *The Urban Condition*. New York: Basic Books, 1963.

24. ELLSWORTH, R., L. FOSTER, B. CHILDERS et al. "Hospital and Community Adjustment as Perceived by Psychiatric Patients, Their Families, and Staff," *J. Consult. Clin. Psychol. Monogr.*, 32 (1968), 1–41.

25. ENDLER, N. and J. McV. HUNT. "S-R Inventories of Hostility and Comparisons of the Proportion of Variance from Persons, Responses, and Situations for Hostility and Anxiousness," *J. Pers. Soc. Psychol.*, 9 (1968), 309–315.

26. ERIKSON, E. *Childhood and Society*. New York: Norton, 1950.

27. FAIRWEATHER, G. *Social Psychology in the Treatment of Mental Illness*. New York: MacMillan, 1963.

28. FELDMAN, K. and T. NEWCOMB. *The Impact of College on Students*. San Francisco. Jossey-Bass, 1969.

29. GALLE, O. R., W. R. GOVE, and J. M. McPHERSON. "Population Density and Pathology: What Are the Relations for Man?" *Science*, 176 (1972), 23–30.

30. GARDNER, J. *Excellence*. New York: Harper & Row, 1961.

31. GERST, M. and R. MOOS. "The Social Ecology of University Student Residences," *J. Educ. Psychol.*, 63 (1972), 513–525.

32. GRIFFITT, W. "Environmental Effects on Interpersonal Affective Behavior: Ambient Effective Temperature and Attraction," *J. Pers. Soc. Psychol.*, 15 (1970), 240–244.

33. GRIFFITT, W. and R. VEITCH. "Hot and Crowded: Influences of Population Density and Temperature on Interpersonal Affective Behavior," *J. Pers. Soc. Psychol.*, 17 (1971), 92–98.

34. GUMP, P., P. SCHOGGEN, and F. REDL. "The Camp Milieu and Its Immediate Effects," *J. Soc. Issues*, 13 (1957), 40–46.

35. ———. "The Behavior of the Same Child in Different Milieus," in R. Barker, ed., *The Stream of Behavior*, pp. 169–202. New York: Appleton-Century-Crofts, 1963.

36. HALPIN, A. and D. CROFT. *The Organizational Climate of Schools*. Chicago: University of Chicago, Midwest Administration Center, 1963.

37. HARTMANN, H. "Ego Psychology and the Problems of Adaptation," in D. Rapaport, ed., *Organization and Pathology of Thought*, pp. 362–396. New York: Columbia University Press, 1959.

38. HOEHN-SARIC, R., J. FRANK, S. IMBER et al. "Systematic Preparation of Patients for Psychotherapy: I. Effects on Therapy Behavior and Outcome," *J. Psychiatr. Res.*, 2 (1964), 267–281.

39. HOLLAND, J. *The Psychology of Vocational Choice*. Waltham, Mass.: Blaisdell, 1966.

40. HOLSTI, O. and R. NORTH. "The History of Human Conflict," in E. McNeil, ed., *The Nature of Human Conflict*. Englewood Cliffs, N.J.: Prentice-Hall, 1965.

41. JANSEN, E. "The Role of the Halfway House in Community Mental Health Programs in the United Kingdom and America," *Am. J. Psychiatry*, 126 (1970), 142–148.

42. JONES, M. *The Therapeutic Community*. New York: Basic Books, 1953.

43. JORDAN, P. "A Real Predicament," *Science*, 175 (1972), 977–978.

44. KASMAR, J. V. "The Development of a Usable Lexicon of Environmental Descriptors," *Environ. Behav.*, 2 (1970), 153–169.

45. KATES, R. and J. WOHLWILL, eds. "Man's Response to the Physical Environment," *J. Soc. Issues*, 22 (1966), 1–140.

46. KATZ, D. and R. KAHN. *The Social Psychology of Organizations*. New York: Wiley, 1966.

47. KELLY, J. "The Coping Process in Varied High School Environments," in M. Feldman, ed., *Studies in Psychotherapy and Behavioral Change*, Vol. 2. Buffalo: State University of New York, 1971.

48. KINZEL, A. F. "Body-Buffer Zone in Violent Prisoners," *Am. J. Psychiatry*, 127 (1970), 99–104.

49. LANSING, J., R. MARANS, and R. ZEHNER. *Planned Residential Environments*. Ann Arbor: University of Michigan, Survey Research Center, Inst. Soc. Res., 1970.

50. LEARY, T. *Interpersonal Diagnosis of Personality*. New York: Ronald, 1957.

51. LEWIN, K. *Field Theory in Social Science*. New York: Harper & Row, 1951.

52. LEWIN, K., R. LIPPITT, and R. WHITE. "Patterns of Aggressive Behavior in Experimentally Created 'Social Climates,'" *J. Soc. Psychol.*, 10 (1939), 271–299.

53. LICHTMAN, C. and R. HUNT. "Personality

and Organizational Theory: A Review of Some Conceptual Literature," *Psychol. Bull.*, 76 (1971), 271–294.

54. LIEBER, A. and C. SHERIN. "Homicides and the Lunar Cycle: Toward a Theory of Lunar Influence on Human Emotional Disturbance," *Am. J. Psychiatry*, 129 (1972), 69–74.

55. LIKERT, R. *The Human Organization: Its Management and Value.* New York: McGraw-Hill, 1967.

56. LINTON, R. *The Cultural Background of Personality.* New York: Century, 1945.

57. McCORD, W., J. McCORD, and I. ZOLA. *Origins of Crime.* New York: Columbia University Press, 1959.

58. MASON, J. "Organization of Psychoendocrine Mechanisms," *Psychosom. Med.*, 30 (1968), 565–808.

59. MARCH, J., ed. *Handbook of Organizations.* Chicago: Rand-McNally, 1965.

60. MASLOW, A. and N. MINITZ. "Effects of Esthetic Surroundings: I. Initial Effects of Three Esthetic Conditions upon Perceiving 'Energy' and 'Well-Being' in Faces," *J. Psychol.*, 41 (1956), 247–254.

61. MICHELSON, W. "Some Like It Hot: Social Participation and Environmental Use as Functions of the Season," *Am. J. Sociol.*, 76 (1971), 1072–1083.

62. MILGRAM, S. "Behavioral Study of Obedience," *J. Abnorm. Soc. Psychol.*, 67 (1963), 371–378.

63. ———. "Group Pressure and Action against a Person," *J. Abnorm. Soc. Psychol.*, 69 (1964), 137–143.

64. ———. "The Experience of Living in Cities," *Science*, 167 (1970), 1461–1468.

65. MILLS, C. *Climate Makes the Man.* New York: Harper & Row, 1942.

66. MISCHEL, W. *Personality and Assessment.* New York: Wiley, 1968.

67. Moos, R. "Sources of Variance in Responses to Questionnaires and in Behavior," *J. Abnorm. Psychol.*, 74 (1969), 405–412.

68. ———. "Assessment of the Psychosocial Environments of Community-Oriented Psychiatric Treatment Programs," *J. Abnorm. Psychol.*, 79 (1972), 9–18.

69. ———. "Changing the Social Milieus of Psychiatric Treatment Settings," *J. Appl. Behav. Sci.*, 9 (1973), 575–593.

70. ———. "Systems for the Assessment and Classification of Human Environments: An Overview," in R. Moos and P. Insel, eds., *Issues in Social Ecology*, pp. 5–28. Palo Alto, Calif.: National Press, 1974.

71. ———. "Psychological Techniques in the Assessment of Adaptive Behavior," in G. Coehlo, D. Hamburg, and J. Adams, eds., *Coping and Adaptive Behavior*, pp. 334–399. New York: Basic Books, 1974.

72. ———. *Evaluating Treatment Environments.* New York: Wiley, 1974.

73. ———. *Evaluating Correctional and Community Settings.* New York: Wiley, 1975.

74. Moos, R. and J. SCHWARTZ. "Treatment Environment and Treatment Outcome," *J. Nerv. Ment. Dis.*, 154 (1972), 264–275.

75. MOYER, K. *The Physiology of Hostility.* Chicago: Markham, 1971.

76. MUECHER, H. and H. UNGEHEUER. "Meteorological Influence on Reaction Time, Flicker Fusion Frequency, Job Accidents, and Use of Medical Treatment," *Percept. Mot. Skills*, 12 (1961), 163–168.

77. OSMOND, H. "Function as a Basis of Psychiatric Ward Design," *Ment. Hosp.*, 8 (1957), 23–39.

78. OTTO, J. and R. Moos. "Evaluating Descriptions of Psychiatric Treatment Programs," *Am. J. Orthopsychiatry*, 43 (1973), 401–410.

79. PACE, R. *College and University Environment Scales.* Tech. Manual, 2nd ed. Princeton: Educational Testing Serv., 1969.

80. PETERSON, R., J. CENTRA, R. HARTNETT et al. *Institutional Functioning Inventory.* Prelim. Tech. Manual. Princeton: Educational Testing Serv., 1970.

81. PORTER, L. and E. LAWLER. "Properties of Organization Structure in Relation to Job Attitudes and Job Behavior," *Psychol. Bull.*, 64 (1965), 23–51.

82. PROSHANSKY, H., W. ITTELSON, and L. RIVLIN, eds. *Environmental Psychology: Man and His Physical Setting.* New York: Holt, Rinehart & Winston, 1970.

83. PUGH, D. "Modern Organization Theory: A Psychological and Sociological Study," *Psychol. Bull.*, 66 (1966), 235–251.

84. PURCELL, K. and K. BRADY. *Assessment of Interpersonal Behavior in Natural Settings.* Final Progr. Rep. Denver: Childrens' Asthma Research Institute and Hospital, 1964.

85. RAUSH, H., A. DITTMAN, and T. TAYLOR.

"Person, Setting, and Change in Social Interaction," *Hum. Rel.*, 12 (1959), 361–378.

86. RIESMAN, D. and C. JENCKS. "The Viability of the American College," in N. Sanford, ed., *The American College*, pp. 74–192. New York: Wiley, 1962.

87. ROBERTS, K. "On Looking at an Elephant: An Evaluation of Cross Cultural Research Related to Organizations," *Psychol. Bull.*, 74 (1970), 327–350.

88. RUSSETT, B. et al. *World Handbook of Political and Social Indicators*. New Haven: Yale University Press, 1964.

89. SCHMID, C. "Urban Crime Areas," *Am. Sociol. Rev.*, 25 (1960), 527, 542, 655–678.

90. SCHOGGEN, P. "Environmental Forces in the Every Day Lives of Children," in R. Barker, ed., *The Stream of Behavior*, pp. 42–69. New York: Appleton-Century-Crofts, 1963.

91. SELLS, S. "Dimensions of Stimulus Situations which Account for Behavior Variance," in S. Sells, ed., *Stimulus Determinants of Behavior*, pp. 1–15. New York: Ronald, 1963.

92. SELLS, S., N. FINDIKYAN, and M. DUKE. *Stress Reviews: Atmosphere*. Tech. Rep. No. 10. Fort Worth: Institute of Behavioral Research, Texas Christian University, 1966.

93. SMITH, M. and N. HOBBS. "The Community and the Community Mental Health Center," *Am. Psychol.*, 21 (1966), 499–501.

94. SOMMER, R. *Personal Space*. Englewood Cliffs, N.J.: Prentice-Hall, 1969.

95. SPEEGLE, J. "College Catalogs: An Investigation of the Congruence of Catalog Descriptions of College Environments with Student Perceptions of the Same Environment as Revealed by the College Characteristics Index." Ph.D dissertation, Syracuse University, 1969.

96. STANTON, A. and M. SCHWARTZ. *The Mental Hospital*. New York: Basic Books, 1954.

97. STERN, G. *People in Context*. New York: Wiley, 1970.

98. SUGIYAMA, Y. "Social Organization of Hanuman Langurs," in S. Altmann, ed., *Social Communications Among Primates*, pp. 221–236. Chicago: University of Chicago Press, 1967.

99. SWIFT, J. W. "Effects of Early Group Experience: The Nursery School and Day Nursery," in M. Hoffman and L. Hoffman, eds., *Child Development Research*, Vol. 1, pp. 249–288. New York: Russell Sage Found., 1964.

100. TRICKETT, E. and R. MOOS. "The Social Environment of Junior High and High School Classrooms," *J. Educ. Psychol.*, 65 (1973), 93–102.

101. WALBERG, H. "Social Environment as a Mediator of Classroom Learning," *J. Educ. Psychol.*, 60 (1969), 443–448.

102. WICKER, A. "Size of Church Membership and Members' Support of Church Behavior Settings," *J. Pers. Soc. Psychol.*, 13 (1969), 278–288.

103. WOLF, R. "The Measure of Environments," in A. Anastasi, ed., *Testing Problems in Perspective*, pp. 491–503. Washington: Am. Council on Education, 1966.

104. WOLFGANG, M. *Patterns in Criminal Homicide*. Philadelphia: University of Pennsylvania, 1958.

105. YALOM, I., P. HOUTS, G. NEWELL et al. "Preparations of Patients for Group Therapy," *Arch. Gen. Psychiatry*, 17 (1967), 416–427.

106. ZLUTNICK, S. and I. ALTMAN. "Crowding and Human Behavior," in J. F. Wohlwill and D. H. Carson, eds., *Environment and the Social Sciences: Perspectives and Applications*, pp. 44–58. Washington: Psychological Assoc., 1972.

CHAPTER 41

PSYCHIATRIC ASPECTS OF THE NAZI PERSECUTION*

Paul Chodoff

ALTHOUGH the lurid light flickering out of the ovens of Auschwitz thirty years ago may seem too far off to illuminate present-day American psychiatry, there are two reasons why the experience of the Jews of Europe under the Nazi terror ought still to engage the interest and concern of psychiatrists. First, although six million Jews were killed, there are some survivors and a significant number of these are now in the United States where they seek out the services of psychiatrists for purposes both of evaluation of their restitution claims and sometimes for treatment of the psychiatric disabilities with which they have been left. Second, since psychiatrists must grapple every day with the effects of various degrees of psychic traumatization on their patients, the concentration-camp experience, by providing a "worst-case"

* This chapter is a revision and expansion of the second half of the chapter, "Effects of Extreme Coercive and Oppressive Forces," that appeared in volume 3 of the 1st edition of this *Handbook*.

example of psychic trauma and its effects, also sheds light on how human beings react to lesser, more ordinary degrees of psychological stress.

In this chapter, I will summarize the main elements of the conditions faced by concentration camp inmates and the adaptive measures employed to deal with these conditions, including in this section an extended account derived from a taped interview with a woman who was a survivor of Auschwitz. I will then deal with the short- and long-term effects of the concentration-camp experience, and with some of the attempts that have been made to conceptualize the long-term sequelae. I will also touch on psychiatric evaluation and treatment of survivors. The material included in the chapter will be based on my own experience with approximately two hundred survivors of the persecution whom I have examined, mostly for purposes of reparations evaluations but also, in a few instances, for more extended treatment purposes, and on references to what has now become a rather voluminous literature.*

The Concentration Camps

The German concentration camps—first established by Heinrich Himmler in 1933 for the internment of enemies of the Third Reich, a category that, of course, included the Jews—followed the Nazi conquests and ultimately formed an extended network throughout the occupied territories, especially in eastern Europe. With the decision for the "final solution" of the Jewish question in 1941, some of the camps (Auschwitz, Treblinka) were designated as extermination camps and were equipped with disguised gas chambers and crematoria; in others (Dachau, Buchenwald) the killing was somewhat less systematic. The concentration camps merged into labor camps that provided a source of slave labor for Nazi industry. However, the differences among all of these categories of camps was only relative and in all of them the conditions were, in the words of A. P. J. Taylor, "loathsome beyond belief." In addition to the out-and-out extermination measures, the physical stresses endured by the prisoners included malnutrition, crowding, sleeplessness, exposure, inadequate clothing, forced labor, beatings, injury, torture, exhaustion, medical experimentation, diarrhea, various epidemic diseases, and the effects of the long "death marches" from the camps in the closing days of the war. The physically depleted state of the prisoners, the brutal and primitive conditions in which they lived, and the entirely inadequate medical facilities were responsible for an extremely high death rate, and also had the effect of increasing the susceptibility of the inmates to the nonphysical stresses they had to face. Chief among these latter was the danger to

* This literature, in addition to articles in various psychiatric journals that will be referred to, included autobiographical accounts by former inmates,[2,6,12] and systematic reviews[10,28] (in English) of various aspects of the problem. Hoppe[23] has prepared a valuable review of the recent literature that includes foreign as well as American sources.

life, ever-present and unavoidable. It is possible, to some degree, for a healthy personality to defend itself against a peril that, though very grave, is predictable and is at least potentially limited in time, as in the case of soldiers in combat who can at least hope for relief and rotation out of the fighting zone. For the concentration-camp inmate however, as has been described by Viktor Frankl[12] from his own experiences in Auschwitz, the absolute uncertainty of his condition was a barrier to the erection of adequate psychological-adaptive measures. In addition to the threat to life, the prisoners had to face the catastrophic trauma of separation from their families and, consequently, to the agonizing uncertainty about their own future, there were added equally agonizing doubts as to whether they would ever see their relatives again. The very least price one had to pay to survive in the camps was to suffer the grossest kind of daily humiliation. Massive frustration of their basic drives had the apparent dual effect of driving the sexual life of the prisoners underground and of rendering the insistent demands of hunger all-dominating, so that fantasies about food occupied much of their conscious awareness. If not himself the victim of casual violence or deliberate cruelty, the prisoner frequently witnessed such exhibitions. Since it was impossible to retaliate effectively, he had to smother his aggressive feelings, for even the appearance of resentment against the torturers could lead to his own destruction. Regimented, imprisoned, without a moment of privacy during each twenty-four hours, the prisoner's human worth, and even his sense of an individual human identity, was under constant and savage assault. His entire environment was designed to impress upon him his utter, his protoplasmic worthlessness, a worthlessness that had no relationship to what he did, only to what he was. Reduced from individual human status to the status of a debased being, identified not by name but by a number and a badge of a particular color, a conviction of his ineluctable inferiority was hammered into the prisoner by the Schutzstaffel (SS) jailers who needed to justify their own behavior by convincing themselves of the inferior, subhuman status of the Jews in their charge. The concentration-camp inmates lived in a Kafkaesque world in which the rules governing their existence were senseless, capricious, and often mutually contradictory, as, for instance, when impossible standards of cleanliness were demanded, while, at the same time, the inadequate opportunities and senseless rules about toileting made even an elementary decency impossible.

At this point, I am going to interpose excerpts from a description—recorded in her own words at my request—of some aspects of life at Auschwitz by a former inmate (Mrs. S) who has also been a patient of mine. This account will convey something of the physical and psychological stresses that confronted the concentration-camp inmate, as well as a suggestion of the adaptive measures called forth by these stresses.

⟨ Life in a Concentration Camp

"We arrived to Auschwitz in the early part of April. That's a story by itself—the arrival and the happenings. We lived in blocks. It's called a block in German, but it's a barracks and it has 1,500 people and the barracks had rows and rows of three-tier bunk beds—they were very poorly built, out of just boards and lumber and each bunk had 12 people—in our case 12 women, and we happened to choose the upper bunk because we thought it would be the best. It was OK for us, but it caused an awful lot of heartache afterward because, as I said, the bunks were not built very well and the boards broke under the weight of us in the beginning before we started losing weight and there were many broken or fractured skulls or bones below us.

"Each person was supposed to have a blanket. It so happened that the blankets were stolen, so we never ended up with enough blankets for all of us. Maybe by the end of the evening we would have two or three blankets left for 12 people. I think the biggest crisis after the day's hardship was finding a blanket

to sleep on and the fights we had keeping the blanket. I must say I was one of the lucky (I say lucky) or exceptional persons who was an assistant to the 'capo.' It came very handy at the time. I suffered an awful lot because of it later, but it gave me protection. Maybe I had the blanket. I don't even remember because all this did not matter.

"Anyway, we got up at two o'clock in the morning. We were awakened by the girls who brought the coffee in big barrels. It was black and it had charcoal in it and maybe chicory. It was rather lukewarm and they thought it was enough to hold us through the day. And no one wanted the coffee. You would rather have an hour sleep or so, but you had to have it. The barracks had to be emptied and we had to get back and line up for the *appel* [roll call] and that was my job, getting people up. I was assigned to three or four bunks and that means I was assigned to wake up approximately 150 to 200 people who did not want to face the day's reality. I mean, because we knew what was coming. So I was up, pulling blankets off of people—'get up', screaming, carrying on, even hitting. Once I hit someone and she looked at me and it was one of my mother's friends. I apologized. I felt terribly bad. I kept on doing it. I got them up. I think the whole process took nearly half an hour, to make 1,500 people get out of the block. We were up, but there was no question of dressing because we got one dress when we entered Auschwitz, and I got a very, very long petticoat. It came all the way down to my ankles. It came in very handy because I was able to use it, little by little, as toilet tissue which was nonexistent, till there was nothing left. So I just had a dress to wear and I think most people, that's all they had, and shoes and a toothbrush that hung around my neck. It was my most prized thing. A toothbrush.

"I know I got out of my bunk a half an hour earlier than anyone else because we were determined to keep clean and we went to the washroom that was at least, oh, two or three bunkers away from us and we stripped ourselves to wash with cold water because we didn't want any lice on us. We checked our clothes for lice, because typhus was spreading already at that time and, anyway, we had to line up for appel—and the 1,500 people were divided into three groups so that means I had 500 people to line up and in each line I think there were maybe 10, 15. I'm not sure. But, somehow, I don't know how, the rumor started, but someone gave the word, that they were going to pick so many people to be cremated. That the first four or five rows are going to be taken to be cremated. Well, I tried to get anyone to get in the first five rows. It was impossible. I had to make them do it. I was shoving and pushing. But we were lined up around two-thirty in the morning and the Germans did not come out till five or six o'clock, I think it was, for the appel and there were 30,000 people in the C lager [camp] and it took them a while. They always miscounted because, after the first counting was over we were being punished for someone was missing. We had to get down on our knees with our hands up and wait till they counted over and over and over. Till they decided that they had a number. But we didn't have the big selections as when Dr. Mengele came around. Just the little officers did their jobs and decided that a girl with a pimple on her face, someone who was a little more run-down than should be, or someone with a little bandage were selected. Naturally, those people were taken out automatically to the crematorium. So we had to be very careful that you shouldn't have any scars showing so you should look fresh and not unwell. Well, by eleven or twelve we were allowed to come in to our bunks and then lunchtime came.

"It is very hard for me to recall food—what we ate or not, because I decided that all those things were unimportant. That I am going to have control over my body, that food is not important. I can't remember. But I think it was one slice of bread and a slice of margarine on it, and some kind of jelly made out of red beets.

"I think in all my eight months that I have been there, maybe twice we were able to take a walk—because we were being punished for one reason or the other and we had to stay in our bunks, or a new transport came in, and they would not allow us out to watch the transport coming in so we were locked in our block or barracks. So the days were spent in the barracks.

"Then came the evening roll call. That started about two o'clock in the afternoon and then again the same circus-lining up, waiting miscounting, and counting, and counting, and counting, and it was seven or eight in the evening before the evening meal came and before we were allowed to come in—sometimes nine-thirty or ten o'clock. If someone was missing, we were punished by kneeling. Otherwise we stood—and we had to stand sometimes in hot sun and sometimes in rain.

"Anyway, evening came around and then we had our meal. The meal consisted of mush. It was some kind of a liquid, thickened with something. It had a few potatoes in the bottom of the barrel and then it had some kind of tranquilizer, but I doubted the Germans spent money on putting tranquilizers in. But another thing, we stopped menstruating and they thought that, whatever chemical taste it had in it, this is the thing that stopped us from menstruating so we didn't menstruate at all.

"Again, I was one of the lucky ones who distributed the food. I think I was fair when it came to distributing food. I did not, I would not allow myself to bring any more up to my bunk than we were allowed to, except for my mother who was quite ill—she had diarrhea and she could not digest the food. She was getting weaker and weaker day by day. You know, she was at that time 43 years old and it is hard to think that I have reached that age. How would I have been able—how would I have reacted under the circumstances that she did at this age? I feel very young, by the way. But she seemed to me very old at that time and well, anyway, evening meal over, we were allowed to take a walk. But, again, when transports were coming in they locked the doors and there was complete curfew and we were not allowed to go out and we were just, well, listening to the screams or the silence or the smell of burning flesh and wondering what tomorrow was going to bring to us. Some were wondering. I knew I was going to make it. The human torture, getting up in the morning and things, smelling the burning flesh and the flying soot. The air was oily, greasy. There were no birds. . . .

"I think they were very worried about our physical well-being and cleanliness. So we had to be shaved. That's right, several times while I stayed in Auschwitz, we were shaved of hair —head, underarms and intimate parts of our body—by Jewish inmates standing. We were standing on a stool so that the Jewish inmates would be able to reach us easier and we were surrounded by SS men who seemed to enjoy it very much. Well, it didn't bother me. I had no feelings, whatsoever. I couldn't care less, at this point of the game. It really didn't matter.

"As I said, we had selections every single day—some just slight—just picking people out, as I mentioned before, because of scars, because of pimples, because, because of being run-down, because of looking tired or because of having a crooked smile, or because someone just didn't like you. But then they were selected either to go to work or to the crematorium, and, in this case, Dr. Mengele was involved in it. He was quite an imposing figure and his presence . . . I don't think everybody was scared, because—rather I wasn't. I was hypnotized by his looks, by his actions.

"The barracks had two massive doors and we were inside. They did not let us out. It was in October and it was rainy. We tried to catch the rain in pots. We didn't sleep because of the rain, because we had to keep ourselves dry. . . . And then the doors swing open quite dramatically . . . great entrance with Mengele in the center accompanied by two SS women and a couple of soldiers. . . . He stands with his whip on one side and his legs apart. It's unbelievable. It looked like Otto Preminger arranged the theme for the whole thing. It seems to me now that it was like a movie.

"Anyway, the capo came out and she gave us orders to undress and line up in front of the barracks. It had two rooms. One was a storage room and one was the capo's room—and Mengele stood in between and he had a switch in the same hand, and while we were lining up, I was able to observe what he was

doing. Till I had to face him, I really had no feelings. I couldn't describe how I felt, but I saw the switch go. It was a horsewhip—left, right, and I noticed that those who were motioned left were in a better condition, physical condition, than the ones who were motioned to go right. Anyway, this went on and on and not a sound, even if it meant life or death. I don't know how other people felt about it, but I was quite well informed, I was accused of being able to face the truth, of being able to know because I had my mother with me. The others said it was easy for me to believe all this because I had my mother with me. I had no great loss. They loved their mothers, they cared, and they wanted to believe their mothers were safe somewhere in another camp. It made them stronger, knowing their parents were not cremated, but I had my mother and I knew my father was OK at that time in another bunk at camp.

"Anyway, my turn came. I had a choice to make. Not only Mengele had a choice to make, I had. I had to make up my mind. Am I going to follow my mother or is this it? Am I going to separate from her? The only way I was able to work out the problem was that I was not going to give myself a chance to decide. I will go ahead in front of my mother— that was unusual, she being my mother, out of courtesy I followed her all the time in any other circumstances—but in this case, I was going first and my mother followed me, and I went. I think my heart was beating quite fast, not because I was afraid—I knew I would come through—but because I was doing something wrong. I was doing something terribly wrong. Anyway, I passed Mengele. I didn't see him. I just passed, and I was sent into the room where I would be kept alive and I turned around and my mother was with me! So this was a very happy ending.

"As I said, in the evenings if I had a chance I went over to talk to my friend . . . to the fence, to the electric fence, and at each end of the fence, they had the watchtowers where the Nazis were able to observe us and, just for the fun of it, the girl who was right next to me—I think they just wanted to see if they could aim well, because I don't know why—

they shot her right in the eye, and she lost her eye. Another time, another girl was at the same place. Her friend threw a package of food over to her, and she ran toward the fence to catch it. And she touched the wire. And there she hung. She looked like Jesus Christ, spread out, with her two arms stuck to the wire. . . .

"In the end, people were losing weight, and they were getting skinnier and skinnier and some of them were just skeletons but I really did not see them. I just wiped the pictures out of my mind. I was able to step over them, and when I came out from the concentration camp, I said I did not see a dead body. I mean, I feel that I didn't see them. Even if I can see them. This is what's killing me now, that I have never felt the strain, the brutality, the physical brutality of the concentration camp. I mean like my aunt, my young aunt. She was 13 or 14 when she was exposed to brutality and death, and she talks with a passion of what they did to her. Then, when I meet another woman who is in her 60's and she will tell me her sufferings, I can't stand them. I broke all the friendships up with them. I don't want them. I can't stand them, because they bore me. I just can't stand listening to them, and I have nothing to do with them."

⟦ Adaptive Behavior in the Camps

What enabled a man or woman to survive such a hell? We have no real answers to this question and must resort to generalizations about the almost miraculous and infinite adaptability of the human species. As far as particular varieties of individual defensive and coping behavior are concerned, there is no doubt that they played a role in whether a prisoner would live or die, but it cannot be emphasized too much that such behavior was far less important than were luck, accident, and chance—where the prisoner happened to be when a selection for the gas chamber was taking place, the quota of victims for that day, the mood of the selector at the time. However,

accounts by survivors[6] do agree on a fairly constant sequence of reactions to concentration-camp life. This sequence began with the universal response of shock and terror on arrest and arrival at the camp since the SS made it their business to impress on the new prisoner their limitless power over him. At the same time, many of the old prisoners displayed the "camp mentality." They were irritable, egotistical, envious, and often cold and unsympathetic to new arrivals. The fright reaction was generally followed by a period of apathy, and, in most cases, by a longer period of mourning and depression. The period of apathy was often psychologically protective,[17] and may be thought of as providing a kind of transitional emotional hibernation. But, in some cases, apathy took over to such an extent that the prisoner became a "Mussulman," who gave up the struggle and did not live very long.

Among those prisoners who continued to struggle for life, certain adaptive measures gradually gained ascendancy and came to be characteristic of the long-term adjustment. Regressive behavior, of a greater or lesser degree, was almost universal, resulting from the overwhelming infantilizing pressures to which prisoners were subjected and their need to stifle aggressive impulses. It has been suggested that such narcissistic regression prepared the ground, among those who survived the camps, for later psychopathological states such as chronic reactive depressions and chronic reactive aggressions.[22] However, it should be pointed out that as a consequence of the complete reversal of values in the camps, regressive behavior probably served an adaptive function, since regressive prisoners, immersed in fantasies, were likely to be docile and submissive toward the SS, and thus have a better chance of escaping retaliatory measures. A consequence of such regression was that many prisoners, like children, became quite dependent on their savage masters, so that attitudes toward the SS were marked more by ambivalence than by conscious overt hostility. Some prisoners went so far as to employ the well-known mechanism of identification with the aggressor, imitating the behavior and taking on the values of the SS. A striking example of the strength of this mechanism and its reality-distorting effects is seen in the dreams of more than one female survivor whom I have examined where SS troopers were always tall, handsome, and godlike. Elements of such a reaction can be seen in Mrs. S's encounter with Dr. Mengele, "the angel of death of Auschwitz" who has been described to me in such awed terms by other survivors of Auschwitz that he can be visualized as a tall, radiant, immaculately dressed figure sitting nonchalantly astride a chair as—like Osiris, the god of the Underworld—he gestures with his riding whip, sending the prisoners lined up in front of him either to life or to death.*

It appears that the most important personality defenses among concentration-camp inmates were denial[2] and isolation of affect, a finding that should not be particularly surprising in view of evidence that these are the two most common and most "normal" personality defenses.[18] Examples of denial are displayed by Mrs. S when she would not see the corpses she was stepping over and in the poignant picture of her fellow inmates who refused to believe that the smoke arising from the crematorium chimneys came from the burning corpses of their mothers. Isolation of affect, which could be so extreme as to involve a kind of emotional anesthesia,[14] seemed to have functioned particularly to protect an inmate's ego against the dangers associated with feelings of hostility toward someone who treats the inmate as if he were an inanimate thing and not a person.[42] This is what Mrs. S was doing when she says, "It didn't bother me, I had no feeling whatsoever" about being shaved while naked in front of SS troopers. When combined with an ability to observe themselves in their surroundings, this kind of tamping down of affect, along with sublimatory processes, helped certain gifted individuals produce remarkably objective reports of

* The real Dr. Mengele, at least as he was after the war, does not quite fit this description. A South American physician who came into contact with Dr. Mengele in 1958–1959, described him in a letter[25] to me as a small, nondescript individual who looked like a frightened rat.

concentration camp life. Some form of companionship with others was indispensable, since a completely isolated individual could not have survived in the camps. But the depth of such companionship was usually limited by the overpowering egotistical demands of self-preservation, except in certain political and religious groups. Daydreams of revenge served the purpose of swallowing up some repressed aggression; some aggression could be discharged in quarrels and angry behavior toward other prisoners, as illustrated by the description of the fighting over food and blankets. Aggression could also be dealt with by projection onto the SS who were then seen as even more formidable, endowed as they thus were with the unexpressed hostility of the prisoners. Since the existence of mental illness of any degree of severity would have been incompatible with survival, one adaptive consequence of imprisonment was that new psychosomatic or psychoneurotic disorders rarely developed while existing ones often markedly improved,[47] and suicide—except under conditions as to be almost indistinguishable from murder—was also an infrequent phenomenon.[6]

(The Postliberation Period

As soon after the end of the war and liberation as recovery of some measure of physical health permitted, most survivors of the concentration camps, as well as those individuals who had managed to evade capture during the war by an "on-the-run"[3] existence, made their way back to their homes primarily for purposes of seeking information about their relatives. More often than not their worse fears were realized: they found their homes destroyed or occupied by strangers, and their communities substantially wiped out. Such frustrating aspects of postliberation reality were powerful factors in the inevitable dissipation of rosy fantasies about postwar life that had blossomed during imprisonment and constituted what Wolfenstein[53] calls the "postdisaster utopia." In their regressed state, such a narcissistic blow, as well as real disappointments in their idealistic hopes for a better world[9] resulted in bitterness, resentment, depression—even, sometimes in temporary flare-ups of antisocial or paranoid behavior.[35] A large number of the liberated prisoners, homeless, alone, bewildered, without resources, took refuge in the displaced persons (D.P.) camps that were set up in various parts of Europe. In some cases, they remained in them for years, with the result that the neurotic symptoms, encouraged by the monotony of D.P. camp life and its fostering of passivity and hypochondrical preoccupation became fixated.[31] In this phase, the flaring up of psychoneurotic and psychosomatic symptoms was due both to undoubted organic factors[26] and to the derepression of hostile impulses that could not be expressed during the concentration-camp period.[14,47]

As the immediate postwar epoch drew to a close, the surviving remnant of concentration-camp prisoners gradually settled themselves in more or less permanent abodes in their countries of origin or elsewhere, especially in the United States and Israel. For this latter group, to the multiple traumas they had endured were added the need to adjust to a new environment, to new customs, to a different language.

(Long-term Effects

At this point, one might expect the grisly story to come to an end for most of the survivors, the passage of time allowing the gradual envelopment of their fears and memories in psychic scar tissue. This is not what happened. In the late 1950s and early 1960s, articles began to appear in the medical literature* of many countries describing features of personality disorder and psychiatric illness still present in a large number of these individuals, in some cases cropping up after a latent period of several years. An important stimulus to the unexpected discovery by psychiatrists of the extent of the problem has undoubtedly been restitu-

* See references 1, 3, 8, 9, 11, 24, 26, 31, 34, 38, 44, 45, 48, 49, 50, and 51.

tion laws enacted by the [West] German Federal Republic during the ten years following the Hitler regime, as a result of which financial compensation was provided for persons in whom a causal relationship between the traumatic experience and an impaired state of health could be established.

Although figures are not available for the overall incidence of psychiatric sequelae among the survivors of the Nazi persecution, it is clear, judging from the reports of many countries including Germany, the United States, Israel, Poland, and Norway, that they are of high frequency and occur not only in concentration-camp survivors but also in those individuals who spent a significantly long period of time in Germany or occupied Europe, either hiding from the Germans or, with the aid of forged papers undertaking the perilous masquerade of assuming non-Jewish identities and becoming a part of the German work force. Illustrative of the high frequency of long-term psychiatric disorders among concentration-camp survivors is the report of Bensheim.[1] He found that in 1960 half of all patients in the neuropsychiatric clinic in Haifa were under treatment for the consequences of Nazi persecution. Even in those individuals who have not sought psychiatric treatment or evaluation and who appear on superficial examination to be well, a more careful scrutiny may reveal evidence that very few of them were left unaffected. For instance, Matussek,[34] in a preliminary report of 130 patients who were believed to have shown no aftereffects of the concentration-camp experience, states that he has not seen a single person who was without pathology, although this may have been covered up. Likewise, Ostwald and Bittner[40] have studied the life adjustment of sixty survivors in California who appeared to have made successful adaptations and found that this had always been attained at a considerable psychic cost.

A remarkable and undoubtedly significant feature of the long-term psychiatric consequences of the concentration-camp experience is the uniformity of these changes as found by observers all over the world including not only the early articles alluded to previously but also the more recent reviews of Krystal and Niederland,[29] Maller,[33] Meerloo,[36] Lederer[30] and Grobin.[19] All observers agree in finding a combination of relatively fixed, unfavorable personality alterations and a group of psychiatric symptoms that can be labeled the "concentration-camp syndrome."*

(Personality Distortions

Personality distortions tend to develop in two widely overlapping ways. In one, there is a tendency toward seclusiveness, social isolation, helplessness, and apathy. The individual is passive, fatalistic and dependent, wanting only to be taken care of and to be let alone by a world whose requirements are too much for him. The other form of personality distortion is typified by the survivor who regards the world with suspicion, hostility, and mistrust. His attitudes toward other people range from quiet, envious bitterness to cynicism and belligerence, sometimes with a distinctly paranoid flavor. Either set of pathologic attitudes, of course, interferes significantly with interpersonal relationships and, thus, in a reverberating fashion, tends to become more extreme as unfavorable experiences pile up. An end point of such a process can be a psychotic development. Thus, in Israel, Eitinger[10] has reported on a group of schizophrenics in whom he regarded the concentration-camp incarceration as causal, while Winnik[52] reported a significant increase in the incidence of affective psychoses among survivors.

(The Concentration-Camp Syndrome

The psychiatric illness that is the most distinctive, long-term consequence of the Nazi persecution is the Concentration-Camp Syndrome. Invariably present in this condition is some degree of felt anxiety, often very marked, along with feelings of tension, motor restless-

* Niederland prefers to refer to the entire picture as the "survivor syndrome."[38]

ness, and a state of what might be called hyperapprehensiveness in which a sudden phone call, an unexpected knock at the door, the sight of a man in uniform, may produce a sudden augmentation of anxiety, sometimes so severe as to constitute a startle reaction. The anxiety may be accompanied by irritability and impatience, with consequent deleterious effects on family and work relationships. Anxiety is often worse at night and is accompanied by various kinds of sleep disturbances such as great difficulty in falling asleep, frequent wakening during the night and, very characteristically, night terrors and nightmares that are either simple or only slightly disguised repetitions of the traumatic experiences endured. Ernest Rappaport[41] has described how his own experience under the persecution continues to produce stimuli for disturbing dreams, even today. Sleep disturbances may be so severe as to be exhausting to the patient and terrifying to his spouse when he wakes up during the night covered with sweat and shouting. Another frequent symptom is psychosomatic involvement of almost all the organ systems, the most common being headaches, weakness, fatigue, and symptoms indicating gastrointestinal disorders. In some instances, phobia formation results in displacement of the anxiety to various symbolic reference points. Anxiety, sleeplessness, and fatigue may result, naturally enough, in difficulty in concentrating and remembering, which may mimic an organic syndrome. A very characteristic symptom is an obsessive-ruminative state characterized by more or less constant preoccupation with recollections of persecutory experiences and, sometimes, with the idealized period of the survivor's life with his family before the persecution began. Interviews with concentration-camp survivors sometimes leave the interviewer with the uncanny sensation that he has been transported in time back to the gray inferno of Auschwitz, so vivid and compelling is the wealth of detail with which survivors describe the events that befell them or that they witnessed. Often the interviewer gets the impression that nothing really significant in their lives has happened since the liberation. Most individuals find these memories unwelcome and obtrusive to such a degree that they may engage in compulsive activity in order to keep their minds free of them. But a few survivors actually seem to derive pleasure from remembering and they look forward to night, when they can lie awake and nurture these dark things from the past. This preoccupation with the past is one of the reasons why concentration-camp survivors often feel alienated, different from others, not really a part of the life around them.

Depression and feelings of guilt are a characteristic phenomenon among concentration-camp survivors. They constitute, along with chronic anxiety and the obsessive-ruminative state previously described, a distinguishing feature of the Concentration-Camp Syndrome. More likely to occur as an unvarying feeling of emptiness, despair, and hopelessness in older people—the "shattered" depression of Levinger[31]—in most other survivors periods of depression occur episodically, particularly at holidays and anniversaries and in connection with events that remind them of the past, such as the Eichmann trial. There is little doubt that such depressive states represent a prolonged and, in a sense, irremedial mourning for lost love objects.[35,39] Feelings that life in the present is meaningless, and even unreal compared with the grim reality of the past, are common, but it is of interest that convictions about the worthlessness of life are seldom accompanied by suicidal preoccupation. On the other hand, quite frequent is a kind of anhedonia, a refusal or inability to take pleasure or satisfaction in those events or occurrences which ordinarily would be gratifying. It is certainly significant that among my own cases there is a clear correlation between depth of depression and magnitude of the object loss of family members, relatives, and friends.[4] However, although it is not difficult to understand why people who have suffered such losses would be chronically or episodically depressed, it does not explain why the depression of concentration-camp survivors is so often tinged by feelings of guilt, either expressed openly or easily to be inferred from their behavior. Here we are dealing with a

special case of the phenomenon of "survivor guilt," which also occurs in so many other settings. Its frequency among concentration-camp survivors varies in different discussions of the subject; it has been put as high as 92 percent of 139 cases studied by Krystal and Niederland.[29] Survivor guilt, however, is not a unitary phenomenon. Concentration-camp survivors may feel guilt because of specific actions on their part that endangered the lives and welfare of others or which the survivors interpreted as having this effect, even though such an interpretation was not true. Mrs. S's behavior in getting into the selection line ahead of her mother is one example. Another example is the guilty preoccupation of a survivor who berated herself for having appropriated the clothes of a woman who had died as her own were falling to pieces. There are other guilty feelings that are related not to particular misdeeds, fancied or real, but, rather, are experienced as a nonspecific, vague, pervasive conviction of having done something wrong and shameful, even though this feeling cannot be connected with any remembered episode. Finally, there is that species of survivor guilt which is attached merely to the fact of having remained alive in the holacaust when so many others had died. This variety of survivor guilt is sometimes linked with expressions of wonderment and incredulity at the vastness of the human tragedy in which the individual had been engulfed, and at the capacity of human beings to behave toward other human beings in the savage manner they witnessed.

([Effects on Children

The effects of the concentration-camp experience differ depending on the age of the individual affected. Studies dealing with the very few surviving individuals who were infants or very young children in the camps are particularly interesting in view of current ideas about the effect of the absence of a mother or a stable relationship with an adult on the personality development of infants. In some instances, as in the case reported by Engel,[11] the effect of such an experience at a very early age, could be catastrophic, producing an almost total arrest in development. Edith Sterba[43] has reported a group of twenty-five displaced children and adolescents who lost both parents and were in concentration camps or in hiding for a period of five years. She describes how her attempts to place these children with foster parents were greatly hampered by the disappointment and dissatisfaction expressed by the children toward whatever was done for them. They displayed a desperate need to cling together, apparently deriving more security from these peer relationships than from even the most benevolent relationships with the adults on whom they displaced all the angry fear engendered in them by the loss of their parents. A somewhat more hopeful view is derived from the fascinating study of Anna Freud and Sophie Dann[13] of a group of six children who had all been in the concentration camp at Theresienstadt before the age of three years. When seen in England after the liberation, these children showed severe emotional disturbances, were hypersensitive, restless, aggressive, and difficult to handle, but they had also evolved a remarkably stable sibling group and a group identity during their internment that seemed to protect them against the worse pathogenic effects of the absence of a maternal figure. A follow-up[15] of the later fates of these children indicates that though they all had stormy experiences during adolescence, most of them achieved some degree of stability by early adulthood. Among my own cases, there were six who were five years of age and younger in 1939 and who, therefore, underwent the experiences of the persecution at an extremely early period of their lives. In addition to various degrees of overt psychoneurotic symptomatology, they are all emotionally volatile people whose moods fluctuate markedly and who react to mild degrees of stress, such as an unexpected event, with an exacerbation of anxiety. Their personalities are marked both by bitter, cynical, pessimistic attitudes toward life and a childlike and total kind of emotional dependency. Although intimacy and closeness are of the greatest importance to them, they tend to show self-defeating patterns of excessive expectation and bitter or despairing withdrawal when these expectations are disappointed. They are extremely sensitive to actual or threatened separation from those on whom they have become dependent. It seems clear that the most damaging consequences to the personality maturation of these individuals resulted from the absence of a reliable and secure interpersonal environment, particularly a lack of adequate mothering in the early years. This applies not only to those children who lost both their natural parents but also to children whose mothers were forced to appear and disappear, actually by force of necessity but in the eyes of the children, cruelly and capriciously.

[The Nature and Causes of the Concentration-Camp Syndrome

The essential features of the Concentration-Camp Syndrome include a core of anxiety complicated by symptomatic defenses against anxiety, an obsessive-ruminative state, psychosomatic symptoms, depression and guilt. While there are those who regard this condition as *sui generis*, comprising a new and hithertofore undescribed entity,[19,32,46] it appears reasonable to regard at least its anxiety core as a special variety of traumatic neurosis. This is especially so if this entity is defined to include any state in which massive and unmistakable external traumas are directly related to the onset and persistence of anxiety symptoms, a typical dream life, and a contraction of the general level of performance in a previously adequately functioning personality. While the Concentration-Camp Syndrome resembles, in some respects, the ordinary combat-stress reaction that is the paradigm of the traumatic neurosis, a more interesting analogy is the Japanese A-bomb disease or neurosis described by Lifton.[32] For many years after the bombing of Hiroshima, the survivors suffered from vague, chronic complaints of fatigue, nervousness, weakness, and various physical ailments, along with characterological changes and feelings of "existential" guilt. Also, although the analogy is not as exact, it is possible without stretching the bounds of imagination too much, to draw significant parallels between certain aspects of the concentration-camp experience and the conditions of life in the poor neighborhoods and ghettoes of our great cities.[4]

A theoretical fallout from study of the Concentration-Camp Syndrome viewed as a traumatic neurosis is to cast serious doubt on the psychoanalytic view—held by Freud and his followers—that objective danger alone cannot give rise to a neurosis without participation of the deeper, unconscious layers of the psychic apparatus, that is, neurosis is impossible without significant childhood predisposition. The ubiquity of the neurotic symptoms occurring in so large a proportion of the survivors, the similarity of the symptom pictures, and the lack of any evidence that these individuals were predisposed to neurotic development indicates that we are dealing with a traumatic neurosis that is almost entirely the result of the trauma itself, although, of course, differences in severity and the variety of complaints can be related to differing, more-or-less healthy character structures. The current literature[16,21,27,39] on the aftermaths of the persecution tends to support this changing view. An ironic consequence of acceptance of the original Freudian view about the linkage connection between earlier psychopathology and traumatic neurosis was its use by certain German forensic psychiatrists to deny the causative role of the persecution when evaluating reparations claims.

There is, of course, no question but that the primary cause of the psychiatric sequelae of the Nazi persecution, including the Concentration-Camp Syndrome is the multiple, massive emotional and physical traumas to which the survivors were subjected. However, these traumas must be mediated and dealt with by a psychic apparatus, so that psychopathological considerations are in order. Also, the survivors came into contact with a whole series of environmental stresses, even after their liberation, and these must be taken into account in attempting to understand the long duration of the symptomatology, and its often-changing character over the years.

Leo Eitinger, one of the foremost investigators of the effects of the persecution, and himself a survivor, was at one time an advocate of the view that organic brain disease incurred during internment as a result of malnutrition, injury, and illness was a significant factor in certain of the chronic symptoms found in survivors.[8] However, Eitinger, as a result of his later investigations, particularly those comparing the long-term effects among a group of Norwegian (non-Jewish) and Israeli survivors, has modified his earlier opinion. He no longer believes that organic factors are so important in most of the Jewish concentration-camp survivors.[10] This view is held by most investigators interested in the subject.

There have been a number of psychoanalytic attempts to explicate the psychodynamics responsible for the persisting symptoms. These attempts are interesting, but the fact that most derive from relatively superficial reparations examinations rather than from intensive psychoanalytic scrutiny vitiate their value. There is general agreement that the massive repression of aggressive impulses which took place in the concentration camps was responsible for later vicissitudes and distortions that seriously impaired the long-term adjustment of many survivors. Guilt and depression particularly can be attributed to this influence. Also of great importance is the extent to which the regressive adaptation so necessary in the camps became fixated in the later personality. Krystal and Niederland[29] feel that the two basic pathogenic forces are survivor guilt and problems of aggression. Grauer[16] emphasizes ego exhaustion and changes in ego–superego boundaries, both factors leading to unmodifiable ego changes and, incidentally, to poor results in treatment. Maller[33] feels that the central phenomenon is "obsessive representations" that, along with other factors, indicate a struggle between cohesion and disillusion in the personality of the survivor.

There is no doubt about the primary role of massive object loss in generating depression and guilt. As noted above, these symptoms can be related to aggressive impulses which had been actually expressed or, more likely, carried out either symbolically or in fantasy. However, such explanations do not seem to me completely to account for all the varieties of survivor guilt that have been described above. I believe that there is a significant component of survivor guilt which serves the purpose of a kind of testimonial. By continuing to suffer himself, the survivor seems to be trying to provide an enduring memorial to his slaughtered friends and relatives.[5]

What happened to a survivor when the war ended and he was liberated could not fail to effect his future emotional health. During this period, the survivor endowed with good material, physical, intellectual, and emotional resources could take advantage of fortunate events and develop a new identity and a new productive life in which symptoms would gradually become attenuated. On the other hand, poor resources of this kind would encourage the development of regressive tendencies, with consequent clinging to symptoms as an unconscious excuse for an inability to live actively, and as a gratification of dependent impulses. Important postwar factors affecting the quality of later adjustments also include the degree of loss of immediate members of family and relatives, of homes and of livelihoods, a dashing of inflated hopes for a postwar utopia, prolonged debilitating residence in displaced persons camps, downward change in socioeconomic status, immigration to and taking up of residence in a strange land with a different language, tempo of life and customs (the "uprooting neurosis" of Hans Strauss[44]).

(**Psychiatric Contact with Survivors**

To deal professionally with survivors, for purposes either of reparations evaluation or psychotherapy is an experience that almost always invokes anxiety and sometimes even guilt in psychiatrists as they listen to the survivors' gothic tales of persecution, each more horrendous and more unbearable than the previous one. This anxiety of the psychiatrist can generate a whole spectrum of defensive behavior, ranging from overidentification with consequent loss of objectivity at one extreme, to reaction formation and denial, appearing as rejection disguised as objectivity at the other. Such attitudes, unless understood and worked through, make even more difficult the already rather artificial task of attempting to assign percentage of disability to survivors as required by the restitution procedures. As for the psychotherapy of survivors, it has been noted that relatively little is being attempted despite the severe and continuing symptoms that the survivors manifest. This phenomenon has been explained by Tanay[46] as due not only to the lack of financial aid from restitution for purposes of psychotherapy but also because the masochistic-regressive personality changes in the survivors were so adaptively necessary as to have become ego-syntonic. He also notes the countertransference attitudes of psychotherapists and their reluctance to undertake the treatment of such seemingly unpromising cases. However, there are an increasing number of articles dealing with psychotherapy of survivors (see Hoppe's review).[23] Some of these are at least cautiously optimistic, but the general tone emphasizes the obstacles and difficulties in the way of successful psychotherapy with these patients. With some exceptions,[7,20,23] there appears to be agreement that goals of psychotherapy should be relatively limited, oriented toward support and symptom relief rather than toward reconstructive goals, a conclusion in accord with my own experience. Although this relative inaccessibility of survivors to intensive psychotherapy can be explained according to various psychodynamic formulations, possibly a more simple and compelling explanation is that the capacity of many of these survivors to trust other human beings has suffered such damage from the horror and rapacity of the Nazi years that they are no longer able to enter into and sustain really reciprocal relationships with other representatives of a species that did them so much harm.

(Bibliography

1. BENSHEIM, H. "Die KZ-Neurose Rassisch Verfolgter," *Nervenarzt*, 31 (1960), 462–469.
2. BETTELHEIM, B. *The Informed Heart*. Glencoe, Ill.: Free Press, 1960.
3. CHODOFF, P. "Late Effects of the Concentration Camp Syndrome," *Arch. Gen. Psychiatry*, 8 (1963), 323–333.
4. ———. "The Nazi Concentration Camp and the American Poverty Ghetto—A Comparison," *J. Contemp. Psychother.*, 1 (1968), 1–8.
5. ———. "Depression and Guilt among Concentration Camp Survivors," *Existential Psychiatry*, 7 (1970), 19–26.
6. COHEN, E. A. *Human Behavior in the Concentration Camp*, New York: Norton, 1953.
7. DEWIND, E. "Persecution, Aggression and Therapy," *Int. J. Psychoanal.* 53 (1972), 173–178.
8. EITINGER, L. "Pathology of Concentration Camp Syndrome," *Arch. Gen. Psychiatry*, 5 (1961), 371–379.
9. ———. "Concentration Camp Survivors in the Post War World," *Am. J. Psychoth.*, 26 (1962), 191.
10. ———. *Concentration Camp Survivors in Norway and Israel*. New York: Humanities Press, 1965.
11. ENGEL, W. "Reflections on the Psychiatric Consequences of Persecution," *Am. J. Psychother.*, 26 (1962), 191–203.
12. FRANKL, V. E. *Man's Search for Meaning*. Boston: Beacon, 1959.
13. FREUD, A. and S. DANN. "An Experiment in Group Upbringing," in *The Psychoanalytic Study of the Child*, Vol. 6, 127–141. New York: International Universities Press, 1951.
14. FRIEDMAN, P. "Some Aspects of Concentration Camp Psychology," *Am. J. Psychiatry*, 105 (1949), 601–605.
15. GOLDBERGER, A. "Follow-Up Notes on the Children from Bulldog Bank," (1964), unpublished.
16. GRAUER, H. "Psychodynamics of the Survivor Syndrome," *Can. Psychiatr. Assoc. J.*, 14 (1969), 617–622.
17. GREENSON, R. R. "The Psychology of Apathy," *Psychoanal. Q.*, 18 (1949), 290–302.
18. GRINKER, R. "Mentally Healthy Young Males (Homoclites)," *Arch. Gen. Psychiatry*, 6 (1962), 405–453.
19. GROBIN, W. "Medical Assessment of Late Effects of National Socialist Persecution," *Can. Med. Assoc. J.*, 92 (1965), 911–917.
20. GYOMROI, E. L. "The Analysis of a Young Concentration Camp Victim," in *The Psychoanalytic Study of the Child*, Vol. 18, pp. 484–491. New York: International Universities Press, 1963.
21. HOCKING, F. "Human Reactions to Extreme Environmental Stress," *Med. J. Aust.*, 2 (1965), 477–483.
22. HOPPE, K. "The Psychodynamics of Concentration Camp Victims," *Psychoanal. Forum*, 1 (1966), 76.
23. ———. "The Aftermath of Nazi Persecution Reflected in Recent Psychiatric Literature," *Int. Psychiatry Clin.*, 8 (1971), 169–204.
24. JACOB, W. "Gesellschaftliche Voraussetzungen zur Überwindung der KZ-Shaden," *Nervenarzt*, 32 (1961), 542–545.
25. JÖRG, M. Personal communication, Aug. 1970.
26. KLEIN, H., J. ZELLERMAYER, and J. SHANAN. "Former Concentration Camp Inmates on a Psychiatric Ward," *Arch. Gen. Psychiatry*, 8 (1963), 334–342.
27. KORANYI, E. "A Theoretical Review of the Survivor Syndrome," *Dis. Nerv. Sys.*, 30 (1969), 115–118.
28. KRYSTAL, H., ed. *Massive Psychic Trauma*. New York: International Universities Press, 1968.
29. KRYSTAL, H. and W. NIEDERLAND. "Clinical Observations on the Survivor Syndrome," in H. Krystal, ed., *Massive Psychic Trauma*, pp. 327–349. New York: International Universities Press, 1968.
30. LEDERER, W. "Persecution and Compensation," *Arch. Gen. Psychiatry*, 12 (1965), 464–474.
31. LEVINGER, L. "Psychiatrische Untersuchungen in Israel an 800 Fällen mit Gesundheitsschaden-Forderungen wegen Nazi Verfolgung," *Nervenarzt*, 33 (1962), 75–80.
32. LIFTON, R. *Death in Life*. New York: Random House, 1967.
33. MALLER, O. "The Late Psychopathology of Former Concentration Camp Inmates," *Psychiatr. Neurol.*, 148 (1967), 140–177.
34. MATUSSEK, P. "Die Kozentrationslagerhaft als Belastungssituation," *Nervenarzt*, 32 (1961), 538–542.
35. MEERLOO, J. "Delayed Mourning in Victims

of Extermination Camps," *J. Hillside Hosp.*, 12 (1963), 96–98.

36. ———. "Persecution Trauma and the Reconditioning of Emotional Life: A Brief Survey," *Am. J. Psychiatry*, 125 (1969), 81–85.

37. NATHAN, T. S., L. EITINGER, and H. Z. WINNIK. "A Psychiatric Study of Survivors of the Nazi Holocaust. A Study in Hospitalized Patients," *Israel Ann. Psychiatry*, 2 (1964), 47–80.

38. NIEDERLAND, W. "The Problem of the Survivor," *J. Hillside Hosp.*, 10 (1961), 237.

39. ———. "Clinical Observations on the Survivor Syndrome," *Int. J. Psychoanal.*, 49 (1968), 313.

40. OSTWALD, P. and E. BITTNER. "Life Adjustment after Severe Persecution," *Am. J. Psychiatry*, 124 (1968), 1393–1400.

41. RAPPAPORT, E. "Beyond Traumatic Neurosis," *Int. J. Psychoanal.*, 49 (1968), 719–731.

42. SARLIN, C. N. "Depersonalization and Derealization," *J. Am. Psychoanal. Assoc.*, 10 (1962), 784–804.

43. STERBA, E. "The Effect of Persecution on Adolescents," in H. Krystal, ed., *Massive Psychic Trauma*, pp. 51–59. New York: International Universities Press, 1968.

44. STRAUSS, H. "Neuropsychiatric Disturbances after Nationalist-Socialist Persecution," *Proc. Virchow Med. Soc.*, 16 (1957), 95–104.

45. STROM, A., S. REFSUM, L. EITINGER et al. "Examination of Norwegian Ex-Concentration Camp Prisoners," *J. Neuropsychiatry*, 4 (1962), 43–62.

46. TANAY, E. "Initiation of Psychotherapy with Survivors of Nazi Persecution," in H. Krystal, ed., *Massive Psychic Trauma*, pp. 219–232. New York: International Universities Press, 1968.

47. TAS, J. "Psychical Disorders among Inmates of Concentration Camps and Repatriates," *Pychiatr. Q.*, 25 (1951), 679–690.

48. TRAUTMAN, E. C. "Psychiatrische Untersuchungen und Überlebenden der National-Socialistischen Vernichtungslager 15 Jahre nach der Befreiung," *Nervenarzt*, 32 (1961), 545–551.

49. ———. "Psychiatric and Sociological Effects of Nazi Atrocities on Survivors of the Extermination Camps," *J. Am. Assoc. Soc. Psychiatry*, Spec. Pub. (Sept.–Dec. 1961), 118–122.

50. VON BAEYER, W. "Erlebnisbedingter Verfolgungsschaden," *Nervenarzt*, 32 (1961), 534–538.

51. WINKLER, G. E. "Neuropsychiatric Symptoms in Survivors of Concentration Camps," *J. Soc. Ther.*, 5 (1959), 281–290.

52. WINNIK, H. "Further Comments Concerning Problems of Late Psychopathological Effects of Nazi Persecution and their Therapy," *Israel Ann. Psychiatry*, 5 (1967), 1–16.

53. WOLFENSTEIN, M. *Disaster*. Glencoe, Ill.: Free Press, 1957.

CHAPTER 42

SOCIAL CHANGES, ECONOMIC STATUS, AND THE PROBLEMS OF AGING

Ewald W. Busse

⟨ Introduction

THE SOCIAL ENVIRONMENT is recognized as one of the three sources that promote or damage the health of the individual. The other two sources are the inherent biological makeup of the individual and the physical environment. Social deprivation in infancy and childhood and social-overload stress in adolescence and adulthood are believed to play a significant role in the etiology of a number of mental disorders. Both types of stress are present in late life and compound the problems of maintaining mental health.[6] Attitudes of social origin underlie many criteria utilized to determine the existence and influence the diagnosis of mental disease. Social relations are important in the treatment of many mental disorders, as sustained improvement cannot be assured unless the adverse social circumstances to which the patient must return are altered. Although our understanding of this complex matter of the relationship between social forces and events and health is far from satisfactory, considerably more is known than is usually acknowledged. Social class with the pathological consequences of social deprivation and hostile social influences upon the infant and the developing child and adolescent have been reported by a number of investigators. Investigation of adults indicates a relationship between lower social class and a higher incidence of disease. The possibility that this is an apparent rather than a real correlation has been considered. Possible explanations that have been suggested include differences in community tolerance, class influences on psychiatric diagnosis, and downward social mobility as a manifestation of mental disease, particularly of biologic etiology. Although it is likely and possible that these explanations have some validity, the additional overload stresses and deprivations encountered in lower classes do appear to be a major contributor to mental disorders.

Definitions

The term "social" in its broadest usage and as applied to human beings "refers to any behavior or attitude that is influenced by past or present experience of the behavior of other people (direct or indirect) or that is oriented (consciously or unconsciously) toward other people. Normally the term is morally neutral."[10] In this chapter dealing with social dimensions in geropsychiatry, it will be necessary not only to look at those social patterns or structures that may be neutral but to try to identify those which promote (mental) health and those that contribute to psychiatric disorders and physical illness.

The field of economics is considered to be an independent area of study and is represented by a specific discipline. However, definitions of economics range from extremely broad to very narrow. All of the definitions do contain evidence that economic structure and process cannot, in Western society, be separated from social dimensions. One definition[16] says "economics is a study of mankind in the ordinary business of life: it examines that part of individual and social action which is most closely connected with the attainment and with the use of the material requisites of well-being." It is clear that the economic condition and economic structure of Western democratic society are key elements in influencing social factors or dimensions that are of major importance to physical and mental health.

Persons 65 years of age and over are commonly referred to as the older population. Brotman[1] recently identified the special characteristics of those 75 years of age and over, referring to these people as "the aged." This subdividing of the older population is of considerable value, as the important health and socioeconomic facts common to a specific group can be lost in the mass of the older population.

"Social gerontology" was first introduced into the literature in 1954 by Clark Tibbitts. Tibbitts defined social gerontology as "a part of the broader field of gerontology which is concerned with biological and physiological aging in all animal and plant species and with the psychological and social cultural aspects of aging in man and society. Social gerontology separates out: (1) the phenomena of aging which are related to man as a member of the social group and of society, and (2) those phenomena which are related to aging in the nature and function of the social system of society itself."[24] Unfortunately, for many individuals this term has been broadened and now includes those occupations which are concerned with delivery of services to elderly people. Hence, when one hears the term social gerontology applied to training fields, it may not be related to the training of persons concerned with the study of the societal aspects of aging, but to the training of various service occupations.

Sociological Theories*

Social scientists are usually concerned with the social role or place (status) of the aged in society. Aging to a social scientist may not only be a decline in social usefulness but may also be related to a change in social and often economic status. Social theories relevant to the aging and the elderly are affected by the structure of society and social change. One such theory—the rapid-change theory—holds that the status of the aged is high in static societies and tends to decline with rapid social change. Another theory is that the status of the aged is high in societies where there are few elderly and that the value and status of the aged decline as they become more numerous. A third theory is that the status and the prestige of the aged are high in those societies in which older people, in spite of physical infirmity, are able to continue to perform useful and socially valued functions. This third theory has a particularly pessimistic quality when

---

* Biological and psychological terms and theories applicable to aging and geriatrics are defined and described in Volume 4, Chapter 3 of this *Handbook*.

applied to Western society, as early retirement plus rapid social change is and will make it increasingly difficult for the elderly person to be involved in socially valued functions, unless provision for their continued participation is rapidly developed. Two recently advanced social theories are called the disengagement theory and the activity theory.[9] The disengagement theory maintains that high satisfaction in old age is usually present in those individuals who accept the inevitability of reduction in social and personal interactions. The activity theory holds that the maintenance of activity is important to most individuals as a basis for obtaining and maintaining satisfaction, self-esteem, and health. Elaborations and modifications on these theories appear in this resume.

(The Elderly—A Minority Group

Social and behavioral scientists define minority groups in a number of ways. It is possible to identify a minority group as a collection of individuals that can be identified by specific characteristics and do not as individuals or a group either voluntarily or by prohibition of the majority participate in all the life experiences of the majority.[5] Furthermore, minority groups do not share all life experiences equally, nor do they have the same responsibilities for or expectancies of certain life experiences. Some minority groups can be in an advantageous position, such as nobility, while others can be in a very deprived relationship to the rest of society. There are some minority groups that elect to bypass opportunities or to reject responsibilities offered by the majority in order to maintain their own value systems. Minority groups can exist in a relatively contented fashion when the advantages offered them by their own group satisfactorily meet their needs; or, if they so elect, when the opportunities of the majority are also open to them. If one accepts the views that have been expressed, then it is evident that the elderly—particularly the retired elderly person—is a member of a deprived minority group. Much of the data presented in this chapter confirms this unsatisfactory social condition.

(Population Changes and Social Problems

Life Expectancy

Life expectancy is a computed projection rather than an observed or estimated phenomenon. The projection is based upon the assumption that the death rate experienced in a single year or the average of experience in a few years will remain completely unchanged in the future. Obviously, any event that influences future death rates, whether it be natural or man-made, automatically affects the accuracy implied in the prognosis of the computed life expectancy. Since the computed life expectancy cannot foresee negative events, it also cannot include positive changes. No assumed positive changes are included, e.g., changes in medical knowledge and care, sanitation and nutrition, reduced mortality in traffic accidents and wars. Longevity is the condition or quality of being long-lived. Longevity is influenced by a complex of interacting factors, including genetic makeup, environmental and nutritional factors, and psychologic, social, and economic influences.

Death Rates

Death rates are the recorded number of deaths occurring in a population for a single calendar year. This type of information is referred to as crude death rate and has very little value when one wants to compare one country with another. The crude death rate reflects the age differences of the population rather than the age-specific death rates. Specific death rates are commonly based upon characteristics such as age, sex, and race and sometimes include marital status, place of residence, income, and other identifiable features. Consequently, they are often referred to as true death rates and are relevant to an understanding of the socioeconomic conditions that are related to life span in a given population.

The recent census concluded by the United States Bureau of the Census has added immeasurably to our understanding of the shifting characteristics of the population and their impact on social issues and planning.

In 1970, 9.9 percent of the population of the United States was age 65 and over. This means that every tenth American is considered to be an older American. One hundred years ago, in 1870, only 2.9 percent was 65 years and over. Between 1960 and 1970, the total population increased 12.5 percent, while those 65 years and over increased 21.1 percent. This percentage increase of older Americans is even more striking when one recognizes that in the same decade (1960–1970) the rate of increase of "the aged," that is, individuals over seventy-five, was almost three times as great as that of the 65- to 74-year-old group.

From state to state there is considerable variation in the percentage of older citizens. The extremes are Florida with 14.5 percent over 65 and Alaska with 2.3 percent. Hawaii ranks next to Alaska with 5.7 percent of its population in the age 65 and over category.[8]

Of particular importance to our society is the growing predominance of women. Even though there are more boy babies than girl babies born, the longer life expectancy for females results in the gradual shift in percentages, so that after the age of 18 there are 105.5 females per every 100 males in the total population. In the U. S. population 65 years and over, there are 138.5 females per 100 males; and after age 75, it moves to 156.2 females to 100 males.

Switzerland has a great discrepancy of aged male and female. In 1970, the ratio was 100 males to 146 females.

Negroes have a shorter life expectancy, as older Negroes compose only 6.9 percent of the total Negro population. The discrepancy in male–female ratio is also apparent in Negroes, as females 65 years and over accounted for 115 to every 100 males in 1960. In 1970, there were 131 black females to every 100 black older males.

⟨ Why Do Women Outlive Men?

In the United States prior to 1900, the average life expectancy favored the male over the female. However, there have been remarkable changes in the status of humans. The pendulum is swinging strongly in favor of women. In many undeveloped countries the unfavorable position in regard to female longevity continues to exist. For example, in India in 1968, the male life expectancy was 41.9 years, while the female expectancy, 40.5 years. In addition to the reduction of maternal mortality, it is claimed that the decline in tuberculosis added substantially to the gain in life expectancy of American females. The question arises as to whether this favorable trend for females is predominantly on a biological basis or whether the socioeconomic environment is the major determinant.[20] The biological explanation is held to be substantiated by the sex differences found in the life span of a number of animals. For those searching for an environmental explanation, one would have to look for groups of men and women with similar social roles and physical environment. A study of male and female Catholics involved in teaching orders indicated that the female religious order has a higher life expectancy than the male.[15] But even this finding is now open to question, as the male members of the Catholic teaching orders apparently are overweight and smoke heavily. Although it will take a number of years to obtain information, it does appear that the current trend of women to assume social roles similar to that of men will throw light on this situation.

The demographic yearbooks published by the United Nations are extremely helpful when one wishes to compare population differences in various countries throughout the world. Little data is available on the population of a number of countries throughout the world. Information regarding Africa is gradually emerging, and it is possible that with the reentry of China into the affairs of the world, knowledge will become available regarding the needs of the elderly adult in this extremely populous country that, for years, is reported to have had a very positive social attitude toward its older citizens.

Living Arrangements

The majority of elderly people are living in the community. Only one in twenty-five lives in an institution such as a rest home, nursing home, or medical facility. There are, however, some striking differences between the way the men and the women live. Two-thirds of the men live with their spouses, but only one-third of the women have husbands. Moreover, only one-sixth of the men live alone or with non-relatives. Less than three-quarters of a million elderly people require some type of institutional care. Consequently, greater emphasis must be given to making certain that the living arrangements for the elderly within the community are conducive to the maintenance of health.

Surveys of older people indicate that they want to live apart from their children but close to at least one of them.[21] Consequently, housing units for the elderly should be conveniently placed so that the old person can have controlled intimacy in terms of frequency and distance. The units should be located so that it is not only possible but relatively easy for old people to see their families often and call upon them for help if and when needed. Unfortunately, a small percentage of older people, probably around 4 percent, have no human contact for as long as a week. This small minority of aged individuals is truly isolated, and although such individuals are few, they are so scattered that they are difficult to find. When found, they are difficult to approach, usually rejecting any offer of assistance.

In a national study of older Americans, 59 percent of those living alone had been visited by an immediate neighbor the previous day, 46 percent by a friend, and 50 percent by relatives, including children.

As indicated above, most older men are married, whereas most older women are widows. There are almost four times as many widows as widowers. It should be noted that about two-fifths of the older married men

have wives under 65 years of age. Furthermore, there are at least 35,000 marriages a year in which the groom, the bride, or both are 65 years of age or over. The number of marriages among elderly people has been steadily increasing.

The difference in married and unmarried status for older patients is of significance to the physician, for it has been noted that the hospital admission rates and stays of unmarried exceed those of the married.[22]

There are about 5 million couples with one partner over the age of 65. In this group 350,000 couples, or 7 percent, have annual incomes of $10,000 or more. Nine hundred and forty thousand couples, that is, 18 percent, have incomes between $5,000 and $10,000. The remainder of such couples, that is, 75 percent, have an annual income of under $5,000, 52 percent under $3,000, and 7 percent under $1000.

Unfortunately, the income distribution of persons age 65 and over who are living alone indicates that the majority are living in poverty. Eighty-nine percent have an annual income of less than $3000, and 62 percent are under $1500. It is evident that men 65 years of age or older not only are likely to have more money than surviving women but are much more likely to have a spouse. Although a man is less likely to live as long as a woman, the years he spends as an older citizen appear to be better ones than the many years spent in old age by a woman.

The marital status of the aged group reflects the social tradition for men to marry younger women. Twice as many aged men as women are married, and only one-third of them have wives 75 and over. About half have wives between 65 and 74 years of age, and one-fifth have wives under 65 years of age.

Of men 75 years of age or older, 33.9 percent are living with their wives. In contrast, of women 75 years of age and older, only 17.8 percent are living with their husbands. Of these women who are 75 years or older, 3 percent have husbands under 65 years of age; roughly 20 percent have younger husbands between the ages of 65 and 74; and the remainder have husbands their own ages or older. Each year approximately 2000 women age 75 or older marry, and 6000 men 75 years or older go to the altar. Both of these groups are usually moving out of widowhood. Of these 8000 marriages, over 4,000 involve partners under age 75.[4]

❮ The Productive and Dependent Aged

Cottrell utilizes a technologic theory base for studying changes in society.[7] He utilizes levels of actual physical energy that flow through the society as a basis for changes in social structure and patterns. He refers to low-energy societies and high-energy societies. Cottrell is providing a measure for differentiation between undeveloped, that is, the low-energy societies, and highly developed nations, the high-energy societies. The high-energy societies depart more from natural energy—an agrarian society—and depend upon man-created energy through the use of technology. This change in energy also alters work patterns so that an increasing number of any population is not required to work, but is dependent on those who by working monitor the increasing energy that has been harnessed by that society. This, then, differentiates the population into the "productive" and "dependent" people. Hence, dependency ratios have appeared. However, dependency ratios clearly are not totally related to the level of energy utilized by the group but also relate to mortality and fertility. Dependency ratios are usually calculated for the part of the population under twenty and over sixty-five as opposed to the productive population that is considered to be between the ages of twenty and sixty-four. The dependency-ratio refinement is actually an outgrowth of the so-called index of aging that is based upon the population sixty years and over and under 15 years, as contrasted with the population between fifteen and sixty. Utilizing the index of aging, Mexico as of 1964 has an index of aging of 12.5 as contrasted to the United States with an index of aging of 41.2.[11] Clearly, this does indicate that the United States has a much higher portion of its population who are relatively nonproductive and who are dependent upon those remaining in the labor force.

❮ Psychoneurotic Reactions to Social Stress

The impression is often conveyed that psychoneurotic reactions in adults are chronic disorders that are sometimes fortuitously alleviated but usually require psychotherapeutic intervention. Longitudinal studies suggest that there are older individuals who, after a period of time, develop psychoneurotic reactions in response to an unfavorable environment. Furthermore, recovery is quite possible if the individual is removed from the stressful life situation or is provided the means of restoring self-esteem.* Two psychoneurotic reactions, depression and hypochondriasis, are frequently found in elderly persons. The possibility of a transient psychoneurotic reaction appears to be especially true of hypochondriasis and mild-to-moderate depressions. Careful evaluations conducted over more than ten years strongly support the view that the signs and symptoms of a psychoneurosis are unconsciously selected by the person so that he can maintain his self-esteem in a particular situation. If the sign or symptom is not an adequate defense in that particular situation, he will abandon that defense mechanism for one that is appropriate to the particular circumstances in which he is living. Hence, some psychoneurotic signs and symptoms "come and go" over a period of time. The exacerbations and remissions are largely determined by an identifiable constellation of socioeconomic conditions. Therefore, in some individuals the hypochondriacal pattern dominates, while in others the depressive attitude is the major factor. In general, the hypochondriacal elderly person is more likely to be a female of low socioeconomic status with little change in her work role, relatively younger and less socially active, with patterns of activities suggesting

* Additional information is presented in Volume 4, Chapter 3 of this *Handbook*.

that they are not conducive to a good adjustment.[14] More specifically, the person is forced into a situation, hopefully temporary, where criticism is the rule and appreciation and work satisfaction are absent. This is compounded by the restricted social activity, so that rewards are few and far between.

It should be mentioned that, in contrast, there are elderly people who utilize a neurotic mechanism of denial; that is, they fail to realistically deal with important physical diseases. This type of person, a persistent optimist, should not automatically be seen as a person with courage, for the courageous person does have a realistic appraisal of the situation. The type of older person who is likely to utilize denial is a male of fairly high economic status who is not burdened with financial responsibility and a demanding work role yet has many and suitable opportunities for social activity.[3,4]

(Economic Influences

Poverty Level in the Aged

According to a working paper prepared for the Special Committee on Aging of the United States Senate and published in 1971, there has been an increase in both the number and proportion of aged poor between 1968 and 1969.[25] In 1969, there were approximately 4.8 million people aged 65 and older who were living in poverty; almost 200,000 more than in 1968. The older poor in 1969 represented 19.7 percent of all persons 65 and older. This was a rise from 8.2 percent found for 1968. Brotman, in another recent report, indicated that only 15 percent of the total poor in 1959 represented the aged population.[2] Brotman also points out that older citizens in 1969 made up approximately 10 percent of the total population, but contributed 20 percent of the poor. Within the older population, every fourth person is poor. Two-thirds of the aged poor in 1969 were women; 85 percent of the aged poor are white. The poverty level for a person of sixty-five or over, living alone or with non-relatives in 1969, averaged $1749 and ranged from $1487 for a woman in a farm area to $1773 for a man in a nonfarm area. The poverty level for a couple, with the head age 65 or over, averaged $2194 in 1969, with a range from $1,861 to $2,217.

A report[12] concerned with the situation of aged blacks states that 50 percent of all Negroes 65 years of age or more live in poverty compared to 23 percent of whites. Approximately 47 percent of aged Negro women and 20 percent of elderly Negro men have annual incomes below one thousand dollars. Another 42 percent of Negro women and 37 percent of Negro men have incomes from $1000 to $1999. The Negro living in a rural area is much harder hit, as two out of every three rural blacks are living in extreme poverty.

The poverty status of older people is not only complicated by the lack of opportunity for employment but by the threat of social-security-benefit reductions if work income exceeds $2520 a year. The elderly person is unlikely to want to accept part-time work in view of this threat, and the employer is reluctant to adjust procedures to accommodate older persons working fewer than forty hours a week.

Standard of Living and Adequacy of Income

No psychiatrist or behavioral scientist would dispute the fact that the social and physical environment in which an individual lives plays a significant role in determining his health and life expectancy. Furthermore, if his health is to improve, the opportunity for upgrading the environment must exist and money is often necessary for an individual to upgrade his standard of living. Unfortunately, although we are willing to accept the fact that we should provide people with an acceptable standard of living, it is most difficult to devise a method of measuring and expressing what constitutes an acceptable standard of living. In this search it has become apparent that certain social patterns that are adverse to health cannot be altered by merely providing money or opportunities for change. This has led, more and more, to oversimplification of an acceptable standard of living by expressing it in terms of an "adequate income."

The difficulties of definition continue when one realizes that the lowest standard of living is expressed by the concept of poverty. Poverty, in turn, is a relative status and cannot be tied solely to income, as income in one area of the United States may be adequate, but in another it would be too little to exist on. This realization has resulted in a gradual refinement of the methodology utilized to designate a poverty level.

One of the first attempts to establish poverty levels was made by the Council on Economic Advisers in January 1964 in their *Economic Report of the President*. This council arbitrarily chose a $3000-per-year family income as the dividing line and analyzed the data on incomes in 1959 as presented in the 1960 census reports. This led quickly to the recognition that this system was inadequate since it did not give consideration to age, size, and composition of the family unit, and its geographic location. Consequently, by 1964 the Department of Agriculture had started to define poverty on the basis of a food budget. Utilizing detailed data collected by it concerning the relationship between expenditures for food and total expenditures for various types of families at low-income levels, the dollar cost of the economic food budgets was multiplied by the appropriate factors to provide an estimate of the total cost for the family unit. These determinations resulted in poverty levels being established for 1964.

Refinements have continued, and by 1968 two major revisions were introduced, in addition to the base determinants of 1964. The first major revision was the use of the percentage change in the total consumer price index over the year for the annual change in the poverty levels rather than change in food prices alone. The second was the computation of farm area poverty levels as 15 percent below the levels for nonfarm areas, rather than the 30 percent differential previously used. It is therefore apparent that it is very difficult for any relatively uninformed individual to appreciate the significance of poverty reports and to know whether the existence of a guaranteed annual income that cannot possibly keep up with inflation will actually substantially alter anything other than the definition of a poverty level.

Using the revised poverty levels, the data regarding poverty has been computed for all years from 1959 to 1969.

Prediction of Longevity

Longitudinal studies of elderly men and women have reinforced the conviction that health and longevity are strongly influenced by the complex interaction of inherent physiological changes and life experiences. Actuarial life expectancy at birth is less than the predicted years of remaining life for those who have achieved advanced age. As birthdays pass, life expectancy lengthens. Therefore, it is important to look at people who have reached a specific age, say sixty-five, and find out why some of these individuals will achieve an age that considerably exceeds the predicted longevity. Multidisciplinary studies of such individuals have given us some important clues as to the relative importance of physical, mental, and social factors in predicting longevity for various age, sex, and race categories. Once a person has reached old age, the theory that longevity runs in families is not sustained. The age at death of the father and the mother showed no correlation with either the longevity index or the longevity quotient as devised by Palmore.[19]

According to Palmore, the six strongest independent variables that affect longevity in late life are: (1) work satisfaction; (2) happiness rating; (3) physical functioning; (4) tobacco use; (5) performance intelligence quotient; and (6) leisure activities.

The work satisfaction score represents a person's reaction to his general usefulness and his ability to perform a meaningful social role. The overall happiness rating is unquestionably influenced by work satisfaction, but reflects a person's general satisfaction with his life situation. The physical function rating is determined by the examining physician, and although it is the third most important factor, it does appear that satisfaction and happiness can compensate for and overcome some physical disability. The use of tobacco is a negative predictor, and it is recognized that it is a complex habit that apparently adversely affects physical functioning yet must play a role in providing some sort of satisfaction to the users. The use of tobacco among the elderly people does show differences between certain age, sex, and racial groups. Tobacco use is a particularly strong negative predictor of longevity among the younger white men and among Negroes. It is probable that both of these groups use a greater amount of tobacco. Palmore concludes that these findings suggest that, in general, the most important ways to increase longevity, once you have moved into the latter part of your life span, are to: (1) maintain a useful and satisfying role in society; (2) maintain a positive view of life; (3) maintain good physical functioning; and (4) avoid smoking.

Lowenthal is concerned with the ambiguities of social stress, particularly the range of responses to what appeared to be stressful events that can be found in elderly people.[13] She points out that certain social events usually considered stressful, such as residential moves or retirement, often produce conflicting results. With respect to these changes she believes that it is necessary to take into account the voluntary or involuntary nature of the event. Furthermore, the characteristic social life style of the individual, that is, how he or she copes with life, is essential to the type of response to stress and whether or not such a response contributes to mental illness. For example, Lowenthal believes that lifelong isolation is not associated with poor adaptation in late life and does not increase the likelihood of developing a mental illness or more accurately be requiring treatment for mental illness. In contrast, lifelong marginal social relationships are associated with poor adaptation, including serious mental illness. However, both patterns are associated with a history of parental deprivation in childhood. One style represents a relatively successful protective pattern, while the other produces excessive strain. These lifelong, marginally socially adjusted individuals constitute a population at serious risk in later life. Lowenthal also contends that some challenging work remains to be done in regard to stressful events that produce negative or decremental results as opposed to those which are neutral, that is, do not seem to alter the individual, or positive ones, those which are actually conducive to a better life adjustment. No doubt there is some validity for this concern. It is evident that individuals can only learn when they are required to adapt to a new stress or demand, but they can be overwhelmed when they lack the capacity to develop coping mechanisms. Lowenthal is also concerned with the issue of physical health status as a stressor or as the result of stress. Obviously, illness can be both, and both features can be present simultaneously in the same individual.

It is of importance to note that when Palmore is using predictors of longevity, he is dealing with many types of variables. For example, the work satisfaction and happiness ratings are types of social adaptation; the use of tobacco, a psychological, physical dimension; and the physical functioning scale, an estimate of health determined by an examining physician. However, his work does suggest that methods of psychosocial adaptation may be more important to longevity than physical habits and physical health.

([Social Position and Retirement

Social Position and Longevity

The disagreement between President Nixon and Congress regarding appointments to the Supreme Court rekindled interest in the apparent longevity of Supreme Court justices, their effectiveness as members of the Supreme Court, and the fact that all federal judges "shall hold their offices during good behavior."

There is little doubt that Supreme Court justices are unusually long-lived men. Since the turn of the century the average age at appointment has been 54.3 years. Chief justices have been appointed at an average age of 57.5 years. Supreme Court justices have remained in office for much longer periods than any other government officials. Exactly half, or forty-eight, of the justices died while on the bench. Twenty-two retired; fourteen resigned; and three became disabled. It would appear that this social role of fulfilling the heavy responsibility of a Supreme Court justice does not actually interfere with longevity. In fact, it obviously encourages it. Lawyers in the United States appear to have only a small advantage over white men in the general population. Furthermore, Supreme Court justices have a considerably better prospect of long lives than do Congressmen and cabinet officers.[17] Since many are drawn from the same pool of professional training and experience, one cannot help but wonder if the position of a justice of the Supreme Court does not in itself make a major contribution to longevity. It would, in this writer's opinion, appear that the prolongation of a useful social role, the continuation of prestige, plus financial security are all major factors in this selective longevity.

Compulsory Retirement

On June 22, 1971, Congressman William Frenzel introduced in the House of Representatives a joint resolution proposing an amendment to the Constitution to provide an age limit and a single six-year term for the president of the United States. The resolution states that "no person who has attained the age of 70 years shall be eligible for election to the office of the President or Vice President." Earlier, on June 14, two senators (C. E. Miller and William Brock) introduced into the Senate Joint Resolution 113, which proposes a constitutional amendment to establish a mandatory age retirement of 72 for senators, representatives, and federal judges. Senator Miller presented to the Senate the following arguments in support of the measure:

Modern day private industry has set the pace when it comes to retirement. The great majority of industrial organizations make retirement mandatory generally at age 65. The reason is that greater efficiency means better profits. Why should not the government adapt a similar policy, recognizing

that the greater efficiency means better service for the people? Of course, a balance should be struck between efficiency and experience, both of which are needed for the best results. But a balance does not now prevail.

The traditional argument against a mandatory retirement age for members of Congress is that if the electorate of a state or congressional district wishes to elect an older person, that is their right. Of course, such an argument has little relevance to federal judges. But there is an answer to the argument as far as members of Congress are concerned; namely, that the right of the electorate within a state or congressional district should not take precedence over the general welfare of the nation, which depends in a considerable degree on the efficiency of Congress. [p. 2.][18]

As of June 1971, there are fifteen congressmen and fourteen senators who are age seventy or over. These individuals would be permitted to complete the term for which they are elected. If over seventy-two, at the end of that term, they could not run for reelection.

It is interesting to note that in his arguments Senator Miller states that there should be a balance between efficiency and experience, but implies that experience does not contribute to efficiency. It is clear to any careful observer that experience is an important component of efficiency, particularly when it relates to including all of the factors in a complex decision process. If the senator means by efficiency speed of response or the energy to work for long periods of time, then these components are indeed important in evaluating final results. No rationale is given for selecting 70 as a turning point for the office of president or vice president nor why it is 72 for senators, representatives, and federal judges. Perhaps it is a compromise of importance of position and greater assurance of efficiency.

Industry is claimed to be setting a pace for retirement that is clearly related to efficiency. This is questionable as no studies are available that indicate young corporate leaders make more or less mistakes than do presidents of corporations older than age 65.

Some determinants setting age of retirement are more rooted in the social sanctions of competitiveness and of achieving financial success (and reward). Certainly, a man who has become the head or a leader in a large industrial organization has accumulated some wealth by the time he has reached the age of 65. There are many young men and women below him who are striving to achieve a similar kind of security as well as an opportunity to spend less time and energy competing and more of both in other activities. Furthermore, one cannot disregard the basic competitiveness and strivings of younger persons to displace older persons. Competitiveness is common throughout most of the animal kingdom and is basic to the free-enterprise system devised by the human animal.

Retirement—Process and Impact

Retirement is both an individual problem and a social pattern of modern industrialized nations. It is the result of a complicated set of factors that has emerged primarily in Western industrialized societies. In the less well-developed social systems, retirement is likely to be the consequences of aging, that is, the development of a disability. In a modern society, retirement is determined by the economic status rather than by the capabilities of the individual. Streib and Schneider have attempted to investigate and differentiate the process of retirement and the actual status of the individual in retirement and its impact upon him.[23] These investigators have attempted to combine the activity and disengagement theories, ending up with what they refer to as "differential disengagement" or changes in roles for the aged that result in "activity within disengagement."

The Streib and Schneider longitudinal study is described as being based upon role theory. Role theory may be described as "through a system of mores, or social norms, society requires that a person enact roles in accordance with his position in the social system." Roles may, in turn, be defined by the subgroups to which a person belongs. Persons often must enact several roles at one time, and it is necessary to integrate these multiple roles and sometimes resolve the conflict between roles. A person may discard a role or define it in ways

that are more congenial to him. There is no doubt that retirement does bring about a redefinition of roles, and these investigators have focused upon this particular aspect. Role theory has two major but overlapping components, one called the structural orientation, and one the interactional or social-psychological orientation. The first is a more static identification of the individual and his relationship to groups and institutions. The other is a study of change and reaction to change.

These investigators conclude that there are two age foci for retirement—age 65 and age 70. Their data indicate that both men and women of higher income levels, higher educational attainments, and higher levels of occupational structure tend to work longer than their counterparts with lower socioeconomic status. Women who are widowed, divorced, or separated are likely to work longer than those who are married. It is also clear that persons who are reluctant to retire are actually able to postpone retirement, while the more one is disposed to retirement, the sooner he is likely to retire. These investigators believe that their data show that the early retirees are more likely to be satisfied than those who retire later. They conclude, "The data tend to support the proposition that one's prior attitude is more important than the mode of retirement, that is, administrative or voluntary, in determining whether a person is satisfied with retirement or with life in general."

E. W. Burgess first described the status of the retired elderly as "a roleless role." Streib et al. claim that the retired individual alters his roles, but is not roleless. There is disengagement from such roles as those associated with work, but they believe that many retirees are capable of coping with this role realignment. Streib and Schneider report that a "clearly defined role is not as important to older persons as it is to younger persons."

As to health, the investigation depended largely upon subjectively rated health. Although a decline in health occurred between age 65 and 70, the authors do not believe that this decline in self-assessment of health was significantly different between those who worked as opposed to those who did not work.

They refute the idea that retirement causes a decline in health. The authors do point out that for certain subgroups, for example, clinical and semiskilled, there does appear to be a decline in health among those who retire as opposed to those who continue working. However, they also believe that the unskilled actually improve in health after retirement. The authors do recognize that their health information is "clearly a subjective self-evaluation measure," but they consider the information sufficiently reliable for their objectives. Although they say that poor health itself may lead to retirement and that those in good health tend to remain employed, this is not thoroughly explored. They do devote considerable effort to looking at health in retirement and do conclude, in general, "that in the impact year, the year after retirement, there is little evidence to suggest that health declines at retirement." They add, "There is a very slight tendency for white-collar occupations to have a decline in reported health in the impact year compared to those in blue-collar occupations." The improved health in the unskilled workers is recognized as possibly related to the fact that these individuals "are more likely to have engaged in more demanding or more onerous physical activity at work then retirement may be viewed as a possible respite and hence an improvement in health may be the result of stopping work." Occupation before retirement influences health after retirement.

⟪ Bibliography

1. BROTMAN, H. Who Are the Aged: A Demographic View. Paper Read at 21st Annu. University of Michigan Conf. Aging. Ann Arbor, Aug. 5, 1968.

2. ———. Facts and Figures on Older Americans—Measuring Adequacy of Income. Washington: Department of Health, Education, and Welfare, 1971.

3. BUSSE, E. W. Therapeutic Implications of Basic Research with the Aged. The Fourth Annual Institute of Pennsylvania Hospital-Award Lecture in Memory of E. A. Strecker. Nutley, N.J.: Roche Labs., 1967.

4. ———. "The Older Population and the Aged Patient," Med. Coll. Va. Q., 5 (1969), 137–139.

5. ———. "The Aged: A Deprived Minority," Editorial, N. Carolina J. Ment. Health, 4 (1970), 3–7.

6. ———. "Psychogeriatrics." Report of a WHO Scientific Group. WHO Technical Report Series no. 507. Geneva: World Health Organization, 1972.

7. COTTRELL, F. "The Technological and Societal Basis of Aging," in Clark Tibbitts, ed., Handbook of Social Gerontology, pp. 92–119. Chicago: University of Chicago Press, 1960.

8. COULTER, O. ed. "Great Variations Found in State Aging Patterns," Aging, 204 (1971), 10–11.

9. CUMMING, E. and W. HENRY. Growing Old. New York: Basic Books, 1961.

10. GOULD, J. and W. KOLB, eds. Dictionary of the Social Sciences. New York: Free Press, 1964.

11. KOLLER, M. Social Gerontology. New York: Random House, 1968.

12. LINDSAY, I. The Multiple Hazards of Age and Race: The Situation of Aged Blacks in the United States. A preliminary survey for the Special Committee on Aging, U.S. Senate. Washington: U.S. Govt. Print. Off., 1971.

13. LOWENTHAL, M. Social Stress and Adaptation toward a Developmental Perspective. Paper Presented at the Task Force on Aging Panel, Developmental Aspects of Aging, Am. Psychol. Assoc., Washington, Sept. 6, 1971.

14. MADDOX, G. L. "Self-assessment of Health Status. A Longitudinal Study of Selected Elderly Subjects," J. Chronic Dis., 17 (1964), 449–460.

15. MADIGAN, F. and R. B. VANCE. "Differential Sex Mortality: A Research Design," Soc. Forces, 35 (1957), 193–199.

16. MARSHALL, A. Principles of Economics, 8th ed., p. 1. London: Macmillan, 1920.

17. METROPOLITAN LIFE STATISTICAL BULLETIN. 52 (1971), 3–4.

18. NATIONAL COUNCIL ON AGING. Industrial Gerontology, Leg. Suppl. (1971), 2.

19. PALMORE, E. "Predicting Longevity—A Follow-up Controlling for Age," The Gerontologist, 9 (1969), 247–250.

20. ROSE, C. "Critique of Longevity Studies," in

E. Palmore and F. Jeffers, eds., *Prediction of Life-Span*, pp. 13–29. Lexington, Mass.: D. C. Heath, 1971.

21. SHANAS, E., P. TOWNSEND, D. WEDDERBURH et al. *Old People in Three Industrial Societies*. New York: Atherton, 1968.

22. SPIEGELMAN, M. "The Changing Demographic Spectrum and Its Implications for Health," *Eugen. Q.*, 10 (1963), 161–174.

23. STREIB, G. and C. J. SCHNEIDER. *Retirement in American Society—Impact and Process.* Ithaca: Cornell University Press, 1971.

24. TIBBITTS, C. *Handbook of Social Gerontology.* Chicago: University of Chicago Press, 1960.

25. UNITED STATES SENATE, SPECIAL COMMITTEE ON AGING. *The Nation's State in the Employment of Middle Aged and Older Persons.* Washington: U.S. Govt. Print. Off., 1971.

CHAPTER 43

THE FEDERAL GOVERNMENT AND MENTAL HEALTH[*]

Lorrin M. Koran, Frank Ochberg, and Bertram S. Brown

(Introduction

THIS CHAPTER describes the Federal Government's structure and organization as related to the mental-health sector, its impact on that sector, and its recent advances and retreats in the mental-health arena. Although complete description of the operations of Government is beyond the scope of this *Handbook*, we hope to shed some light on the intricate processes whereby public will is translated into public policy, and policy is implemented in laws, programs, and procedures.

The forces involved in Federal decision-making include a vast, interacting array of Congressional committees, executive-branch agencies, laws, regulations, judicial decisions, fiscal formulae, individual personalities, and social and historical trends. For example, Congress debated the "health-care crisis" in the United States for decades. The *nonsystem* of care was called inefficient, expensive, unequal, and inhumane. President Truman initiated legislative remedies, but Congress and the American people were reluctant to tamper with the free enterprise of medicine. Most of those early initiatives failed. During Truman's presidency the Public Health Service had a relatively narrow mission—chiefly providing care to merchant seamen and certain other Federal beneficiaries. No coordinated administration of health activity existed. There was no Department of Health, Education, and Welfare (DHEW). During the next twenty-

* The views expressed here are those of the authors and do not necessarily represent the views of their institutions. The authors gratefully acknowledge the assistance of Jeremy Waletsky and Harry Cain in the preparation of this manuscript.

five years citizen concern regarding health care grew and began to be heard. Congress and the executive branch devoted more time and attention to health issues. Finally, specific programs were agreed upon and launched, e.g., the creation of DHEW, the Food and Drug Administration (FDA), and the National Institute of Mental Health (NIMH); Medicare and Medicaid, and programs of manpower development and innovation in health care delivery.

In the past two decades the influence of the Federal Government on psychiatry and the whole field of mental health has been remarkable. In 1959, Daniel Blain wrote an excellent chapter in Volume 2, first ed., of this *Handbook*, "The Organization of Psychiatry in the United States." He noted that the Government would "on occasion assist a [University] psychiatry department in building up its faculty." In Fiscal Year (FY) 1971 on the other hand, the Federal Government provided funds to over half the nation's psychiatry departments and was the largest single source of funds for psychiatric residency training. Moreover, the Federal Government is now the nation's largest supporter of mental-health research and is supplying one-third of the public tax dollars spent for mental-health services (see Community Mental Health Center Program below).

Because the Federal Government has become a major force in the mental-health arena, its decisions have profound influence. It seems prudent now more than ever for mental-health professionals to grasp the basic principles of Federal policy formulation and to sharpen their capacity to contribute to this public process.

(The Structure of the Federal System

The constitutionally mandated branches of the Federal Government are the executive, the legislative, and the judicial. Career civil servants at the level of bureau chief and below (e.g., the Commissioner of the Food and Drug Administration) can be thought of as an informal fourth branch of Government, the bureaucracy, since they do not always carry out the directives of their politically appointed superiors or of the President himself. Frequently they have their own ties and lines of communication to relevant Congressional committee chairmen.[23,47,49]

The Judicial Branch

Judicial branch decisions which influence psychiatry and mental health are not made in the same ways as executive and legislative decisions. Since mental-health professionals influence judicial decisions primarily as technical experts rather than as decision makers or political advocates, we will not discuss the judicial branch in detail. Judicial decisions, however, have shaped the definition of criminal insanity, the right of patients to treatment, the confidentiality of patient records, and the rights of physicians under Federal laws such as the Harrison Narcotic Act, to name but a few important areas of judicial activity. Judicial decisions and broader aspects of forensic psychiatry of importance to mental health professionals are discussed by Overholser,[40] Freedman,[22] Guttmacher,[27] Polier,[43] Robitscher,[45] and King.[28]

Congress

There are four Congressional Committees playing powerful roles in mental health. The House Appropriations Subcommittee on Labor and HEW (Health, Education, and Welfare) and the analogous Senate Subcommittee *appropriate* (or set aside) public funds for mental-health programs. Legislation establishing or affecting mental-health programs may be considered by a number of legislative committees or subcommittees. The two most frequently and directly involved, however, are the House Subcommittee on Public Health and the Environment, (within the Committee on Interstate and Foreign Commerce), and the Senate Subcommittee on Health (within the Committee on Labor and Public Welfare). Legislation establishing mental-health or other programs includes a level of *author-*

ized spending for the program. In each fiscal year, an appropriations subcommittee may appropriate all or a portion of this authorization limit. Several other House and Senate subcommittees consider legislation relevant to mental health. In the House, the Subcommittee on Governmental Activities (within the Government Operations Committee) has held many hearings regarding legislation in the drug-abuse area. The House Ways and Means Committee considers the crucial area of National Health Insurance. In the Senate, subcommittees related to mental-health concerns include the Subcommittee on Acoholism and Narcotics (within Labor and Public Welfare) and the Subcommittee on Drug Abuse in the Armed Forces (within the Armed Services); the Subcommittee on Intergovernmental Relations (within Government Operations); the Subcommittee on Children and Youth; and the Subcommittee on Aging (both within Labor and Public Welfare); and the Subcommittee on Juvenile Delinquency (within Judiciary). In the Senate, the Finance Committee considers health insurance. The Representatives and Senators on these subcommittees wield more influence in mental health areas than most other Congressmen.

The Executive Branch

The executive branch includes not only departments headed by cabinet officers, but also independent regulatory agencies such as the Federal Communications Commission, and organizations and individuals within the Executive Office of the President (EOP). These organizations include the very powerful Office of Management and Budget (OMB), the National Security Council, and the President's personal staff, which consists of counsellors, counsel to the President, communications director, press secretary, appointments secretary, research and writing staff, and numerous administrative assistants and their staff.

The Federal department with the greatest concern for mental health is DHEW. It has over 100,000 employees and a $72 billion budget. The 1974 organizational structure of DHEW is shown in Figure 43-1. The structure has undergone many changes in the past and undoubtedly will change in the future. Within DHEW six health agencies, collectively called the Public Health Service, are supervised by the Assistant Secretary for Health (Fig. 43-2). These agencies are the Alcohol, Drug Abuse, and Mental Health Administration (ADAMHA), which includes the NIMH, the Center for Disease Control, the Food and Drug Administration, the Health Resources Administration, the Health Services Administration, and the National Institutes of Health (NIH). The other major components of DHEW are the Education Division, including the Office of Education, and the National Institute of Education, an Office of Human Development, and two welfare agencies, the Social and Rehabilitation Service (SRS), and the Social Security Administration (SSA). It is highly significant that a major portion of Federal health expenditures pays for services administered by SRS and SSA in the form of Medicaid ($3.4 billion in FY 1972) and Medicare ($9.0 billion in FY 1972). The FY 1973 budget for health research, training, and education was $3 billion.[39]

The focal point for Federal mental-health activity in the executive branch is NIMH, which had an FY 1972 budget of $612 million. From its founding in 1946 under the Mental Health Act (P.L. 79–487) until 1967, NIMH was part of the NIH. On January 1, 1967 NIMH was given the status of an independent Bureau in recognition of its support of service and training programs in addition to the traditional NIH focus on research, and as a result of pressure by constituents and members of the bureaucracy. Less than two years later (October 31, 1968) a reorganization amalgamated NIMH with a number of service-oriented programs into the Health Services and Mental Health Administration (HSMHA), of which NIMH remained the largest part. In 1974 HSMHA was disbanded. Two independent institutes were created from NIMH components—The National Institute on Drug Abuse and the National Institute on Alcoholism and Alcohol abuse—and were joined with NIMH in a new agency, the Alcohol, Drug Abuse and Mental Health Adminis-

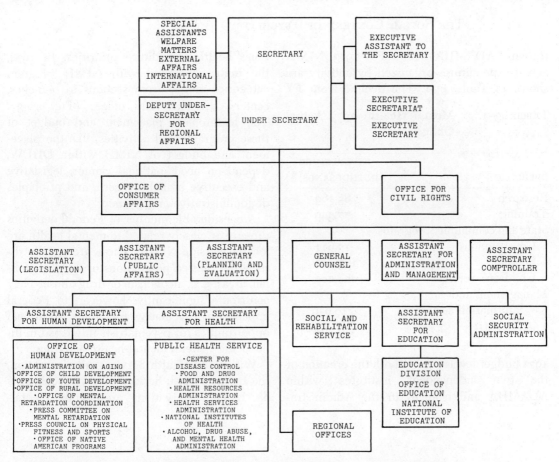

Figure 43–1. The organizational structure of the Department of Health, Education, and Welfare.

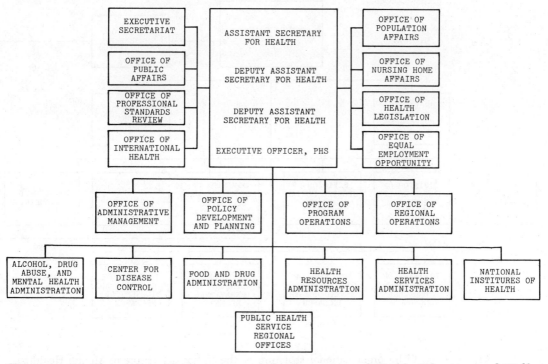

Figure 43–2. The organizational structure of the Department of Health, Education, and Welfare, Public Health Service.

tration (ADAMHA). The FY 1973 NIMH actual expenditures organized by activity are shown in Table 43–1. The decline from FY

TABLE 43–1.   **Mental Health: 1973 Actual Obligations**

OBLIGATION	EXPENDITURE (IN THOUSANDS, $)
Research	85,169
Training	77,349
State and community programs	
Construction	13,611
Staffing	165,100
Children's services	20,000
Management and information services	18,056
Total, NIMH	379,285

1972 budget levels reflects both the creation of the two independent institutes within ADAMHA and changes in the Administra-

tion's health-expenditure priorities. In 1974, the units concerned with NIMH program categories ranged from sections to branches, centers, divisions, and offices (Fig. 43–3). The hierarchical placement and budget of these programs and activities, like the placement and budget of NIMH within DHEW, depend on need, national clamor, legislative and executive branch concern, and principles of administrative management.

A considerable number of Federal activities directly or closely related to mental health are located outside NIMH. These are usually directed at limited populations or specific problem areas, e.g., alcoholism or drug abuse. They contribute significantly, however, to Federal impact on psychiatry and offer additional opportunities for psychiatrists interested in influencing Federal mental-health activities.

Within the Health Services Administration, the Indian Health Service places psychiatrists on Indian reservations and funds mental-

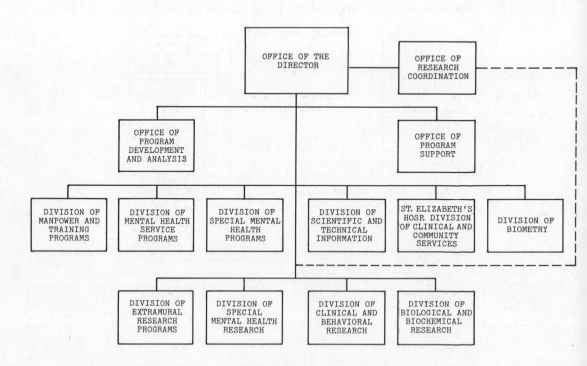

Figure 43–3.   The organizational structure of the National Institute of Mental Health.

health programs for Indians. The Federal Health Programs Service operates Public Health Service hospitals and clinics which provide mental-health services for certain Federal beneficiaries. The Community Health Service funds projects aimed at improving the delivery of health services, including mental-health services, and supports state and area-wide health planning. The Maternal and Child Health Service supports projects which include aid for emotionally disturbed children.

A number of other DHEW agencies also support or influence mental-health programs. The Food and Drug Administration regulates the development and use of all drugs, including drugs used in psychiatry. For example, before lithium was released for clinical use, the FDA evaluated the research on lithium and determined the clinical indications for which there was sufficient evidence of safety and efficacy. Some NIH research institutes, notably the National Institute of Neurological Diseases and Stroke, and the National Institute of Child Health and Human Development, support mental-health related research. In the service area, the SSA and the SRS mentioned above, reimburse citizens who qualify under Medicare and Medicaid for some mental-health expenses. Moreover, SRS, through its Rehabilitation Services Administration and its Youth Development and Delinquency Prevention Administration, funds projects which aid emotionally disturbed and mentally retarded individuals. The Office of Education, primarily through its Bureau for Education of the Handicapped, but also through their other subdivisions, funds projects related to mental health. The Office of Child Development, in the Office of the Secretary, funds service demonstration projects which may include mental health services.

Outside DHEW, mental-health activities exist throughout the executive branch. The Department of Defense supports psychiatric care for active-duty personnel. Psychiatric research is carried out at the Army Medical Center, Walter Reed Hospital, Washington, D. C., and at the Naval Medical Center, Bethesda, Maryland. The Veteran's Administration (VA) had an FY 1972 budget of $2 billion for its network of hospitals and clinics for ex-servicemen; $441 million of this total was devoted to VA psychiatric hospitals. In addition, the VA supports psychiatric training and research in its facilities. The Justice Department investigates and controls the production, distribution, and use of dangerous drugs, including several drugs used in clinical psychiatry through its Drug Enforcement Agency, which includes the former Bureau of Narcotics and Dangerous Drugs (BNDD). Criminal Justice grants from the Justice Department's Law Enforcement Assistance Administration (LEAA) often have mental-health significance. For example, millions of LEAA dollars have gone into drug abuse treatment programs. The Federal Bureau of Prisons employs psychiatrists and supports some mental-health training and research.

Support for mental-health-related services and research also originates in the Model Cities Program of the Department of Housing and Urban Development, the alcohol-prevention program of the Department of Transportation, and other executive branch agencies.

([Characteristics of the Federal Decision-making Process

The process of arriving at budgets, laws, and policies in the executive and legislative branches has certain general characteristics which the politically active mental-health advocate must recognize. These general characteristics, together with the personalities, resources, values, and goals of the individuals involved determine the substance of Federal decisions. Behind almost any particular decision lies a conflict among a number of competing interest groups (some public, some private), each with its own power base and goals. The sources of power include governmental position or access to a powerful official, skill in inter-personal relations, control over patronage positions or projects, past favors, access to the mass media, ability to deliver votes, promises of future cooperation, technical knowledge, prestige, and money.[33,56,59]

Each interest group attempts to influence the others by force of reasoned argument or through bargaining, compromising, and coalition building. Each source of power just mentioned can be used as a bargaining chip. Unwillingness to bargain and compromise frequently means defeat.[7,15]

Federal decision-makers must often act in the face of enormous uncertainties inherent in attempts to deal with social problems. It is often hard to predict the consequences of particular decisions. The consequences of past decisions may provide little guidance not only because they are difficult to assess, but also because social conditions have changed. Alternately, high Government officials may deny or resist information which demonstrates that previous decisions were wrong.[20] Moreover, few problems exist in splendid isolation and their relations to other problems cannot easily be untangled. Unfortunately, intense pressures for rapid decisions and multiple demands on limited numbers of key policy analysts and decision-makers further decreases the amount of analytical intelligence which Federal decision-makers can invest in any particular decision. This limitation, however, creates opportunities for interested individuals outside the Federal government to supply the information and analysis for which Government officials have insufficient time or resources themselves. Because of the complexities and ambiguities facing the decision-maker, and also because of the need to accommodate multiple, competing interests, he often looks for "good enough" or "sufficing" decisions rather than "optimum ones."

Decisions reached by this process are usually temporary ones. Budgets change yearly; laws are amended, repealed or allowed to fade away; policies evolve in response to public and private pressures. The decisions often are not thoroughly consistent, both because of the necessity for compromise and because no single person or agency has the time, information, or power to enforce consistency.

Budget and policy decisions are usually marked by incrementalism, i.e., changes from past practices are made gradually, in small steps.[48,57] Legislative decisions, on the other hand, can be more radical in that wholly new programs (e.g., the Community Mental Health Centers program) or wholly new governmental structures (e.g., the White House Special Action Office for Drug Abuse Prevention) can be created.

With the general characteristics of the Federal decision-making process in mind, let us now examine three specific kinds of Federal decisions: budgets, legislation, and policies.

The Budget Process

Each year the President submits to Congress a budget for the ensuing fiscal year (July 1–June 30) for all Federal organizations and activities. A preliminary draft is drawn up by the Office of Management and Budget (OMB). The OMB is a critical point in governmental decision-making processes. It both prepares the President's budget request, with input from the Departments, and oversees the administration of Federal programs. It may *apportion* (allocate or release) funds *appropriated* by Congress, or may *impound* (withhold wholly or in part) these funds. In FY 1971, for example, the President's budget contained a decrease of $6.7 million in funds for psychiatry training. Congress restored these funds to the budget in the DHEW appropriations bill, but OMB then impounded the restored funds. Only intense lobbying efforts by professional and lay mental-health groups and by DHEW officials convinced OMB to release these funds. Attitudes of OMB staff and OMB evaluations of support for psychiatric residency training and community mental-health centers will continue to influence the future of these two programs.

The OMB planning ceilings for the budget are drawn up in August and submitted to the executive branch departments and agencies for comment and suggested changes. In responding to this draft, a department is more likely to succeed in increasing funds allocated to a particular program than in increasing the total funds allocated to the department. As a result, programs in DHEW, for example, compete more directly for dollars with one another than with programs of another department. The starting point for each year's budget is the previous year's budget. Changes are usually made in small steps so that the effects of previous changes can be observed before larger steps are taken.[48,57] Exceptions to this incrementalism occur when new organizations are created in response to highly visible and politically salient issues. For example, in response to national concern over rising crime rates, Congress gave the Law Enforcement Assistance Administration (LEAA), created in FY 1969, a first-year budget of $60 million. The next three fiscal year budgets for LEAA were $267, $532, and $698 million, respectively. The Office of Economic Opportunity began in FY 1965 with a budget of $237 million. By FY 1970 the OEO budget had grown to $1.8 billion. In FY 1974, however, the Nixon Administration phased OEO out of existence.

In DHEW, the Office of the Secretary analyzes the OMB planning ceilings budget for the department and asks departmental agencies for comments on their budgets. If an agency is not satisfied with its budget allocations, it must argue its case up the departmental hierarchy. The NIMH, for example, must first convince the Administrator of ADAMHA. He in turn must convince the Office of the Secretary. The Secretary must then convince the OMB that the proposed change is desirable in the contexts of the Administration's priorities and the fiscal constraints imposed by estimated revenues and mandatory (uncontrollable) expenditures such as Medicare.[48] The President's budget, in fact, is a statement of the Administration's priorities for expending public funds. All disputes between cabinet officers and the OMB must be settled by December when the President's budget goes to press. In some instances a cabinet officer will take budget issues to the President if he has been unable to convince OMB and believes they are important enough.

The President's budget, together with a budget message explaining the budget rationale and exhorting Congress to agree, is submitted to Congress in January (see, for example, the Budget of the United States Government, Fiscal Year 1973, OMB). In both House and Senate the budget is then examined in a piecemeal fashion by subcommittees of the House and Senate Appropriation Committees. Each subcommittee has jurisdiction over a specific segment of the budget, e.g., defense, DHEW, foreign aid. Unfortunately, Congress does not weigh one budget category against another and thus rarely tries to decide how many guns versus how much butter. Beginning in FY 1977, however, this may change. The House and the Senate have each established a committee to review the budget as a whole in that fiscal year.

The Congressional Appropriations subcommittees provide the best opportunity for the mental-health constituency outside the Federal Government to influence the budgets for mental-health activities. Here, through their professional organizations and as interested citizens, they may legitimately lobby Congressmen regarding funds for mental-health programs. Abuses of "lobbying" have left the word tainted. However, lobbying can be pursued in a completely ethical manner. It derives from the constitutional right of the people to petition the Government for redress of grievances and from the need for citizens to inform their elected representatives of their wishes. Congress as an institution invites lobbying.

The structure, procedure and culture of the Congress tend to obscure the general interest, encourage particularism, and create an environment in which organized interest groups and special pleaders can be assured a sympathetic response. [p. 38][49]

Lobbying involves using the sources of power mentioned above. It takes many forms. An articulate letter or well-reasoned testimony pointing out how and why an expenditure is in the public interest is important. Informal discussions with subcommittee staff or with the staff of the Congressmen on the subcommittee are also useful. Relating the expenditure to problems and programs affecting the Congressman's constituency can be persuasive. Arranging for local or mass media coverage of the issue creates important pressures.

Public statements by respected national organizations carry weight. Recognition of the Congressman's past support and demonstrations of constituency interest are also influential.*

House hearings on the budget usually occur in February, although they may be held as late as April. Senate hearings usually occur about a month after House hearings. The subcommittee's budget figures may be changed by the full committee or by the full House or Senate, and these avenues have sometimes been pursued by lobby groups. The House and Senate vote on the budget in segments, since hearings on budget segments are finished at different times by different subcommittees.

The House and Senate subcommittees on Labor and HEW have voted more funds for certain mental-health programs than were recommended in the President's budget. This contrasts sharply with the action of most other appropriation subcommittees. The Senate appropriation usually exceeds that of the House and the difference is settled by a bargaining process in a House–Senate conference committee. Once Congress has accepted the conference committee report, this segment of budget is returned to the President for signature or veto. President Nixon, for example, vetoed a DHEW budget which he felt was too big for some programs.[38]

In deciding on dollar amounts for the President's budget, and in legislative and policy decisions, conflicts frequently arise between the President's staff, including OMB, and a cabinet officer-bureaucracy partnership. One source of this conflict resides in the different power bases to which these two groups are attuned. While the White House staff seeks to maintain the President's popularity with a national constituency, the cabinet officer, or more often the bureau chief, seeks to advocate the interests of particular groups (such as the mentally ill), and to maintain good relations with limited constituencies (such as mental-health professionals) and select Congressional committee chairmen or committee members.

* See references 10, 23, 33, 53, and 59.

A second reason for the conflict is the different time perspectives of the President's staff and the bureaucracy. While the President's staff has its eye on the two- and four-year cycle of elections, the bureaucracy is focused on maintaining and expanding programs which may take decades to fulfill their social objectives. As Seidman[49] writes:

> The bureaucracy is damned as "uncreative" because it is unable to satisfy the White House appetite for immediate solutions to complex social and economic problems and dramatic imaginative proposals for the legislative program. "Slow moving," "unresponsive," "disloyal" are among the milder epithets used to describe the bureaucracy. [p. 75]

Bureau chiefs who testify before appropriations subcommittees have a limited choice: support the President's budget or resign.

The Legislative Process

There are many steps in the legislative process, but early intervention improves the chances of success. The first step is the introduction of a bill, either by the Administration or any member of Congress. Administration bills and those introduced by the Congressional leadership are much more likely to get attention from the subcommittees. The number of bills introduced is enormous. In the Ninety-second Congress (1971–1972), 17,230 bills were introduced in the House and 4133 in the Senate. The next step is referral of the bill to a committee. Most bills never emerge from the committee; for example, only 11 percent of the bills in the Eighty-eighth Congress (1963–1964) were reported out of committee.[24] Each committee is different. Seidman writes:

> Each committee has its own culture, mode of operations, and set of relationships to executive agencies subject to its oversight, depending on its constituency, its own peculiar traditon, the nature of its legislative jurisdiction, its administrative and legislative processes, and the role and attitude of its chairman. [pp. 38–39][49]

Congressional power resides to a large extent in committee and subcommittee chairmen. A chairman can call meetings, schedule witnesses, recognize members, establish subcommittees, and appoint subcommittee members. He plays a key role in determining which bills get reported out. In the course of considering a bill, hearings may be held and individuals asked to testify. This is a propitious time for input from the mental-health community. Legislators are often weary of hearing from administrators and enjoy clinical reports from practicing professionals.

After a bill has been reported out by the subcommittee and committee, it is placed on the respective calendar in the House and Senate. In the subsequent floor debate, clarifications of the intent of the bill help shape the program which the bill creates or funds. Just as with budgetary bills, other bills passing the House and Senate are nearly always different and go to a House-Senate conference committee so the differences can be ironed out. Sometimes the differences are irreconcilable. An example of a bill that died this way is the extension of the Community Mental-Health Centers Act which passed both the Senate and the House in the closing hours of the Ninety-second Congress. The House bill called for a simple extension, whereas the Senate bill included substantive changes. After the House and Senate have approved a conference report, it goes to the President. If the President vetoes the bill, a two-thirds majority is needed in each chamber to overturn the veto.

The legislative process is one of constant and intense bargaining. Bargaining occurs not only within the Congress, but also between Congress and the President. Sources of information regarding Congressmen and Congressional processes include Bibby and Davidson,[10] Froman,[24] Goodwin,[25] Lees;[32] the Congressional Quarterly's Guide to the Congress,[16] and the Congressional Directory.

The Policy-making Process

Administrative decisions have a large impact on policy. Executive agency decisions take many forms. One form is a written statement (letter or testimony) from a Federal official taking a stand on a substantive issue raised by a private citizen, a Congressman, or a member of the executive branch. For example, Congress asked the Secretary of DHEW to take a stand on whether stimulants should be transferred to a level of stricter controls under P.L. 91–513; he agreed they should.

A second form of policy decision is allocating staff time to particular problems. For example, in FY 1972 the Director of NIMH directed a small group to work on coordinating NIMH service-oriented grants administered by the Drug Division (now the National Institute on Drug Abuse), the National Institute on Alcohol Abuse and Alcoholism (NIAAA), and the Community Mental Health Services Division. Another group was directed to develop a long-term strategy for increasing the nation's mental-health service resources.

Deciding which programs, budgets, or legislative authorities to pursue each fiscal year with the departmental hierarchy and Congress is a third form of policy decision. In FY 1972, for example, NIMH concentrated its attention on psychiatry training, extramural research, and the Community Mental Health Centers Program.

A fourth form of policy decision is changing an agency's organizational structure. For example, growing public and Congressional interest, as well as an increase in budget and responsibilities, led NIMH to elevate its Center for Drug Abuse Studies to the division level. The division was internally divided into branches corresponding to its functional responsibilities, e.g., administering contracts and grants for research, training, education, and services. The Drug Abuse Office and Treatment Act of 1972 (P.L. 92–255) converted the division to an institute in 1974. The institute was then placed on an organizational level equal to NIMH itself.

Finally, policy decisions may take the form of written regulations published in the *Federal Register* describing in detail how a law will be implemented. Although regulations cannot flatly contradict the publicly recorded Congressional intent which adheres to a legislatively created program, they can substantially influence the program's direction. For example, the NIMH drafted regulations spelling out how Public Laws 88–164 and 89–105, which created the Community Mental Health Centers Program, would be carried out. It was these regulations, rather than the law itself, which specified the size of center catchment areas (see p. 971) and required center directors to be members of one of the four core mental-health disciplines. Of course, NIMH did not make these policy decisions by itself. The regulations were written in consultation with the national mental-health organizations which had lobbied for the legislation. Moreover, the regulations had to pass through a series of DHEW clearances beginning at the agency level and ending in the Office of the Secretary. Regulations can be changed at any time. For example, the requirement that center directors be members of the four core disciplines has been expanded to include other disciplines.

In any given day, dozens of policy decisions are made at different agency or department levels. The more far-reaching or controversial the policy, the higher the level at which it is made.*

There are many checks and balances on these powers of administrators. In the mental-health field, one such check is the National Advisory Mental Health Council. It is charged with advising the Secretary of DHEW on programs of the Public Health Service involving mental-health matters. The Council must approve all NIMH grants before they can be awarded. The Council was established by the National Mental Health Act in 1946. It has twelve members who are private citizens and includes distinguished professionals and non-professionals. A second check resides in the fact that administrative decisions must be cleared with higher bureaucratic levels. Constituency groups can influence these levels as well as the initial decisions. Congress exerts additional checks by virtue of its control over the budget.

Thus, through conflict and bargaining among many government and constituency organizations, Federal budgetary, legislative, and policy decisions are made. The decisions, however, are frequently temporary and cer-

* See references 2, 3, 12, 14, 21, 31, and 47.

tain issues return to the center of controversy like the metal ducks which rotate repeatedly through the pond in a shooting gallery. Four mental-health issues which seem certain to rotate for some time are support for psychiatric training, support for community mental-health centers, the place of mental-health coverage in national health insurance, and support for research. These issues are discussed below.

(Current Mental-Health Issues

Support for Psychiatric Training by NIMH

The support of psychiatric training by NIMH began in 1947. Initially, grants were limited to resident stipends and teaching costs, including faculty salaries, in general psychiatry residencies. Over the next decade support became available for specialized psychiatric training in areas such as child psychiatry, geriatrics, and mental retardation. Support for teaching psychiatry to medical students began in 1950. In 1956 grants became available for training psychiatrists for careers in psychiatric education. In 1959 NIMH began supporting psychiatric residency training for general practitioners. In 1960 funds were made available for psychiatrists to undertake postresidency training in research. Support for training in community psychiatry began in 1962.

The objective of all these programs has been to increase the number of psychiatrists and psychiatrically trained physicians working to meet the nation's mental-health needs. By the end of FY 1971 NIMH had supported almost 30,000 man-years of psychiatric residency training. From 1957 to 1971 more than 15,000 medical students pursued extracurricular psychiatric training with NIMH support. From 1947, when NIMH training support began, to 1971, the number of psychiatrists in the nation increased from 3000 to about 25,000.

The intention of the Nixon and Ford administrations to phase out Federal support for psychiatry training has raised serious problems for American psychiatry. The American Psychiatric Association estimates that more than one-third of all psychiatry residency positions will be lost and almost half of the positions in medical schools.[8] No study has been made of how the loss of Federal funds will affect the teaching of psychiatry to medical students, but the effect will be significant. Unlike most other medical specialties, psychiatry cannot rely on patient fees to support residency stipends and teaching costs. Other specialties generate training funds from charges for inpatient and outpatient care which are usually covered by insurance. Insurance coverage for psychiatric services is much more limited than for other medical services, particularly for outpatient care and partial hospitalization, which are increasingly viewed as treatments of choice for most psychiatric conditions. Barton[8] describes the events which followed the Administration's attempt to begin the phase-out in FY 1971. He also presents the arguments against this policy decision. Torrey,[52] in a companion article, presents the other side of the debate. During the struggle to restore the Administration's cuts in the FY 1971 training budget, it became clear that many psychiatrists did not understand the political and governmental processes outlined above, and in particular the relations between the bureaucracy, the appropriations subcommittee chairmen and the OMB. As a result, their analysis of the situation was marred.

The funding of psychiatry training for the late 1970s is uncertain. Federal expenditures have been an important stimulus to the rapid growth in the number and specializations of psychiatrists. The major question for the immediate future is, who will now pay the bill? Since "he who pays the piper calls the tune," shifts in sources of support for psychiatry training are sure to influence the educational experience of the next generation of American psychiatrists. The examination of training methods, priorities, costs, and results which financial uncertainties necessitated was a healthy one. Hopefully, funds needed to apply the lessons learned will be forthcoming.

Community Mental Health Center Program

A 1971 NIMH staff study of the financing of mental-health services put the NIMH financial contribution to mental-health services in perspective. Of an estimated $3.76 billion spent to purchase direct mental-health services in FY 1968 (not including services for the mentally retarded), public funds from tax revenues accounted for almost two-thirds (2.45 billion) and private sources (consumers, private insurance, industry, philanthropy) for one-third (1.31 billion). Of the public funds, state and local governments accounted for two-thirds (1.62 billion) and the Federal Government accounted for one-third (0.83 billion). Thus in FY 1968 the Federal Government accounted for two-ninths or 22 percent of the expenditures on mental-health services. With the growth of Medicare, Medicaid, and the population of veterans eligible for federally supported services, this proportion is probably higher today.

Within the Federal Government, the Veterans Administration accounted for 47 percent of Federal mental-health service expenditures, the Social and Rehabilitation Service (Medicaid and other programs) for 33 percent, the Department of Defense 7 percent, NIMH 6 percent, Medicare 4 percent and other programs 3 percent. The FY 1968 NIMH services budget of $49.3 million was only 2 percent of the public expenditure for mental-health services and little more than 1 percent of all expenditures (public and private) for these services. The NIMH FY 1972 services budget of $150 million represented only slightly higher percentages of these totals.

In view of its small financial leverage, NIMH has had a large impact on patterns of psychiatric care. The bulk of the NIMH services budget has been devoted to construction and staffing grants for community mental health centers (CMHC's). Each center is responsible for providing services to all residents of a geographic area (catchment area) including a population of from 70,000 to 200,000 people. From the inception of the CMHC

Program in 1963 through FY 1970, a total of $365 million was awarded to establish 420 centers, which cover catchment areas with approximately one quarter of the United States population. These catchment areas range from inner city ghettos to farmlands, from affluent suburbs to the poorest counties of Appalachia. There are 66 centers with catchment areas in cities of 500,000 or more, 206 smaller cities, and 148 centers serve large rural areas where mental-health services have previously been virtually unavailable. An index of the acceptance of the CMHC Program is the fact that two-thirds of the cost of centers now in operation is born by state and local governments and private sources. One of the goals of the CMHC Program is to improve the organization and delivery of mental-health services so that effective preventive treatment, and rehabilitative services are available to all the people of the nation. Each center must provide five services: (1) inpatient care; (2) outpatient care; (3) twenty-four-hour emergency service; (4) partial hospitalization; and (5) consultation and education services for community agencies and professional personnel. In addition to these five essential services, centers are encouraged to develop diagnostic services, rehabilitation services, precare and aftercare services (e.g., home visits and halfway houses), training activities, research and evaluation programs, and an administrative organization which will achieve the intent of the program.[30,58] In 1969, only four years after the CMHC Program began, more than 2000 psychiatrists were working part-time or full-time in centers, and centers accounted for more than 10 percent of all inpatient and outpatient psychiatric patient-care episodes.[41] More than 34 percent of new center patients had no previous mental-health service contact, indicating centers are reaching people who might not otherwise have received needed treatment.

Centers have aided the development of new therapeutic concepts such as crisis intervention, partial hospitalization, and outreach to previously underserved groups. The program has also stressed citizen participation in planning center services and formulating center policies. Center staffs are providing consultation to a wide variety of community agencies and caregivers.[42] Nearly one-fourth of consultation efforts are directed toward school personnel, reflecting an emphasis on children and preventive efforts.

Whether the CMHC program will proceed to the goal that some of its originators set— providing centers for the entire United States population—is uncertain. The Nixon and Ford Administrations believe that existing centers provide sufficient models for states and local communities to expand the program if they wish. These Administrations announced their intention to phase out Federal support because they do not favor direct Federal support for health services. So far, the Congress has disagreed and has permitted the CMHC Program to continue growing. The activities of lay and professional groups interested in mental health will have an important influence on the outcome of this Federal policy struggle.

Health Insurance

With mounting public pressure for health care as a right rather than a privilege, changes in the patterns of delivering and financing health services are inevitable. Insurance benefits will play a large role in determining the changes that occur. Coverage for mental illness in present Federal insurance programs varies. Some health programs do not include mental-health services. For example, the Health Maintenance Organization program, being developed as a form of prepaid health care by DHEW, does not require service providers to include mental-health services in their benefit package. The Federal Medicare program includes mental-health services, but limits coverage of inpatient care in psychiatric hospitals to 190 days during a person's lifetime. This limitation does not apply to psychiatric units in general hospitals. Reimbursement for outpatient treatment of mental illness is limited to 50 percent of the cost or $250 per calendar year, whichever is less. This limitation encourages inpatient treatment of older persons who might do equally well or better with outpatient care.[55] In 1971 approximately 20 million Americans were covered by Medicare and 12 million by Medicaid. Psychiatric services, however, accounted for less than 5 percent of Medicare expenditures and less than 10 percent of Medicaid expenditures. The Federal Civilian Health and Medical Program of the Uniformed Services insurance program (CHAMPUS) has been a leader in the coverage of mental-health services and has stimulated demand for similar coverage from private industry. CHAMPUS provides both hospitalization and outpatient care in civilian facilities for approximately 6 million individuals (retired members of the uniformed services and dependents of active-duty, retired, or deceased members). CHAMPUS provides unlimited coverage for outpatient mental-health services and ninety days annually of inpatient care with a renewal option and no lifetime limit. Partial hospitalization is covered under the inpatient part of the program, with two days of partial hospitalization absorbing one day's full hospitalization benefit.

The ongoing debates in Congress and the executive branch regarding health-maintenance organizations, Medicare, Medicaid, and National health insurance are critical points which mental-health professionals and constituent groups can continue to influence. The future pattern of delivery of mental-health services will be shaped in large measure by the funding mechanisms adopted for purchasing these services.*

Federal Support for Mental-Health Research

The Federal Government is the largest source of support for mental-health research. Other government levels and the private sector, however, also contribute to this effort. State governments make a major contribution through their support of State universities, and in some states, research institutes and research units associated with state mental hospitals and other clinical facilities. City and county governments provide indirect support

via funds for hospitals and clinics where research is carried on. The contribution of private foundations and other organizations is also significant; in FY 1968 it was estimated by NIMH to be more than $12 million.

As mentioned above, a number of Federal agencies support mental-health-related research. Federal support is concentrated, however, in the NIMH, which had an FY 1972 research budget of $99 million. In FY 1972 NIMH supported almost 1450 different research studies ranging from the molecular to the cultural level. While it is impossible to catalogue the results which researchers have achieved over the past twenty-five years with NIMH support, the information produced underlies much of today's clinical practice. It includes knowledge regarding neurotransmission mechanisms; increased understanding of drugs to treat anxiety, depression, schizophrenia, mania, hyperkinesis, Parkinsonism, and narcotic addiction; and new perspectives on the relation of culture and social class to the prevalence and forms of mental illness. Researchers supported by NIMH have been active in developing the new treatments which have evolved in the past twenty-five years— group psychotherapy, milieu therapy, behavior therapy, and the use of peer and therapist modeling. They have helped to clarify the genetics of schizophrenia; the effects of early environment on children's social development and intelligence; and the nature of human perception, memory, and judgement. Research is continuing in all these areas and many more, e.g., the nature and functions of sleep, relations between brain and behavior, biological rhythms, biofeedback, psychotherapy, alcoholism, drug abuse, and psychodynamic aspects of attitudes. But Federal support for mental-health research is leveling off rather than growing at a rapid rate. The need to invest research dollars wisely, therefore, is more important than ever.

An NIMH staff task force has examined the entire NIMH research program. The task force asked questions about research substance as well as administrative practices. The issues raised are familiar. How much support for basic research versus applied research? For

* See references 4–6, 13, 26, 35, 44, and 50.

investigator-initiated research versus contract research? Which areas are ripe for breakthroughs in understanding? Which areas have been improperly neglected? Can the field fruitfully absorb more resources? If so, how can they be generated?

Just as in training and service areas, psychiatrists and other mental-health professionals are needed who are willing to engage in the political and governmental processes which determine the nature of Federal support for mental-health research. The concern for humanity and the intellectual vigor which researchers bring to their research are equally valuable in the continuous struggle over public policy.

Finally, we would like to raise a few points of appraisal. The trend in the Federal management of domestic programs is clearly toward decentralization. This does not mean that the Federal experience was in vain, but rather that the same policy-influencing techniques which have been used at the Federal level are needed at the state level. For example, two-thirds of the public-health dollars devoted to mental-health services are currently provided by states and local governments.

Sound evaluation is growing more and more important, not only to justify programs to budget committees, but to help program managers make realistic decisions. If programs are to survive, their advocates must master the language and tools of cost-effectiveness.

The American mental-health movement has come a long way in the past few decades. We have moved from a system of asylums and patchy private care toward a national network of coordinated community services. A highly skilled professional and paraprofessional cadre of mental-health manpower has been developed, although it still falls short of national demands. We are now basing clinical practice on a much firmer foundation of scientific evidence gained from a Federal research effort, intramural and extramural, of unparalleled quality. Our goal must be to ensure that these programs continue. To achieve this we must expand our knowledge base to include a sophisticated understanding of the dynamics of the political process, and the roles of Federal, state and local governments in the mental health arena.

(Bibliography

1. ALINSKY, S. *Rules for Radicals.* New York: Random House, 1971.
2. ALLISON, G. "Conceptual Models and the Cuban Missile Crisis," *Am. Polit. Sci. Rev.,* 63 (1969), 689–718.
3. ALTSHULER, A. *The Politics of the Federal Bureaucracy.* New York: Dodd-Mead, 1968.
4. AMERICAN PSYCHIATRIC ASSOCIATION. *APA Guidlines for Psychiatric Services Covered under Health Insurance Plans,* 2nd ed. Washington: American Psychiatric Association, 1969.
5. AUSTER, S. "Insurance Coverage for Mental and Nervous Problems: Developments and Problems," *Am. J. Psychiatry,* 126 (1969), 698–705.
6. AVNET, H. "Psychiatric Insurance—Ten Years Later," *Am. J. Psychiatry,* 126 (1969), 667–674.
7. BANFIELD, E. *Political Influence.* New York: Free Press, 1965.
8. BARTON, W. "Federal Support of Training of Psychiatrists: A Case Study in Public Policy Formation," *Psychiatr. Ann.,* 2 (1972), 42–59.
9. BERLIN, I. "A Queston of Machiavelli," *N.Y. Rev.,* 15 (1971), 20–32.
10. BIBBY, J. and R. DAVIDSON. *On Capitol Hill: Studies in the Legislative Process.* New York: Holt, Rinehart, & Winston, 1967.
11. BLAIN, D. "The Organization of Psychiatry in the United States," in S. Arieti, ed., *American Handbook of Psychiatry,* Vol. 2, 1st ed., pp. 1960–1982. New York: Basic Books, 1959.
12. BRAYBROOKE, D. and C. LINDBLOOM. *A Strategy of Decision: Policy Evaluation as a Social Process.* New York: Free Press, 1963.
13. BURNS, E. "Health Insurance: Not If, or When, But What Kind?" *Am. J. Public Health,* 61 (1971), 2164–2174.
14. CAIN, H. Doctoral Thesis, Florence Heller School, Tufts University, 1972.
15. CATER, D. *Power in Washington.* New York: Vintage Books, 1964.

16. CONGRESSIONAL QUARTERLY SERVICE. *Congressional Quarterly's Guide to the Congress of the United States: Origin, History, and Procedure.* Washington: Congressional Quarterly Service, 1971.

17. DEPARTMENT OF HEALTH, EDUCATION, AND WELFARE. *Marihuana and Health.* Report to Congress from the Secretary of Health, Education, and Welfare, no. 56–310. Washington: U.S. Govt. Print. Off., 1971.

18. ———. *Marihuana and Health.* Second Annual Report to Congress from the Secretary of Health, Education, and Welfare, HSM 72–9113. Washington: U.S. Govt. Print. Off., 1972.

19. ———. *Alcohol and Health.* First Special Report to U.S. Congress from the Secretary of Health, Education and Welfare, December 1971, HSM 73–9031. Washington: U.S. Govt. Printing Off., 1972.

20. ELLSBERG, D. *Papers on the War.* New York: Simon & Schuster, 1972.

21. FELDMAN, J. and H. KANTER. "Organizational Decision Making," in J. March, ed., *Handbook of Organizations.* Chicago: Rand McNally, 1965.

22. FREEDMAN, L. "Forensic Psychiatry," in A. Freedman and H. Kaplan, eds., *Comprehensive Textbook of Psychiatry.* Baltimore: Williams & Wilkins, 1967.

23. FREEMAN, J. L. *The Political Process: Executive Bureau-Legislative Committee Relations.* New York: Random House, 1965.

24. FROMAN, L. *Congressional Process: Strategies, Rules and Procedures.* Boston: Little, Brown, 1967.

25. GOODWIN, G. *The Little Legislatures: Committees of Congress.* Amherst: University of Massachusetts Press, 1970.

26. GORMAN, M. "The Impact of National Health Insurance on Delivery of Health Care," *Am. J. Public Health,* 61 (1971), 967–971.

27. GUTTMACHER, M. *The Role of Psychiatry in Law.* Springfield, Ill.: Charles C. Thomas, 1968.

28. KING, R. *The Drug Hang-up: America's Fifty Year Folly.* New York: Norton, 1972.

29. KOENIG, L. *The Chief Executive.* New York: Harcourt, Brace and World, 1964.

30. KORAN, L. and B. BROWN. "The Community Mental Health Center—An Approach to Comprehensive Health Services," in L. Corey, et al., eds., *Medicine in a Changing Society.* St. Louis: Mosby, 1972.

31. LACY, A. "The White House Staff Bureaucracy," *Trans. Soc. Sci. Mod. Soc.,* 6 (1969), 50–56.

32. LEES, J. *The Committee System of the United States Congress.* London: Routledge and Kegan Paul, 1967.

33. MCCONNELL, G. *Private Power and American Democracy.* New York: Knopf, 1967.

34. MENINGER, W. *The Crime of Punishment.* New York: Viking Press, 1968.

35. MEYERS, E. "Insurance Coverage for Mental Illness: Present Status and Future Prospects," *Am. J. Public Health,* 60 (1970), 1921–1930.

36. NATIONAL COMMISSION ON MARIHUANA AND DRUG ABUSE, 1st Report. *Marihuana: A Signal of Misunderstanding,* pp. 456–964. Washington: U.S. Govt. Print. Off., 1972.

37. NEUSTADT, R. *Presidential Power.* New York: Wiley, 1960.

38. NIXON, R. M. "Veto Message of Labor-HEW Appropriation Bill," *Congress. Q. Almanac,* 26 (1970), 19A–21A.

39. OFFICE OF MANAGEMENT AND BUDGET. *Special Analyses. The Budget of the United States Government, Fiscal Year 1972,* OMB 4101–0067, pp. 149–173. Washington: U. S. Govt. Print. Off., 1971.

40. OVERHOLSER, W. "Major Principles of Forensic Psychiatry," in S. Arieti, ed., *American Handbook of Psychiatry,* 1st ed., Vol. 2, pp. 1887–1901. New York: Basic Books, 1959.

41. OZARIN, L., C. TAUBE, and F. SPANER. "Operations Indices for Community Mental Health Centers," *Am. J. Psychiatry,* 128 (1972), 1511–1515.

42. PAPANEK, G. "Dynamics of Community Consultation," *Arch. Gen. Psychiatry,* 19 (1968), 189–196.

43. POLIER, J. *The Rule of Law and the Role of Psychiatry,* Baltimore: The Johns Hopkins Press, 1968.

44. REED, L., E. MYERS, and P. SCHEIDEMANDEL. *Health Insurance and Psychiatric Care: Utilization and Cost.* Washington: American Psychiatric Association, 1972.

45. ROBITSCHER, J. *Pursuit of Agreement: Psychiatry and the Law.* Philadelphia: Lippincott, 1966.

46. ROSSITER, C. *The American Presidency.* New York: New American Library, 1956.

47. ROURKE, F. *Bureaucracy, Politics and Public Policy.* Boston: Little, Brown, 1969.

48. SCHULTZE, C. *Setting National Priorities:*

The 1972 Budget. Washington: Brookings Institution, 1971.

49. SEIDMAN, H. *Politics, Position and Power.* London: Oxford University Press, 1970.

50. SOMERS, H. and A. SOMERS. "Major Issues in National Health Insurance," *Milbank Memorial Fund Q.,* 50 (1972), 177–210.

51. SORENSEN, T. *Decision Making in the White House: The Olive Branch and the Arrows.* New York: Columbia University Press, 1963.

52. TORREY, F. F. "Psychiatric Training: The SST of American Medicine," *Psychiatr. Ann.,* 2 (1972), 60–71.

53. TRUMAN, D. *The Governmental Process.* New York: Knopf, 1964.

54. UNITED STATES CONGRESS. *Hearings before the House Subcommittee on Departments of Labor and Health, Education and Welfare,* Ninety-second Congress, First Session. Part 2. Health Services and Mental Health Administration (Testimony on the NIMH Budget), 115–214. Washington: U.S. Govt. Print. Off., 1971.

55. UNITED STATES SOCIAL SECURITY ADMINISTRATION, Office of Research and Statistics. Financing Mental Health Care under Medicare and Medicaid, S/N 1770–0167. Washington: U.S. Govt. Print. Off., 1971.

56. WINTER-BERGER, R. N. *The Washington Pay-off: An Insider's View of Corruption in Government.* New York: Lyle Stuart, 1972.

57. WILDAVSKY, A. *The Politics of the Budget Process.* Boston: Little, Brown, 1964.

58. YOLLES, S. "United States Community Mental Health Program," in A. Freedman, and H. Kaplan, eds., *Comprehensive Textbook of Psychiatry,* pp. 1533–1536. Baltimore: William & Wilkins, 1967.

59. ZIEGLER, H. *Interest Groups in American Society.* Englewood Cliffs, N.J.: Prentice-Hall, 1964.

CHAPTER 44

PSYCHOLOGICAL AND PSYCHIATRIC ASPECTS OF POPULATION PROBLEMS

Warren B. Miller

([Introduction

IN 1615, the population of the world was half a billion. In 1930, it had reached two billion. In 1970, it was three and one-half billion, and, in slightly more than one generation, at the beginning of the twenty-first century, the world population will have reached close to seven billion.[68] The same kind of escalation of population growth has taken place in the United States. In 1790, at the time of the first census, the population was less than four million. By 1860, it was 31 million; by 1900, it was 76 million; and by 1950, it was more than 150 million.[66] Projecting into the future, it is estimated that our population will reach 300 million shortly after the start of the twenty-first century, and, one hundred years from now, depending in large part upon whether American families maintain a two- or three-child average, the population will number between 340 million and almost one billion.[29,158] These figures certainly justify the current wide-spread public concern with population growth, and the problems of bringing it under control. It seems timely, therefore, to discuss in some depth the psychological aspects of current population phenomena, particularly as these have a bearing for the psychologically and behaviorally oriented clinician.

The systematic consideration of the relationship between psychological and demographic variables is a generally new but important endeavor. In the past, demographers implicitly used psychological-level concepts in the process of data collection, or when giving explanation and substance to their broad, normative statements. Psychologists and psychiatrists, on the other hand, used demographic variables to define and describe the degree of heterogeneity of their clinical population. With but a few notable exceptions, there has been comparatively little interdisciplinary work. This chapter will attempt to bridge the gap between these two levels of discourse through a consideration of both psychodemography, the study of the effect of individual decision-making and other psychological processes on population variables, and demopsychology, the study of the effect of population variables on individual behavior. Because these two areas are so broad, the focus of discussion will be primarily, sometimes even exclusively, on clinically relevant variables. It is hoped that such an approach will serve to bring together the basic concepts relevant to both psychological clinicians and demographers, and to outline the current issues and boundaries of knowledge of mutual concern. It should also delineate the modes of action which are available to the clinician and through which he may have an effect on current population problems.

Demography is the study of population phenomena. Historically, it grew out of the very practical need of governments to know some elementary facts about their people. It was based on such data-gathering procedures as the periodic census and the regular registration of vital (life and death) events.[118] Petersen distinguishes between formal demography, or "a gathering, collating, statistical analysis, and technical presentation of population data," and population analysis, which is the "study of population trends and phenomena in relation to their social setting."[118]

This chapter is devoted to the psychological and psychiatric aspects of population analysis. Traditionally, demographers have utilized the basic triad of fertility, mortality, and age composition in the analysis of changes in a given population. In this chapter, an expanded, more psychologically oriented approach will be used to organize discussion. We will distinguish between two types of population variables: structural and dynamic. The structural variables of size, distribution, and composition are inherent aspects of any population. Directly and indirectly, they affect the psychology of each individual member. The dynamic variables of fertility, mortality, and geographic mobility result from, or are affected by, individual decisions and behavior through which they have an aggregate effect on the population. Because it seems to be a completing link in the overall system of variables,[135] we will also consider status mobility among the dynamic properties.

Because of the current focus on fertility and population growth, it is tempting to confine our discussion to this area. However, fertility is greatly affected by the other dynamic and structural elements of the population system defined above and, in turn, has important influences on them. In fact, all of the major elements of demographic analysis are mutually interactive to a significant degree. Since this has been well illustrated by others,[53,135] a single, hypothetical example will serve our purpose here. Let us assume that a small nation, with a stable population, has a crude birth rate of 45 per 1000, and a crude death rate of 25 per 1000 each year, and thus a stable growth rate of 2 percent (close to the average for the world at present). Let us assume that the net migration in and out of this nation is close to zero, and that there is a typical pyramidal social-class structure, with the social mobility rates of individuals from the lower classes upward being matched by the corresponding rates downward from the upper and middle classes. Finally, let us imagine that the nation is largely rural in terms of land area (approximately 85 percent), but that about half the population lives in urban and suburban areas.

Given this situation, it is possible to illustrate how each demographic variable affects the other. For example, if, through the introduction of modern medical techniques, the crude death rate is decreased to 15 per 1000, then the population size will increase more rapidly at the rate of 3 percent per year (close to the average for the developing nations of the world). Since a reduction in infant mortality will be the first and major mortality change, more babies will survive into and through childhood, changing the age composition in the direction of a more youthful population. Initially, this will increase opportunities for work as a result of the expansion of farming and industry in order to meet the growing needs of the young. These work opportunities, in turn, may increase certain types of in-migration. However, in fifteen to twenty years, when the greater numbers surviving infancy and childhood reach working ages, job competition will increase. The economic effects of this may itself depress fertility levels, and it may produce an increase in migration out of the country to areas of greater work opportunity. Finally, since improved mortality would almost certainly favor the lower class, and thus its greater differential growth, there would quite probably be a net increase in upward social mobility as a result of the tendency to maintain similar social-class proportions.

Let us further suppose that, along with the introduction of modern medical technology, there was the successful establishment of a widespread contraceptive-service delivery system and the development of a favorable attitude toward birth control. Let us say this resulted in the reduction of the crude birth rate from 45 to 25 per 1000. This reduction in fertility would have a number of effects. The growth rate of the nation would come down to 1 percent (close to that of the United States at present). There would be a decrease in maternal mortality and a smaller average family size. These, together with a later age at marriage (a probable outcome of increased use of contraception), would increase the availability of women to the labor force. This itself would probably have the ultimate effect of further decreasing fertility. It would also, together with other social forces leading toward urbanization, tend toward the urban migration and upward social mobility of individuals and couples unemcumbered by many children. These latter movements would, in turn, undoubtedly have a major impact upon the spatial and social-class distribution of individuals within the nation.

This brief illustration should provide the reader with a sense of the many, potentially important interconnections between demographic variables. It is for this reason that the following discussion is designed to embrace the whole field of population analysis, rather than focus exclusively on the subject of most obvious, current interest, namely, fertility and fertility control. Such a broad discussion lends itself well to a general systems approach, one which explicitly acknowledges the interconnections on each level of analysis (psychological and demographic) and between levels of analysis. It is the interlevel connections which will be the main topic of this chapter, organized according to the seven fundamental structural and dynamic variables of demography. These variables have themselves been subgrouped into three prominent subsystems, which form the subject for the three main sections which follow. Within the sections, each variable will be discussed with respect to: (1) demographic and psychological concepts which are relevant to it; (2) current issues which bear upon it; and (3) modes of professional action through which psychologically oriented clinicians may affect it. In order to limit the field, and because of the author's greater familiarity with the American scene, the focus of discussion will be on the United States.

⟮ Fertility, Mortality, and Size

The fertility–mortality–size triad forms a natural population subsystem. To be sure, geographic mobility (in the form of migration) often has an important effect upon the size of a particular population, and, in some cases, such as in economically depressed areas, is the most significant determinant of change of population size with time. Nevertheless, geographic mobility interacts more specifically with population distribution, and as may be seen in Figure 44–1, which represents the overall population data for the last forty years for the United States, may have a relatively smaller effect on size than fertility and mortality.

The theory of demographic transition has special relevance to the fertility–mortality–size subsystem. This demographic theory postulates that all societies move from an initial phase of high birth and death rates, through a

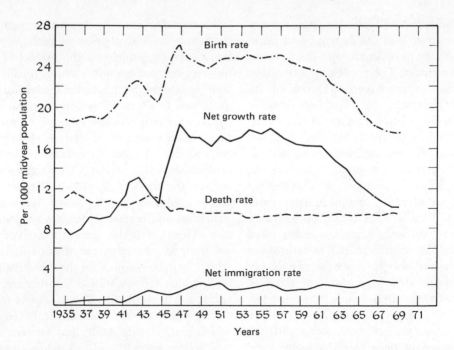

Figure 44–1. Annual rates of births, deaths, net immigration, and net growth in the United States from 1935 to 1969.
Source: United States Department of Commerce, Bureau of the Census, Population Estimates and Projections, Series P–25, No. 442, March 20, 1970.

transitional phase of high birth and low death rates, to a final phase of low birth and death rates. It will be recognized that this sequence roughly parallels the steps through which the hypothetical illustration was carried in the previous section. It is during the transitional phase that the population expands most significantly. Theoretically, at least, during the initial and final phases, the size is more nearly stationary, due to a relatively close balance between births and deaths. Although there are many significant exceptions to this theory, it is one of the best established theories in social science, and still sufficiently useful to find continued application.[85] For our purposes here, it provides a special illustration of the dynamic connectedness of size, fertility, and mortality.

Fertility

RELEVANT CONCEPTS

Because of differences between demographers and biologists in traditional use, there is some general confusion about the meaning of such concepts as fertility and fecundity. For the demographer, fecundity is the biological capacity to have children, while fertility refers to the number of children actually had by an individual or a population. Biologists, on the other hand, often use these concepts in exactly the opposite way. In this discussion, we shall follow the demographic usage. Furthermore, we shall refer to the decreased biological capacity to have children as subfecundity, and to the biological inability to have children (the extreme form of subfecundity) as sterility.

There are a number of important concepts which demarcate the area of fertility behavior at the demographic and psychological levels. We have already made use of an important demographic concept, i.e., the crude birth rate. This expression refers to the ratio of total births to total population during a specific period of time, usually one year. Conventionally, crude birth rate is stated in terms of births per one thousand population. Because the crude birth rate is based on data which include all ages and both sexes in the population, it does not always accurately reflect a population's reproductive behavior. A more refined concept is the general fertility rate, or the number of births per 1000 women in the fecund ages, generally assumed to be between fifteen and forty-five years. A further refinement of this concept, important in that it allows computation of the extent to which a population is replacing itself, is achieved by calculating age-specific fertility rates, often based upon five-year age groupings.

Demographers are interested not only in rates, but also in social norms. With respect to fertility, they are particularly interested in the norms which govern reproduction, especially those concerning family size and birth intervals. In order to measure these norms, demographers look at actual family sizes and birth intervals, and ask people about their ideal, desired, and expected family sizes and birth intervals. These data are gathered through general survey techniques by what must be considered by individually oriented clinicians as somewhat superficial methods. Nevertheless, this kind of approach produces interesting and potentially useful data.[131]

Because of the great social importance of controlling fertility, demographers in their surveys and theoretical work have made distinctions between wanted and unwanted conceptions (also, pregnancies or children). Pohlman[121] has reviewed some of the theoretical and methodological problems inherent in the concept of an unwanted pregnancy by examining such questions as: "Unwanted to whom?," "Unwanted at what psychological level?," and, "Unwanted at what point in time?" His analysis highlights the complexity of the concept of "unwantedness," a complexity which is only confounded by the gathering of data through a survey method. In spite of these problems, Bumpas and Westoff,[17] in a widely quoted article, reported data which they believe indicate the degrees of child-wantedness in the married United States population as a whole. Their method provides what is perhaps best seen as a measure of the "intendedness" or "planfulness" of a conception.

At the psychological level, there is a whole set of behaviors which relate to fertility. These are most readily discussed if they are divided into the following four categories: (1) sexual behavior, or behavior which has sexual stimulation or gratification as part or all of its goal; (2) conceptive behavior, or behavior which has the achievement (proceptive behavior) or the prevention (contraceptive behavior) of conception as its goal; (3) abortion-seeking behavior, or behavior which has the termination of pregnancy as its goal; and, (4) procreational behavior, or behavior which has the bearing and raising of children as its goal.

The author has discussed these categories in some detail in another context.[105] It is noteworthy that sexual, conceptive, and procreational behavior have not always been readily separable in practice. It was only after knowledge of the ovulatory cycle was acquired and effective contraception was developed that sexual and procreative behavior could be separated. It was only with perfection of a coitus-independent method of contraception (for example, the Pill or the IUD) that contraceptive behavior could be separated from sexual behavior. (The same may be said for a coitus-independent method of insemination and proceptive behavior.) Now that these distinctions can be made at a practical level, it is apparent that each set of behaviors is subject to its own social norms and affected by its own group of psychological antecedents.

Social norms regarding these behaviors are undergoing rapid change. For example, sexual norms are becoming less restrictive;[20] contraception is gaining wide acceptance;[168] and family-size norms appear to be becoming significantly smaller.[169] It is likely that such changes will alter the importance of personality variables in the expression of these behaviors; thus, where norms become less restrictive, as they are with regard to premarital sexual behavior, individual factors may assume more importance; where norms become more restrictive, as seems to be happening with family size, they may assume less importance. Changes in the restrictiveness of norms will also alter the type of personality variables which affect fertility behavior; thus, with the relaxation of premarital sexual norms, one might expect a shift away from traits of rebellion and alienation as significant factors in premarital pregnancies, with a shift toward traits perhaps of immaturity and dependency.

In addition to social norms, access to information and to technological means serve to moderate the importance of personality variables in fertility behavior. Without knowledge about sexual and conceptive processes, and without the mechanical and chemical means of contraception, psychological factors which affect decision-making probably have a smaller influence on fertility. For example, in certain lower-income populations, social constraints on access to contraceptive information and contraceptive means appear to play a greater role than motivational factors in the occurrence of out-of-wedlock conceptions. On the other hand, in a community and social-class group where social constraints were much less a factor, a study by the author[108] showed that a group of effective contraceptors and a matched group with unwanted pregnancies were not distinguished by their level of sexual knowledge or their previous use of contraception, although there were significant personality and coping variable differences between them.

What are some of the psychological variables which influence fertility behavior under relatively unrestricted conditions? For sexual behavior, they seem to be, most importantly, feelings about the sexual experience and its associated psychological elements, such as intimacy, trust, and pleasure. For contraceptive behavior, they include attitudes toward the physical effects of particular contraceptive methods (e.g., blood clots or "body pollution" from the pill, decreased genital sensation with the condom) and feelings about the psychological effects of particular methods (e.g., distaste for self-manipulation with the diaphragm, or feeling a lack of personal control with the IUD). Finally, for procreational behavior, they include aspirations regarding family life and feelings about family involvement. These and other relevant psychological dimensions will be discussed more specifically in the next section.

Many of the same considerations apply to the psychological antecedents of abortion-seeking behavior. Lee[89] has discussed the importance of knowledge about abortion and access to it. Her data were generated at a time when illegal abortions were virtually the only type of induced abortion available in this country. However, because of continued societal ambivalence toward induced abortion, social constraints through limitation of access to information about abortion and to the means of achieving it are still major factors affecting abortion-seeking behavior.

Abortion-seeking is also influenced by social norms and personal feelings about having an abortion. As will be discussed in the next section, the social norms are currently undergoing a major change in the United States. Since the decision to obtain an abortion is generally made after consideration of the alternative courses of action, specifically, early marriage, adoption, out-of-wedlock childrearing, abortion-seeking behavior is also influenced by the social norms and personal feelings which govern these other behaviors. Whether personality traits or coping styles, or other psychological factors play an important part in abortion-seeking behavior is still an open question. Some preliminary work has been done in this area,[113,54] but adequate exploration is only just beginning.

CURRENT ISSUES

Let us begin this section by considering some psychological aspects of subfecundity. Whelpton et al., have calculated from a national survey that 31 percent of married couples between the ages of eighteen and thirty-nine are subfecund and that about one third of these (11 percent of all couples) are definitely sterile.[170] About one half of the definitely sterile group have had contraceptive operations (vasectomy or tubal ligation), and about one-third of these (i.e., about 2 percent of the entire sample) had undergone the surgery for other than health reasons. Thus, the psychological antecedents to nonhealth-motivated contraceptive surgery are important for a small but significant proportion of the married population in this country, especially since recently there are definite trends toward an increased use of vasectomy for the purpose of birth control and family-size limitation. These trends appear to be greater in the western United States,[170] where some local communities have reported as much as 16 percent of the married, male population having had vasectomy.[119]

While there is little data to indicate which psychological variables influence the selection or avoidance of surgical contraception, the main motive is to terminate fertility at the end of the procreational career. What psychological consequences does such surgery have on individuals and couples? Although there are many enthusiastic reports and testimonials, the best evidence suggests that some men and women may react to such surgery with feelings of demasculinization or defeminization and some degree of rigid, hypermasculine (or hyperfeminine) behavior.[127] However, the severity and prevalence of this type of reaction is not known and it seems quite likely that, as with abortion, with the change of societal norms toward increased acceptance, this negative psychological reaction will tend to subside.

For those subfecund couples who do not fall in the "definitely sterile" class, there is an important two-directional relationship between subfecundity and contraceptive use. On the one hand, the individuals least likely to use contraception are those who doubt their own ability to conceive for medical reasons, for reasons related to their own experience with conception exposure, or for reasons related primarily to self-image and fantasy. On the other hand, those who use contraception the least are most likely to discover their own subfecundity. For these reasons, there are higher rates of nonuse of contraception among the relatively subfecund. This has special importance during adolescence and menopause. It has been calculated that the percentage of fully fecund adolescents increases from about 5 percent at age thirteen to about 95 percent at age eighteen.[33] Similarly, it has been demonstrated[170] that subfecundity increases from around 5 percent at ages eighteen to nineteen, to about 25 percent around age twenty-nine, to almost 50 percent by age forty. Although not reported in Whelpton's

study, it is well recognized that fecundity drops to virtually zero during the fifth decade. These periods of high subfecundity (below about age sixteen and above age forty) are associated with changing patterns of contraceptive use and a relatively higher rate of overall nonuse of contraception. Thus, these are times of higher risk for unwanted pregnancies.

Turning from the psychological aspects of fecundity to those of fertility, an important contemporary focus has been the running debate among demographers and family planners as to what constitutes the best way to achieve fertility limitation in the United States.* An important issue in that debate has been the question of whether the prevention of unwanted pregnancies alone would suffice to end population growth. Those who say it would, argue that the provision of effective family planning and birth-limitation services, and the efficient use of these by the population, would bring the United States down to a zero rate of growth. Their opponents argue that large numbers of unwanted children is only part of the problem, and that the other part lies in the fact that American couples want too many children. In order to shed some light on this debate and because the distinction between wantedness and unwantedness has obvious relevance to mental health, the discussion in the remainder of this section will focus, first, on unwanted and, second, on wanted pregnancies.

Bumpass' and Westoff's findings[17] leave little doubt that the incidence of unplanned and unwanted pregnancies within marriage in this country is substantial. They analyze and present their data in terms of number failures (i.e., births occurring after a family has had all the children it wants), and timing failures (i.e., births unplanned but not causing a family to exceed its desired family size). They found that approximately 20 percent of all births between 1960 and 1965 were number failures. As might be expected, the percentage varied with birth order, being 5 percent and 8 percent with the first two children respec-

* See references 35, 8, 165, 65, 9, 148, 17, and 79.

tively, and 44 and 50 percent with the fifth and sixth child. The number-failure percentages were found to be significantly higher for the black population, and for the poor and the near-poor. These investigators further found that of the remaining births (the 80 percent which did not represent number failures), 43 percent were timing failures. In their conclusion, they discuss the importance of their findings for the family-planning debate. The usual way of measuring a population's "desired family size" is by asking married women how many children they desire. In 1965, the answers led to an average figure of 3.4 children. Bumpass and Westoff,[17] on the other hand, calculated "desired family size" by subtracting the number of unwanted births (number failures) from the total number of actual births, and arrived at an average figure of 2.5 children. They argue that, since their method tends to underestimate unwantedness, the 2.5 figure is falsely elevated, and the real figure is probably very close to the mean family size of 2.1 which is necessary to achieve zero growth.

Bumpass' and Westoff's data bear only on legitimate childbearing. Unwantedness is of much greater importance with conceptions occurring outside of marriage. Illegitimate births already constituted almost 10 percent of the total fertility[159] in the late 1960s and recently the rate of illegitimacy has been increasing.[32] These trends are, in part a consequence from relaxation of premarital sexual standards and behavior,[20] which result in greater premarital exposure to the chance of conception. They may also reflect, to some degree, relaxation of the social and economic sanctions which work against out-of-wedlock births and child-rearing.

What are some of the psychological antecedents to an unwanted pregnancy? Both within and without marriage, sexual behavior and the individual's feelings about it are of major importance. There is evidence that young, unmarried women who hold values running counter to premarital sexual activity or who experience conflicts in this area of behavior are more likely to have an unwanted pregnancy when they become sexually active.[108] It is as though their values and conflicts prevent them from perceiving themselves as sexual beings and thinking about themselves in adult sexual terms. Sexual behavior within marriage is related to unwantedness in a similar way. Rainwater[123] describes how women who find sex gratifying in marriage are better able to cooperate and communicate with their husbands to achieve effective contraception.

As this last observation suggests, an individual's or couple's actual contraceptive behavior has a great bearing upon the occurrence of unwanted pregnancy. Although the pill, the IUD, and foam have added greatly to our contraceptive armamentarium since the mid-1960s, we are a long way from finding methods that can and will be used effectively by all couples. Each contraceptive method is reacted to differently by individuals,[175] and each method requires a different combination of psychological sets and behavioral skills on the part of the individual for effective use. The author has suggested[104] a group of behavioral dimensions which are essential for the effective use of a particular contraceptive method. These are shown in Table 44–1, where the methods are grouped according to the behavioral prerequisites for effective use which they share. In terms of more traditional personality traits and their effect on contraceptive behavior, there is a growing body of knowledge.[81, 82,108,172] Today, the evidence suggests that effective use of contraception is associated with the following kinds of personality traits: future orientation; internal control, independence, and autonomy; flexibility; and achievement orientation. These findings are very preliminary, especially considering that the investigations have been done almost exclusively with women.

Turning next to procreative behavior and unwanted pregnancy, a major issue is the frequent assertion that unwanted pregnancies often occur as a result of covert motivations for them. The motivational basis has been discussed in terms of the wish for power, dependency, revenge, and a host of other personal meanings[91,176,44] which were viewed as deviant and/or unconscious in origin. Recently,

TABLE 44–1. **Contraceptive Methods, Grouped According to the Common Behavioral Elements on Which Their Effective Use Depends**[104]

CATEGORY OF CONTRACEPTIVE METHOD	METHODS INCLUDED IN CATEGORY	RELEVANT BEHAVIOR DIMENSION	PSYCHOLOGICAL FACTORS WHICH INTERFERE WITH EFFECTIVE USE
Coitus-dependent methods	Diaphragm Foam Condom	Delay of complete sexual response	Poor impulse control Tendency toward rationalization or denial
Abstinence methods	Abstinence Rhythm Withdrawal	Inhibition of complete sexual response	Difficulty coping with partner's sexual demands
Vaginal insertion methods	Diaphragm Foam	Genital manipulation	Distaste for touching own genitals
Methods which invade body integrity	Pill IUD	Attention to body image	Anxiety about bodily function and "side effects"
Methods which involve complex habits and cognitive processes (reasoning and memory)	Pill Rhythm	Use of habit, memory, and independent reasoning	Tendency to perform inconsistently on repetitive tasks Poor memory, reasoning ability Unstable living pattern
Male methods	Condom Withdrawal	Reliance on male partner	Low motivation to protect partner* Tendency to misjudge partner's motivation and reliability†
Coitus-independent methods	Pill IUD	Acquiring new behavior sequences‡	Present orientation Slowness in learning new contraceptive routines

* For men.
† For women.
‡ When one of these methods is discontinued.

the research literature on this subject has included better controls[162] and more prospective design,[117] along with a change in basic assumptions. For example, in a prospective study of pregnant, unmarried teenagers, the question was posed: "Are these girls pregnant because they are different, or different because they are pregnant?" The results of this and other studies[117,48] have lent general support to the latter point of view. There is probably the truth in both positions. We should realize, on the one hand, that all pregnancies are preceded by a complex set of subtle procreational motivations,[44] and, on the other

hand, that "unwanted" pregnancies result primarily from an interplay of chance, situational factors, and nonprocreational motivations.

The author has developed a method for classifying the degree to which a pregnancy is intended. Such a classification provides a way of determining the extent to which procreational (and other) motivations are involved in a particular pregnancy. Using this method, considerable data have been collected from a large heterogeneous population through clinical interviews.[106] All pregnancies of these women were rated on the following scale: Intendedness 1, conception resulted from sustained, active striving; Intendedness 2, conception resulted from ambivalent striving, as demonstrated by intermittent or incomplete efforts; Intendedness 3, conception resulted from the regular nonuse or ineffective use of contraception, with no significant intent to conceive; Intendedness 4, conception resulted from the nonuse or ineffective use of contraception on one occasion or for a brief period, with no significant intent to conceive; Intendedness 5, conception resulted during the effective use of contraception without intent to conceive. Table 44–2 presents selected data from this study, chosen to illustrate several points relevant to this discussion.

If we assume that procreational motives are located predominantly in the Intendedness 1 and 2 categories, and that they are the dominant motives in these categories (assumptions borne out by the content of the clinical interviews), the data in Table 44–2 support the following conclusions: The majority of pregnancies conceived within marriage and wanted sufficiently to be carried to term (column 4) result primarily from procreational motives; on the other hand, over 90 percent of the pregnancies conceived outside of marriage, whether carried to term or terminated (columns 1 and 2), were relatively uninfluenced by procreational motives; the subgroup of pregnancies conceived within marriage which were sufficiently unwanted as to be

terminated (column 3) were less the result of procreational motives than any other group. Stated in another way, the data support the notion that procreational motives play a relatively small part in unwanted pregnancies, when unwantedness is determined by surgical termination and/or premarital conception.

How psychiatric patients compare with the general population on the issues of unwantedness remains to be determined. There is at least one report[57] that psychopathology affects motivations for pregnancy in a major way, and that the occurrence of unwanted pregnancy is more frequent in mentally ill women. However, virtually all of the work on this subject is anecdotal, retrospective, and without appropriate comparison groups. The overall question of the antecedent effect of psychopathology on the occurrence of unwanted pregnancies needs careful exploration.

The psychological consequences of unwanted pregnancy have been the subject of many published observations and impressions, but, again, little has been done in the way of careful research. Pohlman has reviewed much of the general literature on the consequences of unwantedness.[121] Several authors have discussed the same issue from the point of view of the consequences of refused abortion.[120,5,6] It is clear that unwanted conceptions have potentially important psychosomatic effects during pregnancy, labor, and after delivery.

TABLE 44–2.   The Intendedness of Conception by Marital Status at Time of Conception, and Outcome of Pregnancy

| | UNMARRIED AT TIME OF CONCEPTION | | MARRIED AT TIME OF CONCEPTION | |
| | TERMINATED BY THERAPEUTIC ABORTION, PERCENT | CHILD BORN WITHIN MARRIAGE, PERCENT | TERMINATED BY THERAPEUTIC ABORTION, PERCENT | CHILD BORN WITHIN MARRIAGE, PERCENT |
INTENDEDNESS	N = 105	N = 32	N = 31	N = 216
1	1	6	0	58
2	6	3	0	5
3	41	59	19	15
4	28	13	26	13
5	24	19	55	9
	100	100	100	100

Even more important are the potential psychological effects on the child himself of being unwanted and consequently experiencing the gamut of hostile treatment from subtle rejection to outright physical abuse. There are also important effects upon the mother, ranging from postpartum reactions to the "tired-housewife" syndrome. Finally, unwantedness has important consequences for other aspects of family life, including the long-term, cumulative effects on the marital relationship and upon the other children.

Abortion is an increasingly available option for dealing with an unwanted pregnancy. Since the 1960s, revolutionary changes in the public attitude toward abortion have taken place. Gallup polls during the 1960s revealed an overwhelming majority of Americans disapproving of abortion on request,[10] but two polls in the early 1970s have shown a striking reversal of these figures to the extent that the majority now favors abortion on request.[94] The same period has also seen major changes in abortion-seeking behavior. At present, four states have generally unrestricted abortion laws (Alaska, Hawaii, New York, and Washington); eleven others have laws based on the American Law Institute model, or an equivalent, which allows a liberal interpretation of the conditions for induced abortion. As a result, almost 100,000 legal abortions were performed in the first quarter of 1971 in the United States.[22] This compares with an estimated 2000 legal abortions for the same length of time during the 1963–1965 period.[152] It seems very likely that induced abortion will be used increasingly to solve the problem of unwanted pregnancy by those who become pregnant because of contraceptive inefficiency or procreational ambivalence.

The societal trend toward the greater use of induced abortion is generally justified by the behavioral science research regarding the psychological consequences of abortion. In addition to the earlier Scandanavian studies, which showed that many women who were refused abortions had serious psychological problems after carrying an unwanted pregnancy to term,[71] and that children born after refused abortion had more psychological and behavioral difficulties than their controls,[45] the predominant evidence of recent reports* is that the psychological effects of abortion are mild and usually include considerable relief, hopefulness, and positive coping. In considering the relatively small proportion of untoward reactions following abortion, three conclusions stand out: (1) Those who are psychologically at risk for an abortion because of their psychopathology, are equally at risk as a result of an unwanted pregnancy and child; (2) the amount of depression, guilt, and anxiety experienced by the individual woman during and after her abortion is directly related to the attitudes toward her and her actions which are expressed by her family, friends, and medical caretakers; and (3) there is a relatively small but definite proportion of women for whom induced abortion is either contraindicated or highly problematic because of the specific meaning of the particular pregnancy and the resultant ambivalence which they hold regarding the procedure.

Turning to a consideration of wanted fertility, there are a great many different reasons parents offer for their having a child. Pohlman has listed and discussed these at great length.[121] Motivations for a child are closely related to the prospective parent's wishes and feelings in relation to his own parents and childhood, his spouse, his friends and peers, and his aspirations for the prospective child itself. These motivations may be heavily influenced by financial or religious considerations. They also may be influenced by the anticipated effect of a child on the prospective parent's familial role with respect to the spouse and the other children in the family. There are a number of special procreational motivations, such as desiring a child of particular sex, or concern with the maintenance of the family line. There are also a number of idosyncratic motives which are not well defined by social norms. In many instances, these are highly situational and may be ways of coping with family demands or personal

---

* See references 116, 144, 7, 3, and 114.

stresses. These kinds of motives border on the neurotic reasons for wanting a child, where the desire springs from an infantile wish or an unresolved conflict.

In contemporary urban society, the constellation of motives for childbearing tends to be quite different from the constellation seen in more traditional societies. In the latter, the infant mortality rate is generally high, and the child replacement motive is important. In addition, children provide economic security, both by working during childhood and by providing security for the parents in their old age. Thus, there is a strong emphasis on children as a way of preserving and perpetuating self and family. The more modern view is that children are to be enjoyed for themselves, and that parenthood provides self-fulfillment and the enrichment of marriage.

Before proceeding to a discussion of family size and child-spacing preference, we will consider proceptive behavior and the extent to which couples actually control the time sequences in their childbearing. It is surprising how little scientific information has been gathered on this subject. There may never have been any effective demand for knowledge in this area because of the ease of achieving conception relative to the need for preventing it. Whatever the reason, we know relatively little about the psychological antecedents of effective proceptive behavior or the psychological consequences of such behavior when it is ineffective. In this connection, Westoff et al.,[167] found that most couples were unable to speed up conception by orienting their sexual activity to the fertile periods. Only 20 percent of their large, nationally representative sample reported ever even trying to do this, and, of these, only one half had information about the ovulatory cycle which was sufficiently accurate as to give them some chance of success. The increasing complexity of American life, the high degree of geographic mobility of all segments of the population, and the definite ideas which Americans hold regarding birth intervals and child rearing (discussed below), all suggest that mastery over the process of conception through ego control over the psychological and behavioral antecedents to concep-

tion are becoming increasingly important in this country. In spite of this, it appears that the American population is a long way from effective mastery.[105]

Demographic research has defined some of the norms of family size and birth intervals within this country and some of the trends within these norms. For example, Ryder and Westoff[131] have demonstrated a bimodality of desired family size, with two children being the most frequently preferred number, followed closely by four. Some of this demographic bimodality is related to differences between subpopulations. Thus, white non-Catholics and blacks show a strong preference for two, while white Catholics show a strong preference for four children. These investigators hypothesize that some of the bimodality is also a result of the American preference for two and four children over three, and may be related to a desire to keep the offspring balanced for sex or to avoid the problem of coalitions of two children against one by raising children in pairs. They further suggest that the relative unpopularity of a third child may have the same psychological roots as the wish to avoid an only child.

Studies have also been done on desired birth intervals.[166,167,18] It appears that a broad range of intervals between marriage and first birth is acceptable, provided the interval allows time for couples to become adjusted to marriage and financially ready for children, and enjoy each other's company for a time before turning to parental responsibilities. There is also a wide range of acceptable second birth intervals (the interval between the first and second child), and some agreement that spacing children more than four years apart significantly reduces the likelihood of their becoming close companions. The most salient rational consideration in determining the length of the third birth interval (the interval between the second and third child) is allowing the oldest child enough time to develop sufficient independence, so that the mother is not overburdened with dependent demands from three small children at once. In a later interpretation of their data,[18] Westoff and his colleagues suggest that the desired total family size and the desired span of fertility (the period from the first to the last child) are the most important considerations for a couple in determining individual birth intervals. Thus, women who want five, rather than two, children (other things being equal, especially age at marriage), tend to have much shorter birth intervals. These authors also point out that education is negatively related to a woman's span of fertility, suggesting that the more educated woman wishes to complete her childbearing sooner in order to be free for other types of role activities.

These decisions regarding child-spacing and family size have important psychological consequences for the growth and development of all children in the family. In the coming decades, social pressure to control population growth will significantly alter the pattern of these decisions. As a consequence, the average size of the American family will change from three to about two. There will be more childless couples and, probably, more one-child families; there will be far fewer large families of five, six, and seven children. These changes will have direct effects upon the family milieu, particularly upon female roles, and child rearing and development. There will be more first and fewer third and fourth children. So little is known about the effect of ordinal position on personality development that the psychological consequences of this change in family composition cannot be foreseen. However, considering the importance of social learning in most theories about personality development and the genesis of psychopathology, such variables as a child's ordinal position, the size of his family, and density of his sibship may be assumed to have considerable mental-health relevance. Clearly, much investigative work remains to be done in this important area.

A feature of American life which profoundly affects voluntary fertility and which currently seems to be undergoing considerable change is the nature of feminine roles. For example, since World War II, there has been a significant increase in the labor-force participation of American women.[125] While all the implications of this are not certain, the evidence suggests that female labor-force participation and fertility are simultaneously related in at least the following three ways: (1) subfecund women, after a certain period of time, turn to labor for an alternative to family building as a focus of their time and energies; (2) women who have a large number of children relative to the number they can afford, tend to work in order to supplement their family income; and (3) women limit their fertility so that they can go to work in order to supplement their family income or devote themselves to another sphere of creativity.[125,133] In relation to these three possibilities, Whelpton et al.,[170] found that women who worked because they wanted to had fewer children than those working out of necessity, and that the latter, in turn, had fewer children than those who did not work at all. This demographic finding has been extended at the psychological level by the work of Clarkson et al.[26] They found that women who perceived themselves as being high on a cluster of competency traits had fewer children than women who perceived themselves as low on this cluster. Furthermore, only the high self-esteem group was able to work or not work, independently of the number of children they had. The low self-esteem group showed a negative relationship between the number of work years and number of children. These findings suggest that low self-esteem and low general competency may interfere with the processes described under numbers (2) and (3) above. Of course, part of the observed relationship may also be explained by the especially poor self-image associated with depression and withdrawal which may occur in some women as a result of having too many children.

It seems that American women are combining marriage, child-rearing, and work more than ever before,[125] and it may be that recent declines in fertility are directly related to this. These findings may also presage the beginning of a more profound change in the female role and self-image which will significantly alter the corresponding male roles and American family life in general. In that case, not only can we expect more childless or "couple" families,[150] but we can also expect to see increasing periods of nonfamily living during the life cycle (both before and after marriage), increasing use of day centers for infant and child care, and increasing involvement of men in the expressive aspects of family life. Again, the implications that all of these changes have for personality development and the shaping of psychopathology in the child deserve considerable investigation.

Modes of Professional Action

Direct psychological services to women and couples with unwanted pregnancies take a variety of forms and occur in a number of institutions. The majority of such services are designed for the unmarried woman, but, with the recent increase in legal therapeutic abortions, married women with unwanted pregnancies have become an important segment of the population needing such services. Psychological clinicians can provide treatment themselves, especially when they work in an appropriate setting, such as a psychiatric clinic, or with a high-risk population, such as delinquent girls. In addition, they can provide indirect services by consulting with physicians involved with family-planning clinics and abortion services, and with other professionals and paraprofessionals working in schools and colleges, welfare and probation agencies, problem-pregnancy clinics, organizations for unwed mothers, and adoption agencies.

There is also a great need for preventive services. In another context,[104] the author has outlined a series of recurrent hazard points in the sexual and procreational careers of women, at which times they have an increased risk of an unwanted pregnancy. These hazard points are listed below.

1. During early adolescence
   a. When fecundity is absent or low but increasing, and, as a consequence, contraceptive vigilance is incompletely developed.
2. At the start of the sexual career
   a. At the time of the first few intercourses, for which there is typically no contraceptive preparation.

b. During the following three to six months, until the individual recognizes and acknowledges the beginning of her sexual career.
3. In relation to a stable sexual partner
   a. While the relationship is in the stage of development, before a stable sexual and contraceptive pattern has been established.
   b. During conflict and/or separation, when patterns of communication and cooperation are disrupted.
   c. After breakup with a partner with whom a particular sexual and contraceptive pattern has been established.
      (1) When situationally re-exposed to the old partner but without access to the previous contraceptive method.
      (2) When exposed to new partners with different sexual and contraceptive styles.
4. After geographic mobility
   a. When there are major changes in the social field such that sexual and contraceptive norms and opportunities change.
      (1) After moving away from home and nuclear family.
      (2) After moving to a new sociocultural area.
5. In relation to marriage
   a. Just before or just after, when contraceptive vigilance is commonly relaxed.
   b. During conflict and/or separation (same as 3b).
   c. After separation or divorce (same as 3c).
6. After each pregnancy
   a. During the postpartum period, when there is subfecundity, altered sexual activity, and, often, the use of interim contraceptive methods.
   b. When a new level of contraceptive vigilance is required as a result of the demands brought about by a new baby.
7. In relation to the end of childbearing
   a. When the decision to stop having children is being dealt with.
8. During menopause
   a. When fecundity is decreasing and, as a consequence, contraceptive vigilance is waning.

By identifying women with respect to life-cycle stage, these hazard points suggest institutions and help-giving agencies with which the woman is most likely to be in contact, and where preventive counseling and anticipatory guidance may be practiced. As an example, let us consider the hazards which occur at the beginning of a sexual career. In the United States, in spite of the widespread acceptance and use of contraception, it is the exception rather than the rule when an unmarried woman plans and uses contraception on the occasion of her first intercourse. Presumably, this is because of the strong affective meanings attached to this particular act and because of the widely held prohibitive norm regarding premarital intercourse. Thus, by chance alone, one would expect a certain number of unwanted pregnancies occurring around the time of first intercourse. In fact, this is borne out by experience. The author, in a survey of over 1300 women receiving therapeutic abortions at a large, general hospital,[107] found that a small but consistent proportion of the unmarried, adolescent patients reported that they had become pregnant on their first, second, or third intercourse.

After the first few intercourses, a second risk factor becomes important. Most of those who continue sexual activity after their first few experiences with intercourse experience a growing concern with the risks they are taking. Some of these young women are precipitated into taking action by the high anxiety generated by a perceived near miss, that is when there is a slight delay in the onset of one of their menstrual periods during the first few months after the initiation of sexual activity. Others respond to an increasing amount of peer-group advice. Still others act simply as a result of the growing realization that they have, in fact, begun an active sexual life. However, there are some women who disregard these social, psychological, and physiological warnings. Encouraged by their failure to become pregnant after a few unprotected exposures (often a result of adolescent subfecundity), they become less and less anxious during the next few months of unprotected intercourse.

The first type of risk-taking behavior results from conflicted feelings about sexual activity and poorly defined self-expectations. The second type is a result of the way some adolescents cope with threat and anxiety through denial and suppression, thus failing to progress to the normal stage of taking precautionary action. Since a large proportion of these two kinds of risk-taking will occur among women who are in high school or college, it should be possible to launch preventive counseling and educational programs geared to deal with these specific hazard points.[107]

Preventive work can also be done through health and educational outreach programs in the communities where poverty and social disorganization retard the development of adequate sources of information regarding sex, contraception, and pregnancy planning, and prevent the effective delivery of related services. For the psychological clinician, such work may involve the training and supervision of paraprofessionals regarding the emotional and interpersonal aspects of fertility behavior, helping in the development of meaningful programs designed to influence that behavior, and actively participating in concept development, research, and program evaluation.

In addition to work in the area of unwanted pregnancies, the psychological clinician can affect decision-making and planning of wanted pregnancies. This can be accomplished by helping individuals with decisions regarding a particular pregnancy or regarding "background" decisions which lead to marriage or significantly affect sex roles. These same choice points can be affected if the clinician works to provide indirect services and at the level of program development and evaluation. In these ways, he can help to maximize the wantedness of pregnancies in a given community.

This section is summarized in Table 44–3, indicating the many different kinds of counseling which can affect fertility, and placing them in a rational framework based upon the kinds of decisions being made. Such a framework, organized according to dominant life-cycle processes and focal issues, suggests the most appropriate timing and focus of intervention.

TABLE 44–3.   **Typology of Counseling**

TYPES OF COUNSELING	FOCUS OF CONCERN
Sexual	Decisions and problems related to sexual behavior
Virginal	The decision to initiate sexual activity and the associated problems
Nonmarital	Decisions and problems related to nonmarital sexual behavior, especially for adolescent and postmarital individuals
Marital	Decisions and problems related to marital sexual behavior
Contraceptive	Decisions and problems related to contraceptive behavior
Marriage	Decisions and problems related to marriage, the marriage partner, and family life
Premarital	The decision to marry and the associated problems
Marital	Problems and conflicts within marriage
Divorce	The decision to divorce and the associated problems
Procreational	Decisions and problems related to planning for childbearing
Genetic	Decisions and problems associated with the prevention of genetically determined undesirable characteristics and the selection of genetically determined desirable characteristics
Birth-planning	Decisions and problems related to planning for the number and timing of children
Proceptive	Decisions and problems associated with efforts to conceive
Pregnancy	Processes and problems associated with pregnancy
Infertility	Problems leading to and resulting from infertility
Adoption	Decisions and problems associated with adoption
Sterilization	Decisions and problems associated with permanent termination of the procreational period through sterilization
Problem-pregnancy	Decisions and problems related to an unwanted or ambivalently regarded pregnancy
Abortion	Decisions and problems associated with seeking and having an induced abortion
Child-placement	Decisions and problems associated with the placement of an unwanted child

Mortality

RELEVANT CONCEPTS

The most elementary mortality concept is that of the crude death rate, or the number of deaths per year per 1000 persons in the population. This measure is analogous to the fertility measure of crude birth rate, and, as with the latter, there are more refined kinds of mortality rates which are specific for age and sex. These are useful to demographers because they allow more accurate comparisons between populations with different age compositions. Another useful way of conceptualizing mortality is in terms of life expectancy, most commonly expressed as the average expectation of life at birth. The figures for the United States in 1966 were 66.7 years for males, and 73.8 years for females.[161] Life expectancies at all ages are calculated from statistical tables known as "life tables."

There are other ways of making death rates more specific and thus more useful. For example, the United Nations has classified the causes of death into five major types, according to their responsiveness to public-health and medical-care programs.[155] This makes it possible to compare death rates for these five groups and draw conclusions about societal needs for health programs. For psychodemographic purposes, it may be useful to develop a more behaviorally oriented classification, where categories would be determined by similar psychological antecedents. For example, without substantial modification of the present system for the collection of data on causes of death, such a classification might be as follows: death resulting from (1) nonpreventable illness, adequately treated; (2) nonpreventable illness, inadequately treated; (3) preventable illness, adequately treated; (4) preventable illness, inadequately treated; (5) accident; (6) suicide; (7) homicide; and (8) war. While the psychological and psychiatric relevance of such a scheme is apparent, the concepts developed below should make it even clearer.

The following are some of the broad areas of behavior relevant to mortality. Because of limitation of space, these will not be discussed in detail, and consideration will be limited to the psychological antecedents of mortality.

1. *Health-maintenance and health-compromising behavior.* These two aspects of behavior may be distinguished conceptually. However, they are here discussed together because of considerable overlap in the practical application. In health-maintenance behavior health is a positive goal, and the individual acts to maximize his physical fitness and subjective well-being by such activities as appropriate exercise and rest, appropriate feeding, and pursuit of preventive health care. In health-compromising behavior, on the other hand, physical health is risked for the sake of some competing goal. Examples of such behavior include smoking, eating a high-fat diet, driving at high speeds, certain high-risk sports, working under sustained high-pressure conditions, etc. These two subcategories of behaviors are influenced by the relative salience for the individual of competing health and non-health goals, and the ways that these are inte-

grated by him, as determined especially by his coping and life styles.

2. *Illness behavior.* This category includes an individual's behavior in reaction to an illness, in seeking help for it, in readjusting during recovery, and in adapting to a residual disability or chronic illness. These types of behavior have been discussed at some length by Mechanic.[99] He hypothesizes a set of psychological characteristics which influence illness behavior. Somewhat modified for our purposes here, these include: (1) the individual's perception of deviant physical signs and symptoms; (2) his knowledge of or assumptions about their meaning; (3) the extent to which these signs and symptoms pose a psychological threat or disrupt ongoing functions; (4) the individual's coping or defensive style in the face of physical threat or disability; and (5) the relative psychological benefits and costs of seeking help and (in the case of chronic illness) continuing to use it.

3. *Accident behavior.* This category includes behavior which tends to involve an individual in an accident in a specific situation or in accidents generally. Some behaviors included here, such as certain kinds of risk-taking, are special instances of health-compromising behavior. However, because of the high accident mortality in this country and because of the importance of formulating a behavioral approach to this subject,[59] accident behavior is included here under a separate category.

4. and 5. *Suicide and homicide behavior.* These are the behaviors disposing individuals to suicide and homicide and preceding such actions. Both of these, especially suicide behavior, have long been of special interest to psychological clinicians. Homicide behavior includes the behavior of both the victim and the perpetrator of the homicidal act. It is noteworthy that both of these individuals are well-known to each other in the majority of murders and both seem to participate in the homicide process.[149] In many cases, the victim's behavior seems to be a type of suicide equivalent. Many behavioral scientists have devoted their attention to suicide and homicide behavior, and recent reviews discuss the

various theoretical approaches and the complex psychological antecedents to these two types of violent death.[124,4,34]

In this brief discussion of the behavioral concepts relevant to mortality, we have focused on individual psychological antecedents and have not commented upon interpersonal or dyadic factors. Such an exclusion is most obviously deficient in connection with homicide, where, in a fashion parallel to fertility, there is a "doer" and a "done to," and, in many instances, dyadic psychology is essential to an understanding of the process. Dyadic psychology has some importance in other categories of mortality as well. Many suicide deaths closely involve the psychology of a significant other person and many preventable medical deaths are contributed to by family members or physicians who participate with a patient in his denial of illness or the mismanagement of his medical condition.

CURRENT ISSUES

A major issue with respect to population growth is the question of what will happen to the death rate in the United States in the future. Petersen has calculated that the average life expectancy doubled from prehistoric times to the Middle Ages, then remained more or less the same until the nineteenth century. In the last 100 years, it has doubled again.[118] In the United States, the crude death rate per 1000 has dropped from about 17 in 1900 to between 9 and 10 in the 1960s.[157,160] This decrease occurred before 1950. Subsequently, the death rate has been level or even slightly increasing. These trends suggest that the death rate in the United States will not significantly decrease in the future, barring some unforeseen medical developments, even though it has not reached the low points achieved in other nations (7.6 and 7.2 per 1000 in Canada and Russia, respectively, in 1964). Whereas in 1900, the leading causes of death were influenza, pneumonia, tuberculosis, and gastroenteritis, these diseases have been replaced by heart disease, cancer, and stroke. These are all diseases of late life or secondary to degenerative processes. Even though these diseases appear to be less influenced by psychological and behav-

ioral antecedents than some of the causes of death dominant earlier in the century, there is still ample room for the development of knowledge regarding the role of health-maintenance, health-compromising, and illness behavior in the mortality of these diseases. This knowledge will become increasingly important as our population ages.

An examination of the causes of death in specific age groups suggests one group in which the psychological antecedents to death play an unusually prominent role. Accidents are the leading cause of death from age one to thirty-four, and account for more than one half of all deaths in the age group fifteen to twenty-four. In this latter group, homicide and suicide are the fourth and fifth leading causes of death. Were there to be a major societal effort at death control through an investigation of the psychological antecedents to death, this late adolescent to early adult age group would very likely be a primary target.

Another important issue for mortality behavior is the lack of a comprehensive approach to death control. One way of conceptually unifying the psychological antecedents to mortality is through consideration along the wanted-unwanted continuum, as was done above with fertility. Shneidman has pioneered discussion of the roles that individuals play in their own demise and has offered a schema for classification.[141] Such a schema can be used to classify the degree and type of individual intention, thus providing some measure of the extent and character of psychological antecedents. The following categories, which parallel the ones used in the discussion of fertility, classify death according to the intendedness of the antecedent behavior: Intendedness 1, where death was sought and brought about with definite conscious intent; Intendedness 2, where death was sought and brought about with clear ambivalence, as demonstrated by considerable vacillation in deciding or by an impulsive decision; Intendedness 3, where there was a regular exposure to a significant possibility of death with little or no adequate protection against that possibility but no conscious intent; Intendedness 4, where there was a situational exposure to a significant possibility of death without adequate precaution and no conscious intent; and Intendedness 5, where death resulted from factors totally outside the control of the individual.

In this schema, suicides would generally be included in categories 1 and 2. The same would be true of homicides with respect to the perpetrator. "Manslaughter," commonly conceptualized as an accident, would be included in categories 3 and 4. With respect to victims, homicidal deaths would generally be included in categories 3 through 5. Many accidental deaths would fall into category 5, but those which represent self-exposure to unusual risk[30] would be included in categories 3 and 4. Of course, when a death should be considered accidental is not always clear, and a certain number of accidental deaths are, in fact, consciously intended suicides, putting them in categories 1 and 2. Finally, deaths which result from a delay of help-seeking in response to the development of threatening physical signs and symptoms, or from mismanagement on the part of the patient of his chronic medical condition represent a form of category 3 and 4; as with accidents, some of these cases may actually fall into categories 1 and 2.

Modes of Professional Action

Psychological clinicians provide a number of direct and indirect services in connection with mortality behavior. In the general hospital and in medical clinics, much work is done with medically ill patients through the mode of psychiatric or psychological consultation and psychotherapy in an effort to intervene against self-destructive illness behavior. While there is a great deal of indirect (consultative) work done with suicidal and homicidal individuals in nonpsychiatric facilites, a large number of cases, especially of suicidal patients, are handled in direct care. Often, accident victims receive consultation and therapy for help with psychological consequences of an accident. In some instances, this work is expanded when, after his injury, the patient recognizes his own role in the "accident."

Preventive action to help in death control is another aspect of the psychological clinician's role. Through informational and educational programs, the public can be made more aware of the concept of self-destructive behavior and of its social-communicational features (i.e., as "a cry for help"). Then they may be made aware of the community services which are available to provide such help. There are also preventive health programs which emphasize positive health goals, some of which deal with health risks, such as those associated with smoking, poor diet, or promiscuous sexual activity, and some of which focus on the early detection and treatment of serious disease. Finally, with respect to accident prevention, there are numerous informational and educational programs in industry and the community in general.

The psychological clinician is also essential in the study of mortality behavior. He may participate in the development of concepts for research and the evaluation of programs which help with death control. However, professional action in this area is consuming of resources, and, at this point in time, the psychological clinician must weigh the relative personal and demographic merit of commitment to behavioral research in the area of death control rather than birth control.

(Population Size

In this section, we shall consider briefly the effect of population size upon individual psychology. For discussion purposes, we shall distinguish between direct effects, where the individual is aware of population size and is affected through his perception, and indirect effects, where the individual is affected by aspects of the social environment which are themselves influenced by population size.

Considering first the indirect effects, there are two aspects of the social environment which seem to be influenced by population size: the size and types of social institutions and the number and types of interpersonal contacts. Although much has been written which touches on these two areas, we shall limit ourselves by drawing only upon a few recent publications. Barker has reviewed the literature on the effect of institutional size upon individual psychology.[2] On the basis of this review and his own research, he found that there was a negative relationship between group and organizational size and the amount of participation, involvement, and satisfaction which the individual developed during his activities within that group or organization. If we assume that larger populations generate larger and more complex social institutions, then it may be concluded that, as a population grows, individuals tend to experience these decreased amounts of participation, involvement, and satisfaction.

With respect to the effect of population size upon interpersonal relations, Milgram has discussed three aspects of a city's population which affect interpersonal experience: the number, density, and heterogeneity of people.[100] He suggests that all three of these variables affect the city dweller, producing, when they are pronounced, a tendency toward noninvolvement, impersonality and competitiveness, and a functional approach to interpersonal relationships. He explains this effect in terms of adaptation to a stimulus overload, suggesting that city dwellers adjust their personal relations to high social-field input by various interpersonal screening and inhibitory processes.

Such indirect effects of population size almost certainly have mental-health implications. For example, Cassel has pointed out that most cross-cultural blood-pressure studies show that individuals living in small, cohesive societies tend to have blood pressures which are low and not positively correlated with age.[21] He hypothesizes that, in part, this is because people living in such small societies have been subjected to less stress. However, convincing studies are lacking, and whether there is a positive relationship between population size and stress remains to be established.

The direct effects of population size upon individual psychology have not been widely studied. One way to conceptualize this relationship is to consider the largest social or demographic unit with which an individual identifies himself. Over fifty years ago, before the development of modern means of communication and transportation, it was not unusual for individuals to identify themselves primarily with relatively small demographic units, namely, the family, the clan, or the town. The nation itself was an upper limit of reference for most and often a relatively weak one. Today, identification at the level of smaller units continues to be important, but many people also identify themselves readily with regional, national, and international units. For some, there is even a somewhat urgently felt identification with the whole human race, vividly suggested by the "spaceship earth" concept. Much of this broadening of the population base of identification, self-reference, and community feeling has been augmented by technological advances, especially in the areas of communication and transportation. Nevertheless, it is clear that individuals have concerns and fantasies about the population of which they feel a part, and that the size of that population will affect these psychological states together with the level and nature of involvement in their community.

(Distribution and Geographic Mobility

In this section, we shall be concerned with the structural and dynamic aspects of the way a population is located in space. The two main variables, population distribution and geographic mobility, constitute a second population subsystem. Because population distribution is a structural variable and has some demopsychological properties in common with the topic of population size, we shall maintain continuity with the preceding section by considering distribution first before turning to the dynamic variable, geographic mobility.

Some aspects of the recent relationships between the geographical distribution of the American population and its geographical movement are illustrated in Figure 44-2, which shows the relative growth and decline of the three basic community types in the

United States during the last three decades. Much of this changing pattern of population distribution has been accomplished through geographic mobility. Since rural, urban, and suburban areas have different characteristic densities, the pattern also represents relative changes in population density.

Distribution

The population density in the United States varies greatly. This is well demonstrated in Table 44–4, which shows data illustrating the continuum between the average national population density and one of the most densely populated areas in the world, residential Manhattan. In order to consider the other end of the density spectrum, one need only recall that there remain a number of very large wilderness areas within the United States, and that many states contain hundreds of square miles which are totally uninhabited.

At present, the public is concerned with overpopulated areas and crowding, and we shall emphasize these problems in our discus-sion. However, in keeping with the systems theme of this chapter, it should be kept in mind that large sections of our country are becoming depopulated and perhaps under-populated. Thus, during the discussion of the relationship between high population density, on the one hand, and such psychological vari-ables as personal values, subjective states, and psychological stress, on the other, it is impor-tant to keep in mind that there are important, corresponding relationships between low pop-ulation density and similar psychological vari-ables.

There are both positive and negative as-pects of either increasing or high population density. As Winsborough has discussed,[174] the advantages and disadvantages are epit-omized by the historically opposed theoretical positions of two sociological groups—the be-haviorally oriented group associated with Georg Simmel, and the structuralist group associated with Émile Durkheim. The behav-iorists, on the one hand, have argued that high density leads to high psychological and physi-ological strain. The structuralists, on the other

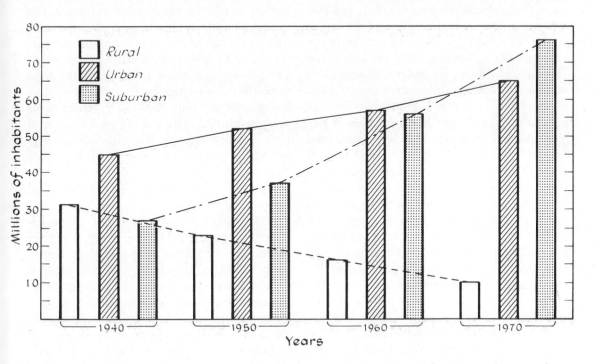

Figure 44–2.　The population in rural, urban, and suburban areas for each decade, 1940 to 1970. **Source:** Population Bulletin 27 (October 1971), 2.[156]

TABLE 44–4.   The portion of the United States population density spectrum lying between the middle range (the U.S. average) and the upper limit (one of the most compacted cities in the country).[149]

	UNITED STATES	NEW YORK METROPOLITAN AREA	NEW YORK CITY	MANHATTAN	RESIDENTIAL MANHATTAN
Population density, in persons per square mile	50	3,000	25,000	90,000	380,000

hand, have argued that high density leads to a refined development of the division of labor, thus allowing greater expression of each individual's aptitudes and needs. These opposing points of view serve to illustrate, at the beginning of our discussion, that a particular population density, or the movement of a population with time from one density to another, cannot be adequately measured or evaluated along one or even a few simple dimensions.

RELEVANT CONCEPTS

There are several demographic measures or expressions of density: (1) persons per unit space (e.g., people per square mile); (2) persons per functional unit (e.g., people per room or per household); (3) functional units per unit space (e.g., housing units per acre); and (4) functional units per functional unit (e.g., housing units per building structure).[49] Each of these ratios measures a different facet of population density and has a different demo-pyschological meaning. This is substantiated by the work of Galle et al.,[49] who demonstrated that, in the Chicago area, measures of social pathology, such as juvenile delinquency or public assistance rates, were best correlated, first with persons per room, and second with housing units per structure, while mental hospitalization rates were best correlated with rooms per housing unit. We can understand this finding if we assume that a high number of persons per room promotes intrafamily stress, that a high number of housing units per structure promotes interfamily stress, and that a low number of rooms per housing unit promotes a situation where there are many people living alone.

A somewhat distinct population density measure is that of population potential.[70] This is a summed, person-to-distance ratio which takes into account the number of people not only in the particular area under study but in all contiguous areas. This sort of concept may be helpful in exploring the role that open areas in and around highly populated areas play in relieving the distressful aspects of high density.

Factors other than spatial density may be important in relating population distribution to individual psychology. Although we will not consider them in detail, some of the following may be important parallel measures to spatial density: (1) temporal density, measured in terms of the number of persons per unit time to whom individuals are exposed; (2) privacy, measured in terms of the total available private space or the private-to-public space ratio per individual); (3) social isolation, measured in terms of the total number of close relationships or the ratio of close-to-superficial relationships per individual; and (4) use-intensity,[50] measured in terms of the amount of interpersonal contact per individual per subarea of space.

It is probable that a number of social-ecological aspects of the community buffer or accentuate the effect of population density upon individual psychology. A list of such variables would include, at the very least, some of the physical properties of the environment, such as noise, light, visual qualities, and the architectural use of space.[60] It would also include social institutions, together with certain important dimensions along which they vary. Important among these institutions might be the family, especially as it varies along the nuclear extended dimension; work institutions, especially as they vary along the role-development dimension; political-governmental institutions, especially as they vary along the dimension of individual involvement alienation; and, ultimately, the overall culture or subculture, especially as it varies along the dimensions of homogeneity and cohesion of norms and values. Another set of ecological variables which may moderate density effects deals with the interaction between environment potential and individual or group needs. These are important because it appears likely that density effects are greater where the environment constrains, inhibits, or is, in other ways, incongruent with behavior. Barker's concepts of a behavior setting, and the degree to which it is over- or undermanned is an example of this type of moderating variable.[2] Finally, since increased density is frequently associated with the increased complexity of role behavior, some of the concepts of social-role theory, such as role differentiation, role complexity, and role strain may provide moderating variables which are useful in studying how density affects individual psychology.

Among the most fundamental psychological concepts relevant to the study of population distribution are the concepts of personal space. Horowitz has developed the concept of the body-buffer zone, a small area extending from the surface of an individual's body which is perceived as an extension of his body into the space around him and which affects the way he spaces himself with respect to other people and objects.[73] The anthropologist, Hall, has discussed personal space in terms of four types of distances that people maintain between themselves and other peole, depending upon the situation.[60] He has called these distances intimate, personal, social, and public. They vary from close, i.e., with body contact, to distant, i.e., with 25 feet or more between persons, and each has a definite function. Another aspect of personal space is dealt with in the concept of territory.[74,69,60] While this concept was originally developed from observations of animal behavior, humans also develop a sense of territory, both spatially

(e.g., at home or at work) and symbolically (e.g., in fields of competence), and there is little doubt that the concept has some useful application to man as well.

The psychological concepts of importance to density effects are not limited to the area of space. Also important are the effects upon arousal and related behavior of other people's presence, including social facilitation[177] and social-stimulus overload.[100] Additional kinds of concepts of some relevance are those which refer to interpersonal traits, such as Murray's need affiliation and autonomy, and those which bear on individual-institution and individual-culture interaction, such as internal versus external control,[129] modernity,[146] and inner-directedness versus other-directedness.[126] Finally, because it appears that high density can be stressful, the gamut of psychological concepts of coping and adaptation are relevant.

The concepts of crowding and overcrowding are commonly used in discussions of density. At the psychological level, these represent subjective states in response to social and physical conditions. Exactly which conditions are perceived as crowded depends greatly on cultural values and conventions regarding interpersonal transactions,[23] customary stimulation levels, and the duration, location, and purposes of density exposure. The Great Plains farmer probably feels crowded in Manhattan. Many Americans do not feel crowded in a tightly packed sports stadium until it is time to go home. The exact relationship between stress and feeling crowded, or between the latter and pathological behavior, is an unresolved question.

CURRENT ISSUES

The major current issue, a direct outgrowth of rapid population growth and the concentration of peoples in subareas of the nation, is the question of the extent to which high density has a detrimental effect upon the quality of life. This is an extremely difficult issue to resolve. First of all, it is hard to separate out density as a variable from other social, economic, and political factors. Secondly, the "quality of life" is itself complex, including some elements which, because they depend upon personal values, are unanswerable by scientific method, and including others which depend upon answers from a wide spectrum of social and behavioral science research. In fact, relatively little careful research has been done in this area. In spite of these difficulties, the following discussion will approach the quality-of-life issue by an examination of how high density may affect psychological stress and adaptation.

Some important animal studies have probed the relationships between population density and behavior. Calhoun allowed a population of wild Norway rats to increase in a confined space with unlimited food and water.[19] After the density had reached a very high level (much higher than ordinarily experienced by man), the population stabilized. Under these conditions, he found marked disturbances in feeding and social behaviors, including territoriality, dominance, and aggression. He also found numerous sexual aberrations and frequent disturbances of pregnancy and maternal behavior which resulted in high maternal and infant mortality. Other investigators have observed similar behavioral changes in other animals under more normal conditions[25] and have also noted disturbances at the physiological level, particularly involving the endocrine systems.

There have also been important contributions regarding the effects of density from sociological studies of human communities. In a study of the community areas of Chicago, Winsborough showed strong statistical associations between density and a group of social pathology variables which were suggested by Calhoun's animal work.[174] However, these relationships disappeared for adults when socioeconomic status, quality of housing, and migration were statistically controlled. Other investigators[134] have found strong relationships between population density and social breakdown variables which did not disappear when levels of education and income were controlled. Galle,[49] studying the same areas in Chicago as Winsborough but using other measures of density, found significant correlations which also did not disappear when controlled

for social structural variables. Other evidence on these questions comes from experience with slum clearance[164] and studies of the effects of housing on stress, physical and mental health, life satisfactions, values, family activities, and friendship patterns.[136] In general, the findings suggest that crowding may, indeed, cause stress, but that people can adapt to a wide variety of density conditions, depending upon environmental conditions and their own behavior and value systems.

There have been some recent experimental studies of people under relatively controlled laboratory conditions to determine the effects of density. One series of investigations involved placing groups of various sizes in the same room and observing their behavior over a period of several hours. These studies suggest that room density does not affect individual or group-task performance,[46] although it does seem to affect interpersonal processes and affective responses.[56,37] Griffitt found that subjects evaluated themselves, others, and the room more negatively in a high-density room.[56] Ehrlich reports that men in all-male groups became significantly more competitive, severe, and unfriendly in high-density rooms, whereas women became more cooperative, lenient, and friendly. There was no differential effect of density with mixed groups. In a different type of investigation, where subjects placed human figures in a small-scale room with different assumed social contexts, Desor was able to support the hypothesis that the sense of "being crowded" was more related to space.[36] Finally, in a third type of investigation,[1] pairs of subjects were isolated for nine days in a 12-foot by 12-foot room, and their territorial behavior was studied. Among other observations, it was noted that dyad incompatibility on the personality dimensions of dominance and affiliation, but not on achievement and dogmatism, led to an increased rigidity and possessiveness of territorial behavior.

Cassel summarized what is known about the effects of population density upon health.[21] He reiterated a familiar theme, namely, that the effects of density on health depended, in some cases, on the association of density with other variables, such as poverty, poor nutrition, and poor housing. He further stated that density effects are apparent only during the period of adjustment following an individual's or a subpopulation's change in living conditions and density exposure. He also noted that the effect of density on health varies according to the degree to which an individual has membership in a supportive social group (i.e., high density is more detrimental for "marginal" people) and according to his particular status within the hierarchy of that group.

Certain themes emerge from the above observations and research on density. These themes are summarized in the general statements listed below and illustrated in Figure 44–3. (It is assumed that stress and personal distress appear at the low end of the density continuum as well as at the high end. The evidence for this has not been discussed but some of it appears in the references cited above.)

1. For each individual, there is an optimum range of population density beyond which, in either direction, he begins to experience stress, represented by the set of U-shaped curves in Figure 44-3.

2. This range varies according to the type of activity in which the individual is participating, the duration of the activity, some personal characteristics of the individual, some cultural or subcultural characteristics of his group, the nature of his relationship to the group, and some social-ecological characteristics of his environment.

3. The disruptive effects of density extremes occur within a narrower range for some psychological-behavioral dimensions (for example, affective interpersonal behavior) than for other dimensions (for example, task performance).

4. In a large population, the range of population densities to which different individuals can adjust is wide, as represented by the solid U-shaped curve in Figure 44–3.

5. For a given individual, or subpopulation, as represented by the dotted lines A and B in Figure 44–3, the range of nonstressful densities is more restrictive.

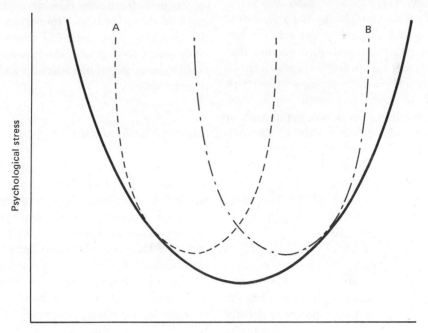

Figure 44–3.   Hypothetical curves representing the postulated curvilinear relationship between population density and psychological stress.

6. Moving an individual or subpopulation along the density dimension to a point outside his usual experience, such as from A to B in Figure 44–3, creates stress which is relieved with time with adaptation to the new conditions.

There are many density issues which have been left untouched in this discussion, in part because of their relative unimportance for clinical matters, and in part because of the absence of data regarding them. For example, we know relatively little about what Americans' density preferences are, how these may have changed during this century, and how they change during the life cycle. We know little about the importance for the relief of density stress of the public-to-private space ratio, about how large homes or single-family dwellings compensate for crowded communities, or about how the provision of wilderness areas is psychologically important to a crowded population.

As mentioned earlier, we know relatively little about the psychological impact and mental-health relevance of low and decreasing population density. The extent of such depopulation is not insignificant. During the 1960s, over half of the counties in the nation actually lost population.[67] It is reasonable to assume that areas undergoing this process suffer a form of demoralization, especially in view of our cultural emphasis upon a growth psychology. Since depopulation affects the population of an area differentially, such as through the relatively greater loss of youth, there may be other important changes in psychosocial climate associated with this process. Clearly, a great deal of work deserves to be done on the psychological impact of these trends.

MODES OF PROFESSIONAL ACTION

Psychological clinicians have an obvious role to play in the treatment of distress and interpersonal disturbance associated with the two extreme ends of the population density continuum. On the preventive and public-health side, psychological clinicians can work with community planners[90] and others who are involved in the redesign of old communi-

ties and the creation of new ones. If the continued growth of the three megapolitan areas is to be arrested, the increase in the United States' population over the next fifty years must be absorbed into small cities, secondary growth centers, and new towns.[156] It seems entirely reasonable that psychological clinicians should take part in the design of these communities, including the use of public and private space. Lemkau gives an interesting account of a psychiatrist's role in the construction of an entirely new city.[90]

Psychological clinicians are sufficiently sensitized to the various uses of space in individual and group psychotherapy, and are familiar with the effects of space arrangements on lives and communities from their experiences with therapeutic milieus. Expanding these impressions through investigation, it has been possible to demonstrate how schizophrenic patients have enlarged and distorted body-buffer zones[72] and to confirm that a patient's behavior in an inpatient unit is significantly affected by territorial considerations.[77] A growing appreciation of the important connection between self-esteem and territory has led to new treatment considerations.[28] As a result of these kinds of experiences with spatial issues, the psychological clinician is specially suited to help with the investigation and evaluation of population-density and distribution problems.

Geographic Mobility

Geographic mobility is a major feature of American life. It has been estimated that one out of five Americans changes residence every year and, during the same time period, one out of sixteen migrates to another county or region of the country.[11] Considering the same phenomena longitudinally, it is estimated that the average American will migrate between three and four times in a lifetime and may change his residence as much as thirteen times.[171] As is suggested by Figure 44–3, rural, urban, and suburban shifts represent an important segment of such geographic mobility. The three major directions of such shifts are from rural to urban, from urban to sub-urban, and from suburban to suburban areas.[13,67]

RELEVANT CONCEPTS

There are numerous types of geographic mobility, such as the wandering and ranging of primitive people, the impelled or forced movement of groups of slaves, refugees, or disaster victims, and the pioneer migration of individuals and small groups to frontier areas.[118] In this discussion, we shall consider the three important types of geographic mobility in the United States, i.e. local moving, intranational migration, and international migration. The former refers to a local change of residence, while the two latter refer to the crossing of some geographical, legal, or cultural boundary. Intranational migration includes moving to another county, state, or region within the United States.

Motivation for geographic mobility has traditionally been discussed in terms of the "push" factors which make an individual want to get away from his present location, the "pull" factors which attract him to another location, and the intervening factors.[11] Demographers have considered the "push" and "pull" factors in socioeconomic, sociopolitical, occupational, and life-cycle terms and they have viewed the intervening factors as determined by physical, cultural, and financial barriers. This approach has had refinements[88] but has essentially remained in the form of a simple hydraulic model.

Psychological and personality factors in migration have been largely unexplored. There is some reference in the migration literature to motives[76,51] and attempts to seek significance in such primitive personality qualities as wanderlust and sedentary preference (sitzlust).[118] A more refined approach to the psychological aspects of mobility behavior would have to deal with both the psychological antecedents and consequences of geographic mobility. The psychological antecedents include the factors which lead up to the decision to move, and on when, how, and where to move. In studying these decision processes, it would be important to consider an individual's intrapsychic and interpersonal methods of reaching a decision, including his perception and evaluation of his present living situation, his information-gathering and evaluation processes concerning the various alternative situations, distress-relieving and resource-mobilization techniques, and ways of planning his course of action. The psychological consequences of geographic mobility proceed from the individual's separation from his present living situation, continue with the impact of the physical move itself, and conclude with the problems of adaptation to the new setting. Here, again, information-gathering, evaluational, tension-reducing, resource-mobilizing, and planning processes are important variables. This outline for understanding mobility behavior is essentially a coping model.[62,143,63] It underscores that geographic mobility is "a process, not an event,"[15] in which the psychological antecedents and consequences are largely adaptational.

A concept of importance for mobility behavior is that of migratory selection, i.e., the tendency for individuals with certain traits to be more or less migratory than others. This concept frequently applies demographically, as is demonstrated by the tendency for migrants to be young, unmarried men. However, psychological and personality traits, as well as demographic ones, may also be assumed to affect migratory selection. As an example, it would be interesting to see how mobility behavior is related to Kelly's[83] four types of coping behavior: anticipation, exploration, locus of control, and social effectiveness. Some other personality traits which might differentially affect mobility behavior are need achievement, tolerance of ambiguity,[14] and sensation-seeking.[178]

While these and other psychological variables may be helpful in explaining both variability within the norm of geographic mobility and behavior which deviates from that norm, the interaction of psychological traits with other variables must be taken into account in attempting more adequate explanation. For example, persons with high need for achievement will tend to stay in one location or move to another, depending upon the relative opportunity structure of the two places. Unless the individual's perception of the opportunity structure is taken into account, the relationship between the need for achievement and mobility behavior may be obscured. Variable interaction is also crucial when psychological variables are themselves strongly linked to demographic variables. For example, since geographic mobility in the early adult years is strongly work-related, and in the late adult years is more health- and retirement-related, it is likely that need for achievement would be predictive of mobility only in the early adult years.

CURRENT ISSUES

Geographic mobility in industrially developed countries such as the United States is believed to be motivated most commonly by economic and vocational considerations (search for work, changing jobs, promotions), and next most commonly by family life considerations (marriage, family expansion, divorce). In the last several decades, as demonstrated by migration streams into Florida and the Southwestern United States, health and retirement considerations have gained in importance.* From the point of view of the distance moved, the mobility motivations for most local moves are related to family, house, and neighborhood; for most migrations they are related to work.[128,110]

Virtually no studies of these phenomena have made use of psychological assessment tools beyond general survey techniques. While it is understandable that work and economic motives have accounted for a large part of the variance in mobility behavior, the relative importance of personality traits, especially as facilitatory and inhibitory factors, cannot be stated at this time.

What are the mental-health implications of geographic mobility? While moving represents for many people an opportunity and not a problem, in order to discuss the mental-health relevance of mobility behavior, it will be helpful to approach it using a stress model. There are four main stress points in the process of

moving: (1) the experience of life events antecedent to and influencing the decision to move; (2) separation from one's family, one's social network, and one's home; (3) moving itself, i.e., the process of travel, temporary lodging, transport of one's family and possessions, and contact with unfamiliar social groups and norms; and (4) establishment in a new area, including finding a new home and achieving economic and social assimilation into a new social system. These four stress points have had differential treatment in the psychological and psychiatric literature.

1. The kinds of stressful events which are antecedent to geographic mobility are numerous. They include all the events which mark the major transitions in family life, education, and work. To the author's knowledge, there has not been any significant psychological study of the impact of life events upon geographic mobility and the decision to move.

2. It has been reasonably well demonstrated that forced relocation can cause considerable stress and grieving for the lost home.[58] When the relocation is not forced, however, there may be relatively few serious psychosocial sequellae,[173] provided the mover is not prevented from replacing his lost social organization.[61] When the individual's family remains behind, some migrant groups rely appreciably upon that "stem family" as a source of support via the mechanism of return migration.[16]

3. The stress of the actual move has the greatest importance when the migratory period is long. However, in this country, as a result of the norm of geographic mobility, the moving and motel industries have standardized the moving process and made it relatively tolerable. Therefore, this type of stress is probably greatest with international migration.

4. Establishment in a new area is stressful in proportion to the differences of the new community from the home community; its distance from the home community (thus affecting return migration); the extent to which the migrant has family or friends in the new community;[16] the amount of family burden the migrant brings with him; the extent to

---

* See references 12, 76, 51, 62, 128, 92, and 67.

which the move is associated with social mobility (according to Gutman,[58] either upward or downward social mobility makes geographic mobility more stressful); the new community's attitude toward the migrant and its resources for him; the availability of work;[64] and the migrant's health.[64]

While the above material helps to clarify the psychological stresses upon geographically mobile individuals, apart from very general factors, such as ego-strength, we have little information about what specific personality traits and coping styles may help migrants to cope with such stress.

Another way of exploring the stressfulness of migration is through its association with mental illness. Following the development in this country of the "melting-pot" philosophy and coincident with the growing financial rewards to workers for international and intranational migration, it was noted by some state officials that mental hospitalization rates for foreign-born immigrants and native-born migrants from other states were higher than the rates for the native-born, nonmigrant population.[112,96,80] Two general hypotheses have been suggested to explain these findings, namely, a social-causation hypothesis which was based on the assumption that migration was more stressful than nonmigration and thus resulted in a greater incidence of mental illness, and a social-selection hypothesis which assumed that the mentally ill were affected by migratory selection and migrated in greater numbers than the nonmentally ill. Neither one of these hypotheses has been well substantiated. In a long and careful review of the literature, Sanua demonstrated that the observed relationships between migration and mental illness disappear or hold only for a very specific and limited subpopulation when the study includes adequate controls.[132] It is important to control the following variables: demographic, such as sex, age, race, occupation, and social class; origin-destination differences, such as occur in rural-urban or cross-cultural migration; individual motivations, such as occur along the forced-voluntary move dimension; and social-system supports, such as the type of family life of the migrant, the

dominant attitudes toward him, and the services available in the host community. There are other serious reasons for questioning the meaning of the association between mental hospitalization rates and migration. In the first place, most investigations are limited because they compare a migrant group with a nonmigrant group in the place of destination and not simultaneously with a nonmigrant group in the place of origin. In the second place, for a variety of reasons, the tendency for a migrant group to use psychiatric services or to be labeled as psychiatric patients may vary substantially with respect to the comparison group.

At its best, the relationship between psychiatric disease and mobility behavior is a complex one, and the two main hypotheses appear much too simplistic. In some situations, geographic mobility results from the avoidance of responsibility, and, in others, from the avoidance of undue stress. Certain types of mental disturbance may incline people toward moving, while other types may incline them away from moving. Migrants who move into an area may be more stressed than people already there, but they may be less stressed than they were before they came and better able to cope than the population already at hand.

MODES OF PROFESSIONAL ACTION

Psychological clinicians may become involved with geographically mobile individuals and families at three different points in the movement process, namely, in the communities of origin, transition, and destination. In the latter two, if his area has significant numbers of geographically mobile individuals, the psychological clinician can provide direct service within his own practice or as a staff member of a mental-health center or some equivalent institution. The mental-health center offers a better organized and more extensive service, which is especially important in those high-movement areas where impoverishment and social disorganization prevent the establishment of an effective social and economic network for transient and incoming migrants. Brody discusses various interventions which may be aimed at the migrant and the "host" society.[16] Such activity varies from the provision of direct mental-health services through the training of migrant counselors, to consultation with community leaders, gate-keeping agencies, and the dominant institutions in the "host" society. In general, because there is such a lack of clinically relevant knowledge, psychiatric and psychological insights need considerable further development, and a great deal of overall clinical investigation of this subject is warranted.

In the community of origin, psychological clinicians can work preventively, especially through anticipatory guidance for those about to move. To aid in this work, a life-cycle chart should be developed similar to that presented earlier for unwanted pregnancy, outlining mobility-prone points and suggesting those life events and personal characteristics which are likely to make geographic mobility hazardous. On the basis of extensive study of migration within the United States, several authors[12,142] have identified specific subpopulations who are especially disposed to migrate. These include the following: men and women just beginning or just ending college; men beginning and ending military service; women at the time of marriage; men, and often their dependent families, in relation to career development or unemployment; couples at the time of family expansion; men and women following separation and divorce; men and women following death of an important family member; aged men and women with failing health. Such life-cycle patterns are different for different subcultures. The identification of mobility- and hazard-prone individuals and families would allow different types of preventive intervention through educational and counseling services aimed at helping such people to anticipate and cope with problems of their projected move.

(Status Mobility and Composition

The composition of a population is determined by the distribution of a variety of demographic and social statuses or traits within it. The statuses of greatest interest to demographers are age, sex, marital status, religion, education, occupation, race, and social class. Composition, a structural or cross-sectional aspect of a population, changes with time as a result of the four dynamic aspects of population mentioned in the introduction. The most important of these for our present consideration is status mobility, which, together with composition, will be treated as forming a third demographic subsystem.

Status mobility refers to the movement of individuals through social and psychological space, from one status to another. Status mobility, like fertility, mortality, and geographic mobility, is a descriptive and not a capacity concept, i.e., it refers to actual and not to potential movement across social statuses. Thus defined, status mobility denotes what some writers call "social mobility" in its general sense.[136] To avoid confusion in this chapter, the more specific and limited meaning of social mobility will be adhered to, namely, movement across social strata, typically the class strata, and it will be considered to represent one type of status mobility. Because of the natural and potentially useful parallels between status and geographic mobility, we shall maintain continuity with the previous section by treating status and social mobility first, moving then to a discussion of composition.

Status Mobility

This large subject area includes movement across such statuses as marital, educational, occupational, religious, and social-class statuses. Although of minor demographic significance, it has recently even become possible for movement to occur across sex statuses. All such movement—as a result of intention and decision-making—has important psychological antecedents. Together with the movement across age statuses, these kinds of movements have equally important psychological consequences. Any one of these status movements can be analyzed and investigated with much the same approach as geographic movement.

Occupational mobility provides a concrete example. Table 44–5 presents selected data in percentage form which show the work force composition of four occupational categories of American men, cross-tabulated with the work-force participation of (1) these same men at the time of their first jobs; and (2) their fathers when these same men were sixteen years old. Thus, the table presents information regarding the intragenerational and the intergenerational occupational mobility of a group of American men. Such movement could be studied with reference to a psychological "push-pull" theory by exploring those factors which

made the individual want to leave his old occupation and those which attracted him to his new one. Here again, however, the hydraulic model is too simplistic, and it would be more useful to employ an adaptational-coping model which utilizes (1) a life-cycle approach, including an elucidation of mobile- and hazard-prone points; (2) a description of relevant motivational clusters; (3) a determination of those personality factors which influenced the adaptive or maladaptive expression of motivation; and (4) an account of the coping styles and tactics used in response to the stresses of occupational transition. Hope-

TABLE 44–5.   Data Showing the Intergenerational and Intragenerational Occupational Mobility of American Men

FATHER'S OCCUPATION / OWN OCCUPATION AT FIRST JOB	PROFESSIONAL, TECHNICAL WORKER	MANAGER, OFFICIAL, PROPRIETOR	SALES WORKER	CLERICAL WORKER	CRAFTSMAN, FOREMAN	OPERATIVE WORKER	SERVICE WORKER	NON-FARM LABORER	FARMER, FARM MANAGER	FARM LABORER, FOREMAN	NOT WORKING	TOTAL PERCENT
Professional, technical, and kindred workers	39	17	9	7	8	10	3	2	1	0	5	101*
	63	17	3	5	4	2	1	1	1	0	4	101*
Clerical and kindred workers	26	16	7	9	5	8	6	3	1	0	8	100
	15	23	9	18	11	10	4	3	1	0	6	100
Operatives and kindred workers	11	11	4	6	22	24	5	7	1	1	8	100
	6	3	4	5	25	26	5	6	2	1	7	100
Farm laborers and foremen	2	7	2	3	19	24	7	12	6	9	8	99*
	2	7	2	3	18	20	6	9	19	7	8	101*

LEGEND: Data from a large sample of American men showing the types and percentages of change in four occupation categories from (1) father's occupation to own current occupation (intergenerational occupational mobility) and (2) own initial occupation to own current occupation (intragenerational occupational mobility). Shaded boxes are those which represent no occupational mobility. Boxes to the left of these generally indicate upward mobility, and to the right, downward mobility.
* Total percentages in some cases are not equal to 100 due to rounding.
  Source: P. M. Blau, and O. D. Duncan. *The American Occupational Structure*, New York: Wiley, 1967.

fully, some of the more detailed discussion of earlier sections will help the reader to picture the potential behind this brief sketch.

The same adaptational model could be applied equally to most of the other major status movements with a likelihood of high yield for demography and psychological clinicians. Because of the extent and complexity of these topics, we will confine further illustration of this subject area to a focused and limited discussion of social mobility and its association with psychiatric conditions.

Social Mobility

RELEVANT CONCEPTS

As previously discussed, social mobility refers principally to movement up and down the social-class strata. Unfortunately, there are no clearly established criteria for measuring social-class stratification, and several different measurement methods have arisen, including determination by occupation, education, housing, or income, all taken alone or in some combination. As an example, the occupations in Table 44-5 are generally arranged—moving from left to right—along a continuum from high to low social status. Thus, they provide one type of measure of social mobility. The table also illustrates the conceptual difference between intra- and intergenerational mobility, a difference which is probably of considerable importance with regard to both the psychological antecedents and consequences of mobility.

The methodological problems posed by the absence of clear criteria for social class are major and may account, in part, for the conflicting and limited findings of psychological and psychiatric investigations. Unlike occupational or marital mobility, it is not clear to what extent social mobility even exists as an independent and significant psychological phenomenon in American society. Nonetheless, several authors have reviewed the literature on the psychological aspects of the subject[31,93] and more work continues.[38,153,163] The psychological dimensions most frequently mentioned as having important antecedents to social mobility behavior are intel-

ligence, need for achievement, and the ability to defer gratification. Both inner-directed, self-reliant individuals and other-directed, affiliative individuals tend to be upwardly mobile, suggesting that Gough's personality dimensions of achievement-via-conformance and achievement-via-independence[55] may have important bearings upon social-mobility behavior. With regard to the consequences of social mobility, the psychological factors most frequently mentioned are those of personal fulfillment and intrapsychic strain.[40]

CURRENT ISSUES

There are two ways in which psychiatric illness may be associated with social-mobility behavior. On the one hand, specific kinds of psychiatric illness may predispose toward upward or downward social mobility (social selection); on the other hand, social mobility, in either direction, may result in stress and specific kinds of psychiatric illness (social causation). In either of these cases, a pooling of specific psychiatric illnesses in certain social classes would be expected. In fact, the frequent discovery of such pooling has been explained not only by the social-selection or -causation hypotheses just mentioned, but also by the particular stress effects of life in those social classes (independent of social mobility). Thus, the finding of schizophrenic individuals pooled in the lowest social stratum of a population can be understood only by determining to what extent this pooling was the result of selective downward mobility, to what extent it was caused by the stress of downward mobility, and to what extent it was the result of the relatively greater stress of life in the lowest stratum. A fourth process must be considered in the assessment of such pooling, i.e., the differential societal reaction to mental illness. Thus, more schizophrenic individuals may be identified in the lowest stratum because of a relatively poorer family-support system for the psychotic individual in that class or because of a qualitatively different medical care system, with quicker hospitalization for psychotic illness. In a study by Rushing,[130] in which he summarizes most of these considerations, the distribution of mental-hospitalization rates across social classes was found to have at least two discrete but super-imposed patterns, presumably resulting from two different processes and suggesting that the pooling of types of psychiatric illness in certain social classes is a multidetermined process. The relative importance of social mobility in this pooling is, as yet, unclarified. In general, what we know about the psychiatric antecedents to social mobility suggests that neuroticism is an antecedent to upward movement,[*] while psychotic conditions predispose to both intergenerational downward movement and intragenerational downward "drift,"[†] although the evidence for the downward consequences of psychoticism is not uniform.[27]

The stress effects and psychiatric consequences of social mobility are of equal interest, although only a few studies present actual data on the subject.[40,87,84] In general, stress is believed to be associated with both upward and downward social mobility, although the evidence is conflicting. Kleiner and Parker have reviewed much of the research in this area and concluded that results will not be more meaningful until investigators (1) standardize the measure of social mobility (they point out that the relationships between occupational, educational, and income mobility, on the one hand, and mental disorder, on the other, are each different); (2) examine the direction, speed, and degree of social mobility independently; and (3) consider the differential effects of social mobility for different subpopulations through such moderating variables as social class, racial or ethnic group, diagnostic category, etc.[87,115]

Modes of Professional Action

With respect to social mobility, psychological clinicians are probably most involved in working to prevent the downward drift of their most disturbed patients through their engagement in therapy and broad, community-based treatment programs. However, clinicians can also take a preventive approach by helping in the identification of those who are at risk for social-mobility hazards, and by con-

[*] See references 31, 93, 39, 148, and 84.
[†] See references 154, 148, 52, 109, and 95.

sulting to institutions and organizations who can significantly influence the social-mobility process.

Composition

In the study of composition, a population is broken into subpopulations, based on the way individuals are distributed across status categories. One of the most fundamental categories for demographers is age. It is important because of its biological base and because of the major relationship that the age structure of a population inevitably bears to the dynamic processes of fertility and mortality. Figure 44–4 depicts the age distribution for the United States for each decade between 1930 and 1970.

The half-pyramids clearly reflect the changes in the American age structure which resulted from the decrease of fertility during the depression years of the thirties, the increase in fertility as a result of the marriage and baby "boom" of the late forties and fifties, and the declining fertility of the sixties. As Bogue has said,[11] this represents one of the most extraordinary transformations of a population's age structure ever to have occurred, apart from the devastation of a population by war or large-scale migration. Such change can occur only when there is widespread knowledge and use of methods of fertility control in a population.

Relevant Concepts

It is possible to determine the composition of a population with respect to any of the statuses already mentioned in this chapter. This allows an examination of the differential effect of each status category upon behavior, especially that behavior which is important demographically. To illustrate, it is possible to examine how religious status affects fertility, how marital status affects mortality, how occupational status affects geographic mobility, and how racial status affects status mobility. Of parallel interest is the determination of how demographic behavior affects status distributions in the population.

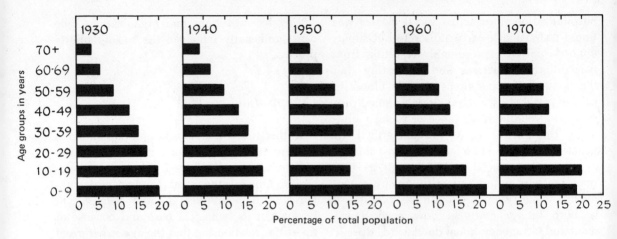

Figure 44–4. The age structure of the United States for each decade 1930 to 1970.
Source: United States Department of Commerce, Bureau of the Census, General Population Characteristics, 1970 Census, United States Summary, PC(1)–B1.

At the psychological level, both the antecedents and consequences of population composition and its change are of interest. A complete discussion of this subject would obviously be impossible in this chapter. Therefore, in the following section, we will confine our attention to two areas of current interest which illustrate the interaction of psychological variables and population composition through the common factor of fertility behavior.

The distribution in a population of psychological traits or statuses is another aspect of composition. Any of the psychological variables discussed earlier in this chapter, which have an important relationship to one or more of the demographically significant behavior areas, may be used for this type of analysis. Thus, we could select such traits as intelligence, modernism, or need for achievement and study the way these are distributed through a population, and then the way subpopulations, grouped according to these dimensions, behave demographically. Of particular interest to psychological clinicians is the psychiatric status composition of a population and the way psychiatric statuses differentially affect demographic behavior. We shall also consider some examples of this in the next section.

CURRENT ISSUES

Man's growing ability to influence the phenotypal characteristics of his offspring through gamete selection and modification illustrates how psychological factors can affect population composition. The most imminent and potentially significant example of this type of influence lies in sex preselection.[41] Should this become technologically feasible within the next decade, evidence regarding the current attitudes toward sex selection[97] suggests that a significant portion of the American population would immediately accept and even use this procedure, and that eventually, with public dissemination of information, it could gain widespread acceptance and use. Considering the significant preference for male offspring, the option for parents to choose the sex of their children would have major consequences for family planning and composition. Markle[97] estimates that the sex ratio would change from 105 to 122 males born for every 100 females, a change which would have an obvious cumulative effect upon the sex composition of the United States' population. Etzioni has discussed the societal consequences of such a sex composition change, noting the potential effect of excess males upon such activities as church attendance, criminal behavior, voting patterns, marital behavior, and sexual behavior.[41] Furthermore, it is quite possible that there would be dynamic, compensatory changes in sex preferences which would fluctuate with time as a result of the changing sex composition. This process might result in fluctuations in the sex structure matching in magnitude and significance the changes for age structure illustrated in Figure 44-4.

The effect of population composition on individual psychology can be illustrated by the changes which will result from the current societal press for zero-population growth. The achievement by this country of a stationary population, with little or no change in size, will be accompanied by a significant change in age structure. The mean age will change from twenty-eight to forty, the proportion of those under fifteen years from 30 to 20 percent and of those over sixty-five from 10 to 20 percent. In short, the population will be older. This will mean a shift in aggregate values, beliefs, and behavioral traits away from those associated with youth toward those dominant in mid- and late life. Individual behavior will be affected, generally by modification of the predominant value system, and specifically by alterations in the tempo of life, the rate of social change, the process of job advancement, the importance of seniority, the nature of education, the types of available recreation, etc.

A third and final compositional issue, of special significance to psychological clinicians, involves the differential effects upon demographic behavior of psychiatric status. It has been suggested that the community mental-health centers and other psychiatric agencies have some responsibility for the fertility behavior of the psychiatric subpopulations which they serve.[137] It was argued that the center should provide case finding, education, referral, and, in some cases, direct contraceptive aid as a form of preventive psychiatric service. This argument may be extended for psychiatric subpopulations to other forms of demographic behavior, underscoring the importance of knowing more about the effect of psychiatric status on all of these behaviors. Unfortunately, relatively little systematic work

has been done in this area, and what has been done is difficult to synthesize because of the different definitions of psychiatric status which have been used. For example, some studies focus exclusively on that subpopulation which has had a psychiatric hospitalization; others focus on one which has had some form of psychiatric treatment; and others focus on one which has a certain level of psychiatric impairment or symptomatology irrespective of whether or not there has been a treatment contact.

In some of the earlier studies on the fertility of hospitalized mental patients, this subpopulation was observed to have a lower overall fertility than the general population. This relationship, however, may have been confounded by the effects of marital status, since married women have greater fertility but also have a lower rate of hospitalization for psychiatric illness.[86] Slater investigated the fertility of a large sample of male and female psychiatric-clinic patients and inpatients in England.[144] In this investigation, the subpopulation was divided into diagnostic groups, i.e., those with schizophrenia, manic depression, personality disorders, obsessional neurosis, and other neuroses. For all diagnostic categories, the number ever married was lower, and the number separated and divorced was greater than for the general population. Furthermore, marital fertility for all diagnostic groups was markedly depressed, compared with the general population.

The mortality of the psychiatric population appears to be different from the general population where information is available. There is some evidence that suicide rates are higher among current and former mental-hospital patients.[151] Within the psychiatric subpopulation, suicide rates are highest among those with a diagnosis of depression.[122] It may be that homicide rates for psychiatric patients are higher, but evidence regarding this is inadequate. The evidence is stronger regarding accident-death rates. For example, the presence of severe psychopathology has been associated with the occurrence of fatal auto accidents.[139,140] For all causes of death, evidence indicates that psychiatric patients—

both those hospitalized and, to a lesser extent, those formerly hospitalized—have higher death rates, although the responsible behavioral factors have not been well delineated.[75,111]

Faris and Dunham were among the first to observe that psychiatric status was affected by geographic distribution.[42] They noted that the subpopulation of individuals requiring hospitalization for a psychiatric condition, specifically those diagnosed as schizophrenic, tended to be concentrated in the more densely populated and socially disorganized central city. They considered both a social causation and a social selection hypothesis, and concluded that this concentration of schizophrenic patients was caused by the social conditions in the central city and did not result from the most disturbed psychiatric subpopulation drifting into those areas. In a more contemporary study, Jaco also found a higher incidence of mental disorder in urban, as opposed to rural areas, although he did observe extremely divergent rates between the two highly industrialized communities within the overall area of study.[78]

The effect of psychiatric status upon geographic mobility has yet to be clearly delineated, mostly because only a few investigators[112] have completed studies which compare a migrant population with a nonmigrant population. However, it appears that the relationship between psychiatric status and geographic mobility depends upon the social norms governing migration. As Sanua has suggested, in the United States and other countries where geographic mobility is the norm and thus relatively easy, individuals may be freer to express their psychopathology through moving.[132] Regarding the effect of psychiatric status upon the social mobility, as already cited, the evidence indicates that the neurotic subgroup has a higher rate of upward movement than the general population, and the psychotic subgroup a higher rate of downward movement. Because of space considerations, other kinds of status mobility will not be discussed here. However, it seems very likely that psychiatric subpopulations are different from the general population in some of these other areas, such as occupational or marital-status mobility, as well.

MODES OF PROFESSIONAL ACTION

A great deal is unknown regarding the psychological antecedents and consequences of population composition and its change. Similarly, much is unknown regarding the demographic behavior of psychiatric subpopulations. Thus, one of the first orders of business is further investigation. Pending the development of more information, the chief modes of professional action will be the treatment and prevention services outlined in the previous sections with regard to the specific categories of demographic behavior.

❰ Final Comment

While the scope of this essay is admittedly very broad, it is hoped that the general and sometimes abstract level of discussion will be compensated for by assembling a large number of concepts and pieces of information which heretofore have been considered separately but which are, in fact, systematically and dynamically related. Treated in more detail, this subject area can easily extend to several volumes. However, enough of the material presented here is in its early development as to justify a limited, comprehensive treatment in an effort to sketch the outlines of a single field of study.

Such a field is a step in the direction of the integration of the life sciences through a general-systems approach.[101-103] Such an approach is essential in the case of population problems because of the dynamic interplay of events and processes, not only at the two levels under consideration—the demographic and the psychological—but also between these levels. In the past, there has been a tendency for each level to be treated independently, as a separate field. Hopefully, the importance of interlevel considerations has been effectively demonstrated in the body of this essay.

In the next decade, government at all levels will be under increasing pressure to develop and implement population policies designed to influence the behavior of the public. Such policies will be strongly affected by population theories and extant knowledge in the field. There are major aspects of population policy which depend upon input at the psychological level[43] and the behavioral scientist who hopes to influence population policy formation and implementation needs to be aware of the many interlevel (psychological-demographic) relationships. Through his effective participation in the solving of social and political problems made necessary by growing population pressures, the quality of human life may be protected and even enhanced.

⟪ Bibliography

1. ALTMAN, I. and W. W. HAYTHORN. "The Ecology of Isolated Groups," *Behav. Sci.*, 12 (1967), 169–182.

2. BARKER, R. *Ecological Psychology*. Stanford: Stanford University Press, 1968.

3. BARNES, A. B., E. COHEN, J. D. STOECKLE et al. "Therapeutic Abortion: Medical and Social Sequels," *Ann. Intern. Med.*, 75 (1971), 881–886.

4. BEALL, L. "The Dynamics of Suicide: A Review of the Literature, 1897–1965," *Bull. Suicidol.* (March, 1969), 2–16.

5. BECK, M. B. "Abortion: The Mental Health Consequences of Unwantedness," *Semin. Psychiatry*, 2 (1970), 263–274.

6. BECK, M. B., S. H. NEWMAN, and S. LEWIT. "Abortion: A National Public and Mental Health Problem—Past, Present, and Proposed Research," *Am. J. Public Health*, 59 (1969), 2131–2143.

7. BERNSTEIN, N. R. and C. B. TINKHAM. "Group Therapy Following Abortion," *J. Nerv. Ment. Dis.*, 152 (1971), 303–314.

8. BLAKE, J. "Population Policy for Americans: Is the Government Being Misled?" *Science*, 164 (1969), 522–529.

9. ———. "Family Planning and Public Policy: Who Is Misleading Whom?" *Science*, 165 (1969), 1203.

10. ———. "Abortion and Public Opinion," *Science*, 171 (1971), 540–549.

11. BOGUE, D. J. *Principles of Demography*. New York: Wiley, 1969.

12. BOGUE, D. J., M. J. HAGOOD, and G. K. BOWLES. *Differential Migration in the Corn and Cotton Belts*, Vol. 2. Oxford, Ohio: Scripps Foundation for Research in Population Problems, Miami University, 1957.

13. BOGUE, D. J., H. S. SHRYOCK, JR., and S. A. HOERMANN. *Streams of Migration Between Subregions*, Vol. 1. Oxford, Ohio: Scripps Foundation for Research in Population Problems, Miami University, 1953.

14. BRIM, O. G. and D. B. HOFF. "Individual and Situational Differences in Desire for Certainty," *J. Abnorm. Soc. Psychol.*, 54 (1957), 225–229.

15. BRODY, E. B. "Migration and Adaptation: The Nature of the Problem," in E. B. Brody, ed., *Behavior in New Environments*, pp. 13–21. Beverly Hills: Sage Publications, 1969.

16. ———. "Preventive Planning and Strategies of Intervention: An Overview," in E. G. Brody, ed., *Behavior in New Environments*, pp. 437–443. Beverly Hills: Sage Publications, 1969.

17. BUMPASS, L. and C. F. WESTOFF. "The 'Perfect Contraceptive' Population," *Science*, 169 (1970), 1177–1182.

18. ———. *The Later Years of Childbearing*. Princeton, N.J.: Princeton University Press, 1970.

19. CALHOUN, J. B. "Population Density and Social Pathology," *Sci. Am.*, 206 (1962), 139–148.

20. CANNON, K. L. and R. LONG. "Premarital Sexual Behavior in the Sixties," *J. Marriage Fam.*, 33 (1971), 36–49.

21. CASSEL, J. "Health Consequences of Population Density and Crowding," in *Rapid Population Growth*, pp. 462–478. Prepared by a Study Committee of the Office of the Foreign Secretary, National Academy of Sciences. Baltimore: The Johns Hopkins Press, 1971.

22. CENTER FOR DISEASE CONTROL. Abortion Surveillance Report, January-March 1971; Atlanta, March 1972. Washington: U.S. Govt. Print. Off., 1972.

23. CHOLDIN, H. M. "Population Density and Social Relations," Paper presented at Meeting of the Population Association of America, Toronto, April 14, 1972.

24. CHRISTENSEN, H. T. and G. R. CARPENTER. "Value-Behavior Discrepancies Regarding Premarital Coitus in Three Western Cultures," *Am. Sociol. Rev.*, 27 (1962), 66–74.

25. CHRISTIAN, J. J. "The Pathology of Over-population," *Milit. Med.*, 128 (1963), 571–603.

26. CLARKSON, F. E., S. R. VOGEL, I. K. BRAVERMAN et al. "Family Size and Sex-Role Stereotypes," *Science*, 167 (1970), 390–392.

27. CLAUSEN, J. A. and M. L. KOHN. "Relation of Schizophrenia to the Social Structure of a Small City," in B. Pasamanick, ed., *Epidemiology of Mental Disorder*, Publication Number 60. Washington: American Association for the Advancement of Science, 1959.

28. COLMAN, A. D. "Territoriality in Man: A Comparison of Behavior in Home and Hospital," *Am. J. Orthopsychiatry*, 38 (1968), 464–468.

29. COMMISSION ON POPULATION GROWTH AND THE AMERICAN FUTURE. *An Interim Report to the President and the Congress*. Washington: U.S. Govt. Print. Off., 1971.

30. CONGER, J. J. and H. S. GASKILL. "Accident Proneness," in A. M. Freeman and H. I. Kaplan, eds., *Comprehensive Textbook of Psychiatry*, pp. 1107–1110. Baltimore: Williams & Wilkins, 1967.

31. CROCKETT, H. J., JR. "Psychological Origins of Mobility," in N. J. Smelser and S. M. Lipset, eds., *Social Structure and Mobility in Economic Development*, pp. 280–309. Chicago: Aldine, 1966.

32. CUTRIGHT, P. "Illegitimacy: Myths, Causes and Cures," *Fam. Plann. Perspect.*, 3 (1971), 25–48.

33. ———. "The Teenage Sexual Revolution and the Myth of an Abstinent Past," *Fam. Plann. Perspect.*, 4 (1972), 24–31.

34. DANIELS, D., M. F. GILULA, and F. M. OCHBERG, eds., *Violence and the Struggle for Existence*. Boston: Little, Brown, 1970.

35. DAVIS, K. "Population Policy: Will Current Programs Succeed?" *Science*, 158 (1967), 730–739.

36. DESOR, J. A. "Toward a Psychological Theory of Crowding," *J. Pers. Soc. Psychol.*, 21 (1972), 79–83.

37. EHRLICH, P. R., and J. FREEDMAN. "Population, Crowding, and Human Behavior," *N. Scient. Sci. J.*, 50 (1971), 10–14.

38. ELDER, G. H. "Achievement Motivation and Intelligence in Occupational Mobility: A Longitudinal Analysis," *Sociometry*, 31 (1968), 327–354.

39. ELLIS, E. "Social Psychological Correlates of Upward Social Mobility Among Unmarried Career Women," *Am. Sociol. Rev.*, 17 (1952), 558–563.

40. ELLIS, R. A. and C. W. LANE. "Social Mobility and Social Isolation: A Test of Sorokin's Dissociative Hypothesis," *Am. Sociol. Rev.*, 32 (1967), 237–253.

41. ETZIONI, A. "Sex Control, Science and Society," *Science*, 161 (1968), 1107–1112.

42. FARIS, R. E. L. and H. W. DUNHAM. *Mental Disorders in Urban Areas*. Chicago: University of Chicago Press, 1939.

43. FAWCETT, J. T. *Psychology and Population*. New York: Population Council, 1970.

44. FLAPAN, M. "A Paradigm for the Analysis of Childbearing Motivations of Married Women Prior to Birth of the First Child," *Am. J. Orthopsychiatry*, 39 (1969), 402–417.

45. FORSSMAN, H. and I. THUWE. "One Hundred and Twenty Children Born after Application for Abortion Refused," *Acta Psychiatr. Scand.*, 42 (1966), 71–88.

46. FREEDMAN, J., L. S. KLEVANSKY, and P. R. EHRLICH. "The Effect of Crowding on Human Task Performance," *J. Appl. Soc. Psychol.*, 1 (1971), 7–25.

47. FRIED, M. "Grieving for a Lost Home," in L. J. Duhl, ed., *The Urban Condition*, pp. 151–171. New York: Basic Books, 1963.

48. FURSTENBERG, F., JR., L. GORDIS, and M. MARKOWITZ. "Birth Control Knowledge and Attitudes among Unmarried Pregnant Adolescents: A Preliminary Report," *J. Marriage Fam.*, 31 (1969), 34–42.

49. GALLE, O. R., W. R. GROVE, and J. M. MCPHERSON. "Population Density and Pathology: What Are the Relations for Man?" *Science*, 176 (1972), 23–30.

50. GANS, H. J. *People and Plans*, p. 8. New York: Basic Books, 1968.

51. GIRARD, A., H. BASTIDE, and G. POURCHER. "Geographic Mobility and Urban Concentration in France: A Study of the Provinces," in C. J. Jansen, ed., *Readings in the Sociology of Migration*, pp. 203–253. New York: Pergamon, 1970.

52. GOLDBERG, E. M. and S. L. MORRISON. "Schizophrenia and Social Class," *Br. J. Psychiatry*, 109 (1963), 785–802.

53. GOLDSCHEIDER, C. *Population Modernization and Social Structure*. Boston: Little, Brown, 1971.

54. GOLDSMITH, S., M. O. GABRIELSON, I. GABRIELSON et al. "Teenagers, Sex, and Con-

traception," *Fam. Plann. Perspect.*, 4 (1972), 31–38.

55. GOUGH, H. G. *Manual for California Psychological Inventory*, rev. Palo Alto: Conculting Psychologists Press, 1969.

56. GRIFFITT, W. and R. VEITCH. "Hot and Crowded: Influences of Population Density and Temperature on Interpersonal Affective Behavior," *J. Pers. Soc. Psychol.*, 17 (1971), 92–98.

57. GRUNEBAUM, H. V., V. D. ABERNETHY, E. S. ROFMAN et al. "The Family Planning Attitudes, Practices and Motivations of Mental Patients," *Am. J. Psychiatry*, 128 (1971), 740–744.

58. GUTMAN, R. "Population Mobility in the Middle Class," in L. J. Duhl, ed., *The Urban Condition*, pp. 172–183. New York: Basic Books, 1963.

59. HADDON, W., E. SUCHMAN, and D. KLEIN. *Accident Research and Approaches*. New York: Harper, 1964.

60. HALL, E. T. *The Hidden Dimension*. Garden City, N.Y.: Doubleday, 1966.

61. ———. "Environmental Communication," in A. H. Esser, ed., *Behavior and Environment: The Use of Space by Animals and Men*, pp. 247–256. New York: Plenum, 1971.

62. HAMBURG, D. A. and J. E. ADAMS. "A Perspective on Coping Behavior: Seeking and Utilizing Information in Major Transitions," *Arch. Gen. Psychiatry*, 17 (1967), 227–284.

63. HAMBURG, D. A., G. V. COELHO, and J. E. ADAMS, eds., *Coping and Adaptation*. New York: Basic Books, 1974.

64. HANSON, R. C. and O. G. SIMMONS. "Differential Experience Paths of Rural Migrants to the City," in E. B. Brody, ed., *Behavior in New Environments*, pp. 145–166. Beverly Hills: Sage Publications, 1969.

65. HARKAVY, O., F. S. JAFFE, and S. M. WISHIK. "Family Planning and Public Policy: Who is Misleading Whom?" *Science*, 165 (1969), 367–373.

66. HAUSER, P. M. "The Population of the United States, Retrospect and Prospect," in P. M. Hauser, ed., *Population Dilemma*, 2nd ed., pp. 85–105. Englewood Cliffs, N.J.: Prentice Hall, 1969.

67. ———. "The Census of 1970," *Sci. Am.*, 225 (1971), 17–25.

68. ———. "World Population: Retrospect and Prospect," in *Rapid Population Growth*, pp. 103–122. Prepared by a Study Committee of the Office of the Foreign Secretary, National Academy of Sciences. Baltimore: The Johns Hopkins Press, 1971.

69. HEDIGER, H. *Studies of Psychology and Behavior of Captive Animals in Zoos and Circuses*. New York: Criterion Books, 1955.

70. HEER, D. M. and J. W. BOYTON. "A Multivariate Regression Analysis of Differences in Fertility of U. S. Counties," *Soc. Biol.*, 17 (1970), 180–194.

71. HÖÖK, K. "Refused Abortion," *Acta Psychiatr. Scand.*, 41 (1965), 87–110.

72. HOROWITZ, M. J. "Spatial Behavior and Psychopathology," *J. Nerv. Ment. Dis.*, 146 (1968), 24–35.

73. HOROWITZ, M. J., D. F. DUFF, and L. O. STRATTON. "Personal Space and the Body-Buffer Zone," *Arch. Gen. Psychiatry*, 11 (1964), 651–656.

74. HOWARD, H. E. *Territory in Bird Life*. London: Collins, 1920.

75. HUSSAR, A. E. "Leading Causes of Death in Institutionalized Chronic Schizophrenic Patients: A Study of 1,275 Autopsy Protocols," *J. Nerv. Ment. Dis.*, 142 (1966), 45–57.

76. ILLSLEY, R., A. FINLAYSON, and B. THOMPSON. "The Motivation and Characteristics of Internal Migrants: A Socio-Medical Study of Young Migrants in Scotland," in C. J. Jansen, ed., *Readings in the Sociology of Migration*, pp. 123–156. New York: Pergamon, 1970.

77. ITTELSON, W. H., H. M. PROSHANSKY, and L. G. RIVLIN. "The Environmental Psychology of the Psychiatric Ward," in H. M. Proshansky, W. H. Ittelson, and L. G. Rivlin, eds., *Environmental Psychology*, pp. 419–439. New York: Holt, Rinehart & Winston, 1970.

78. JACO, E. G. *The Social Epidemiology of Mental Disorders*. New York: Russell Sage Foundation, 1960.

79. JAFFE, F. S. "Toward the Reduction of Unwanted Pregnancy," *Science*, 174 (1971), 119–127.

80. KANTOR, M. B., ed., *Mobility and Mental Health*. Springfield, Ill.: Charles C. Thomas, 1963.

81. KAR, S. B. "Individual Aspirations as Related to Early and Late Acceptance of Contraception," *J. Soc. Psychiatry*, 83 (1971), 235–245.

82. KELLER, A. B., J. H. SIMS, W. E. HENRY

et al. "Psychological Sources of 'Resistance' to Family Planning," *Merrill-Palmer Q.*, 16 (1970), 286–302.

83. KELLY, J. "Adaptive Behavior in Varied High School Environments." Ann Arbor, Mich.: Institute for Social Research, University of Michigan, 1968. Unpublished manuscript.

84. KESSIN, K. "Social and Psychological Consequences of Intergenerational Occupational Mobility," *Am. J. Sociol.*, 77 (1971), 1–18.

85. KIRK, D. "A New Demographic Transition?" in *Rapid Population Growth*, pp. 123–147. Prepared by a Study Committee of the Office of the Foreign Secretary, National Academy of Sciences. Baltimore: The Johns Hopkins Press, 1971.

86. KISER, C. V., W. H. GRABIL, and A. A. CAMPBELL. *Trends and Variations in Fertility in the United States.* Cambridge: Harvard University Press, 1968.

87. KLEINER, R. J. and S. PARKER. "Social-Psychological Aspects of Migration and Mental Disorder in the Negro Population," in E. G. Brody, ed., *Behavior in New Environments*, pp. 353–374. Beverly Hills: Sage Publications, 1969.

88. LEE, E. S. "A Theory of Migration," *Demography*, 3 (1966), 47–57.

89. LEE, N. H. *The Search for an Abortionist.* Chicago: University of Chicago Press, 1969.

90. LEMKAU, P. V. "The Planning Project for Columbia," in M. F. Shore and F. V. Mannino, eds., *Mental Health and the Community: Problems, Programs, and Strategies.* New York: Behavioral Publications, 1969.

91. LERNER, B., R. RASKIN, and E. B. DAVIS, "On the Need To Be Pregnant," *Int. J. Psycho-Anal.*, 48 (1967), 288–297.

92. LESLIE, G. R. and RICHARDSON, A. H. "Life-Cycle, Career Pattern, and the Decision to Move," *Am. Sociol. Rev.*, 26 (1961), 894–902.

93. LIPSET, S. M. and R. BENDIX. *Social Mobility in Industrial Society.* Berkeley: University of California Press, 1959.

94. LIPSON, G. and D. WOLMAN. "Polling Americans on Birth Control and Population," *Fam. Plann. Perspect.*, 4 (1972), 39–42.

95. LYSTAD, M. H. "Social Mobility among Selected Groups of Schizophrenic Pa-

tients," *Am. Sociol. Rev.*, 22 (1957), 288–292.

96. McCAROLL, J. R. and W. HADDON, JR. "A Controlled Study of Fatal Automobile Accidents in New York City," *J. Chronic Dis.*, 15 (1962), 811–826.

97. MALZBERG, B. and E. S. LEE. *Migration and Mental Disease.* New York: Social Science Research Council, 1956.

98. MARKLE, G. E. and C. B. NAM. "Sex Predetermination: Its Impact on Fertility," *Soc. Biol.*, 18 (1971), 73–83.

99. MECHANIC, D. *Medical Sociology.* New York: Free Press, 1968.

100. MILGRAM, S. "The Experience of Living in Cities," *Science*, 167 (1967), 1461–1468.

101. MILLER, J. G. "Living Systems: Basic Concepts," *Behav. Sci.*, 10 (1965), 193–237.

102. ———. "Living Systems: Structure and Process," *Behav. Sci.*, 10 (1965), 337–379.

103. ———. "Living Systems: Cross-Level Hypotheses," *Behav. Sci.*, 10 (1965), 380–411.

104. MILLER, W. B. *Personality and Ego Factors Relative to Family Planning and Population Control.* Proceedings of A Conference on Psychological Measurement in the Study of Population Problems, University of California, Berkeley, February 26–27, 1971, pp. 41–51.

105. ———. "Conception Mastery; Ego Control of the Psychological and Behavioral Antecedents to Conception," *Comments Contemp. Psychiatry*, 1 (1973), 157–177.

106. ———. "Relationships between the Intendedness of Conception and the Wantedness of Pregnancy," in *J. Nerv. Ment. Dis.*, 159 (1974), 396–406.

107. ———. Psychological Antecedents to Conception among Abortion Seekers," *West. J. Med.*, 122 (1975), 12–19.

108. MILLER, W. B. and A. E. WEISZ. Psychosocial Aspects of Unwanted Pregnancy, Stanford: Stanford University, December, 1970. Unpublished paper.

109. MORRIS, J. N. "Health and Social Class," *Lancet*, 1 (1959), 303–305.

110. MORRISON, P. A. "The Role of Migration in California's Growth," in K. Davis and F. G. Styles, eds., *California's Twenty Million: Research Contributions to Population Policy*, pp. 33–60. Berkeley: Institute of International Studies, 1971.

111. NISWANDER, G. D., G. M. HASLERUD, and G. D. MITCHELL. "Changes in Cause of Death of Schizophrenic Patients," *Arch. Gen. Psychiatry*, 9 (1963), 229–234.

112. ODEGAARD, O. "Emigration and Insanity," *Acta Psychiatr. Neurol., Suppl.* 4 (1932), 9–206.

113. OLLEY, P. C. "Age, Marriage, Personality and Distress: A Study of Personality Factors in Women Referred for Therapeutic Abortion," *Semin. Psychiatry*, 2 (1970), 341–351.

114. OSOFSKY, J. D. and H. J. OSOFSKY. "The Psychological Reaction of Patients to Legalized Abortion," *Am. J. Orthopsychiatry*, 42 (1972), 48–60.

115. PARKER, S. and R. J. KLEINER. *Mental Illness in the Urban Negro Community*. New York: Free Press, 1966.

116. PATT, S. L., R. G. RAPPAPORT, and P. BARGLOW. "Followup of Therapeutic Abortion," *Arch. Gen. Psychiatry*, 20 (1969), 408–414.

117. PAUKER, J. D. "Girls Pregnant Out of Wedlock," in *The Double Jeopardy, The Triple Crisis—Illegitimacy Today*, pp. 47–68. New York: National Council on Illegitimacy, 1969.

118. PETERSEN, W. *Population*. London: Macmillan, 1969.

119. PHILLIPS, N. "The Prevalence of Surgical Sterilization in a Suburban Population," *Demography*, 8 (1971), 261–270.

120. POHLMAN, E. "The Child Born after Denial of Abortion Request," in S. H. Newman, M. B. Beck, and S. Lewit, eds., *Abortion, Obtained and Denied: Research Approaches*, pp. 59–73. New York: Population Council, 1971.

121. POHLMAN, E. and J. M. POHLMAN. *The Psychology of Birth Planning*. Cambridge, Mass.: Schenkman, 1969.

122. POKORNY, A. D. "Myths About Suicide," in H. L. P. Resnik, ed., *Suicidal Behaviors: Diagnosis and Management*, pp. 57–72. Boston: Little, Brown & Co., 1968.

123. RAINWATER, L. *Family Design: Marital Sexuality, Family Size, and Family Planning*. Chicago: Aldine, 1965.

124. RESNICK, H. L. P., ed. *Suicidal Behaviors: Diagnosis and Management*. Boston: Little, Brown, 1968.

125. RIDLEY, J. C. "The Changing Position of American Women: Education, Labor Force Participation, and Fertility," in Fogarty International Center Proceedings, no. 3, *The Family in Transition*, pp. 199–236. Washington: U.S. Govt. Print. Off., Nov. 1969.

126. RIESMAN, D., R. DENNEY, and N. GLAZER. *The Lonely Crowd*, p. 17. New Haven: Yale University Press, 1950.

127. RODGERS, D. A. and F. J. ZIEGLER. "Psychological Reactions to Surgical Contraception," in J. T. Fawcett, ed., *Psychological Perspectives on Population*, pp. 306–326. New York: Basic Books, 1972.

128. ROSSI, P. H. *Why Families Move*. Glencoe, Ill.: Free Press, 1955.

129. ROTTER, J. B. "Generalized Expectancies for Internal Versus External Control of Reinforcement," *Psychol. Monogr.*, 80 (1966), 1–28.

130. RUSHING, W. A. "Two Patterns in the Relationship between Social Class and Mental Hospitalization," *Am. Sociol. Rev.*, 34 (1969), 533–541.

131. RYDER, N. B. and C. F. WESTOFF. *Relationships among Intended, Expected, Desired, and Ideal Family Size: United States, 1965*. Princeton, N.J.: Center for Population Research, Princeton University, March, 1969.

132. SANUA, V. D. "Immigration, Migration and Mental Illness: A Review of the Literature with Special Emphasis on Schizophrenia," in E. G. Brody, ed., *Behavior in New Environments*, pp. 291–352. Beverly Hills: Sage Publications, 1969.

133. SCANZONI, J. and M. McMURRY. "Continuities in the Explanation of Fertility Control," *J. Marriage Fam.*, 34 (1972), 315–322.

134. SCHMITT, R. C. "Density, Health, and Social Disorganization," *J. Am. Inst. Plann.*, 32 (1966), 38–40.

135. SCHNORE, L. F. "Social Mobility in Demographic Perspective," *Am. Sociol. Rev.*, 26 (1961), 407–423.

136. SCHORR, A. L. "Housing and Its Effects," in *Slums and Social Insecurity*. U.S. Dept. of Health, Education, and Welfare, Social Security Administration Division of Research and Statistics, Research Report no. 1, pp. 7–31. Washington: U.S. Govt. Print. Off., 1966.

137. SCHWARTZ, R. A. "The Role of Family Planning in the Primary Prevention of

Mental Illness," *Am. J. Psychiatry*, 125 (1969), 1711–1717.

138. Schwarzweller, H. K. and J. S. Brown. "Social Class Origins and the Economic Social and Psychological Adjustments of Kentucky Mountain Migrants: A Case Study," in E. G. Brody, ed., *Behavior in New Environments*, pp. 117–144. Beverly Hills: Sage Publications, 1969.

139. Selzer, M. L. "Alcoholism, Mental Illness, and Stress in 96 Drivers Causing Fatal Accidents," *Behav. Sci.*, 14 (1969), 1–10.

140. Selzer, M. L., J. E. Rogers, and S. Kern. "Fatal Accidents: The Role of Psychopathology, Social Stress, and Acute Disturbance," *Am. J. Psychiatry*, 124 (1968), 1028–1036.

141. Shneidman, E. S. "Orientation Towards Death: A Vital Aspect of the Study of Lives," in R. W. White, ed., *The Study of Lives*, pp. 201–227. New York: Atherton Press, 1964.

142. Shryock, H. S. *Population Mobility within the United States*, pp. 411. Chicago: Family and Community Study Center, 1964.

143. Sidle, A. C., R. H. Moos, J. E. Adams et al. "Development of a Coping Scale," *Arch. Gen. Psychiatry*, 20 (1969), 226–232.

144. Slater, E., E. H. Hare, and J. S. Price. "Marriage and Fertility of Psychiatric Patients Compared with National Data," *Soc. Biol.*, 18 (1971), S60–S94.

145. Sloane, B. R. "Unwanted Pregnancy," *N. Engl. J. Med.*, 280 (1969), 1206–1213.

146. Smith, D. H. and A. Inkeles. "The OM Scale: A Comparative Sociopsychological Measure of Individual Modernity," *Sociometry*, 21 (1966), 353–377.

147. Spengler, J. J. "Population Problem: In Search of a Solution," *Science*, 166 (1969), 1234–1238.

148. Srole, T., T. S. Langner, S. T. Michael et al. *Mental Health in the Metropolis: The Midtown Manhattan Study*. New York: McGraw-Hill, 1962.

149. Taeuber, I. B. "Change and Transition in Family Structures," in Fogarty International Center Proceedings, no. 3, *The Family in Transition*, pp. 35–97. Washington: U.S. Govt. Print. Off., November 3–6, 1969.

150. Tanay, E. "Psychiatric Aspects of Homicide Prevention," *Am. J. Psychiatry*, 128 (1972), 815–818.

151. Temoche, A., T. F. Pugh, and B. Mac-

Mahon. "Suicide Rates among Current and Former Mental Institution Patients," *J. Nerv. Ment. Dis.*, 138 (1964), 124–130.

152. Tietze, C. "Therapeutic Abortions in the United States," *Am. J. Obstetr. Gynecol.*, 101 (1968), 784–787.

153. Toppen, J. T. "Underemployment: Economic or Psychological," *Psychol. Rep.*, 28 (1971), 111–122.

154. Turner, R. J. and M. O. Wagenfield. "Occupational Mobility and Schizophrenia: An Assessment of the Social Causation and Social Selection Hypothesis," *Am. Sociol. Rev.*, 32 (1967), 104–113.

155. United Nations. "Recent Trends of Mortality in the World," *Population Bull.*, 6 (1962), 73–75.

156. ———. "Where will the Next 50 Million Americans Live?" *Population Bull.*, 27 (1971), 2–30.

157. United States Department of Commerce, Bureau of the Census. "Estimates of the Population of the United States and Components of Change: 1940 to 1970," *Current Population Rep.*, Ser. P-25, no. 442, pp. 1–8. Washington: U.S. Govt. Print. Off., 1970.

158. ———. "Projections of the Population of the United States, by Age and Sex (Interim revision): 1970 to 2020," *Current Population Rep.*, Ser. P-25, no. 448. pp. 1–50. Washington: U.S. Govt. Print. Off., 1970.

159. ———. "Fertility Indicators, 1970," *Current Population Rep.*, Special Studies, Ser. P-23, no. 36, pp. 41–46. Washington: U.S. Govt. Print. Off., April 16, 1971.

160. United States Public Health Service. *Vital Statistics of the United States*, 1964. Washington: U.S. Govt. Print. Off., 1966.

161. ———. *Vital Statistics of the United States*, 1966, Vol. 2, Sec. 5, Life Tables. Washington: U.S. Govt. Print. Off., 1966.

162. Vincent, C. E. *Unmarried Mothers*. New York: Free Press, 1961.

163. Waller, J. H. "Achievement and Social Mobility: Relationships among IQ Score, Education and Occupation in Two Generations," *Soc. Biol.*, 18 (1971), 252–259.

164. Weaver, R. C. "Major Factors in Urban Planning," in Duhl, L. J., ed., *The Urban Condition*, pp. 97–112. New York: Basic Books, 1963.

165. Weissman, M. M. "Birth Control—Population Policy," *Science*, 165 (1969), 121.

166. WESTOFF, C. F., R. G. POTTER, JR., P. C. SAGI et al. *Family Growth in Metropolitan America.* Princeton, N.J.: Princeton University Press, 1961.

167. ———. *The Third Child.* Princeton, N.J.: Princeton University Press, 1963.

168. WESTOFF, C. F. and N. B. RYDER. "Recent Trends in Attitudes Toward Fertility Control and in the Practice of Contraception in the United States," in S. J. Behrman, L. Corsa, Jr., and R. Freedman, eds., *Fertility and Family Planning: A World View,* pp. 388–412. Ann Arbor: University of Michigan, 1969.

169. WESTOFF, L. A. and C. F. WESTOFF. *From Now to Zero.* Boston: Little, Brown, 1968.

170. WHELPTON, P. K., A. A. CAMPBELL, and J. E. PATTERSON. *Fertility and Family Planning in the United States.* Princeton, N.J.: Princeton University Press, 1966.

171. WILBUR, G. "Migration on Expectancy in the United States," *J. Am. Statist. Assoc.,* 58 (1963), 444–453.

172. WILLIAMSON, J. B. "Subjective Efficacy and Ideal Family Size as Predictors of Favorability Toward Birth Control," *Demography,* 7 (1970), 329–339.

173. WILNER, D. M. and R. P. WALKLEY. "Effects of Housing on Health and Performance," in L. J. Duhl, ed., *The Urban Condition,* pp. 215–228. New York: Basic Books, 1963.

174. WINSBOROUGH, H. H. "The Social Consequences of High Population Density," *Immigr. Law Contemp. Probl.,* 30 (1965), 120–126.

175. WOOD, C., J. LEETON, B. DOWNING et al. "Emotional Attitudes to Contraceptive Methods," *Contraception,* 2 (1970), 113–126.

176. YOUNG, L. *Out of Wedlock.* New York: McGraw-Hill, 1954.

177. ZAJONC, R. B. "Social Facilitation," *Science,* 149 (1965), 269–274.

178. ZUCKERMAN, M., E. KOLIN, L. PRICE et al. "Development of a Sensation Seeking Scale," *J. Consult. Psychol.,* 28 (1964), 477–482.

EDITOR-IN-CHIEF'S
CONCLUDING REMARKS

Silvano Arieti

WITH THIS VOLUME the second edition of the *American Handbook of Psychiatry*, comes to a conclusion. A reading of its various tables of contents, or even a cursory perusal of a few sections, is sufficient to reveal its scope and magnitude.

If for a few seconds we suspend our scientific judgment and give our human propensity for metaphor free rein, what may come to mind is the building of a Medieval cathedral. In this *Handbook*, as in the cathedral, many people from different fields participated. They were united in the hard and long work by a common vision and aim, which we hope has been achieved, of giving an adequate representation of contemporary psychiatry. But here our metaphor ends. Instead of a unity of style and the all-embracing synthesis of the cathedral, we have a wealth of styles, many approaches, and a diversity of method with which to explore the human psyche and relieve its suffering.

When the first edition of the *Handbook* ap-

peared in 1959, no comparable work existed in the United States. Several textbooks of psychiatry, written by one or two authors, had been published, but a handbook like the present one, the work of many contributors, had not seemed feasible in the United States. This was not the case in Germany, where the renowned handbook of psychiatry edited by Oswald Bumke had remained the undisputed authority for several generations of psychiatrists. There was an apparently logical reason why works of this type appeared possible in Germany but not in the United States. Although minor dissident groups existed in Germany, the majority of German psychiatrists belonged to a single school of thought, the neuropsychiatric approach, which acquired prominence expecially under the leadership of Wilhelm Griesinger. Thus whatever was presented in a German textbook was more or less consistent with this approach.

How could we achieve such consistency in America, where so many schools of thought, so many approaches, so many treatments—often in theoretical opposition to one another—were adopted? Were we to present so many disparate and controversial points of view, would we not be in danger of confusing the student and discouraging the beginner? Because this situation prevailed in American psychiatry, many teachers and professionals used small textbooks by one or two authors, conceived within a single frame of reference.

The idea came to me that in the field of psychiatry the need to be consistent had to be abandoned. It had to be replaced by the concept of plurality. All the reputable schools of thought and therapeutic approaches should be presented to students and professionals, who eventually would have to choose and pave their own ways either toward eclecticism, plurality, or a given orientation. This idea, which seems so simple as to be taken for granted today, was an innovation then. It also required open-mindedness on the part of the publisher, Arthur Rosenthal, then president of Basic Books to accept this editorial revolution. It was by no means a Copernican revolution, but only an innovation that was immediately appreciated and very soon imitated. It is to the merit of Mr. Rosenthal's successor, Mr. Erwin Glikes, and to Mr. Herbert Reich, Director of the Behavioral Sciences Program of Basic Books, that they have given their full support to the preparation of the second edition with the same pioneering spirit and for the readiness to accept the necessary expansion. The whole staff of Basic Books has cooperated with unusual devotion. Special praise must go to Jamelia Saied, who as staff editor of the entire project, has shown a rare degree of skill and dedication.

It would be redundant to enumerate here the innovations presented in the first edition. I shall only mention a few of the new concepts introduced in this new edition. Among the many foundations of psychiatry and several contributions from related fields, Volume One offers, for the first time in a textbook of psychiatry, a detailed analysis of the normal life cycle and its common, not necessarily pathological, vicissitudes. Knowledge of the normal life cycle has always been taken for granted.

Thus a gap in the preparation of the psychiatrist has been perpetuated from generation to generation. Volume Two, in addition to much enlarged sections on child and adolescence psychiatry, offers extensive sections on new aspects of sociocultural and community psychiatry. Volume Three, among the many other expanded presentations of clinical entities, offers an unusual coverage of schizophrenia from genetic, biochemical, psychodynamic, psychostructural, pharmacological, and psychotherapeutic approaches. The affective psychoses are examined from a general biological aspect as well as from a specific psychological one. Volume Four, in addition to covering the usual organic psychiatric disorders, has a very informative chapter on physical illness in relation to psychiatry and two chapters on the problem of aphasia and its psychiatric implications. The section on psychosomatic medicine describes many recent breakthroughs in that field. Volume Five reports the newest findings in the ever-expanding field of drug therapy and a compendium of the various types of psychotherapies from the classic psychoanalytic method to many new ones, including brief psychotherapy. Finally, Volume Six opens new horizons, too many to be mentioned here.

The amount of material in these six volumes is immense; yet some readers can justifiably point out that certain topics were left out. Omissions and selections are unavoidable. Curiosities, or conditions or methods which have become obsolete or which would interest only an infinitesimal part of the readership, have been left out. Were we to include these areas, we would have been compelled to put together a work almost of the size of the *Encyclopaedia Britannica*, with unnecessary added cost for the vast majority of readers. Others may wonder why we have not allotted more space to neurological diseases accompanied by mental symptoms. In fact, the first edition had a chapter on brain tumors, which has been omitted in the second. It was not the Editor's intention for the student to overlook the possibility of brain tumors in mental disorders, but a short chapter on this and other organic subjects would not do justice to what is better treated in neurological textbooks. The reader is alerted to the possibility of brain tumors in Chapter 9 of Volume Four on focal lesions of the central nervous system and in other chapters. On the whole, Part I of Volume Four, on organic conditions, has been greatly expanded from what was presented in the first edition.

In a book of this size, and in a discipline like psychiatry where sharp demarcations are not possible between one subject and another, some overlapping is unavoidable. We have tried to keep it to a minimum. In some cases the apparent overlapping was actually a way of offering more than one approach to very important subjects. For instance, alcoholism is presented in Chapter 48 of Volume Two by Chafetz and Demone; in Chapter 18 of Volume Three by Chafetz, Hertzman, and Berenson; and in Chapter 14 of Volume Four by Mello and Mendelson. All aspects of alcoholism are covered and different approaches described. Classic psychoanalysis is presented separately by Drellich and Greenson in the two sections of Chapter 37 of Volume One, and again by Nemiah in Chapter 9 of Volume Five. Aphasia is presented by Mohr and Sidman, by Brown, and briefly by Benson and Geschwind.

Can we at this point give an answer to the question "Where do we go from here?" What will psychiatry be in the future? The human being being what he is—subject not only to biological nature but to an environment that is rapidly changing its multiple systems of symbols, feelings, and values—predictions are impossible except for the immediate future. For us it will be sufficient to have given an adequate representation of psychiatry in our own time.

NAME INDEX

Note: Bold face figures indicate chapter pages.

SUBJECT INDEX

897; recent advances in, 843–850

Behavior-modification programs: alpha feedback in, 79; consent in, 684

Behavior therapy, 719; computerized, 830; federal research in, 973; habituation in, 57

Belief systems: biological superiority in, 283; communication and, 896; computer simulation of, 832; drug attitudes and, 553; drug use and, 569, 596; LSD use and, 604–605; self-conception and, 213

Bennett Amendment to Social Security Act, 757, 768–771

Benzoquinolazine: depression and, 452; structure-activity relationships in, 438–439

Betaine, 493

Beta-phenylethylamine, and depression, 470

Beta waves: definition of, 76; EEG recording of, 75

Bias in drug researchers, 563, 570

Bias-setting mechanism, in neuroendocrinology, 102

Bible, 238, 741

Bicêtre hospital, 718

Bigotry: blue-collar youth and, 402; social behavior theories and, 284

Bilirubin levels, and hemolysis, 647

Binet test results, and race of administrator, 278

Binocular vision: light deprivation experiments on, 56; neuronal mechanisms in, 49–54

Biochemistry, 266, 352, 536; amphetamine in, 419; androgen and, 348; behavioral modification studies with, 61; depression and, 655; drug abuse and, 598; evolution theory and, 4, 5; genetic research and, 375; medical education and, 881, 886; primate studies of, 326–330; psychiatric illness and, 636; psychiatry and, 260; psychopathology and, 310, 634; psychopharmacological agents and, 537; rapid-eye-movement (REM) sleep and, 146, 147, 155; schizophrenia and, 268; sensitization in, 62; separation studies and, 326; sleep in, 164–166, 177; socially induced syndromes and, 329–330; sociological processes and, 634; systems approach to, 261

Biofeedback: federal research in, 973; sexual dysfunction treatment and, 677

Biogenetics: general systems theory and, 253; schizophrenia and, 267

Biological factors: aggression and, 10; alcoholism and, 364; attachment and, 295; behavior and, 44–45, 260; bipolar individuals

and, 506–507; communication and, 896; creativity and, 245; criminality and, 364; dependence and, 295; disadvantaged and, 716; homosexuality and, 674; intelligence and, 277; isolation and, 316; mania and, 510–513; neuroleptic drugs and, 445; night terrors and, 176; poverty and, 284–286; psychopathic illness and, 634; schizophrenia and, 267, 373

Biological sciences: medical education and, 881, 886; medicine and, 840, 841; psychoanalysis and, 263; reductionistic approach to, 251

Biology: as an adaptive mechanism, 11; homeostasis and, 258; information theory and, 897; molecular, see Molecular biology; psychiatry and, 259; psychology and, 44–45; revolution in, 387; see also Neurobiology

Biomedical profession, 389

Biophysics, 335

Biopsy, in genetic counseling, 647, 658

Biopsychosocial system, and schizophrenia, 269

Bipedal locomotion, see Walking

Bipolar illness, 461; affective disorders and, 518; age of onset of, 505; catechol-o-methyl transferase in, 470, 506; characteristics of, 505–507; clinical and psychological characteristics of, 505–506; familial transmission of, 504–505; genetic factors in, 367–368; homovanillic acid (HVA) and, 466; 5-hydroindoleacetic acid (5HIAA) in, 471; lithium in, 510, 544; mania and, 502, 503–507; mania switch process in, 515; monamine oxidase activity in, 476, 547; pharmacologic individuals and, 507; psychophysiological and biological characteristics of, 506–507; x-linked transmission of, 368

Birds: attachment behavior in, 295; imprinting in, 280, 293; sleep research in, 139, 143

Birmingham, Alabama, 741

Birth, 695; attachment behavior and trauma at, 299; health and, 264; intelligence at, 276; intervals between, 988–989; mental retardation and difficulties at, 358; schizophrenia and complications at, 374

Birth control, 979; attitudes toward child-bearing and, 403; delivery systems for, 548; see also Contraception

Birth defects, risk for, 643, 644

Birth order: childhood psychoses

and, 362; dyslexia and, 361; homosexuality and, 366

Birth rate: crude, 980–981; demographic aspects of, 979–980; increase in total youth population and, 395–396; intelligence and, 283; shrinking family size and, 392; women's attitudes toward child-bearing and, 403

Birth weight: gestational age and, 80–81; minimal brain dysfunction and, 361; schizophrenia and, 373

Bisexuality, 675

Biting behavior: blindness and, 696; Klüver-Bucy syndrome and, 101

Black culture, 716

Black English, 279

Black Muslim movement, 287

Black nationalism: family planning and, 283; self-image and, 287–288

Black Panther movement, 401

Black power movement, 400

Blacks: aged poor among, 953; blue-collar youth and, 402; civil-rights movement and, 398–399; college enrollment among, 396; developmental failure among, 287; drug use among, 563; English language and, 279; family structure of, 286; heroin use among, 556, 576–577, 582; heterosexual-homosexual differences and, 679; income level of, 286; intelligence measurement in, 276–277; life expectancy among, 950; medical education and, 881, 882–883; population and test differences among, 280; race of test administrator and, 278; self-evaluation studies among, 214–218, 222–223, 225, 226; sickle-cell anemia in, 651; student movement and, 400–401; test performance by, 276; unemployment among, 282

Black studies programs, 287–288, 400

Blindness: children and, 696–697; color, see Color blindness; light deprivation studies resulting in, 55; psychoanalytic theory on, 696–697; sexual behavior and, 681

Blocking, and LSD, 600

Blood: brain barrier with, 547; catechol o-methyl transferase in, 470; drug absorption processes and, 547; hormone circulation in, 199; psychopharmacology and, 547; sugar concentration in, and circadian rhythms, 167; tyrosine in, and depression, 467

Blood flow, during rapid-eye-movement (REM) sleep, 141

Blood group, in twin studies, 357

Blood pressure: coital activity and, 681; computers and, 812; sleep research and, 177

Blue-collar class: black movement and, 401; drug use in, 583; generation gap and, 391; retirement and, 958; youth in, 401–402

Blue Collar Project, New York, 698–699

Blue Cross, 746

Body behavior: homosexuality treatment and, 679; sleep research and, 176

Body-buffer zone, 999, 1002

Body image: contraception and, 985; intersexed children and, 668

Body language, 903

Body temperature: circadian rhythms and, 167; pseudoinsomnia and, 175; sleep and, 168; stress and, 336

Body weight: alcoholism and, 364; stress and, 629

Bonding, 626; psychiatric process disturbances and, 633; roles and, 625

Bone sodium, and mania, 512

Bonnet macaques (Macaca radiata), in separation studies, 321, 323–324

Books: child-rearing, 390; drug use and, 559; nuclear-family model in, 673; violence in, 404

Borderline schizophrenia, 371n

Borderline syndrome: children and, 696; drug use and, 579, 580, 592; mania and, 508; systems approach to, 260

Boredom: contingent negative variation (CNV) reduced by, 82; drug use and, 568–569, 581; narcolepsy and, 148

Boston, 666

Boston State Hospital, 796–800

Boundaries: general systems theory and, 255, 260; social systems and, 258

Boundary conditions concept, 204

Boundary confusion, and LSD use, 601

Brain: as adaptation organ, 11; Australopithecine, 7, 8; biological insult in poverty and, 284–286; bipedal locomotion and size increases in, 34; blood barrier with, 547; cellular techniques in study of, 49; components of, 199; conscious experience and information about, 192; double dissociation of signs of trauma to, 112; euphorigens in, 495; evolution and structure of, 8; evolutionary theories on, 7; federal research in, 973; Homo erectus, 7; language in relation to, 11; learning of skills and, 9; machine intelligence and, 197; malnutrition and development of, 284–

285; mania switch from direct stimulation of, 517; metabolic studies in, 329; minimal damage in, see Minimal brain damage; neurons in, 199–200; self-association of cells in, 70; speech and, 38; split brain experiments in, 207–208; stereotaxic placement of medication in, 548; stimulation and development of, 342; tumors in, and headaches, 173; see also Specific areas of brain

Brain and Conscious Experience (Sperry), 197

Brain-damaged states, and EEG, 78; see also Minimal brain damage

Brain Information Service, University of California at Los Angeles, 131, 137

Brain Mechanisms and Intelligence (Lashley), 111

Brain scans, 81

Brain stem: associative functions of, 120; consciousness and, 208; efferent partitioning in, 123; 5-hydroxyindoleacetic acid (5HIAA) in, 473; limbic lobe and, 97; limbic system and, 94, 97, 102; medial forebrain bundle and, 98; monoamine pathways in, 415, 428, 430; olfaction and, 100; PGO spikes and, 150; sleep and, 133, 165; tricyclic uptake studies in, 441

Brain Trust, 397

Branching ability of computers, 828, 829, 831

Breath shortness, and psychosomatic evaluation, 227

Breeding programs, and heritability, 355

Brief group therapy, 708

Brief Psychiatric Rating Scale, 824

Bromide, 542

Brothers: affectionate bonds between, in early man, 40; chimpanzee, and bonding, 25; depression and, 368; homosexuality and, 366; stuttering among, 357

Brushing hair, and social grooming, 38

Buchenwald concentration camp, 933

Buddhism, 79

Budget processes, federal, 965, 966–968, 970

Bufotenin (N, N-dimethyleserotonin): euphorigenic properties of, 490, 492, 493, 495; methylated amines in, 544

Bunney-Hamburg scale, 506

Bureaucracy: apathy and, 288; college, 397; community mental health center movement and, 764; comprehensiveness and, 773–774; federal mental health pro-

grams and, 961, 968; health-center movement and, 762; health system, 717–718; medical education and, 890–891; poverty and, 717; psychiatric, 718; staffing and, 761

Bureau for Education of the Handicapped, 965

Bureau of Narcotics and Dangerous Drugs (BNDD), 965

Bushmen of Kalahari: aggression among, 29; communication among, 39; tool-using among, 19

Business, and systems approach, 257

Butyrophenones: depression and, 451; dopaminergic systems and, 436, 545; mania and, 517; mechanisms of action of, 415, 416, 417; specificity of action of, 445

Cabinet, and mental health programs, 962, 967, 968

Cable television, 404

Caffeine, 542

Calcium: lithium and, 517; sponge cell self-association and, 70; neurotransmission with, 48, 542

Calculus, 279

California, 685; abortion laws in, 658; group therapy movement in, 703; peer review program in, 770–771

California Rehabilitation Center Program, 593

Calmness, and serotonin systems, 437

Cambridge University, 880

Cameroons, 19

Canada, 563, 994

Cancer, and death rates, 994

Cannabis plant, 536

Cannulae: push-pull, and tricyclic uptake studies, 441; sleep research with, 177

Canon of Medicine (Avicenna), 878

Capillaries, and retinal fibers, 54

Carbachol, 438

Carbazole, and structure-activity relationships, 440

Carbohydrate binding protein, and slime-mold cell self-association, 71

Carbohydrate metabolism: mania and, 512; mental retardation and, 358

Carbonic anhydrase, and chimpanzee-human differences, 4

Carcinoid syndrome, and parachlorophenylalanine, 470

Carcinomas: colonic, 659; prostatic, 684

Cardiology, 835

Cardiovascular system; apnea and, 173; Dopa and, 468; drub abuse and, 599; monoamine oxidase in-

Communication (*continued*)
  self-help groups and, 593; drug use and, 555, 575, 582; erroneous timing in, 903; evolution of, 9–10; family's role in, 264; feedback distortions in, 904; function of, 895; health-illness system and, 265; historical note on, 893–895; hospital and, 787, 820; information sciences and, 893–913; language and speech difficulties and, 904; mathematical theory of, 897; mental-health programs and, 728; message discrepant with stimulus in, 904; mind-body dichotomy in, 901–903; nonverbal, *see* Nonverbal communication; overload and underload in, 903; self-destructive behavior and, 995; sexual, 676; within systems, 255–256, 260; systems analysis and operations research in, 899–901; therapeutic, 906–907, 909; threatening content in, 905; transactional, 256
Communism, 398–399, 762
Community: assessment research into drug use in, 560; chimpanzee, 16; community mental health centers and, 730, 761; day-care programs in, 786; drug-abuse treatment and, 587, 588; drug education and, 589; drug use and, 566, 573, 590, 596; elderly people in, 951; geographical mobility and, 996–997; health-center movement and, 762; health services delivery and, 724; health services evaluation and, 748; hospitalization and dangers toward, 784–785; medical education and, 887; nuclear family and, 391; physician in, 890; preventive health programs and, 995; retirement, 394; state hospitals and, 719; structural isolation of family and, 392–393
Community care: Louisville Experiment on, 802–803; Social Breakdown Syndrome (SBS) and, 808
Community Health Service, 965
Community Mental Health Centers Act of 1963, 715–716, 720, 730, 761, 969
Community mental health programs, 756, 757, 781; clinical-audit method to assess, 749–750; as coordinating mechanism, 761; emergency services in, 727; evaluation in, 730; federal support of, 720–721, 966, 970, 971–972; health-center movement and, 763; historical note on, 761–763; impact of, on community, 730; legislation for, 715–716, 759; manpower in, 729; primary function of, 761; psychoanalysis in, 698; public mental hospitals

and, 782; reception for, 760; social ecology and, 925; state mental hospitals and, 760; systems approach to, 266
Community Mental Health Services Division, 969
Community psychiatry, 763; federal support for, 970; psychoanalysis in, 698; social ecology and, 925; systems approach to, 265–267, 269
Community therapy, in systems approach, 262
Compassion, and youth, 571
Compensatory programs, for disadvantaged children, 288
Competence: adaptation and, 213; life-cycle stage correlated to, 224–226; self-evaluation of, 212–229; sex education and, 686
Competition: blue-collar youth and, 401; chimpanzee tool-using behavior and, 17; group therapy and, 706, 709; health consumers and, 721; homeostasis and, 258; homosexual men and, 669; language acquisition and, 39; many-to-many communication in, 895; public and private hospitals in, 783
Competitiveness: amphetamines and, 605; drug abuse and, 591; LSD use and, 604; population size and, 996; retirement and, 956–957
Complexity, role, 999
Complications in pregnancy: childhood morbidity and, 282; height of mothers and, 284
Composition of populations: current issues in, 1010–1012; modes of professional action in, 1012; relevant concepts in, 1009–1010
Compulsive behavior: amphetamines and, 419; animal studies of, 312; creative processes and, 232; drug use and, 561; Lesch-Nyhan syndrome and, 651
Computers: boundary conditions concept in, 204; coding in, 125; concepts in, 811–813; data banks in, 813–815; diagnosis with, 822–823; EEG recordings and, 77, 78; evaluation of health services and, 749; genetic linkage methods with, 657–658; health services and, 737; information theory and, 897, 898; interviewing by, 828–830; logical decision-tree approach in, 822–823, 825; machine intelligence and, 197–201; pattern vision experiments with, 123; Planning-Program-Budget Systems (PPBS) and, 776; psychiatry and, 811–839; psychological tests and, 826–828; research uses of, 832–834; sleep research with, 177; statistics and,

816–820; technology and, 390; therapy by, 830–831; training and, 831–832; treatment recommendations from, 823–825
Computers and Brains (Schade and Smith), 197
Computer technicians, in medicine, 746
COMT, *see* Catechol-o-methyl-transferase (COMT)
Concentration, and amphetamines, 598
Concentration camps: adaptive behavior in, 937–938; children in, 281, 941–942; concentration camp syndrome and, 940–941, 942–944; long-term effects of, 939–940; personal accounts of, 934–937; personality disorders in, 939, 940; psychiatric aspects of persecution in, 932–946; psychiatric contact with survivors of, 944
Conceptive behavior, 981
Concepts: knowing and, 256; perceptualization of, 243
Conceptualization, and learning to talk, 38
Concordance rates in twin studies, 357
Concreteness, 833
Concretization, and creativity, 233, 235
Condensation, and primary process thinking, 232
Condenser charging averagers, in evoked potentials, 80
Conditioning: Alpha feedback in, 79; drug dependence models with, 583–585; drug screening programs with, 534–535; drug use and, 554, 590–591, 608; experimental neurosis with, 312; frontal cortical lesions and, 117–118; homosexuality treatment with, 680; recovery cycles and, 81; sex differences in, 667; social isolation studies and, 315; sociopathic behavior and, 633
Cones, retinal, 49
Confidence, and attachment, 298
Confidentiality of records: computers and, 814, 820; judicial decisions on, 961
Conflicts: adolescent, 697; animal studies of, 312; creativity and replaying of, 247–248; delivery of mental health services and, 777; drug use and, 562, 579, 580, 590; homeostasis and, 258; LSD use and, 601, 602; mania and, 513; poverty and, 717; psychoanalysis and, 263; role, 625; schizophrenia and, 258; sexual identity and, 672–673; status and, 29, 626
Conformity: generation gap and,

and, 343, 345, 346; male development and, 666; old age and, 682

Estrus: child-care patterns and, 37; chimpanzee community organization and, 16; chimpanzee feeding behavior and, 21; chimpanzee, first, during adolescence, 26; chimpanzee mating behavior and, 35

Ethical problems: clinical trials and, 794–795; drug-abuse programs and, 594, 596; genetic counseling and, 652, 653; sex offender treatment and, 684; sexual identity conflict treatment and, 672–673; treatment of homosexuality and, 679

Ethics: evolution theory and, 3; homeostasis and, 258; moral worth and, 213; systems and, 253

Ethnic groups: agricultural workers' migration and, 389; alcoholism and, 364; gene distribution and, 284; individual differences and, 358; inheritance and, 355; nuclear family and, 391; occupational status and, 220, 223–224; psychometric measurements and, 276; self-conception development and, 213; self-evaluation studies among, 214–218, 219–220, 223–224, 226; youth and, 572

Ethology: attachment theory and, 292, 293; drug research and, 555

Ethological zoology, and model criteria, 313

Ethoxybutamoxane, 446

Ethylene, 417

Etiocholanolone, and homosexuality, 674, 675

Eugenics movement, 283

Eugranular cortex, and reinforcement, 119

Euphoria: cultural factors in, 489; definition of, 490; depression and, 504; direct brain stimulation and, 517; L-Dopa and, 468; drug use and, 585; hypomania and, 515; mania and, 507, 508, 515, 516, 517; neurobiology of, 488–501

Euphorigens: adaptive mechanisms in, 495–498; *cannabis* plant compounds and, 536; cultural factors in use of, 489; naturally occurring, 492–495; structure and effects in, 490–492

Europe: dyslexia in, 361; *Homo erectus* in, 8; sex offender treatment in, 684

European-American neonates, and differences, 358

Evaluation, 756; ambulatory care and, 750; clinical-audit method for, 749–750; clinical trial in, 794–796; communication and,

903–904; computers and, 832; cross-country studies of, 750–751; delivery in, 765; federal programs for, 760; goal-attainment model in, 747–748, 750; indices for, 740–741; individual treatment programs and, 787; interdisciplinary team approach to, 776–777; interpretation of data in, 795–796; legislation and, 736; manpower and, 744, 745–746; medical education and, 889; mental health delivery systems and, 730; peer review programs for, 770–771; preventive trial in, 796; Professional Standards Review Organizations (PSRO) as, 768–771; program-planning-budgeting system (PPBS) for, 736; research in, 793–794; statistical models in, 749; system model for, 748; value systems in, 792

Evangelical religious sects, 595

Evoked potential, *see* Potential

Evolution, 352–353, 385, 386; ability to learn in, 9–10; acceptance of theory of, 3; apes and men in, 4–6; behavior and anatomy and, 5–6; brain and, 8; creative process theory in, 244; culture and, 352–353; environmental influence and, 342; hair loss during, 30; hierarchies in, 255; homeostasis and, 258; language as unique achievement of, 38; learning of skills in, 8–9; molecular clues to, 4–5; rate of, 5; social systems and, 257–258; stages of, 8; systems and, 256

Excitantia, 490

Excitation, in rapid-eye-movement (REM) sleep, 138

Excitatory postsynaptic potentials (EPSPs), 46, 75

Excitement: chimpanzee hunting behavior and, 31, 32; nonverbal communication during, 27

Executive Branch, and mental health programs, 960, 962–964, 965, 969, 973

Exhibitionism, 683, 784

Existential crisis, 489

Existentialism, and psychiatry, 259

Expectancy: contingent negative variation (CNV) and, 83; remembering and, 124

Expectations: adolescent, 697; attachment and, 297–298; consumer, 778; drug-abuse treatment and, 591, 593; drug use and, 572, 574, 576, 586, 603; educational, 280, 282; expansion of health services and, 745; LSD use and, 599; marijuana and, 606; poverty and, 717; revolution of rising, 389; role and, 624–625; social ecology and, 915; stereotyping and self-image

and, 287; university education and, 398

Expeditors, mental health, 729

Experience, 626; blind children and, 696; creative processes and, 231, 232; development and, 341–342; differences and, 358; drug dependence and, 584; drug use .and, 572; EEG arousal and, 78; erotica and, 683; erotic arousal patterns and, 678; genetic factors and, 253; health-illness system and, 265; intelligence measurement and, 276, 277; intersexed children and, 667; knowing and, 256; LSD use and, 599; psychopathic illness and, 634; response specificity to, 267; schizophrenia and, 373; scientific concepts of nature and, 192–211; sexual behavior and, 101; stress and, 855–859; systems approach to, 261; television and, 403; test results and, 284

Experimental design, in sleep research, 177–178

Experimentation, in drug use, 561, 565, 575, 588

Exploratory behavior: blind children and, 696; dopaminergic systems and, 437; drug screening programs and, 534; independence training and, 394; mania and, 519; peer separation and, 326; reserpine and, 328; social isolation and, 315, 317

Exposure data, in drug use, 564

Extended family, 390; black family as, 286; shrinking family size and, 392

Extinction: drug use and, 584, 590–591; frontal cortical lesions and, 118

Extrasensory perception, 197

Extraversion, and mania, 510

Extrinsic cortex, 108–110; afferent-efferent overlap in, 111; behavior classes and, 125–126; efferent control mechanisms and, 123; transcortical model of organization and, 119–120

Eyes: alpha waves and, 79; conscious experiences and appearance of, 192, 196; EEG recordings of movement of, 75; extrinsic cortical system and movement of, 120; Lesch-Nyhan syndrome and, 360; neonatal rapid movements of, 153; opening of, 341; sleep movements of, 132, 177; status and contact with, 627

Face validity assessment, 227

Facial expressions: alpha-methylparatyrosine and, 469; brain processing of, 208; conscious experi-

proach to, 252; self-evaluation correlation with, 213, 214, 219–220, 225; sex differences in self-evaluation of, 219, 220–223, 224; systems approach to, 254, 260

Life expectancy: aging and, 949; chimpanzee, 16; living arrangements and, 951–952

Life of Reason, The (Santayana), 757

Light: deprivation of, 55–57; mania and, 509; photoreceptor cells for, 69; response to intensity of, 50, 53

Light microscopy, 434

Limb girdle muscular dystrophy, 371

Limbic lobe, 97

Limbic system, 89–106; ability to learn and, 10; amygdaloid nuclear complex in, 96; anatomical considerations in, 94–99; behavior aspects and, 100–101; definitions in, 93–94; early work on, 89, 97; electrical stimulation of, 545; endocrine system and, 101–102; functional considerations in, 99–103; habenular complex in, 98; hippocampal formation in, 94–95; limbic lobe in, 97; memory in, 102–103; monoamine pathways in, 415; neocortex in, 98–99; olfactory structures and, 95–96; speech learning and, 9; use of term, 92–93, 93–94, 96, 99

Limbs: flexion withdrawal reflex of, 58; rapid-eye-movement (REM) sleep and, 142; restless legs syndrome and, 173–174

Lincoln Hospital Community Mental Health Center, 760–761

Lincoln (Nebraska) Insane Asylum, 781n

Linear properties of visual stimuli, 50

Line cross analysis, in EEG, 76

Line of Balance (LOB) techniques, in delivery of mental health services, 775

Linguistics: communication of information described by, 255; computational, 833

Linkage workers, mental health, 729

Lipid metabolism, in Tay-Sachs disease, 358

Lips, in Lesch-Nyhan syndrome, 360

LISP (computer language), 812

Lisping, 904

List-produced language (LISP), 812

Literature: cultural factors in, 245; role conflicts in, 625

Lithium carbonate, 824, 965; augmenting-reducing and, 85, 506; bipolar individuals and, 506, 507;

depression and, 367–368, 460; discovery of, 502–503, 534, 536; dosage for, 517; EEG activity and, 76; future directions in use of, 544; glucose utilization and, 512; mania and, 460, 507, 510, 517, 518; manic-depressive treatment with, 417; 3-methoxy-4-hydroxyphenylglycol (MHPG) and, 466; neurotransmission with, 542; norepinephrine and, 477; primate studies of, 327; response prediction for, 547; sodium depletion with, 512; stress from discontinuance of, 514

Little Hans case, and phobia, 303

Liver: monoamine oxidase (MAO) inhibitors in, 541; phenylketonuria and, 656; phorphyrias and, 656, 657; self-association of cells in, 70

Living arrangements, and life expectancy, 951–952

Lobster stomatogastric ganglion, 68

Local government: coordination and, 766; health services programs of, 757, 765; regional planning and, 772; state review programs and, 771, 772; training in, 778

Locked wards, 781

Locomotion: alpha-methyl-para-tyrosine (AMPT) and, 328; amphetamines and, 419; anatomy and, 6; bipedal, *see* Walking; blindness and, 696–697; dopaminergic systems and, 446; *Drosophilia* mutation studies on, 69; mother-child dependence and, 21; peer separation and, 326; play and, 22; reserpine and, 328; social isolation and, 315, 316, 317, 319; spinal cord mediation in, 58

Locus coeruleus: amphetamine and, 419; norepinephrine systems and, 430, 437; rapid-eye-movement (REM) sleep and, 148

Logic: communication and, 255; computer and, 812, 813; creative process and, 231; systems approach to, 257; wit and, 236–237, 340

Logical decision-tree approach in computers, 822–823, 825

London, 555

Lonely Crowd, The (Riesman), 570

Longevity: definition of, 949; prediction of, 954–955

Long-term memory, 61, 62–63

Lordosis, rat, 343, 344–346

Los Angeles, 923

Loss: anger at, 300–301; anxiety and, 295; drug use and, 582; mania and, 502; mourning and, 304–305; studies in, 843–849

Loudness, and insular-temporal cortex, 122

Louisville, Kentucky, hospitalization study, 802–803, 805

Love: attachment behavior and, 295; creativity and, 233; deprivation of, 693; drug use and, 583; group therapy and, 707; intergroup marriages and, 26; language and, 38; physical contact and, 38; youth and, 571

Lower classes: adolescence in, 287; biological insult and, 284; childhood morbidity in, 282; child-rearing practices in, 286; generation gap and, 391; health care and, 284, 285; heroin use in, 556; higher incidence of disease in, 947; hypochondriasis among, 952; infant mortality and, 740, 741; intelligence tests and, 277; language competence in, 279; leisure activities among, 223; medical education and, 884; political exploitation of, 289; pregnancy problems and, 284; race of test administrator, 278; sex education in, 686; state hospitals and, 719

Loyalty oaths, 498

LSD (lysergic acid diethylamide), 594; acute reactions to, 599–600; adverse reactions to, 599–603; animal abuse studies on, 585; attitude, belief and value change with, 604–605; creativity and, 246; cultural factors in, 570–571; group interaction and, 572; historical overview of use of, 557–559; ideas of reference in, 606; introduction of, 420; mechanisms of action of, 419–420, 421; neurological effects of, 597, 598; organicity of, 598; PGO waves in, 161; precipitants in use of, 576–577; prolonged reactions to, 600–601; psychedelic state of, 419; schizophrenia and, 578–579; serotonin and, 540; speech patterns in, 833; spontaneous recurrences with, 603–604; therapeutic uses of, 560; tolerance to, 498; toxic effects of, 597; treatment for reactions to, 601; variability of, 581

"LSD and the Psychedelic Syndrome" (Smith), 600

Lumbar cerebrospinal fluid: 5-hydroxyindoleacetic acid (5HIAA) and, 471–472, 473; 3-methoxy-4-hydroxyphenylglycol (MHPG) and, 465–466, 467, 468; rapid-eye-movement (REM) sleep and, 148

Lust, and limbic system, 101

Luteinizing hormone, and limbic system, 102

in, 282; child-rearing in, 286; college education and mobility of, 398; developmental studies of, 214; drug use in, 563, 574, 582–583; generation gap and, 391; heroin use in, 556; intelligence tests and, 277; linguistic competence of children of, 279; psychotherapy and, 719–720; verbal abilities of, 717

Middle ear muscle activity during sleep, 141, 142, 152

Middle East, 577

Midwestern states, 398

Migration: agricultural workers and, 389; chimpanzee, 31; communication during, 895; modes of professional action in, 1005–1006; poverty and, 717; stress and, 1004–1005; youth and, 571

Milbank Memorial Fund, 805

Milieus, see Social ecology

Milieu therapy: evolution of, 719, 758; interaction of drugs with, 796–800

Military life: drug abuse research and, 562; gonadal hormones and, 675; marginal draftees in, 281; organization in, 896; psychiatric work in, 758; see also Soldiers

Milk, and chimpanzee infants, 22

Milk depots, 761

Mind, and matter, 195–196

Minimal brain damage: genetic factors in, 360–361; LSD use and, 598

Minnesota-Hartford Personality Assay, 824

Minnesota Multiphasic Personality Inventory (MMPI): bipolar individuals on, 506; computers and, 824, 826; sleep disturbances on, 174

Minority groups: class and, 286; creativity in, 249; drug use and, 567, 593; elderly as, 949; family planning in, 283–284; medical education and, 886; poverty and, 716; self-image in, 287; test performance in, 276; universities and, 401

Miocene Era, 6

Mirror tracing, and EEG recordings, 76

Miscarriages: amniocentesis and, 644–645; progestin and, 654

Missouri Standard System of Psychiatry, 815, 816, 820, 822

MMPI, see Minnesota Multiphasic Personality Inventory (MMPI)

Mobility: computer data banks and, 814; demography and, 978, 979; distribution of population and, 997–998; downward, 947, 1005; geographic, 996–97, 1002–1003; occupational, and education, 286; shrinking family size

and, 392; social, see Social mobility; upward, 401, 1005

Model Cities Program, 965

Modeling, in homosexuality treatment, 679

Models: animal, criteria for, 313–314; behavior study with, 44, 45; of central nerve cells, 48–49; in chimpanzee tool-using, 18; computer simulation of, 898; computer testing of, 832; of general systems, 256; goal attainment, in evaluation, 747–748, 750; of human body, 877–878; medical school, 884; of neuronal functioning, 46; nuclear family, 673; psychiatry and, 260; schizophrenia and, 268–269; threshold genetic, 356–357

Molecular biology: behavior study with, 63; evolution theory and, 4–5; genetics theories in, 3

Molecules: drug use and, 554, 607; systems approach to, 254

Molluscs: identified neuron structure in, 68; nerve system studies in, 58

Moloch, 238

Mongolism, see Down's syndrome

Monist view of social systems, 775, 776

Monitoring: automated record systems and, 815, 816; behavior therapy and, 830; computer, 899; pregnancy, 658–659

Monkeys: alpha-methyl-p-tyrosine in, 413; amphetamine studies in, 605–606; axonal pathways in, 430; behavior and anatomy in, 5–6; biochemical studies in, 326–330; biological reversal of abnormal behavior in, 330; cortical ablation experiments in, 111; criticism of experimental use of, 311; discrimination task studies in, 113–116; drug dependence studies with, 584; evolution rates in, 5; experimental psychopathology in, 310–314; fear in, 297; frontal cortical lesions in, 118–119; Harlow vertical chamber in studies on, 316–319; hormone studies in, 653; labeling in studies in, 311; learning of skills by, 9; man's relation to, 4–5; maternal and peer interaction in, 56; maternal deprivation studies on, 281, 293, 339; methylamphetamine studies in, 597; molecular biology in evolution theory and, 4; pattern vision in, 123; penile tumescence during sleep in, 145; PGO waves in, 161, 162; separation studies in, 320–327; sleep stages in, 138; social isolation studies in, 314–316; social rewards among, 10; visual discrimination in, 52;

visual efferent control mechanisms in, 121–122; voluntary movement experiments on, 207

Monoamine oxidase: bipolar individuals and, 506–507; depressions and, 475–477, 478; Dopa and, 468; histochemical analysis of, 415; major terminals of, 431; neuroanatomic techniques for, 428, 429–430; primate studies of, 328; probenecid and, 372; putative transmitters and, 412; reserpine and, 413

Monoamine oxidase inhibitors (MAOI): antidepressant effect of, 417; depressions and, 368, 460, 543; discovery of, 535; Dopa and, 468; dopaminergic systems and, 446; enzyme inhibition with, 414; euphorigens and, 493; genetic factors in response to, 374; homovanillic acid (HVA) and, 447; mania and, 460, 510, 511, 516; norepinephrine and, 538, 539; phenylethylamine and, 470; rapid-eye-movement (REM) sleep and, 146–147, 148, 155, 164; regulation by, 496; schizophrenia and, 474; screening procedures and, 546; serotonin and, 540; specificity of, 547; synaptic transmission and, 537

Monogamy: primates and, 35; sexual attractiveness and, 36

Monomethyl, 493

Monopolar recordings, in EEG, 75

Monotony, and narcolepsy, 148

Monozygotic twin studies: alcoholism and, 363; childhood psychosis and, 362; criminality in, 364; dyslexia in, 361; genetic studies of, 357–358; homosexuality in, 366; hyperkinesis in, 361; intrapair differences in, 358; mania and, 504–505; manic-depressive illness in, 367, 368; mental retardation in, 358; minimal brain dysfunction in, 360; nortriptyline in, 546; schizophrenia and, 368–369, 373; sex reassignment studies in, 669; threshold characteristics in, 356; see also Twin studies

Monte Cassino monastery, 878

Moodiness, and drug use, 577

Moods: chimpanzee, 29; mania and swings in, 503

Moon phases, and murder rates, 923

Morality: responses to crime and, 287; youth and, 571, 572

Moral treatment of insane, 718

Moral worth, and self-evaluation, 212–229

Morbidity, 553; abortion and, 659; childhood, 282; cross-country studies of, 751; drug abuse and,

Physicians *(continued)*
574–575; geographic distribution of, 890; marijuana use by, 563; patient ratio to, 745–746

Physics, 200, 201

Physiological sociology, 633–636

Physiology, 901; androgen and brain, 348; behavior and, 635; cerebral mantle functions in, 107; computers in, 834; criminality and, 366; dreaming and, 155; fetal, 658; genetic research into, 375; medical education and, 878, 879, 881; night terrors and, 176; population density and, 1000; psychiatry and, 260; schizophrenia and, 268; sexual receptivity and, 36; sleep research and, 138–139; stress and, 851–866; synaptic, 537; *see also* Neurophysiology; Psychophysiology

Physostigmine, 438, 450; depressions and, 478, 545; mania and, 545; stereotype with, 450

Pickwickian syndrome, and apnea, 172

Pigs, in behavioral studies, 312

Pigtail monkeys (*Macaca nemestrina*): separation studies in, 321, 322; social isolation studies with, 314

Pilocarpine, 548

Pimozide: dopamine systems and, 446–447, 449, 453; norepinephrine and, 449; PGO waves and, 161

Piriform cortex, 96

Pitch discrimination, and cortex, 122

Pituitary: afferents controlling, 101–102; dopamine systems and, 447; habenular complex and, 98; homosexuality and, 675; limbic system and, 101; regulation function of, 254; stress and, 336, 337, 338–341

Placenta, and amniocentesis, 644

Planning, 756, 764; federal timetables for, 760; regional, 772–773; social aspects of, 914

Plant extracts, 535–536

Plasma studies: criminality and, 365; homosexuality and, 366; hormone studies with, 666; mania and, 512, 513; predicting drug response and, 546; socially-induced syndromes and, 330

Plasticity: averaged evoked potentials (AEP) and, 83–84; human, 626

Plastic membrane for drug delivery, 548

Platelets: amine metabolism and, 547; depression and, 368; lithium and, 517; monoamine oxidase activity and, 476

Play: aggression and, 666; attachment and, 293; atypical sex-role behavior and, 669, 670; chim-

panzee adolescence and, 26; chimpanzee mother-child relationship and, 23, 24; chimpanzee nonverbal communication and, 29; chimpanzee tool-using and, 18; early man and, 40; gonadal hormones and, 665; hunting practice in, 10; observational learning during, 22–23; separation and, 322, 325; sex differences in, 66, 667; social isolation and, 315, 316; wish fulfillment in, 231

Playmates, as significant others, 215

Pleasure: drug abuse and, 553, 575; intoxication and, 566; puritanical attitudes toward, 499

Plethysmography, 677, 678

Plovers, and fear behavior, 297

Pluralist view of social systems, 775

Poetics (Aristotle), 139

Poetry, and creative processes, 239–244, 245

Poisoning, 553; accidental, 285, 695; lead, 285; paleologic thinking and, 235

Police: amphetamine use and, 557; blue-collar youth and, 402; drug use and, 577; heroin use and, 556; illegal sexual behavior and, 685; mental health services and, 727; social psychiatry and, 267

Poliomyelitis, 31, 33, 738

Political factors: acceptance of poverty and, 275, 276; blue-collar youth and, 402; delivery of health services and, 724; drug abuse and, 552, 572; drug abuse treatment and, 560; gin epidemic and, 555; health care movement and, 762; health services evaluation and, 750; marijuana and, 572; lower classes and, 289; mental health services and, 757, 776; population and, 999; student movement and, 398, 399

Political groups, and drug use, 563

Political science: as academic division, 11; drug use research and, 555; systems approach to, 257

Politics: cultural factors in, 245; health, 737; women in, 389

Polls, *see* Public opinion polls

Polydipsia, and social isolation, 315

Polygraphy, in sleep research, 134, 154, 174, 177

Polyposis of colon, 659

Pompe's type of glycogen storage disease, 647, 650

Pons: monoamine pathways and, 429; norepinephrine systems and, 430, 437; sleep studies on, 141, 165, 166; tricyclic uptake studies in, 442

Poorhouses, 758

Population: aging and changes in, 949–950; composition of, 1009–1012; current issues in, 999–

1002; distribution of, 997–998; individual behavior and, 995–996; intelligence test differences and differences in, 280; in 1950s, 388; in 1920s, 388–389; in 1950s, 390; psychological and psychiatric aspects of problems of, 977–1019; relevant concepts in, 998–999; youth, 395–396

Population biology, 352

Porphobilinogen, 657

Porphyrias, 656–657

Porteus maze, 279

Positive feedback, in systems approach, 254

Positive reinforcements, in computers, 830, 831

Postindustrial society, 386, 390

Postpartum affective disorders, 505

Post-tetanic potentiation, 71

Posture: circadian rhythms and, 167; 3-methoxy-4-hydroxy phenylglycol (MHPG) and, 465; nonverbal communication and, 27; reserpine and, 328; sleep and, 168; spinal cord mediation in, 58; status and, 627

Potassium, 544; electrophysiological neuronal studies of, 46–47, 48; lithium and, 517; mania and, 512

Potassium chloride, 45

Potential: averaged evoked, *see* Averaged evoked potentials (AEP); chemical processes and, 200; cognition and, 81–83; computers in, 834–835; contingent negative variation (CNV) and, 82–83; cortical organization and, 109–110; dendrites in, 75; depression and, 367; EEG physiology and, 75; excitatory postsynaptic (EPSP), 46; eye movement in sleep and, 136; gill withdrawal in *Aplysia* and, 59; habituation and, 60; hippocampal, 100; importance of, 205; inhibitory postsynaptic (IPSP), 46; ionic hypothesis for, 46–47; LSD use and, 598; mania and, 510; microiontophoresis in, 415; phasic-integrated muscle potential (PIP) in, 143, 145; post-tetanic, 71; potassium-equilibrium, 47; recovery cycles in, 81; repression and, 85; resting-membrane, 45–47; variability in, 84; visual system and, 49

Poverty: achievement and, 278; aged and, 951, 953; biological insult and, 284–286; child development and, 275–291; community mental health programs and, 266; cultural factors in, 286–288; culture of, 286–287, 389, 716–718; data interpretation in, 276–282; depression and, 389; drug use and, 574; explanatory hypothesis for, 282–288; future directions

Sleep research (continued)
stages in, 137–138; standard sleep recording in, 176

Sleep Research (journal), 131

"Sleep Reviews," 131

Sleepwalking: psychiatric interest in, 176; research into, 173

Slide rule, and intelligence, 200–201

Slime mold cell self-association, 70

Slow-wave sleep, 139

Slums: changes in, 289; health-center movement and, 761; maternal development and, 685; skills for survival in, 279

Small-town life, 388, 392–393

Smell, see Olfaction

Smiling: attachment and, 292; nonverbal communication with, 28

Smoking, opium, 555, 556

SNCC (Student Non-Violent Coordinating Committee), 400

Snoring, in apnea, 173

Sociability, and bipolar individuals, 506

Social agencies: community psychiatry and, 267; consultation and education programs in, 756; drug abuse research by, 566; drug education by, 589; drug use and, 559; morphine use and, 556

Social and Rehabilitation Service (SRS), 962, 965

Social behavior: alpha-methylparatyrosine and, 469; catecholamines in, 632–633; Huntington's chorea and, 657; monkey studies in, 311; olfaction in, 100; social isolation and, 315; status and, 626

Social Breakdown Syndrome (SBS), 807–808

Social change, 759, 764; aging and, 947–959; black student movement and, 400–401; blue-collar youth in, 401–402; childrearing and, 390–395; computer simulations of, 811; decline in parental authority and, 393; delegation of parental authority and, 394–395; drug use and, 568, 574, 575; generation gap and, 391; group therapy and 705; Hawthorne Effect and, 799; historical overview of, 385–386; increase in total youth population and, 395–396; independence training of children and, 394; in 1900s, 388; in 1920s, 388–390; in 1970s, 390; paternal deprivation and, 393–394; problems of youth and, 384–408; psychotherapy and, 707–708; public mental health hospital and, 782; role conflicts and, 625; shrinking family size and, 392; social ecology and, 925, 926; social psychiatry and, 288; status and, 628;

structural isolation of family and, 392–393; youth and sex roles and, 402–403; youth and television and, 403–404; youth and universities and, 397–400

Social communication, see Communication

Social context of psychiatry, 875–1019

Social depreciation: achievement and, 278; biological insult and, 284–286; child development and, 275–291; cultural factors in, 286–288; data interpretation in, 276–282; explanatory hypothesis for, 282–288; future directions for change in, 288–289; genetic theories on, 282–284; intelligence tests and, 276–278; permanence of deficits due to, 280–281; population and test differences in, 280; test differences and, 278–282

Social ecology, 914–931; behavioral settings and, 917, 918–919; conceptualization of, 915–922; ecological dimensions in, 917–918; functional or reinforcement analysis of, 921–922; organizational structure of, 919; psychosocial characteristics in, 920–921; see also Environment

Social factors: ability to learn and, 10; abortion and, 660, 661; aggression and, 10; alcoholism and, 364; amphetamine use and, 556–557; behavior and, 260; chimpanzee behavior and, 30; creativity and, 248; drug abuse treatment programs and, 594, 596; drug use and, 552, 553, 555, 561, 565, 566, 567, 569, 570–572, 575, 581, 585, 590, 599, 608–609; drug use research and, 560; genetic counseling and, 652, 653, 660–661; genetic research and, 375; health and, 264; health care and, 652; intravenous drug use and, 599; learning of skills and, 9; longevity and, 743, 949, 955; mental health services and, 772–773; mental illness and, 758; mourning and, 305; peyote use and, 602; poverty and, 721; rewards in learning and, 10; sexual receptivity and, 36; tomboyish traits and, 654

Social gerontology, 948

Social interaction: attachment behavior and, 295; drug use and, 568; hypomania and, 515; infant development and, 56; machine, 201; role reciprocity and, 625; self-esteem in, 213; separation and, 323; status and, 627; structural isolation of family and, 392–393; studies of, 692

Socialism, 398, 762

Socialization, 387, 693; atypical sex-role behavior and, 670, 671; bisexuality and, 675; drug use and, 573; intersexed children and, 668; maternal development and, 696; novelty in environment and, 387; roles and, 221, 222; self-conception changes and, 214; sexual identity and, 669; social change and, 394; status and, 627, 628; XXY chromosomal anomaly and, 669; youth and, 387, 398

Social mobility: college education and, 398; current issues in, 1008–1009; modes of professional action in, 1009; relevant concepts in, 1008

Social model of psychiatry, 265

Social psychiatry: individual development and, 288–289; systems approach to, 266–267, 269

Social psychology: group therapy and, 703; psychology and, 45

Social sciences: balance theories in, 623; drug abuse and, 552, 555, 560; general systems applicability to, 257–269; humanistic approaches to, 252; medical education and, 881; primitive ways of thinking in, 11; psychiatry and, 259; psychoanalysis and, 263

Social Security Act, Bennett Amendment, 757, 768–771

Social Security Administration (SSA), 962, 965

Social security benefiits: national health insurance proposals and, 767, 768; work income and, 953

Social status, see Status

Social system: chimpanzee, 15–16; computer simulation of, 898–899; Homo sapiens, 8; monist view of, 775, 776; personality conglomerates in, 266; pluralist view of, 775; self-esteem in, 212, 213; systems approach to, 254

Social work: health work and, 762; individual focus in, 763–764

Social workers, in team approach, 729

Society: age segregation in, 394; biological quality and success in, 283; black nationalism movement and, 288; change in, see Social change; consumer, 571; creativity and, 233; crime and, 287; culture and, 387; cybernetics and, 897; drug abuse cost to, 596; drug attitudes in, 553; early man and, 40; family of 1950s and, 392; health-illness system and, 265; hierarchies in, 255; learning disorders and, 360; mythologizing of youth in,

Vestibular stimulation, and evoked responses, 81

Veterans Administration (VA), 415, 826, 965, 971

Vice Presidency, 956

Vicki (chimpanzee), and language, 39

Videotape methods: drug programs with, 593; medical education with, 883; patient interviews with, 832; research interviews with, 798; sexual dysfunction treatment with, 676

Vienna Medical School, 879

Vietnam War: blue-collar youth and, 402; college enrollment and, 397; drug use in, 572; protest movement against, 399; youth and, 387, 570

Violence: amphetamine and, 557; black student movement and, 400, 401; blue-collar youth and, 402; children and, 693; civil-rights movement and, 398, 399; criminality and, 364, 365; drug use and, 585, 597; learning and, 10; sex crimes against women and, 684; social change and, 386; social ecology and, 914, 922–925; television and, 404; by whites against blacks, 287; youth and, 570, 571

Viral infections, and schizophrenia, 372

Visceral brain, use of term, 93, 96, 99

Visionary mode, and creativity, 232, 233

Visiting nurses, 729

Visual cortex: input from, 120; light deprivation and, 55–56; rapid-eye-movement (REM) sleep and, 141

Visual stimulation: averaged evoked potential (AEP) and, 83–84; bipolar individuals and, 506; evoked responses in, 81; LSD use and, 598; mania and, 509, 510; separation studies and, 322; verbal response to, 206–207

Visual system: amphetamine and, 606; binocular interactions in, 49–54; development of connections in, 54–55; discrimination in, 52; EEG recordings in, 76; efferent control mechanism in, 120–122; extrinsic and intrinsic cortex in, 120; eye movements in, 153; hand autonomy in, 696; hierarchal processing in, 52–53; inferior temporal cortex in, 113; light deprivation in, 55–57; moment of sleep and fixation in, 144; mutations in study of, 63; neocortex and, 99; neuronal mechanisms in, 49–57; pursuit differences in, 358; reserpine and, 328; split brain experiments with, 207–208; striate cortex and, 111, 120

Vital brain, use of term, 92, 99

Vital depression, 461, 472

Vitalism, 256

Vitamin B6, and depression, 473

Vitamin E8, in restless legs syndrome, 174

Vita Nuova, La (Dante), 241, 242–243

VMA, *see* 3-methoxy-4-hydroxy-mandelic acid (VMA)

Vocabulary, in test construction, 277, 278

Volitional activity, in mechanical man concept, 193

Voltage, in EEG, 75

Voluntary hospitalization, 787, 789; drug treatment with, 587; legal aspects of, 784–785

Voluntary movement: experimental methods for, 207; rapid-eye-movement (REM) sleep and, 140

Volunteer work, 762

Voting, 289, 388; blacks and, 402; women and, 389; youth and, 402

Voyeurism, 683, 686, 784

Vultures, as scavengers, 32

Waika Indians, and mouthing behavior, 38

Wakefulness: brain stem and, 208; circadian rhythms and, 168; rapid-eye-movement (REM) sleep and, 141; transition to sleep from, 176–177

Walk-in clinics, 727

Walking, 901; anatomy and, 6; bipedal posture in, 33–34, 40; blind children and, 696; chimpanzee-human differences in, 30, 33–35; hunting and, 30; language acquisition and, 39

Walter Reed Hospital, 965

Wards: locked, 781; monitoring of, 816; open, 784, 787, 804–805; psychosocial characteristics and, 920, 921, 923

Wars: primitive societies and, 10; regulation mechanisms and, 255; significance of games related to, 198

Washington, D.C., 402, 651

Washington State, 658, 987

Washoe (chimpanzee), and language, 38, 39

Wastes, and environmental problems, 284

Water: as element, 11; hypothalamic regulation of intake of, 101; lithium and, 517; mania and metabolism of, 512, 513

Wave forms, sleep, 135

Ways and Means Committee, House, 962

Weaning: chimpanzee, 22; weight and, 341

Weapons: bipedal locomotion and, 34, 35; hunting and, 32, 33

Weather, and behavior, 923

Weaving, 279

Weight: alcoholism and, 364; amphetamine control of, 575; birth, *see* Birth weight; brain, and stimulation, 342; infant mortality by, 741; mania and, 513; parachlorophenylalanine and, 470; status and, 628; stimulation and, 341

Welfare-rights organizations, 283

Welfare system: college students and, 398; delegation of parental authority for, 394; family size and, 283; federal, 962; focus on individual in, 763; health-center movement and, 762; matriarchal family structure and, 286; mental hospital patients and, 781; neighborhood health centers and, 747; public mental hospitals and, 782; reform in, 717; working mothers and, 403

Wepman Auditory Discrimination Test, 278

Wernicke-Korsakoff encephalopathy, 102

Western states, 388, 563, 574

Western tradition countries: creativity in, 248; drug use in, 553, 569; Industrial Revolution in, 386; manic-depressive illness in, 366; mourning in, 304

West Germany, 597, 677, 939

Wheat production, and fertilizers, 283

White-collar class: generation gap and, 391; retirement and, 958

White House Conference on Children, 1973, 403

White House Special Action Office for Drug Abuse Prevention, 966

Whites: black student movement and, 401; college enrollment and, 396; cystic fibrosis in, 651; developmental studies in, 214; drug use in, 582–583; family structure in, 286; heterosexual-homosexual differences in, 679; income levels in, 286; infant mortality for, 740–741; intelligence in, 276–277; LSD use in, 557; marijuana and, 562, 563; mobility of, 398; population and test differences in, 280; poverty in, 716; self-evaluation studies in, 214–218, 222, 223, 226; sense of superiority in, 289; stereotyping of, 287; test performance by, 276; unemployment in, 282

Widowers, 304, 951